2016 ANNUAL ICD-10-PCS

The Educational Annotation of ICD-10-PCS

CRAIG D. PUCKETT

**2016 ICD-10-PCS
Procedure Index, Tables, and Appendices**

Complete Official ICD-10-PCS Text, 2016 VERSION
as standardized by
U.S. DEPARTMENT OF HEALTH AND HUMAN SERVICES
CENTERS FOR MEDICARE AND MEDICAID SERVICES

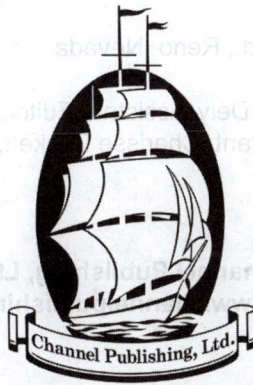

Channel Publishing, Ltd.
Reno, Nevada
1-800-248-2882
www.channelpublishing.com

Publishing Quality
ICD Code Books
Since 1986

DISCLAIMER

Every effort has been made to ensure the accuracy and reliability of the information contained in this publication. However, complete accuracy cannot be guaranteed. The editor and publisher will not be held responsible or liable for any errors.

Corrections Identification and Reporting

In an effort to provide our customers with the best code books possible, Channel Publishing has added a "Channel Errata Page" for each of its ICD-10-PCS code books on its web site: www.channelpublishing.com. These Channel Errata Pages will be updated promptly whenever an error is identified. Check the appropriate web page periodically for any changes to your Channel Publishing ICD-10-PCS.

In addition, if at any time you identify a potential error, please copy the page and fax/mail/e-mail it to: Channel Publishing, Ltd., Attn: ICD-10-PCS Book Production Department, 4750 Longley Lane, Suite 110, Reno, NV 89502. FAX (775) 825-5633. E-mail: info@channelpublishing.com

---

ICD-10-PCS, Version 2016.PCS – Published August 2015

© 2015 CHANNEL PUBLISHING, LTD.

All rights reserved. This book is protected by copyright. No part of it, including but not limited to, the unique, distinctive graphic design and arrangement of the displayed information and other distinctive graphic elements that enhance the usefulness of this publication, may not be used, copied, imitated, replicated, or reproduced in any form or by any means, including photocopying, electronic, mechanical, recording, or utilized by any information storage and retrieval system without prior written permission from the copyright owner.

This edition contains the Complete, Official ICD-10-PCS Text, 2016 Version as standardized by the U.S. Department of Health and Human Services, Centers for Medicare and Medicaid Services.

Published by CHANNEL PUBLISHING, Ltd., Reno, Nevada

Produced by Craig Puckett, Editor; Susan Dely, Assistant Editor;
Jo Ann Jones, RHIA, CCS, Editorial Assistant; Charisse Puckett, Editorial Assistant

Printed in the United States of America

Additional sets may be ordered from Channel Publishing, Ltd., 4750 Longley Lane, Suite 110, Reno, Nevada 89502, 1-800-248-2882, www.channelpublishing.com

ISBN: 978-1-933053-69-1

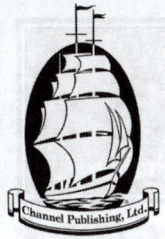

Channel Publishing, Ltd.

Publishers of
"THE EDUCATIONAL ANNOTATION OF ICD-10-CM/PCS"

August 2015

Dear ICD-10 Colleague:

    First, I would like to personally thank each and every Channel Publishing customer who has purchased and enjoyed our ICD-9-CM coding products and services over these past 29 years.

    Thank you for purchasing Channel Publishing's *2016 The Educational Annotation ICD-10-PCS* code book. I trust you will enjoy the new, innovative design, layout, and new, coder-helpful features that we have created for you. I would also like to thank everyone who shared their ICD-10 comments and suggestions over the years from our "Preparing for ICD-10" seminars fifteen years ago, to those of you who called or wrote in, and those who stopped by our booth at AHIMA. We listened and made note of those comments and suggestions to bring you what we believe is an excellent ICD-10-PCS code book, and at an incredibly low price.

    In addition to this *2016 Educational Annotation of ICD-10-PCS* code book, I'd like to remind you about all our ICD-10 products and services. I strongly believe that the ICD-10 products and services we've developed will make this transition easier for you, both from a learning point of view and a budget point of view. Please visit our web site www.channelpublishing.com for details and sample content.

    Once again, thank you for your purchase and I look forward to providing quality ICD-10 products and services to you in the years to come.

Sincerely,

Craig D. Puckett

Craig D. Puckett,
President, and Publisher

4750 Longley Lane, Suite 110 • Reno, NV 89502-5977 • (775) 825-0880 • Customer Service 1-800-248-2882 • FAX (775) 825-5633
WEB SITE: www.channelpublishing.com • E-MAIL: info@channelpublishing.com

You Asked for ...
AFFORDABLE ICD-10 CODE BOOKS
...we delivered!!!

2016 ICD-10-CM

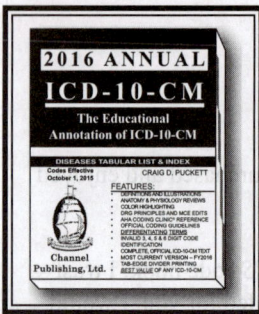

2016 Annual Version
- Paperback bound
- Same content as SoftCover
- Buy new book each year

Only $64.95

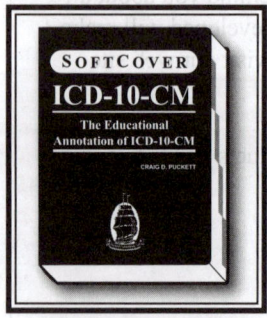

2016 SoftCover
- Loose-leaf, updateable
- Same content as Annual
- Yearly full-text replacement (Future updates 30% below new book regular price)
- Optional tab-divider set

Only $69.95

ICD-10-CM ANNOTATED/ENHANCED FEATURES
- ✓ Color Highlighting of Text & Symbols
- ✓ Definitions
- ✓ Illustrations
- ✓ Anatomy Reviews
- ✓ Physiology Reviews
- ✓ DRG Principles
- ✓ Medicare Code Edits
- ✓ AHA Coding Clinic® Reference Notations
- ✓ Highlighted Term Differentiation
- ✓ Further use of Placeholder "x"
- ✓ Further use of Dashes (-)
- ✓ Excludes ● Graphic
- ✓ Excludes 1 and Excludes ● Key
- ✓ Highlighted 7th Digit Subclassifications
- ✓ Official Coding Guidelines
- ✓ Invalid Code Identification Symbols
- ✓ Complete, Official Text
- ✓ Color Tab-Edge Printing

Compare our Products/Features/Prices to others!!

See Web Site for Sample Pages

2016 ICD-10-PCS

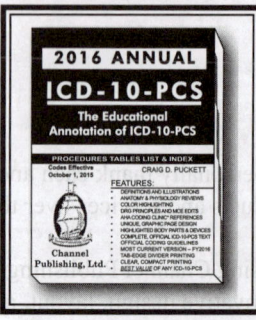

2016 Annual Version
- Paperback bound
- Same content as SoftCover
- Buy new book each year

Only $54.95

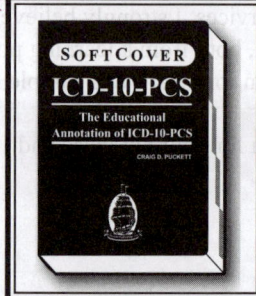

2016 SoftCover
- Loose-leaf, updateable
- Same content as Annual
- Yearly full-text replacement (Future updates 30% below new book regular price)
- Optional tab-divider set

Only $59.95

ICD-10-PCS ANNOTATED/ENHANCED FEATURES
- ✓ Color Highlighting of Text, Tables & Symbols
- ✓ Definitions
- ✓ Illustrations
- ✓ Anatomy Reviews
- ✓ Physiology Reviews
- ✓ DRG Principles
- ✓ Medicare Code Edits
- ✓ AHA Coding Clinic® Reference Notations
- ✓ Unique, Enhanced Table Design
- ✓ Root Operation:
  - Definition
  - Example
  - Brief Explanation
- ✓ Unique, Graphic Page Design
- ✓ First 3 Digits Highlighted in Index
- ✓ Highlighted Body Part and Device Terms
- ✓ Body Part, Device & Aggregation Keys
- ✓ Official Coding Guidelines
- ✓ Complete, Official Text
- ✓ Color Tab-Edge Printing

SEMINAR-IN-A-BOX ICD-10-CM & PCS TRAINING

SEMINAR-IN-A-BOX ICD-10 TRAINING PROGRAMS

- ❖ **Professional Version** – Learning ICD-10-CM (Step 1) — Sale $559.95
  - Additional Workbook & ICD-10-CM Book Packages — $65.95
- ❖ **Professional Version** – Learning ICD-10-PCS (Step 1) — Sale $649.95
  - Additional Workbook & ICD-10-PCS Book Packages — $55.95
- ❖ **Individual Version** – Learning ICD-10-CM (Step 1) — Sale $269.95
  - (12 CEUs)
- ❖ **Individual Version** – Learning ICD-10-PCS (Step 1) — Sale $359.95
  - (20 CEUs)

Professional Versions Include: PowerPoint Slides, Instructor's Manual, DVD Set, Workbook & Code Book

Individual Versions Include: DVD Set, Workbook & Code Book

ICD-10 TRAINING BOOKS & ADDITIONAL PRODUCTS

- ❖ 2015 Mastering ICD-10-CM Exercise Book (Step 2) — $59.95
- ❖ 2015 Mastering ICD-10-PCS Exercise Book (Step 2) — $59.95
- ❖ 2015 Mastering ICD-10-CM Guidelines Exercise Book (Step 3) — $59.95
- ❖ 2015 Mastering ICD-10-PCS Guidelines Exercise Book (Step 3) — $59.95
- ❖ The Last Word on ICD-10 (Step 4) — $69.95
- ❖ 2016 Clinotes for ICD-10-CM — Sale $29.95
- ❖ 2016 Expanded ICD-10-CM Table of Drugs & Chemicals — Sale $29.95

Sale Prices Expire 12/31/15

www.channelpublishing.com • 800-248-2882

2015 ICD-10 FALL SALE ORDER FORM
Sale Prices Expire 12/31/15

1. CUSTOMER INFORMATION (Ship books to address below)

☐ Organization or ☐ Individual   ATTN: Name/Title/Dept.   Customer ID #   Order Date

Shipping Address (Street address required for FedEx delivery)   E-Mail Address

City   State   Zip   Telephone   Fax

2. ORDER INFORMATION

Quantity	Product — See Web Site for Complete Product Descriptions	Regular Price	Fall Sale Price Exp. 12/31/15	Total(s)
	2016 ICD-10 CODE BOOK PRODUCTS			
	2016 ICD-10-CM, The Educational Annotation of ICD-10-CM			
	Annual Version ICD-10-CM (Paperback) (ISBN: 9781933053-68-4)	$64.95 ea.	—	
	SoftCover Version ICD-10-CM (Vinyl cover, updateable) (ISBN: 9781933053-70-7)	$69.95 ea.	—	
	Tab Set for ICD-10-CM (SoftCover only) (ITEM: TABCM)	$17.95 ea.	—	
	2016 ICD-10-PCS, The Educational Annotation of ICD-10-PCS			
	Annual Version ICD-10-PCS (Paperback) (ISBN: 9781933053-69-1)	$54.95 ea.	—	
	SoftCover Version ICD-10-PCS (Vinyl cover, updateable) (ISBN: 9781933053-71-4)	$59.95 ea.	—	
	Tab Set for ICD-10-PCS (SoftCover only) (ITEM: TABPCS)	$17.95 ea.	—	
	ICD-10 CODING TRAINING – SEMINAR-IN-A-BOX PROGRAMS			
	(Professional Version – Includes: PowerPoint Slides, Instructor's Manual, DVD set, Workbook & Code Book) (Individual Version – Includes: DVD set, Workbook & Code Book - CM-12 CEUs, PCS-20 CEUs)			
	Professional Version – Learning ICD-10-CM (Step 1) (ITEM: SBCM-P)	$599.95 ea.	$559.95 ea.	
	Additional Learning ICD-10-CM Workbook & Book Packages (ITEM: GCM15W)	$65.95 ea.	—	
	Professional Version – Learning ICD-10-PCS (Step 1) (ITEM: SBPCS-P)	$699.95 ea.	$649.95 ea.	
	Additional Learning ICD-10-PCS Workbook & Book Packages (ITEM: GPCS15W)	$55.95 ea.	—	
	Individual Version – Learning ICD-10-CM (Step 1) (12 CEUs) (ITEM: SBCM-I)	$299.95 ea.	$269.95 ea.	
	Individual Version – Learning ICD-10-PCS (Step 1) (20 CEUs) (ITEM: SBPCS-I)	$399.95 ea.	$359.95 ea.	
	ICD-10 CODING TRAINING – ADDITIONAL LEARNING PRODUCTS			
	2015 Mastering ICD-10-CM Exercise Book (Step 2) (ISBN: 9781933053-64-6)	$59.95 ea.	—	
	2015 Mastering ICD-10-PCS Exercise Book (Step 2) (ISBN: 9781933053-66-0)	$59.95 ea.	—	
	2015 Mastering ICD-10-CM Guidelines Exercise Book (Step 3) (ISBN: 9781933053-65-3)	$59.95 ea.	—	
	2015 Mastering ICD-10-PCS Guidelines Exercise Book (Step 3) (ISBN: 9781933053-67-7)	$59.95 ea.	—	
	The Last Word on ICD-10 (Step 4) (ISBN: 9781933053-61-5)	$69.95 ea.	—	
	ICD-10 ADDITIONAL PRODUCTS AND ACCESSORIES			
	2016 Clinotes for ICD-10-CM (ISBN: 9781933053-59-2)	$39.95 ea.	$29.95 ea.	
	2016 Expanded ICD-10-CM Table of Drugs & Chemicals (ISBN: 9781933053-60-8)	$39.95 ea.	$29.95 ea.	
	Acrylic Bookstand ☐ One-piece (ITEM: BSOP) ☐ Two-piece (ITEM: BSTP)	$34.95 ea.		

- OUTSIDE CONTINENTAL U.S.: Call for rates and shipping options. U.S. Dollars.
- EXPRESS SHIPPING: Call for delivery options and rates.

Fall Sale Prices Expire 12/31/15

Continental U.S. Shipping & Handling
Less than $50. . . . . . $7
$50-$99 . . . . $12
$100-$199 . . . . $19
$200-$299. . . . .$29
$300+. $39

Product Subtotal
Shipping & Handling
Nevada Res. Only Add Local Sales Tax
Total Order Amount

3. PAYMENT METHOD
☐ Purchase Order (Attach copy)   ☐ Check Enclosed
☐ Credit Card: MC, VISA, DISC, AMEX (Charged date order received)

__ __ __ __ — __ __ __ __ — __ __ __ __ — __ __ __ __
__ __ / __ __
Exp. Date   Sec. Code   Authorized Cardholder Signature

Billing Address (Street number or PO Box and Zip Code)   ☐ Same as shipping

MAKE CHECKS PAYABLE AND MAIL TO:
Channel Publishing, Ltd.
4750 Longley Lane, Suite 110
Reno, NV 89502-5977
1-800-248-2882
(775) 825-0880
Fax (775) 825-5633
E-Mail: info@channelpublishing.com
Web Site: www.channelpublishing.com

THANK YOU FOR YOUR ORDER   FS99095

INTRODUCTION – 2016 ICD-10-PCS

TABLE OF CONTENTS

Introduction to ICD-10-PCS vii
ICD-10-PCS Official Coding Guidelines CG-1
Procedure Index 1

Procedure Tabular – Medical and Surgical Section (Section 0)

Body System (Chapter)

0	Central Nervous System	85
1	Peripheral Nervous System	105
2	Heart and Great Vessels	121
3	Upper Arteries	147
4	Lower Arteries	171
5	Upper Veins	195
6	Lower Veins	211
7	Lymphatic and Hemic Systems	229
8	Eye	245
9	Ear, Nose, Sinus	265
B	Respiratory System	289
C	Mouth and Throat	309
D	Gastrointestinal System	331
F	Hepatobiliary System and Pancreas	363
G	Endocrine System	381
H	Skin and Breast	393
J	Subcutaneous Tissue and Fascia	413
K	Muscles	435
L	Tendons	451
M	Bursae and Ligaments	463
N	Head and Facial Bones	481
P	Upper Bones	499
Q	Lower Bones	521
R	Upper Joints	543
S	Lower Joints	567
T	Urinary System	589
U	Female Reproductive System	611
V	Male Reproductive System	637
W	Anatomical Regions, General	655
X	Anatomical Regions, Upper Extremities	671
Y	Anatomical Regions, Lower Extremities	683

Procedure Tabular – Medical/Surgical Related Sections

1	Obstetrics	695
2	Placement	705
3	Administration	713
4	Measurement and Monitoring	735
5	Extracorporeal Assistance and Performance	743
6	Extracorporeal Therapies	747
7	Osteopathic	753
8	Other Procedures	757
9	Chiropractic	761

Procedure Tabular – Ancillary Sections

B	Imaging	765
C	Nuclear Medicine	807
D	Radiation Therapy	823
F	Physical Rehabilitation and Diagnostic Audiology	845
G	Mental Health	867
H	Substance Abuse	873
X	New Technology	879

Appendices

A	Root Operations of the Medical and Surgical Section	883
B	Approach Definitions of the Medical and Surgical Section	891
C	Body Part Key	893
D	Device Key	905
E	Device Aggregation Table	912
F	Physical Rehabilitation and Diagnostic Audiology Qualifier Key	913
G	Mental Health Qualifier Key	919
H	Substance Key	921
I	New Technology Key	922

INTRODUCTION TO ICD-10-PCS

THE INTERNATIONAL CLASSIFICATION OF DISEASES Tenth Revision Procedure Coding System (ICD-10-PCS) was created to accompany the World Health Organization's (WHO) ICD-10 diagnosis classification. The new procedure coding system was developed to replace ICD-9-CM procedure codes for reporting inpatient procedures.

Unlike the ICD-9-CM classification, ICD-10-PCS was designed to enable each code to have a standard structure and be very descriptive, and yet flexible enough to accommodate future needs.

This Introduction contains the following parts:
- What is ICD-10-PCS?
- ICD-10-PCS code structure
- ICD-10-PCS system organization
- ICD-10-PCS design
- ICD-10-PCS additional characteristics
- ICD-10-PCS applications

WHAT IS ICD-10-PCS?

ICD-10-PCS is a procedure coding system that will be used to collect data, determine payment, and support the electronic health record for all inpatient procedures performed in the United States.

History of ICD-10-PCS

The World Health Organization has maintained the International Classification of Diseases (ICD) for recording cause of death since 1893. It has updated the ICD periodically to reflect new discoveries in epidemiology and changes in medical understanding of disease.

The International Classification of Diseases Tenth Revision (ICD-10), published in 1992, is the latest revision of the ICD. The WHO authorized the National Center for Health Statistics (NCHS) to develop a clinical modification of ICD-10 for use in the United States. This version of ICD-10 is called ICD-10-CM. ICD-10-CM is intended to replace the previous U.S. clinical modification, ICD-9-CM, that has been in use since 1979. ICD-9-CM contains a procedure classification; ICD-10-CM does not.

The Centers for Medicare and Medicaid Services, the agency responsible for maintaining the inpatient procedure code set in the U.S., contracted with 3M Health Information Systems in 1993 to design and then develop a procedure classification system to replace Volume 3 of ICD-9-CM. ICD-10-PCS is the result. ICD-10-PCS was initially released in 1998. It has been updated annually since that time.

ICD-9-CM Volume 3 Compared with ICD-10-PCS

With ICD-10 implementation, the U.S. clinical modification of the ICD will not include a procedure classification based on the same principles of organization as the diagnosis classification. Instead, a separate procedure coding system has been developed to meet the rigorous and varied demands that are made of coded data in the healthcare industry. This represents a significant step toward building a health information infrastructure that functions optimally in the electronic age.

The following table highlights basic differences between ICD-9-CM Volume 3 and ICD-10-PCS.

ICD-9-CM Volume 3	ICD-10-PCS
Follows ICD structure (designed for diagnosis coding)	Designed/developed to meet healthcare needs for a procedure code system
Codes available as a fixed/finite set in list form	Codes constructed from flexible code components (values) using tables
Codes are numeric	Codes are alphanumeric
Codes are 3 through 4 digits long	All codes are seven characters long

ICD-10-PCS CODE STRUCTURE

Undergirding ICD-10-PCS is a logical, consistent structure that informs the system as a whole, down to the level of a single code. This means that the process of constructing codes in ICD-10-PCS is also logical and consistent: individual letters and numbers, called "values," are selected in sequence to occupy the seven spaces of the code, called "characters."

Characters

All codes in ICD-10-PCS are seven characters long. Each character in the seven-character code represents an aspect of the procedure, as shown in the following diagram of characters from the main section of ICD-10-PCS, called MEDICAL AND SURGICAL.

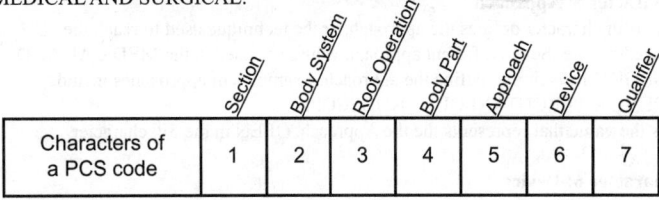

An ICD-10-PCS code is best understood as the result of a process rather than as an isolated, fixed quantity. The process consists of assigning values from among the valid choices for that part of the system, according to the rules governing the construction of codes.

Values

One of 34 possible values can be assigned to each character in a code: the numbers 0 through 9 and the alphabet (except I and O, because they are easily confused with the numbers 1 and 0). A finished code looks like the example below.

$$0\ 2\ 1\ 0\ 3\ D\ 4$$

This code is derived by choosing a specific value for each of the seven characters. Based on details about the procedure performed, values for each character specifying the section, body system, root operation, body part, approach, device, and qualifier are assigned.

Because the definition of each character is a function of its physical position in the code, the same value placed in a different position in the code means something different. The value 0 in the first character means something different than 0 in the second character, or 0 in the third character, and so on.

Code Structure: Medical and Surgical Section

The following character explanations define each character using the code 0 L B 5 0 Z Z, "Excision of right lower arm and wrist tendon, open approach" as an example. This example comes from the MEDICAL AND SURGICAL section of ICD-10-PCS.

Character 1: Section

The first character in the code determines the broad procedure category, or section, where the code is found. In this example, the section is MEDICAL AND SURGICAL.
0 is the value that represents MEDICAL AND SURGICAL in the 1ST character.

Character 2: Body System

The second character defines the body system—the general physiological system or anatomical region involved. Examples of body systems include LOWER ARTERIES, CENTRAL NERVOUS SYSTEM, and RESPIRATORY SYSTEM.
L is the value that represents the Body System, TENDONS in the 2ND character.

Character 3: Root Operation

The third character defines the root operation, or the objective of the procedure. Some examples of root operations are BYPASS, DRAINAGE, and REATTACHMENT. In the sample code below, the root operation is EXCISION.
B is the value that represents the Root Operation, EXCISION in the 3RD character.

INTRODUCTION – 2016 ICD-10-PCS

Character 4: Body Part
The fourth character defines the body part, or specific anatomical site where the procedure was performed. The body system (second character) provides only a general indication of the procedure site. The body part and body system values together provide a precise description of the procedure site.

Examples of body parts are KIDNEY, TONSILS, and THYMUS. When the second character is L, the value 5 when used in the fourth character of the code represents the right lower arm and wrist tendon.
5 is the value that represents the Body Part, LOWER ARM AND WRIST, RIGHT in the 4TH character.

Character 5: Approach
The fifth character defines the approach, or the technique used to reach the procedure site. Seven different approach values are used in the MEDICAL AND SURGICAL section to define the approach. Examples of approaches include OPEN and PERCUTANEOUS ENDOSCOPIC.
0 is the value that represents the the Approach, OPEN in the 5TH character.

Character 6: Device
Depending on the procedure performed, there may or may not be a device left in place at the end of the procedure. The sixth character defines the device. Device values fall into four basic categories:
- Grafts and Prostheses
- Implants
- Simple or Mechanical Appliances
- Electronic Appliances

In this example, there is no device used in the procedure. The value Z is used to represent NO DEVICE, as shown below.
Z is the value that represents the Device, NO DEVICE in the 6TH character.

Character 7: Qualifier
The seventh character defines a qualifier for the code. A qualifier specifies an additional attribute of the procedure, if applicable.

Examples of qualifiers include DIAGNOSTIC and STEREOTACTIC. Qualifier choices vary depending on the previous values selected. In this example, there is no specific qualifier applicable to this procedure.
Z is the value that represents the Qualifier, NO QUALIFIER in the 7TH character.

0 L B 5 0 Z Z is the complete specification of the above procedure:
"Excision of right lower arm and wrist tendon, open approach."

ICD-10-PCS SYSTEM ORGANIZATION

The ICD-10-PCS system is organized in three parts: the Tables, the Index, and the Definitions.

Tables (see example below)
The Tables are organized in a series, beginning with section 0, MEDICAL AND SURGICAL, and body system 0, CENTRAL NERVOUS SYSTEM, and proceeding in numerical order. Sections 0 through 9 are followed by sections B through D and F through H and X. The same convention is followed within each table for the second through the seventh characters—numeric values in order first, followed by alphabetical values in order.

The following examples use the MEDICAL AND SURGICAL section to describe the organization and format of the ICD-10-PCS Tables.

The MEDICAL AND SURGICAL section (first character 0) is organized by its 31 body system values. Each body system subdivision in the MEDICAL AND SURGICAL section contains tables that list the valid root operations for that body system. These are the root operation tables that form the the system. These tables provide the valid choices of values available to construct a code.

The root operation tables consist of four columns and a varying number of rows, as in the following example of the root operation EXCISION, in the TENDONS body system.

The values for characters 1 through 3 are provided at the top of each table. Four columns contain the applicable values for characters 4 through 7, given the values in characters 1 through 3.

A table may be separated into rows to specify the valid choices of values in characters 4 through 7. A code built using values from more than one row of a table is not a valid code.

For the complete list of ICD-10-PCS Official Coding Guidelines, please refer to the Official Coding Guidelines following this Introduction.

See Tables above for Table explanation.

EXCISION GROUP: Excision, Resection, Destruction, (Extraction), (Detachment)
Root Operations that take out some or all of a body part.

1ST - **0** Medical and Surgical (Section)	EXAMPLE: Ganglionectomy tendon sheath CMS Ex: Liver biopsy
2ND - **L** Tendons (Body System)	**EXCISION:** Cutting out or off, without replacement, a portion of a body part.
3RD - **B** EXCISION (Root Operation)	EXPLANATION: Qualifier "X Diagnostic" indicates biopsy ...

Body Part – 4TH				Approach – 5TH	Device – 6TH	Qualifier – 7TH
0	Head and Neck Tendon	F	Abdomen Tendon, Right	0 Open	Z No device	X Diagnostic
1	Shoulder Tendon, Right	G	Abdomen Tendon, Left	3 Percutaneous		Z No qualifier
2	Shoulder Tendon, Left	H	Perineum Tendon	4 Percutaneous endoscopic		
3	Upper Arm Tendon, Right	J	Hip Tendon, Right			
4	Upper Arm Tendon, Left	K	Hip Tendon, Left			
5	Lower Arm and Wrist Tendon, Right	L	Upper Leg Tendon, Right			
		M	Upper Leg Tendon, Left			
6	Lower Arm and Wrist Tendon, Left	N	Lower Leg Tendon, Right			
		P	Lower Leg Tendon, Left			
7	Hand Tendon, Right	Q	Knee Tendon, Right			
8	Hand Tendon, Left	R	Knee Tendon, Left			
9	Trunk Tendon, Right	S	Ankle Tendon, Right			
B	Trunk Tendon, Left	T	Ankle Tendon, Left			

Sections

ICD-10-PCS is composed of 17 sections, represented by the numbers 0 through 9 and the letters B through D, F through H, and X. The broad procedure categories contained in these sections range from surgical procedures to new technology.

The 17 sections are divided into three groups:
- Medical and Surgical Section
- Medical/Surgical Related Sections
- Ancillary Sections

Medical and Surgical Section

The first section, and the only section in the first group, MEDICAL AND SURGICAL, contains the great majority of procedures typically reported in an inpatient setting. As shown in the previous section discussing ICD-10-PCS code structure, all procedure codes in the MEDICAL AND SURGICAL section begin with the section value 0.

For a complete list of the Body Systems (Character 2) in the MEDICAL AND SURGICAL section, please see the Table of Contents located on page vi.

Medical/Surgical Related Sections

Sections 1 through 9 of ICD-10-PCS comprise the Medical and Surgical-related sections. These sections include obstetrical procedures, administration of substances, measurement and monitoring of body functions, and extracorporeal therapies, as listed below:

Section Value	Section Title
1	Obstetrics
2	Placement
3	Administration
4	Measurement and Monitoring
5	Extracorporeal Assistance and Performance
6	Extracorporeal Therapies
7	Osteopathic
8	Other Procedures
9	Chiropractic

In sections 1 and 2, all seven characters define the same aspects of the procedure as in the MEDICAL AND SURGICAL section.

Codes in sections 3 through 9 are structured for the most part like their counterparts in the MEDICAL AND SURGICAL section, with a few exceptions. For example, in sections 5 and 6, the fifth character is defined as duration instead of approach.

Additional differences include these uses of the sixth character:
- Section 3 defines the sixth character as substance.
- Sections 4 and 5 define the sixth character as function.
- Sections 7 through 9 define the sixth character as method.

Ancillary Sections

Sections B through D, F through H, and X comprise the ancillary sections of ICD-10-PCS. These seven sections include imaging procedures, nuclear medicine, and substance abuse treatment, as listed below:

Section Value	Section Title
B	Imaging
C	Nuclear Medicine
D	Radiation Therapy
F	Physical Rehabilitation and Diagnostic Audiology
G	Mental Health
H	Substance Abuse Treatment
X	New Technology

The definitions of some characters in the ancillary sections differs from that seen in previous sections. In the IMAGING section, the third character is defined as type, and the fifth and sixth characters define contrast and contrast/qualifier respectively.

Additional differences include:
- Section C defines the fifth character as radionuclide.
- Section D defines the fifth character as modality qualifier and the sixth character as isotope.
- Section F defines the fifth character as type qualifier and the sixth character as equipment.
- Sections G and H define the third character as a type qualifier.

Index

The ICD-10-PCS Index can be used to access the Tables. The Index mirrors the structure of the Tables, so it follows a consistent pattern of organization and use of hierarchies.

The Index is organized as an alphabetic lookup. Two types of main terms are listed in the Index:
- Based on the value of the third character (e.g., Root Operation, Root Type)
- Common procedure terms (e.g., Cholecystectomy)

Also included in the Index are the body parts identified in the Body Part Key and the devices identified in the Device Key.

Main Terms

For the MEDICAL AND SURGICAL and related sections, the root operation values are used as main terms in the Index. In other sections, the values representing the general type of procedure performed, such as nuclear medicine or imaging type, are listed as main terms.

For the MEDICAL AND SURGICAL and related sections, values such as EXCISION, BYPASS, and TRANSPLANTATION are included as main terms in the Index. The applicable body system entries are listed beneath the main term, and refer to a specific table. For the ancillary sections, values such as FLUOROSCOPY and POSITRON EMISSION TOMOGRAPHY are listed as main terms.

In the example below, the index entry "Bypass" refers to the MEDICAL AND SURGICAL section tables for all applicable body systems, including ANATOMICAL REGIONS and CENTRAL NERVOUS SYSTEM.

Bypass
   Cavity, Cranial 0W110J-
   Cerbral Ventricle 0016-

Common Procedure Terms

The second type of term listed in the Index uses procedure names, such as "appendectomy" or "fundoplication." These entries are listed as main terms, and refer to the possible valid Root Operations by using a "see" instruction, as shown in the following example.

Cholecystectomy
   – see Excision, Gallbladder 0FB4-
   – see Resection, Gallbladder 0FT4-

Definitions

The ICD-10-PCS Definitions contain the official definitions of ICD-10-PCS values in characters 3 through 7 of the seven-character code, and may also provide additional explanation or examples. The definitions are arranged in section order, and designate the section and the character within the section being defined.

The Medical and Surgical section body part value definitions refer from the body part value to corresponding anatomical terms. The Medical and Surgical section device definitions refer from the device value to corresponding device terms or manufacturer's names. The Substance value definitions in the Administration section refer from the substance value to a common substance name or manufacturer's substance name. These definitions are also sorted by common term and listed separately as the Body Part Key, Device Key, and Substance Key respectively.

The ICD-10-PCS Device Aggregation Table contains entries that correlate a specific ICD-10-PCS device value with a general device value to be used in tables containing only general device values.

Tabular Order File

The ICD-10-PCS Order file contains a unique "order number" for each valid code or table "header," a flag distinguishing valid codes from headers, and both long and short descriptions combined in a single file.

The code descriptions are generated using rules that produce standardized, complete, and easy-to-read code descriptions.

ICD-10-PCS DESIGN

ICD-10-PCS is fundamentally different from ICD-9-CM in its structure, organization, and capabilities. It was designed and developed to adhere to recommendations made by the National Committee on Vital and Health Statistics (NCVHS). It also incorporates input from a wide range of organizations, individual physicians, healthcare professionals, and researchers.

Several structural attributes were recommended for a new procedure coding system. These attributes include:
- Multiaxial structure
- Completeness
- Expandability

Multiaxial structure

The key attribute that provides the framework for all other structural attributes is multiaxial code structure. Multiaxial code structure makes it possible for the ICD-10-PCS to be complete, expandable, and to provide a high degree of flexibility and functionality.

As mentioned earlier, ICD-10-PCS codes are composed of seven characters. Each character represents a category of information that can be specified about the procedure performed. A character defines both the category of information and its physical position in the code.

A character's position can be understood as a semi-independent axis of classification that allows different specific values to be inserted into that space, and whose physical position remains stable. Within a defined code range, a character retains the general meaning that it confers on any value in that position. For example, the fifth character retains the general meaning "approach" in sections 0 through 4 and 7 through 9 of the system. Any specific value in the fifth character will define a specific approach, such as OPEN.

Each group of values for a character contains all of the valid choices in relation to the other characters of the code, giving the system completeness. In the fifth character, for example, each significantly distinct approach is assigned its own approach value and all applicable approach values are included to represent the possible versions of a procedure.

Each group of values for a character can be added to as needed, giving the system expandability. If a significantly distinct approach is used to perform procedures, a new approach value can be added to the system.

Each group of values is confined to its own character, giving ICD-10-PCS a stable, predictable readability across a wide range of codes. In sections 0 through 4 and 7 through 9 of the system, for example, the fifth character always represents the approach.

ICD-10-PCS' multiaxial structure houses its capacity for completeness, expandability, and flexibility, giving it a high degree of functionality for multiple uses.

Completeness

Completeness is considered a key structural attribute for a new procedure coding system. The specific recommendation for completeness includes these characteristics:
- A unique code is available for each significantly different procedure.
- Each code retains its unique definition. Codes are not reused.

In Volume 3 of ICD-9-CM, procedures performed on many different body parts using different approaches or devices may be assigned to the same procedure code. In ICD-10-PCS, a unique code can be constructed for every significantly different procedure.

Within each section, a character defines a consistent component of a code, and contains all applicable values for that character. The values define individual expressions (open, percutaneous) of the character's general meaning (approach) that are then used to construct unique procedure codes.

Because all approaches by which a procedure is performed are assigned a separate approach value in the system, every procedure which uses a different approach will have its own unique code. This is true of the other characters as well. The same procedure performed on a different body part has its own unique code, the same procedure performed using a different device has its own unique code, and so on.

Because ICD-10-PCS codes are constructed of individual values rather than lists of fixed codes and text descriptions, the unique, stable definition of a code in the system is retained. New values may be added to the system to represent a specific new approach or device or qualifier, but whole codes by design cannot be given new meanings and reused.

Expandability

Expandability was also recommended as a key structural attribute. The specific recommendation for expandability includes these characteristics:
- Accommodate new procedures and technologies
- Add new codes without disrupting the existing structure

ICD-10-PCS is designed to be easily updated as new codes are required for new procedures and new techniques. Changes to ICD-10-PCS can all be made within the existing structure, because whole codes are not added. Instead, one of two possible changes is made to the system:
- A new value for a character is added as needed to the system
- An existing value for a character is added to a table(s) in the system

ICD-10-PCS update: PICVA

An example of how the updating of ICD-10-PCS works can be seen in the coronary artery bypass procedure called Percutaneous in-situ coronary venous arterialization (PICVA). This procedure is no more invasive than a percutaneous coronary angioplasty, but achieves the benefits of a bypass procedure by placing a specialized stent into the diseased coronary artery, through its wall into the adjacent coronary vein, and diverting blood flow through the stent into the artery past the blockage.

ICD-10-PCS was updated in 2004 to include an appropriate range of codes for the PICVA procedure (16 possible codes). This was accomplished simply by adding another row to the relevant table (as shown in the example below) containing two approach values for the non-invasive approach, two device values for the possible types of stent, and a single qualifier defining the coronary vein as the source of the new blood flow, as in the example below.

The values for characters 1 through 3 at the top of each table are:
0: MEDICAL AND SURGICAL (Section)
2: HEART AND GREAT VESSELS (Body system)
1: BYPASS: Altering the route of passage of the contents of a tubular body part

Body Part Character 4	Approach Character 5	Device Character 6	Qualifier Character 7
0 Coronary Artery, One Site 1 Coronary Artery, Two Sites 2 Coronary Artery, Three Sites 3 Coronary Artery, Four or More Sites	3 Percutaneous 4 Percutaneous Endoscopic	4 Drug-eluting Intraluminal Device D Intraluminal Device	D Coronary Vein

Structural integrity

As shown in the previous example, ICD-10-PCS can be easily expanded without disrupting the structure of the system.
In the PICVA example, one new value—the qualifier value Coronary Vein—was added to the system to effect this change. All other values in the new row are existing values used to create unique, new codes.
This type of updating can be replicated anywhere in the system when a change is required. ICD-10-PCS allows unique new codes to be added to the system because values for the seven characters that make up a code can be combined as needed. The system can evolve as medical technology and clinical practice evolve, without disrupting the ICD-10-PCS structure.

ICD-10-PCS ADDITIONAL CHARACTERISTICS

ICD-10-PCS possesses several additional characteristics in response to government and industry recommendations. These characteristics are:
- Standardized terminology within the coding system
- Standardized level of specificity
- No diagnostic information
- No explicit "not otherwise specified" (NOS) code options
- Limited use of "not elsewhere classified" (NEC) code options

Standardized Terminology
Words commonly used in clinical vocabularies may have multiple meanings. This can cause confusion and result in inaccurate data. ICD-10-PCS is standardized and self-contained. Characters and values used in the system are defined in the system.

For example, the word "excision" is used to describe a wide variety of surgical procedures. In ICD-10-PCS, the word "excision" describes a single, precise surgical objective, defined as "Cutting out or off, without replacement, a portion of a body part."

No Eponyms or Common Procedure Names
The terminology used in ICD-10-PCS is standardized to provide precise and stable definitions of all procedures performed. This standardized terminology is used in all ICD-10-PCS code descriptions.

As a result, ICD-10-PCS code descriptions do not include eponyms or common procedure names. Two examples from ICD-9-CM are 22.61, "Excision of lesion of maxillary sinus with Caldwell-Luc approach," and 51.10, "Endoscopic retrograde cholangiopancreatography [ERCP]." In ICD-10-PCS, physicians' names are not included in a code description, nor are procedures identified by common terms or acronyms such as appendectomy or CABG. Instead, such procedures are coded to the root operation that accurately identifies the objective of the procedure.

The procedures described in the preceding paragraph by ICD-9-CM codes are coded in ICD-10-PCS according to the root operation that matches the objective of the procedure. Here the ICD-10-PCS equivalents would be EXCISION and INSPECTION respectively. By relying on the universal objectives defined in root operations rather than eponyms or specific procedure titles that change or become obsolete, ICD-10-PCS preserves the capacity to define past, present, and future procedures accurately using stable terminology in the form of characters and values.

No Combination Codes
With rare exceptions, ICD-10-PCS does not define multiple procedures with one code. This is to preserve standardized terminology and consistency across the system. Procedures that are typically performed together but are distinct procedures may be defined by a single "combination code" in ICD-9-CM. An example of a combination code in ICD-9-CM is 28.3, "Tonsillectomy with adenoidectomy."

A procedure that meets the reporting criteria for a separate procedure is coded separately in ICD-10-PCS. This allows the system to respond to changes in technology and medical practice with the maximum degree of stability and flexibility.

Standardized Level of Specificity
In ICD-9-CM, one code with its description and includes notes may encompass a vast number of procedure variations while another code defines a single specific procedure. ICD-10-PCS provides a standardized level of specificity for each code, so that each code represents a single procedure variation.

The ICD-9-CM code 39.31, "Suture of artery," does not specify the artery, whereas the code range 38.40 through 38.49, "Resection of artery with replacement," provides a fourth-digit subclassification for specifying the artery by anatomical region (thoracic, abdominal, etc.).

In ICD-10-PCS, the codes identifying all artery suture and artery replacement procedures possess the same degree of specificity. The ICD-9-CM examples above coded to their ICD-10-PCS equivalents would use the same artery body part values in all codes identifying the respective procedures.

In general, ICD-10-PCS code descriptions are much more specific than their ICD-9-CM counterparts, but sometimes an ICD-10-PCS code description is actually less specific. In most cases this is because the ICD-9-CM code contains diagnosis information. The standardized level of code specificity in ICD-10-PCS cannot always take account of these fluctuations in ICD-9-CM level of specificity. Instead, ICD-10-PCS provides a standardized level of specificity that can be predicted across the system.

Diagnosis Information Excluded
Another key feature of ICD-10-PCS is that information pertaining to a diagnosis is excluded from the code descriptions.

ICD-9-CM often contains information about the diagnosis in its procedure codes. Adding diagnosis information limits the flexibility and functionality of a procedure coding system. It has the effect of placing a code "off limits" because the diagnosis in the medical record does not match the diagnosis in the procedure code description. The code cannot be used even though the procedural part of the code description precisely matches the procedure performed.

Diagnosis information is not contained in any ICD-10-PCS code. The diagnosis codes, not the procedure codes, will specify the reason the procedure is performed.

NOS Code Options Restricted
ICD-9-CM often designates codes as "unspecified" or "not otherwise specified" codes. By contrast, the standardized level of specificity designed into ICD-10-PCS restricts the use of broadly applicable NOS or unspecified code options in the system. A minimal level of specificity is required to construct a valid code.

In ICD-10-PCS, each character defines information about the procedure and all seven characters must contain a specific value obtained from a single row of a table to build a valid code. Even values such as the sixth-character value Z, NO DEVICE and the seventh-character value Z, NO QUALIFIER, provide important information about the procedure performed.

Limited NEC Code Options
ICD-9-CM often designates codes as "not elsewhere classified" or "other specified" versions of a procedure throughout the code set. NEC options are also provided in ICD-10-PCS, but only for specific, limited use.

In the MEDICAL AND SURGICAL section, two significant "not elsewhere classified" options are the root operation value Q, REPAIR and the device value Y, OTHER DEVICE.

The root operation REPAIR is a true NEC value. It is used only when the procedure performed is not one of the other root operations in the MEDICAL AND SURGICAL section.

OTHER DEVICE, on the other hand, is intended to be used to temporarily define new devices that do not have a specific value assigned, until one can be added to the system. No categories of medical or surgical devices are permanently classified to OTHER DEVICE.

ICD-10-PCS APPLICATIONS

ICD-10-PCS code structure results in qualities that optimize the performance of the system in electronic applications, and maximize the usefulness of the coded healthcare data. These qualities include:
- Optimal search capability
- Consistent character definitions
- Consistent values wherever possible
- Code readability

Some have argued that, in the world of the electronic health record, the classification system as we know it is outmoded, that classification doesn't matter because a computer is able to find a code with equal ease whether the code has been generated at random or is part of a classification scheme. While this may be true from an IT perspective, assignment of randomly generated code numbers makes it impossible to aggregate data according to related ranges of codes. This is a critical capability for providers, payers, and researchers to make meaningful use of the data.

Optimal Search Capability
ICD-10-PCS is designed for maximum versatility in the ability to aggregate coded data. Values belonging to the same character as defined in a section or sections can be easily compared, since they occupy the same position in a code. This provides a high degree of flexibility and functionality for data mining.

For example, the body part value 6, STOMACH, retains its meaning for all codes in the MEDICAL AND SURGICAL section that define procedures performed on the stomach. Because the body part value is dependent for its meaning on the body system in which it is found, the body system value D, GASTROINTESTINAL, must also be included in the search.

A person wishing to examine data regarding all medical and surgical procedures performed on the stomach could do so simply by searching the following code range: 0D*6***

Consistent Characters and Values
In the previous example, the value 6 means STOMACH only when the body system value is D, GASTROINTESTINAL. In many other cases, values retain their meaning across a much broader range of codes. This provides consistency and readability.

For example, the value 0 in the fifth character defines the approach OPEN and the value 3 in the fifth character defines the approach PERCUTANEOUS across sections 0 through 4 and 7 through 9, where applicable. As a result, all open and percutaneous procedures represented by codes in sections 0-4 and 7-9 can be compared based on a single character—approach—by conducting a query on the following code ranges:
[0 through 4,7 through 9]***0** vs. [0 through 4,7 through 9]***3**

Searches can be progressively refined by adding specific values. For example, one could search on a body system value or range of body system values, plus a body part value or range of body part values, plus a root operation value or range of root operation values.

To refine the search above, one could add the body system value for GASTROINTESTINAL and the body part value for STOMACH to limit the search to open vs. percutaneous procedures performed on the stomach: 0D*60** vs. 0D*63**

To refine the search even further and limit the comparison to open and percutaneous biopsies of the stomach, one could add the third-character value for the root operation EXCISION and the seventh-character qualifier DIAGNOSTIC, as follows: 0DB60*X vs. 0DB63*X

Stability of characters and values across vast ranges of codes provides the maximum degree of functionality and flexibility for the collection and analysis of data. The search capabilities demonstrated above function equally well for all uses of healthcare data: investigating quality of care, resource utilization, risk management, conducting research, determining reimbursement, and many others.

Because the character definition is consistent, and only the individual values assigned to that character differ as needed, meaningful comparisons of data over time can be conducted across a virtually infinite range of procedures.

Code readability
ICD-10-PCS resembles a language in the sense that it is made up of semi-independent values combined by following the rules of the system, much the way a sentence is formed by combining words and following the rules of grammar and syntax. As with words in their context, the meaning of any single value is a combination of its position in the code and any preceding values on which it may be dependent.

For example, in the MEDICAL AND SURGICAL section, a body part value is always dependent for its meaning on the body system in which it is found. It cannot stand alone as a letter or a number and be meaningful. A fourth-character value of 6 by itself can mean 31 different things, but a fourth-character value of 6 in the context of a second-character value of D means one thing only—STOMACH.

On the other hand, a root operation value is not dependent on any character but the section for its meaning, and identifies a single consistent objective wherever the third character is defined as root operation. For example, the third-character value T identifies the root operation RESECTION in both the MEDICAL AND SURGICAL and OBSTETRICS sections.

The approach value also identifies a single consistent approach wherever the fifth character is defined as approach. The fifth-character value 3 identifies the approach PERCUTANEOUS in the MEDICAL AND SURGICAL section, the OBSTETRICS section, the ADMINISTRATION section, and others.

The sixth-character device value or seventh-character qualifier value identifies the same device or qualifier in the context of the body system where it is found. Although there may be consistencies across body systems or within whole sections, this is not true in all cases.

Values in their designated context have a precise meaning, like words in a language. As seen in the code example which began this chapter, 0LB50ZZ represents the text description of the specific procedure "Excision of right lower arm and wrist tendon, open approach." Since ICD-10-PCS values in context have a single, precise meaning, a complete, valid code can be read and understood without its accompanying text description, much like one would read a sentence.

Please see the Appendices following the Ancillary Sections for further detailed information on ICD-10-PCS and its components.

Channel Publishing 2016 ICD-10-PCS Additional *Enhanced* Features

Unique, Enhanced Table Design

The basic PCS tables have been significantly enhanced (graphic design) to help coders clearly and quickly identify the components of each PCS code table.

Inclusion of Example and Brief Explanation in PCS Table design

The addition of root operation examples and a brief explanation of the root operation (in addition to the root operation definition) helps coders understand each root operation without referring to a table in the appendices.

Unique, Graphic Page Design

The unique, graphic page design clearly identifies which PCS code tables are located on that page and helps coders stay focused on the particular root operation for that body system. In addition, code tables that are too extensive for one page have that continued information very clearly identified.

Highlighted First 3 Digits in Index

The first 3 digits of each code in the Alphabetic Index are in boldface type to help coders identify and search for the correct 3-digit PCS code table in the Tabular Table sections.

Highlighted Body Part & Device Terms

The body part and device terms in the index have gray screen bars placed over them to help coders more easily differentiate between standard index entries and the body part and device terms.

Body Part, Device & Device Aggregation Keys

The body part, device, and device aggregation keys (tables) are listed in separate appendices following the Tabular Table sections.

All 7 Characters Clearly Identified

All 7 characters of a PCS code are clearly identified in each PCS code table to help coders learn and properly select the appropriate character for each digit.

Tab-Edge Printing

Chapter-by-chapter, and section-by-section stair-stepped, tab-edge printing helps coders locate the correct section quickly.

Clear, Compact Type Face Printing

The use of clear, compact type face to allow coders to clearly and easily locate and read all text in the Alphabetic Index and Tabular Tables.

Clear, Compact Guidewords at the Top of Each Page

The use of clear, compact guidewords allow coders to clearly and easily locate the correct page in the Alphabetic Index and Tabular Tables.

Channel Publishing Additional 2016 *Enhanced* Features

Educational Annotations for Each Body System and Section

Anatomy and Physiology Reviews
Anatomy and physiology reviews that help coders understand the anatomical structures and physiology of the various systems.

Illustrations
Anatomical illustrations with call outs of body parts.

Definitions
Medical definitions of common procedures written by a coder for coders.

AHA Coding Clinic® Reference Notations
Identifies AHA Coding Clinic® articles and Q&As (with descriptive title) that have relevant information for certain codes or code categories.

Body Part Key Listings
Identifies the Body Part Key listings specific for that body system or section.

Device Key Listings
Identifies the Device Key listings specific for that body system or section.

Device Aggregation Table Listings
Identifies the Device Aggregation Table listings specific for that body system or section.

Coding Guidelines
Lists the Official Coding Guidelines specific for that body system or section.

PCS Reference Manual Exercises
Lists the exercises found in the PCS Reference Manual specific for that body system or section.

Tab-Edge Printing for Educational Annotations Pages
The Educational Annotations pages are identified by two digits in the screen bar: First digit – Section, Second digit – Body System.

Additional 2016 Features

Groups of Similar Root Operations
At the top of each table is a list of similar Root Operations that includes that table's Root Operation. The screened-out Root Operations are Root Operations that are not included in that Body System.

Body System Specific Root Operation Examples
Each table identifies the CMS general Root Operation example and a Channel Publishing created Body System Specific example.

Medicare Code Editor Edits
Identifies codes that are edit-reviewed for age and sex-related discrepancies and principal diagnosis criteria.

Color Highlighting
Color highlighting of Index:
- Guide words – Burgundy
- Continued headers – Burgundy
- Highlighted Body Part Key terms – Screened Blue
- Highlighted Device Key terms – Screened Blue
- Tab-Edge Printing – Blue

Color highlighting of Tables:
- Tables – Blue
- Root Operation Definitions – Burgundy
- Similar Root Operation Groupings – Green
- Medicare Code Editor Edits – Blue
- Tab-Edge Printing – Blue

INTRODUCTION – 2016 ICD-10-PCS [2016.PCS]

INTRODUCTION TO AHA CODING CLINIC® REFERENCE NOTATIONS

BACKGROUND

AHA Coding Clinic® is a registered trademark of the American Hospital Association. AHA Coding Clinic® Reference Notations is not a product of the American Hospital Association, and Channel Publishing, Ltd. is not affiliated with or endorsed by the American Hospital Association. The American Hospital coding website can be accessed at www.ahacentraloffice.org.

The AHA Coding Clinic® for ICD-10-CM/PCS is published quarterly by the American Hospital Association. The *Coding Clinic* is the official publication for *ICD-10-CM/PCS* coding guidelines and advice as designated by the four cooperating parties. The cooperating parties listed below have final approval of the coding advice provided in the *Coding Clinic*: American Hospital Association, American Health Information Management Association, Centers for Medicare and Medicaid Services, National Center for Health Statistics.

The *Coding Clinic* provides specific information and guidelines that are helpful for determining proper coding, and is used by CMS in reviewing claims. The goal of the *Coding Clinic* is to provide coding advice, official coding decisions, and news. It promotes accuracy and consistency in the use of ICD-10-CM/PCS. It offers coding guidelines and advice based on adherence to the statistical classification scheme of ICD-10-CM/PCS and the definitions specified in the Uniform Hospital Discharge Data Set (UHDDS).

INTRODUCTION

Channel Publishing has developed the AHA Coding Clinic® Reference Notations to help coders access the official coding advice found throughout all issues of the *Coding Clinic*. This information has been referenced in three ways: 1) at the Educational Annotations portion of each Body System/Section, 2) at the identified Coding Guideline, and 3) a categorical index of articles (see below) that are too broad in scope to be assigned to 1) or 2). Any comments regarding these reference notations should be directed to: *Coding Clinic* Reference Notations, c/o Channel Publishing, Ltd., 4750 Longley Lane, Suite 110, Reno, Nevada 89502.

GUIDANCE IN USE

Coders are encouraged to reference all relevant information contained in the *Coding Clinic* to promote the most accurate coding possible for their organization. It is important to understand the basic criteria for assigning the *Coding Clinic* Reference Notations. The basic criteria consists of: Assignment to codes with direct or indirect information concerning the proper use of each particular code, assignment to a code category when the information is relevant to all codes in that category, and assignment to codes where a coder might commonly attempt to use a code in error.

MISCELLANEOUS AHA CODING CLINIC® REFERENCE NOTATIONS INDEX

APPROACHES (MEDICAL AND SURGICAL SECTION)
MISC
    Minimally invasive approaches .... AHA 13:4Q:p108
OPEN - 0
    Open approach value not an option .... AHA 13:2Q:p34
    .... AHA 14:4Q:p34
    Repair of second degree perineal laceration including muscle .... AHA 13:4Q:p120
PERCUTANEOUS - 3
PERCUTANEOUS ENDOSCOPIC - 4
    Hand-assisted laparoscopy .... AHA 14:3Q:p16
VIA NATURAL OR ARTIFICIAL OPENING - 7
    Percutaneous endoscopic gastrostomy (PEG) placement .... AHA 13:4Q:p117
VIA NATURAL OR ARTIFICIAL OPENING ENDOSCOPIC - 8
VIA NATURAL OR ARTIFICIAL OPENING PERCUTANEOUS ENDOSCOPIC ASSISTANCE - F
EXTERNAL - X
    Removal of left eye .... AHA 15:2Q:p12
    Wide local excision of soft palate with placement of a maxillary
        surgical obturator .... AHA 14:3Q:p25
DEVICE VALUE ISSUES
    Autograft, allograft, and BMP .... AHA 13:1Q:p23
    Biologically derived skin substitutes .... AHA 14:2Q:p5
    Gelfoam embolization of uterine artery .... AHA 15:2Q:p27
    Intraoral graft using Oasis® acellular matrix .... AHA 14:2Q:p5,6
    Material classified as device or substance .... AHA 14:2Q:p12
    Placement of Ioban™ drape (antimicrobial barrier) .... AHA 15:2Q:p29
    Zooplastic not a device option .... AHA 14:4Q:p37
BODY PART ISSUES
    Cricotracheal resection .... AHA 15:1Q:p15
    Incision and drainage of femoral region wound infection .... AHA 15:1Q:p22
    Incision and drainage of inguinal region wound infection .... AHA 15:1Q:p22
    Polyp excision in ileal loop (neobladder) .... AHA 14:2Q:p8
    Restenosis of saphenous vein coronary artery bypass graft using a stent .... AHA 14:2Q:p4
    Use "Face" when "Eyebrow" is not designated body part .... AHA 15:1Q:p31
AHA MISC
    Documentation issues .... AHA 14:1Q:p11
    Use of clinical information published in Coding Clinic for ICD-9-CM
        when coding in ICD-10 .... AHA 14:1Q:p11
    Separation of conjoined twins .... AHA 13:4Q:p109
    Supplement can be used as "Repair with device NEC" .... AHA 15:1Q:p28

OFFICIAL CODING GUIDELINES – 2016 ICD-10-PCS

IMPORTANT NOTES REGARDING THESE PRINTED GUIDELINES

These guidelines are effective for the 2016 version (April 2015 posting) of ICD-10-PCS. A newer version may become available after this book has been printed. Coders should periodically check the Centers for Medicare and Medicaid Services (CMS) web site for the most current version. CMS Web Site: www.cms.gov

Any text printed in red represents an addition, deletion, or revision from the 2015 Official Guidelines.

Some Body System specific Guidelines have been reprinted on the Educational Annotations pages for those Body Systems. However, they are not a substitute for using the entire set of Official Coding Guidelines.

Channel Publishing, Ltd.

2016 ICD-10-PCS Official Guidelines for Coding and Reporting

The Centers for Medicare and Medicaid Services (CMS) and the National Center for Health Statistics (NCHS), two departments within the U.S. Federal Government's Department of Health and Human Services (DHHS) provide the following guidelines for coding and reporting using the International Classification of Diseases, 10th Revision, Procedure Coding System (ICD-10-PCS). These guidelines should be used as a companion document to the official version of the ICD-10-PCS as published on the CMS website. The ICD-10-PCS is a procedure classification published by the United States for classifying procedures performed in hospital inpatient health care settings.

These guidelines have been approved by the four organizations that make up the Cooperating Parties for the ICD-10-PCS: the American Hospital Association (AHA), the American Health Information Management Association (AHIMA), CMS, and NCHS.

These guidelines are a set of rules that have been developed to accompany and complement the official conventions and instructions provided within the ICD-10-PCS itself. The instructions and conventions of the classification take precedence over guidelines. These guidelines are based on the coding and sequencing instructions in the Tables, Index and Definitions of ICD-10-PCS, but provide additional instruction. Adherence to these guidelines when assigning ICD-10-PCS procedure codes is required under the Health Insurance Portability and Accountability Act (HIPAA). The procedure codes have been adopted under HIPAA for hospital inpatient healthcare settings. A joint effort between the healthcare provider and the coder is essential to achieve complete and accurate documentation, code assignment, and reporting of diagnoses and procedures. These guidelines have been developed to assist both the healthcare provider and the coder in identifying those procedures that are to be reported. The importance of consistent, complete documentation in the medical record cannot be overemphasized. Without such documentation accurate coding cannot be achieved.

Table of Contents

A. Conventions	CG-1
B. Medical and Surgical Section Guidelines	CG-2
2. Body System	CG-2
3. Root Operation	CG-2
4. Body Part	CG-4
5. Approach	CG-5
6. Device	CG-5
C. Obstetrics Section Guidelines	CG-6
D. New Technology Section Guidelines	CG-6
Selection of Principal Procedure	CG-6

Conventions

A1
ICD-10-PCS codes are composed of seven characters. Each character is an axis of classification that specifies information about the procedure performed. Within a defined code range, a character specifies the same type of information in that axis of classification.
Example: The fifth axis of classification specifies the approach in sections 0 through 4 and 7 through 9 of the system.

A2
One of 34 possible values can be assigned to each axis of classification in the seven-character code: they are the numbers 0 through 9 and the alphabet (except I and O because they are easily confused with the numbers 1 and 0). The number of unique values used in an axis of classification differs as needed.
Example: Where the fifth axis of classification specifies the approach, seven different approach values are currently used to specify the approach.

A3
The valid values for an axis of classification can be added to as needed.
Example: If a significantly distinct type of device is used in a new procedure, a new device value can be added to the system.

A4
As with words in their context, the meaning of any single value is a combination of its axis of classification and any preceding values on which it may be dependent.
Example: The meaning of a body part value in the Medical and Surgical section is always dependent on the body system value. The body part value 0 in the Central Nervous body system specifies Brain and the body part value 0 in the Peripheral Nervous body system specifies Cervical Plexus.

A5
As the system is expanded to become increasingly detailed, over time more values will depend on preceding values for their meaning.
Example: In the Lower Joints body system, the device value 3 in the root operation Insertion specifies Infusion Device and the device value 3 in the root operation Replacement specifies Ceramic Synthetic Substitute.

A6
The purpose of the alphabetic index is to locate the appropriate table that contains all information necessary to construct a procedure code. The PCS Tables should always be consulted to find the most appropriate valid code.

A7
It is not required to consult the index first before proceeding to the tables to complete the code. A valid code may be chosen directly from the tables.
AHA Coding Clinic® Reference Notation(s) — Coding Guideline A7
Reconstruction, main index term .... AHA 14:2Q:p10

A8
All seven characters must be specified to be a valid code. If the documentation is incomplete for coding purposes, the physician should be queried for the necessary information.

A9
Within a PCS table, valid codes include all combinations of choices in characters 4 through 7 contained in the same row of the table. In the example below, 0JHT3VZ is a valid code, and 0JHW3VZ is *not* a valid code.

EXAMPLE: Placement pacemaker generator

1ST- **0** Medical and Surgical
2ND- **J** Subcutaneous Tissue and Fascia
3RD- **H** INSERTION

INSERTION: Putting in a nonbiological appliance that monitors, assists, performs, or prevents a physiological function but does not physically take the place of a body part.

EXPLANATION: None

4TH Body Part	5TH Approach	6TH Device	7TH Qualifier
S Subcutaneous Tissue and Fascia, Head and Neck V Subcutaneous Tissue and Fascia, Upper Extremity **W Subcutaneous Tissue and Fascia, Lower Extremity**	0 Open 3 Percutaneous	1 Radioactive Element 3 Infusion Device	Z No Qualifier
T Subcutaneous Tissue and Fascia, Trunk	0 Open 3 Percutaneous	1 Radioactive Element 3 Infusion Device **V Infusion Pump**	Z No Qualifier

OFFICIAL CODING GUIDELINES – 2016 ICD-10-PCS [2016.PCS]

A10
"And," when used in a code description, means "and/or."
Example: Lower Arm and Wrist Muscle means lower arm and/or wrist muscle.

A11
Many of the terms used to construct PCS codes are defined within the system. It is the coder's responsibility to determine what the documentation in the medical record equates to in the PCS definitions. The physician is not expected to use the terms used in PCS code descriptions, nor is the coder required to query the physician when the correlation between the documentation and the defined PCS terms is clear.
Example: When the physician documents "partial resection" the coder can independently correlate "partial resection" to the root operation Excision without querying the physician for clarification.

Medical and Surgical Section Guidelines (Section 0)

B2. Body System

General guidelines

B2.1a
The procedure codes in the general anatomical regions body systems should only be used when the procedure is performed on an anatomical region rather than a specific body part (e.g., root operations Control and Detachment, Drainage of a body cavity) or on the rare occasion when no information is available to support assignment of a code to a specific body part.
Example: Control of postoperative hemorrhage is coded to the root operation Control found in the general anatomical regions body systems.

B2.1b
Where the general body part values "upper" and "lower" are provided as an option in the Upper Arteries, Lower Arteries, Upper Veins, Lower Veins, Muscles and Tendons body systems, "upper" and "lower" specifies body parts located above or below the diaphragm respectively.
Example: Vein body parts above the diaphragm are found in the Upper Veins body system; vein body parts below the diaphragm are found in the Lower Veins body system.

AHA Coding Clinic® Reference Notation(s) — Coding Guideline B2.1b
Upper or lower veins body system ....AHA 14:3Q:p25

B3. Root Operation

General guidelines

B3.1a
In order to determine the appropriate root operation, the full definition of the root operation as contained in the PCS Tables must be applied.

B3.1b
Components of a procedure specified in the root operation definition and explanation are not coded separately. Procedural steps necessary to reach the operative site and close the operative site, including anastomosis of a tubular body part, are also not coded separately.
Example: Resection of a joint as part of a joint replacement procedure is included in the root operation definition of Replacement and is not coded separately. Laparotomy performed to reach the site of an open liver biopsy is not coded separately. In a resection of sigmoid colon with anastomosis of descending colon to rectum, the anastomosis is not coded separately.

AHA Coding Clinic® Reference Notation(s) — Coding Guideline B3.1b
Components in fusion procedures included in Fusion root operation .... AHA 14:3Q:p30
Coronary artery release prior to bypass .... AHA 13:2Q:p37
Debridement considered as procedure preparation .... AHA 14:3Q:p31
FloSeal on small bleeder during cholecystectomy .... AHA 13:3Q:p22
Injection of substances with vitrectomy .... AHA 15:2Q:p24
Lysis of adhesions, integral or code separately .... AHA 14:1Q:p3
Omental bleeding repair during cholecystectomy .... AHA 13:3Q:p23
Orthotopic liver transplant with end-to-side cavoplasty and choledochostomy AHA 14:3Q:p13

CG-2

Multiple procedures

B3.2

During the same operative episode, multiple procedures are coded if:
a. The same root operation is performed on different body parts as defined by distinct values of the body part character.
Example: Diagnostic excision of liver and pancreas are coded separately.
b. The same root operation is repeated in multiple body parts, and those body parts are separate and distinct body parts classified to a single ICD-10-PCS body part value.
AHA Coding Clinic® Reference Notation(s) — Coding Guideline B3.2b
Coil embolization of gastroduodenal artery, and chemoembolization of hepatic artery .... AHA 14:3Q:p26
Uterine fibroids, multiple .... AHA 14:4Q:p16
Example: Excision of the sartorius muscle and excision of the gracilis muscle are both included in the upper leg muscle body part value, and multiple procedures are coded.
c. Multiple root operations with distinct objectives are performed on the same body part.
Example: Destruction of sigmoid lesion and bypass of sigmoid colon are coded separately.
AHA Coding Clinic® Reference Notation(s) — Coding Guideline B3.2c
Laminoplasty with two distinct objectives .... AHA 15:2Q:p20
d. The intended root operation is attempted using one approach, but is converted to a different approach.
Example: Laparoscopic cholecystectomy converted to an open cholecystectomy is coded as percutaneous endoscopic Inspection and open Resection.
AHA Coding Clinic® Reference Notation(s) — Coding Guideline B3.2d
Laparoscopic procedure converted to open .... AHA 15:1Q:p33

Discontinued procedures

B3.3

If the intended procedure is discontinued, code the procedure to the root operation performed. If a procedure is discontinued before any other root operation is performed, code the root operation Inspection of the body part or anatomical region inspected.
Example: A planned aortic valve replacement procedure is discontinued after the initial thoracotomy and before any incision is made in the heart muscle, when the patient becomes hemodynamically unstable. This procedure is coded as an open Inspection of the mediastinum.

Biopsy procedures

B3.4a

Biopsy procedures are coded using the root operations Excision, Extraction, or Drainage and the qualifier Diagnostic. ~~The qualifier Diagnostic is used only for biopsies.~~
Example: Fine needle aspiration biopsy of lung is coded to the root operation Drainage with the qualifier Diagnostic. Biopsy of bone marrow is coded to the root operation Extraction with the qualifier Diagnostic. Lymph node sampling for biopsy is coded to the root operation Excision with the qualifier Diagnostic.

Biopsy followed by more definitive treatment

B3.4b

If a diagnostic Excision, Extraction, or Drainage procedure (biopsy) is followed by a more definitive procedure, such as Destruction, Excision or Resection at the same procedure site, both the biopsy and the more definitive treatment are coded.
Example: Biopsy of breast followed by partial mastectomy at the same procedure site, both the biopsy and the partial mastectomy procedure are coded.

Overlapping body layers

B3.5

If the root operations Excision, Repair or Inspection are performed on overlapping layers of the musculoskeletal system, the body part specifying the deepest layer is coded.
Example: Excisional debridement that includes skin and subcutaneous tissue and muscle is coded to the muscle body part.
AHA Coding Clinic® Reference Notation(s) — Coding Guideline B3.5
Deepest layer coded .... AHA 14:3Q:p14

Bypass procedures

B3.6a

Bypass procedures are coded by identifying the body part bypassed "from" and the body part bypassed "to." The fourth character body part specifies the body part bypassed from, and the qualifier specifies the body part bypassed to.
Example: Bypass from stomach to jejunum, stomach is the body part and jejunum is the qualifier.
AHA Coding Clinic® Reference Notation(s) — Coding Guideline B3.6a
Creation of percutaneous cutaneoperitoneal fistula for peritoneal dialysis ...... AHA 13:4Q:p126

B3.6b

Coronary arteries are classified by number of distinct sites treated, rather than number of coronary arteries or anatomic name of a coronary artery (e.g., left anterior descending). Coronary artery bypass procedures are coded differently than other bypass procedures as described in the previous guideline. Rather than identifying the body part bypassed from, the body part identifies the number of coronary artery sites bypassed to, and the qualifier specifies the vessel bypassed from.
Example: Aortocoronary artery bypass of one site on the left anterior descending coronary artery and one site on the obtuse marginal coronary artery is classified in the body part axis of classification as two coronary artery sites and the qualifier specifies the aorta as the body part bypassed from.
AHA Coding Clinic® Reference Notation(s) — Coding Guideline B3.6b
Distinct coronary lesion sites treated .... AHA 15:2Q:p3-5

B3.6c

If multiple coronary artery sites are bypassed, a separate procedure is coded for each coronary artery site that uses a different device and/or qualifier.
Example: Aortocoronary artery bypass and internal mammary coronary artery bypass are coded separately.

Control vs. more definitive root operations

B3.7

The root operation Control is defined as, "Stopping, or attempting to stop, postprocedural bleeding." If an attempt to stop postprocedural bleeding is initially unsuccessful, and to stop the bleeding requires performing any of the definitive root operations Bypass, Detachment, Excision, Extraction, Reposition, Replacement, or Resection, then that root operation is coded instead of Control.
Example: Resection of spleen to stop postprocedural bleeding is coded to Resection instead of Control.

Excision vs. Resection

B3.8

PCS contains specific body parts for anatomical subdivisions of a body part, such as lobes of the lungs or liver and regions of the intestine. Resection of the specific body part is coded whenever all of the body part is cut out or off, rather than coding Excision of a less specific body part.
Example: Left upper lung lobectomy is coded to Resection of Upper Lung Lobe, Left rather than Excision of Lung, Left.

Excision for graft

B3.9

If an autograft is obtained from a different body part in order to complete the objective of the procedure, a separate procedure is coded.
Example: Coronary bypass with excision of saphenous vein graft, excision of saphenous vein is coded separately.
AHA Coding Clinic® Reference Notation(s) — Coding Guideline B3.9
Harvesting of fat graft from abdomen .... AHA 14:3Q:p22

Fusion procedures of the spine

B3.10a

The body part coded for a spinal vertebral joint(s) rendered immobile by a spinal fusion procedure is classified by the level of the spine (e.g. thoracic). There are distinct body part values for a single vertebral joint and for multiple vertebral joints at each spinal level.
Example: Body part values specify Lumbar Vertebral Joint, Lumbar Vertebral Joints, 2 or More and Lumbosacral Vertebral Joint.
AHA Coding Clinic® Reference Notation(s) — Coding Guideline B3.10a
Fusion, level of spine .... AHA 13:1Q:p29
Fusion of multiple vertebral joints... AHA 13:1Q:p21

B3.10b

If multiple vertebral joints are fused, a separate procedure is coded for each vertebral joint that uses a different device and/or qualifier.
Example: Fusion of lumbar vertebral joint, posterior approach, anterior column and fusion of lumbar vertebral joint, posterior approach, posterior column are coded separately.

B3.10c

Combinations of devices and materials are often used on a vertebral joint to render the joint immobile. When combinations of devices are used on the same vertebral joint, the device value coded for the procedure is as follows:
- If an interbody fusion device is used to render the joint immobile (alone or containing other material like bone graft), the procedure is coded with the device value Interbody Fusion Device
- If bone graft is the *only* device used to render the joint immobile, the procedure is coded with the device value Nonautologous Tissue Substitute or Autologous Tissue Substitute
- If a mixture of autologous and nonautologous bone graft (with or without biological or synthetic extenders or binders) is used to render the joint immobile, code the procedure with the device value Autologous Tissue Substitute

Examples: Fusion of a vertebral joint using a cage style interbody fusion device containing morsellized bone graft is coded to the device Interbody Fusion Device.
Fusion of a vertebral joint using a bone dowel interbody fusion device made of cadaver bone and packed with a mixture of local morsellized bone and demineralized bone matrix is coded to the device Interbody Fusion Device.
Fusion of a vertebral joint using both autologous bone graft and bone bank bone graft is coded to the device Autologous Tissue Substitute.
AHA Coding Clinic® Reference Notation(s) — Coding Guideline B3.10c
Interbody fusion device .... AHA 13:1Q:p29
Bone graft with mixture of autologous and nonautologous bone ..... AHA 13:3Q:p25
Fusion of multiple vertebral joints... AHA 13:1Q:p21

Inspection procedures

B3.11a

Inspection of a body part(s) performed in order to achieve the objective of a procedure is not coded separately.
Example: Fiberoptic bronchoscopy performed for irrigation of bronchus, only the irrigation procedure is coded.

B3.11b

If multiple tubular body parts are inspected, the most distal body part ~~inspected~~ (the body part furthest from the starting point of the inspection) is coded. If multiple non-tubular body parts in a region are inspected, the body part that specifies the entire area inspected is coded.
Examples: Cystoureteroscopy with inspection of bladder and ureters is coded to the ureter body part value.
Exploratory laparotomy with general inspection of abdominal contents is coded to the peritoneal cavity body part value.

B3.11c

When both an Inspection procedure and another procedure are performed on the same body part during the same episode, if the Inspection procedure is performed using a different approach than the other procedure, the Inspection procedure is coded separately.
Example: Endoscopic Inspection of the duodenum is coded separately when open Excision of the duodenum is performed during the same procedural episode.

Occlusion vs. Restriction for vessel embolization procedures

B3.12

If the objective of an embolization procedure is to completely close a vessel, the root operation Occlusion is coded. If the objective of an embolization procedure is to narrow the lumen of a vessel, the root operation Restriction is coded.
Examples: Tumor embolization is coded to the root operation Occlusion, because the objective of the procedure is to cut off the blood supply to the vessel.
Embolization of a cerebral aneurysm is coded to the root operation Restriction, because the objective of the procedure is not to close off the vessel entirely, but to narrow the lumen of the vessel at the site of the aneurysm where it is abnormally wide.

Release procedures

B3.13

In the root operation Release, the body part value coded is the body part being freed and not the tissue being manipulated or cut to free the body part.
Example: Lysis of intestinal adhesions is coded to the specific intestine body part value.
AHA Coding Clinic® Reference Notation(s) — Coding Guideline B3.13
Lysis of adhesions, integral or code separately................................. AHA 14:1Q:p3

Release vs. Division

B3.14

If the sole objective of the procedure is freeing a body part without cutting the body part, the root operation is Release. If the sole objective of the procedure is separating or transecting a body part, the root operation is Division.
Examples: Freeing a nerve root from surrounding scar tissue to relieve pain is coded to the root operation Release. Severing a nerve root to relieve pain is coded to the root operation Division.

Reposition for fracture treatment

B3.15

Reduction of a displaced fracture is coded to the root operation Reposition and the application of a cast or splint in conjunction with the Reposition procedure is not coded separately. Treatment of a nondisplaced fracture is coded to the procedure performed.
Examples: Putting a pin in a nondisplaced fracture is coded to the root operation Insertion.
Casting of a nondisplaced fracture is coded to the root operation Immobilization in the Placement section.

Transplantation vs. Administration

B3.16

Putting in a mature and functioning living body part taken from another individual or animal is coded to the root operation Transplantation. Putting in autologous or nonautologous cells is coded to the Administration section.
Example: Putting in autologous or nonautologous bone marrow, pancreatic islet cells or stem cells is coded to the Administration section.

B4. Body Part

General guidelines

B4.1a

If a procedure is performed on a portion of a body part that does not have a separate body part value, code the body part value corresponding to the whole body part.
Example: A procedure performed on the alveolar process of the mandible is coded to the mandible body part.

B4.1b

If the prefix "peri" is combined with a body part to identify the site of the procedure, and the site of the procedure is not further specified, then the procedure is coded to the body part named. This guideline applies only when a more specific body part value is not available.
Examples: A procedure site identified as perirenal is coded to the kidney body part when the site of the procedure is not further specified.
A procedure site described in the documentation as peri-urethral, and the documentation also indicates that it is the vulvar tissue and not the urethral tissue that is the site of the procedure, then the procedure is coded to the vulva body part.

AHA Coding Clinic® Reference Notation(s) — Coding Guideline B4.1b
Catheter ablation of peripulmonary veins to target the conduction pathway
  of left atrium ....AHA 14:4Q:p47
Periurethral obstetric laceration repair ....AHA 14:4Q:p18

Branches of body parts

B4.2

Where a specific branch of a body part does not have its own body part value in PCS, the body part is coded to the closest proximal branch that has a specific body part value.
Example: A procedure performed on the mandibular branch of the trigeminal nerve is coded to the trigeminal nerve body part value.

Bilateral body part values

B4.3

Bilateral body part values are available for a limited number of body parts. If the identical procedure is performed on contralateral body parts, and a bilateral body part value exists for that body part, a single procedure is coded using the bilateral body part value. If no bilateral body part value exists, each procedure is coded separately using the appropriate body part value.
Example: The identical procedure performed on both fallopian tubes is coded once using the body part value Fallopian Tubes, Bilateral. The identical procedure performed on both knee joints is coded twice using the body part values Knee Joint, Right and Knee Joint, Left.

AHA Coding Clinic® Reference Notation(s) — Coding Guideline B4.3
Repair of midline diaphragm (paraesophageal) hernia ....AHA 14:3Q:p28

Coronary arteries

B4.4

The coronary arteries are classified as a single body part that is further specified by number of sites treated and not by name or number of arteries. Separate body part values are used to specify the number of sites treated when the same procedure is performed on multiple sites in the coronary arteries.
Examples: Angioplasty of two distinct sites in the left anterior descending coronary artery with placement of two stents is coded as Dilation of Coronary Arteries, Two Sites, with Intraluminal Device.
Angioplasty of two distinct sites in the left anterior descending coronary artery, one with stent placed and one without, is coded separately as Dilation of Coronary Artery, One Site with Intraluminal Device, and Dilation of Coronary Artery, One Site with no device.

Tendons, ligaments, bursae and fascia near a joint

B4.5

Procedures performed on tendons, ligaments, bursae and fascia supporting a joint are coded to the body part in the respective body system that is the focus of the procedure. Procedures performed on joint structures themselves are coded to the body part in the joint body systems.
Example: Repair of the anterior cruciate ligament of the knee is coded to the knee bursae and ligament body part in the bursae and ligaments body system. Knee arthroscopy with shaving of articular cartilage is coded to the knee joint body part in the Lower Joints body system.

Skin, subcutaneous tissue and fascia overlying a joint

B4.6

If a procedure is performed on the skin, subcutaneous tissue or fascia overlying a joint, the procedure is coded to the following body part:
- Shoulder is coded to Upper Arm
- Elbow is coded to Lower Arm
- Wrist is coded to Lower Arm
- Hip is coded to Upper Leg
- Knee is coded to Lower Leg
- Ankle is coded to Foot

Fingers and toes

B4.7

If a body system does not contain a separate body part value for fingers, procedures performed on the fingers are coded to the body part value for the hand. If a body system does not contain a separate body part value for toes, procedures performed on the toes are coded to the body part value for the foot.
Example: Excision of finger muscle is coded to one of the hand muscle body part values in the Muscles body system.

Upper and lower intestinal tract

B4.8

In the Gastrointestinal body system, the general body part values Upper Intestinal Tract and Lower Intestinal Tract are provided as an option for the root operations Change, Inspection, Removal and Revision. Upper Intestinal Tract includes the portion of the gastrointestinal tract from the esophagus down to and including the duodenum, and Lower Intestinal Tract includes the portion of the gastrointestinal tract from the jejunum down to and including the rectum and anus.
Example: In the root operation Change table, change of a device in the jejunum is coded using the body part Lower Intestinal Tract.

B5. Approach

Open approach with percutaneous endoscopic assistance

B5.2

Procedures performed using the open approach with percutaneous endoscopic assistance are coded to the approach Open.
Example: Laparoscopic-assisted sigmoidectomy is coded to the approach Open.

External approach

B5.3a

Procedures performed within an orifice on structures that are visible without the aid of any instrumentation are coded to the approach External.
Example: Resection of tonsils is coded to the approach External.

B5.3b

Procedures performed indirectly by the application of external force through the intervening body layers are coded to the approach External.
Example: Closed reduction of fracture is coded to the approach External.

Percutaneous procedure via device

B5.4
Procedures performed percutaneously via a device placed for the procedure are coded to the approach Percutaneous.
Example: Fragmentation of kidney stone performed via percutaneous nephrostomy is coded to the approach Percutaneous.

B6. Device

General guidelines

B6.1a
A device is coded only if a device remains after the procedure is completed. If no device remains, the device value No Device is coded.

B6.1b
Materials such as sutures, ligatures, radiological markers and temporary post-operative wound drains are considered integral to the performance of a procedure and are not coded as devices.
AHA Coding Clinic® Reference Notation(s) — Coding Guideline B6.1b
Bronchoscopic placement of fiducial marker..................................AHA 14:1Q:p20
Fluoroscopic guided fiducial marker placement ....AHA 14:1Q:p20

B6.1c
Procedures performed on a device only and not on a body part are specified in the root operations Change, Irrigation, Removal and Revision, and are coded to the procedure performed.
Example: Irrigation of percutaneous nephrostomy tube is coded to the root operation Irrigation of indwelling device in the Administration section.
AHA Coding Clinic® Reference Notation(s) — Coding Guideline B6.1c
Replacement of arterial conduit is not coded as Removal of device ....AHA 14:3Q:p30

Drainage device

B6.2
A separate procedure to put in a drainage device is coded to the root operation Drainage with the device value Drainage Device.

Obstetric Section Guidelines (Section 1)

C. Obstetrics Section

Products of conception

C1
Procedures performed on the products of conception are coded to the Obstetrics section. Procedures performed on the pregnant female other than the products of conception are coded to the appropriate root operation in the Medical and Surgical section.
Example: Amniocentesis is coded to the products of conception body part in the Obstetrics section. Repair of obstetric urethral laceration is coded to the urethra body part in the Medical and Surgical section.

Procedures following delivery or abortion

C2
Procedures performed following a delivery or abortion for curettage of the endometrium or evacuation of retained products of conception are all coded in the Obstetrics section, to the root operation Extraction and the body part Products of Conception, Retained. Diagnostic or therapeutic dilation and curettage performed during times other than the postpartum or post-abortion period are all coded in the Medical and Surgical section, to the root operation Extraction and the body part Endometrium.

New Technology Section Guidelines (Section X)

D. New Technology Section

General guidelines

D1
Section X codes are standalone codes. They are not supplemental codes. Section X codes fully represent the specific procedure described in the code title, and do not require any additional codes from other sections of ICD-10-PCS. When section X contains a code title which describes a specific new technology procedure, only that X code is reported for the procedure. There is no need to report a broader, non-specific code in another section of ICD-10-PCS.
Example: XW04321 Introduction of Ceftazidime-Avibactam Anti-infective into Central Vein, Percutaneous Approach, New Technology Group 1, can be coded to indicate that Ceftazidime-Avibactam Anti-infective was administered via a central vein. A separate code from table 3E0 in the Administration section of ICD-10-PCS is not coded in addition to this code.

Selection of Principal Procedure

Selection of Principal Procedure

The following instructions should be applied in the selection of principal procedure and clarification on the importance of the relation to the principal diagnosis when more than one procedure is performed:

1. Procedure performed for definitive treatment of both principal diagnosis and secondary diagnosis;
    a. Sequence procedure performed for definitive treatment most related to principal diagnosis as principal procedure.
2. Procedure performed for definitive treatment and diagnostic procedures performed for both principal and secondary diagnosis;
    a. Sequence procedure performed for definitive treatment most related to principal diagnosis as principal procedure.
3. A diagnostic procedure was performed for the principal diagnosis and a procedure is performed for definitive treatment of a secondary diagnosis;
    a. Sequence diagnostic procedure as principal procedure, since the procedure most related to the principal diagnosis takes precedence.
4. No procedures performed that are related to principal diagnosis; procedures performed for definitive treatment and diagnostic procedures were performed for secondary diagnosis;
    a. Sequence procedure performed for definitive treatment of secondary diagnosis as principal procedure, since there are no procedures (definitive or nondefinitive treatment) related to principal diagnosis.

AHA Coding Clinic® Reference Notation(s) — Coding Guideline Selection of Principal Procedure
Sequencing of mechanical ventilation with other procedures ....AHA 14:4Q:p11

INDEX TO PROCEDURES – 2016 ICD-10-PCS

A

3f (Aortic) Bioprosthesis valve
 use Zooplastic Tissue in Heart and Great Vessels
Abdominal aortic plexus
 use Nerve, Abdominal Sympathetic
Abdominal esophagus
 use Esophagus, Lower
Abdominohysterectomy
 see Resection, Cervix 0UTC-
 see Resection, Uterus 0UT9-
Abdominoplasty
 see Alteration, Abdominal Wall 0W0F-
 see Repair, Abdominal Wall 0WQF-
 see Supplement, Abdominal Wall 0WUF-
Abductor hallucis muscle
 use Muscle, Foot, Left
 use Muscle, Foot, Right
AbioCor® Total Replacement Heart
 use Synthetic Substitute
Ablation see Destruction
Abortion
 Products of Conception 10A0-
 Abortifacient 10A07ZX
 Laminaria 10A07ZW
 Vacuum 10A07Z6
Abrasion see Extraction
Absolute Pro Vascular (OTW) Self-Expanding Stent System
 use Intraluminal Device
Accessory cephalic vein
 use Vein, Cephalic, Left
 use Vein, Cephalic, Right
Accessory obturator nerve
 use Nerve, Lumbar Plexus
Accessory phrenic nerve
 use Nerve, Phrenic
Accessory spleen
 use Spleen
Acculink (RX) Carotid Stent System
 use Intraluminal Device
Acellular Hydrated Dermis
 use Nonautologous Tissue Substitute
Acetabular cup
 use Liner in Lower Joints
Acetabulectomy
 see Excision, Lower Bones 0QB-
 see Resection, Lower Bones 0QT-
Acetabulofemoral joint
 use Joint, Hip, Left
 use Joint, Hip, Right
Acetabuloplasty
 see Repair, Lower Bones 0QQ-
 see Replacement, Lower Bones 0QR-
 see Supplement, Lower Bones 0QU-
Achilles tendon
 use Tendon, Lower Leg, Left
 use Tendon, Lower Leg, Right
Achillorrhaphy see Repair, Tendons 0LQ-
Achillotenotomy, achillotomy
 see Division, Tendons 0L8-
 see Drainage, Tendons 0L9-
Acromioclavicular ligament
 use Bursa and Ligament, Shoulder, Left
 use Bursa and Ligament, Shoulder, Right
Acromion (process)
 use Scapula, Left
 use Scapula, Right
Acromionectomy
 see Excision, Upper Joints 0RB-
 see Resection, Upper Joints 0RT-
Acromioplasty
 see Repair, Upper Joints 0RQ-
 see Replacement, Upper Joints 0RR-
 see Supplement, Upper Joints 0RU-

Activa PC neurostimulator
 use Stimulator Generator, Multiple Array in 0JH-
Activa RC neurostimulator
 use Stimulator Generator, Multiple Array Rechargeable in 0JH-
Activa SC neurostimulator
 use Stimulator Generator, Single Array in 0JH-
Activities of Daily Living Assessment F02-
Activities of Daily Living Treatment F08-
ACUITY™ Steerable Lead
 use Cardiac Lead, Defibrillator in 02H-
 use Cardiac Lead, Pacemaker in 02H-
Acupuncture
 Breast
  Anesthesia 8E0H300
  No Qualifier 8E0H30Z
 Integumentary System
  Anesthesia 8E0H300
  No Qualifier 8E0H30Z
Adductor brevis muscle
 use Muscle, Upper Leg, Left
 use Muscle, Upper Leg, Right
Adductor hallucis muscle
 use Muscle, Foot, Left
 use Muscle, Foot, Right
Adductor longus muscle
 use Muscle, Upper Leg, Left
 use Muscle, Upper Leg, Right
Adductor magnus muscle
 use Muscle, Upper Leg, Left
 use Muscle, Upper Leg, Right
Adenohypophysis
 use Gland, Pituitary
Adenoidectomy
 see Excision, Adenoids 0CBQ-
 see Resection, Adenoids 0CTQ-
Adenoidotomy see Drainage, Adenoids 0C9Q-
Adhesiolysis see Release
Administration
 Blood products see Transfusion
 Other substance see Introduction of substance in or on
Adrenalectomy
 see Excision, Endocrine System 0GB-
 see Resection, Endocrine System 0GT-
Adrenalorrhaphy see Repair, Endocrine System 0GQ-
Adrenalotomy see Drainage, Endocrine System 0G9-
Advancement
 see Reposition
 see Transfer
Advisa (MRI)
 use Pacemaker, Dual Chamber in 0JH-
AIGISRx Antibacterial Envelope
 use Anti-Infective Envelope
Alar ligament of axis
 use Bursa and Ligament, Head and Neck
Alimentation see Introduction of substance in or on
Alteration
 Abdominal Wall 0W0F-
 Ankle Region
  Left 0Y0L-
  Right 0Y0K-
 Arm
  Lower
   Left 0X0F-
   Right 0X0D-
  Upper
   Left 0X09-
   Right 0X08-
 Axilla
  Left 0X05-
  Right 0X04-

Alteration — continued
 Back
  Lower 0W0L-
  Upper 0W0K-
 Breast
  Bilateral 0H0V-
  Left 0H0U-
  Right 0H0T-
 Buttock
  Left 0Y01-
  Right 0Y00-
 Chest Wall 0W08-
 Ear
  Bilateral 0902-
  Left 0901-
  Right 0900-
 Elbow Region
  Left 0X0C-
  Right 0X0B-
 Extremity
  Lower
   Left 0Y0B-
   Right 0Y09-
  Upper
   Left 0X07-
   Right 0X06-
 Eyelid
  Lower
   Left 080R-
   Right 080Q-
  Upper
   Left 080P-
   Right 080N-
 Face 0W02-
 Head 0W00-
 Jaw
  Lower 0W05-
  Upper 0W04-
 Knee Region
  Left 0Y0G-
  Right 0Y0F-
 Leg
  Lower
   Left 0Y0J-
   Right 0Y0H-
  Upper
   Left 0Y0D-
   Right 0Y0C-
 Lip
  Lower 0C01X-
  Upper 0C00X-
 Neck 0W06-
 Nose 090K-
 Perineum
  Female 0W0N-
  Male 0W0M-
 Shoulder Region
  Left 0X03-
  Right 0X02-
 Subcutaneous Tissue and Fascia
  Abdomen 0J08-
  Back 0J07-
  Buttock 0J09-
  Chest 0J06-
  Face 0J01-
  Lower Arm
   Left 0JOH-
   Right 0J0G-
  Lower Leg
   Left 0J0P-
   Right 0J0N-
  Neck
   Anterior 0J04-
   Posterior 0J05-
  Upper Arm
   Left 0J0F-
   Right 0J0D-
  Upper Leg
   Left 0J0M-
   Right 0J0L-

Alteration — continued
 Wrist Region
  Left 0X0H-
  Right 0X0G-
Alveolar process of mandible
 use Mandible, Left
 use Mandible, Right
Alveolar process of maxilla
 use Maxilla, Left
 use Maxilla, Right
Alveolectomy
 see Excision, Head and Facial Bones 0NB-
 see Resection, Head and Facial Bones 0NT-
Alveoloplasty
 see Repair, Head and Facial Bones 0NQ-
 see Replacement, Head and Facial Bones 0NR-
 see Supplement, Head and Facial Bones 0NU-
Alveolotomy
 see Division, Head and Facial Bones 0N8-
 see Drainage, Head and Facial Bones 0N9-
Ambulatory cardiac monitoring 4A12X45
Amniocentesis see Drainage, Products of Conception 1090-
Amnioinfusion see Introduction of substance in or on, Products of Conception 3E0E-
Amnioscopy 10J08ZZ
Amniotomy see Drainage, Products of Conception 1090-
AMPLATZER® Muscular VSD Occluder
 use Synthetic Substitute
Amputation see Detachment
AMS 800® Urinary Control System
 use Artificial Sphincter in Urinary System
Anal orifice
 use Anus
Analog radiography see Plain Radiography
Analog radiology see Plain Radiography
Anastomosis see Bypass
Anatomical snuffbox
 use Muscle, Lower Arm and Wrist, Left
 use Muscle, Lower Arm and Wrist, Right
AneuRx® AAA Advantage®
 use Intraluminal Device
Angiectomy
 see Excision, Heart and Great Vessels 02B-
 see Excision, Lower Arteries 04B-
 see Excision, Lower Veins 06B-
 see Excision, Upper Arteries 03B-
 see Excision, Upper Veins 05B-
Angiocardiography
 Combined right and left heart see Fluoroscopy, Heart, Right and Left B216-
 Left Heart see Fluoroscopy, Heart, Left B215-
 Right Heart see Fluoroscopy, Heart, Right B214-
 SPY see Fluoroscopy, Heart B21-
Angiography
 see Plain Radiography, Heart B20-
 see Fluoroscopy, Heart B21-
Angioplasty
 see Dilation, Heart and Great Vessels 027-
 see Dilation, Lower Arteries 047-

Angioplasty

Angioplasty — *continued*
- *see* Dilation, Upper Arteries **037**-
- *see* Repair, Heart and Great Vessels **02Q**-
- *see* Repair, Lower Arteries **04Q**-
- *see* Repair, Upper Arteries **03Q**-
- *see* Replacement, Heart and Great Vessels **02R**-
- *see* Replacement, Lower Arteries **04R**-
- *see* Replacement, Upper Arteries **03R**-
- *see* Supplement, Heart and Great Vessels **02U**-
- *see* Supplement, Lower Arteries **04U**-
- *see* Supplement, Upper Arteries **03U**-

Angiorrhaphy
- *see* Repair, Heart and Great Vessels **02Q**-
- *see* Repair, Lower Arteries **04Q**-
- *see* Repair, Upper Arteries **03Q**-

Angioscopy
- **02JY4ZZ**
- **03JY4ZZ**
- **04JY4ZZ**

Angiotripsy
- *see* Occlusion, Lower Arteries **04L**-
- *see* Occlusion, Upper Arteries **03L**-

Angular artery
- *use* Artery, Face

Angular vein
- *use* Vein, Face, Left
- *use* Vein, Face, Right

Annular ligament
- *use* Bursa and Ligament, Elbow, Left
- *use* Bursa and Ligament, Elbow, Right

Annuloplasty
- *see* Repair, Heart and Great Vessels **02Q**-
- *see* Supplement, Heart and Great Vessels **02U**-

Annuloplasty ring
- *use* Synthetic Substitute

Anoplasty
- *see* Repair, Anus **0DQQ**-
- *see* Supplement, Anus **0DUQ**-

Anorectal junction
- *use* Rectum

Anoscopy 0DJD8ZZ

Ansa cervicalis
- *use* Nerve, Cervical Plexus

Antabuse therapy HZ93ZZZ

Antebrachial fascia
- *use* Subcutaneous Tissue and Fascia, Lower Arm, Left
- *use* Subcutaneous Tissue and Fascia, Lower Arm, Right

Anterior (pectoral) lymph node
- *use* Lymphatic, Axillary, Left
- *use* Lymphatic, Axillary, Right

Anterior cerebral artery
- *use* Artery, Intracranial

Anterior cerebral vein
- *use* Vein, Intracranial

Anterior choroidal artery
- *use* Artery, Intracranial

Anterior circumflex humeral artery
- *use* Artery, Axillary, Left
- *use* Artery, Axillary, Right

Anterior communicating artery
- *use* Artery, Intracranial

Anterior cruciate ligament (ACL)
- *use* Bursa and Ligament, Knee, Left
- *use* Bursa and Ligament, Knee, Right

Anterior crural nerve
- *use* Nerve, Femoral

Anterior facial vein
- *use* Vein, Face, Left
- *use* Vein, Face, Right

Anterior intercostal artery
- *use* Artery, Internal Mammary, Left
- *use* Artery, Internal Mammary, Right

Anterior interosseous nerve
- *use* Nerve, Median

Anterior lateral malleolar artery
- *use* Artery, Anterior Tibial, Left
- *use* Artery, Anterior Tibial, Right

Anterior lingual gland
- *use* Gland, Minor Salivary

Anterior medial malleolar artery
- *use* Artery, Anterior Tibial, Left
- *use* Artery, Anterior Tibial, Right

Anterior spinal artery
- *use* Artery, Vertebral, Left
- *use* Artery, Vertebral, Right

Anterior tibial recurrent artery
- *use* Artery, Anterior Tibial, Left
- *use* Artery, Anterior Tibial, Right

Anterior ulnar recurrent artery
- *use* Artery, Ulnar, Left
- *use* Artery, Ulnar, Right

Anterior vagal trunk
- *use* Nerve, Vagus

Anterior vertebral muscle
- *use* Muscle, Neck, Left
- *use* Muscle, Neck, Right

Antihelix
- *use* Ear, External, Bilateral
- *use* Ear, External, Left
- *use* Ear, External, Right

Antimicrobial envelope
- *use* Anti-Infective Envelope

Antitragus
- *use* Ear, External, Bilateral
- *use* Ear, External, Left
- *use* Ear, External, Right

Antrostomy *see* Drainage, Ear, Nose, Sinus **099**-

Antrotomy *see* Drainage, Ear, Nose, Sinus **099**-

Antrum of Highmore
- *use* Sinus, Maxillary, Left
- *use* Sinus, Maxillary, Right

Aortic annulus
- *use* Valve, Aortic

Aortic arch
- *use* Aorta, Thoracic

Aortic intercostal artery
- *use* Aorta, Thoracic

Aortography
- *see* Fluoroscopy, Lower Arteries **B41**-
- *see* Fluoroscopy, Upper Arteries **B31**-
- *see* Plain Radiography, Lower Arteries **B40**-
- *see* Plain Radiography, Upper Arteries **B30**-

Aortoplasty
- *see* Repair, Aorta, Abdominal **04Q0**-
- *see* Repair, Aorta, Thoracic **02QW**-
- *see* Replacement, Aorta, Abdominal **04R0**-
- *see* Replacement, Aorta, Thoracic **02RW**-
- *see* Supplement, Aorta, Abdominal **04U0**-
- *see* Supplement, Aorta, Thoracic **02UW**-

Apical (subclavicular) lymph node
- *use* Lymphatic, Axillary, Left
- *use* Lymphatic, Axillary, Right

Apneustic center
- *use* Pons

Appendectomy
- *see* Excision, Appendix **0DBJ**-
- *see* Resection, Appendix **0DTJ**-

Appendicolysis *see* Release, Appendix **0DNJ**-

Appendicotomy *see* Drainage, Appendix **0D9J**-

Application *see* Introduction of substance in or on

Aquapheresis 6A550Z3

Aqueduct of Sylvius
- *use* Cerebral Ventricle

Aqueous humour
- *use* Anterior Chamber, Left
- *use* Anterior Chamber, Right

Arachnoid mater, intracranial
- *use* Cerebral Meninges

Arachnoid mater, spinal
- *use* Spinal Meninges

Arcuate artery
- *use* Artery, Foot, Left
- *use* Artery, Foot, Right

Areola
- *use* Nipple, Left
- *use* Nipple, Right

AROM (artificial rupture of membranes) 10907ZC

Arterial canal (duct)
- *use* Artery, Pulmonary, Left

Arterial pulse tracing *see* Measurement, Arterial **4A03**-

Arteriectomy *see* Excision, Heart and Great Vessels **02B**-
- *see* Excision, Lower Arteries **04B**-
- *see* Excision, Upper Arteries **03B**-

Arteriography
- *see* Fluoroscopy, Heart **B21**-
- *see* Fluoroscopy, Lower Arteries **B41**-
- *see* Fluoroscopy, Upper Arteries **B31**-
- *see* Plain Radiography, Heart **B20**-
- *see* Plain Radiography, Lower Arteries **B40**-
- *see* Plain Radiography, Upper Arteries **B30**-

Arterioplasty
- *see* Repair, Heart and Great Vessels **02Q**-
- *see* Repair, Lower Arteries **04Q**-
- *see* Repair, Upper Arteries **03Q**-
- *see* Replacement, Heart and Great Vessels **02R**-
- *see* Replacement, Lower Arteries **04R**-
- *see* Replacement, Upper Arteries **03R**-
- *see* Supplement, Heart and Great Vessels **02U**-
- *see* Supplement, Lower Arteries **04U**-
- *see* Supplement, Upper Arteries **03U**-

Arteriorrhaphy
- *see* Repair, Heart and Great Vessels **02Q**-
- *see* Repair, Lower Arteries **04Q**-
- *see* Repair, Upper Arteries **03Q**-

Arterioscopy
- **02JY4ZZ**
- **03JY4ZZ**
- **04JY4ZZ**

Arthrectomy
- *see* Excision, Lower Joints **0SB**-
- *see* Excision, Upper Joints **0RB**-
- *see* Resection, Lower Joints **0ST**-
- *see* Resection, Upper Joints **0RT**-

Arthrocentesis
- *see* Drainage, Lower Joints **0S9**-
- *see* Drainage, Upper Joints **0R9**-

Arthrodesis
- *see* Fusion, Lower Joints **0SG**-
- *see* Fusion, Upper Joints **0RG**-

Arthrography
- *see* Plain Radiography, Non-Axial Lower Bones **BQ0**-
- *see* Plain Radiography, Non-Axial Upper Bones **BP0**-
- *see* Plain Radiography, Skull and Facial Bones **BN0**-

Arthrolysis
- *see* Release, Lower Joints **0SN**-
- *see* Release, Upper Joints **0RN**-

Arthropexy
- *see* Repair, Lower Joints **0SQ**-
- *see* Repair, Upper Joints **0RQ**-
- *see* Reposition, Lower Joints **0SS**-
- *see* Reposition, Upper Joints **0RS**-

Arthroplasty
- *see* Repair, Lower Joints **0SQ**-
- *see* Repair, Upper Joints **0RQ**-
- *see* Replacement, Lower Joints **0SR**-
- *see* Replacement, Upper Joints **0RR**-
- *see* Supplement, Lower Joints **0SU**-
- *see* Supplement, Upper Joints **0RU**-

Arthroscopy
- *see* Inspection, Lower Joints **0SJ**-
- *see* Inspection, Upper Joints **0RJ**-

Arthrotomy
- *see* Drainage, Lower Joints **0S9**-
- *see* Drainage, Upper Joints **0R9**-

Artificial anal sphincter (AAS)
- *use* Artificial Sphincter in Gastrointestinal System

Artificial bowel sphincter (neosphincter)
- *use* Artificial Sphincter in Gastrointestinal System

Artificial Sphincter
Insertion of device in
- Anus **0DHQ**
- Bladder **0THB**-
- Bladder Neck **0THC**-
- Urethra **0THD**-

Removal of device from
- Anus **0DPQ**
- Bladder **0TPB**-
- Urethra **0TPD**-

Revision of device in
- Anus **0DWQ**
- Bladder **0TWB**-
- Urethra **0TWD**-

Artificial urinary sphincter (AUS)
- *use* Artificial Sphincter in Urinary System

Aryepiglottic fold
- *use* Larynx

Arytenoid cartilage
- *use* Larynx

Arytenoid muscle
- *use* Muscle, Neck, Left
- *use* Muscle, Neck, Right

Arytenoidectomy *see* Excision, Larynx **0CBS**-

Arytenoidopexy
- *see* Repair, Larynx **0CQS**-

Ascenda Intrathecal Catheter
- *use* Infusion Device

Ascending aorta
- *use* Aorta, Thoracic

Ascending palatine artery
- *use* Artery, Face

Ascending pharyngeal artery
- *use* Artery, External Carotid, Left
- *use* Artery, External Carotid, Right

Aspiration, fine needle
Fluid or gas *see* Drainage
Tissue *see* Excision

Assessment
Activities of daily living *see* Activities of Daily Living Assessment, Rehabilitation **F02**-
Hearing *see* Hearing Assessment, Diagnostic Audiology **F13**-
Hearing aid *see* Hearing Aid Assessment, Diagnostic Audiology **F14**-
Motor function *see* Motor Function Assessment, Rehabilitation **F01**-
Nerve function *see* Motor Function Assessment, Rehabilitation **F01**-
Speech *see* Speech Assessment, Rehabilitation **F00**-
Vestibular *see* Vestibular Assessment, Diagnostic Audiology **F15**-
Vocational *see* Activities of Daily Living Treatment, Rehabilitation **F08**-

INDEX TO PROCEDURES – 2016 ICD-10-PCS

Assistance
Cardiac
  Continuous
    Balloon Pump **5A02210**
    Impeller Pump **5A0221D**
    Other Pump **5A02216**
    Pulsatile Compression **5A02215**
  Intermittent
    Balloon Pump **5A02110**
    Impeller Pump **5A0211D**
    Other Pump **5A02116**
    Pulsatile Compression **5A02115**
Circulatory
  Continuous
    Hyperbaric **5A05221**
    Supersaturated **5A0522C**
  Intermittent
    Hyperbaric **5A05121**
    Supersaturated **5A0512C**
Respiratory
  24-96 Consecutive Hours
    Continuous Negative Airway Pressure **5A09459**
    Continuous Positive Airway Pressure **5A09457**
    Intermittent Negative Airway Pressure **5A0945B**
    Intermittent Positive Airway Pressure **5A09458**
    No Qualifier **5A0945Z**
  Greater than 96 Consecutive Hours
    Continuous Negative Airway Pressure **5A09559**
    Continuous Positive Airway Pressure **5A09557**
    Intermittent Negative Airway Pressure **5A0955B**
    Intermittent Positive Airway Pressure **5A09558**
    No Qualifier **5A0955Z**
  Less than 24 Consecutive Hours
    Continuous Negative Airway Pressure **5A09359**
    Continuous Positive Airway Pressure **5A09357**
    Intermittent Negative Airway Pressure **5A0935B**
    Intermittent Positive Airway Pressure **5A09358**
    No Qualifier **5A0935Z**

Assurant (Cobalt) stent
use Intraluminal Device

Atherectomy
see Extirpation, Heart and Great Vessels **02C-**
see Extirpation, Lower Arteries **04C-**
see Extirpation, Upper Arteries **03C-**

Atlantoaxial joint
use Joint, Cervical Vertebral

Atmospheric Control **6A0Z-**

Atrioseptoplasty
see Repair, Heart and Great Vessels **02Q-**
see Replacement, Heart and Great Vessels **02R-**
see Supplement, Heart and Great Vessels **02U-**

Atrioventricular node
use Conduction Mechanism

Atrium dextrum cordis
use Atrium, Right

Atrium pulmonale
use Atrium, Left

Attain Ability® lead
use Cardiac Lead, Defibrillator in **02H-**
use Cardiac Lead, Pacemaker in **02H-**

Attain StarFix® (OTW) lead
use Cardiac Lead, Defibrillator in **02H-**
use Cardiac Lead, Pacemaker in **02H-**

Audiology, diagnostic
see Hearing Aid Assessment, Diagnostic Audiology **F14-**
see Hearing Assessment, Diagnostic Audiology **F13-**
see Vestibular Assessment, Diagnostic Audiology **F15-**

Audiometry *see* Hearing Assessment, Diagnostic Audiology **F13-**

Auditory tube
use Eustachian Tube, Left
use Eustachian Tube, Right

Auerbach's (myenteric) plexus
use Nerve, Abdominal Sympathetic

Auricle
use Ear, External, Bilateral
use Ear, External, Left
use Ear, External, Right

Auricularis muscle
use Muscle, Head

Autograft
use Autologous Tissue Substitute

Autologous artery graft
use Autologous Arterial Tissue in Heart and Great Vessels
use Autologous Arterial Tissue in Lower Arteries
use Autologous Arterial Tissue in Lower Veins
use Autologous Arterial Tissue in Upper Arteries
use Autologous Arterial Tissue in Upper Veins

Autologous vein graft
use Autologous Venous Tissue in Heart and Great Vessels
use Autologous Venous Tissue in Lower Arteries
use Autologous Venous Tissue in Lower Veins
use Autologous Venous Tissue in Upper Arteries
use Autologous Venous Tissue in Upper Veins

Autotransfusion *see* Transfusion

Autotransplant
Adrenal tissue *see* Reposition, Endocrine System **0GS-**
Kidney *see* Reposition, Urinary System **0TS-**
Pancreatic tissue *see* Reposition, Pancreas **0FSG-**
Parathyroid tissue *see* Reposition, Endocrine System **0GS-**
Thyroid tissue *see* Reposition, Endocrine System **0GS-**
Tooth *see* Reattachment, Mouth and Throat **0CM-**

Avulsion *see* Extraction

Axial Lumbar Interbody Fusion System
use Interbody Fusion Device in Lower Joints

AxiaLIF® System
use Interbody Fusion Device in Lower Joints

Axillary fascia
use Subcutaneous Tissue and Fascia, Upper Arm, Left
use Subcutaneous Tissue and Fascia, Upper Arm, Right

Axillary nerve
use Nerve, Brachial Plexus

B

BAK/C® Interbody Cervical Fusion System
use Interbody Fusion Device in Upper Joints

BAL (bronchial alveolar lavage), diagnostic
see Drainage, Respiratory System **0B9-**

Balanoplasty
see Repair, Penis **0VQS-**
see Supplement, Penis **0VUS-**

Balloon Pump
Continuous, Output **5A02210**
Intermittent, Output **5A02110**

Bandage, Elastic *see* Compression

Banding
see Occlusion
see Restriction

Bard® Composix® (E/X) (LP) mesh
use Synthetic Substitute

Bard® Composix® Kugel® patch
use Synthetic Substitute

Bard® Dulex™ mesh
use Synthetic Substitute

Bard® Ventralex™ hernia patch
use Synthetic Substitute

Barium swallow *see* Fluoroscopy, Gastrointestinal System **BD1-**

Baroreflex Activation Therapy® (BAT®)
use Stimulator Generator in Subcutaneous Tissue and Fascia
use Stimulator Lead in Upper Arteries

Bartholin's (greater vestibular) gland
use Gland, Vestibular

Basal (internal) cerebral vein
use Vein, Intracranial

Basal metabolic rate (BMR) *see* Measurement, Physiological Systems **4A0Z-**

Basal nuclei
use Basal Ganglia

Basilar artery
use Artery, Intracranial

Basis pontis
use Pons

Beam Radiation
Abdomen **DW03-**
  Intraoperative **DW033Z0**
Adrenal Gland **DG02-**
  Intraoperative **DG023Z0**
Bile Ducts **DF02-**
  Intraoperative **DF023Z0**
Bladder **DT02-**
  Intraoperative **DT023Z0**
Bone
  Intraoperative **DP0C3Z0**
  Other **DP0C-**
Bone Marrow **D700-**
  Intraoperative **D7003Z0**
Brain **D000-**
  Intraoperative **D0003Z0**
Brain Stem **D001-**
  Intraoperative **D0013Z0**
Breast
  Left **DM00-**
    Intraoperative **DM003Z0**
  Right **DM01-**
    Intraoperative **DM013Z0**
Bronchus **DB01-**
  Intraoperative **DB013Z0**
Cervix **DU01-**
  Intraoperative **DU013Z0**
Chest **DW02-**
  Intraoperative **DW023Z0**
Chest Wall **DB07-**
  Intraoperative **DB073Z0**

Beam Radiation — *continued*
Colon **DD05-**
  Intraoperative **DD053Z0**
Diaphragm **DB08-**
  Intraoperative **DB083Z0**
Duodenum **DD02-**
  Intraoperative **DD023Z0**
Ear **D900-**
  Intraoperative **D9003Z0**
Esophagus **DD00-**
  Intraoperative **DD003Z0**
Eye **D800-**
  Intraoperative **D8003Z0**
Femur **DP09-**
  Intraoperative **DP093Z0**
Fibula **DP0B-**
  Intraoperative **DP0B3Z0**
Gallbladder **DF01-**
  Intraoperative **DF013Z0**
Gland
  Adrenal **DG02-**
    Intraoperative **DG023Z0**
  Parathyroid **DG04-**
    Intraoperative **DG043Z0**
  Pituitary **DG00-**
    Intraoperative **DG003Z0**
  Thyroid **DG05-**
    Intraoperative **DG053Z0**
Glands
  Intraoperative **D9063Z0**
  Salivary **D906-**
Head and Neck **DW01**
  Intraoperative **DW013Z0**
Hemibody **DW04-**
  Intraoperative **DW043Z0**
Humerus **DP06-**
  Intraoperative **DP063Z0**
Hypopharynx **D903-**
  Intraoperative **D9033Z0**
Ileum **DD04-**
  Intraoperative **DD043Z0**
Jejunum **DD03-**
  Intraoperative **DD033Z0**
Kidney **DT00-**
  Intraoperative **DT003Z0**
Larynx **D90B-**
  Intraoperative **D90B3Z0**
Liver **DF00-**
  Intraoperative **DF003Z0**
Lung **DB02-**
  Intraoperative **DB023Z0**
Lymphatics
  Abdomen **D706-**
    Intraoperative **D7063Z0**
  Axillary **D704-**
    Intraoperative **D7043Z0**
  Inguinal **D708-**
    Intraoperative **D7083Z0**
  Neck **D703-**
    Intraoperative **D7033Z0**
  Pelvis **D707-**
    Intraoperative **D7073Z0**
  Thorax **D705-**
    Intraoperative **D7053Z0**
Mandible **DP03-**
  Intraoperative **DP033Z0**
Maxilla **DP02-**
  Intraoperative **DP023Z0**
Mediastinum **DB06-**
  Intraoperative **DB063Z0**
Mouth **D904-**
  Intraoperative **D9043Z0**
Nasopharynx **D90D-**
  Intraoperative **D90D3Z0**
Neck and Head **DW01-**
  Intraoperative **DW013Z0**
Nerve
  Intraoperative **D0073Z0**
  Peripheral **D007-**
Nose **D901-**
  Intraoperative **D9013Z0**

Beam — INDEX TO PROCEDURES – 2016 ICD-10-PCS

Beam Radiation — *continued*
- Oropharynx **D90F**-
  - Intraoperative **D90F3Z0**
- Ovary **DU00**-
  - Intraoperative **DU003Z0**
- Palate
  - Hard **D908**-
    - Intraoperative **D9083Z0**
  - Soft **D909**-
    - Intraoperative **D9093Z0**
- Pancreas **DF03**-
  - Intraoperative **DF033Z0**
- Parathyroid Gland **DG04**-
  - Intraoperative **DG043Z0**
- Pelvic Bones **DP08**-
  - Intraoperative **DP083Z0**
- Pelvic Region **DW06**-
  - Intraoperative **DW063Z0**
- Pineal Body **DG01**-
  - Intraoperative **DG013Z0**
- Pituitary Gland **DG00**-
  - Intraoperative **DG003Z0**
- Pleura **DB05**-
  - Intraoperative **DB053Z0**
- Prostate **DV00**-
  - Intraoperative **DV003Z0**
- Radius **DP07**-
  - Intraoperative **DP073Z0**
- Rectum **DD07**-
  - Intraoperative **DD073Z0**
- Rib **DP05**-
  - Intraoperative **DP053Z0**
- Sinuses **D907**-
  - Intraoperative **D9073Z0**
- Skin
  - Abdomen **DH08**-
    - Intraoperative **DH083Z0**
  - Arm **DH04**-
    - Intraoperative **DH043Z0**
  - Back **DH07**-
    - Intraoperative **DH073Z0**
  - Buttock **DH09**-
    - Intraoperative **DH093Z0**
  - Chest **DH06**-
    - Intraoperative **DH063Z0**
  - Face **DH02**-
    - Intraoperative **DH023Z0**
  - Leg **DH0B**-
    - Intraoperative **DH0B3Z0**
  - Neck **DH03**-
    - Intraoperative **DH033Z0**
- Skull **DP00**-
  - Intraoperative **DP003Z0**
- Spinal Cord **D006**-
  - Intraoperative **D0063Z0**
- Spleen **D702**-
  - Intraoperative **D7023Z0**
- Sternum **DP04**-
  - Intraoperative **DP043Z0**
- Stomach **DD01**-
  - Intraoperative **DD013Z0**
- Testis **DV01**-
  - Intraoperative **DV013Z0**
- Thymus **D701**-
  - Intraoperative **D7013Z0**
- Thyroid Gland **DG05**-
  - Intraoperative **DG053Z0**
- Tibia **DP0B**-
  - Intraoperative **DP0B3Z0**
- Tongue **D905**-
  - Intraoperative **D9053Z0**
- Trachea **DB00**-
  - Intraoperative **DB003Z0**
- Ulna **DP07**-
  - Intraoperative **DP073Z0**
- Ureter **DT01**-
  - Intraoperative **DT013Z0**
- Urethra **DT03**-
  - Intraoperative **DT033Z0**
- Uterus **DU02**-
  - Intraoperative **DU023Z0**

Beam Radiation — *continued*
- Whole Body **DW05**-
  - Intraoperative **DW053Z0**

Bedside swallow F00ZJWZ

Berlin Heart Ventricular Assist Device
- *use* Implantable Heart Assist System in Heart and Great Vessels

Biceps brachii muscle
- *use* Muscle, Upper Arm, Left
- *use* Muscle, Upper Arm, Right

Biceps femoris muscle
- *use* Muscle, Upper Leg, Left
- *use* Muscle, Upper Leg, Right

Bicipital aponeurosis
- *use* Subcutaneous Tissue and Fascia, Lower Arm, Left
- *use* Subcutaneous Tissue and Fascia, Lower Arm, Right

Bicuspid valve
- *use* Valve, Mitral

Bililite therapy *see* Ultraviolet Light Therapy, Skin **6A80**-

Bioactive embolization coil(s)
- *use* Intraluminal Device, Bioactive in Upper Arteries

Biofeedback GZC9ZZZ

Biopsy
- *see* Drainage with qualifier Diagnostic
- *see* Excision with qualifier Diagnostic
- Bone Marrow *see* Extraction with qualifier Diagnostic

BiPAP *see* Assistance, Respiratory **5A09**-

Bisection *see* Division

Biventricular external heart assist system
- *use* External Heart Assist System in Heart and Great Vessels

Blepharectomy
- *see* Excision, Eye **08B**-
- *see* Resection, Eye **08T**-

Blepharoplasty
- *see* Repair, Eye **08Q**-
- *see* Replacement, Eye **08R**-
- *see* Reposition, Eye **08S**-
- *see* Supplement, Eye **08U**-

Blepharorrhaphy *see* Repair, Eye **08Q**-

Blepharotomy *see* Drainage, Eye **089**-

Blinatumomab antineoplastic immunothrerapy XW0-

Block, Nerve, anesthetic injection 3E0T3CZ

Blood glucose monitoring system
- *use* Monitoring Device

Blood pressure *see* Measurement, Arterial **4A03**-

BMR (basal metabolic rate) *see* Measurement, Physiological Systems **4A0Z**-

Body of femur
- *use* Femoral Shaft, Left
- *use* Femoral Shaft, Right

Body of fibula
- *use* Fibula, Left
- *use* Fibula, Right

Bone anchored hearing device
- *use* Hearing Device, Bone Conduction in 09H-
- *use* Hearing Device in Head and Facial Bones

Bone bank bone graft
- *use* Nonautologous Tissue Substitute

Bone growth stimulator
- Insertion of device in
  - Bone
    - Facial **0NHW**-
    - Lower **0QHY**-
    - Nasal **0NHB**-
    - Upper **0PHY**-
    - Skull **0NH0**-

Bone growth stimulator — *continued*
- Removal of device from
  - Bone
    - Facial **0NPW**-
    - Lower **0QPY**-
    - Nasal **0NPB**-
    - Upper **0PPY**-
    - Skull **0NP0**-
- Revision of device in
  - Bone
    - Facial **0NWW**-
    - Lower **0QWY**-
    - Nasal **0NWB**-
    - Upper **0PWY**-
    - Skull **0NW0**-

Bone marrow transplant *see* Transfusion

Bone morphogenetic protein 2 (BMP 2)
- *use* Recombinant Bone Morphogenetic Protein

Bone screw (interlocking) (lag) (pedicle) (recessed)
- *use* Internal Fixation Device in Head and Facial Bones
- *use* Internal Fixation Device in Lower Bones
- *use* Internal Fixation Device in Upper Bones

Bony labyrinth
- *use* Ear, Inner, Left
- *use* Ear, Inner, Right

Bony orbit
- *use* Orbit, Left
- *use* Orbit, Right

Bony vestibule
- *use* Ear, Inner, Left
- *use* Ear, Inner, Right

Botallo's duct
- *use* Artery, Pulmonary, Left

Bovine pericardial valve
- *use* Zooplastic Tissue in Heart and Great Vessels

Bovine pericardium graft
- *use* Zooplastic Tissue in Heart and Great Vessels

BP (blood pressure) *see* Measurement, Arterial **4A03**-

Brachial (lateral) lymph node
- *use* Lymphatic, Axillary, Left
- *use* Lymphatic, Axillary, Right

Brachialis muscle
- *use* Muscle, Upper Arm, Left
- *use* Muscle, Upper Arm, Right

Brachiocephalic artery
- *use* Artery, Innominate

Brachiocephalic trunk
- *use* Artery, Innominate

Brachiocephalic vein
- *use* Vein, Innominate, Left
- *use* Vein, Innominate, Right

Brachioradialis muscle
- *use* Muscle, Lower Arm and Wrist, Left
- *use* Muscle, Lower Arm and Wrist, Right

Brachytherapy
- Abdomen **DW13**-
- Adrenal Gland **DG12**-
- Bile Ducts **DF12**-
- Bladder **DT12**-
- Bone Marrow **D710**-
- Brain **D010**-
- Brain Stem **D011**-
- Breast
  - Left **DM10**-
  - Right **DM11**-
- Bronchus **DB11**-
- Cervix **DU11**-
- Chest **DW12**-
- Chest Wall **DB17**-

Brachytherapy — *continued*
- Colon **DD15**-
- Diaphragm **DB18**-
- Duodenum **DD12**-
- Ear **D910**-
- Esophagus **DD10**-
- Eye **D810**-
- Gallbladder **DF11**-
- Gland
  - Adrenal **DG12**-
  - Parathyroid **DG14**-
  - Pituitary **DG10**-
  - Thyroid **DG15**-
- Glands, Salivary **D916**-
- Head and Neck **DW11**-
- Hypopharynx **D913**-
- Ileum **DD14**-
- Jejunum **DD13**-
- Kidney **DT10**-
- Larynx **D91B**-
- Liver **DF10**-
- Lung **DB12**-
- Lymphatics
  - Abdomen **D716**-
  - Axillary **D714**-
  - Inguinal **D718**-
  - Neck **D713**-
  - Pelvis **D717**-
  - Thorax **D715**-
- Mediastinum **DB16**-
- Mouth **D914**-
- Nasopharynx **D91D**-
- Neck and Head **DW11**-
- Nerve, Peripheral **D017**-
- Nose **D911**-
- Oropharynx **D91F**-
- Ovary **DU10**-
- Palate
  - Hard **D918**-
  - Soft **D919**-
- Pancreas **DF13**-
- Parathyroid Gland **DG14**-
- Pelvic Region **DW16**-
- Pineal Body **DG11**-
- Pituitary Gland **DG10**-
- Pleura **DB15**-
- Prostate **DV10**-
- Rectum **DD17**-
- Sinuses **D917**-
- Spinal Cord **D016**-
- Spleen **D712**-
- Stomach **DD11**-
- Testis **DV11**-
- Thymus **D711**-
- Thyroid Gland **DG15**-
- Tongue **D915**-
- Trachea **DB10**-
- Ureter **DT11**-
- Urethra **DT13**-
- Uterus **DU12**-

Brachytherapy seeds
- *use* Radioactive Element

Broad ligament
- *use* Uterine Supporting Structure

Bronchial artery
- *use* Aorta, Thoracic

Bronchography
- *see* Fluoroscopy, Respiratory System **BB1**-
- *see* Plain Radiography, Respiratory System **BB0**-

Bronchoplasty
- *see* Repair, Respiratory System **0BQ**-
- *see* Supplement, Respiratory System **0BU**-

Bronchorrhaphy *see* Repair, Respiratory System **0BQ**-

Bronchoscopy 0BJ08ZZ

Bronchotomy *see* Drainage, Respiratory System **0B9**-

BRYAN® Cervical Disc System
- *use* Synthetic Substitute

Buccal gland
  use Buccal Mucosa
Buccinator lymph node
  use Lymphatic, Head
Buccinator muscle
  use Muscle, Facial
Buckling, scleral with implant *see* Supplement, Eye 08U-
Bulbospongiosus muscle
  use Muscle, Perineum
Bulbourethral (Cowper's) gland
  use Urethra
Bundle of His
  use Conduction Mechanism
Bundle of Kent
  use Conduction Mechanism
Bunionectomy *see* Excision, Lower Bones 0QB-
Bursectomy
  see Excision, Bursae and Ligaments 0MB-
  see Resection, Bursae and Ligaments 0MT-
Bursocentesis *see* Drainage, Bursae and Ligaments 0M9-
Bursography
  see Plain Radiography, Non-Axial Lower Bones BQ0-
  see Plain Radiography, Non-Axial Upper Bones BP0-
Bursotomy
  see Division, Bursae and Ligaments 0M8-
  see Drainage, Bursae and Ligaments 0M9-
BVS 5000 Ventricular Assist Device
  use External Heart Assist System in Heart and Great Vessels
Bypass
  Anterior Chamber
    Left 08133-
    Right 08123-
  Aorta
    Abdominal 0410-
    Thoracic 021W-
  Artery
    Axillary
      Left 03160-
      Right 03150-
    Brachial
      Left 03180-
      Right 03170-
    Common Carotid
      Left 031J0-
      Right 031H0-
    Common Iliac
      Left 041D-
      Right 041C-
    Coronary
      One Site 0210-
      Two Sites 0211-
      Three Sites 0212-
      Four or More Sites 0213-
    External Carotid
      Left 031N0-
      Right 031M0-
    External Iliac
      Left 041J-
      Right 041H-
    Femoral
      Left 041L-
      Right 041K-
    Innominate 03120-
    Internal Carotid
      Left 031L0-
      Right 031K0-
    Internal Iliac
      Left 041F-
      Right 041E-
    Intracranial 031G0-

Bypass — *continued*
Artery — *continued*
  Popliteal
    Left 041N-
    Right 041M-
  Radial
    Left 031C0-
    Right 031B0-
  Splenic 0414-
  Subclavian
    Left 03140-
    Right 03130-
  Temporal
    Left 031T0-
    Right 031S0-
  Ulnar
    Left 031A0-
    Right 03190-
Atrium
  Left 0217-
  Right 0216-
Bladder 0T1B-
Cavity, Cranial 0W110J-
Cecum 0D1H-
Cerebral Ventricle 0016-
Colon
  Ascending 0D1K-
  Descending 0D1M-
  Sigmoid 0D1N-
  Transverse 0D1L-
Duct
  Common Bile 0F19-
  Cystic 0F18-
  Hepatic
    Left 0F16-
    Right 0F15-
  Lacrimal
    Left 081Y-
    Right 081X-
  Pancreatic 0F1D-
    Accessory 0F1F-
Duodenum 0D19-
Ear
  Left 091E0-
  Right 091D0-
Esophagus 0D15-
  Lower 0D13-
  Middle 0D12-
  Upper 0D11-
Fallopian Tube
  Left 0U16-
  Right 0U15-
Gallbladder 0F14-
Ileum 0D1B-
Jejunum 0D1A-
Kidney Pelvis
  Left 0T14-
  Right 0T13-
Pancreas 0F1G-
Pelvic Cavity 0W1J-
Peritoneal Cavity 0W1G-
Pleural Cavity
  Left 0W1B-
  Right 0W19-
Spinal Canal 001U-
Stomach 0D16-
Trachea 0B11-
Ureter
  Left 0T17-
  Right 0T16-
Ureters, Bilateral 0T18-
Vas Deferens
  Bilateral 0V1Q-
  Left 0V1P-
  Right 0V1N-
Vein
  Axillary
    Left 0518-
    Right 0517-
  Azygos 0510-

Bypass — *continued*
Vein — *continued*
  Basilic
    Left 051C-
    Right 051B-
  Brachial
    Left 051A-
    Right 0519-
  Cephalic
    Left 051F-
    Right 051D-
  Colic 0617-
  Common Iliac
    Left 061D-
    Right 061C-
  Esophageal 0613-
  External Iliac
    Left 061G-
    Right 061F-
  External Jugular
    Left 051Q-
    Right 051P-
  Face
    Left 051V-
    Right 051T-
  Femoral
    Left 061N-
    Right 061M-
  Foot
    Left 061V-
    Right 061T-
  Gastric 0612-
  Greater Saphenous
    Left 061Q-
    Right 061P-
  Hand
    Left 051H-
    Right 051G-
  Hemiazygos 0511-
  Hepatic 0614-
  Hypogastric
    Left 061J-
    Right 061H-
  Inferior Mesenteric 0616-
  Innominate
    Left 0514-
    Right 0513-
  Internal Jugular
    Left 051N-
    Right 051M-
  Intracranial 051L-
  Lesser Saphenous
    Left 061S-
    Right 061R-
  Portal 0618-
  Renal
    Left 061B-
    Right 0619-
  Splenic 0611-
  Subclavian
    Left 0516-
    Right 0515-
  Superior Mesenteric 0615-
  Vertebral
    Left 051S-
    Right 051R-
  Vena Cava
    Inferior 0610-
    Superior 021V-
  Ventricle
    Left 021L-
    Right 021K-
Bypass, cardiopulmonary 5A1221Z

C

Caesarean section *see* Extraction, Products of Conception 10D0-
Calcaneocuboid joint
  use Joint, Tarsal, Left
  use Joint, Tarsal, Right
Calcaneocuboid ligament
  use Bursa and Ligament, Foot, Left
  use Bursa and Ligament, Foot, Right
Calcaneofibular ligament
  use Bursa and Ligament, Ankle, Left
  use Bursa and Ligament, Ankle, Right
Calcaneus
  use Tarsal, Left
  use Tarsal, Right
Cannulation
  see Bypass
  see Dilation
  see Drainage
  see Irrigation
Canthorrhaphy *see* Repair, Eye 08Q-
Canthotomy *see* Release, Eye 08N-
Capitate bone
  use Carpal, Left
  use Carpal, Right
Capsulectomy, lens *see* Excision, Eye 08B-
Capsulorrhaphy, joint
  see Repair, Lower Joints 0SQ-
  see Repair, Upper Joints 0RQ-
Cardia
  use Esophagogastric Junction
Cardiac contractility modulation lead
  use Cardiac Lead in Heart and Great Vessels
Cardiac event recorder
  use Monitoring Device
Cardiac Lead
  Defibrillator
    Atrium
      Left 02H7-
      Right 02H6-
    Pericardium 02HN-
    Vein, Coronary 02H4-
    Ventricle
      Left 02HL-
      Right 02HK-
  Insertion of device in
    Atrium
      Left 02H7-
      Right 02H6-
    Pericardium 02HN-
    Vein, Coronary 02H4-
    Ventricle
      Left 02HL-
      Right 02HK-
  Pacemaker
    Atrium
      Left 02H7-
      Right 02H6-
    Pericardium 02HN-
    Vein, Coronary 02H4-
    Ventricle
      Left 02HL-
      Right 02HK-
  Removal of device from, Heart 02PA-
  Revision of device in, Heart 02WA-
Cardiac plexus
  use Nerve, Thoracic Sympathetic
Cardiac Resynchronization Defibrillator Pulse Generator
  Abdomen 0JH8-
  Chest 0JH6-
Cardiac Resynchronization Pacemaker Pulse Generator
  Abdomen 0JH8-
  Chest 0JH6-

Cardiac resynchronization

Cardiac resynchronization therapy (CRT) lead
use Cardiac Lead, Defibrillator in 02H-
use Cardiac Lead, Pacemaker in 02H-

Cardiac Rhythm Related Device
Insertion of device in
 Abdomen 0JH8-
 Chest 0JH6-
Removal of device from, Subcutaneous Tissue and Fascia, Trunk 0JPT-
Revision of device in, Subcutaneous Tissue and Fascia, Trunk 0JWT-

Cardiocentesis see Drainage, Pericardial Cavity 0W9D-

Cardioesophageal junction
use Esophagogastric Junction

Cardiolysis see Release, Heart and Great Vessels 02N-

CardioMEMS® pressure sensor
use Monitoring Device, Pressure Sensor in 02H-

Cardiomyotomy see Division, Esophagogastric Junction 0D84-

Cardioplegia see Introduction of substance in or on, Heart 3E08-

Cardiorrhaphy see Repair, Heart and Great Vessels 02Q-

Cardioversion 5A2204Z

Caregiver Training F0FZ

Caroticotympanic artery
use Artery, Internal Carotid, Left
use Artery, Internal Carotid, Right

Carotid (artery) sinus (baroreceptor) lead
use Stimulator Lead in Upper Arteries

Carotid glomus
use Carotid Bodies, Bilateral
use Carotid Body, Left
use Carotid Body, Right

Carotid sinus
use Artery, Internal Carotid, Left
use Artery, Internal Carotid, Right

Carotid sinus nerve
use Nerve, Glossopharyngeal

Carotid WALLSTENT® Monorail® Endoprosthesis
use Intraluminal Device

Carpectomy
see Excision, Upper Bones 0PB-
see Resection, Upper Bones 0PT-

Carpometacarpal (CMC) joint
use Joint, Metacarpocarpal, Left
use Joint, Metacarpocarpal, Right

Carpometacarpal ligament
use Bursa and Ligament, Hand, Left
use Bursa and Ligament, Hand, Right

Casting see Immobilization

CAT scan see Computerized Tomography (CT Scan)

Catheterization
see Dilation
see Drainage
see Insertion of device in
see Irrigation
Heart see Measurement, Cardiac 4A02-
Umbilical vein, for infusion 06H033T

Cauda equina
use Spinal Cord, Lumbar

Cauterization
see Destruction
see Repair

Cavernous plexus
use Nerve, Head and Neck Sympathetic

Cecectomy
see Excision, Cecum 0DBH-
see Resection, Cecum 0DTH-

Cecocolostomy
see Bypass, Gastrointestinal System 0D1-
see Drainage, Gastrointestinal System 0D9-

Cecopexy
see Repair, Cecum 0DQH-
see Reposition, Cecum 0DSH-

Cecoplication see Restriction, Cecum 0DVH-

Cecorrhaphy see Repair, Cecum 0DQH-

Cecostomy
see Bypass, Cecum 0D1H-
see Drainage, Cecum 0D9H-

Cecotomy see Drainage, Cecum 0D9H-

Ceftazidime-avibactam anti-infective XW0-

Celiac (solar) plexus
use Nerve, Abdominal Sympathetic

Celiac ganglion
use Nerve, Abdominal Sympathetic

Celiac lymph node
use Lymphatic, Aortic

Celiac trunk
use Artery, Celiac

Central axillary lymph node
use Lymphatic, Axillary, Left
use Lymphatic, Axillary, Right

Central venous pressure see Measurement, Venous 4A04-

Centrimag® Blood Pump
use External Heart Assist System in Heart and Great Vessels

Cephalogram BN00ZZZ

Cerclage see Restriction

Cerebral aqueduct (Sylvius)
use Cerebral Ventricle

Cerebrum
use Brain

Cervical esophagus
use Esophagus, Upper

Cervical facet joint
use Joint, Cervical Vertebral
use Joint, Cervical Vertebral, 2 or more

Cervical ganglion
use Nerve, Head and Neck Sympathetic

Cervical interspinous ligament
use Bursa and Ligament, Head and Neck

Cervical intertransverse ligament
use Bursa and Ligament, Head and Neck

Cervical ligamentum flavum
use Bursa and Ligament, Head and Neck

Cervical lymph node
use Lymphatic, Neck, Left
use Lymphatic, Neck, Right

Cervicectomy
see Excision, Cervix 0UBC-
see Resection, Cervix 0UTC-

Cervicothoracic facet joint
use Joint, Cervicothoracic Vertebral

Cesarean section see Extraction, Products of Conception 10D0-

Change device in
Abdominal Wall 0W2FX-
Back
 Lower 0W2LX-
 Upper 0W2KX-
Bladder 0T2BX-
Bone
 Facial 0N2WX-
 Lower 0Q2YX-
 Nasal 0N2BX-
 Upper 0P2YX-
Bone Marrow 072TX-
Brain 0020X-
Breast
 Left 0H2UX-
 Right 0H2TX-

Change device in — continued
Bursa and Ligament
 Lower 0M2YX-
 Upper 0M2XX-
Cavity, Cranial 0W21X-
Chest Wall 0W28X-
Cisterna Chyli 072LX-
Diaphragm 0B2TX-
Duct
 Hepatobiliary 0F2BX-
 Pancreatic 0F2DX-
Ear
 Left 092JX-
 Right 092HX-
Epididymis and Spermatic Cord 0V2MX-
Extremity
 Lower
  Left 0Y2BX-
  Right 0Y29X-
 Upper
  Left 0X27X-
  Right 0X26X-
Eye
 Left 0821X-
 Right 0820X-
Face 0W22X-
Fallopian Tube 0U28X-
Gallbladder 0F24X-
Gland
 Adrenal 0G25X-
 Endocrine 0G2SX-
 Pituitary 0G20X-
 Salivary 0C2AX-
Head 0W20X-
Intestinal Tract
 Lower 0D2DXUZ
 Upper 0D20XUZ
Jaw
 Lower 0W25X-
 Upper 0W24X-
Joint
 Lower 0S2YX-
 Upper 0R2YX-
Kidney 0T25X-
Larynx 0C2SX-
Liver 0F20X-
Lung
 Left 0B2LX-
 Right 0B2KX-
Lymphatic 072NX-
 Thoracic Duct 072KX-
Mediastinum 0W2CX-
Mesentery 0D2VX-
Mouth and Throat 0C2YX-
Muscle
 Lower 0K2YX-
 Upper 0K2XX-
Neck 0W26X-
Nerve
 Cranial 002EX-
 Peripheral 012YX-
Nose 092KX-
Omentum 0D2UX-
Ovary 0U23X-
Pancreas 0F2GX-
Parathyroid Gland 0G2RX-
Pelvic Cavity 0W2JX-
Penis 0V2SX-
Pericardial Cavity 0W2DX-
Perineum
 Female 0W2NX-
 Male 0W2MX-
Peritoneal Cavity 0W2GX-
Peritoneum 0D2WX-
Pineal Body 0G21X-
Pleura 0B2QX-
Pleural Cavity
 Left 0W2BX-
 Right 0W29X-
Products of Conception 10207-
Prostate and Seminal Vesicles 0V24X-

Change device in — continued
Retroperitoneum 0W2HX-
Scrotum and Tunica Vaginalis 0V28X-
Sinus 092YX-
Skin 0H2PX-
Skull 0N20X-
Spinal Canal 002UX-
Spleen 072PX-
Subcutaneous Tissue and Fascia
 Head and Neck 0J2SX-
 Lower Extremity 0J2WX-
 Trunk 0J2TX-
 Upper Extremity 0J2VX-
Tendon
 Lower 0L2YX-
 Upper 0L2XX-
Testis 0V2DX-
Thymus 072MX-
Thyroid Gland 0G2KX-
Trachea 0B21-
Tracheobronchial Tree 0B20X-
Ureter 0T29X-
Urethra 0T2DX-
Uterus and Cervix 0U2DXHZ
Vagina and Cul-de-sac 0U2HXGZ
Vas Deferens 0V2RX-
Vulva 0U2MX-

Change device in or on
Abdominal Wall 2W03X-
Anorectal 2Y03X5Z
Arm
 Lower
  Left 2W0DX-
  Right 2W0CX-
 Upper
  Left 2W0BX-
  Right 2W0AX-
Back 2W05X-
Chest Wall 2W04X-
Ear 2Y02X5Z
Extremity
 Lower
  Left 2W0MX-
  Right 2W0LX-
 Upper
  Left 2W09X-
  Right 2W08X-
Face 2W01X-
Finger
 Left 2W0KX-
 Right 2W0JX-
Foot
 Left 2W0TX-
 Right 2W0SX-
Genital Tract, Female 2Y04X5Z
Hand
 Left 2W0FX-
 Right 2W0EX-
Head 2W00X-
Inguinal Region
 Left 2W07X-
 Right 2W06X-
Leg
 Lower
  Left 2W0RX-
  Right 2W0QX-
 Upper
  Left 2W0PX-
  Right 2W0NX-
Mouth and Pharynx 2Y00X5Z
Nasal 2Y01X5Z
Neck 2W02X-
Thumb
 Left 2W0HX-
 Right 2W0GX-
Toe
 Left 2W0VX-
 Right 2W0UX-
Urethra 2Y05X5Z

INDEX TO PROCEDURES – 2016 ICD-10-PCS

Chemoembolization see Introduction of substance in or on
Chemosurgery, Skin 3E00XTZ
Chemothalamectomy see Destruction, Thalamus 0059-
Chemotherapy, Infusion for cancer see Introduction of substance in or on
Chest x-ray see Plain Radiography, Chest BW03-
Chiropractic Manipulation
  Abdomen 9WB9X-
  Cervical 9WB1X-
  Extremities
    Lower 9WB6X-
    Upper 9WB7X-
  Head 9WB0X-
  Lumbar 9WB3X-
  Pelvis 9WB5X-
  Rib Cage 9WB8X-
  Sacrum 9WB4X-
  Thoracic 9WB2X-
Choana
  use Nasopharynx
Cholangiogram
  see Fluoroscopy, Hepatobiliary System and Pancreas BF1-
  see Plain Radiography, Hepatobiliary System and Pancreas BF0-
Cholecystectomy
  see Excision, Gallbladder 0FB4-
  see Resection, Gallbladder 0FT4-
Cholecystojejunostomy
  see Bypass, Hepatobiliary System and Pancreas 0F1-
  see Drainage, Hepatobiliary System and Pancreas 0F9-
Cholecystopexy
  see Repair, Gallbladder 0FQ4-
  see Reposition, Gallbladder 0FS4-
Cholecystoscopy 0FJ44ZZ
Cholecystostomy
  see Drainage, Gallbladder 0F94-
  see Bypass, Gallbladder 0F14-
Cholecystotomy see Drainage, Gallbladder 0F94-
Choledochectomy
  see Excision, Hepatobiliary System and Pancreas 0FB-
  see Resection, Hepatobiliary System and Pancreas 0FT-
Choledocholithotomy see Extirpation, Duct, Common Bile 0FC9-
Choledochoplasty
  see Repair, Hepatobiliary System and Pancreas 0FQ-
  see Replacement, Hepatobiliary System and Pancreas 0FR-
  see Supplement, Hepatobiliary System and Pancreas 0FU-
Choledochoscopy 0FJB8ZZ
Choledochotomy see Drainage, Hepatobiliary System and Pancreas 0F9-
Cholelithotomy see Extirpation, Hepatobiliary System and Pancreas 0FC-
Chondrectomy
  see Excision, Lower Joints 0SB-
  see Excision, Upper Joints 0RB-
  Knee see Excision, Lower Joints 0SB-
  Semilunar cartilage see Excision, Lower Joints 0SB-
Chondroglossus muscle
  use Muscle, Tongue, Palate, Pharynx
Chorda tympani
  use Nerve, Facial
Chordotomy see Division, Central Nervous System 008-
Choroid plexus
  use Cerebral Ventricle

Choroidectomy
  see Excision, Eye 08B-
  see Resection, Eye 08T-
Ciliary body
  use Eye, Left
  use Eye, Right
Ciliary ganglion
  use Nerve, Head and Neck Sympathetic
Circle of Willis
  use Artery, Intracranial
Circumcision 0VTTXZZ
Circumflex iliac artery
  use Artery, Femoral, Left
  use Artery, Femoral, Right
Clamp and rod internal fixation system (CRIF)
  use Internal Fixation Device in Lower Bones
  use Internal Fixation Device in Upper Bones
Clamping see Occlusion
Claustrum
  use Basal Ganglia
Claviculectomy
  see Excision, Upper Bones 0PB-
  see Resection, Upper Bones 0PT-
Claviculotomy
  see Division, Upper Bones 0P8-
  see Drainage, Upper Bones 0P9-
Clipping, aneurysm see Restriction using Extraluminal Device
Clitorectomy, clitoridectomy
  see Excision, Clitoris 0UBJ-
  see Resection, Clitoris 0UTJ-
Clolar
  use Clofarabine
Closure
  see Occlusion
  see Repair
Clysis see Introduction of substance in or on
Coagulation see Destruction
CoAxia NeuroFlo catheter
  use Intraluminal Device
Cobalt/chromium head and polyethylene socket
  use Synthetic Substitute, Metal on Polyethylene in 0SR-
Cobalt/chromium head and socket
  use Synthetic Substitute, Metal in 0SR-
Coccygeal body
  use Coccygeal Glomus
Coccygeus muscle
  use Muscle, Trunk, Left
  use Muscle, Trunk, Right
Cochlea
  use Ear, Inner, Left
  use Ear, Inner, Right
Cochlear implant (CI), multiple channel (electrode)
  use Hearing Device, Multiple Channel Cochlear Prosthesis in 09H-
Cochlear implant (CI), single channel (electrode)
  use Hearing Device, Single Channel Cochlear Prosthesis in 09H-
Cochlear Implant Treatment F0BZ0
Cochlear nerve
  use Nerve, Acoustic
COGNIS® CRT-D
  use Cardiac Resynchronization Defibrillator Pulse Generator in 0JH-
Colectomy
  see Excision, Gastrointestinal System 0DB-
  see Resection, Gastrointestinal System 0DT-
Collapse see Occlusion

Collection from
  Breast, Breast Milk 8E0HX62
  Indwelling Device
    Circulatory System
      Blood 8C02X6K
      Other Fluid 8C02X6L
    Nervous System
      Cerebrospinal Fluid 8C01X6J
      Other Fluid 8C01X6L
  Integumentary System, Breast Milk 8E0HX62
  Reproductive System, Male, Sperm 8E0VX63
Colocentesis see Drainage, Gastrointestinal System 0D9-
Colofixation
  see Repair, Gastrointestinal System 0DQ-
  see Reposition, Gastrointestinal System 0DS-
Cololysis see Release, Gastrointestinal System 0DN-
Colonic Z-Stent®
  use Intraluminal Device
Colonoscopy 0DJD8ZZ
Colopexy
  see Repair, Gastrointestinal System 0DQ-
  see Reposition, Gastrointestinal System 0DS-
Coloplication see Restriction, Gastrointestinal System 0DV-
Coloproctectomy
  see Excision, Gastrointestinal System 0DB-
  see Resection, Gastrointestinal System 0DT-
Coloproctostomy
  see Bypass, Gastrointestinal System 0D1-
  see Drainage, Gastrointestinal System 0D9-
Colopuncture see Drainage, Gastrointestinal System 0D9-
Colorrhaphy see Repair, Gastrointestinal System 0DQ-
Colostomy
  see Bypass, Gastrointestinal System 0D1-
  see Drainage, Gastrointestinal System 0D9-
Colpectomy
  see Excision, Vagina 0UBG-
  see Resection, Vagina 0UTG-
Colpocentesis see Drainage, Vagina 0U9G-
Colpopexy
  see Repair, Vagina 0UQG-
  see Reposition, Vagina 0USG-
Colpoplasty
  see Repair, Vagina 0UQG-
  see Supplement, Vagina 0UUG-
Colporrhaphy see Repair, Vagina 0UQG-
Colposcopy 0UJH8ZZ
Columella
  use Nose
Common digital vein
  use Vein, Foot, Left
  use Vein, Foot, Right
Common facial vein
  use Vein, Face, Left
  use Vein, Face, Right
Common fibular nerve
  use Nerve, Peroneal
Common hepatic artery
  use Artery, Hepatic
Common iliac (subaortic) lymph node
  use Lymphatic, Pelvis
Common interosseous artery
  use Artery, Ulnar, Left
  use Artery, Ulnar, Right

Common peroneal nerve
  use Nerve, Peroneal
Complete (SE) stent
  use Intraluminal Device
Compression
  see Restriction
  Abdominal Wall 2W13X-
  Arm
    Lower
      Left 2W1DX-
      Right 2W1CX-
    Upper
      Left 2W1BX-
      Right 2W1AX-
  Back 2W15X-
  Chest Wall 2W14X-
  Extremity
    Lower
      Left 2W1MX-
      Right 2W1LX-
    Upper
      Left 2W19X-
      Right 2W18X-
  Face 2W11X-
  Finger
    Left 2W1KX-
    Right 2W1JX-
  Foot
    Left 2W1TX-
    Right 2W1SX-
  Hand
    Left 2W1FX-
    Right 2W1EX-
  Head 2W10X-
  Inguinal Region
    Left 2W17X-
    Right 2W16X-
  Leg
    Lower
      Left 2W1RX-
      Right 2W1QX-
    Upper
      Left 2W1PX-
      Right 2W1NX-
  Neck 2W12X-
  Thumb
    Left 2W1HX-
    Right 2W1GX-
  Toe
    Left 2W1VX-
    Right 2W1UX-
Computer Assisted Procedure
  Extremity
    Lower
      No Qualifier 8E0YXBZ
      With Computerized Tomography 8E0YXBG
      With Fluoroscopy 8E0YXBF
      With Magnetic Resonance Imaging 8E0YXBH
    Upper
      No Qualifier 8E0XXBZ
      With Computerized Tomography 8E0XXBG
      With Fluoroscopy 8E0XXBF
      With Magnetic Resonance Imaging 8E0XXBH
  Head and Neck Region
    No Qualifier 8E09XBZ
    With Computerized Tomography 8E09XBG
    With Fluoroscopy 8E09XBF
    With Magnetic Resonance Imaging 8E09XBH
  Trunk Region
    No Qualifier 8E0WXBZ
    With Computerized Tomography 8E0WXBG
    With Fluoroscopy 8E0WXBF
    With Magnetic Resonance Imaging 8E0WXBH

Computerized   **INDEX TO PROCEDURES – 2016 ICD-10-PCS**   [2016.PCS]

Computerized Tomography (CT Scan)
- Abdomen **BW20-**
- Chest and Pelvis **BW25-**
- Abdomen and Chest **BW24-**
- Abdomen and Pelvis **BW21-**
- Airway, Trachea **BB2F-**
- Ankle
  - Left **BQ2H-**
  - Right **BQ2G-**
- Aorta
  - Abdominal **B420-**
    - Intravascular Optical Coherence **B420Z2Z**
  - Thoracic **B320-**
    - Intravascular Optical Coherence **B320Z2Z**
- Arm
  - Left **BP2F-**
  - Right **BP2E-**
- Artery
  - Celiac **B421-**
    - Intravascular Optical Coherence **B421Z2Z**
  - Common Carotid
    - Bilateral **B325-**
      - Intravascular Optical Coherence **B325Z2Z**
  - Coronary
    - Bypass Graft
      - Multiple **B223-**
        - Intravascular Optical Coherence **B223Z2Z**
    - Multiple **B221-**
      - Intravascular Optical Coherence **B221Z2Z**
  - Internal Carotid
    - Bilateral **B328-**
      - Intravascular Optical Coherence **B328Z2Z**
  - Intracranial **B32R-**
    - Intravascular Optical Coherence **B32RZ2Z**
  - Lower Extremity
    - Bilateral **B42H-**
      - Intravascular Optical Coherence **B42HZ2Z**
    - Left **B42G-**
      - Intravascular Optical Coherence **B42GZ2Z**
    - Right **B42F-**
      - Intravascular Optical Coherence **B42FZ2Z**
  - Pelvic **B42C-**
    - Intravascular Optical Coherence **B42CZ2Z**
  - Pulmonary
    - Left **B32T-**
      - Intravascular Optical Coherence **B32TZ2Z**
    - Right **B32S-**
      - Intravascular Optical Coherence **B32SZ2Z**
  - Renal
    - Bilateral **B428-**
      - Intravascular Optical Coherence **B428Z2Z**
    - Transplant **B42M-**
      - Intravascular Optical Coherence **B42MZ2Z**
  - Superior Mesenteric **B424-**
    - Intravascular Optical Coherence **B424Z2Z**
  - Vertebral
    - Bilateral **B32G-**
      - Intravascular Optical Coherence **B32GZ2Z**

Computerized Tomography (CT Scan) — *continued*
- Bladder **BT20-**
- Bone
  - Facial **BN25-**
  - Temporal **BN2F-**
- Brain **B020-**
- Calcaneus
  - Left **BQ2K-**
  - Right **BQ2J-**
- Cerebral Ventricle **B028-**
- Chest, Abdomen and Pelvis **BW25-**
- Chest and Abdomen **BW24-**
- Cisterna **B027-**
- Clavicle
  - Left **BP25-**
  - Right **BP24-**
- Coccyx **BR2F-**
- Colon **BD24-**
- Ear **B920-**
- Elbow
  - Left **BP2H-**
  - Right **BP2G-**
- Extremity
  - Lower
    - Left **BQ2S-**
    - Right **BQ2R-**
  - Upper
    - Bilateral **BP2V-**
    - Left **BP2U-**
    - Right **BP2T-**
- Eye
  - Bilateral **B827-**
  - Left **B826-**
  - Right **B825-**
- Femur
  - Left **BQ24-**
  - Right **BQ23-**
- Fibula
  - Left **BQ2C-**
  - Right **BQ2B-**
- Finger
  - Left **BP2S-**
  - Right **BP2R-**
- Foot
  - Left **BQ2M-**
  - Right **BQ2L-**
- Forearm
  - Left **BP2K-**
  - Right **BP2J-**
- Gland
  - Adrenal, Bilateral **BG22-**
  - Parathyroid **BG23-**
  - Parotid, Bilateral **B926-**
  - Salivary, Bilateral **B92D-**
  - Submandibular, Bilateral **B929-**
  - Thyroid **BG24-**
- Hand
  - Left **BP2P-**
  - Right **BP2N-**
- Hands and Wrists, Bilateral **BP2Q-**
- Head **BW28-**
- Head and Neck **BW29-**
- Heart
  - Intravascular Optical Coherence **B226Z2Z**
  - Right and Left **B226-**
- Hepatobiliary System, All **BF2C-**
- Hip
  - Left **BQ21-**
  - Right **BQ20-**
- Humerus
  - Left **BP2B-**
  - Right **BP2A-**
- Intracranial Sinus **B522-**
  - Intravascular Optical Coherence **B522Z2Z**

Computerized Tomography (CT Scan) — *continued*
- Joint
  - Acromioclavicular, Bilateral **BP23-**
  - Finger
    - Left **BP2DZZZ**
    - Right **BP2CZZZ**
  - Foot
    - Left **BQ2Y-**
    - Right **BQ2X-**
  - Hand
    - Left **BP2DZZZ**
    - Right **BP2CZZZ**
  - Sacroiliac **BR2D-**
  - Sternoclavicular
    - Bilateral **BP22-**
    - Left **BP21-**
    - Right **BP20-**
  - Temporomandibular, Bilateral **BN29-**
  - Toe
    - Left **BQ2Y-**
    - Right **BQ2X-**
- Kidney
  - Bilateral **BT23-**
  - Left **BT22-**
  - Right **BT21-**
  - Transplant **BT29-**
- Knee
  - Left **BQ28-**
  - Right **BQ27-**
- Larynx **B92J-**
- Leg
  - Left **BQ2F-**
  - Right **BQ2D-**
- Liver **BF25-**
- Liver and Spleen **BF26-**
- Lung, Bilateral **BB24-**
- Mandible **BN26-**
- Nasopharynx **B92F-**
- Neck **BW2F-**
- Neck and Head **BW29-**
- Orbit, Bilateral **BN23-**
- Oropharynx **B92F-**
- Pancreas **BF27-**
- Patella
  - Left **BQ2W-**
  - Right **BQ2V-**
- Pelvic Region **BW2G-**
- Pelvis **BR2C-**
  - Chest and Abdomen **BW25-**
- Pelvis and Abdomen **BW21-**
- Pituitary Gland **B029-**
- Prostate **BV23-**
- Ribs
  - Left **BP2Y-**
  - Right **BP2X-**
- Sacrum **BR2F-**
- Scapula
  - Left **BP27-**
  - Right **BP26-**
- Sella Turcica **B029-**
- Shoulder
  - Left **BP29-**
  - Right **BP28-**
- Sinus
  - Intracranial **B522-**
    - Intravascular Optical Coherence **B522Z2Z**
  - Paranasal **B922-**
- Skull **BN20-**
- Spinal Cord **B02B-**
- Spine
  - Cervical **BR20-**
  - Lumbar **BR29-**
  - Thoracic **BR27-**
- Spleen and Liver **BF26-**
- Thorax **BP2W-**

Computerized Tomography (CT Scan) — *continued*
- Tibia
  - Left **BQ2C-**
  - Right **BQ2B-**
- Toe
  - Left **BQ2Q-**
  - Right **BQ2P-**
- Trachea **BB2F-**
- Tracheobronchial Tree
  - Bilateral **BB29-**
  - Left **BB28-**
  - Right **BB27-**
- Vein
  - Pelvic (Iliac)
    - Left **B52G-**
      - Intravascular Optical Coherence **B52GZ2Z**
    - Right **B52F-**
      - Intravascular Optical Coherence **B52FZ2Z**
  - Pelvic (Iliac) Bilateral **B52H-**
    - Intravascular Optical Coherence **B52HZ2Z**
  - Portal **B52T-**
    - Intravascular Optical Coherence **B52TZ2Z**
  - Pulmonary
    - Bilateral **B52S-**
      - Intravascular Optical Coherence **B52SZ2Z**
    - Left **B52R-**
      - Intravascular Optical Coherence **B52RZ2Z**
    - Right **B52Q-**
      - Intravascular Optical Coherence **B52QZ2Z**
  - Renal
    - Bilateral **B52L-**
      - Intravascular Optical Coherence **B52LZ2Z**
    - Left **B52K-**
      - Intravascular Optical Coherence **B52KZ2Z**
    - Right **B52J-**
      - Intravascular Optical Coherence **B52JZ2Z**
  - Spanchnic **B52T-**
    - Intravascular Optical Coherence **B52TZ2Z**
  - Vena Cava
    - Inferior **B529-**
      - Intravascular Optical Coherence **B529Z2Z**
    - Superior **B528-**
      - Intravascular Optical Coherence **B528Z2Z**
- Ventricle, Cerebral **B028-**
- Wrist
  - Left **BP2M-**
  - Right **BP2L-**

Concerto II CRT-D
- *use* Cardiac Resynchronization Defibrillator Pulse Generator **0JH-**

Condylectomy
- *see* Excision, Head and Facial Bones **0NB-**
- *see* Excision, Lower Bones **0QB-**
- *see* Excision, Upper Bones **0PB-**

Condyloid process
- *use* Mandible, Left
- *use* Mandible, Right

Condylotomy
- *see* Division, Head and Facial Bones **0N8-**
- *see* Division, Lower Bones **0Q8-**
- *see* Division, Upper Bones **0P8-**
- *see* Drainage, Head and Facial Bones **0N9-**
- *see* Drainage, Lower Bones **0Q9-**
- *see* Drainage, Upper Bones **0P9-**

Condylysis
　see Release, Head and Facial Bones 0NN-
　see Release, Lower Bones 0QN-
　see Release, Upper Bones 0PN-
Conization, cervix see Excision, Uterus 0UB9-
Conjunctivoplasty
　see Repair, Eye 08Q-
　see Replacement, Eye 08R-
CONSERVE® PLUS Total Resurfacing Hip System
　use Resurfacing Device in Lower Joints
Construction
　Auricle, ear see Replacement, Ear, Nose, Sinus 09R-
　Ileal conduit see Bypass, Urinary System 0T1
Consulta CRT-D
　use Cardiac Resynchronization Defibrillator Pulse Generator in 0JH-
Consulta CRT-P
　use Cardiac Resynchronization Pacemaker Pulse Generator in 0JH-
Contact Radiation
　Abdomen DWY37ZZ
　Adrenal Gland DGY27ZZ
　Bile Ducts DFY27ZZ
　Bladder DTY27ZZ
　Bone, Other DPYC7ZZ
　Brain D0Y07ZZ
　Brain Stem D0Y17ZZ
　Breast
　　Left DMY07ZZ
　　Right DMY17ZZ
　Bronchus DBY17ZZ
　Cervix DUY17ZZ
　Chest DWY27ZZ
　Chest Wall DBY77ZZ
　Colon DDY57ZZ
　Diaphragm DBY87ZZ
　Duodenum DDY27ZZ
　Ear D9Y07ZZ
　Esophagus DDY07ZZ
　Eye D8Y07ZZ
　Femur DPY97ZZ
　Fibula DPYB7ZZ
　Gallbladder DFY17ZZ
　Gland
　　Adrenal DGY27ZZ
　　Parathyroid DGY47ZZ
　　Pituitary DGY07ZZ
　　Thyroid DGY57ZZ
　Glands, Salivary D9Y67ZZ
　Head and Neck DWY17ZZ
　Hemibody DWY47ZZ
　Humerus DPY67ZZ
　Hypopharynx D9Y37ZZ
　Ileum DDY47ZZ
　Jejunum DDY37ZZ
　Kidney DTY07ZZ
　Larynx D9YB7ZZ
　Liver DFY07ZZ
　Lung DBY27ZZ
　Mandible DPY37ZZ
　Maxilla DPY27ZZ
　Mediastinum DBY67ZZ
　Mouth D9Y47ZZ
　Nasopharynx D9YD7ZZ
　Neck and Head DWY17ZZ
　Nerve, Peripheral D0Y77ZZ
　Nose D9Y17ZZ
　Oropharynx D9YF7ZZ
　Ovary DUY07ZZ
　Palate
　　Hard D9Y87ZZ
　　Soft D9Y97ZZ
　Pancreas DFY37ZZ
　Parathyroid Gland DGY47ZZ

Contact Radiation — continued
　Pelvic Bones DPY87ZZ
　Pelvic Region DWY67ZZ
　Pineal Body DGY17ZZ
　Pituitary Gland DGY07ZZ
　Pleura DBY57ZZ
　Prostate DVY07ZZ
　Radius DPY77ZZ
　Rectum DDY77ZZ
　Rib DPY57ZZ
　Sinuses D9Y77ZZ
　Skin
　　Abdomen DHY87ZZ
　　Arm DHY47ZZ
　　Back DHY77ZZ
　　Buttock DHY97ZZ
　　Chest DHY67ZZ
　　Face DHY27ZZ
　　Leg DHYB7ZZ
　　Neck DHY37ZZ
　Skull DPY07ZZ
　Spinal Cord D0Y67ZZ
　Sternum DPY47ZZ
　Stomach DDY17ZZ
　Testis DVY17ZZ
　Thyroid Gland DGY57ZZ
　Tibia DPYB7ZZ
　Tongue D9Y57ZZ
　Trachea DBY07ZZ
　Ulna DPY77ZZ
　Ureter DTY17ZZ
　Urethra DTY37ZZ
　Uterus DUY27ZZ
　Whole Body DWY57ZZ
CONTAK RENEWAL® 3 RF (HE) CRT-D
　use Cardiac Resynchronization Defibrillator Pulse Generator in 0JH-
Contegra Pulmonary Valved Conduit
　use Zooplastic Tissue in Heart and Great Vessels
Continuous Glucose Monitoring (CGM) device
　use Monitoring Device
Continuous Negative Airway Pressure
　24-96 Consecutive Hours, Ventilation 5A09459
　Greater than 96 Consecutive Hours, Ventilation 5A09559
　Less than 24 Consecutive Hours, Ventilation 5A09359
Continuous Positive Airway Pressure
　24-96 Consecutive Hours, Ventilation 5A09457
　Greater than 96 Consecutive Hours, Ventilation 5A09557
　Less than 24 Consecutive Hours, Ventilation 5A09357
Contraceptive Device
　Change device in, Uterus and Cervix 0U2DXHZ
　Insertion of device in
　　Cervix 0UHC-
　　Subcutaneous Tissue and Fascia
　　　Abdomen 0JH8-
　　　Chest 0JH6-
　　　Lower Arm
　　　　Left 0JHH-
　　　　Right 0JHG-
　　　Lower Leg
　　　　Left 0JHP-
　　　　Right 0JHN-
　　　Upper Arm
　　　　Left 0JHF-
　　　　Right 0JHD-

Contraceptive Device — continued
　Insertion of device in — continued
　　Subcutaneous Tissue and Fascia — continued
　　　Upper Leg
　　　　Left 0JHM-
　　　　Right 0JHL-
　　Uterus 0UH9-
　Removal of device from
　　Subcutaneous Tissue and Fascia
　　　Lower Extremity 0JPW-
　　　Trunk 0JPT-
　　　Upper Extremity 0JPV-
　　Uterus and Cervix 0UPD-
　Revision of device in
　　Subcutaneous Tissue and Fascia
　　　Lower Extremity 0JWW-
　　　Trunk 0JWT-
　　　Upper Extremity 0JWV-
　　Uterus and Cervix 0UWD-
Contractility Modulation Device
　Abdomen 0JH8-
　Chest 0JH6-
Control postprocedural bleeding in
　Abdominal Wall 0W3F-
　Ankle Region
　　Left 0Y3L-
　　Right 0Y3K-
　Arm
　　Lower
　　　Left 0X3F-
　　　Right 0X3D-
　　Upper
　　　Left 0X39-
　　　Right 0X38-
　Axilla
　　Left 0X35-
　　Right 0X34-
　Back
　　Lower 0W3L-
　　Upper 0W3K-
　Buttock
　　Left 0Y31-
　　Right 0Y30-
　Cavity, Cranial 0W31-
　Chest Wall 0W38-
　Elbow Region
　　Left 0X3C-
　　Right 0X3B-
　Extremity
　　Lower
　　　Left 0Y3B-
　　　Right 0Y39-
　　Upper
　　　Left 0X37-
　　　Right 0X36-
　Face 0W32-
　Femoral Region
　　Left 0Y38-
　　Right 0Y37-
　Foot
　　Left 0Y3N-
　　Right 0Y3M-
　Gastrointestinal Tract 0W3P-
　Genitourinary Tract 0W3R-
　Hand
　　Left 0X3K-
　　Right 0X3J-
　Head 0W30-
　Inguinal Region
　　Left 0Y36-
　　Right 0Y35-
　Jaw
　　Lower 0W35-
　　Upper 0W34-
　Knee Region
　　Left 0Y3G-
　　Right 0Y3F-

Control postprocedural bleeding in — continued
　Leg
　　Lower
　　　Left 0Y3J-
　　　Right 0Y3H-
　　Upper
　　　Left 0Y3D-
　　　Right 0Y3C-
　Mediastinum 0W3C-
　Neck 0W36-
　Oral Cavity and Throat 0W33-
　Pelvic Cavity 0W3J-
　Pericardial Cavity 0W3D-
　Perineum
　　Female 0W3N-
　　Male 0W3M-
　Peritoneal Cavity 0W3G-
　Pleural Cavity
　　Left 0W3B-
　　Right 0W39-
　Respiratory Tract 0W3Q-
　Retroperitoneum 0W3H-
　Shoulder Region
　　Left 0X33-
　　Right 0X32-
　Wrist Region
　　Left 0X3H-
　　Right 0X3G-
Conus arteriosus
　use Ventricle, Right
Conus medullaris
　use Spinal Cord, Lumbar
Conversion
　Cardiac rhythm 5A2204Z
　Gastrostomy to jejunostomy feeding device see Insertion of device in, Jejunum 0DHA-
Coracoacromial ligament
　use Bursa and Ligament, Shoulder, Left
　use Bursa and Ligament, Shoulder, Right
Coracobrachialis muscle
　use Muscle, Upper Arm, Left
　use Muscle, Upper Arm, Right
Coracoclavicular ligament
　use Bursa and Ligament, Shoulder, Left
　use Bursa and Ligament, Shoulder, Right
Coracohumeral ligament
　use Bursa and Ligament, Shoulder, Left
　use Bursa and Ligament, Shoulder, Right
Coracoid process
　use Scapula, Left
　use Scapula, Right
Cordotomy see Division, Central Nervous System 008-
Core needle biopsy see Excision with qualifier Diagnostic
CoreValve transcatheter aortic valve
　use Zooplastic Tissue in Heart and Great Vessels
Cormet Hip Resurfacing System
　use Resurfacing Device in Lower Joints
Corniculate cartilage
　use Larynx
CoRoent® XL
　use Interbody Fusion Device in Lower Joints
Coronary arteriography
　see Fluoroscopy, Heart B21-
　see Plain Radiography, Heart B20-

Corox — INDEX TO PROCEDURES – 2016 ICD-10-PCS

Corox OTW (Bipolar) Lead
use Cardiac Lead, Defibrillator in 02H-
use Cardiac Lead, Pacemaker in 02H-

Corpus callosum
use Brain

Corpus cavernosum
use Penis

Corpus spongiosum
use Penis

Corpus striatum
use Basal Ganglia

Corrugator supercilii muscle
use Muscle, Facial

Cortical strip neurostimulator lead
use Neurostimulator Lead in Central Nervous System

Costatectomy
see Excision, Upper Bones 0PB-
see Resection, Upper Bones 0PT-

Costectomy
see Excision, Upper Bones 0PB-
see Resection, Upper Bones 0PT-

Costocervical trunk
use Artery, Subclavian, Left
use Artery, Subclavian, Right

Costochondrectomy
see Excision, Upper Bones 0PB-
see Resection, Upper Bones 0PT-

Costoclavicular ligament
use Bursa and Ligament, Shoulder, Left
use Bursa and Ligament, Shoulder, Right

Costosternoplasty
see Repair, Upper Bones 0PQ-
see Replacement, Upper Bones 0PR-
see Supplement, Upper Bones 0PU-

Costotomy
see Division, Upper Bones 0P8-
see Drainage, Upper Bones 0P9-

Costotransverse joint
use Joint, Thoracic Vertebral

Costotransverse ligament
use Bursa and Ligament, Thorax, Left
use Bursa and Ligament, Thorax, Right

Costovertebral joint
use Joint, Thoracic Vertebral

Costoxiphoid ligament
use Bursa and Ligament, Thorax, Left
use Bursa and Ligament, Thorax, Right

Counseling
Family, for substance abuse, Other Family Counseling HZ63ZZZ
Group
  12-Step HZ43ZZZ
  Behavioral HZ41ZZZ
  Cognitive HZ40ZZZ
  Cognitive-Behavioral HZ42ZZZ
  Confrontational HZ48ZZZ
  Continuing Care HZ49ZZZ
  Infectious Disease
    Post-Test HZ4CZZZ
    Pre-Test HZ4CZZZ
  Interpersonal HZ44ZZZ
  Motivational Enhancement HZ47ZZZ
  Psychoeducation HZ46ZZZ
  Spiritual HZ4BZZZ
  Vocational HZ45ZZZ

Counseling — continued
Individual
  12-Step HZ33ZZZ
  Behavioral HZ31ZZZ
  Cognitive HZ30ZZZ
  Cognitive-Behavioral HZ32ZZZ
  Confrontational HZ38ZZZ
  Continuing Care HZ39ZZZ
  Infectious Disease
    Post-Test HZ3CZZZ
    Pre-Test HZ3CZZZ
  Interpersonal HZ34ZZZ
  Motivational Enhancement HZ37ZZZ
  Psychoeducation HZ36ZZZ
  Spiritual HZ3BZZZ
  Vocational HZ35ZZZ
Mental Health Services
  Educational GZ60ZZZ
  Other Counseling GZ63ZZZ
  Vocational GZ61ZZZ

Countershock, cardiac 5A2204Z

Cowper's (bulbourethral) gland
use Urethra

CPAP (continuous positive airway pressure)
see Assistance, Respiratory 5A09-

Craniectomy
see Excision, Head and Facial Bones 0NB-
see Resection, Head and Facial Bones 0NT-

Cranioplasty
see Repair, Head and Facial Bones 0NQ-
see Replacement, Head and Facial Bones 0NR-
see Supplement, Head and Facial Bones 0NU-

Craniotomy
see Division, Head and Facial Bones 0N8-
see Drainage, Central Nervous System 009-
see Drainage, Head and Facial Bones 0N9-

Creation
Female 0W4N0-
Male 0W4M0-

Cremaster muscle
use Muscle, Perineum

Cribriform plate
use Bone, Ethmoid, Left
use Bone, Ethmoid, Right

Cricoid cartilage
use Trachea

Cricoidectomy see Excision, Larynx 0CBS-

Cricothyroid artery
use Artery, Thyroid, Left
use Artery, Thyroid, Right

Cricothyroid muscle
use Muscle, Neck, Left
use Muscle, Neck, Right

Crisis Intervention GZ2ZZZZ

Crural fascia
use Subcutaneous Tissue and Fascia, Upper Leg, Left
use Subcutaneous Tissue and Fascia, Upper Leg, Right

Crushing, nerve
Cranial see Destruction, Central Nervous System 005-
Peripheral see Destruction, Peripheral Nervous System 015-

Cryoablation see Destruction

Cryotherapy see Destruction

Cryptorchidectomy
see Excision, Male Reproductive System 0VB-
see Resection, Male Reproductive System 0VT-

Cryptorchiectomy
see Excision, Male Reproductive System 0VB-
see Resection, Male Reproductive System 0VT-

Cryptotomy
see Division, Gastrointestinal System 0D8-
see Drainage, Gastrointestinal System 0D9-

CT scan see Computerized Tomography (CT Scan)

CT sialogram see Computerized Tomography (CT Scan), Ear, Nose, Mouth and Throat B92-

Cubital lymph node
use Lymphatic, Upper Extremity, Left
use Lymphatic, Upper Extremity, Right

Cubital nerve
use Nerve, Ulnar

Cuboid bone
use Tarsal, Left
use Tarsal, Right

Cuboideonavicular joint
use Joint, Tarsal, Left
use Joint, Tarsal, Right

Culdocentesis see Drainage, Cul-de-sac 0U9F-

Culdoplasty
see Repair, Cul-de-sac 0UQF-
see Supplement, Cul-de-sac 0UUF-

Culdoscopy 0UJH8ZZ

Culdotomy see Drainage, Cul-de-sac 0U9F-

Culmen
use Cerebellum

Cultured epidermal cell autograft
use Autologous Tissue Substitute

Cuneiform cartilage
use Larynx

Cuneonavicular joint
use Joint, Tarsal, Left
use Joint, Tarsal, Right

Cuneonavicular ligament
use Bursa and Ligament, Foot, Left
use Bursa and Ligament, Foot, Right

Curettage
see Excision
see Extraction

Cutaneous (transverse) cervical nerve
use Nerve, Cervical Plexus

CVP (central venous pressure) see Measurement, Venous 4A04-

Cyclodiathermy see Destruction, Eye 085-

Cyclophotocoagulation see Destruction, Eye 085-

CYPHER® Stent
use Intraluminal Device, Drug-eluting in Heart and Great Vessels

Cystectomy
see Excision, Bladder 0TBB-
see Resection, Bladder 0TTB-

Cystocele repair see Repair, Subcutaneous Tissue and Fascia, Pelvic Region 0JQC-

Cystography
see Fluoroscopy, Urinary System BT1-
see Plain Radiography, Urinary System BT0-

Cystolithotomy see Extirpation, Bladder 0TCB-

Cystopexy
see Repair, Bladder 0TQB-
see Reposition, Bladder 0TSB-

Cystoplasty
see Repair, Bladder 0TQB-
see Replacement, Bladder 0TRB-
see Supplement, Bladder 0TUB-

Cystorrhaphy see Repair, Bladder 0TQB-

Cystoscopy 0TJB8ZZ

Cystostomy see Bypass, Bladder 0T1B-

Cystostomy tube
use Drainage Device

Cystotomy see Drainage, Bladder 0T9B-

Cystourethrography
see Fluoroscopy, Urinary System BT1-
see Plain Radiography, Urinary System BT0-

Cystourethroplasty
see Repair, Urinary System 0TQ-
see Replacement, Urinary System 0TR-
see Supplement, Urinary System 0TU-

INDEX TO PROCEDURES – 2016 ICD-10-PCS

D

DBS lead
 use Neurostimulator Lead in Central Nervous System
DeBakey Left Ventricular Assist Device
 use Implantable Heart Assist System in Heart and Great Vessels
Debridement
 Excisional see Excision
 Non-excisional see Extraction
Decompression, Circulatory 6A15-
Decortication, lung see Extraction, Respiratory System 0BD-
Deep brain neurostimulator lead
 use Neurostimulator Lead in Central Nervous System
Deep cervical fascia
 use Subcutaneous Tissue and Fascia, Neck, Anterior
Deep cervical vein
 use Vein, Vertebral, Left
 use Vein, Vertebral, Right
Deep circumflex iliac artery
 use Artery, External Iliac, Left
 use Artery, External Iliac, Right
Deep facial vein
 use Vein, Face, Left
 use Vein, Face, Right
Deep femoral (profunda femoris) vein
 use Vein, Femoral, Left
 use Vein, Femoral, Right
Deep femoral artery
 use Artery, Femoral, Left
 use Artery, Femoral, Right
Deep Inferior Epigastric Artery Perforator Flap
 Bilateral 0HRV077
 Left 0HRU077
 Right 0HRT077
Deep palmar arch
 use Artery, Hand, Left
 use Artery, Hand, Right
Deep transverse perineal muscle
 use Muscle, Perineum
Deferential artery
 use Artery, Internal Iliac, Left
 use Artery, Internal Iliac, Right
Defibrillator Generator
 Abdomen 0JH8-
 Chest 0JH6-
Delivery
 Cesarean see Extraction, Products of Conception 10D0-
 Forceps see Extraction, Products of Conception 10D0-
 Manually assisted 10E0XZZ
 Products of Conception 10E0XZZ
 Vacuum assisted see Extraction, Products of Conception 10D0-
Delta frame external fixator
 use External Fixation Device, Hybrid in 0PH-
 use External Fixation Device, Hybrid in 0PS-
 use External Fixation Device, Hybrid in 0QH-
 use External Fixation Device, Hybrid in 0QS-
Delta III Reverse shoulder prosthesis
 use Synthetic Substitute, Reverse Ball and Socket in 0RR-

Deltoid fascia
 use Subcutaneous Tissue and Fascia, Upper Arm, Left
 use Subcutaneous Tissue and Fascia, Upper Arm, Right
Deltoid ligament
 use Bursa and Ligament, Ankle, Left
 use Bursa and Ligament, Ankle, Right
Deltoid muscle
 use Muscle, Shoulder, Left
 use Muscle, Shoulder, Right
Deltopectoral (infraclavicular) lymph node
 use Lymphatic, Upper Extremity, Left
 use Lymphatic, Upper Extremity, Right
Denervation
 Cranial nerve see Destruction, Central Nervous System 005-
 Peripheral nerve see Destruction, Peripheral Nervous System 015-
Densitometry
 Plain Radiography
  Femur
   Left BQ04ZZ1
   Right BQ03ZZ1
  Hip
   Left BQ01ZZ1
   Right BQ00ZZ1
  Spine
   Cervical BR00ZZ1
   Lumbar BR09ZZ1
   Thoracic BR07ZZ1
   Whole BR0GZZ1
 Ultrasonography
  Elbow
   Left BP4HZZ1
   Right BP4GZZ1
  Hand
   Left BP4PZZ1
   Right BP4NZZ1
  Shoulder
   Left BP49ZZ1
   Right BP48ZZ1
  Wrist
   Left BP4MZZ1
   Right BP4LZZ1
Denticulate (dentate) ligament
 use Spinal Meninges
Depressor anguli oris muscle
 use Muscle, Facial
Depressor labii inferioris muscle
 use Muscle, Facial
Depressor septi nasi muscle
 use Muscle, Facial
Depressor supercilii muscle
 use Muscle, Facial
Dermabrasion see Extraction, Skin and Breast 0HD-
Dermis
 use Skin
Descending genicular artery
 use Artery, Femoral, Left
 use Artery, Femoral, Right
Destruction
 Acetabulum
  Left 0Q55-
  Right 0Q54-
 Adenoids 0C5Q-
 Ampulla of Vater 0F5C-
 Anal Sphincter 0D5R-
 Anterior Chamber
  Left 08533ZZ
  Right 08523ZZ
 Anus 0D5Q-
 Aorta
  Abdominal 0450-
  Thoracic 025W-
 Aortic Body 0G5D-
 Appendix 0D5J-

Destruction — continued
 Artery
  Anterior Tibial
   Left 045Q-
   Right 045P-
  Axillary
   Left 0356-
   Right 0355-
  Brachial
   Left 0358-
   Right 0357-
  Celiac 0451-
  Colic
   Left 0457-
   Middle 0458-
   Right 0456-
  Common Carotid
   Left 035J-
   Right 035H-
  Common Iliac
   Left 045D-
   Right 045C-
  External Carotid
   Left 035N-
   Right 035M-
  External Iliac
   Left 045J-
   Right 045H-
  Face 035R-
  Femoral
   Left 045L-
   Right 045K-
  Foot
   Left 045W-
   Right 045V-
  Gastric 0452-
  Hand
   Left 035F-
   Right 035D-
  Hepatic 0453-
  Inferior Mesenteric 045B-
  Innominate 0352-
  Internal Carotid
   Left 035L-
   Right 035K-
  Internal Iliac
   Left 045F-
   Right 045E-
  Internal Mammary
   Left 0351-
   Right 0350-
  Intracranial 035G-
  Lower 045Y-
  Peroneal
   Left 045U-
   Right 045T-
  Popliteal
   Left 045N-
   Right 045M-
  Posterior Tibial
   Left 045S-
   Right 045R-
  Pulmonary
   Left 025R-
   Right 025Q-
  Pulmonary Trunk 025P-
  Radial
   Left 035C-
   Right 035B-
  Renal
   Left 045A-
   Right 0459-
  Splenic 0454-
  Subclavian
   Left 0354-
   Right 0353-
  Superior Mesenteric 0455-

Destruction — continued
 Artery — continued
  Temporal
   Left 035T-
   Right 035S-
  Thyroid
   Left 035V-
   Right 035U-
  Ulnar
   Left 035A-
   Right 0359-
  Upper 035Y-
  Vertebral
   Left 035Q-
   Right 035P-
 Atrium
  Left 0257-
  Right 0256-
 Auditory Ossicle
  Left 095A0ZZ
  Right 09590ZZ
 Basal Ganglia 0058-
 Bladder 0T5B-
 Bladder Neck 0T5C-
 Bone
  Ethmoid
   Left 0N5G-
   Right 0N5F-
  Frontal
   Left 0N52-
   Right 0N51-
  Hyoid 0N5X-
  Lacrimal
   Left 0N5J-
   Right 0N5H-
  Nasal 0N5B-
  Occipital
   Left 0N58-
   Right 0N57-
  Palatine
   Left 0N5L-
   Right 0N5K-
  Parietal
   Left 0N54-
   Right 0N53-
  Pelvic
   Left 0Q53-
   Right 0Q52-
  Sphenoid
   Left 0N5D-
   Right 0N5C-
  Temporal
   Left 0N56-
   Right 0N55-
  Zygomatic
   Left 0N5N-
   Right 0N5M-
 Brain 0050-
 Breast
  Bilateral 0H5V-
  Left 0H5U-
  Right 0H5T-
 Bronchus
  Lingula 0B59-
  Lower Lobe
   Left 0B5B-
   Right 0B56-
  Main
   Left 0B57-
   Right 0B53-
  Middle Lobe, Right 0B55-
  Upper Lobe
   Left 0B58-
   Right 0B54-
 Buccal Mucosa 0C54-

Destruction
INDEX TO PROCEDURES – 2016 ICD-10-PCS

Destruction — *continued*
- Bursa and Ligament
  - Abdomen
    - Left 0M5J-
    - Right 0M5H-
  - Ankle
    - Left 0M5R-
    - Right 0M5Q-
  - Elbow
    - Left 0M54-
    - Right 0M53-
  - Foot
    - Left 0M5T-
    - Right 0M5S-
  - Hand
    - Left 0M58-
    - Right 0M57-
  - Head and Neck 0M50-
  - Hip
    - Left 0M5M-
    - Right 0M5L-
  - Knee
    - Left 0M5P-
    - Right 0M5N-
  - Lower Extremity
    - Left 0M5W-
    - Right 0M5V-
  - Perineum 0M5K-
  - Shoulder
    - Left 0M52-
    - Right 0M51-
  - Thorax
    - Left 0M5G-
    - Right 0M5F-
  - Trunk
    - Left 0M5D-
    - Right 0M5C-
  - Upper Extremity
    - Left 0M5B-
    - Right 0M59-
  - Wrist
    - Left 0M56-
    - Right 0M55-
- Carina 0B52-
- Carotid Bodies, Bilateral 0G58-
- Carotid Body
  - Left 0G56-
  - Right 0G57-
- Carpal
  - Left 0P5N-
  - Right 0P5M-
- Cecum 0D5H-
- Cerebellum 005C-
- Cerebral Hemisphere 0057-
- Cerebral Meninges 0051-
- Cerebral Ventricle 0056-
- Cervix 0U5C-
- Chordae Tendineae 0259-
- Choroid
  - Left 085B-
  - Right 085A-
- Cisterna Chyli 075L-
- Clavicle
  - Left 0P5B-
  - Right 0P59-
- Clitoris 0U5J-
- Coccygeal Glomus 0G5B-
- Coccyx 0Q5S-
- Colon
  - Ascending 0D5K-
  - Descending 0D5M-
  - Sigmoid 0D5N-
  - Transverse 0D5L-
- Conduction Mechanism 0258-
- Conjunctiva
  - Left 085TXZZ
  - Right 085SXZZ

Destruction — *continued*
- Cord
  - Bilateral 0V5H-
  - Left 0V5G-
  - Right 0V5F-
- Cornea
  - Left 0859XZZ
  - Right 0858XZZ
- Cul-de-sac 0U5F-
- Diaphragm
  - Left 0B5S-
  - Right 0B5R-
- Disc
  - Cervical Vertebral 0R53-
  - Cervicothoracic Vertebral 0R55-
  - Lumbar Vertebral 0S52-
  - Lumbosacral 0S54-
  - Thoracic Vertebral 0R59-
  - Thoracolumbar Vertebral 0R5B-
- Duct
  - Common Bile 0F59-
  - Cystic 0F58-
  - Hepatic
    - Left 0F56-
    - Right 0F55-
  - Lacrimal
    - Left 085Y-
    - Right 085X-
  - Pancreatic 0F5D-
    - Accessory 0F5F-
  - Parotid
    - Left 0C5C-
    - Right 0C5B-
- Duodenum 0D59-
- Dura Mater 0052-
- Ear
  - External
    - Left 0951-
    - Right 0950-
  - External Auditory Canal
    - Left 0954-
    - Right 0953-
  - Inner
    - Left 095E0ZZ
    - Right 095D0ZZ
  - Middle
    - Left 09560ZZ
    - Right 09550ZZ
- Endometrium 0U5B-
- Epididymis
  - Bilateral 0V5L-
  - Left 0V5K-
  - Right 0V5J-
- Epiglottis 0C5R-
- Esophagogastric Junction 0D54-
- Esophagus 0D55-
  - Lower 0D53-
  - Middle 0D52-
  - Upper 0D51-
- Eustachian Tube
  - Left 095G-
  - Right 095F-
- Eye
  - Left 0851XZZ
  - Right 0850XZZ
- Eyelid
  - Lower
    - Left 085R-
    - Right 085Q-
  - Upper
    - Left 085P-
    - Right 085N-
- Fallopian Tube
  - Left 0U56-
  - Right 0U55-
- Fallopian Tubes, Bilateral 0U57-
- Femoral Shaft
  - Left 0Q59-
  - Right 0Q58-

Destruction — *continued*
- Femur
  - Lower
    - Left 0Q5C-
    - Right 0Q5B-
  - Upper
    - Left 0Q57-
    - Right 0Q56-
- Fibula
  - Left 0Q5K-
  - Right 0Q5J-
- Finger Nail 0H5QXZZ
- Gallbladder 0F54-
- Gingiva
  - Lower 0C56-
  - Upper 0C55-
- Gland
  - Adrenal
    - Bilateral 0G54-
    - Left 0G52-
    - Right 0G53-
  - Lacrimal
    - Left 085W-
    - Right 085V-
  - Minor Salivary 0C5J-
  - Parotid
    - Left 0C59-
    - Right 0C58-
  - Pituitary 0G50-
  - Sublingual
    - Left 0C5F-
    - Right 0C5D-
  - Submaxillary
    - Left 0C5H-
    - Right 0C5G-
  - Vestibular 0U5L-
- Glenoid Cavity
  - Left 0P58-
  - Right 0P57-
- Glomus Jugulare 0G5C-
- Humeral Head
  - Left 0P5D-
  - Right 0P5C-
- Humeral Shaft
  - Left 0P5G-
  - Right 0P5F-
- Hymen 0U5K-
- Hypothalamus 005A-
- Ileocecal Valve 0D5C-
- Ileum 0D5B-
- Intestine
  - Large 0D5E-
    - Left 0D5G-
    - Right 0D5F-
  - Small 0D58-
- Iris
  - Left 085D3ZZ
  - Right 085C3ZZ
- Jejunum 0D5A-
- Joint
  - Acromioclavicular
    - Left 0R5H-
    - Right 0R5G-
  - Ankle
    - Left 0S5G-
    - Right 0S5F-
  - Carpal
    - Left 0R5R-
    - Right 0R5Q-
  - Cervical Vertebral 0R51-
  - Cervicothoracic Vertebral 0R54-
  - Coccygeal 0S56-
  - Elbow
    - Left 0R5M-
    - Right 0R5L-
  - Finger Phalangeal
    - Left 0R5X-
    - Right 0R5W-

Destruction — *continued*
- Joint — *continued*
  - Hip
    - Left 0S5B-
    - Right 0S59-
  - Knee
    - Left 0S5D-
    - Right 0S5C-
  - Lumbar Vertebral 0S50-
  - Lumbosacral 0S53-
  - Metacarpocarpal
    - Left 0R5T-
    - Right 0R5S-
  - Metacarpophalangeal
    - Left 0R5V-
    - Right 0R5U-
  - Metatarsal-Phalangeal
    - Left 0S5N-
    - Right 0S5M-
  - Metatarsal-Tarsal
    - Left 0S5L-
    - Right 0S5K-
  - Occipital-cervical 0R50-
  - Sacrococcygeal 0S55-
  - Sacroiliac
    - Left 0S58-
    - Right 0S57-
  - Shoulder
    - Left 0R5K-
    - Right 0R5J-
  - Sternoclavicular
    - Left 0R5F-
    - Right 0R5E-
  - Tarsal
    - Left 0S5J-
    - Right 0S5H-
  - Temporomandibular
    - Left 0R5D-
    - Right 0R5C-
  - Thoracic Vertebral 0R56-
  - Thoracolumbar Vertebral 0R5A-
  - Toe Phalangeal
    - Left 0S5Q-
    - Right 0S5P-
  - Wrist
    - Left 0R5P-
    - Right 0R5N-
- Kidney
  - Left 0T51-
  - Right 0T50-
- Kidney Pelvis
  - Left 0T54-
  - Right 0T53-
- Larynx 0C5S-
- Lens
  - Left 085K3ZZ
  - Right 085J3ZZ
- Lip
  - Lower 0C51-
  - Upper 0C50-
- Liver 0F50-
  - Left Lobe 0F52-
  - Right Lobe 0F51-
- Lung
  - Bilateral 0B5M-
  - Left 0B5L-
  - Lower Lobe
    - Left 0B5J-
    - Right 0B5F-
  - Middle Lobe, Right 0B5D-
  - Right 0B5K-
  - Upper Lobe
    - Left 0B5G-
    - Right 0B5C-
- Lung Lingula 0B5H-

12

Destruction — continued
Lymphatic
  Aortic 075D-
  Axillary
    Left 0756-
    Right 0755-
  Head 0750-
  Inguinal
    Left 075J-
    Right 075H-
  Internal Mammary
    Left 0759-
    Right 0758-
  Lower Extremity
    Left 075G-
    Right 075F-
  Mesenteric 075B-
  Neck
    Left 0752-
    Right 0751-
  Pelvis 075C-
  Thoracic Duct 075K-
  Thorax 0757-
  Upper Extremity
    Left 0754-
    Right 0753-
Mandible
  Left 0N5V-
  Right 0N5T-
Maxilla
  Left 0N5S-
  Right 0N5R-
Medulla Oblongata 005D-
Mesentery 0D5V-
Metacarpal
  Left 0P5Q-
  Right 0P5P-
Metatarsal
  Left 0Q5P-
  Right 0Q5N-
Muscle
  Abdomen
    Left 0K5L-
    Right 0K5K-
  Extraocular
    Left 085M-
    Right 085L-
  Facial 0K51-
  Foot
    Left 0K5W-
    Right 0K5V-
  Hand
    Left 0K5D-
    Right 0K5C-
  Head 0K50-
  Hip
    Left 0K5P-
    Right 0K5N-
  Lower Arm and Wrist
    Left 0K5B-
    Right 0K59-
  Lower Leg
    Left 0K5T-
    Right 0K5S-
  Neck
    Left 0K53-
    Right 0K52-
  Papillary 025D-
  Perineum 0K5M-
  Shoulder
    Left 0K56-
    Right 0K55-
  Thorax
    Left 0K5J-
    Right 0K5H-
  Tongue, Palate, Pharynx 0K54-
  Trunk
    Left 0K5G-
    Right 0K5F-

Destruction — continued
Muscle — continued
  Upper Arm
    Left 0K58-
    Right 0K57-
  Upper Leg
    Left 0K5R-
    Right 0K5Q-
Nasopharynx 095N-
Nerve
  Abdominal Sympathetic 015M-
  Abducens 005L-
  Accessory 005R-
  Acoustic 005N-
  Brachial Plexus 0153-
  Cervical 0151-
  Cervical Plexus 0150-
  Facial 005M-
  Femoral 015D-
  Glossopharyngeal 005P-
  Head and Neck Sympathetic 015K-
  Hypoglossal 005S-
  Lumbar 015B-
  Lumbar Plexus 0159-
  Lumbar Sympathetic 015N-
  Lumbosacral Plexus 015A-
  Median 0155-
  Oculomotor 005H-
  Olfactory 005F-
  Optic 005G-
  Peroneal 015H-
  Phrenic 0152-
  Pudendal 015C-
  Radial 0156-
  Sacral 015R-
  Sacral Plexus 015Q-
  Sacral Sympathetic 015P-
  Sciatic 015F-
  Thoracic 0158-
  Thoracic Sympathetic 015L-
  Tibial 015G-
  Trigeminal 005K-
  Trochlear 005J-
  Ulnar 0154-
  Vagus 005Q-
Nipple
  Left 0H5X-
  Right 0H5W-
Nose 095K-
Omentum
  Greater 0D5S-
  Lesser 0D5T-
Orbit
  Left 0N5Q-
  Right 0N5P-
Ovary
  Bilateral 0U52-
  Left 0U51-
  Right 0U50-
Palate
  Hard 0C52-
  Soft 0C53-
Pancreas 0F5G-
Para-aortic Body 0G59-
Paraganglion Extremity 0G5F-
Parathyroid Gland 0G5R-
  Inferior
    Left 0G5P-
    Right 0G5N-
  Multiple 0G5Q-
  Superior
    Left 0G5M-
    Right 0G5L-
Patella
  Left 0Q5F-
  Right 0Q5D-
Penis 0V5S-
Pericardium 025N-
Peritoneum 0D5W-

Destruction — continued
Phalanx
  Finger
    Left 0P5V-
    Right 0P5T-
  Thumb
    Left 0P5S-
    Right 0P5R-
  Toe
    Left 0Q5R-
    Right 0Q5Q-
Pharynx 0C5M-
Pineal Body 0G51-
Pleura
  Left 0B5P-
  Right 0B5N-
Pons 005B-
Prepuce 0V5T-
Prostate 0V50-
Radius
  Left 0P5J-
  Right 0P5H-
Rectum 0D5P-
Retina
  Left 085F3ZZ
  Right 085E3ZZ
Retinal Vessel
  Left 085H3ZZ
  Right 085G3ZZ
Rib
  Left 0P52-
  Right 0P51-
Sacrum 0Q51-
Scapula
  Left 0P56-
  Right 0P55-
Sclera
  Left 0857XZZ
  Right 0856XZZ
Scrotum 0V55-
Septum
  Atrial 0255-
  Nasal 095M-
  Ventricular 025M-
Sinus
  Accessory 095P-
  Ethmoid
    Left 095V-
    Right 095U-
  Frontal
    Left 095T-
    Right 095S-
  Mastoid
    Left 095C-
    Right 095B-
  Maxillary
    Left 095R-
    Right 095Q-
  Sphenoid
    Left 095X-
    Right 095W-
Skin
  Abdomen 0H57XZ-
  Back 0H56XZ-
  Buttock 0H58XZ-
  Chest 0H55XZ-
  Ear
    Left 0H53XZ-
    Right 0H52XZ-
  Face 0H51XZ-
  Foot
    Left 0H5NXZ-
    Right 0H5MXZ-
  Genitalia 0H5AXZ-
  Hand
    Left 0H5GXZ-
    Right 0H5FXZ-
  Lower Arm
    Left 0H5EXZ-
    Right 0H5DXZ-

Destruction — continued
Skin — continued
  Lower Leg
    Left 0H5LXZ-
    Right 0H5KXZ-
  Neck 0H54XZ-
  Perineum 0H59XZ-
  Scalp 0H50XZ-
  Upper Arm
    Left 0H5CXZ-
    Right 0H5BXZ-
  Upper Leg
    Left 0H5JXZ-
    Right 0H5HXZ-
Skull 0N50-
Spinal Cord
  Cervical 005W-
  Lumbar 005Y-
  Thoracic 005X-
Spinal Meninges 005T-
Spleen 075P-
Sternum 0P50-
Stomach 0D56-
  Pylorus 0D57-
Subcutaneous Tissue and Fascia
  Abdomen 0J58-
  Back 0J57-
  Buttock 0J59-
  Chest 0J56-
  Face 0J51-
  Foot
    Left 0J5R-
    Right 0J5Q-
  Hand
    Left 0J5K-
    Right 0J5J-
  Lower Arm
    Left 0J5H-
    Right 0J5G-
  Lower Leg
    Left 0J5P-
    Right 0J5N-
  Neck
    Anterior 0J54-
    Posterior 0J55-
  Pelvic Region 0J5C-
  Perineum 0J5B-
  Scalp 0J50-
  Upper Arm
    Left 0J5F-
    Right 0J5D-
  Upper Leg
    Left 0J5M-
    Right 0J5L-
Tarsal
  Left 0Q5M-
  Right 0Q5L-
Tendon
  Abdomen
    Left 0L5G-
    Right 0L5F-
  Ankle
    Left 0L5T-
    Right 0L5S-
  Foot
    Left 0L5W-
    Right 0L5V-
  Hand
    Left 0L58-
    Right 0L57-
  Head and Neck 0L50-
  Hip
    Left 0L5K-
    Right 0L5J-
  Knee
    Left 0L5R-
    Right 0L5Q-
  Lower Arm and Wrist
    Left 0L56-
    Right 0L55-

Destruction

Destruction — *continued*
Tendon — *continued*
Lower Leg
Left 0L5P-
Right 0L5N-
Perineum 0L5H-
Shoulder
Left 0L52-
Right 0L51-
Thorax
Left 0L5D-
Right 0L5C-
Trunk
Left 0L5B-
Right 0L59-
Upper Arm
Left 0L54-
Right 0L53-
Upper Leg
Left 0L5M-
Right 0L5L-
Testis
Bilateral 0V5C-
Left 0V5B-
Right 0V59-
Thalamus 0059-
Thymus 075M-
Thyroid Gland 0G5K-
Left Lobe 0G5G-
Right Lobe 0G5H-
Tibia
Left 0Q5H-
Right 0Q5G-
Toe Nail 0H5RXZZ
Tongue 0C57-
Tonsils 0C5P-
Tooth
Lower 0C5X-
Upper 0C5W-
Trachea 0B51-
Tunica Vaginalis
Left 0V57-
Right 0V56-
Turbinate, Nasal 095L-
Tympanic Membrane
Left 0958-
Right 0957-
Ulna
Left 0P5L-
Right 0P5K-
Ureter
Left 0T57-
Right 0T56-
Urethra 0T5D-
Uterine Supporting Structure 0U54-
Uterus 0U59-
Uvula 0C5N-
Vagina 0U5G-
Valve
Aortic 025F-
Mitral 025G-
Pulmonary 025H-
Tricuspid 025J-
Vas Deferens
Bilateral 0V5Q-
Left 0V5P-
Right 0V5N-
Vein
Axillary
Left 0558-
Right 0557-
Azygos 0550-
Basilic
Left 055C-
Right 055B-
Brachial
Left 055A-
Right 0559-

Destruction — *continued*
Vein — *continued*
Cephalic
Left 055F-
Right 055D-
Colic 0657-
Common Iliac
Left 065D-
Right 065C-
Coronary 0254-
Esophageal 0653-
External Iliac
Left 065G-
Right 065F-
External Jugular
Left 055Q-
Right 055P-
Face
Left 055V-
Right 055T-
Femoral
Left 065N-
Right 065M-
Foot
Left 065V-
Right 065T-
Gastric 0652-
Greater Saphenous
Left 065Q-
Right 065P-
Hand
Left 055H-
Right 055G-
Hemiazygos 0551-
Hepatic 0654-
Hypogastric
Left 065J-
Right 065H-
Inferior Mesenteric 0656-
Innominate
Left 0554-
Right 0553-
Internal Jugular
Left 055N-
Right 055M-
Intracranial 055L-
Lesser Saphenous
Left 065S-
Right 065R-
Lower 065Y-
Portal 0658-
Pulmonary
Left 025T-
Right 025S-
Renal
Left 065B-
Right 0659-
Splenic 0651-
Subclavian
Left 0556-
Right 0555-
Superior Mesenteric 0655-
Upper 055Y-
Vertebral
Left 055S-
Right 055R-
Vena Cava
Inferior 0650-
Superior 025V-
Ventricle
Left 025L-
Right 025K-
Vertebra
Cervical 0P53-
Lumbar 0Q50-
Thoracic 0P54-
Vesicle
Bilateral 0V53-
Left 0V52-
Right 0V51-

Destruction — *continued*
Vitreous
Left 08553ZZ
Right 08543ZZ
Vocal Cord
Left 0C5V-
Right 0C5T-
Vulva 0U5M-
Detachment
Arm
Lower
Left 0X6F0Z-
Right 0X6D0Z-
Upper
Left 0X690Z-
Right 0X680Z-
Elbow Region
Left 0X6C0ZZ
Right 0X6B0ZZ
Femoral Region
Left 0Y680ZZ
Right 0Y670ZZ
Finger
Index
Left 0X6P0Z-
Right 0X6N0Z-
Little
Left 0X6W0Z-
Right 0X6V0Z-
Middle
Left 0X6R0Z-
Right 0X6Q0Z-
Ring
Left 0X6T0Z-
Right 0X6S0Z-
Foot
Left 0Y6N0Z-
Right 0Y6M0Z-
Forequarter
Left 0X610ZZ
Right 0X600ZZ
Hand
Left 0X6K0Z-
Right 0X6J0Z-
Hindquarter
Bilateral 0Y640ZZ
Left 0Y630ZZ
Right 0Y620ZZ
Knee Region
Left 0Y6G0ZZ
Right 0Y6F0ZZ
Leg
Lower
Left 0Y6J0Z-
Right 0Y6H0Z-
Upper
Left 0Y6D0Z-
Right 0Y6C0Z-
Shoulder Region
Left 0X630ZZ
Right 0X620ZZ
Thumb
Left 0X6M0Z-
Right 0X6L0Z-
Toe
1st
Left 0Y6Q0Z-
Right 0Y6P0Z-
2nd
Left 0Y6S0Z-
Right 0Y6R0Z-
3rd
Left 0Y6U0Z-
Right 0Y6T0Z-
4th
Left 0Y6W0Z-
Right 0Y6V0Z-
5th
Left 0Y6Y0Z-
Right 0Y6X0Z-

Determination, Mental status
GZ14ZZZ
Detorsion
see Release
see Reposition
Detoxification Services, for substance abuse HZ2ZZZZ
Device Fitting F0DZ-
Diagnostic Audiology *see* Audiology, Diagnostic
Diagnostic imaging *see* Imaging, Diagnostic
Diagnostic radiology *see* Imaging, Diagnostic
Dialysis
Hemodialysis 5A1D00Z
Peritoneal 3E1M39Z
Diaphragma sellae
use Dura Mater
Diaphragmatic pacemaker generator
use Stimulator Generator in Subcutaneous Tissue and Fascia
Diaphragmatic Pacemaker Lead
Insertion of device in
Left 0BHS-
Right 0BHR-
Removal of device from, Diaphragm 0BPT-
Revision of device in, Diaphragm 0BWT-
Digital radiography, plain *see* Plain Radiography
Dilation
Ampulla of Vater 0F7C-
Anus 0D7Q-
Aorta
Abdominal 0470-
Thoracic 027W-
Artery
Anterior Tibial
Left 047Q-
Right 047P-
Axillary
Left 0376-
Right 0375-
Brachial
Left 0378-
Right 0377-
Celiac 0471-
Colic
Left 0477-
Middle 0478-
Right 0476-
Common Carotid
Left 037J-
Right 037H-
Common Iliac
Left 047D-
Right 047C-
Coronary
One Site 0270-
Two Sites 0271-
Three Sites 0272-
Four or More Sites 0273-
External Carotid
Left 037N-
Right 037M-
External Iliac
Left 047J-
Right 047H-
Face 037R-
Femoral
Left 047L-
Right 047K-
Foot
Left 047W-
Right 047V-
Gastric 0472-

INDEX TO PROCEDURES – 2016 ICD-10-PCS

Dilation — *continued*
 Artery — *continued*
  Hand
   Left 037F-
   Right 037D-
  Hepatic 0473-
  Inferior Mesenteric 047B-
  Innominate 0372-
  Internal Carotid
   Left 037L-
   Right 037K-
  Internal Iliac
   Left 047F-
   Right 047E-
  Internal Mammary
   Left 0371-
   Right 0370-
  Intracranial 037G-
  Lower 047Y-
  Peroneal
   Left 047U-
   Right 047T-
  Popliteal
   Left 047N-
   Right 047M-
  Posterior Tibial
   Left 047S-
   Right 047R-
  Pulmonary
   Left 027R-
   Right 027Q-
  Pulmonary Trunk 027P-
  Radial
   Left 037C-
   Right 037B-
  Renal
   Left 047A-
   Right 0479-
  Splenic 0474-
  Subclavian
   Left 0374-
   Right 0373-
  Superior Mesenteric 0475-
  Temporal
   Left 037T-
   Right 037S-
  Thyroid
   Left 037V-
   Right 037U-
  Ulnar
   Left 037A-
   Right 0379-
  Upper 037Y-
  Vertebral
   Left 037Q-
   Right 037P-
 Bladder 0T7B-
 Bladder Neck 0T7C-
 Bronchus
  Lingula 0B79-
  Lower Lobe
   Left 0B7B-
   Right 0B76-
  Main
   Left 0B77-
   Right 0B73-
  Middle Lobe, Right 0B75-
  Upper Lobe
   Left 0B78-
   Right 0B74-
 Carina 0B72-
 Cecum 0D7H-
 Cervix 0U7C-
 Colon
  Ascending 0D7K-
  Descending 0D7M-
  Sigmoid 0D7N-
  Transverse 0D7L-

Dilation — *continued*
 Duct
  Common Bile 0F79-
  Cystic 0F78-
  Hepatic
   Left 0F76-
   Right 0F75-
  Lacrimal
   Left 087Y-
   Right 087X-
  Pancreatic 0F7D-
   Accessory 0F7F-
  Parotid
   Left 0C7C-
   Right 0C7B-
 Duodenum 0D79-
 Esophagogastric Junction 0D74-
 Esophagus 0D75-
  Lower 0D73-
  Middle 0D72-
  Upper 0D71-
 Eustachian Tube
  Left 097G-
  Right 097F-
 Fallopian Tube
  Left 0U76-
  Right 0U75-
 Fallopian Tubes, Bilateral 0U77-
 Hymen 0U7K-
 Ileocecal Valve 0D7C-
 Ileum 0D7B-
 Intestine
  Large 0D7E-
   Left 0D7G-
   Right 0D7F-
  Small 0D78-
 Jejunum 0D7A-
 Kidney Pelvis
  Left 0T74-
  Right 0T73-
 Larynx 0C7S-
 Pharynx 0C7M-
 Rectum 0D7P-
 Stomach 0D76-
  Pylorus 0D77-
 Trachea 0B71-
 Ureter
  Left 0T77-
  Right 0T76-
 Ureters, Bilateral 0T78-
 Urethra 0T7D-
 Uterus 0U79-
 Vagina 0U7G-
 Valve
  Aortic 027F-
  Mitral 027G-
  Pulmonary 027H-
  Tricuspid 027J-
 Vas Deferens
  Bilateral 0V7Q-
  Left 0V7P-
  Right 0V7N-
 Vein
  Axillary
   Left 0578-
   Right 0577-
  Azygos 0570-
  Basilic
   Left 057C-
   Right 057B-
  Brachial
   Left 057A-
   Right 0579-
  Cephalic
   Left 057F-
   Right 057D-
  Colic 0677-
  Common Iliac
   Left 067D-
   Right 067C-

Dilation — *continued*
 Vein — *continued*
  Esophageal 0673-
  External Iliac
   Left 067G-
   Right 067F-
  External Jugular
   Left 057Q-
   Right 057P-
  Face
   Left 057V-
   Right 057T-
  Femoral
   Left 067N-
   Right 067M-
  Foot
   Left 067V-
   Right 067T-
  Gastric 0672-
  Greater Saphenous
   Left 067Q-
   Right 067P-
  Hand
   Left 057H-
   Right 057G-
  Hemiazygos 0571-
  Hepatic 0674-
  Hypogastric
   Left 067J-
   Right 067H-
  Inferior Mesenteric 0676-
  Innominate
   Left 0574-
   Right 0573-
  Internal Jugular
   Left 057N-
   Right 057M-
  Intracranial 057L-
  Lesser Saphenous
   Left 067S-
   Right 067R-
  Lower 067Y-
  Portal 0678-
  Pulmonary
   Left 027T-
   Right 027S-
  Renal
   Left 067B-
   Right 0679-
  Splenic 0671-
  Subclavian
   Left 0576-
   Right 0575-
  Superior Mesenteric 0675-
  Upper 057Y-
  Vertebral
   Left 057S-
   Right 057R-
  Vena Cava
   Inferior 0670-
   Superior 027V-
  Ventricle, Right 027K-
Direct Lateral Interbody Fusion (DLIF) device
 use Interbody Fusion Device in Lower Joints
Disarticulation *see* Detachment
Discectomy, diskectomy
 see Excision, Lower Joints 0SB-
 see Excision, Upper Joints 0RB-
 see Resection, Lower Joints 0ST-
 see Resection, Upper Joints 0RT-
Discography
 see Fluoroscopy, Axial Skeleton, Except Skull and Facial Bones BR1-
 see Plain Radiography, Axial Skeleton, Except Skull and Facial Bones BR0-
Distal humerus
 use Humeral Shaft, Left
 use Humeral Shaft, Right

Distal humerus, involving joint
 use Joint, Elbow, Left
 use Joint, Elbow, Right
Distal radioulnar joint
 use Joint, Wrist, Left
 use Joint, Wrist, Right
Diversion *see* Bypass
Diverticulectomy *see* Excision, Gastrointestinal System 0DB-
Division
 Acetabulum
  Left 0Q85-
  Right 0Q84-
 Anal Sphincter 0D8R-
 Basal Ganglia 0088-
 Bladder Neck 0T8C-
 Bone
  Ethmoid
   Left 0N8G-
   Right 0N8F-
  Frontal
   Left 0N82-
   Right 0N81-
  Hyoid 0N8X-
  Lacrimal
   Left 0N8J-
   Right 0N8H-
  Nasal 0N8B-
  Occipital
   Left 0N88-
   Right 0N87-
  Palatine
   Left 0N8L-
   Right 0N8K-
  Parietal
   Left 0N84-
   Right 0N83-
  Pelvic
   Left 0Q83-
   Right 0Q82-
  Sphenoid
   Left 0N8D-
   Right 0N8C-
  Temporal
   Left 0N86-
   Right 0N85-
  Zygomatic
   Left 0N8N-
   Right 0N8M-
 Brain 0080-
 Bursa and Ligament
  Abdomen
   Left 0M8J-
   Right 0M8H-
  Ankle
   Left 0M8R-
   Right 0M8Q-
  Elbow
   Left 0M84-
   Right 0M83-
  Foot
   Left 0M8T-
   Right 0M8S-
  Hand
   Left 0M88-
   Right 0M87-
  Head and Neck 0M80-
  Hip
   Left 0M8M-
   Right 0M8L-
  Knee
   Left 0M8P-
   Right 0M8N-
  Lower Extremity
   Left 0M8W-
   Right 0M8V-
  Perineum 0M8K-
  Shoulder
   Left 0M82-
   Right 0M81-

Division

PROCEDURE INDEX

15

INDEX TO PROCEDURES – 2016 ICD-10-PCS

Division — continued
 Bursa and Ligament — continued
  Thorax
   Left 0M8G-
   Right 0M8F-
  Trunk
   Left 0M8D-
   Right 0M8C-
  Upper Extremity
   Left 0M8B-
   Right 0M89-
  Wrist
   Left 0M86-
   Right 0M85-
 Carpal
  Left 0P8N-
  Right 0P8M-
 Cerebral Hemisphere 0087-
 Chordae Tendineae 0289-
 Clavicle
  Left 0P8B-
  Right 0P89-
 Coccyx 0Q8S-
 Conduction Mechanism 0288-
 Esophagogastric Junction 0D84-
 Femoral Shaft
  Left 0Q89-
  Right 0Q88-
 Femur
  Lower
   Left 0Q8C-
   Right 0Q8B-
  Upper
   Left 0Q87-
   Right 0Q86-
 Fibula
  Left 0Q8K-
  Right 0Q8J-
 Gland, Pituitary 0G80-
 Glenoid Cavity
  Left 0P88-
  Right 0P87-
 Humeral Head
  Left 0P8D-
  Right 0P8C-
 Humeral Shaft
  Left 0P8G-
  Right 0P8F-
 Hymen 0U8K-
 Kidneys, Bilateral 0T82-
 Mandible
  Left 0N8V-
  Right 0N8T-
 Maxilla
  Left 0N8S-
  Right 0N8R-
 Metacarpal
  Left 0P8Q-
  Right 0P8P-
 Metatarsal
  Left 0Q8P-
  Right 0Q8N-
 Muscle
  Abdomen
   Left 0K8L-
   Right 0K8K-
  Facial 0K81-
  Foot
   Left 0K8W-
   Right 0K8V-
  Hand
   Left 0K8D-
   Right 0K8C-
  Head 0K80-
  Hip
   Left 0K8P-
   Right 0K8N-
  Lower Arm and Wrist
   Left 0K8B-
   Right 0K89-

Division — continued
 Muscle — continued
  Lower Leg
   Left 0K8T-
   Right 0K8S-
  Neck
   Left 0K83-
   Right 0K82-
  Papillary 028D-
  Perineum 0K8M-
  Shoulder
   Left 0K86-
   Right 0K85-
  Thorax
   Left 0K8J-
   Right 0K8H-
  Tongue, Palate, Pharynx 0K84-
  Trunk
   Left 0K8G-
   Right 0K8F-
  Upper Arm
   Left 0K88-
   Right 0K87-
  Upper Leg
   Left 0K8R-
   Right 0K8Q-
 Nerve
  Abdominal Sympathetic 018M-
  Abducens 008L-
  Accessory 008R-
  Acoustic 008N-
  Brachial Plexus 0183-
  Cervical 0181-
  Cervical Plexus 0180-
  Facial 008M-
  Femoral 018D-
  Glossopharyngeal 008P-
  Head and Neck Sympathetic 018K-
  Hypoglossal 008S-
  Lumbar 018B-
  Lumbar Plexus 0189-
  Lumbar Sympathetic 018N-
  Lumbosacral Plexus 018A-
  Median 0185-
  Oculomotor 008H-
  Olfactory 008F-
  Optic 008G-
  Peroneal 018H-
  Phrenic 0182-
  Pudendal 018C-
  Radial 0186-
  Sacral 018R-
  Sacral Plexus 018Q-
  Sacral Sympathetic 018P-
  Sciatic 018F-
  Thoracic 0188-
  Thoracic Sympathetic 018L-
  Tibial 018G-
  Trigeminal 008K-
  Trochlear 008J-
  Ulnar 0184-
  Vagus 008Q-
 Orbit
  Left 0N8Q-
  Right 0N8P-
 Ovary
  Bilateral 0U82-
  Left 0U81-
  Right 0U80-
 Pancreas 0F8G-
 Patella
  Left 0Q8F-
  Right 0Q8D-
 Perineum, Female 0W8NXZZ
 Phalanx
  Finger
   Left 0P8V-
   Right 0P8T-
  Thumb
   Left 0P8S-
   Right 0P8R-

Division — continued
 Phalanx — continued
  Toe
   Left 0Q8R-
   Right 0Q8Q-
 Radius
  Left 0P8J-
  Right 0P8H-
 Rib
  Left 0P82-
  Right 0P81-
 Sacrum 0Q81-
 Scapula
  Left 0P86-
  Right 0P85-
 Skin
  Abdomen 0H87XZZ
  Back 0H86XZZ
  Buttock 0H88XZZ
  Chest 0H85XZZ
  Ear
   Left 0H83XZZ
   Right 0H82XZZ
  Face 0H81XZZ
  Foot
   Left 0H8NXZZ
   Right 0H8MXZZ
  Genitalia 0H8AXZZ
  Hand
   Left 0H8GXZZ
   Right 0H8FXZZ
  Lower Arm
   Left 0H8EXZZ
   Right 0H8DXZZ
  Lower Leg
   Left 0H8LXZZ
   Right 0H8KXZZ
  Neck 0H84XZZ
  Perineum 0H89XZZ
  Scalp 0H80XZZ
  Upper Arm
   Left 0H8CXZZ
   Right 0H8BXZZ
  Upper Leg
   Left 0H8JXZZ
   Right 0H8HXZZ
 Skull 0N80-
 Spinal Cord
  Cervical 008W-
  Lumbar 008Y-
  Thoracic 008X-
 Sternum 0P80-
 Stomach, Pylorus 0D87-
 Subcutaneous Tissue and Fascia
  Abdomen 0J88-
  Back 0J87-
  Buttock 0J89-
  Chest 0J86-
  Face 0J81-
  Foot
   Left 0J8R-
   Right 0J8Q-
  Hand
   Left 0J8K-
   Right 0J8J-
  Head and Neck 0J8S-
  Lower Arm
   Left 0J8H-
   Right 0J8G-
  Lower Extremity 0J8W-
  Lower Leg
   Left 0J8P-
   Right 0J8N-
  Neck
   Anterior 0J84-
   Posterior 0J85-
  Pelvic Region 0J8C-
  Perineum 0J8B-
  Scalp 0J80-

Division — continued
 Subcutaneous Tissue and Fascia — continued
  Trunk 0J8T-
  Upper Arm
   Left 0J8F-
   Right 0J8D-
  Upper Extremity 0J8V-
  Upper Leg
   Left 0J8M-
   Right 0J8L-
 Tarsal
  Left 0Q8M-
  Right 0Q8L-
 Tendon
  Abdomen
   Left 0L8G-
   Right 0L8F-
  Ankle
   Left 0L8T-
   Right 0L8S-
  Foot
   Left 0L8W-
   Right 0L8V-
  Hand
   Left 0L88-
   Right 0L87-
  Head and Neck 0L80-
  Hip
   Left 0L8K-
   Right 0L8J-
  Knee
   Left 0L8R-
   Right 0L8Q-
  Lower Arm and Wrist
   Left 0L86-
   Right 0L85-
  Lower Leg
   Left 0L8P-
   Right 0L8N-
  Perineum 0L8H-
  Shoulder
   Left 0L82-
   Right 0L81-
  Thorax
   Left 0L8D-
   Right 0L8C-
  Trunk
   Left 0L8B-
   Right 0L89-
  Upper Arm
   Left 0L84-
   Right 0L83-
  Upper Leg
   Left 0L8M-
   Right 0L8L-
 Thyroid Gland Isthmus 0G8J-
 Tibia
  Left 0Q8H-
  Right 0Q8G-
 Turbinate, Nasal 098L-
 Ulna
  Left 0P8L-
  Right 0P8K-
 Uterine Supporting Structure 0U84-
 Vertebra
  Cervical 0P83-
  Lumbar 0Q80-
  Thoracic 0P84-
Doppler study see Ultrasonography
Dorsal digital nerve
 use Nerve, Radial
Dorsal metacarpal vein
 use Vein, Hand, Left
 use Vein, Hand, Right
Dorsal metatarsal artery
 use Artery, Foot, Left
 use Artery, Foot, Right

INDEX TO PROCEDURES – 2016 ICD-10-PCS

Drainage

Dorsal metatarsal vein
 use Vein, Foot, Left
 use Vein, Foot, Right
Dorsal scapular artery
 use Artery, Subclavian, Left
 use Artery, Subclavian, Right
Dorsal scapular nerve
 use Nerve, Brachial Plexus
Dorsal venous arch
 use Vein, Foot, Left
 use Vein, Foot, Right
Dorsalis pedis artery
 use Artery, Anterior Tibial, Left
 use Artery, Anterior Tibial, Right
Drainage
 Abdominal Wall 0W9F-
 Acetabulum
  Left 0Q95-
  Right 0Q94-
 Adenoids 0C9Q-
 Ampulla of Vater 0F9C-
 Anal Sphincter 0D9R-
 Ankle Region
  Left 0Y9L-
  Right 0Y9K-
 Anterior Chamber
  Left 0893-
  Right 0892-
 Anus 0D9Q-
 Aorta, Abdominal 0490-
 Aortic Body 0G9D-
 Appendix 0D9J-
 Arm
  Lower
   Left 0X9F-
   Right 0X9D-
  Upper
   Left 0X99-
   Right 0X98-
 Artery
  Anterior Tibial
   Left 049Q-
   Right 049P-
  Axillary
   Left 0396-
   Right 0395-
  Brachial
   Left 0398-
   Right 0397-
  Celiac 0491-
  Colic
   Left 0497-
   Middle 0498-
   Right 0496-
  Common Carotid
   Left 039J-
   Right 039H-
  Common Iliac
   Left 049D-
   Right 049C-
  External Carotid
   Left 039N-
   Right 039M-
  External Iliac
   Left 049J-
   Right 049H-
  Face 039R-
  Femoral
   Left 049L-
   Right 049K-
  Foot
   Left 049W-
   Right 049V-
  Gastric 0492-
  Hand
   Left 039F-
   Right 039D-
  Hepatic 0493-
  Inferior Mesenteric 049B-

Drainage — continued
 Artery — continued
  Innominate 0392-
  Internal Carotid
   Left 039L-
   Right 039K-
  Internal Iliac
   Left 049F-
   Right 049E-
  Internal Mammary
   Left 0391-
   Right 0390-
  Intracranial 039G-
  Lower 049Y-
  Peroneal
   Left 049U-
   Right 049T-
  Popliteal
   Left 049N-
   Right 049M-
  Posterior Tibial
   Left 049S-
   Right 049R-
  Radial
   Left 039C-
   Right 039B-
  Renal
   Left 049A-
   Right 0499-
  Splenic 0494-
  Subclavian
   Left 0394-
   Right 0393-
  Superior Mesenteric 0495-
  Temporal
   Left 039T-
   Right 039S-
  Thyroid
   Left 039V-
   Right 039U-
  Ulnar
   Left 039A-
   Right 0399-
  Upper 039Y-
  Vertebral
   Left 039Q-
   Right 039P-
 Auditory Ossicle
  Left 099A-
  Right 0999-
 Axilla
  Left 0X95-
  Right 0X94-
 Back
  Lower 0W9L-
  Upper 0W9K-
 Basal Ganglia 0098-
 Bladder 0T9B-
 Bladder Neck 0T9C-
 Bone
  Ethmoid
   Left 0N9G-
   Right 0N9F-
  Frontal
   Left 0N92-
   Right 0N91-
  Hyoid 0N9X-
  Lacrimal
   Left 0N9J-
   Right 0N9H-
  Nasal 0N9B-
  Occipital
   Left 0N98-
   Right 0N97-
  Palatine
   Left 0N9L-
   Right 0N9K-
  Parietal
   Left 0N94-
   Right 0N93-

Drainage — continued
 Bone — continued
  Pelvic
   Left 0Q93-
   Right 0Q92-
  Sphenoid
   Left 0N9D-
   Right 0N9C-
  Temporal
   Left 0N96-
   Right 0N95-
  Zygomatic
   Left 0N9N-
   Right 0N9M-
 Bone Marrow 079T-
 Brain 0090-
 Breast
  Bilateral 0H9V-
  Left 0H9U-
  Right 0H9T-
 Bronchus
  Lingula 0B99-
  Lower Lobe
   Left 0B9B-
   Right 0B96-
  Main
   Left 0B97-
   Right 0B93-
  Middle Lobe, Right 0B95-
  Upper Lobe
   Left 0B98-
   Right 0B94-
 Buccal Mucosa 0C94-
 Bursa and Ligament
  Abdomen
   Left 0M9J-
   Right 0M9H-
  Ankle
   Left 0M9R-
   Right 0M9Q-
  Elbow
   Left 0M94-
   Right 0M93-
  Foot
   Left 0M9T-
   Right 0M9S-
  Hand
   Left 0M98-
   Right 0M97-
  Head and Neck 0M90-
  Hip
   Left 0M9M-
   Right 0M9L-
  Knee
   Left 0M9P-
   Right 0M9N-
  Lower Extremity
   Left 0M9W-
   Right 0M9V-
  Perineum 0M9K-
  Shoulder
   Left 0M92-
   Right 0M91-
  Thorax
   Left 0M9G-
   Right 0M9F-
  Trunk
   Left 0M9D-
   Right 0M9C-
  Upper Extremity
   Left 0M9B-
   Right 0M99-
  Wrist
   Left 0M96-
   Right 0M95-
 Buttock
  Left 0Y91-
  Right 0Y90-
 Carina 0B92-
 Carotid Bodies, Bilateral 0G98-

Drainage — continued
 Carotid Body
  Left 0G96-
  Right 0G97-
 Carpal
  Left 0P9N-
  Right 0P9M-
 Cavity, Cranial 0W91-
 Cecum 0D9H-
 Cerebellum 009C-
 Cerebral Hemisphere 0097-
 Cerebral Meninges 0091-
 Cerebral Ventricle 0096-
 Cervix 0U9C-
 Chest Wall 0W98-
 Choroid
  Left 089B-
  Right 089A-
 Cisterna Chyli 079L-
 Clavicle
  Left 0P9B-
  Right 0P99-
 Clitoris 0U9J-
 Coccygeal Glomus 0G9B-
 Coccyx 0Q9S-
 Colon
  Ascending 0D9K-
  Descending 0D9M-
  Sigmoid 0D9N-
  Transverse 0D9L-
 Conjunctiva
  Left 089T-
  Right 089S-
 Cord
  Bilateral 0V9H-
  Left 0V9G-
  Right 0V9F-
 Cornea
  Left 0899-
  Right 0898-
 Cul-de-sac 0U9F-
 Diaphragm
  Left 0B9S-
  Right 0B9R-
 Disc
  Cervical Vertebral 0R93-
  Cervicothoracic Vertebral 0R95-
  Lumbar Vertebral 0S92-
  Lumbosacral 0S94-
  Thoracic Vertebral 0R99-
  Thoracolumbar Vertebral 0R9B-
 Duct
  Common Bile 0F99-
  Cystic 0F98-
  Hepatic
   Left 0F96-
   Right 0F95-
  Lacrimal
   Left 089Y-
   Right 089X-
  Pancreatic 0F9D-
   Accessory 0F9F-
  Parotid
   Left 0C9C-
   Right 0C9B-
 Duodenum 0D99-
 Dura Mater 0092-
 Ear
  External
   Left 0991-
   Right 0990-
  External Auditory Canal
   Left 0994-
   Right 0993-
  Inner
   Left 099E-
   Right 099D-
  Middle
   Left 0996-
   Right 0995-

17

Drainage

Drainage — continued
- Elbow Region
  - Left 0X9C-
  - Right 0X9B-
- Epididymis
  - Bilateral 0V9L-
  - Left 0V9K-
  - Right 0V9J-
- Epidural Space 0093-
- Epiglottis 0C9R-
- Esophagogastric Junction 0D94-
- Esophagus 0D95-
  - Lower 0D93-
  - Middle 0D92-
  - Upper 0D91-
- Eustachian Tube
  - Left 099G-
  - Right 099F-
- Extremity
  - Lower
    - Left 0Y9B-
    - Right 0Y99-
  - Upper
    - Left 0X97-
    - Right 0X96-
- Eye
  - Left 0891-
  - Right 0890-
- Eyelid
  - Lower
    - Left 089R-
    - Right 089Q-
  - Upper
    - Left 089P-
    - Right 089N-
- Face 0W92-
- Fallopian Tube
  - Left 0U96-
  - Right 0U95-
- Fallopian Tubes, Bilateral 0U97-
- Femoral Region
  - Left 0Y98-
  - Right 0Y97-
- Femoral Shaft
  - Left 0Q99-
  - Right 0Q98-
- Femur
  - Lower
    - Left 0Q9C-
    - Right 0Q9B-
  - Upper
    - Left 0Q97-
    - Right 0Q96-
- Fibula
  - Left 0Q9K-
  - Right 0Q9J-
- Finger Nail 0H9Q-
- Foot
  - Left 0Y9N-
  - Right 0Y9M-
- Gallbladder 0F94-
- Gingiva
  - Lower 0C96-
  - Upper 0C95-
- Gland
  - Adrenal
    - Bilateral 0G94-
    - Left 0G92-
    - Right 0G93-
  - Lacrimal
    - Left 089W-
    - Right 089V-
  - Minor Salivary 0C9J-
  - Parotid
    - Left 0C99-
    - Right 0C98-
  - Pituitary 0G90-
  - Sublingual
    - Left 0C9F-
    - Right 0C9D-

Drainage — continued
- Gland — continued
  - Submaxillary
    - Left 0C9H-
    - Right 0C9G-
  - Vestibular 0U9L-
- Glenoid Cavity
  - Left 0P98-
  - Right 0P97-
- Glomus Jugulare 0G9C-
- Hand
  - Left 0X9K-
  - Right 0X9J-
- Head 0W90-
- Humeral Head
  - Left 0P9D-
  - Right 0P9C-
- Humeral Shaft
  - Left 0P9G-
  - Right 0P9F-
- Hymen 0U9K-
- Hypothalamus 009A-
- Ileocecal Valve 0D9C-
- Ileum 0D9B-
- Inguinal Region
  - Left 0Y96-
  - Right 0Y95-
- Intestine
  - Large 0D9E-
    - Left 0D9G-
    - Right 0D9F-
  - Small 0D98-
- Iris
  - Left 089D-
  - Right 089C-
- Jaw
  - Lower 0W95-
  - Upper 0W94-
- Jejunum 0D9A-
- Joint
  - Acromioclavicular
    - Left 0R9H-
    - Right 0R9G-
  - Ankle
    - Left 0S9G-
    - Right 0S9F-
  - Carpal
    - Left 0R9R-
    - Right 0R9Q-
  - Cervical Vertebral 0R91-
  - Cervicothoracic Vertebral 0R94-
  - Coccygeal 0S96-
  - Elbow
    - Left 0R9M-
    - Right 0R9L-
  - Finger Phalangeal
    - Left 0R9X-
    - Right 0R9W-
  - Hip
    - Left 0S9B-
    - Right 0S99-
  - Knee
    - Left 0S9D-
    - Right 0S9C-
  - Lumbar Vertebral 0S90-
  - Lumbosacral 0S93-
  - Metacarpocarpal
    - Left 0R9T-
    - Right 0R9S-
  - Metacarpophalangeal
    - Left 0R9V-
    - Right 0R9U-
  - Metatarsal-Phalangeal
    - Left 0S9N-
    - Right 0S9M-
  - Metatarsal-Tarsal
    - Left 0S9L-
    - Right 0S9K-
  - Occipital-cervical 0R90-
  - Sacrococcygeal 0S95-

Drainage — continued
- Joint — continued
  - Sacroiliac
    - Left 0S98-
    - Right 0S97-
  - Shoulder
    - Left 0R9K-
    - Right 0R9J-
  - Sternoclavicular
    - Left 0R9F-
    - Right 0R9E-
  - Tarsal
    - Left 0S9J-
    - Right 0S9H-
  - Temporomandibular
    - Left 0R9D-
    - Right 0R9C-
  - Thoracic Vertebral 0R96-
  - Thoracolumbar Vertebral 0R9A-
  - Toe Phalangeal
    - Left 0S9Q-
    - Right 0S9P-
  - Wrist
    - Left 0R9P-
    - Right 0R9N-
- Kidney
  - Left 0T91-
  - Right 0T90-
- Kidney Pelvis
  - Left 0T94-
  - Right 0T93-
- Knee Region
  - Left 0Y9G-
  - Right 0Y9F-
- Larynx 0C9S-
- Leg
  - Lower
    - Left 0Y9J-
    - Right 0Y9H-
  - Upper
    - Left 0Y9D-
    - Right 0Y9C-
- Lens
  - Left 089K-
  - Right 089J-
- Lip
  - Lower 0C91-
  - Upper 0C90-
- Liver 0F90-
  - Left Lobe 0F92-
  - Right Lobe 0F91-
- Lung
  - Bilateral 0B9M-
  - Left 0B9L-
  - Lower Lobe
    - Left 0B9J-
    - Right 0B9F-
  - Middle Lobe, Right 0B9D-
  - Right 0B9K-
  - Upper Lobe
    - Left 0B9G-
    - Right 0B9C-
- Lung Lingula 0B9H-
- Lymphatic
  - Aortic 079D-
  - Axillary
    - Left 0796-
    - Right 0795-
  - Head 0790-
  - Inguinal
    - Left 079J-
    - Right 079H-
  - Internal Mammary
    - Left 0799-
    - Right 0798-
  - Lower Extremity
    - Left 079G-
    - Right 079F-
  - Mesenteric 079B-

Drainage — continued
- Lymphatic — continued
  - Neck
    - Left 0792-
    - Right 0791-
  - Pelvis 079C-
  - Thoracic Duct 079K-
  - Thorax 0797-
  - Upper Extremity
    - Left 0794-
    - Right 0793-
- Mandible
  - Left 0N9V-
  - Right 0N9T-
- Maxilla
  - Left 0N9S-
  - Right 0N9R-
- Mediastinum 0W9C-
- Medulla Oblongata 009D-
- Mesentery 0D9V-
- Metacarpal
  - Left 0P9Q-
  - Right 0P9P-
- Metatarsal
  - Left 0Q9P-
  - Right 0Q9N-
- Muscle
  - Abdomen
    - Left 0K9L-
    - Right 0K9K-
  - Extraocular
    - Left 089M-
    - Right 089L-
  - Facial 0K91-
  - Foot
    - Left 0K9W-
    - Right 0K9V-
  - Hand
    - Left 0K9D-
    - Right 0K9C-
  - Head 0K90-
  - Hip
    - Left 0K9P-
    - Right 0K9N-
  - Lower Arm and Wrist
    - Left 0K9B-
    - Right 0K99-
  - Lower Leg
    - Left 0K9T-
    - Right 0K9S-
  - Neck
    - Left 0K93-
    - Right 0K92-
  - Perineum 0K9M-
  - Shoulder
    - Left 0K96-
    - Right 0K95-
  - Thorax
    - Left 0K9J-
    - Right 0K9H-
  - Tongue, Palate, Pharynx 0K94-
  - Trunk
    - Left 0K9G-
    - Right 0K9F-
  - Upper Arm
    - Left 0K98-
    - Right 0K97-
  - Upper Leg
    - Left 0K9R-
    - Right 0K9Q-
- Nasopharynx 099N-
- Neck 0W96-
- Nerve
  - Abdominal Sympathetic 019M-
  - Abducens 009L-
  - Accessory 009R-
  - Acoustic 009A-
  - Brachial Plexus 0193-
  - Cervical 0191-
  - Cervical Plexus 0190-

INDEX TO PROCEDURES – 2016 ICD-10-PCS

Drainage

Drainage — continued
Nerve — continued
- Facial 009M-
- Femoral 019D-
- Glossopharyngeal 009P-
- Head and Neck Sympathetic 019K-
- Hypoglossal 009S-
- Lumbar 019B-
- Lumbar Plexus 0199-
- Lumbar Sympathetic 019N-
- Lumbosacral Plexus 019A-
- Median 0195-
- Oculomotor 009H-
- Olfactory 009F-
- Optic 009G-
- Peroneal 019H-
- Phrenic 0192-
- Pudendal 019C-
- Radial 0196-
- Sacral 019R-
- Sacral Plexus 019Q-
- Sacral Sympathetic 019P-
- Sciatic 019F-
- Thoracic 0198-
- Thoracic Sympathetic 019L-
- Tibial 019G-
- Trigeminal 009K-
- Trochlear 009J-
- Ulnar 0194-
- Vagus 009Q-

Nipple
- Left 0H9X-
- Right 0H9W-

Nose 099K-

Omentum
- Greater 0D9S-
- Lesser 0D9T-

Oral Cavity and Throat 0W93-

Orbit
- Left 0N9Q-
- Right 0N9P-

Ovary
- Bilateral 0U92-
- Left 0U91-
- Right 0U90-

Palate
- Hard 0C92-
- Soft 0C93-

Pancreas 0F9G-

Para-aortic Body 0G99-

Paraganglion Extremity 0G9F-

Parathyroid Gland 0G9R-
- Inferior
  - Left 0G9P-
  - Right 0G9N-
- Multiple 0G9Q-
- Superior
  - Left 0G9M-
  - Right 0G9L-

Patella
- Left 0Q9F-
- Right 0Q9D-

Pelvic Cavity 0W9J-

Penis 0V9S-

Pericardial Cavity 0W9D-

Perineum
- Female 0W9N-
- Male 0W9M-

Peritoneal Cavity 0W9G-

Peritoneum 0D9W-

Phalanx
- Finger
  - Left 0P9V-
  - Right 0P9T-
- Thumb
  - Left 0P9S-
  - Right 0P9R-
- Toe
  - Left 0Q9R-
  - Right 0Q9Q-

Drainage — continued
Pharynx 0C9M-
Pineal Body 0G91-
Pleura
- Left 0B9P-
- Right 0B9N-

Pleural Cavity
- Left 0W9B-
- Right 0W99-

Pons 009B-
Prepuce 0V9T-

Products of Conception
- Amniotic Fluid
  - Diagnostic 1090-
  - Therapeutic 1090-
- Fetal Blood 1090-
- Fetal Cerebrospinal Fluid 1090-
- Fetal Fluid, Other 1090-
- Fluid, Other 1090-

Prostate 0V90-

Radius
- Left 0P9J-
- Right 0P9H-

Rectum 0D9P-

Retina
- Left 089F-
- Right 089E-

Retinal Vessel
- Left 089H-
- Right 089G-

Retroperitoneum 0W9H-

Rib
- Left 0P92-
- Right 0P91-

Sacrum 0Q91-

Scapula
- Left 0P96-
- Right 0P95-

Sclera
- Left 0897-
- Right 0896-

Scrotum 0V95-

Septum, Nasal 099M-

Shoulder Region
- Left 0X93-
- Right 0X92-

Sinus
- Accessory 099P-
- Ethmoid
  - Left 099V-
  - Right 099U-
- Frontal
  - Left 099T-
  - Right 099S-
- Mastoid
  - Left 099F-
  - Right 099B-
- Maxillary
  - Left 099R-
  - Right 099Q-
- Sphenoid
  - Left 099X-
  - Right 099W-

Skin
- Abdomen 0H97-
- Back 0H96-
- Buttock 0H98-
- Chest 0H95-
- Ear
  - Left 0H93-
  - Right 0H92-
- Face 0H91-
- Foot
  - Left 0H9N-
  - Right 0H9M-
- Genitalia 0H9A-
- Hand
  - Left 0H9G-
  - Right 0H9F-

Drainage — continued
Skin — continued
- Lower Arm
  - Left 0H9E-
  - Right 0H9D-
- Lower Leg
  - Left 0H9L-
  - Right 0H9K-
- Neck 0H94-
- Perineum 0H99-
- Scalp 0H90-
- Upper Arm
  - Left 0H9C-
  - Right 0H9B-
- Upper Leg
  - Left 0H9J-
  - Right 0H9H-

Skull 0N90-
Spinal Canal 009U-

Spinal Cord
- Cervical 009W-
- Lumbar 009Y-
- Thoracic 009X-

Spinal Meninges 009T-
Spleen 079P-
Sternum 0P90-
Stomach 0D96-
- Pylorus 0D97-

Subarachnoid Space 0095-

Subcutaneous Tissue and Fascia
- Abdomen 0J98-
- Back 0J97-
- Buttock 0J99-
- Chest 0J96-
- Face 0J91-
- Foot
  - Left 0J9R-
  - Right 0J9Q-
- Hand
  - Left 0J9K-
  - Right 0J9J-
- Lower Arm
  - Left 0J9H-
  - Right 0J9G-
- Lower Leg
  - Left 0J9P-
  - Right 0J9N-
- Neck
  - Anterior 0J94-
  - Posterior 0J95-
- Pelvic Region 0J9C-
- Perineum 0J9B-
- Scalp 0J90-
- Upper Arm
  - Left 0J9F-
  - Right 0J9D-
- Upper Leg
  - Left 0J9M-
  - Right 0J9L-

Subdural Space 0094-

Tarsal
- Left 0Q9M-
- Right 0Q9L-

Tendon
- Abdomen
  - Left 0L9G-
  - Right 0L9F-
- Ankle
  - Left 0L9T-
  - Right 0L9S-
- Foot
  - Left 0L9W-
  - Right 0L9V-
- Hand
  - Left 0L98-
  - Right 0L97-
- Head and Neck 0L90-
- Hip
  - Left 0L9K-
  - Right 0L9J-

Drainage — continued
Tendon — continued
- Knee
  - Left 0L9R-
  - Right 0L9Q-
- Lower Arm and Wrist
  - Left 0L96-
  - Right 0L95-
- Lower Leg
  - Left 0L9P-
  - Right 0L9N-
- Perineum 0L9H-
- Shoulder
  - Left 0L92-
  - Right 0L91-
- Thorax
  - Left 0L9D-
  - Right 0L9C-
- Trunk
  - Left 0L9B-
  - Right 0L99-
- Upper Arm
  - Left 0L94-
  - Right 0L93-
- Upper Leg
  - Left 0L9M-
  - Right 0L9L-

Testis
- Bilateral 0V9C-
- Left 0V9B-
- Right 0V99-

Thalamus 0099-
Thymus 079M-

Thyroid Gland 0G9K-
- Left Lobe 0G9G-
- Right Lobe 0G9H-

Tibia
- Left 0Q9H-
- Right 0Q9G-

Toe Nail 0H9R-
Tongue 0C97-
Tonsils 0C9P-

Tooth
- Lower 0C9X-
- Upper 0C9W-

Trachea 0B91-

Tunica Vaginalis
- Left 0V97-
- Right 0V96-

Turbinate, Nasal 099L-

Tympanic Membrane
- Left 0998-
- Right 0997-

Ulna
- Left 0P9L-
- Right 0P9K-

Ureter
- Left 0T97-
- Right 0T96-

Ureters, Bilateral 0T98-
Urethra 0T9D-
Uterine Supporting Structure 0U94-
Uterus 0U99-
Uvula 0C9N-
Vagina 0U9G-

Vas Deferens
- Bilateral 0V9Q-
- Left 0V9P-
- Right 0V9N-

Vein
- Axillary
  - Left 0598-
  - Right 0597-
- Azygos 0590-
- Basilic
  - Left 059C-
  - Right 059B-
- Brachial
  - Left 059A-
  - Right 0599-

Drainage

Drainage — continued
Vein — continued
Cephalic
Left **059F-**
Right **059D-**
Colic **0697-**
Common Iliac
Left **069D-**
Right **069C-**
Esophageal **0693-**
External Iliac
Left **069G-**
Right **069F-**
External Jugular
Left **059Q-**
Right **059P-**
Face
Left **059V-**
Right **059T-**
Femoral
Left **069N-**
Right **069M-**
Foot
Left **069V-**
Right **069T-**
Gastric **0692-**
Greater Saphenous
Left **069Q-**
Right **069P-**
Hand
Left **059H-**
Right **059G-**
Hemiazygos **0591-**
Hepatic **0694-**
Hypogastric
Left **069J-**
Right **069H-**
Inferior Mesenteric **0696-**
Innominate
Left **0594-**
Right **0593-**
Internal Jugular
Left **059N-**
Right **059M-**
Intracranial **059L-**
Lesser Saphenous
Left **069S-**
Right **069R-**
Lower **069Y-**
Portal **0698-**
Renal
Left **069B-**
Right **0699-**
Splenic **0691-**
Subclavian
Left **0596-**
Right **0595-**
Superior Mesenteric **0695-**
Upper **059Y-**
Vertebral
Left **059S-**
Right **059R-**
Vena Cava, Inferior **0690-**
Vertebra
Cervical **0P93-**
Lumbar **0Q90-**
Thoracic **0P94-**
Vesicle
Bilateral **0V93-**
Left **0V92-**
Right **0V91-**
Vitreous
Left **0895-**
Right **0894-**
Vocal Cord
Left **0C9V-**
Right **0C9T-**
Vulva **0U9M-**
Wrist Region
Left **0X9H-**
Right **0X9G-**

Dressing
Abdominal Wall **2W23X4Z**
Arm
Lower
Left **2W2DX4Z**
Right **2W2CX4Z**
Upper
Left **2W2BX4Z**
Right **2W2AX4Z**
Back **2W25X4Z**
Chest Wall **2W24X4Z**
Extremity
Lower
Left **2W2MX4Z**
Right **2W2LX4Z**
Upper
Left **2W29X4Z**
Right **2W28X4Z**
Face **2W21X4Z**
Finger
Left **2W2KX4Z**
Right **2W2JX4Z**
Foot
Left **2W2TX4Z**
Right **2W2SX4Z**
Hand
Left **2W2FX4Z**
Right **2W2EX4Z**
Head **2W20X4Z**
Inguinal Region
Left **2W27X4Z**
Right **2W26X4Z**
Leg
Lower
Left **2W2RX4Z**
Right **2W2QX4Z**
Upper
Left **2W2PX4Z**
Right **2W2NX4Z**
Neck **2W22X4Z**
Thumb
Left **2W2HX4Z**
Right **2W2GX4Z**
Toe
Left **2W2VX4Z**
Right **2W2UX4Z**
Driver stent (RX) (OTW)
  use Intraluminal Device
Drotrecogin alfa *see* Introduction of Recombinant Human-activated Protein C
Duct of Santorini
  use Duct, Pancreatic, Accessory
Duct of Wirsung
  use Duct, Pancreatic
Ductogram, mammary *see* Plain Radiography, Skin, Subcutaneous Tissue and Breast **BH0-**
Ductography, mammary *see* Plain Radiography, Skin, Subcutaneous Tissue and Breast **BH0-**
Ductus deferens
  use Vas Deferens
  use Vas Deferens, Bilateral
  use Vas Deferens, Left
  use Vas Deferens, Right
Duodenal ampulla
  use Ampulla of Vater
Duodenectomy
  see Excision, Duodenum **0DB9-**
  see Resection, Duodenum **0DT9-**
Duodenocholedochotomy *see* Drainage, Gallbladder **0F94-**
Duodenocystostomy
  see Bypass, Gallbladder **0F14-**
  see Drainage, Gallbladder **0F94-**
Duodenoenterostomy
  see Bypass, Gastrointestinal System **0D1-**
  see Drainage, Gastrointestinal System **0D9-**

Duodenojejunal flexure
  use Jejunum
Duodenolysis *see* Release, Duodenum **0DN9-**
Duodenorrhaphy *see* Repair, Duodenum **0DQ9-**
Duodenostomy
  see Bypass, Duodenum **0D19-**
  see Drainage, Duodenum **0D99-**
Duodenotomy *see* Drainage, Duodenum **0D99-**
Dura mater, intracranial
  use Dura Mater
Dura mater, spinal
  use Spinal Meninges
DuraHeart Left Ventricular Assist System
  use Implantable Heart Assist System in Heart and Great Vessels
Dural venous sinus
  use Vein, Intracranial
Durata® Defibrillation Lead
  use Cardiac Lead, Defibrillator in **02H-**
Dynesys® Dynamic Stabilization System
  use Spinal Stabilization Device, Pedicle-Based in **0RH-**
  use Spinal Stabilization Device, Pedicle-Based in **0SH-**

E

E-Luminexx™ (Biliary) (Vascular) Stent
  use Intraluminal Device
Earlobe
  use Ear, External, Bilateral
  use Ear, External, Left
  use Ear, External, Right
Echocardiogram *see* Ultrasonography, Heart **B24-**
Echography *see* Ultrasonography
ECMO *see* Performance, Circulatory **5A15-**
EEG (electroencephalogram) *see* Measurement, Central Nervous **4A00-**
EGD (esophagogastroduodenoscopy) 0DJ08ZZ
Eighth cranial nerve
  use Nerve, Acoustic
Ejaculatory duct
  use Vas Deferens
  use Vas Deferens, Bilateral
  use Vas Deferens, Left
  use Vas Deferens, Right
EKG (electrocardiogram) *see* Measurement, Cardiac **4A02-**
Electrical bone growth stimulator (EBGS)
  use Bone Growth Stimulator in Head and Facial Bones
  use Bone Growth Stimulator in Lower Bones
  use Bone Growth Stimulator in Upper Bones
Electrical muscle stimulation (EMS) lead
  use Stimulator Lead in Muscles
Electrocautery
  Destruction *see* Destruction
  Repair *see* Repair
Electroconvulsive Therapy
  Bilateral-Multiple Seizure **GZB3ZZZ**
  Bilateral-Single Seizure **GZB2ZZZ**
  Electroconvulsive Therapy, Other **GZB4ZZZ**
  Unilateral-Multiple Seizure **GZB1ZZZ**
  Unilateral-Single Seizure **GZB0ZZZ**
Electroencephalogram (EEG) *see* Measurement, Central Nervous **4A00-**
Electromagnetic Therapy
  Central Nervous **6A22-**
  Urinary **6A21-**
Electronic muscle stimulator lead
  use Stimulator Lead in Muscles
Electrophysiologic stimulation (EPS) *see* Measurement, Cardiac **4A02-**
Electroshock therapy *see* Electroconvulsive Therapy
Elevation, bone fragments, skull *see* Reposition, Head and Facial Bones **0NS-**
Eleventh cranial nerve
  use Nerve, Accessory
E-Luminexx™ (Biliary) (Vascular) Stent
  use Intraluminal Device
Embolectomy *see* Extirpation
Embolization
  see Occlusion
  see Restriction
Embolization coil(s)
  use Intraluminal Device
EMG (electromyogram) *see* Measurement, Musculoskeletal **4A0F-**
Encephalon
  use Brain

INDEX TO PROCEDURES – 2016 ICD-10-PCS

Endarterectomy
 see Extirpation, Lower Arteries 04C-
 see Extirpation, Upper Arteries 03C-
Endeavor® (III) (IV) (Sprint) Zotarolimus-eluting Coronary Stent System
 use Intraluminal Device, Drug-eluting in Heart and Great Vessels
EndoSure® sensor
 use Monitoring Device, Pressure Sensor in 02H-
ENDOTAK RELIANCE® (G) Defibrillation Lead
 use Cardiac Lead, Defibrillator in 02H-
Endotracheal tube (cuffed) (double-lumen)
 use Intraluminal Device, Endotracheal Airway in Respiratory System
Endurant® Endovascular Stent Graft
 use Intraluminal Device
Enlargement
 see Dilation
 see Repair
EnRhythm
 use Pacemaker, Dual Chamber 0JH-
Enterorrhaphy see Repair, Gastrointestinal System 0DQ-
Enterra gastric neurostimulator
 use Stimulator Generator, Multiple Array in 0JH-
Enucleation
 Eyeball see Resection, Eye 08T-
 Eyeball with prosthetic implant see Replacement, Eye 08R-
Ependyma
 use Cerebral Ventricle
Epicel® cultured epidermal autograft
 use Autologous Tissue Substitute
Epic™ Stented Tissue Valve (aortic)
 use Zooplastic Tissue in Heart and Great Vessels
Epidermis
 use Skin
Epididymectomy
 see Excision, Male Reproductive System 0VB-
 see Resection, Male Reproductive System 0VT-
Epididymoplasty
 see Repair, Male Reproductive System 0VQ-
 see Supplement, Male Reproductive System 0VU-
Epididymorrhaphy see Repair, Male Reproductive System 0VQ-
Epididymotomy see Drainage, Male Reproductive System 0V9-
Epidural space, intracranial
 use Epidural Space
Epidural space, spinal
 use Spinal Canal
Epiphysiodesis
 see Fusion, Lower Joints 0SG-
 see Fusion, Upper Joints 0RG-
Epiploic foramen
 use Peritoneum
Epiretinal Visual Prosthesis
 Left 08H105Z
 Right 08H005Z
Episiorrhaphy see Repair, Perineum, Female 0WQN-
Episiotomy see Division, Perineum, Female 0W8N-
Epithalamus
 use Thalamus
Epitrochlear lymph node
 use Lymphatic, Upper Extremity, Left
 use Lymphatic, Upper Extremity, Right

EPS (electrophysiologic stimulation) see Measurement, Cardiac 4A02-
Eptifibatide, infusion see Introduction of Platelet Inhibitor
ERCP (endoscopic retrograde cholangiopancreatography) see Fluoroscopy, Hepatobiliary System and Pancreas BF1-
Erector spinae muscle
 use Muscle, Trunk, Left
 use Muscle, Trunk, Right
Esophageal artery
 use Aorta, Thoracic
Esophageal obturator airway (EOA)
 use Intraluminal Device, Airway in Gastrointestinal System
Esophageal plexus
 use Nerve, Thoracic Sympathetic
Esophagectomy
 see Excision, Gastrointestinal System 0DB-
 see Resection, Gastrointestinal System 0DT-
Esophagocoloplasty
 see Repair, Gastrointestinal System 0DQ-
 see Supplement, Gastrointestinal System 0DU-
Esophagoenterostomy
 see Bypass, Gastrointestinal System 0D1-
 see Drainage, Gastrointestinal System 0D9-
Esophagoesophagostomy
 see Bypass, Gastrointestinal System 0D1-
 see Drainage, Gastrointestinal System 0D9-
Esophagogastrectomy
 see Excision, Gastrointestinal System 0DB-
 see Resection, Gastrointestinal System 0DT-
Esophagogastroduodenscopy (EGD) 0DJ08ZZ
Esophagogastroplasty
 see Repair, Gastrointestinal System 0DQ-
 see Supplement, Gastrointestinal System 0DU-
Esophagogastroscopy 0DJ68ZZ
Esophagogastrostomy
 see Bypass, Gastrointestinal System 0D1-
 see Drainage, Gastrointestinal System 0D9-
Esophagojejunoplasty see Supplement, Gastrointestinal System 0DU-
Esophagojejunostomy
 see Bypass, Gastrointestinal System 0D1-
 see Drainage, Gastrointestinal System 0D9-
Esophagomyotomy see Division, Esophagogastric Junction 0D84-
Esophagoplasty
 see Repair, Gastrointestinal System 0DQ-
 see Replacement, Esophagus 0DR5-
 see Supplement, Gastrointestinal System 0DU-
Esophagoplication see Restriction, Gastrointestinal System 0DV-
Esophagorrhaphy see Repair, Gastrointestinal System 0DQ-
Esophagoscopy 0DJ08ZZ
Esophagotomy see Drainage, Gastrointestinal System 0D9-

Esteem® implantable hearing system
 use Hearing Device in Ear, Nose, Sinus
ESWL (extracorporeal shock wave lithotripsy) see Fragmentation
Ethmoidal air cell
 use Sinus, Ethmoid, Left
 use Sinus, Ethmoid, Right
Ethmoidectomy
 see Excision, Ear, Nose, Sinus 09B-
 see Excision, Head and Facial Bones 0NB-
 see Resection, Ear, Nose, Sinus 09T-
 see Resection, Head and Facial Bones 0NT-
Ethmoidotomy see Drainage, Ear, Nose, Sinus 099-
Evacuation
 Hematoma see Extirpation
 Other Fluid see Drainage
Evera (XT) (S) (DR/VR)
 use Defibrillator Generator in 0JH-
Everolimus-eluting coronary stent
 use Intraluminal Device, Drug-eluting in Heart and Great Vessels
Evisceration
 Eyeball see Resection, Eye 08T-
 Eyeball with prosthetic implant see Replacement, Eye 08R-
Ex-PRESS™ mini glaucoma shunt
 use Synthetic Substitute
Examination see Inspection
Exchange see Change device in
Excision
 Abdominal Wall 0WBF-
 Acetabulum
  Left 0QB5-
  Right 0QB4-
 Adenoids 0CBQ-
 Ampulla of Vater 0FBC-
 Anal Sphincter 0DBR-
 Ankle Region
  Left 0YBL-
  Right 0YBK-
 Anus 0DBQ-
 Aorta
  Abdominal 04B0-
  Thoracic 02BW-
 Aortic Body 0GBD-
 Appendix 0DBJ-
 Arm
  Lower
   Left 0XBF-
   Right 0XBD-
  Upper
   Left 0XB9-
   Right 0XB8-
 Artery
  Anterior Tibial
   Left 04BQ-
   Right 04BP-
  Axillary
   Left 03B6-
   Right 03B5-
  Brachial
   Left 03B8-
   Right 03B7-
  Celiac 04B1-
  Colic
   Left 04B7-
   Middle 04B8-
   Right 04B6-
  Common Carotid
   Left 03BJ-
   Right 03BH
  Common Iliac
   Left 04BD-
   Right 04BC-
  External Carotid
   Left 03BN-
   Right 03BM-

Excision — *continued*
 Artery — *continued*
  External Iliac
   Left 04BJ-
   Right 04BH-
  Face 03BR-
  Femoral
   Left 04BL-
   Right 04BK-
  Foot
   Left 04BW-
   Right 04BV-
  Gastric 04B2-
  Hand
   Left 03BF-
   Right 03BD-
  Hepatic 04B3-
  Inferior Mesenteric 04BB-
  Innominate 03B2-
  Internal Carotid
   Left 03BL-
   Right 03BK-
  Internal Iliac
   Left 04BF-
   Right 04BE-
  Internal Mammary
   Left 03B1-
   Right 03B0-
  Intracranial 03BG-
  Lower 04BY-
  Peroneal
   Left 04BU-
   Right 04BT-
  Popliteal
   Left 04BN-
   Right 04BM-
  Posterior Tibial
   Left 04BS-
   Right 04BR-
  Pulmonary
   Left 02BR-
   Right 02BQ-
  Pulmonary Trunk 02BP-
  Radial
   Left 03BC-
   Right 03BB-
  Renal
   Left 04BA-
   Right 04B9-
  Splenic 04B4-
  Subclavian
   Left 03B4-
   Right 03B3-
  Superior Mesenteric 04B5-
  Temporal
   Left 03BT-
   Right 03BS-
  Thyroid
   Left 03BV-
   Right 03BU-
  Ulnar
   Left 03BA-
   Right 03B9-
  Upper 03BY-
  Vertebral
   Left 03BQ-
   Right 03BP-
 Atrium
  Left 02B7-
  Right 02B6-
 Auditory Ossicle
  Left 09BA0Z-
  Right 09B90Z-
 Axilla
  Left 0XB5-
  Right 0XB4-
 Back
  Lower 0WBL-
  Upper 0WBK-
 Basal Ganglia 00B8-
 Bladder 0TBB-
 Bladder Neck 0TBC-

Excision — continued
- Bone
  - Ethmoid
    - Left 0NBG-
    - Right 0NBF-
  - Frontal
    - Left 0NB2-
    - Right 0NB1-
  - Hyoid 0NBX-
  - Lacrimal
    - Left 0NBJ-
    - Right 0NBH-
  - Nasal 0NBB-
  - Occipital
    - Left 0NB8-
    - Right 0NB7-
  - Palatine
    - Left 0NBL-
    - Right 0NBK-
  - Parietal
    - Left 0NB4-
    - Right 0NB3-
  - Pelvic
    - Left 0QB3-
    - Right 0QB2-
  - Sphenoid
    - Left 0NBD-
    - Right 0NBC-
  - Temporal
    - Left 0NB6-
    - Right 0NB5-
  - Zygomatic
    - Left 0NBN-
    - Right 0NBM-
- Brain 00B0-
- Breast
  - Bilateral 0HBV-
  - Left 0HBU-
  - Right 0HBT-
  - Supernumerary 0HBY-
- Bronchus
  - Lingula 0BB9-
  - Lower Lobe
    - Left 0BBB-
    - Right 0BB6-
  - Main
    - Left 0BB7-
    - Right 0BB3-
  - Middle Lobe, Right 0BB5-
  - Upper Lobe
    - Left 0BB8-
    - Right 0BB4-
- Buccal Mucosa 0CB4-
- Bursa and Ligament
  - Abdomen
    - Left 0MBJ-
    - Right 0MBH-
  - Ankle
    - Left 0MBR-
    - Right 0MBQ-
  - Elbow
    - Left 0MB4-
    - Right 0MB3-
  - Foot
    - Left 0MBT-
    - Right 0MBS-
  - Hand
    - Left 0MB8-
    - Right 0MB7-
  - Head and Neck 0MB0-
  - Hip
    - Left 0MBM-
    - Right 0MBL-
  - Knee
    - Left 0MBP-
    - Right 0MBN-
  - Lower Extremity
    - Left 0MBW-
    - Right 0MBV-
  - Perineum 0MBK-

Excision — continued
- Bursa and Ligament — continued
  - Shoulder
    - Left 0MB2-
    - Right 0MB1-
  - Thorax
    - Left 0MBG-
    - Right 0MBF-
  - Trunk
    - Left 0MBD-
    - Right 0MBC-
  - Upper Extremity
    - Left 0MBB-
    - Right 0MB9-
  - Wrist
    - Left 0MB6-
    - Right 0MB5-
- Buttock
  - Left 0YB1-
  - Right 0YB0-
- Carina 0BB2-
- Carotid Bodies, Bilateral 0GB8-
- Carotid Body
  - Left 0GB6-
  - Right 0GB7-
- Carpal
  - Left 0PBN-
  - Right 0PBM-
- Cecum 0DBH-
- Cerebellum 00BC-
- Cerebral Hemisphere 00B7-
- Cerebral Meninges 00B1-
- Cerebral Ventricle 00B6-
- Cervix 0UBC-
- Chest Wall 0WB8-
- Chordae Tendineae 02B9-
- Choroid
  - Left 08BB-
  - Right 08BA-
- Cisterna Chyli 07BL-
- Clavicle
  - Left 0PBB-
  - Right 0PB9-
- Clitoris 0UBJ-
- Coccygeal Glomus 0GBB-
- Coccyx 0QBS-
- Colon
  - Ascending 0DBK-
  - Descending 0DBM-
  - Sigmoid 0DBN-
  - Transverse 0DBL-
- Conduction Mechanism 02B8-
- Conjunctiva
  - Left 08BTXZ-
  - Right 08BSXZ-
- Cord
  - Bilateral 0VBH-
  - Left 0VBG-
  - Right 0VBF-
- Cornea
  - Left 08B9XZ-
  - Right 08B8XZ-
- Cul-de-sac 0UBF-
- Diaphragm
  - Left 0BBS-
  - Right 0BBR-
- Disc
  - Cervical Vertebral 0RB3-
  - Cervicothoracic Vertebral 0RB5-
  - Lumbar Vertebral 0SB2-
  - Lumbosacral 0SB4-
  - Thoracic Vertebral 0RB9-
  - Thoracolumbar Vertebral 0RBB-
- Duct
  - Common Bile 0FB9-
  - Cystic 0FB8-
  - Hepatic
    - Left 0FB6-
    - Right 0FB5-
  - Lacrimal
    - Left 08BY-
    - Right 08BX-

Excision — continued
- Duct — continued
  - Pancreatic 0FBD-
    - Accessory 0FBF-
  - Parotid
    - Left 0CBC-
    - Right 0CBB-
- Duodenum 0DB9-
- Dura Mater 00B2-
- Ear
  - External
    - Left 09B1-
    - Right 09B0-
  - External Auditory Canal
    - Left 09B4-
    - Right 09B3-
  - Inner
    - Left 09BE0Z-
    - Right 09BD0Z-
  - Middle
    - Left 09B60Z-
    - Right 09B50Z-
- Elbow Region
  - Left 0XBC-
  - Right 0XBB-
- Epididymis
  - Bilateral 0VBL-
  - Left 0VBK-
  - Right 0VBJ-
- Epiglottis 0CBR-
- Esophagogastric Junction 0DB4-
- Esophagus 0DB5-
  - Lower 0DB3-
  - Middle 0DB2-
  - Upper 0DB1-
- Eustachian Tube
  - Left 09BG-
  - Right 09BF-
- Extremity
  - Lower
    - Left 0YBB-
    - Right 0YB9-
  - Upper
    - Left 0XB7-
    - Right 0XB6-
- Eye
  - Left 08B1-
  - Right 08B0-
- Eyelid
  - Lower
    - Left 08BR-
    - Right 08BQ-
  - Upper
    - Left 08BP-
    - Right 08BN-
- Face 0WB2-
- Fallopian Tube
  - Left 0UB6-
  - Right 0UB5-
- Fallopian Tubes, Bilateral 0UB7-
- Femoral Region
  - Left 0YB8-
  - Right 0YB7-
- Femoral Shaft
  - Left 0QB9-
  - Right 0QB8-
- Femur
  - Lower
    - Left 0QBC-
    - Right 0QBB-
  - Upper
    - Left 0QB7-
    - Right 0QB6-
- Fibula
  - Left 0QBK-
  - Right 0QBJ-
- Finger Nail 0HBQXZ-
- Foot
  - Left 0YBN-
  - Right 0YBM-
- Gallbladder 0FB4-

Excision — continued
- Gingiva
  - Lower 0CB6-
  - Upper 0CB5-
- Gland
  - Adrenal
    - Bilateral 0GB4-
    - Left 0GB2-
    - Right 0GB3-
  - Lacrimal
    - Left 08BW-
    - Right 08BV-
  - Minor Salivary 0CBJ-
  - Parotid
    - Left 0CB9-
    - Right 0CB8-
  - Pituitary 0GB0-
  - Sublingual
    - Left 0CBF-
    - Right 0CBD-
  - Submaxillary
    - Left 0CBH-
    - Right 0CBG-
  - Vestibular 0UBL-
- Glenoid Cavity
  - Left 0PB8-
  - Right 0PB7-
- Glomus Jugulare 0GBC-
- Hand
  - Left 0XBK-
  - Right 0XBJ-
- Head 0WB0-
- Humeral Head
  - Left 0PBD-
  - Right 0PBC-
- Humeral Shaft
  - Left 0PBG-
  - Right 0PBF-
- Hymen 0UBK-
- Hypothalamus 00BA-
- Ileocecal Valve 0DBC-
- Ileum 0DBB-
- Inguinal Region
  - Left 0YB6-
  - Right 0YB5-
- Intestine
  - Large 0DBE-
    - Left 0DBG-
    - Right 0DBF-
  - Small 0DB8-
- Iris
  - Left 08BD3Z-
  - Right 08BC3Z-
- Jaw
  - Lower 0WB5-
  - Upper 0WB4-
- Jejunum 0DBA-
- Joint
  - Acromioclavicular
    - Left 0RBH-
    - Right 0RBG-
  - Ankle
    - Left 0SBG-
    - Right 0SBF-
  - Carpal
    - Left 0RBR-
    - Right 0RBQ-
  - Cervical Vertebral 0RB1-
  - Cervicothoracic Vertebral 0RB4-
  - Coccygeal 0SB6-
  - Elbow
    - Left 0RBM-
    - Right 0RBL-
  - Finger Phalangeal
    - Left 0RBX-
    - Right 0RBW-
  - Hip
    - Left 0SBB-
    - Right 0SB9-
  - Knee
    - Left 0SBD-
    - Right 0SBC-

INDEX TO PROCEDURES – 2016 ICD-10-PCS

Excision

Excision — *continued*
Joint — *continued*
  Lumbar Vertebral 0SB0-
  Lumbosacral 0SB3-
  Metacarpocarpal
    Left 0RBT-
    Right 0RBS-
  Metacarpophalangeal
    Left 0RBV-
    Right 0RBU-
  Metatarsal-Phalangeal
    Left 0SBN-
    Right 0SBM-
  Metatarsal-Tarsal
    Left 0SBL-
    Right 0SBK-
  Occipital-cervical 0RB0-
  Sacrococcygeal 0SB5-
  Sacroiliac
    Left 0SB8-
    Right 0SB7-
  Shoulder
    Left 0RBK-
    Right 0RBJ-
  Sternoclavicular
    Left 0RBF-
    Right 0RBE-
  Tarsal
    Left 0SBJ-
    Right 0SBH-
  Temporomandibular
    Left 0RBD-
    Right 0RBC-
  Thoracic Vertebral 0RB6-
  Thoracolumbar Vertebral 0RBA-
  Toe Phalangeal
    Left 0SBQ-
    Right 0SBP-
  Wrist
    Left 0RBP-
    Right 0RBN-
Kidney
  Left 0TB1-
  Right 0TB0-
Kidney Pelvis
  Left 0TB4-
  Right 0TB3-
Knee Region
  Left 0YBG-
  Right 0YBF-
Larynx 0CBS-
Leg
  Lower
    Left 0YBJ-
    Right 0YBH-
  Upper
    Left 0YBD-
    Right 0YBC-
Lens
  Left 08BK3Z-
  Right 08BJ3Z-
Lip
  Lower 0CB1-
  Upper 0CB0-
Liver 0FB0-
  Left Lobe 0FB2-
  Right Lobe 0FB1-
Lung
  Bilateral 0BBM-
  Left 0BBL-
  Lower Lobe
    Left 0BBJ-
    Right 0BBF-
  Middle Lobe, Right 0BBD-
  Right 0BBK-
  Upper Lobe
    Left 0BBG-
    Right 0BBC-
Lung Lingula 0BBH-
Lymphatic
  Aortic 07BD-

Excision — *continued*
Lymphatic — *continued*
  Axillary
    Left 07B6-
    Right 07B5-
  Head 07B0-
  Inguinal
    Left 07BJ-
    Right 07BH-
  Internal Mammary
    Left 07B9-
    Right 07B8-
  Lower Extremity
    Left 07BG-
    Right 07BF-
  Mesenteric 07BB-
  Neck
    Left 07B2-
    Right 07B1-
  Pelvis 07BC-
  Thoracic Duct 07BK-
  Thorax 07B7-
  Upper Extremity
    Left 07B4-
    Right 07B3-
Mandible
  Left 0NBV-
  Right 0NBT-
Maxilla
  Left 0NBS-
  Right 0NBR-
Mediastinum 0WBC-
Medulla Oblongata 00BD-
Mesentery 0DBV-
Metacarpal
  Left 0PBQ-
  Right 0PBP-
Metatarsal
  Left 0QBP-
  Right 0QBN-
Muscle
  Abdomen
    Left 0KBL-
    Right 0KBK-
  Extraocular
    Left 08BM-
    Right 08BL-
  Facial 0KB1-
  Foot
    Left 0KBW-
    Right 0KBV-
  Hand
    Left 0KBD-
    Right 0KBC-
  Head 0KB0-
  Hip
    Left 0KBP-
    Right 0KBN-
  Lower Arm and Wrist
    Left 0KBB-
    Right 0KB9-
  Lower Leg
    Left 0KBT-
    Right 0KBS-
  Neck
    Left 0KB3-
    Right 0KB2-
  Papillary 02BD-
  Perineum 0KBM-
  Shoulder
    Left 0KB6-
    Right 0KB5-
  Thorax
    Left 0KBJ-
    Right 0KBH-
  Tongue, Palate, Pharynx 0KB4-
  Trunk
    Left 0KBG-
    Right 0KBF-
  Upper Arm
    Left 0KB8-
    Right 0KB7-

Excision — *continued*
Muscle — *continued*
  Upper Leg
    Left 0KBR-
    Right 0KBQ-
Nasopharynx 09BN-
Neck 0WB6-
Nerve
  Abdominal Sympathetic 01BM-
  Abducens 00BL-
  Accessory 00BR-
  Acoustic 00BN-
  Brachial Plexus 01B3-
  Cervical 01B1-
  Cervical Plexus 01B0-
  Facial 00BM-
  Femoral 01BD-
  Glossopharyngeal 00BP-
  Head and Neck Sympathetic 01BK-
  Hypoglossal 00BS-
  Lumbar 01BB-
  Lumbar Plexus 01B9-
  Lumbar Sympathetic 01BN-
  Lumbosacral Plexus 01BA-
  Median 01B5-
  Oculomotor 00BH-
  Olfactory 00BF-
  Optic 00BG-
  Peroneal 01BH-
  Phrenic 01B2-
  Pudendal 01BC-
  Radial 01B6-
  Sacral 01BR-
  Sacral Plexus 01BQ-
  Sacral Sympathetic 01BP-
  Sciatic 01BF-
  Thoracic 01B8-
  Thoracic Sympathetic 01BL-
  Tibial 01BG-
  Trigeminal 00BK-
  Trochlear 00BJ-
  Ulnar 01B4-
  Vagus 00BQ-
Nipple
  Left 0HBX-
  Right 0HBW-
Nose 09BK-
Omentum
  Greater 0DBS-
  Lesser 0DBT-
Orbit
  Left 0NBQ-
  Right 0NBP-
Ovary
  Bilateral 0UB2-
  Left 0UB1-
  Right 0UB0-
Palate
  Hard 0CB2-
  Soft 0CB3-
Pancreas 0FBG-
Para-aortic Body 0GB9-
Paraganglion Extremity 0GBF-
Parathyroid Gland 0GBR-
  Inferior
    Left 0GBP-
    Right 0GBN-
  Multiple 0GBQ-
  Superior
    Left 0GBM-
    Right 0GBL-
Patella
  Left 0QBF-
  Right 0QBD-
Penis 0VBS-
Pericardium 02BN-
Perineum
  Female 0WBN-
  Male 0WBM-
Peritoneum 0DBW-

Excision — *continued*
Phalanx
  Finger
    Left 0PBV-
    Right 0PBT-
  Thumb
    Left 0PBS-
    Right 0PBR-
  Toe
    Left 0QBR-
    Right 0QBQ-
Pharynx 0CBM-
Pineal Body 0GB1-
Pleura
  Left 0BBP-
  Right 0BBN-
Pons 00BB-
Prepuce 0VBT-
Prostate 0VB0-
Radius
  Left 0PBJ-
  Right 0PBH-
Rectum 0DBP-
Retina
  Left 08BF3Z-
  Right 08BE3Z-
Retroperitoneum 0WBH-
Rib
  Left 0PB2-
  Right 0PB1-
Sacrum 0QB1-
Scapula
  Left 0PB6-
  Right 0PB5-
Sclera
  Left 08B7XZ-
  Right 08B6XZ-
Scrotum 0VB5-
Septum
  Atrial 02B5-
  Nasal 09BM-
  Ventricular 02BM-
Shoulder Region
  Left 0XB3-
  Right 0XB2-
Sinus
  Accessory 09BP-
  Ethmoid
    Left 09BV-
    Right 09BU-
  Frontal
    Left 09BT-
    Right 09BS-
  Mastoid
    Left 09BC-
    Right 09BB-
  Maxillary
    Left 09BR-
    Right 09BQ-
  Sphenoid
    Left 09BX-
    Right 09BW-
Skin
  Abdomen 0HB7XZ-
  Back 0HB6XZ-
  Buttock 0HB8XZ-
  Chest 0HB5XZ-
  Ear
    Left 0HB3XZ-
    Right 0HB2XZ-
  Face 0HB1XZ-
  Foot
    Left 0HBNXZ-
    Right 0HBMXZ-
  Genitalia 0HBAXZ-
  Hand
    Left 0HBGXZ-
    Right 0HBFXZ-
  Lower Arm
    Left 0HBEXZ-
    Right 0HBDXZ-

Excision — *continued*
  Skin — *continued*
    Lower Leg
      Left 0HBLXZ-
      Right 0HBKXZ-
    Neck 0HB4XZ-
    Perineum 0HB9XZ-
    Scalp 0HB0XZ-
    Upper Arm
      Left 0HBCXZ-
      Right 0HBBXZ-
    Upper Leg
      Left 0HBJXZ-
      Right 0HBHXZ-
  Skull 0NB0-
  Spinal Cord
    Cervical 00BW-
    Lumbar 00BY-
    Thoracic 00BX-
  Spinal Meninges 00BT-
  Spleen 07BP-
  Sternum 0PB0-
  Stomach 0DB6-
    Pylorus 0DB7-
  Subcutaneous Tissue and Fascia
    Abdomen 0JB8-
    Back 0JB7-
    Buttock 0JB9-
    Chest 0JB6-
    Face 0JB1-
    Foot
      Left 0JBR-
      Right 0JBQ-
    Hand
      Left 0JBK-
      Right 0JBJ-
    Lower Arm
      Left 0JBH-
      Right 0JBG-
    Lower Leg
      Left 0JBP-
      Right 0JBN-
    Neck
      Anterior 0JB4-
      Posterior 0JB5-
    Pelvic Region 0JBC-
    Perineum 0JBB-
    Scalp 0JB0-
    Upper Arm
      Left 0JBF-
      Right 0JBD-
    Upper Leg
      Left 0JBM-
      Right 0JBL-
  Tarsal
    Left 0QBM-
    Right 0QBL-
  Tendon
    Abdomen
      Left 0LBG-
      Right 0LBF-
    Ankle
      Left 0LBT-
      Right 0LBS-
    Foot
      Left 0LBW-
      Right 0LBV-
    Hand
      Left 0LB8-
      Right 0LB7-
    Head and Neck 0LB0-
    Hip
      Left 0LBK-
      Right 0LBJ-
    Knee
      Left 0LBR-
      Right 0LBQ-
    Lower Arm and Wrist
      Left 0LB6-
      Right 0LB5-

Excision — *continued*
  Tendon — *continued*
    Lower Leg
      Left 0LBP-
      Right 0LBN-
    Perineum 0LBH-
    Shoulder
      Left 0LB2-
      Right 0LB1-
    Thorax
      Left 0LBD-
      Right 0LBC-
    Trunk
      Left 0LBB-
      Right 0LB9-
    Upper Arm
      Left 0LB4-
      Right 0LB3-
    Upper Leg
      Left 0LBM-
      Right 0LBL-
  Testis
    Bilateral 0VBC-
    Left 0VBB-
    Right 0VB9-
  Thalamus 00B9-
  Thymus 07BM-
  Thyroid Gland
    Left Lobe 0GBG-
    Right Lobe 0GBH-
  Tibia
    Left 0QBH-
    Right 0QBG-
  Toe Nail 0HBRXZ-
  Tongue 0CB7-
  Tonsils 0CBP-
  Tooth
    Lower 0CBX-
    Upper 0CBW-
  Trachea 0BB1-
  Tunica Vaginalis
    Left 0VB7-
    Right 0VB6-
  Turbinate, Nasal 09BL-
  Tympanic Membrane
    Left 09B8-
    Right 09B7-
  Ulna
    Left 0PBL-
    Right 0PBK-
  Ureter
    Left 0TB7-
    Right 0TB6-
  Urethra 0TBD-
  Uterine Supporting Structure 0UB4-
  Uterus 0UB9-
  Uvula 0CBN-
  Vagina 0UBG-
  Valve
    Aortic 02BF-
    Mitral 02BG-
    Pulmonary 02BH-
    Tricuspid 02BJ-
  Vas Deferens
    Bilateral 0VBQ-
    Left 0VBP-
    Right 0VBN-
  Vein
    Axillary
      Left 05B8-
      Right 05B7-
    Azygos 05B0-
    Basilic
      Left 05BC-
      Right 05BB-
    Brachial
      Left 05BA-
      Right 05B9-
    Cephalic
      Left 05BF-
      Right 05BD-
    Colic 06B7-

Excision — *continued*
  Vein — *continued*
    Common Iliac
      Left 06BD-
      Right 06BC-
    Coronary 02B4-
    Esophageal 06B3-
    External Iliac
      Left 06BG-
      Right 06BF-
    External Jugular
      Left 05BQ-
      Right 05BP-
    Face
      Left 05BV-
      Right 05BT-
    Femoral
      Left 06BN-
      Right 06BM-
    Foot
      Left 06BV-
      Right 06BT-
    Gastric 06B2-
    Greater Saphenous
      Left 06BQ-
      Right 06BP-
    Hand
      Left 05BH-
      Right 05BG-
    Hemiazygos 05B1-
    Hepatic 06B4-
    Hypogastric
      Left 06BJ-
      Right 06BH-
    Inferior Mesenteric 06B6-
    Innominate
      Left 05B4-
      Right 05B3-
    Internal Jugular
      Left 05BN-
      Right 05BM-
    Intracranial 05BL-
    Lesser Saphenous
      Left 06BS-
      Right 06BR-
    Lower 06BY-
    Portal 06B8-
    Pulmonary
      Left 02BT-
      Right 02BS-
    Renal
      Left 06BB-
      Right 06B9-
    Splenic 06B1-
    Subclavian
      Left 05B6-
      Right 05B5-
    Superior Mesenteric 06B5-
    Upper 05BY-
    Vertebral
      Left 05BS-
      Right 05BR-
  Vena Cava
    Inferior 06B0-
    Superior 02BV-
  Ventricle
    Left 02BL-
    Right 02BK-
  Vertebra
    Cervical 0PB3-
    Lumbar 0QB0-
    Thoracic 0PB4-
  Vesicle
    Bilateral 0VB3-
    Left 0VB2-
    Right 0VB1-
  Vitreous
    Left 08B53Z-
    Right 08B43Z-
  Vocal Cord
    Left 0CBV-
    Right 0CBT-

Excision — *continued*
  Vulva 0UBM-
  Wrist Region
    Left 0XBH-
    Right 0XBG-
Exclusion, Left atrial appendage (LAA) *see* Occlusion, Atrium, Left 02L7-
Exercise, rehabilitation *see* Motor Treatment, Rehabilitation F07-
Exploration *see* Inspection
Express® (LD) Premounted Stent System
  use Intraluminal Device
Express® Biliary SD Monorail® Premounted Stent System
  use Intraluminal Device
Ex-PRESS™ mini glaucoma shunt
  use Synthetic Substitute
Express® SD Renal Monorail® Premounted Stent System
  use Intraluminal Device
Extensor carpi radialis muscle
  use Muscle, Lower Arm and Wrist, Left
  use Muscle, Lower Arm and Wrist, Right
Extensor carpi ulnaris muscle
  use Muscle, Lower Arm and Wrist, Left
  use Muscle, Lower Arm and Wrist, Right
Extensor digitorum brevis muscle
  use Muscle, Foot, Left
  use Muscle, Foot, Right
Extensor digitorum longus muscle
  use Muscle, Lower Leg, Left
  use Muscle, Lower Leg, Right
Extensor hallucis brevis muscle
  use Muscle, Foot, Left
  use Muscle, Foot, Right
Extensor hallucis longus muscle
  use Muscle, Lower Leg, Left
  use Muscle, Lower Leg, Right
External anal sphincter
  use Anal Sphincter
External auditory meatus
  use Ear, External Auditory Canal, Left
  use Ear, External Auditory Canal, Right
External fixator
  use External Fixation Device in Head and Facial Bones
  use External Fixation Device in Lower Bones
  use External Fixation Device in Lower Joints
  use External Fixation Device in Upper Bones
  use External Fixation Device in Upper Joints
External maxillary artery
  use Artery, Face
External naris
  use Nose
External oblique aponeurosis
  use Subcutaneous Tissue and Fascia, Trunk
External oblique muscle
  use Muscle, Abdomen, Left
  use Muscle, Abdomen, Right
External popliteal nerve
  use Nerve, Peroneal
External pudendal artery
  use Artery, Femoral, Left
  use Artery, Femoral, Right
External pudendal vein
  use Vein, Greater Saphenous, Left
  use Vein, Greater Saphenous, Right
External urethral sphincter
  use Urethra

INDEX TO PROCEDURES – 2016 ICD-10-PCS

Extirpation

Extirpation
- Acetabulum
  - Left 0QC5-
  - Right 0QC4-
- Adenoids 0CCQ-
- Ampulla of Vater 0FCC-
- Anal Sphincter 0DCR-
- Anterior Chamber
  - Left 08C3-
  - Right 08C2-
- Anus 0DCQ-
- Aorta
  - Abdominal 04C0-
  - Thoracic 02CW-
- Aortic Body 0GCD-
- Appendix 0DCJ-
- Artery
  - Anterior Tibial
    - Left 04CQ-
    - Right 04CP-
  - Axillary
    - Left 03C6-
    - Right 03C5-
  - Brachial
    - Left 03C8-
    - Right 03C7-
  - Celiac 04C1-
  - Colic
    - Left 04C7-
    - Middle 04C8-
    - Right 04C6-
  - Common Carotid
    - Left 03CJ-
    - Right 03CH-
  - Common Iliac
    - Left 04CD-
    - Right 04CC-
  - Coronary
    - One Site 02C0-
    - Two Sites 02C1-
    - Three Sites 02C2-
    - Four or More Sites 02C3-
  - External Carotid
    - Left 03CN-
    - Right 03CM-
  - External Iliac
    - Left 04CJ-
    - Right 04CH-
  - Face 03CR-
  - Femoral
    - Left 04CL-
    - Right 04CK-
  - Foot
    - Left 04CW-
    - Right 04CV-
  - Gastric 04C2-
  - Hand
    - Left 03CF-
    - Right 03CD-
  - Hepatic 04C3-
  - Inferior Mesenteric 04CB-
  - Innominate 03C2-
  - Internal Carotid
    - Left 03CL-
    - Right 03CK-
  - Internal Iliac
    - Left 04CF-
    - Right 04CE-
  - Internal Mammary
    - Left 03C1-
    - Right 03C0-
  - Intracranial 03CG-
  - Lower 04CY-
  - Peroneal
    - Left 04CU-
    - Right 04CT-

Extirpation — continued
- Artery — continued
  - Popliteal
    - Left 04CN-
    - Right 04CM-
  - Posterior Tibial
    - Left 04CS-
    - Right 04CR-
  - Pulmonary
    - Left 02CR-
    - Right 02CQ-
  - Pulmonary Trunk 02CP-
  - Radial
    - Left 03CC-
    - Right 03CB-
  - Renal
    - Left 04CA-
    - Right 04C9-
  - Splenic 04C4-
  - Subclavian
    - Left 03C4-
    - Right 03C3-
  - Superior Mesenteric 04C5-
  - Temporal
    - Left 03CT-
    - Right 03CS-
  - Thyroid
    - Left 03CV-
    - Right 03CU-
  - Ulnar
    - Left 03CA-
    - Right 03C9-
  - Upper 03CY-
  - Vertebral
    - Left 03CQ-
    - Right 03CP-
- Atrium
  - Left 02C7-
  - Right 02C6-
- Auditory Ossicle
  - Left 09CA0ZZ
  - Right 09C90ZZ
- Basal Ganglia 00C8-
- Bladder 0TCB-
- Bladder Neck 0TCC-
- Bone
  - Ethmoid
    - Left 0NCG-
    - Right 0NCF-
  - Frontal
    - Left 0NC2-
    - Right 0NC1-
  - Hyoid 0NCX-
  - Lacrimal
    - Left 0NCJ-
    - Right 0NCH-
  - Nasal 0NCB-
  - Occipital
    - Left 0NC8-
    - Right 0NC7-
  - Palatine
    - Left 0NCL-
    - Right 0NCK-
  - Parietal
    - Left 0NC4-
    - Right 0NC3-
  - Pelvic
    - Left 0QC3-
    - Right 0QC2-
  - Sphenoid
    - Left 0NCD-
    - Right 0NCC-
  - Temporal
    - Left 0NC6-
    - Right 0NC5-
  - Zygomatic
    - Left 0NCN-
    - Right 0NCM-

Extirpation — continued
- Brain 00C0-
- Breast
  - Bilateral 0HCV-
  - Left 0HCU-
  - Right 0HCT-
- Bronchus
  - Lingula 0BC9-
  - Lower Lobe
    - Left 0BCB-
    - Right 0BC6-
  - Main
    - Left 0BC7-
    - Right 0BC3-
  - Middle Lobe, Right 0BC5-
  - Upper Lobe
    - Left 0BC8-
    - Right 0BC4-
- Buccal Mucosa 0CC4-
- Bursa and Ligament
  - Abdomen
    - Left 0MCJ-
    - Right 0MCH-
  - Ankle
    - Left 0MCR-
    - Right 0MCQ-
  - Elbow
    - Left 0MC4-
    - Right 0MC3-
  - Foot
    - Left 0MCT-
    - Right 0MCS-
  - Hand
    - Left 0MC8-
    - Right 0MC7-
  - Head and Neck 0MC0-
  - Hip
    - Left 0MCM-
    - Right 0MCL-
  - Knee
    - Left 0MCP-
    - Right 0MCN-
  - Lower Extremity
    - Left 0MCW-
    - Right 0MCV-
  - Perineum 0MCK-
  - Shoulder
    - Left 0MC2-
    - Right 0MC1-
  - Thorax
    - Left 0MCG-
    - Right 0MCF-
  - Trunk
    - Left 0MCD-
    - Right 0MCC-
  - Upper Extremity
    - Left 0MC8-
    - Right 0MC9-
  - Wrist
    - Left 0MC6-
    - Right 0MC5-
- Carina 0BC2-
- Carotid Bodies, Bilateral 0GC8-
- Carotid Body
  - Left 0GC6-
  - Right 0GC7-
- Carpal
  - Left 0PCN-
  - Right 0PCM-
- Cavity, Cranial 0WC1-
- Cecum 0DCH-
- Cerebellum 00CC-
- Cerebral Hemisphere 00C7-
- Cerebral Meninges 00C1-
- Cerebral Ventricle 00C6-
- Cervix 0UCC-
- Chordae Tendineae 02C9-
- Choroid
  - Left 08CB-
  - Right 08CA-

Extirpation — continued
- Cisterna Chyli 07CL-
- Clavicle
  - Left 0PCB-
  - Right 0PC9-
- Clitoris 0UCJ-
- Coccygeal Glomus 0GCB-
- Coccyx 0QCS-
- Colon
  - Ascending 0DCK-
  - Descending 0DCM-
  - Sigmoid 0DCN-
  - Transverse 0DCL-
- Conduction Mechanism 02C8-
- Conjunctiva
  - Left 08CTXZZ
  - Right 08CSXZZ
- Cord
  - Bilateral 0VCH-
  - Left 0VCG-
  - Right 0VCF-
- Cornea
  - Left 08C9XZZ
  - Right 08C8XZZ
- Cul-de-sac 0UCF-
- Diaphragm
  - Left 0BCS-
  - Right 0BCR-
- Disc
  - Cervical Vertebral 0RC3-
  - Cervicothoracic Vertebral 0RC5-
  - Lumbar Vertebral 0SC2-
  - Lumbosacral 0SC4-
  - Thoracic Vertebral 0RC9-
  - Thoracolumbar Vertebral 0RCB-
- Duct
  - Common Bile 0FC9-
  - Cystic 0FC8-
  - Hepatic
    - Left 0FC6-
    - Right 0FC5-
  - Lacrimal
    - Left 08CY-
    - Right 08CX-
  - Pancreatic 0FCD-
    - Accessory 0FCF-
  - Parotid
    - Left 0CCC-
    - Right 0CCB-
- Duodenum 0DC9-
- Dura Mater 00C2-
- Ear
  - External
    - Left 09C1-
    - Right 09C0-
  - External Auditory Canal
    - Left 09C4-
    - Right 09C3-
  - Inner
    - Left 09CE0ZZ
    - Right 09CD0ZZ
  - Middle
    - Left 09C60ZZ
    - Right 09C50ZZ
- Endometrium 0UCB-
- Epididymis
  - Bilateral 0VCL-
  - Left 0VCK-
  - Right 0VCJ-
- Epidural Space 00C3-
- Epiglottis 0CCR-
- Esophagogastric Junction 0DC4-
- Esophagus 0DC5-
  - Lower 0DC3-
  - Middle 0DC2-
  - Upper 0DC1-

Extirpation — *continued*
  Eustachian Tube
    Left 09CG-
    Right 09CF-
  Eye
    Left 08C1XZZ
    Right 08C0XZZ
  Eyelid
    Lower
      Left 08CR-
      Right 08CQ-
    Upper
      Left 08CP-
      Right 08CN-
  Fallopian Tube
    Left 0UC6-
    Right 0UC5-
  Fallopian Tubes, Bilateral 0UC7-
  Femoral Shaft
    Left 0QC9-
    Right 0QC8-
  Femur
    Lower
      Left 0QCC-
      Right 0QCB-
    Upper
      Left 0QC7-
      Right 0QC6-
  Fibula
    Left 0QCK-
    Right 0QCJ-
  Finger Nail 0HCQXZZ
  Gallbladder 0FC4-
  Gastrointestinal Tract 0WCP-
  Genitourinary Tract 0WCR-
  Gingiva
    Lower 0CC6-
    Upper 0CC5-
  Gland
    Adrenal
      Bilateral 0GC4-
      Left 0GC2-
      Right 0GC3-
    Lacrimal
      Left 08CW-
      Right 08CV-
    Minor Salivary 0CCJ-
    Parotid
      Left 0CC9-
      Right 0CC8-
    Pituitary 0GC0-
    Sublingual
      Left 0CCF-
      Right 0CCD-
    Submaxillary
      Left 0CCH-
      Right 0CCG-
    Vestibular 0UCL-
  Glenoid Cavity
    Left 0PC8-
    Right 0PC7-
  Glomus Jugulare 0GCC-
  Humeral Head
    Left 0PCD-
    Right 0PCC-
  Humeral Shaft
    Left 0PCG-
    Right 0PCF-
  Hymen 0UCK-
  Hypothalamus 00CA-
  Ileocecal Valve 0DCC-
  Ileum 0DCB-
  Intestine
    Large 0DCE-
      Left 0DCG-
      Right 0DCF-
    Small 0DC8-

Extirpation — *continued*
  Iris
    Left 08CD-
    Right 08CC-
  Jejunum 0DCA-
  Joint
    Acromioclavicular
      Left 0RCH-
      Right 0RCG-
    Ankle
      Left 0SCG-
      Right 0SCF-
    Carpal
      Left 0RCR-
      Right 0RCQ-
    Cervical Vertebral 0RC1-
    Cervicothoracic Vertebral 0RC4-
    Coccygeal 0SC6-
    Elbow
      Left 0RCM-
      Right 0RCL-
    Finger Phalangeal
      Left 0RCX-
      Right 0RCW-
    Hip
      Left 0SCB-
      Right 0SC9-
    Knee
      Left 0SCD-
      Right 0SCC-
    Lumbar Vertebral 0SC0-
    Lumbosacral 0SC3-
    Metacarpocarpal
      Left 0RCT-
      Right 0RCS-
    Metacarpophalangeal
      Left 0RCV-
      Right 0RCU-
    Metatarsal-Phalangeal
      Left 0SCN-
      Right 0SCM-
    Metatarsal-Tarsal
      Left 0SCL-
      Right 0SCK-
    Occipital-cervical 0RC0-
    Sacrococcygeal 0SC5-
    Sacroiliac
      Left 0SC8-
      Right 0SC7-
    Shoulder
      Left 0RCK-
      Right 0RCJ-
    Sternoclavicular
      Left 0RCF-
      Right 0RCE-
    Tarsal
      Left 0SCJ-
      Right 0SCH-
    Temporomandibular
      Left 0RCD-
      Right 0RCC-
    Thoracic Vertebral 0RC6-
    Thoracolumbar Vertebral 0RCA-
    Toe Phalangeal
      Left 0SCQ-
      Right 0SCP-
    Wrist
      Left 0RCP-
      Right 0RCN-
  Kidney
    Left 0TC1-
    Right 0TC0-
  Kidney Pelvis
    Left 0TC4-
    Right 0TC3-

Extirpation — *continued*
  Larynx 0CCS-
  Lens
    Left 08CK-
    Right 08CJ-
  Lip
    Lower 0CC1-
    Upper 0CC0-
  Liver 0FC0-
    Left Lobe 0FC2-
    Right Lobe 0FC1-
  Lung
    Bilateral 0BCM-
    Left 0BCL-
    Lower Lobe
      Left 0BCJ-
      Right 0BCF-
    Middle Lobe, Right 0BCD-
    Right 0BCK-
    Upper Lobe
      Left 0BCG-
      Right 0BCC-
  Lung Lingula 0BCH-
  Lymphatic
    Aortic 07CD-
    Axillary
      Left 07C6-
      Right 07C5-
    Head 07C0-
    Inguinal
      Left 07CJ-
      Right 07CH-
    Internal Mammary
      Left 07C9-
      Right 07C8-
    Lower Extremity
      Left 07CG-
      Right 07CF-
    Mesenteric 07CB-
    Neck
      Left 07C2-
      Right 07C1-
    Pelvis 07CC-
    Thoracic Duct 07CK-
    Thorax 07C7-
    Upper Extremity
      Left 07C4-
      Right 07C3-
  Mandible
    Left 0NCV-
    Right 0NCT-
  Maxilla
    Left 0NCS-
    Right 0NCR-
  Mediastinum 0WCC-
  Medulla Oblongata 00CD-
  Mesentery 0DCV-
  Metacarpal
    Left 0PCQ-
    Right 0PCP-
  Metatarsal
    Left 0QCP-
    Right 0QCN-
  Muscle
    Abdomen
      Left 0KCL-
      Right 0KCK-
    Extraocular
      Left 08CM-
      Right 08CL-
    Facial 0KC1-
    Foot
      Left 0KCW-
      Right 0KCV-
    Hand
      Left 0KCD-
      Right 0KCC-
    Head 0KC0-
    Hip
      Left 0KCP-
      Right 0KCN-

Extirpation — *continued*
  Muscle — *continued*
    Lower Arm and Wrist
      Left 0KCB-
      Right 0KC9-
    Lower Leg
      Left 0KCT-
      Right 0KCS-
    Neck
      Left 0KC3-
      Right 0KC2-
    Papillary 02CD-
    Perineum 0KCM-
    Shoulder
      Left 0KC6-
      Right 0KC5-
    Thorax
      Left 0KCJ-
      Right 0KCH-
    Tongue, Palate, Pharynx 0KC4-
    Trunk
      Left 0KCG-
      Right 0KCF-
    Upper Arm
      Left 0KC8-
      Right 0KC7-
    Upper Leg
      Left 0KCR-
      Right 0KCQ-
  Nasopharynx 09CN-
  Nerve
    Abdominal Sympathetic 01CM-
    Abducens 00CL-
    Accessory 00CR-
    Acoustic 00CN-
    Brachial Plexus 01C3-
    Cervical 01C1-
    Cervical Plexus 01C0-
    Facial 00CM-
    Femoral 01CD-
    Glossopharyngeal 00CP-
    Head and Neck Sympathetic 01CK-
    Hypoglossal 00CS-
    Lumbar 01CB-
    Lumbar Plexus 01C9-
    Lumbar Sympathetic 01CN-
    Lumbosacral Plexus 01CA-
    Median 01C5-
    Oculomotor 00CH-
    Olfactory 00CF-
    Optic 00CG-
    Peroneal 01CH-
    Phrenic 01C2-
    Pudendal 01CC-
    Radial 01C6-
    Sacral 01CR-
    Sacral Plexus 01CQ-
    Sacral Sympathetic 01CP-
    Sciatic 01CF-
    Thoracic 01C8-
    Thoracic Sympathetic 01CL-
    Tibial 01CG-
    Trigeminal 00CK-
    Trochlear 00CJ-
    Ulnar 01C4-
    Vagus 00CQ-
  Nipple
    Left 0HCX-
    Right 0HCW-
  Nose 09CK-
  Omentum
    Greater 0DCS-
    Lesser 0DCT-
  Oral Cavity and Throat 0WC3-
  Orbit
    Left 0NCQ-
    Right 0NCP-
  Orbital Atherectomy Technology X2C-

Extirpation

Extirpation — *continued*
- Ovary
  - Bilateral 0UC2-
  - Left 0UC1-
  - Right 0UC0-
- Palate
  - Hard 0CC2-
  - Soft 0CC3-
- Pancreas 0FCG-
- Para-aortic Body 0GC9-
- Paraganglion Extremity 0GCF-
- Parathyroid Gland 0GCR-
  - Inferior
    - Left 0GCP-
    - Right 0GCN-
  - Multiple 0GCQ-
  - Superior
    - Left 0GCM-
    - Right 0GCL-
- Patella
  - Left 0QCF-
  - Right 0QCD-
- Pelvic Cavity 0WCJ-
- Penis 0VCS-
- Pericardial Cavity 0WCD-
- Pericardium 02CN-
- Peritoneal Cavity 0WCG-
- Peritoneum 0DCW-
- Phalanx
  - Finger
    - Left 0PCV-
    - Right 0PCT-
  - Thumb
    - Left 0PCS-
    - Right 0PCR-
  - Toe
    - Left 0QCR-
    - Right 0QCQ-
- Pharynx 0CCM-
- Pineal Body 0GC1-
- Pleura
  - Left 0BCP-
  - Right 0BCN-
- Pleural Cavity
  - Left 0WCB-
  - Right 0WC9-
- Pons 00CB-
- Prepuce 0VCT-
- Prostate 0VC0-
- Radius
  - Left 0PCJ-
  - Right 0PCH-
- Rectum 0DCP-
- Respiratory Tract 0WCQ-
- Retina
  - Left 08CF-
  - Right 08CE-
- Retinal Vessel
  - Left 08CH-
  - Right 08CG-
- Rib
  - Left 0PC2-
  - Right 0PC1-
- Sacrum 0QC1-
- Scapula
  - Left 0PC6-
  - Right 0PC5-
- Sclera
  - Left 08C7XZZ
  - Right 08C6XZZ
- Scrotum 0VC5-
- Septum
  - Atrial 02C5-
  - Nasal 09CM-
  - Ventricular 02CM-

Extirpation — *continued*
- Sinus
  - Accessory 09CP-
  - Ethmoid
    - Left 09CV-
    - Right 09CU-
  - Frontal
    - Left 09CT-
    - Right 09CS-
  - Mastoid
    - Left 09CC-
    - Right 09CB-
  - Maxillary
    - Left 09CR-
    - Right 09CQ-
  - Sphenoid
    - Left 09CX-
    - Right 09CW-
- Skin
  - Abdomen 0HC7XZZ
  - Back 0HC6XZZ
  - Buttock 0HC8XZZ
  - Chest 0HC5XZZ
  - Ear
    - Left 0HC3XZZ
    - Right 0HC2XZZ
  - Face 0HC1XZZ
  - Foot
    - Left 0HCNXZZ
    - Right 0HCMXZZ
  - Genitalia 0HCAXZZ
  - Hand
    - Left 0HCGXZZ
    - Right 0HCFXZZ
  - Lower Arm
    - Left 0HCEXZZ
    - Right 0HCDXZZ
  - Lower Leg
    - Left 0HCLXZZ
    - Right 0HCKXZZ
  - Neck 0HC4XZZ
  - Perineum 0HC9XZZ
  - Scalp 0HC0XZZ
  - Upper Arm
    - Left 0HCCXZZ
    - Right 0HCBXZZ
  - Upper Leg
    - Left 0HCJXZZ
    - Right 0HCHXZZ
- Spinal Cord
  - Cervical 00CW-
  - Lumbar 00CY-
  - Thoracic 00CX-
- Spinal Meninges 00CT-
- Spleen 07CP-
- Sternum 0PC0-
- Stomach 0DC6-
  - Pylorus 0DC7-
- Subarachnoid Space 00C5-
- Subcutaneous Tissue and Fascia
  - Abdomen 0JC8-
  - Back 0JC7-
  - Buttock 0JC9-
  - Chest 0JC6-
  - Face 0JC1-
  - Foot
    - Left 0JCR-
    - Right 0JCQ-
  - Hand
    - Left 0JCK-
    - Right 0JCJ-
  - Lower Arm
    - Left 0JCH-
    - Right 0JCG-
  - Lower Leg
    - Left 0JCP-
    - Right 0JCN-

Extirpation — *continued*
- Subcutaneous Tissue and Fascia — *continued*
  - Neck
    - Anterior 0JC4-
    - Posterior 0JC5-
  - Pelvic Region 0JCC-
  - Perineum 0JCB-
  - Scalp 0JC0-
  - Upper Arm
    - Left 0JCF-
    - Right 0JCD-
  - Upper Leg
    - Left 0JCM-
    - Right 0JCL-
- Subdural Space 00C4-
- Tarsal
  - Left 0QCM-
  - Right 0QCL-
- Tendon
  - Abdomen
    - Left 0LCG-
    - Right 0LCF-
  - Ankle
    - Left 0LCT-
    - Right 0LCS-
  - Foot
    - Left 0LCW-
    - Right 0LCV-
  - Hand
    - Left 0LC8-
    - Right 0LC7-
  - Head and Neck 0LC0-
  - Hip
    - Left 0LCK-
    - Right 0LCJ-
  - Knee
    - Left 0LCR-
    - Right 0LCQ-
  - Lower Arm and Wrist
    - Left 0LC6-
    - Right 0LC5-
  - Lower Leg
    - Left 0LCP-
    - Right 0LCN-
  - Perineum 0LCH-
  - Shoulder
    - Left 0LC2-
    - Right 0LC1-
  - Thorax
    - Left 0LCD-
    - Right 0LCC-
  - Trunk
    - Left 0LCB-
    - Right 0LC9-
  - Upper Arm
    - Left 0LC4-
    - Right 0LC3-
  - Upper Leg
    - Left 0LCM-
    - Right 0LCL-
- Testis
  - Bilateral 0VCC-
  - Left 0VCB-
  - Right 0VC9-
- Thalamus 00C9-
- Thymus 07CM-
- Thyroid Gland 0GCK-
  - Left Lobe 0GCG-
  - Right Lobe 0GCH-
- Tibia
  - Left 0QCH-
  - Right 0QCG-
- Toe Nail 0HCRXZZ
- Tongue 0CC7-
- Tonsils 0CCP-
- Tooth
  - Lower 0CCX-
  - Upper 0CCW-

Extirpation — *continued*
- Trachea 0BC1-
- Tunica Vaginalis
  - Left 0VC7-
  - Right 0VC6-
- Turbinate, Nasal 09CL-
- Tympanic Membrane
  - Left 09C8-
  - Right 09C7-
- Ulna
  - Left 0PCL-
  - Right 0PCK-
- Ureter
  - Left 0TC7-
  - Right 0TC6-
- Urethra 0TCD-
- Uterine Supporting Structure 0UC4-
- Uterus 0UC9-
- Uvula 0CCN-
- Vagina 0UCG-
- Valve
  - Aortic 02CF-
  - Mitral 02CG-
  - Pulmonary 02CH-
  - Tricuspid 02CJ-
- Vas Deferens
  - Bilateral 0VCQ-
  - Left 0VCP-
  - Right 0VCN-
- Vein
  - Axillary
    - Left 05C8-
    - Right 05C7-
  - Azygos 05C0-
  - Basilic
    - Left 05CC-
    - Right 05CB-
  - Brachial
    - Left 05CA-
    - Right 05C9-
  - Cephalic
    - Left 05CF-
    - Right 05CD-
  - Colic 06C7-
  - Common Iliac
    - Left 06CD-
    - Right 06CC-
  - Coronary 02C4-
  - Esophageal 06C3-
  - External Iliac
    - Left 06CG-
    - Right 06CF-
  - External Jugular
    - Left 05CQ-
    - Right 05CP-
  - Face
    - Left 05CV-
    - Right 05CT-
  - Femoral
    - Left 06CN-
    - Right 06CM-
  - Foot
    - Left 06CV-
    - Right 06CT-
  - Gastric 06C2-
  - Greater Saphenous
    - Left 06CQ-
    - Right 06CP-
  - Hand
    - Left 05CH-
    - Right 05CG-
  - Hemiazygos 05C1-
  - Hepatic 06C4-
  - Hypogastric
    - Left 06CJ-
    - Right 06CH-
  - Inferior Mesenteric 06C6-
  - Innominate
    - Left 05C4-
    - Right 05C3-

Extirpation

Extirpation — *continued*
- Vein — *continued*
  - Internal Jugular
    - Left 05CN-
    - Right 05CM-
  - Intracranial 05CL-
  - Lesser Saphenous
    - Left 06CS-
    - Right 06CR-
  - Lower 06CY-
  - Portal 06C8-
  - Pulmonary
    - Left 02CT-
    - Right 02CS-
  - Renal
    - Left 06CB-
    - Right 06C9-
  - Splenic 06C1-
  - Subclavian
    - Left 05C6-
    - Right 05C5-
  - Superior Mesenteric 06C5-
  - Upper 05CY-
  - Vertebral
    - Left 05CS-
    - Right 05CR-
- Vena Cava
  - Inferior 06C0-
  - Superior 02CV-
- Ventricle
  - Left 02CL-
  - Right 02CK-
- Vertebra
  - Cervical 0PC3-
  - Lumbar 0QC0-
  - Thoracic 0PC4-
- Vesicle
  - Bilateral 0VC3-
  - Left 0VC2-
  - Right 0VC1-
- Vitreous
  - Left 08C5-
  - Right 08C4-
- Vocal Cord
  - Left 0CCV-
  - Right 0CCT-
- Vulva 0UCM-

Extracorporeal shock wave lithotripsy *see* Fragmentation

Extracranial-intracranial bypass (EC-IC) *see* Bypass, Upper Arteries 031-

Extraction
- Auditory Ossicle
  - Left 09DA0ZZ
  - Right 09D90ZZ
- Bone Marrow
  - Iliac 07DR-
  - Sternum 07DQ-
  - Vertebral 07DS-
- Bursa and Ligament
  - Abdomen
    - Left 0MDJ-
    - Right 0MDH-
  - Ankle
    - Left 0MDR-
    - Right 0MDQ-
  - Elbow
    - Left 0MD4-
    - Right 0MD3-
  - Foot
    - Left 0MDT-
    - Right 0MDS-
  - Hand
    - Left 0MD8-
    - Right 0MD7-
  - Head and Neck 0MD0-
  - Hip
    - Left 0MDM-
    - Right 0MDL-

Extraction — *continued*
- Bursa and Ligament — *continued*
  - Knee
    - Left 0MDP-
    - Right 0MDN-
  - Lower Extremity
    - Left 0MDW-
    - Right 0MDV-
  - Perineum 0MDK-
  - Shoulder
    - Left 0MD2-
    - Right 0MD1-
  - Thorax
    - Left 0MDG-
    - Right 0MDF-
  - Trunk
    - Left 0MDD-
    - Right 0MDC-
  - Upper Extremity
    - Left 0MDB-
    - Right 0MD9-
  - Wrist
    - Left 0MD6-
    - Right 0MD5-
- Cerebral Meninges 00D1-
- Cornea
  - Left 08D9XZ-
  - Right 08D8XZ-
- Dura Mater 00D2-
- Endometrium 0UDB-
- Finger Nail 0HDQXZZ
- Hair 0HDSXZZ
- Kidney
  - Left 0TD1-
  - Right 0TD0-
- Lens
  - Left 08DK3ZZ
  - Right 08DJ3ZZ
- Nerve
  - Abdominal Sympathetic 01DM-
  - Abducens 00DL-
  - Accessory 00DR-
  - Acoustic 00DN-
  - Brachial Plexus 01D3-
  - Cervical 01D1-
  - Cervical Plexus 01D0-
  - Facial 00DM-
  - Femoral 01DD-
  - Glossopharyngeal 00DP-
  - Head and Neck Sympathetic 01DK-
  - Hypoglossal 00DS-
  - Lumbar 01DB-
  - Lumbar Plexus 01D9-
  - Lumbar Sympathetic 01DN-
  - Lumbosacral Plexus 01DA-
  - Median 01D5-
  - Oculomotor 00DH-
  - Olfactory 00DF-
  - Optic 00DG-
  - Peroneal 01DH-
  - Phrenic 01D2-
  - Pudendal 01DC-
  - Radial 01D6-
  - Sacral 01DR-
  - Sacral Plexus 01DQ-
  - Sacral Sympathetic 01DP-
  - Sciatic 01DF-
  - Thoracic 01D8-
  - Thoracic Sympathetic 01DL-
  - Tibial 01DG-
  - Trigeminal 00DK-
  - Trochlear 00DJ-
  - Ulnar 01D4-
  - Vagus 00DQ-
- Ova 0UDN-
- Pleura
  - Left 0BDP-
  - Right 0BDN-

Extraction — *continued*
- Products of Conception
  - Classical 10D00Z0
  - Ectopic 10D2-
  - Extraperitoneal 10D00Z2
  - High Forceps 10D07Z5
  - Internal Version 10D07Z7
  - Low Cervical 10D00Z1
  - Low Forceps 10D07Z3
  - Mid Forceps 10D07Z4
  - Other 10D07Z8
  - Retained 10D1-
  - Vacuum 10D07Z6
- Septum, Nasal 09DM-
- Sinus
  - Accessory 09DP-
  - Ethmoid
    - Left 09DV-
    - Right 09DU-
  - Frontal
    - Left 09DT-
    - Right 09DS-
  - Mastoid
    - Left 09DC-
    - Right 09DB-
  - Maxillary
    - Left 09DR-
    - Right 09DQ-
  - Sphenoid
    - Left 09DX-
    - Right 09DW-
- Skin
  - Abdomen 0HD7XZZ
  - Back 0HD6XZZ
  - Buttock 0HD8XZZ
  - Chest 0HD5XZZ
  - Ear
    - Left 0HD3XZZ
    - Right 0HD2XZZ
  - Face 0HD1XZZ
  - Foot
    - Left 0HDNXZZ
    - Right 0HDMXZZ
  - Genitalia 0HDAXZZ
  - Hand
    - Left 0HDGXZZ
    - Right 0HDFXZZ
  - Lower Arm
    - Left 0HDEXZZ
    - Right 0HDDXZZ
  - Lower Leg
    - Left 0HDLXZZ
    - Right 0HDKXZZ
  - Neck 0HD4XZZ
  - Perineum 0HD9XZZ
  - Scalp 0HD0XZZ
  - Upper Arm
    - Left 0HDCXZZ
    - Right 0HDBXZZ
  - Upper Leg
    - Left 0HDJXZZ
    - Right 0HDHXZZ
- Spinal Meninges 00DT-
- Subcutaneous Tissue and Fascia
  - Abdomen 0JD8-
  - Back 0JD7-
  - Buttock 0JD9-
  - Chest 0JD6-
  - Face 0JD1-
  - Foot
    - Left 0JDR-
    - Right 0JDQ-
  - Hand
    - Left 0JDK-
    - Right 0JDJ-
  - Lower Arm
    - Left 0JDH-
    - Right 0JDG-
  - Lower Leg
    - Left 0JDP-
    - Right 0JDN-

Extraction — *continued*
- Subcutaneous Tissue and Fascia — *continued*
  - Neck
    - Anterior 0JD4-
    - Posterior 0JD5-
  - Pelvic Region 0JDC-
  - Perineum 0JDB-
  - Scalp 0JD0-
  - Upper Arm
    - Left 0JDF-
    - Right 0JDD-
  - Upper Leg
    - Left 0JDM-
    - Right 0JDL-
- Toe Nail 0HDRXZZ
- Tooth
  - Lower 0CDXXZ-
  - Upper 0CDWXZ-
- Turbinate, Nasal 09DL-
- Tympanic Membrane
  - Left 09D8-
  - Right 09D7-
- Vein
  - Basilic
    - Left 05DC-
    - Right 05DB-
  - Brachial
    - Left 05DA-
    - Right 05D9-
  - Cephalic
    - Left 05DF-
    - Right 05DD-
  - Femoral
    - Left 06DN-
    - Right 06DM-
  - Foot
    - Left 06DV-
    - Right 06DT-
  - Greater Saphenous
    - Left 06DQ-
    - Right 06DP-
  - Hand
    - Left 05DH-
    - Right 05DG-
  - Lesser Saphenous
    - Left 06DS-
    - Right 06DR-
  - Lower 06DY-
  - Upper 05DY-
- Vocal Cord
  - Left 0CDV-
  - Right 0CDT-

Extradural space, intracranial
use Epidural Space

Extradural space, spinal
use Spinal Canal

EXtreme Lateral Interbody Fusion (XLIF) device
use Interbody Fusion Device in Lower Joints

INDEX TO PROCEDURES – 2016 ICD-10-PCS

F

Face lift see Alteration, Face 0W02-
Facet replacement spinal stabilization device
  use Spinal Stabilization Device, Facet Replacement in 0RH-
  use Spinal Stabilization Device, Facet Replacement in 0SH-
Facial artery
  use Artery, Face
False vocal cord
  use Larynx
Falx cerebri
  use Dura Mater
Fascia lata
  use Subcutaneous Tissue and Fascia, Upper Leg, Left
  use Subcutaneous Tissue and Fascia, Upper Leg, Right
Fasciaplasty, fascioplasty
  see Repair, Subcutaneous Tissue and Fascia 0JQ-
  see Replacement, Subcutaneous Tissue and Fascia 0JR-
Fasciectomy see Excision, Subcutaneous Tissue and Fascia 0JB-
Fasciorrhaphy see Repair, Subcutaneous Tissue and Fascia 0JQ-
Fasciotomy
  see Division, Subcutaneous Tissue and Fascia 0J8-
  see Drainage, Subcutaneous Tissue and Fascia 0J9-
Feeding Device
  Change device in
    Lower 0D2DXUZ
    Upper 0D20XUZ
  Insertion of device in
    Duodenum 0DH9-
    Esophagus 0DH5-
    Ileum 0DHB-
    Intestine, Small 0DH8-
    Jejunum 0DHA-
    Stomach 0DH6-
  Removal of device from
    Esophagus 0DP5-
    Intestinal Tract
      Lower 0DPD-
      Upper 0DP0-
    Stomach 0DP6-
  Revision of device in
    Intestinal Tract
      Lower 0DWD-
      Upper 0DW0-
    Stomach 0DW6-
Femoral head
  use Femur, Upper, Left
  use Femur, Upper, Right
Femoral lymph node
  use Lymphatic, Lower Extremity, Left
  use Lymphatic, Lower Extremity, Right
Femoropatellar joint
  use Joint, Knee, Left
  use Joint, Knee, Right
  use Joint, Knee, Left, Femoral Surface
  use Joint, Knee, Right, Femoral Surface
Femorotibial joint
  use Joint, Knee, Left
  use Joint, Knee, Right
  use Joint, Knee, Left, Tibial Surface
  use Joint, Knee, Right, Tibial Surface
Fibular artery
  use Artery, Peroneal, Left
  use Artery, Peroneal, Right
Fibularis brevis muscle
  use Muscle, Lower Leg, Left
  use Muscle, Lower Leg, Right

Fibularis longus muscle
  use Muscle, Lower Leg, Left
  use Muscle, Lower Leg, Right
Fifth cranial nerve
  use Nerve, Trigeminal
Fimbriectomy
  see Excision, Female Reproductive System 0UB-
  see Resection, Female Reproductive System 0UT-
Fine needle aspiration
  Fluid or gas see Drainage
  Tissue see Excision
First cranial nerve
  use Nerve, Olfactory
First intercostal nerve
  use Nerve, Brachial Plexus
Fistulization
  see Bypass
  see Drainage
  see Repair
Fitting
  Arch bars, for fracture reduction see Reposition, Mouth and Throat 0CS-
  Arch bars, for immobilization see Immobilization, Face 2W31-
  Artificial limb see Device Fitting, Rehabilitation F0D-
  Hearing aid see Device Fitting, Rehabilitation F0D-
  Ocular prosthesis F0DZ8UZ
  Prosthesis, limb see Device Fitting, Rehabilitation F0D-
  Prosthesis, ocular F0DZ8UZ
Fixation, bone
  External, with fracture reduction see Reposition
  External, without fracture reduction see Insertion
  Internal, with fracture reduction see Reposition
  Internal, without fracture reduction see Insertion
FLAIR® Endovascular Stent Graft
  use Intraluminal Device
Flexible Composite Mesh
  use Synthetic Substitute
Flexor carpi radialis muscle
  use Muscle, Lower Arm and Wrist, Left
  use Muscle, Lower Arm and Wrist, Right
Flexor carpi ulnaris muscle
  use Muscle, Lower Arm and Wrist, Left
  use Muscle, Lower Arm and Wrist, Right
Flexor digitorum brevis muscle
  use Muscle, Foot, Left
  use Muscle, Foot, Right
Flexor digitorum longus muscle
  use Muscle, Lower Leg, Left
  use Muscle, Lower Leg, Right
Flexor hallucis brevis muscle
  use Muscle, Foot, Left
  use Muscle, Foot, Right
Flexor hallucis longus muscle
  use Muscle, Lower Leg, Left
  use Muscle, Lower Leg, Right
Flexor pollicis longus muscle
  use Muscle, Lower Arm and Wrist, Left
  use Muscle, Lower Arm and Wrist, Right
Fluoroscopy
  Abdomen and Pelvis BW11-
  Airway, Upper BB1DZZZ
  Ankle
    Left BQ1H-
    Right BQ1G-

Fluoroscopy — continued
  Aorta
    Abdominal B410-
      Laser, Intraoperative B410-
    Thoracic B310-
      Laser, Intraoperative B310-
    Thoraco-Abdominal B31P-
      Laser, Intraoperative B31P-
  Aorta and Bilateral Lower Extremity Arteries B41D-
      Laser, Intraoperative B41D-
  Arm
    Left BP1FZZZ
    Right BP1EZZZ
  Artery
    Brachiocephalic-Subclavian
      Laser, Intraoperative B311-
      Right B311-
    Bronchial B31L-
      Laser, Intraoperative B31L-
    Bypass Graft, Other B21F-
    Cervico-Cerebral Arch B31Q-
      Laser, Intraoperative B31Q-
    Common Carotid
      Bilateral B315-
        Laser, Intraoperative B315-
      Left B314-
        Laser, Intraoperative B314-
      Right B313-
        Laser, Intraoperative B313-
    Coronary
      Bypass Graft
        Multiple B213-
          Laser, Intraoperative B213-
        Single B212-
          Laser, Intraoperative B212-
      Multiple B211-
        Laser, Intraoperative B211-
      Single B210-
        Laser, Intraoperative B210-
    External Carotid
      Bilateral B31C-
        Laser, Intraoperative B31C-
      Left B31B-
        Laser, Intraoperative B31B-
      Right B319-
        Laser, Intraoperative B319-
    Hepatic B412-
      Laser, Intraoperative B412-
    Inferior Mesenteric B415-
      Laser, Intraoperative B415-
    Intercostal B31L-
      Laser, Intraoperative B31L-
    Internal Carotid
      Bilateral B318-
        Laser, Intraoperative B318-
      Left B317-
        Laser, Intraoperative B317-
      Right B316-
        Laser, Intraoperative B316-
    Internal Mammary Bypass Graft
      Left B218-
      Right B217-
    Intra-Abdominal
      Other B41B-
        Laser, Intraoperative B41B-
    Intracranial B31R-
      Laser, Intraoperative B31R-
    Lower
      Other B41J-
        Laser, Intraoperative B41J-
    Lower Extremity
      Bilateral and Aorta B41D-
        Laser, Intraoperative B41D-
      Left B41G-
        Laser, Intraoperative B41G-
      Right B41F-
        Laser, Intraoperative B41F-
    Lumbar B419-
      Laser, Intraoperative B419-
    Pelvic B41C-
      Laser, Intraoperative B41C-

Fluoroscopy — continued
  Artery — continued
    Pulmonary
      Left B31T-
        Laser, Intraoperative B31T-
      Right B31S-
        Laser, Intraoperative B31S-
    Renal
      Bilateral B418-
        Laser, Intraoperative B418-
      Left B417-
        Laser, Intraoperative B417-
      Right B416-
        Laser, Intraoperative B416-
    Spinal B31M-
      Laser, Intraoperative B31M-
    Splenic B413-
      Laser, Intraoperative B413-
    Subclavian
      Left B312-
        Laser, Intraoperative B312-
    Superior Mesenteric B414-
      Laser, Intraoperative B414-
    Upper
      Laser, Intraoperative B31N-
      Other B31N-
    Upper Extremity
      Bilateral B31K-
        Laser, Intraoperative B31K-
      Left B31J-
        Laser, Intraoperative B31J-
      Right B31H-
        Laser, Intraoperative B31H-
    Vertebral
      Bilateral B31G-
        Laser, Intraoperative B31G-
      Left B31F-
        Laser, Intraoperative B31F-
      Right B31D-
        Laser, Intraoperative B31D-
  Bile Duct BF10-
    Pancreatic Duct and Gallbladder BF14-
  Bile Duct and Gallbladder BF13-
  Biliary Duct BF11-
  Bladder BT10-
    Kidney and Ureter BT14-
    Left BT1F-
    Right BT1D-
  Bladder and Urethra BT1B-
  Bowel, Small BD1-
  Calcaneus
    Left BQ1KZZZ
    Right BQ1JZZZ
  Clavicle
    Left BP15ZZZ
    Right BP14ZZZ
  Coccyx BR1F-
  Colon BD14-
  Corpora Cavernosa BV10-
  Dialysis Fistula B51W-
  Dialysis Shunt B51W-
  Diaphragm BB16ZZZ-
  Disc
    Cervical BR11-
    Lumbar BR13-
    Thoracic BR12-
  Duodenum BD19-
  Elbow
    Left BP1H-
    Right BP1G-
  Epiglottis B91G-
  Esophagus BD11-
  Extremity
    Lower BW1C-
    Upper BW1J-
  Facet Joint
    Cervical BR14-
    Lumbar BR16-
    Thoracic BR15-

Fluoroscopy — continued
  Fallopian Tube
    Bilateral **BU12-**
    Left **BU11-**
    Right **BU10-**
  Fallopian Tube and Uterus **BU18-**
  Femur
    Left **BQ14ZZZ**
    Right **BQ13ZZZ**
  Finger
    Left **BP1SZZZ**
    Right **BP1RZZZ**
  Foot
    Left **BQ1MZZZ**
    Right **BQ1LZZZ**
  Forearm
    Left **BP1KZZZ**
    Right **BP1JZZZ**
  Gallbladder **BF12-**
    Bile Duct and Pancreatic Duct **BF14-**
  Gallbladder and Bile Duct **BF13-**
  Gastrointestinal, Upper **BD1-**
  Hand
    Left **BP1PZZZ**
    Right **BP1NZZZ**
  Head and Neck **BW19-**
  Heart
    Left **B215-**
    Right **B214-**
    Right and Left **B216-**
  Hip
    Left **BQ11-**
    Right **BQ10-**
  Humerus
    Left **BP1BZZZ**
    Right **BP1AZZZ**
  Ileal Diversion Loop **BT1C-**
  Ileal Loop, Ureters and Kidney **BT1G-**
  Intracranial Sinus **B512-**
  Joint
    Acromioclavicular, Bilateral **BP13ZZZ**
    Finger
      Left **BP1D-**
      Right **BP1C-**
    Foot
      Left **BQ1Y-**
      Right **BQ1X-**
    Hand
      Left **BP1D-**
      Right **BP1C-**
    Lumbosacral **BR1B-**
    Sacroiliac **BR1D-**
    Sternoclavicular
      Bilateral **BP12ZZZ**
      Left **BP11ZZZ**
      Right **BP10ZZZ**
    Temporomandibular
      Bilateral **BN19-**
      Left **BN18-**
      Right **BN17-**
    Thoracolumbar **BR18-**
    Toe
      Left **BQ1Y-**
      Right **BQ1X-**
  Kidney
    Bilateral **BT13-**
    Ileal Loop and Ureter **BT1G-**
    Left **BT12-**
    Right **BT11-**
    Ureter and Bladder **BT14-**
      Left **BT1F-**
      Right **BT1D-**
  Knee
    Left **BQ18-**
    Right **BQ17-**
  Larynx **B91J-**
  Leg
    Left **BQ1FZZZ**
    Right **BQ1DZZZ**

Fluoroscopy — continued
  Lung
    Bilateral **BB14ZZZ**
    Left **BB13ZZZ**
    Right **BB12ZZZ**
  Mediastinum **BB1CZZZ**
  Mouth **BD1B-**
  Neck and Head **BW19-**
  Oropharynx **BD1B-**
  Pancreatic Duct **BF1-**
    Gallbladder and Bile Duct **BF14-**
  Patella
    Left **BQ1WZZZ**
    Right **BQ1VZZZ**
  Pelvis **BR1C-**
  Pelvis and Abdomen **BW11-**
  Pharynix **B91G-**
  Ribs
    Left **BP1YZZZ**
    Right **BP1XZZZ**
  Sacrum **BR1F-**
  Scapula
    Left **BP17ZZZ**
    Right **BP16ZZZ**
  Shoulder
    Left **BP19-**
    Right **BP18-**
  Sinus, Intracranial **B512-**
  Spinal Cord **B01B-**
  Spine
    Cervical **BR10-**
    Lumbar **BR19-**
    Thoracic **BR17-**
    Whole **BR1G-**
  Sternum **BR1H-**
  Stomach **BD12-**
  Toe
    Left **BQ1QZZZ**
    Right **BQ1PZZZ**
  Tracheobronchial Tree
    Bilateral **BB19YZZ**
    Left **BB18YZZ**
    Right **BB17YZZ**
  Ureter
    Ileal Loop and Kidney **BT1G-**
    Kidney and Bladder **BT14-**
      Left **BT1F-**
      Right **BT1D-**
    Left **BT17-**
    Right **BT16-**
  Urethra **BT15-**
  Urethra and Bladder **BT1B-**
  Uterus **BU16-**
  Uterus and Fallopian Tube **BU18-**
  Vagina **BU19-**
  Vasa Vasorum **BV18-**
  Vein
    Cerebellar **B511-**
    Cerebral **B511-**
    Epidural **B510-**
    Jugular Bilateral **B515-**
      Left **B514-**
      Right **B513-**
    Lower Extremity
      Bilateral **B51D-**
      Left **B51C-**
      Right **B51B-**
    Other **B51V-**
    Pelvic (Iliac)
      Left **B51G-**
      Right **B51F-**
    Pelvic (Iliac) Bilateral **B51H-**
    Portal **B51T-**
    Pulmonary
      Bilateral **B51S-**
      Left **B51R-**
      Right **B51Q-**
    Renal
      Bilateral **B51L-**
      Left **B51K-**
      Right **B51J-**
    Spanchnic **B51T-**

Fluoroscopy — continued
  Vein — continued
    Subclavian
      Left **B517-**
      Right **B516-**
    Upper Extremity
      Bilateral **B51P-**
      Left **B51N-**
      Right **B51M-**
    Vena Cava
      Inferior **B519-**
      Superior **B518-**
  Wrist
    Left **BP1M-**
    Right **BP1L-**
Fluoroscopy, laser intraoperative
  see Fluoroscopy, Heart **B21-**
  see Fluoroscopy, Lower Arteries **B41-**
  see Fluoroscopy, Upper Arteries **B31-**
Flushing *see* Irrigation
Foley catheter
  use Drainage Device
Foramen magnum
  use Bone, Occipital, Left
  use Bone, Occipital, Right
Foramen of Monro (intraventricular)
  use Cerebral Ventricle
Foreskin
  use Prepuce
Formula™ Balloon-Expandable Renal Stent System
  use Intraluminal Device
Fossa of Rosenmuller
  use Nasopharynx
Fourth cranial nerve
  use Nerve, Trochlear
Fourth ventricle
  use Cerebral Ventricle
Fovea
  use Retina, Left
  use Retina, Right
Fragmentation
  Ampulla of Vater **0FFC-**
  Anus **0DFQ-**
  Appendix **0DFJ-**
  Bladder **0TFB-**
  Bladder Neck **0TFC-**
  Bronchus
    Lingula **0BF9-**
    Lower Lobe
      Left **0BFB-**
      Right **0BF6-**
    Main
      Left **0BF7-**
      Right **0BF3-**
    Middle Lobe, Right **0BF5-**
    Upper Lobe
      Left **0BF8-**
      Right **0BF4-**
  Carina **0BF2-**
  Cavity, Cranial **0WF1-**
  Cecum **0DFH-**
  Cerebral Ventricle **00F6-**
  Colon
    Ascending **0DFK-**
    Descending **0DFM-**
    Sigmoid **0DFN-**
    Transverse **0DFL-**
  Duct
    Common Bile **0FF9-**
    Cystic **0FF8-**
    Hepatic
      Left **0FF6-**
      Right **0FF5-**
    Pancreatic **0FFD-**
      Accessory **0FFF-**
    Parotid
      Left **0CFC-**
      Right **0CFB-**
  Duodenum **0DF9-**
  Epidural Space **00F3-**

Fragmentation — continued
  Esophagus **0DF5-**
  Fallopian Tube
    Left **0UF6-**
    Right **0UF5-**
  Fallopian Tubes, Bilateral **0UF7-**
  Gallbladder **0FF4-**
  Gastrointestinal Tract **0WFP-**
  Genitourinary Tract **0WFR-**
  Ileum **0DFB-**
  Intestine
    Large **0DFE-**
      Left **0DFG-**
      Right **0DFF-**
    Small **0DF8-**
  Jejunum **0DFA-**
  Kidney Pelvis
    Left **0TF4-**
    Right **0TF3-**
  Mediastinum **0WFC-**
  Oral Cavity and Throat **0WF3-**
  Pelvic Cavity **0WFJ-**
  Pericardial Cavity **0WFD-**
  Pericardium **02FN-**
  Peritoneal Cavity **0WFG-**
  Pleural Cavity
    Left **0WFB-**
    Right **0WF9-**
  Rectum **0DFP-**
  Respiratory Tract **0WFQ-**
  Spinal Canal **00FU-**
  Stomach **0DF6-**
  Subarachnoid Space **00F5-**
  Subdural Space **00F4-**
  Trachea **0BF1-**
  Ureter
    Left **0TF7-**
    Right **0TF6-**
  Urethra **0TFD-**
  Uterus **0UF9-**
  Vitreous
    Left **08F5-**
    Right **08F4-**
Freestyle (Stentless) Aortic Root Bioprosthesis
  use Zooplastic Tissue in Heart and Great Vessels
Frenectomy
  see Excision, Mouth and Throat **0CB-**
  see Resection, Mouth and Throat **0CT-**
Frenoplasty, frenuloplasty
  see Repair, Mouth and Throat **0CQ-**
  see Replacement, Mouth and Throat **0CR-**
  see Supplement, Mouth and Throat **0CU-**
Frenotomy
  see Drainage, Mouth and Throat **0C9-**
  see Release, Mouth and Throat **0CN-**
Frenulotomy
  see Drainage, Mouth and Throat **0C9-**
  see Release, Mouth and Throat **0CN-**
Frenulum labii inferioris
  use Lip, Lower
Frenulum labii superioris
  use Lip, Upper
Frenulum linguae
  use Tongue
Frenulumectomy
  see Excision, Mouth and Throat **0CB-**
  see Resection, Mouth and Throat **0CT-**
Frontal lobe
  use Cerebral Hemisphere
Frontal vein
  use Vein, Face, Left
  use Vein, Face, Right

Fulguration see Destruction
Fundoplication, gastroesophageal see Restriction, Esophagogastric Junction 0DV4-
Fundus uteri
 use Uterus
Fusion
 Acromioclavicular
  Left 0RGH-
  Right 0RGG-
 Ankle
  Left 0SGG-
  Right 0SGF-
 Carpal
  Left 0RGR-
  Right 0RGQ-
 Cervical Vertebral 0RG1-
  2 or more 0RG2-
 Cervicothoracic Vertebral 0RG4-
 Coccygeal 0SG6-
 Elbow
  Left 0RGM-
  Right 0RGL-
 Finger Phalangeal
  Left 0RGX-
  Right 0RGW-
 Hip
  Left 0SGB-
  Right 0SG9-
 Knee
  Left 0SGD-
  Right 0SGC-
 Lumbar Vertebral 0SG0-
  2 or more 0SG1-
 Lumbosacral 0SG3-
 Metacarpocarpal
  Left 0RGT-
  Right 0RGS-
 Metacarpophalangeal
  Left 0RGV-
  Right 0RGU-
 Metatarsal-Phalangeal
  Left 0SGN-
  Right 0SGM-
 Metatarsal-Tarsal
  Left 0SGL-
  Right 0SGK-
 Occipital-cervical 0RG0-
 Sacrococcygeal 0SG5-
 Sacroiliac
  Left 0SG8-
  Right 0SG7-
 Shoulder
  Left 0RGK-
  Right 0RGJ-
 Sternoclavicular
  Left 0RGF-
  Right 0RGE-
 Tarsal
  Left 0SGJ-
  Right 0SGH-
 Temporomandibular
  Left 0RGD-
  Right 0RGC-
 Thoracic Vertebral 0RG6-
  2 to 7 0RG7-
  8 or more 0RG8-
 Thoracolumbar Vertebral 0RGA-
 Toe Phalangeal
  Left 0SGQ-
  Right 0SGP-
 Wrist
  Left 0RGP-
  Right 0RGN-
Fusion screw (compression) (lag) (locking)
 use Internal Fixation Device in Lower Joints
 use Internal Fixation Device in Upper Joints

G

Gait training see Motor Treatment, Rehabilitation F07-
Galea aponeurotica
 use Subcutaneous Tissue and Fascia, Scalp
Ganglion impar (ganglion of Walther)
 use Nerve, Sacral Sympathetic
Ganglionectomy
 Destruction of lesion see Destruction
 Excision of lesion see Excision
Gasserian ganglion
 use Nerve, Trigeminal
Gastrectomy
 Partial see Excision, Stomach 0DB6-
 Total see Resection, Stomach 0DT6-
 Vertical (sleeve) see Excision, Stomach 0DB6-
Gastric electrical stimulation (GES) lead
 use Stimulator Lead in Gastrointestinal System
Gastric lymph node
 use Lymphatic, Aortic
Gastric pacemaker lead
 use Stimulator Lead in Gastrointestinal System
Gastric plexus
 use Nerve, Abdominal Sympathetic
Gastrocnemius muscle
 use Muscle, Lower Leg, Left
 use Muscle, Lower Leg, Right
Gastrocolic ligament
 use Omentum, Greater
Gastrocolic omentum
 use Omentum, Greater
Gastrocolostomy
 see Bypass, Gastrointestinal System 0D1-
 see Drainage, Gastrointestinal System 0D9-
Gastroduodenal artery
 use Artery, Hepatic
Gastroduodenectomy
 see Excision, Gastrointestinal System 0DB-
 see Resection, Gastrointestinal System 0DT-
Gastroduodenoscopy 0DJ08ZZ
Gastroenteroplasty
 see Repair, Gastrointestinal System 0DQ-
 see Supplement, Gastrointestinal System 0DU-
Gastroenterostomy
 see Bypass, Gastrointestinal System 0D1-
 see Drainage, Gastrointestinal System 0D9-
Gastroesophageal (GE) junction
 use Esophagogastric Junction
Gastrogastrostomy
 see Bypass, Stomach 0D16-
 see Drainage, Stomach 0D96-
Gastrohepatic omentum
 use Omentum, Lesser
Gastrojejunostomy
 see Bypass, Stomach 0D16-
 see Drainage, Stomach 0D96-
Gastrolysis see Release, Stomach 0DN6-
Gastropexy
 see Repair, Stomach 0DQ6-
 see Reposition, Stomach 0DS6-
Gastrophrenic ligament
 use Omentum, Greater
Gastroplasty
 see Repair, Stomach 0DQ6-
 see Supplement, Stomach 0DU6-
Gastroplication see Restriction, Stomach 0DV6-
Gastropylorectomy see Excision, Gastrointestinal System 0DB-
Gastrorrhaphy see Repair, Stomach 0DQ6-
Gastroscopy 0DJ68ZZ
Gastrosplenic ligament
 use Omentum, Greater
Gastrostomy
 see Bypass, Stomach 0D16-
 see Drainage, Stomach 0D96-
Gastrotomy see Drainage, Stomach 0D96-
Gemellus muscle
 use Muscle, Hip, Left
 use Muscle, Hip, Right
Geniculate ganglion
 use Nerve, Facial
Geniculate nucleus
 use Thalamus
Genioglossus muscle
 use Muscle, Tongue, Palate, Pharynx
Genioplasty see Alteration, Jaw, Lower 0W05-
Genitofemoral nerve
 use Nerve, Lumbar Plexus
Gingivectomy see Excision, Mouth and Throat 0CB-
Gingivoplasty
 see Repair, Mouth and Throat 0CQ-
 see Replacement, Mouth and Throat 0CR-
 see Supplement, Mouth and Throat 0CU-
Glans penis
 use Prepuce
Glenohumeral joint
 use Joint, Shoulder, Left
 use Joint, Shoulder, Right
Glenohumeral ligament
 use Bursa and Ligament, Shoulder, Left
 use Bursa and Ligament, Shoulder, Right
Glenoid fossa (of scapula)
 use Glenoid Cavity, Left
 use Glenoid Cavity, Right
Glenoid ligament (labrum)
 use Shoulder Joint, Left
 use Shoulder Joint, Right
Globus pallidus
 use Basal Ganglia
Glomectomy
 see Excision, Endocrine System 0GB-
 see Resection, Endocrine System 0GT-
Glossectomy
 see Excision, Tongue 0CB7-
 see Resection, Tongue 0CT7-
Glossoepiglottic fold
 use Epiglottis
Glossopexy
 see Repair, Tongue 0CQ7-
 see Reposition, Tongue 0CS7-
Glossoplasty
 see Repair, Tongue 0CQ7-
 see Replacement, Tongue 0CR7-
 see Supplement, Tongue 0CU7-
Glossorrhaphy see Repair, Tongue 0CQ7-
Glossotomy see Drainage, Tongue 0C97-
Glottis
 use Larynx
Gluteal Artery Perforator Flap
 Bilateral 0HRV079
 Left 0HRU079
 Right 0HRT079

Gluteal lymph node
 use Lymphatic, Pelvis
Gluteal vein
 use Vein, Hypogastric, Left
 use Vein, Hypogastric, Right
Gluteus maximus muscle
 use Muscle, Hip, Left
 use Muscle, Hip, Right
Gluteus medius muscle
 use Muscle, Hip, Left
 use Muscle, Hip, Right
Gluteus minimus muscle
 use Muscle, Hip, Left
 use Muscle, Hip, Right
GORE® DUALMESH®
 use Synthetic Substitute
Gracilis muscle
 use Muscle, Upper Leg, Left
 use Muscle, Upper Leg, Right
Graft
 see Replacement
 see Supplement
Great auricular nerve
 use Nerve, Cervical Plexus
Great cerebral vein
 use Vein, Intracranial
Great saphenous vein
 use Vein, Greater Saphenous, Left
 use Vein, Greater Saphenous, Right
Greater alar cartilage
 use Nose
Greater occipital nerve
 use Nerve, Cervical
Greater splanchnic nerve
 use Nerve, Thoracic Sympathetic
Greater superficial petrosal nerve
 use Nerve, Facial
Greater trochanter
 use Femur, Upper, Left
 use Femur, Upper, Right
Greater tuberosity
 use Humeral Head, Left
 use Humeral Head, Right
Greater vestibular (Bartholin's) gland
 use Gland, Vestibular
Greater wing
 use Bone, Sphenoid, Left
 use Bone, Sphenoid, Right
Guedel airway
 use Intraluminal Device, Airway in Mouth and Throat
Guidance, catheter placement
 EKG see Measurement, Physiological Systems 4A0-
 Fluoroscopy see Fluoroscopy, Veins B51-
 Ultrasound see Ultrasonography, Veins B54-

Hallux INDEX TO PROCEDURES – 2016 ICD-10-PCS [2016.PCS]

H

Hallux
use Toe, 1st, Left
use Toe, 1st, Right
Hamate bone
use Carpal, Left
use Carpal, Right
Hancock Bioprosthesis (aortic) (mitral) valve
use Zooplastic Tissue in Heart and Great Vessels
Hancock Bioprosthetic Valved Conduit
use Zooplastic Tissue in Heart and Great Vessels
Harvesting, stem cells see Pheresis, Circulatory 6A55-
Head of fibula
use Fibula, Left
use Fibula, Right
Hearing Aid Assessment F14Z-
Hearing Assessment F13Z-
Hearing Device
Bone Conduction
Left 09HE-
Right 09HD-
Insertion of device in
Left 0NH6-
Right 0NH5-
Multiple Channel Cochlear Prosthesis
Left 09HE-
Right 09HD-
Removal of device from, Skull 0NP0-
Revision of device in, Skull 0NW0-
Single Channel Cochlear Prosthesis
Left 09HE-
Right 09HD-
Hearing Treatment F09Z-
Heart Assist System
External
Insertion of device in, Heart 02HA-
Removal of device from, Heart 02PA-
Revision of device in, Heart 02WA-
Implantable
Insertion of device in, Heart 02HA-
Removal of device from, Heart 02PA-
Revision of device in, Heart 02WA-
HeartMate II® Left Ventricular Assist Device (LVAD)
use Implantable Heart Assist System in Heart and Great Vessels
HeartMate XVE® Left Ventricular Assist Device (LVAD)
use Implantable Heart Assist System in Heart and Great Vessels
HeartMate® implantable heart assist system see Insertion of device in, Heart 02HA-
Helix
use Ear, External, Bilateral
use Ear, External, Left
use Ear, External, Right
Hemicolectomy see Resection, Gastrointestinal System 0DT-
Hemicystectomy see Excision, Urinary System 0TB-
Hemigastrectomy see Excision, Gastrointestinal System 0DB-
Hemiglossectomy see Excision, Mouth and Throat 0CB-
Hemilaminectomy
see Excision, Lower Bones 0QB-
see Excision, Upper Bones 0PB-

Hemilaminotomy
see Drainage, Lower Bones 0Q9-
see Drainage, Upper Bones 0P9-
see Excision, Lower Bones 0QB-
see Excision, Upper Bones 0PB-
see Release, Central Nervous System 00N-
see Release, Lower Bones 0QN-
see Release, Peripheral Nervous System 01N-
see Release, Upper Bones 0PN-
Hemilaryngectomy see Excision, Larynx 0CBS-
Hemimandibulectomy see Excision, Head and Facial Bones 0NB-
Hemimaxillectomy see Excision, Head and Facial Bones 0NB-
Hemipylorectomy see Excision, Gastrointestinal System 0DB-
Hemispherectomy
see Excision, Central Nervous System 00B-
see Resection, Central Nervous System 00T-
Hemithyroidectomy
see Excision, Endocrine System 0GB-
see Resection, Endocrine System 0GT-
Hemodialysis 5A1D00Z
Hepatectomy
see Excision, Hepatobiliary System and Pancreas 0FB-
see Resection, Hepatobiliary System and Pancreas 0FT-
Hepatic artery proper
use Artery, Hepatic
Hepatic flexure
use Colon, Ascending
Hepatic lymph node
use Lymphatic, Aortic
Hepatic plexus
use Nerve, Abdominal Sympathetic
Hepatic portal vein
use Vein, Portal
Hepaticoduodenostomy
see Bypass, Hepatobiliary System and Pancreas 0F1-
see Drainage, Hepatobiliary System and Pancreas 0F9-
Hepaticotomy see Drainage, Hepatobiliary System and Pancreas 0F9-
Hepatocholedochostomy see Drainage, Duct, Common Bile 0F99-
Hepatogastric ligament
use Omentum, Lesser
Hepatopancreatic ampulla
use Ampulla of Vater
Hepatopexy
see Repair, Hepatobiliary System and Pancreas 0FQ-
see Reposition, Hepatobiliary System and Pancreas 0FS-
Hepatorrhaphy see Repair, Hepatobiliary System and Pancreas 0FQ-
Hepatotomy see Drainage, Hepatobiliary System and Pancreas 0F9-
Herculink (RX) Elite Renal Stent System
use Intraluminal Device

Herniorrhaphy
see Repair, Anatomical Regions, General 0WQ-
see Repair, Anatomical Regions, Lower Extremities 0YQ-
With synthetic substitute
see Supplement, Anatomical Regions, General 0WU-
see Supplement, Anatomical Regions, Lower Extremities 0YU-
Hip (joint) liner
use Liner in Lower Joints
Holter monitoring 4A12X45
Holter valve ventricular shunt
use Synthetic Substitute
Humeroradial joint
use Joint, Elbow, Left
use Joint, Elbow, Right
Humeroulnar joint
use Joint, Elbow, Left
use Joint, Elbow, Right
Humerus, distal
use Humeral Shaft, Left
use Humeral Shaft, Right
Hydrocelectomy see Excision, Male Reproductive System 0VB-
Hydrotherapy
Assisted exercise in pool see Motor Treatment, Rehabilitation F07-
Whirlpool see Activities of Daily Living Treatment, Rehabilitation F08-
Hymenectomy
see Excision, Hymen 0UBK-
see Resection, Hymen 0UTK-
Hymenoplasty
see Repair, Hymen 0UQK-
see Supplement, Hymen 0UUK-
Hymenorrhaphy see Repair, Hymen 0UQK-
Hymenotomy
see Division, Hymen 0U8K-
see Drainage, Hymen 0U9K-
Hyoglossus muscle
use Muscle, Tongue, Palate, Pharynx
Hyoid artery
use Artery, Thyroid, Left
use Artery, Thyroid, Right
Hyperalimentation see Introduction of substance in or on
Hyperbaric oxygenation
Decompression sickness treatment see Decompression, Circulatory 6A15-
Wound treatment see Assistance, Circulatory 5A05-
Hyperthermia
Radiation Therapy
Abdomen DWY38ZZ
Adrenal Gland DGY28ZZ
Bile Ducts DFY28ZZ
Bladder DTY28ZZ
Bone, Other DPYC8ZZ
Bone Marrow D7Y08ZZ
Brain D0Y08ZZ
Brain Stem D0Y18ZZ
Breast
Left DMY08ZZ
Right DMY18ZZ
Bronchus DBY18ZZ
Cervix DUY18ZZ
Chest DWY28ZZ
Chest Wall DBY78ZZ
Colon DDY58ZZ
Diaphragm DBY88ZZ
Duodenum DDY28ZZ
Ear D9Y08ZZ
Esophagus DDY08ZZ
Eye D8Y08ZZ
Femur DPY98ZZ
Fibula DPYB8ZZ
Gallbladder DFY18ZZ

Hyperthermia — continued
Radiation Therapy — continued
Gland
Adrenal DGY28ZZ
Parathyroid DGY48ZZ
Pituitary DGY08ZZ
Thyroid DGY58ZZ
Glands, Salivary D9Y68ZZ
Head and Neck DWY18ZZ
Hemibody DWY48ZZ
Humerus DPY68ZZ
Hypopharynx D9Y38ZZ
Ileum DDY48ZZ
Jejunum DDY38ZZ
Kidney DTY08ZZ
Larynx D9YB8ZZ
Liver DFY08ZZ
Lung DBY28ZZ
Lymphatics
Abdomen D7Y68ZZ
Axillary D7Y48ZZ
Inguinal D7Y88ZZ
Neck D7Y38ZZ
Pelvis D7Y78ZZ
Thorax D7Y58ZZ
Mandible DPY38ZZ
Maxilla DPY28ZZ
Mediastinum DBY68ZZ
Mouth D9Y48ZZ
Nasopharynx D9YD8ZZ
Neck and Head DWY18ZZ
Nerve, Peripheral D0Y78ZZ
Nose D9Y18ZZ
Oropharynx D9YF8ZZ
Ovary DUY08ZZ
Palate
Hard D9Y88ZZ
Soft D9Y98ZZ
Pancreas DFY38ZZ
Parathyroid Gland DGY48ZZ
Pelvic Bones DPY88ZZ
Pelvic Region DWY68ZZ
Pineal Body DGY18ZZ
Pituitary Gland DGY08ZZ
Pleura DBY58ZZ
Prostate DVY08ZZ
Radius DPY78ZZ
Rectum DDY78ZZ
Rib DPY58ZZ
Sinuses D9Y78ZZ
Skin
Abdomen DHY88ZZ
Arm DHY48ZZ
Back DHY78ZZ
Buttock DHY98ZZ
Chest DHY68ZZ
Face DHY28ZZ
Leg DHYB8ZZ
Neck DHY38ZZ
Skull DPY08ZZ
Spinal Cord D0Y68ZZ
Spleen D7Y28ZZ
Sternum DPY48ZZ
Stomach DDY18ZZ
Testis DVY18ZZ
Thymus D7Y18ZZ
Thyroid Gland DGY58ZZ
Tibia DPYB8ZZ
Tongue D9Y58ZZ
Trachea DBY08ZZ
Ulna DPY78ZZ
Ureter DTY18ZZ
Urethra DTY38ZZ
Uterus DUY28ZZ
Whole Body DWY58ZZ
Whole Body 6A3Z-
Hypnosis GZFZZZZ
Hypogastric artery
use Artery, Internal Iliac, Left
use Artery, Internal Iliac, Right
Hypopharynx
use Pharynx

32

Hypophysectomy
 see Excision, Gland, Pituitary **0GB0-**
 see Resection, Gland, Pituitary **0GT0-**
Hypophysis
 use Gland, Pituitary
Hypothalamotomy see Destruction, Thalamus **0059-**
Hypothenar muscle
 use Muscle, Hand, Left
 use Muscle, Hand, Right
Hypothermia, Whole Body 6A4Z-
Hysterectomy
 Supracervical
  see Resection, Uterus **0UT9-**
 Total
  see Resection, Cervix **0UTC-**
  see Resection, Uterus **0UT9-**
Hysterolysis see Release, Uterus **0UN9-**
Hysteropexy
 see Repair, Uterus **0UQ9-**
 see Reposition, Uterus **0US9-**
Hysteroplasty see Repair, Uterus **0UQ9-**
Hysterorrhaphy see Repair, Uterus **0UQ9-**
Hysteroscopy 0UJD8ZZ
Hysterotomy see Drainage, Uterus **0U99-**
Hysterotrachelectomy
 see Resection, Cervix **0UTC-**
 see Resection, Uterus **0UT9-**
Hysterotracheloplasty see Repair, Uterus **0UQ9-**
Hysterotrachelorrhaphy see Repair, Uterus **0UQ9-**

IABP (Intra-aortic balloon pump)
 see Assistance, Cardiac **5A02-**
IAEMT (Intraoperative anesthetic effect monitoring and titration) see Monitoring, Central Nervous **4A10-**
Idarucizumab, Dabigatran reversal agent XW0-
Ileal artery
 use Artery, Superior Mesenteric
Ileectomy
 see Excision, Ileum **0DBB-**
 see Resection, Ileum **0DTB-**
Ileocolic artery
 use Artery, Superior Mesenteric
Ileocolic vein
 use Vein, Colic
Ileopexy
 see Repair, Ileum **0DQB-**
 see Reposition, Ileum **0DSB-**
Ileorrhaphy see Repair, Ileum **0DQB-**
Ileoscopy 0DJD8ZZ
Ileostomy
 see Bypass, Ileum **0D1B-**
 see Drainage, Ileum **0D9B-**
Ileotomy see Drainage, Ileum **0D9B-**
Ileoureterostomy see Bypass, Urinary System **0T1-**
Iliac crest
 use Bone, Pelvic, Left
 use Bone, Pelvic, Right
Iliac fascia
 use Subcutaneous Tissue and Fascia, Upper Leg, Left
 use Subcutaneous Tissue and Fascia, Upper Leg, Right
Iliac lymph node
 use Lymphatic, Pelvis
Iliacus muscle
 use Muscle, Hip, Left
 use Muscle, Hip, Right
Iliofemoral ligament
 use Bursa and Ligament, Hip, Left
 use Bursa and Ligament, Hip, Right
Iliohypogastric nerve
 use Nerve, Lumbar Plexus
Ilioinguinal nerve
 use Nerve, Lumbar Plexus
Iliolumbar artery
 use Artery, Internal Iliac, Left
 use Artery, Internal Iliac, Right
Iliolumbar ligament
 use Bursa and Ligament, Trunk, Left
 use Bursa and Ligament, Trunk, Right
Iliotibial tract (band)
 use Subcutaneous Tissue and Fascia, Upper Leg, Left
 use Subcutaneous Tissue and Fascia, Upper Leg, Right
Ilium
 use Bone, Pelvic, Left
 use Bone, Pelvic, Right
Ilizarov external fixator
 use External Fixation Device, Ring in **0PH-**
 use External Fixation Device, Ring in **0PS-**
 use External Fixation Device, Ring in **0QH-**
 use External Fixation Device, Ring in **0QS-**
Ilizarov-Vecklich device
 use External Fixation Device, Limb Lengthening in **0PH-**
 use External Fixation Device, Limb Lengthening in **0QH-**

Imaging, diagnostic
 see Computerized Tomography (CT Scan)
 see Fluoroscopy
 see Magnetic Resonance Imaging (MRI)
 see Plain Radiography
 see Ultrasonography
Immobilization
 Abdominal Wall **2W33X-**
 Arm
  Lower
   Left **2W3DX-**
   Right **2W3CX-**
  Upper
   Left **2W3BX-**
   Right **2W3AX-**
 Back **2W35X-**
 Chest Wall **2W34X-**
 Extremity
  Lower
   Left **2W3MX-**
   Right **2W3LX-**
  Upper
   Left **2W39X-**
   Right **2W38X-**
 Face **2W31X-**
 Finger
  Left **2W3KX-**
  Right **2W3JX-**
 Foot
  Left **2W3TX-**
  Right **2W3SX-**
 Hand
  Left **2W3FX-**
  Right **2W3EX-**
 Head **2W30X-**
 Inguinal Region
  Left **2W37X-**
  Right **2W36X-**
 Leg
  Lower
   Left **2W3RX-**
   Right **2W3QX-**
  Upper
   Left **2W3PX-**
   Right **2W3NX-**
 Neck **2W32X-**
 Thumb
  Left **2W3HX-**
  Right **2W3GX-**
 Toe
  Left **2W3VX-**
  Right **2W3UX-**
Immunization see Introduction of Serum, Toxoid, and Vaccine
Immunotherapy see Introduction of Immunotherapeutic Substance
Immunotherapy, antineoplastic
 Interferon see Introduction of Low-dose Interleukin-2
 Interleukin-2, high-dose see Introduction of High-dose Interleukin-2
 Interleukin-2, low-dose see Introduction of Low-dose Interleukin-2
 Monoclonal antibody see Introduction of Monoclonal Antibody
 Proleukin, high-dose see Introduction of High-dose Interleukin-2
 Proleukin, low-dose see Introduction of Low-dose Interleukin-2
Impeller Pump
 Continuous, Output **5A0221D**
 Intermittent, Output **5A0211D**
Implantable cardioverter-defibrillator (ICD)
 use Defibrillator Generator in **0JH-**

Implantable drug infusion pump (anti-spasmodic) (chemotherapy) (pain)
 use Infusion Device, Pump in Subcutaneous Tissue and Fascia
Implantable gastric pacemaker generator
 use Stimulator Generator in Subcutaneous Tissue and Fascia
Implantable glucose monitoring device
 use Monitoring Device
Implantable hemodynamic monitor (IHM)
 use Monitoring Device, Hemodynamic in **0JH-**
Implantable hemodynamic monitoring system (IHMS)
 use Monitoring Device, Hemodynamic in **0JH-**
Implantable Miniature Telescope™ (IMT)
 use Synthetic Substitute, Intraocular Telescope in **08R-**
Implantation
 see Insertion
 see Replacement
Implanted (venous) (access) port
 use Vascular Access Device, Reservoir in Subcutaneous Tissue and Fascia
IMV (intermittent mandatory ventilation) see Assistance, Respiratory **5A09-**
In Vitro Fertilization 8E0ZXY1
Incision, abscess see Drainage
Incudectomy
 see Excision, Ear, Nose, Sinus **09B-**
 see Resection, Ear, Nose, Sinus **09T-**
Incudopexy
 see Repair, Ear, Nose, Sinus **09Q-**
 see Reposition, Ear, Nose, Sinus **09S-**
Incus
 use Auditory Ossicle, Left
 use Auditory Ossicle, Right
Induction of labor
 Artificial rupture of membranes see Drainage, Pregnancy **109-**
 Oxytocin see Introduction of Hormone
InDura, intrathecal catheter (1P) (spinal)
 use Infusion Device
Inferior cardiac nerve
 use Nerve, Thoracic Sympathetic
Inferior cerebellar vein
 use Vein, Intracranial
Inferior cerebral vein
 use Vein, Intracranial
Inferior epigastric artery
 use Artery, External Iliac, Left
 use Artery, External Iliac, Right
Inferior epigastric lymph node
 use Lymphatic, Pelvis
Inferior genicular artery
 use Artery, Popliteal, Left
 use Artery, Popliteal, Right
Inferior gluteal artery
 use Artery, Internal Iliac, Left
 use Artery, Internal Iliac, Right
Inferior gluteal nerve
 use Nerve, Sacral Plexus
Inferior hypogastric plexus
 use Nerve, Abdominal Sympathetic
Inferior labial artery
 use Artery, Face
Inferior longitudinal muscle
 use Muscle, Tongue, Palate, Pharynx
Inferior mesenteric ganglion
 use Nerve, Abdominal Sympathetic
Inferior mesenteric lymph node
 use Lymphatic, Mesenteric

Inferior mesenteric

Inferior mesenteric plexus
  use Nerve, Abdominal Sympathetic
Inferior oblique muscle
  use Muscle, Extraocular, Left
  use Muscle, Extraocular, Right
Inferior pancreaticoduodenal artery
  use Artery, Superior Mesenteric
Inferior phrenic artery
  use Aorta, Abdominal
Inferior rectus muscle
  use Muscle, Extraocular, Left
  use Muscle, Extraocular, Right
Inferior suprarenal artery
  use Artery, Renal, Left
  use Artery, Renal, Right
Inferior tarsal plate
  use Eyelid, Lower, Left
  use Eyelid, Lower, Right
Inferior thyroid vein
  use Vein, Innominate, Left
  use Vein, Innominate, Right
Inferior tibiofibular joint
  use Joint, Ankle, Left
  use Joint, Ankle, Right
Inferior turbinate
  use Turbinate, Nasal
Inferior ulnar collateral artery
  use Artery, Brachial, Left
  use Artery, Brachial, Right
Inferior vesical artery
  use Artery, Internal Iliac, Left
  use Artery, Internal Iliac, Right
Infraauricular lymph node
  use Lymphatic, Head
Infraclavicular (deltopectoral) lymph node
  use Lymphatic, Upper Extremity, Left
  use Lymphatic, Upper Extremity, Right
Infrahyoid muscle
  use Muscle, Neck, Left
  use Muscle, Neck, Right
Infraparotid lymph node
  use Lymphatic, Head
Infraspinatus fascia
  use Subcutaneous Tissue and Fascia, Upper Arm, Left
  use Subcutaneous Tissue and Fascia, Upper Arm, Right
Infraspinatus muscle
  use Muscle, Shoulder, Left
  use Muscle, Shoulder, Right
Infundibulopelvic ligament
  use Uterine Supporting Structure
Infusion see Introduction of substance in or on
Infusion Device, Pump
  Insertion of device in
    Abdomen 0JH8-
    Back 0JH7-
    Chest 0JH6-
    Lower Arm
      Left 0JHH-
      Right 0JHG-
    Lower Leg
      Left 0JHP-
      Right 0JHN-
    Trunk 0JHT-
    Upper Arm
      Left 0JHF-
      Right 0JHD-
    Upper Leg
      Left 0JHM-
      Right 0JHL-
  Removal of device from
    Lower Extremity 0JPW-
    Trunk 0JPT-
    Upper Extremity 0JPV-
  Revision of device in
    Lower Extremity 0JWW-
    Trunk 0JWT-
    Upper Extremity 0JWV-

Infusion, glucarpidase
  Central vein 3E043GQ
  Peripheral vein 3E033GQ
Inguinal canal
  use Inguinal Region, Bilateral
  use Inguinal Region, Left
  use Inguinal Region, Right
Inguinal triangle
  use Inguinal Region, Bilateral
  use Inguinal Region, Left
  use Inguinal Region, Right
Injection see Introduction of substance in or on
Injection reservoir, port
  use Vascular Access Device, Reservoir in Subcutaneous Tissue and Fascia
Injection reservoir, pump
  use Infusion Device, Pump in Subcutaneous Tissue and Fascia
Insemination, artificial 3E0P7LZ
Insertion
  Antimicrobial envelope see Introduction of Anti-infective
  Aqueous drainage shunt
    see Bypass, Eye 081-
    see Drainage, Eye 089-
  Products of Conception 10H0-
  Spinal Stabilization Device
    see Insertion of device in, Lower Joints 0SH-
    see Insertion of device in, Upper Joints 0RH-
Insertion of device in
  Abdominal Wall 0WHF-
  Acetabulum
    Left 0QH5-
    Right 0QH4-
  Anal Sphincter 0DHR-
  Ankle Region
    Left 0YHL-
    Right 0YHK-
  Anus 0DHQ-
  Aorta
    Abdominal 04H0-
    Thoracic 02HW-
  Arm
    Lower
      Left 0XHF-
      Right 0XHD-
    Upper
      Left 0XH9-
      Right 0XH8-
  Artery
    Anterior Tibial
      Left 04HQ-
      Right 04HP-
    Axillary
      Left 03H6-
      Right 03H5-
    Brachial
      Left 03H8-
      Right 03H7-
    Celiac 04H1-
    Colic
      Left 04H7-
      Middle 04H8-
      Right 04H6-
    Common Carotid
      Left 03HJ-
      Right 03HH-
    Common Iliac
      Left 04HD-
      Right 04HC-
    External Carotid
      Left 03HN-
      Right 03HM-
    External Iliac
      Left 04HJ-
      Right 04HH-
    Face 03HR-

Insertion of device in — *continued*
  Artery — *continued*
    Femoral
      Left 04HL-
      Right 04HK-
    Foot
      Left 04HW-
      Right 04HV-
    Gastric 04H2-
    Hand
      Left 03HF-
      Right 03HD-
    Hepatic 04H3-
    Inferior Mesenteric 04HB-
    Innominate 03H2-
    Internal Carotid
      Left 03HL-
      Right 03HK-
    Internal Iliac
      Left 04HF-
      Right 04HE-
    Internal Mammary
      Left 03H1-
      Right 03H0-
    Intracranial 03HG-
    Lower 04HY-
    Peroneal
      Left 04HU-
      Right 04HT-
    Popliteal
      Left 04HN-
      Right 04HM-
    Posterior Tibial
      Left 04HS-
      Right 04HR-
    Pulmonary
      Left 02HR-
      Right 02HQ-
    Pulmonary Trunk 02HP-
    Radial
      Left 03HC-
      Right 03HB-
    Renal
      Left 04HA-
      Right 04H9-
    Splenic 04H4-
    Subclavian
      Left 03H4-
      Right 03H3-
    Superior Mesenteric 04H5-
    Temporal
      Left 03HT-
      Right 03HS-
    Thyroid
      Left 03HV-
      Right 03HU-
    Ulnar
      Left 03HA-
      Right 03H9-
    Upper 03HY-
    Vertebral
      Left 03HQ-
      Right 03HP-
  Atrium
    Left 02H7-
    Right 02H6-
  Axilla
    Left 0XH5-
    Right 0XH4-
  Back
    Lower 0WHL-
    Upper 0WHK-
  Bladder 0THB-
  Bladder Neck 0THC-
  Bone
    Ethmoid
      Left 0NHG-
      Right 0NHF-
    Facial 0NHW-
    Frontal
      Left 0NH2-
      Right 0NH1-

Insertion of device in — *continued*
  Bone — *continued*
    Hyoid 0NHX-
    Lacrimal
      Left 0NHJ-
      Right 0NHH-
    Lower 0QHY-
    Nasal 0NHB-
    Occipital
      Left 0NH8-
      Right 0NH7-
    Palatine
      Left 0NHL-
      Right 0NHK-
    Parietal
      Left 0NH4-
      Right 0NH3-
    Pelvic
      Left 0QH3-
      Right 0QH2-
    Sphenoid
      Left 0NHD-
      Right 0NHC-
    Temporal
      Left 0NH6-
      Right 0NH5-
    Upper 0PHY-
    Zygomatic
      Left 0NHN-
      Right 0NHM-
  Brain 00H0-
  Breast
    Bilateral 0HHV-
    Left 0HHU-
    Right 0HHT-
  Bronchus
    Lingula 0BH9-
    Lower Lobe
      Left 0BHB-
      Right 0BH6-
    Main
      Left 0BH7-
      Right 0BH3-
    Middle Lobe, Right 0BH5-
    Upper Lobe
      Left 0BH8-
      Right 0BH4-
  Buttock
    Left 0YH1-
    Right 0YH0-
  Carpal
    Left 0PHN-
    Right 0PHM-
  Cavity, Cranial 0WH1-
  Cerebral Ventricle 00H6-
  Cervix 0UHC-
  Chest Wall 0WH8-
  Cisterna Chyli 07HL-
  Clavicle
    Left 0PHB-
    Right 0PH9-
  Coccyx 0QHS-
  Cul-de-sac 0UHF-
  Diaphragm
    Left 0BHS-
    Right 0BHR-
  Disc
    Cervical Vertebral 0RH3-
    Cervicothoracic Vertebral 0RH5-
    Lumbar Vertebral 0SH2-
    Lumbosacral 0SH4-
    Thoracic Vertebral 0RH9-
    Thoracolumbar Vertebral 0RHB-
  Duct
    Hepatobiliary 0FHB-
    Pancreatic 0FHD-
  Duodenum 0DH9-
  Ear
    Left 09HE-
    Right 09HD-

INDEX TO PROCEDURES – 2016 ICD-10-PCS

Insertion of

Insertion of device in — *continued*
Elbow Region
  Left 0XHC-
  Right 0XHB-
Epididymis and Spermatic Cord 0VHM-
Esophagus 0DH5-
Extremity
  Lower
    Left 0YHB-
    Right 0YH9-
  Upper
    Left 0XH7-
    Right 0XH6-
Eye
  Left 08H1-
  Right 08H0-
Face 0WH2-
Fallopian Tube 0UH8-
Femoral Region
  Left 0YH8-
  Right 0YH7-
Femoral Shaft
  Left 0QH9-
  Right 0QH8-
Femur
  Lower
    Left 0QHC-
    Right 0QHB-
  Upper
    Left 0QH7-
    Right 0QH6-
Fibula
  Left 0QHK-
  Right 0QHJ-
Foot
  Left 0YHN-
  Right 0YHM-
Gallbladder 0FH4-
Gastrointestinal Tract 0WHP-
Genitourinary Tract 0WHR-
Gland, Endocrine 0GHS-
Glenoid Cavity
  Left 0PH8-
  Right 0PH7-
Hand
  Left 0XHK-
  Right 0XHJ-
Head 0WH0-
Heart 02HA-
Humeral Head
  Left 0PHD-
  Right 0PHC-
Humeral Shaft
  Left 0PHG-
  Right 0PHF-
Ileum 0DHB-
Inguinal Region
  Left 0YH6-
  Right 0YH5-
Intestine
  Large 0DHE-
  Small 0DH8-
Jaw
  Lower 0WH5-
  Upper 0WH4-
Jejunum 0DHA-
Joint
  Acromioclavicular
    Left 0RHH-
    Right 0RHG-
  Ankle
    Left 0SHG-
    Right 0SHF-
  Carpal
    Left 0RHR-
    Right 0RHQ-
  Cervical Vertebral 0RH1-
  Cervicothoracic Vertebral 0RH4-
  Coccygeal 0SH6-
  Elbow
    Left 0RHM-
    Right 0RHL-

Insertion of device in — *continued*
Joint — *continued*
  Finger Phalangeal
    Left 0RHX-
    Right 0RHW-
  Hip
    Left 0SHB-
    Right 0SH9-
  Knee
    Left 0SHD-
    Right 0SHC-
  Lumbar Vertebral 0SH0-
  Lumbosacral 0SH3-
  Metacarpocarpal
    Left 0RHT-
    Right 0RHS-
  Metacarpophalangeal
    Left 0RHV-
    Right 0RHU-
  Metatarsal-Phalangeal
    Left 0SHN-
    Right 0SHM-
  Metatarsal-Tarsal
    Left 0SHL-
    Right 0SHK-
  Occipital-cervical 0RH0-
  Sacrococcygeal 0SH5-
  Sacroiliac
    Left 0SH8-
    Right 0SH7-
  Shoulder
    Left 0RHK-
    Right 0RHJ-
  Sternoclavicular
    Left 0RHF-
    Right 0RHE-
  Tarsal
    Left 0SHJ-
    Right 0SHH-
  Temporomandibular
    Left 0RHD-
    Right 0RHC-
  Thoracic Vertebral 0RH6-
  Thoracolumbar Vertebral 0RHA-
  Toe Phalangeal
    Left 0SHQ-
    Right 0SHP-
  Wrist
    Left 0RHP-
    Right 0RHN-
Kidney 0TH5-
Knee Region
  Left 0YHG-
  Right 0YHF-
Leg
  Lower
    Left 0YHJ-
    Right 0YHH-
  Upper
    Left 0YHD-
    Right 0YHC-
Liver 0FH0-
  Left Lobe 0FH2-
  Right Lobe 0FH1-
Lung
  Left 0BHL-
  Right 0BHK-
Lymphatic 07HN-
  Thoracic Duct 07HK-
Mandible
  Left 0NHV-
  Right 0NHT
Maxilla
  Left 0NHS-
  Right 0NHR-
Mediastinum 0WHC-
Metacarpal
  Left 0PHQ-
  Right 0PHP-
Metatarsal
  Left 0QHP-
  Right 0QHN-

Insertion of device in — *continued*
Mouth and Throat 0CHY-
Muscle
  Lower 0KHY-
  Upper 0KHX-
Nasopharynx 09HN-
Neck 0WH6-
Nerve
  Cranial 00HE-
  Peripheral 01HY-
Nipple
  Left 0HHX-
  Right 0HHW-
Oral Cavity and Throat 0WH3-
Orbit
  Left 0NHQ-
  Right 0NHP-
Ovary 0UH3-
Pancreas 0FHG-
Patella
  Left 0QHF-
  Right 0QHD-
Pelvic Cavity 0WHJ-
Penis 0VHS-
Pericardial Cavity 0WHD-
Pericardium 02HN-
Perineum
  Female 0WHN-
  Male 0WHM-
Peritoneal Cavity 0WHG-
Phalanx
  Finger
    Left 0PHV-
    Right 0PHT-
  Thumb
    Left 0PHS-
    Right 0PHR-
  Toe
    Left 0QHR-
    Right 0QHQ-
Pleural Cavity
  Left 0WHB-
  Right 0WH9-
Prostate 0VH0-
Prostate and Seminal Vesicles 0VH4-
Radius
  Left 0PHJ-
  Right 0PHH-
Rectum 0DHP-
Respiratory Tract 0WHQ-
Retroperitoneum 0WHH-
Rib
  Left 0PH2-
  Right 0PH1-
Sacrum 0QH1-
Scapula
  Left 0PH6-
  Right 0PH5-
Scrotum and Tunica Vaginalis 0VH8-
Shoulder Region
  Left 0XH3-
  Right 0XH2-
Skull 0NH0-
Spinal Canal 00HU-
Spinal Cord 00HV-
Spleen 07HP-
Sternum 0PH0-
Stomach 0DH6-
Subcutaneous Tissue and Fascia
  Abdomen 0JH8-
  Back 0JH7-
  Buttock 0JH9-
  Chest 0JH6-
  Face 0JH1-
  Foot
    Left 0JHR-
    Right 0JHQ-
  Hand
    Left 0JHK-
    Right 0JHJ-
  Head and Neck 0JHS-

Insertion of device in — *continued*
Subcutaneous Tissue and Fascia — *continued*
  Lower Arm
    Left 0JHH-
    Right 0JHG-
  Lower Extremity 0JHW-
  Lower Leg
    Left 0JHP-
    Right 0JHN-
  Neck
    Anterior 0JH4-
    Posterior 0JH5-
  Pelvic Region 0JHC-
  Perineum 0JHB-
  Scalp 0JH0-
  Trunk 0JHT-
  Upper Arm
    Left 0JHF-
    Right 0JHD-
  Upper Extremity 0JHV-
  Upper Leg
    Left 0JHM-
    Right 0JHL-
Tarsal
  Left 0QHM-
  Right 0QHL-
Testis 0VHD-
Thymus 07HM-
Tibia
  Left 0QHH-
  Right 0QHG-
Tongue 0CH7-
Trachea 0BH1-
Tracheobronchial Tree 0BH0-
Ulna
  Left 0PHL-
  Right 0PHK-
Ureter 0TH9-
Urethra 0THD-
Uterus 0UH9-
Uterus and Cervix 0UHD-
Vagina 0UHG-
Vagina and Cul-de-sac 0UHH-
Vas Deferens 0VHR-
Vein
  Axillary
    Left 05H8-
    Right 05H7-
  Azygos 05H0-
  Basilic
    Left 05HC-
    Right 05HB-
  Brachial
    Left 05HA-
    Right 05H9-
  Cephalic
    Left 05HF-
    Right 05HD-
  Colic 06H7-
  Common Iliac
    Left 06HD-
    Right 06HC-
  Coronary 02H4-
  Esophageal 06H3-
  External Iliac
    Left 06HG-
    Right 06HF-
  External Jugular
    Left 05HQ-
    Right 05HP-
  Face
    Left 05HV-
    Right 05HT-
  Femoral
    Left 06HN-
    Right 06HM-
  Foot
    Left 06HV-
    Right 06HT-
  Gastric 06H2-

Insertion of — INDEX TO PROCEDURES – 2016 ICD-10-PCS

Insertion of device in — *continued*
- Vein — *continued*
  - Greater Saphenous
    - Left 06HQ-
    - Right 06HP-
  - Hand
    - Left 05HH-
    - Right 05HG-
  - Hemiazygos 05H1-
  - Hepatic 06H4-
  - Hypogastric
    - Left 06HJ-
    - Right 06HH-
  - Inferior Mesenteric 06H6-
  - Innominate
    - Left 05H4-
    - Right 05H3-
  - Internal Jugular
    - Left 05HN-
    - Right 05HM-
  - Intracranial 05HL-
  - Lesser Saphenous
    - Left 06HS-
    - Right 06HR-
  - Lower 06HY-
  - Portal 06H8-
  - Pulmonary
    - Left 02HT-
    - Right 02HS-
  - Renal
    - Left 06HB-
    - Right 06H9-
  - Splenic 06H1-
  - Subclavian
    - Left 05H6-
    - Right 05H5-
  - Superior Mesenteric 06H5-
  - Upper 05HY-
  - Vertebral
    - Left 05HS-
    - Right 05HR-
- Vena Cava
  - Inferior 06H0-
  - Superior 02HV-
- Ventricle
  - Left 02HL-
  - Right 02HK-
- Vertebra
  - Cervical 0PH3-
  - Lumbar 0QH0-
  - Thoracic 0PH4-
- Wrist Region
  - Left 0XHH-
  - Right 0XHG-

Inspection
- Abdominal Wall 0WJF-
- Ankle Region
  - Left 0YJL-
  - Right 0YJK-
- Arm
  - Lower
    - Left 0XJF-
    - Right 0XJD-
  - Upper
    - Left 0XJ9-
    - Right 0XJ8-
- Artery
  - Lower 04JY-
  - Upper 03JY-
- Axilla
  - Left 0XJ5-
  - Right 0XJ4-
- Back
  - Lower 0WJL-
  - Upper 0WJK-
- Bladder 0TJB-
- Bone
  - Facial 0NJW-
  - Lower 0QJY-
  - Nasal 0NJB-
  - Upper 0PJY-

Inspection — *continued*
- Bone Marrow 07JT-
- Brain 00J0-
- Breast
  - Left 0HJU-
  - Right 0HJT-
- Bursa and Ligament
  - Lower 0MJY-
  - Upper 0MJX-
- Buttock
  - Left 0YJ1-
  - Right 0YJ0-
- Cavity, Cranial 0WJ1-
- Chest Wall 0WJ8-
- Cisterna Chyli 07JL-
- Diaphragm 0BJT-
- Disc
  - Cervical Vertebral 0RJ3-
  - Cervicothoracic Vertebral 0RJ5-
  - Lumbar Vertebral 0SJ2-
  - Lumbosacral 0SJ4-
  - Thoracic Vertebral 0RJ9-
  - Thoracolumbar Vertebral 0RJB-
- Duct
  - Hepatobiliary 0FJB-
  - Pancreatic 0FJD-
- Ear
  - Inner
    - Left 09JE-
    - Right 09JD-
  - Left 09JJ-
  - Right 09JH-
- Elbow Region
  - Left 0XJC-
  - Right 0XJB-
- Epidydimis and Spermatic Cord 0VJM-
- Extremity
  - Lower
    - Left 0YJB-
    - Right 0YJ9-
  - Upper
    - Left 0XJ7-
    - Right 0XJ6-
- Eye
  - Left 08J1XZZ
  - Right 08J0XZZ
- Face 0WJ2-
- Fallopian Tube 0UJ8-
- Femoral Region
  - Bilateral 0YJE-
  - Left 0YJ8-
  - Right 0YJ7-
- Finger Nail 0HJQXZZ
- Foot
  - Left 0YJN-
  - Right 0YJM-
- Gallbladder 0FJ4-
- Gastrointestinal Tract 0WJP
- Genitourinary Tract 0WJR
- Gland
  - Adrenal 0GJ5-
  - Endocrine 0GJS-
  - Pituitary 0GJ0-
  - Salivary 0CJA-
- Great Vessel 02JY-
- Hand
  - Left 0XJK-
  - Right 0XJJ-
- Head 0WJ0-
- Heart 02JA-
- Inguinal Region
  - Bilateral 0YJA-
  - Left 0YJ6-
  - Right 0YJ5-
- Intestinal Tract
  - Lower 0DJD-
  - Upper 0DJ0-
- Jaw
  - Lower 0WJ5-
  - Upper 0WJ4-

Inspection — *continued*
- Joint
  - Acromioclavicular
    - Left 0RJH-
    - Right 0RJG-
  - Ankle
    - Left 0SJG-
    - Right 0SJF-
  - Carpal
    - Left 0RJR-
    - Right 0RJQ-
  - Cervical Vertebral 0RJ1-
  - Cervicothoracic Vertebral 0RJ4-
  - Coccygeal 0SJ6-
  - Elbow
    - Left 0RJM-
    - Right 0RJL-
  - Finger Phalangeal
    - Left 0RJX-
    - Right 0RJW-
  - Hip
    - Left 0SJB-
    - Right 0SJ9-
  - Knee
    - Left 0SJD-
    - Right 0SJC-
  - Lumbar Vertebral 0SJ0-
  - Lumbosacral 0SJ3-
  - Metacarpocarpal
    - Left 0RJT-
    - Right 0RJS-
  - Metacarpophalangeal
    - Left 0RJV-
    - Right 0RJU-
  - Metatarsal-Phalangeal
    - Left 0SJN-
    - Right 0SJM-
  - Metatarsal-Tarsal
    - Left 0SJL-
    - Right 0SJK-
  - Occipital-cervical 0RJ0-
  - Sacrococcygeal 0SJ5-
  - Sacroiliac
    - Left 0SJ8-
    - Right 0SJ7-
  - Shoulder
    - Left 0RJK-
    - Right 0RJJ-
  - Sternoclavicular
    - Left 0RJF-
    - Right 0RJE-
  - Tarsal
    - Left 0SJJ-
    - Right 0SJH-
  - Temporomandibular
    - Left 0RJD-
    - Right 0RJC-
  - Thoracic Vertebral 0RJ6-
  - Thoracolumbar Vertebral 0RJA-
  - Toe Phalangeal
    - Left 0SJQ-
    - Right 0SJP-
  - Wrist
    - Left 0RJP-
    - Right 0RJN-
- Kidney 0TJ5-
- Knee Region
  - Left 0YJG-
  - Right 0YJF-
- Larynx 0CJS-
- Leg
  - Lower
    - Left 0YJJ-
    - Right 0YJH-
  - Upper
    - Left 0YJD-
    - Right 0YJC-
- Lens
  - Left 08JKXZZ
  - Right 08JJXZZ
- Liver 0FJ0-

Inspection — *continued*
- Lung
  - Left 0BJL-
  - Right 0BJK-
- Lymphatic 07JN-
  - Thoracic Duct 07JK-
- Mediastinum 0WJC-
- Mesentery 0DJV-
- Mouth and Throat 0CJY-
- Muscle
  - Extraocular
    - Left 08JM-
    - Right 08JL-
  - Lower 0KJY-
  - Upper 0KJX-
- Neck 0WJ6-
- Nerve
  - Cranial 00JE-
  - Peripheral 01JY-
- Nose 09JK-
- Omentum 0DJU-
- Oral Cavity and Throat 0WJ3-
- Ovary 0UJ3-
- Pancreas 0FJG-
- Parathyroid Gland 0GJR-
- Pelvic Cavity 0WJJ-
- Penis 0VJS-
- Pericardial Cavity 0WJD-
- Perineum
  - Female 0WJN-
  - Male 0WJM-
- Peritoneal Cavity 0WJG-
- Peritoneum 0DJW-
- Pineal Body 0GJ1-
- Pleura 0BJQ-
- Pleural Cavity
  - Left 0WJB-
  - Right 0WJ9-
- Products of Conception 10J0-
  - Ectopic 10J2-
  - Retained 10J1-
- Prostate and Seminal Vesicles 0VJ4-
- Respiratory Tract 0WJQ-
- Retroperitoneum 0WJH-
- Scrotum and Tunica Vaginalis 0VJ8-
- Shoulder Region
  - Left 0XJ3-
  - Right 0XJ2-
- Sinus 09JY-
- Skin 0HJPXZZ
- Skull 0NJ0-
- Spinal Canal 00JU-
- Spinal Cord 00JV-
- Spleen 07JP-
- Stomach 0DJ6-
- Subcutaneous Tissue and Fascia
  - Head and Neck 0JJS-
  - Lower Extremity 0JJW-
  - Trunk 0JJT-
  - Upper Extremity 0JJV-
- Tendon
  - Lower 0LJY-
  - Upper 0LJX-
- Testis 0VJD-
- Thymus 07JM-
- Thyroid Gland 0GJK-
- Toe Nail 0HJRXZZ
- Trachea 0BJ1-
- Tracheobronchial Tree 0BJ0-
- Tympanic Membrane
  - Left 09J8-
  - Right 09J7-
- Ureter 0TJ9-
- Urethra 0TJD-
- Uterus and Cervix 0UJD-
- Vagina and Cul-de-sac 0UJH-
- Vas Deferens 0VJR-
- Vein
  - Lower 06JY-
  - Upper 05JY-
- Vulva 0UJM-

Inspection — *continued*
Wrist Region
Left 0XJH-
Right 0XJG-
Instillation *see* Introduction of substance in or on
Insufflation *see* Introduction of substance in or on
Interatrial septum
use Septum, Atrial
Interbody fusion (spine) cage
use Interbody Fusion Device in Lower Joints
use Interbody Fusion Device in Upper Joints
Intercarpal joint
use Joint, Carpal, Left
use Joint, Carpal, Right
Intercarpal ligament
use Bursa and Ligament, Hand, Left
use Bursa and Ligament, Hand, Right
Interclavicular ligament
use Bursa and Ligament, Shoulder, Left
use Bursa and Ligament, Shoulder, Right
Intercostal lymph node
use Lymphatic, Thorax
Intercostal muscle
use Muscle, Thorax, Left
use Muscle, Thorax, Right
Intercostal nerve
use Nerve, Thoracic
Intercostobrachial nerve
use Nerve, Thoracic
Intercuneiform joint
use Joint, Tarsal, Left
use Joint, Tarsal, Right
Intercuneiform ligament
use Bursa and Ligament, Foot, Left
use Bursa and Ligament, Foot, Right
Intermediate cuneiform bone
use Tarsal, Left
use Tarsal, Right
Intermittent mandatory ventilation *see* Assistance, Respiratory 5A09-
Intermittent Negative Airway Pressure
24-96 Consecutive Hours, Ventilation 5A0945B
Greater than 96 Consecutive Hours, Ventilation 5A0955B
Less than 24 Consecutive Hours, Ventilation 5A0935B
Intermittent Positive Airway Pressure
24-96 Consecutive Hours, Ventilation 5A09458
Greater than 96 Consecutive Hours, Ventilation 5A09558
Less than 24 Consecutive Hours, Ventilation 5A09358
Intermittent positive pressure breathing *see* Assistance, Respiratory 5A09-
Internal (basal) cerebral vein
use Vein, Intracranial
Internal anal sphincter
use Anal Sphincter
Internal carotid plexus
use Nerve, Head and Neck Sympathetic
Internal iliac vein
use Vein, Hypogastric, Left
use Vein, Hypogastric, Right
Internal maxillary artery
use Artery, External Carotid, Left
use Artery, External Carotid, Right
Internal naris
use Nose

Internal oblique muscle
use Muscle, Abdomen, Left
use Muscle, Abdomen, Right
Internal pudendal artery
use Artery, Internal Iliac, Left
use Artery, Internal Iliac, Right
Internal pudendal vein
use Vein, Hypogastric, Left
use Vein, Hypogastric, Right
Internal thoracic artery
use Artery, Internal Mammary, Left
use Artery, Internal Mammary, Right
use Artery, Subclavian, Left
use Artery, Subclavian, Right
Internal urethral sphincter
use Urethra
Interphalangeal (IP) joint
use Joint, Finger Phalangeal, Left
use Joint, Finger Phalangeal, Right
use Joint, Toe Phalangeal, Left
use Joint, Toe Phalangeal, Right
Interphalangeal ligament
use Bursa and Ligament, Foot, Left
use Bursa and Ligament, Foot, Right
use Bursa and Ligament, Hand, Left
use Bursa and Ligament, Hand, Right
Interrogation, cardiac rhythm related device
Interrogation only *see* Measurement, Cardiac 4B02-
With cardiac function testing *see* Measurement, Cardiac 4A02-
Interruption *see* Occlusion
Interspinalis muscle
use Muscle, Trunk, Left
use Muscle, Trunk, Right
Interspinous ligament
use Bursa and Ligament, Head and Neck
use Bursa and Ligament, Trunk, Left
use Bursa and Ligament, Trunk, Right
Interspinous process spinal stabilization device
use Spinal Stabilization Device, Interspinous Process in 0RH-
use Spinal Stabilization Device, Interspinous Process in 0SH-
InterStim® Therapy lead
use Neurostimulator Lead in Peripheral Nervous System
InterStim® Therapy neurostimulator
use Stimulator Generator, Single Array in 0JH-
Intertransversarius muscle
use Muscle, Trunk, Left
use Muscle, Trunk, Right
Intertransverse ligament
use Bursa and Ligament, Trunk, Left
use Bursa and Ligament, Trunk, Right
Interventricular foramen (Monro)
use Cerebral Ventricle
Interventricular septum
use Septum, Ventricular
Intestinal lymphatic trunk
use Cisterna Chyli
Intraluminal Device
Airway
Esophagus 0DH5-
Mouth and Throat 0CHY-
Nasopharynx 09HN-
Bioactive
Occlusion
Common Carotid
Left 03LJ-
Right 03LH-
External Carotid
Left 03LN-
Right 03LM-

Intraluminal Device — *continued*
Bioactive — *continued*
Occlusion — *continued*
Internal Carotid
Left 03LL-
Right 03LK-
Intracranial 03LG-
Vertebral
Left 03LQ-
Right 03LP-
Restriction
Common Carotid
Left 03VJ-
Right 03VH-
External Carotid
Left 03VN-
Right 03VM-
Internal Carotid
Left 03VL-
Right 03VK-
Intracranial 03VG-
Vertebral
Left 03VQ-
Right 03VP-
Endobronchial Valve
Lingula 0BH9-
Lower Lobe
Left 0BHB-
Right 0BHF-
Main
Left 0BH7-
Right 0BH3-
Middle Lobe, Right 0BH5-
Upper Lobe
Left 0BH8-
Right 0BH4-
Endotracheal Airway
Change device in, Trachea 0B21XEZ
Insertion of device in, Trachea 0BH1-
Pessary
Change device in, Vagina and Cul-de-sac 0U2HXGZ
Insertion of device in Cul-de-sac 0UHF-
Vagina 0UHG-
Intramedullary (IM) rod (nail)
use Internal Fixation Device, Intramedullary in Lower Bones
use Internal Fixation Device, Intramedullary in Upper Bones
Intramedullary skeletal kinetic distractor (ISKD)
use Internal Fixation Device, Intramedullary in Lower Bones
use Internal Fixation Device, Intramedullary in Upper Bones
Intraocular Telescope
Left 08RK30Z
Right 08RJ30Z
Intraoperative knee replacement sensor XR2
Intraoperative Radiation Therapy (IORT)
Anus DDY8CZZ
Bile Ducts DFY2CZZ
Bladder DTY2CZZ
Cervix DUY1CZZ
Colon DDY5CZZ
Duodenum DDY2CZZ
Gallbladder DFY1CZZ
Ileum DDY4CZZ
Jejunum DDY3CZZ
Kidney DTY0CZZ
Larynx D9YBCZZ
Liver DFY0CZZ
Mouth D9Y4CZZ
Nasopharynx D9YDCZZ
Ovary DUY0CZZ
Pancreas DFY3CZZ
Pharynx D9YCCZZ

Intraoperative Radiation Therapy (IORT) — *continued*
Prostate DVY0CZZ
Rectum DDY7CZZ
Stomach DDY1CZZ
Ureter DTY1CZZ
Urethra DTY3CZZ
Uterus DUY2CZZ
Intrauterine device (IUD)
use Contraceptive Device in Female Reproductive System
Introduction of substance in or on
Artery
Central 3E06-
Analgesics 3E06-
Anesthetic, Intracirculatory 3E06-
Antiarrhythmic 3E06-
Anti-infective 3E06-
Anti-inflammatory 3E06-
Antineoplastic 3E06-
Destructive Agent 3E06-
Diagnostic Substance, Other 3E06-
Electrolytic Substance 3E06-
Hormone 3E06-
Hypnotics 3E06-
Immunotherapeutic 3E06-
Nutritional Substance 3E06-
Platelet Inhibitor 3E06-
Radioactive Substance 3E06-
Sedatives 3E06-
Serum 3E06-
Thrombolytic 3E06-
Toxoid 3E06-
Vaccine 3E06-
Vasopressor 3E06-
Water Balance Substance 3E06-
Coronary 3E07-
Diagnostic Substance, Other 3E07-
Platelet Inhibitor 3E07-
Thrombolytic 3E07-
Peripheral 3E05-
Analgesics 3E05-
Anesthetic, Intracirculatory 3E05-
Antiarrhythmic 3E05-
Anti-infective 3E05-
Anti-inflammatory 3E05-
Antineoplastic 3E05-
Destructive Agent 3E05-
Diagnostic Substance, Other 3E05-
Electrolytic Substance 3E05-
Hormone 3E05-
Hypnotics 3E05-
Immunotherapeutic 3E05-
Nutritional Substance 3E05-
Platelet Inhibitor 3E05-
Radioactive Substance 3E05-
Sedatives 3E05-
Serum 3E05-
Thrombolytic 3E05-
Toxoid 3E05-
Vaccine 3E05-
Vasopressor 3E05-
Water Balance Substance 3E05-
Biliary Tract 3E0J-
Analgesics 3E0J-
Anesthetic, Local 3E0J-
Anti-infective 3E0J
Anti-inflammatory 3E0J
Antineoplastic 3E0J-
Destructive Agent 3E0J-
Diagnostic Substance, Other 3E0J-
Electrolytic Substance 3E0J-
Gas 3E0J-
Hypnotics 3E0J-
Islet Cells, Pancreatic 3E0J-
Nutritional Substance 3E0J-
Radioactive Substance 3E0J-
Sedatives 3E0J-
Water Balance Substance 3E0J-

Introduction to Procedures – 2016 ICD-10-PCS

Introduction of substance in or on — *continued*

Bone 3E0V-
- Analgesics 3E0V3NZ
- Anesthetic, Local 3E0V3BZ
- Anti-infective 3E0V32-
- Anti-inflammatory 3E0V33Z
- Antineoplastic 3E0V30-
- Destructive Agent 3E0V3TZ
- Diagnostic Substance, Other 3E0V3KZ
- Electrolytic Substance 3E0V37Z
- Hypnotics 3E0V3NZ
- Nutritional Substance 3E0V36Z
- Radioactive Substance 3E0V3HZ
- Sedatives 3E0V3NZ
- Water Balance Substance 3E0V37Z

Bone Marrow 3E0A3GC
- Antineoplastic 3E0A30-

Brain 3E0Q3GC
- Analgesics 3E0Q3NZ
- Anesthetic, Local 3E0Q3BZ
- Anti-infective 3E0Q32-
- Anti-inflammatory 3E0Q33Z
- Antineoplastic 3E0Q-
- Destructive Agent 3E0Q3TZ
- Diagnostic Substance, Other 3E0Q3KZ
- Electrolytic Substance 3E0Q37Z
- Gas 3E0Q-
- Hypnotics 3E0Q3NZ
- Nutritional Substance 3E0Q36Z
- Radioactive Substance 3E0Q3HZ
- Sedatives 3E0Q3NZ
- Stem Cells
  - Embryonic 3E0Q-
  - Somatic 3E0Q-
- Water Balance Substance 3E0Q37Z

Cranial Cavity 3E0Q3GC
- Analgesics 3E0Q3NZ
- Anesthetic, Local 3E0Q3BZ
- Anti-infective 3E0Q32-
- Anti-inflammatory 3E0Q33Z
- Antineoplastic 3E0Q-
- Destructive Agent 3E0Q3TZ
- Diagnostic Substance, Other 3E0Q3KZ
- Electrolytic Substance 3E0Q37Z
- Gas 3E0Q-
- Hypnotics 3E0Q3NZ
- Nutritional Substance 3E0Q36Z
- Radioactive Substance 3E0Q3HZ
- Sedatives 3E0Q3NZ
- Stem Cells
  - Embryonic 3E0Q-
  - Somatic 3E0Q-
- Water Balance Substance 3E0Q37Z

Ear 3E0B
- Analgesics 3E0B-
- Anesthetic, Local 3E0B-
- Anti-infective 3E0B-
- Anti-inflammatory 3E0B-
- Antineoplastic 3E0B-
- Destructive Agent 3E0B-
- Diagnostic Substance, Other 3E0B-
- Hypnotics 3E0B-
- Radioactive Substance 3E0B-
- Sedatives 3E0B-

Epidural Space 3E0S3GC
- Analgesics 3E0S3NZ
- Anesthetic
  - Local 3E0S3BZ
  - Regional 3E0S3CZ
- Anti-infective 3E0S32-
- Anti-inflammatory 3E0S33Z
- Antineoplastic 3E0S30-
- Destructive Agent 3E0S3TZ

Introduction of substance in or on — *continued*

Epidural Space 3E0S3GC — *continued*
- Diagnostic Substance, Other 3E0S3KZ
- Electrolytic Substance 3E0S37Z
- Gas 3E0S-
- Hypnotics 3E0S3NZ
- Nutritional Substance 3E0S36Z
- Radioactive Substance 3E0S3HZ
- Sedatives 3E0S3NZ
- Water Balance Substance 3E0S37Z

Eye 3E0C
- Analgesics 3E0C-
- Anesthetic, Local 3E0C-
- Anti-infective 3E0C-
- Anti-inflammatory 3E0C-
- Antineoplastic 3E0C-
- Destructive Agent 3E0C-
- Diagnostic Substance, Other 3E0C-
- Gas 3E0C-
- Hypnotics 3E0C-
- Pigment 3E0C-
- Radioactive Substance 3E0C-
- Sedatives 3E0C-

Gastrointestinal Tract
- Lower 3E0H-
  - Analgesics 3E0H-
  - Anesthetic, Local 3E0H-
  - Anti-infective 3E0H-
  - Anti-inflammatory 3E0H-
  - Antineoplastic 3E0H-
  - Destructive Agent 3E0H-
  - Diagnostic Substance, Other 3E0H-
  - Electrolytic Substance 3E0H-
  - Gas 3E0H-
  - Hypnotics 3E0H-
  - Nutritional Substance 3E0H-
  - Radioactive Substance 3E0H-
  - Sedatives 3E0H-
  - Water Balance Substance 3E0H-
- Upper 3E0G-
  - Analgesics 3E0G-
  - Anesthetic, Local 3E0G-
  - Anti-infective 3E0G-
  - Anti-inflammatory 3E0G-
  - Antineoplastic 3E0G-
  - Destructive Agent 3E0G-
  - Diagnostic Substance, Other 3E0G-
  - Electrolytic Substance 3E0G-
  - Gas 3E0G-
  - Hypnotics 3E0G-
  - Nutritional Substance 3E0G-
  - Radioactive Substance 3E0G-
  - Sedatives 3E0G-
  - Water Balance Substance 3E0G-

Genitourinary Tract 3E0K-
- Analgesics 3E0K-
- Anesthetic, Local 3E0K-
- Anti-infective 3E0K-
- Anti-inflammatory 3E0K-
- Antineoplastic 3E0K-
- Destructive Agent 3E0K-
- Diagnostic Substance, Other 3E0K-
- Electrolytic Substance 3E0K-
- Gas 3E0K-
- Hypnotics 3E0K-
- Nutritional Substance 3E0K-
- Radioactive Substance 3E0K-
- Sedatives 3E0K-
- Water Balance Substance 3E0K-

Heart 3E08-
- Diagnostic Substance, Other 3E08-
- Platelet Inhibitor 3E08-
- Thrombolytic 3E08-

Introduction of substance in or on — *continued*

Joint 3E0U-
- Analgesics 3E0U3NZ
- Anesthetic, Local 3E0U3BZ
- Anti-infective 3E0U-
- Anti-inflammatory 3E0U33Z
- Antineoplastic 3E0U30-
- Destructive Agent 3E0U3TZ
- Diagnostic Substance, Other 3E0U3KZ
- Electrolytic Substance 3E0U37Z
- Gas 3E0U3SF
- Hypnotics 3E0U3NZ
- Nutritional Substance 3E0U36Z
- Radioactive Substance 3E0U3HZ
- Sedatives 3E0U3NZ
- Water Balance Substance 3E0U37Z

Lymphatic 3E0W3GC
- Analgesics 3E0W3NZ
- Anesthetic, Local 3E0W3BZ
- Anti-infective 3E0W32-
- Anti-inflammatory 3E0W33Z
- Antineoplastic 3E0W30-
- Destructive Agent 3E0W3TZ
- Diagnostic Substance, Other 3E0W3KZ
- Electrolytic Substance 3E0W37Z
- Hypnotics 3E0W3NZ
- Nutritional Substance 3E0W36Z
- Radioactive Substance 3E0W3HZ
- Sedatives 3E0W3NZ
- Water Balance Substance 3E0W37Z

Mouth 3E0D-
- Analgesics 3E0D-
- Anesthetic, Local 3E0D-
- Antiarrhythmic 3E0D-
- Anti-infective 3E0D-
- Anti-inflammatory 3E0D-
- Antineoplastic 3E0D-
- Destructive Agent 3E0D-
- Diagnostic Substance, Other 3E0D-
- Electrolytic Substance 3E0D-
- Hypnotics 3E0D-
- Nutritional Substance 3E0D-
- Radioactive Substance 3E0D-
- Sedatives 3E0D-
- Serum 3E0D-
- Toxoid 3E0D-
- Vaccine 3E0D-
- Water Balance Substance 3E0D-

Mucous Membrane 3E00XGC
- Analgesics 3E00XNZ
- Anesthetic, Local 3E00XBZ
- Anti-infective 3E00X2-
- Anti-inflammatory 3E00X3Z
- Antineoplastic 3E00X0-
- Destructive Agent 3E00XTZ
- Diagnostic Substance, Other 3E00XKZ
- Hypnotics 3E00XNZ
- Pigment 3E00XMZ
- Sedatives 3E00XNZ
- Serum 3E00X4Z
- Toxoid 3E00X4Z
- Vaccine 3E00X4Z

Muscle 3E023GC
- Analgesics 3E023NZ
- Anesthetic, Local 3E023BZ
- Anti-infective 3E0232-
- Anti-inflammatory 3E0233Z
- Antineoplastic 3E0230-
- Destructive Agent 3E023TZ
- Diagnostic Substance, Other 3E023KZ
- Electrolytic Substance 3E0237Z
- Hypnotics 3E023NZ
- Nutritional Substance 3E0236Z
- Radioactive Substance 3E023HZ
- Sedatives 3E023NZ

Introduction of substance in or on — *continued*

Muscle 3E023GC — *continued*
- Serum 3E0234Z
- Toxoid 3E0234Z
- Vaccine 3E0234Z
- Water Balance Substance 3E0237Z

Nerve
- Cranial 3E0X3GC
  - Anesthetic
    - Local 3E0X3BZ
    - Regional 3E0X3CZ
  - Anti-inflammatory 3E0X33Z
  - Destructive Agent 3E0X3TZ
- Peripheral 3E0T3GC
  - Anesthetic
    - Local 3E0T3BZ
    - Regional 3E0T3CZ
  - Anti-inflammatory 3E0T33Z
  - Destructive Agent 3E0T3TZ
- Plexus 3E0T3GC
  - Anesthetic
    - Local 3E0T3BZ
    - Regional 3E0T3CZ
  - Anti-inflammatory 3E0T33Z
  - Destructive Agent 3E0T3TZ

Nose 3E09-
- Analgesics 3E09-
- Anesthetic, Local 3E09-
- Anti-infective 3E09-
- Anti-inflammatory 3E09-
- Antineoplastic 3E09-
- Destructive Agent 3E09-
- Diagnostic Substance, Other 3E09-
- Hypnotics 3E09-
- Radioactive Substance 3E09-
- Sedatives 3E09-
- Serum 3E09-
- Toxoid 3E09-
- Vaccine 3E09-

Pancreatic Tract 3E0J-
- Analgesics 3E0J-
- Anesthetic, Local 3E0J-
- Anti-infective 3E0J-
- Anti-inflammatory 3E0J-
- Antineoplastic 3E0J-
- Destructive Agent 3E0J-
- Diagnostic Substance, Other 3E0J-
- Electrolytic Substance 3E0J-
- Gas 3E0J-
- Hypnotics 3E0J-
- Islet Cells, Pancreatic 3E0J-
- Nutritional Substance 3E0J-
- Radioactive Substance 3E0J-
- Sedatives 3E0J-
- Water Balance Substance 3E0J-

Pericardial Cavity 3E0Y3GC
- Analgesics 3E0Y3NZ
- Anesthetic, Local 3E0Y3BZ
- Anti-infective 3E0Y32-
- Anti-inflammatory 3E0Y33Z
- Antineoplastic 3E0Y-
- Destructive Agent 3E0Y3TZ
- Diagnostic Substance, Other 3E0Y3KZ
- Electrolytic Substance 3E0Y37Z
- Gas 3E0Y-
- Hypnotics 3E0Y3NZ
- Nutritional Substance 3E0Y36Z
- Radioactive Substance 3E0Y3HZ
- Sedatives 3E0Y3NZ
- Water Balance Substance 3E0Y37Z

Peritoneal Cavity 3E0M3GC
- Adhesion Barrier 3E0M05Z
- Analgesics 3E0M3NZ
- Anesthetic, Local 3E0M3BZ
- Anti-infective 3E0M32-
- Anti-inflammatory 3E0M33Z
- Antineoplastic 3E0M-
- Destructive Agent 3E0M3TZ

Introduction of substance in or on — *continued*
  Peritoneal Cavity 3E0M3GC — *continued*
    Diagnostic Substance, Other 3E0M3KZ
    Electrolytic Substance 3E0M37Z
    Gas 3E0M-
    Hypnotics 3E0M3NZ
    Nutritional Substance 3E0M36Z
    Radioactive Substance 3E0M3HZ
    Sedatives 3E0M3NZ
    Water Balance Substance 3E0M37Z
  Pharynx 3E0D-
    Analgesics 3E0D-
    Anesthetic, Local 3E0D-
    Antiarrhythmic 3E0D-
    Anti-infective 3E0D-
    Anti-inflammatory 3E0D-
    Antineoplastic 3E0D-
    Destructive Agent 3E0D-
    Diagnostic Substance, Other 3E0D-
    Electrolytic Substance 3E0D-
    Hypnotics 3E0D-
    Nutritional Substance 3E0D-
    Radioactive Substance 3E0D-
    Sedatives 3E0D-
    Serum 3E0D-
    Toxoid 3E0D-
    Vaccine 3E0D-
    Water Balance Substance 3E0D-
  Pleural Cavity 3E0L3GC
    Adhesion Barrier 3E0L05Z
    Analgesics 3E0L3NZ
    Anesthetic, Local 3E0L3BZ
    Anti-infective 3E0L32-
    Anti-inflammatory 3E0L33Z
    Antineoplastic 3E0L-
    Destructive Agent 3E0L3TZ
    Diagnostic Substance, Other 3E0L3KZ
    Electrolytic Substance 3E0L37Z
    Gas 3E0L-
    Hypnotics 3E0L3NZ
    Nutritional Substance 3E0L36Z
    Radioactive Substance 3E0L3HZ
    Sedatives 3E0L3NZ
    Water Balance Substance 3E0L37Z
  Products of Conception 3E0E-
    Analgesics 3E0E-
    Anesthetic, Local 3E0E-
    Anti-infective 3E0E-
    Anti-inflammatory 3E0E-
    Antineoplastic 3E0E-
    Destructive Agent 3E0E-
    Diagnostic Substance, Other 3E0E-
    Electrolytic Substance 3E0E-
    Gas 3E0E-
    Hypnotics 3E0E-
    Nutritional Substance 3E0E-
    Radioactive Substance 3E0E-
    Sedatives 3E0E-
    Water Balance Substance 3E0E-
  Reproductive
    Female 3E0P-
      Adhesion Barrier 3E0P05Z
      Analgesics 3E0P-
      Anesthetic, Local 3E0P-
      Anti-infective 3E0P-
      Anti-inflammatory 3E0P-
      Antineoplastic 3E0P-
      Destructive Agent 3E0P-
      Diagnostic Substance, Other 3E0P-
      Electrolytic Substance 3E0P-
      Gas 3E0P-
      Hypnotics 3E0P-
      Nutritional Substance 3E0P-
      Ovum, Fertilized 3E0P-
      Radioactive Substance 3E0P-

Introduction of substance in or on — *continued*
  Reproductive — *continued*
    Female 3E0P- — *continued*
      Sedatives 3E0P-
      Sperm 3E0P-
      Water Balance Substance 3E0P-
    Male 3E0N-
      Analgesics 3E0N-
      Anesthetic, Local 3E0N-
      Anti-infective 3E0N-
      Anti-inflammatory 3E0N-
      Antineoplastic 3E0N-
      Destructive Agent 3E0N-
      Diagnostic Substance, Other 3E0N-
      Electrolytic Substance 3E0N-
      Gas 3E0N-
      Hypnotics 3E0N-
      Nutritional Substance 3E0N-
      Radioactive Substance 3E0N-
      Sedatives 3E0N-
      Water Balance Substance 3E0N-
  Respiratory Tract 3E0F-
    Analgesics 3E0F-
    Anesthetic
      Inhalation 3E0F-
      Local 3E0F-
    Anti-infective 3E0F-
    Anti-inflammatory 3E0F-
    Antineoplastic 3E0F-
    Destructive Agent 3E0F-
    Diagnostic Substance, Other 3E0F-
    Electrolytic Substance 3E0F-
    Gas 3E0F-
    Hypnotics 3E0F-
    Nutritional Substance 3E0F-
    Radioactive Substance 3E0F-
    Sedatives 3E0F-
    Water Balance Substance 3E0F-
  Skin 3E00XGC
    Analgesics 3E00XNZ
    Anesthetic, Local 3E00XBZ
    Anti-infective 3E00X2-
    Anti-inflammatory 3E00X3Z
    Antineoplastic 3E00X0-
    Destructive Agent 3E00XTZ
    Diagnostic Substance, Other 3E00XKZ
    Hypnotics 3E00XNZ
    Pigment 3E00XMZ
    Sedatives 3E00XNZ
    Serum 3E00X4Z
    Toxoid 3E00X4Z
    Vaccine 3E00X4Z
  Spinal Canal 3E0R3GC
    Analgesics 3E0R3NZ
    Anesthetic
      Local 3E0R3BZ
      Regional 3E0R3CZ
    Anti-infective 3E0R32-
    Anti-inflammatory 3E0R33Z
    Antineoplastic 3E0R30-
    Destructive Agent 3E0R3TZ
    Diagnostic Substance, Other 3E0R3KZ
    Electrolytic Substance 3E0R37Z
    Gas 3E0R-
    Hypnotics 3E0R3NZ
    Nutritional Substance 3E0R36Z
    Radioactive Substance 3E0R3HZ
    Sedatives 3E0R3NZ
    Stem Cells
      Embryonic 3E0R-
      Somatic 3E0R-
    Water Balance Substance 3E0R37Z
  Subcutaneous Tissue 3E013GC
    Analgesics 3E013NZ
    Anesthetic, Local 3E013BZ
    Anti-infective 3E01-
    Anti-inflammatory 3E0133Z

Introduction of substance in or on — *continued*
  Subcutaneous Tissue 3E013GC — *continued*
    Antineoplastic 3E0130-
    Destructive Agent 3E013TZ
    Diagnostic Substance, Other 3E013KZ
    Electrolytic Substance 3E0137Z
    Hormone 3E013V-
    Hypnotics 3E013NZ
    Nutritional Substance 3E0136Z
    Radioactive Substance 3E013HZ
    Sedatives 3E013NZ
    Serum 3E0134Z
    Toxoid 3E0134Z
    Vaccine 3E0134Z
    Water Balance Substance 3E0137Z
  Vein
    Central 3E04-
      Analgesics 3E04-
      Anesthetic, Intracirculatory 3E04-
      Antiarrhythmic 3E04-
      Anti-infective 3E04-
      Anti-inflammatory 3E04-
      Antineoplastic 3E04-
      Destructive Agent 3E04-
      Diagnostic Substance, Other 3E04-
      Electrolytic Substance 3E04-
      Hormone 3E04-
      Hypnotics 3E04-
      Immunotherapeutic 3E04-
      Nutritional Substance 3E04-
      Platelet Inhibitor 3E04-
      Radioactive Substance 3E04-
      Sedatives 3E04-
      Serum 3E04-
      Thrombolytic 3E04-
      Toxoid 3E04-
      Vaccine 3E04-
      Vasopressor 3E04-
      Water Balance Substance 3E04-
    Peripheral 3E03-
      Analgesics 3E03-
      Anesthetic, Intracirculatory 3E03-
      Antiarrhythmic 3E03-
      Anti-infective 3E03-
      Anti-inflammatory 3E03-
      Antineoplastic 3E03-
      Destructive Agent 3E03-
      Diagnostic Substance, Other 3E03-
      Electrolytic Substance 3E03-
      Hormone 3E03-
      Hypnotics 3E03-
      Immunotherapeutic 3E03-
      Islet Cells, Pancreatic 3E03-
      Nutritional Substance 3E03-
      Platelet Inhibitor 3E03-
      Radioactive Substance 3E03-
      Sedatives 3E03-
      Serum 3E03-
      Thrombolytic 3E03-
      Toxoid 3E03-
      Vaccine 3E03-
      Vasopressor 3E03-
      Water Balance Substance 3E03-
Intubation
  Airway
    see Insertion of device in, Esophagus 0DH5-
    see Insertion of device in, Mouth and Throat 0CHY-
    see Insertion of device in, Trachea 0BH1-
  Drainage device *see* Drainage
  Feeding Device *see* Insertion of device in, Gastrointestinal System 0DH-

IPPB (intermittent positive pressure breathing) *see* Assistance, Respiratory 5A09-
Iridectomy
  see Excision, Eye 08B-
  see Resection, Eye 08T-
Iridoplasty
  see Repair, Eye 08Q-
  see Replacement, Eye 08R-
  see Supplement, Eye 08U-
Iridotomy *see* Drainage, Eye 089-
Irrigation
  Biliary Tract, Irrigating Substance 3E1J-
  Brain, Irrigating Substance 3E1Q38Z
  Cranial Cavity, Irrigating Substance 3E1Q38Z
  Ear, Irrigating Substance 3E1B-
  Epidural Space, Irrigating Substance 3E1S38Z
  Eye, Irrigating Substance 3E1C-
  Gastrointestinal Tract
    Lower, Irrigating Substance 3E1H-
    Upper, Irrigating Substance 3E1G-
  Genitourinary Tract, Irrigating Substance 3E1K-
  Irrigating Substance 3C1ZX8Z
  Joint, Irrigating Substance 3E1U38Z
  Mucous Membrane, Irrigating Substance 3E10-
  Nose, Irrigating Substance 3E19-
  Pancreatic Tract, Irrigating Substance 3E1J-
  Pericardial Cavity, Irrigating Substance 3E1Y38Z
  Peritoneal Cavity
    Dialysate 3E1M39Z
    Irrigating Substance 3E1M38Z
  Pleural Cavity, Irrigating Substance 3E1L38Z
  Reproductive
    Female, Irrigating Substance 3E1P-
    Male, Irrigating Substance 3E1N-
  Respiratory Tract, Irrigating Substance 3E1F-
  Skin, Irrigating Substance 3E10-
  Spinal Canal, Irrigating Substance 3E1R38Z
Isavuconazole anti-infective XW0-
Ischiatic nerve
  use Nerve, Sciatic
Ischiocavernosus muscle
  use Muscle, Perineum
Ischiofemoral ligament
  use Bursa and Ligament, Hip, Left
  use Bursa and Ligament, Hip, Right
Ischium
  use Bone, Pelvic, Left
  use Bone, Pelvic, Right
Isolation 8E0ZXY6
Isotope Administration, Whole Body DWY5G-
Itrel (3) (4) neurostimulator
  use Stimulator Generator, Single Array in 0JH-

J

Jejunal artery
  use Artery, Superior Mesenteric
Jejunectomy
  see Excision, Jejunum 0DBA-
  see Resection, Jejunum 0DTA-
Jejunocolostomy
  see Bypass, Gastrointestinal System 0D1-
  see Drainage, Gastrointestinal System 0D9-
Jejunopexy
  see Repair, Jejunum 0DQA-
  see Reposition, Jejunum 0DSA-
Jejunostomy
  see Bypass, Jejunum 0D1A-
  see Drainage, Jejunum 0D9A-
Jejunotomy see Drainage, Jejunum 0D9A-
Joint fixation plate
  use Internal Fixation Device in Lower Joints
  use Internal Fixation Device in Upper Joints
Joint liner (insert)
  use Liner in Lower Joints
Joint spacer (antibiotic)
  use Spacer in Lower Joints
  use Spacer in Upper Joints
Jugular body
  use Glomus Jugulare
Jugular lymph node
  use Lymphatic, Neck, Left
  use Lymphatic, Neck, Right

K

Kappa
  use Pacemaker, Dual Chamber in 0JH-
Kcentra
  use 4-Factor Prothrombin Complex Concentrate
Keratectomy, kerectomy
  see Excision, Eye 08B-
  see Resection, Eye 08T-
Keratocentesis see Drainage, Eye 089-
Keratoplasty
  see Repair, Eye 08Q-
  see Replacement, Eye 08R-
  see Supplement, Eye 08U-
Keratotomy
  see Drainage, Eye 089-
  see Repair, Eye 08Q-
Kirschner wire (K-wire)
  use Internal Fixation Device in Head and Facial Bones
  use Internal Fixation Device in Lower Bones
  use Internal Fixation Device in Lower Joints
  use Internal Fixation Device in Upper Bones
  use Internal Fixation Device in Upper Joints
Knee (implant) insert
  use Liner in Lower Joints
KUB x-ray see Plain Radiography, Kidney, Ureter and Bladder BT04-
Kuntscher nail
  use Internal Fixation Device, Intramedullary in Lower Bones
  use Internal Fixation Device, Intramedullary in Upper Bones

L

Labia majora
  use Vulva
Labia minora
  use Vulva
Labial gland
  use Lip, Lower
  use Lip, Upper
Labiectomy
  see Excision, Female Reproductive System 0UB-
  see Resection, Female Reproductive System 0UT-
Lacrimal canaliculus
  use Duct, Lacrimal, Left
  use Duct, Lacrimal, Right
Lacrimal punctum
  use Duct, Lacrimal, Left
  use Duct, Lacrimal, Right
Lacrimal sac
  use Duct, Lacrimal, Left
  use Duct, Lacrimal, Right
Laminectomy
  see Excision, Lower Bones 0QB-
  see Excision, Upper Bones 0PB-
Laminotomy
  see Drainage, Lower Bones 0Q9-
  see Drainage, Upper Bones 0P9-
  see Excision, Lower Bones 0QB-
  see Excision, Upper Bones 0PB-
  see Release, Central Nervous System 00N-
  see Release, Lower Bones 0QN-
  see Release, Peripheral Nervous System 01N-
  see Release, Upper Bones 0PN-
LAP-BAND® adjustable gastric banding system
  use Extraluminal Device
Laparoscopy see Inspection
Laparotomy
  Drainage see Drainage, Peritoneal Cavity 0W9G-
  Exploratory see Inspection, Peritoneal Cavity 0WJG-
Laryngectomy
  see Excision, Larynx 0CBS-
  see Resection, Larynx 0CTS-
Laryngocentesis see Drainage, Larynx 0C9S-
Laryngogram see Fluoroscopy, Larynx B91J-
Laryngopexy see Repair, Larynx 0CQS-
Laryngopharynx
  use Pharynx
Laryngoplasty
  see Repair, Larynx 0CQS-
  see Replacement, Larynx 0CRS-
  see Supplement, Larynx 0CUS-
Laryngorrhaphy see Repair, Larynx 0CQS-
Laryngoscopy 0CJS8ZZ
Laryngotomy see Drainage, Larynx 0C9S-
Laser Interstitial Thermal Therapy
  Adrenal Gland DGY2KZZ
  Anus DDY8KZZ
  Bile Ducts DFY2KZZ
  Brain D0Y0KZZ
  Brain Stem D0Y1KZZ
  Breast
    Left DMY0KZZ
    Right DMY1KZZ
  Bronchus DBY1KZZ
  Chest Wall DBY7KZZ
  Colon DDY5KZZ
  Diaphragm DBY8KZZ
  Duodenum DDY2KZZ
  Esophagus DDY0KZZ

Laser Interstitial Thermal Therapy — continued
  Gallbladder DFY1KZZ
  Gland
    Adrenal DGY2KZZ
    Parathyroid DGY4KZZ
    Pituitary DGY0KZZ
    Thyroid DGY5KZZ
  Ileum DDY4KZZ
  Jejunum DDY3KZZ
  Liver DFY0KZZ
  Lung DBY2KZZ
  Mediastinum DBY6KZZ
  Nerve, Peripheral D0Y7KZZ
  Pancreas DFY3KZZ
  Parathyroid Gland DGY4KZZ
  Pineal Body DGY1KZZ
  Pituitary Gland DGY0KZZ
  Pleura DBY5KZZ
  Prostate DVY0KZZ
  Rectum DDY7KZZ
  Spinal Cord D0Y6KZZ
  Stomach DDY1KZZ
  Thyroid Gland DGY5KZZ
  Trachea DBY0KZZ
Lateral (brachial) lymph node
  use Lymphatic, Axillary, Left
  use Lymphatic, Axillary, Right
Lateral canthus
  use Eyelid, Upper, Left
  use Eyelid, Upper, Right
Lateral collateral ligament (LCL)
  use Bursa and Ligament, Knee, Left
  use Bursa and Ligament, Knee, Right
Lateral condyle of femur
  use Femur, Lower, Left
  use Femur, Lower, Right
Lateral condyle of tibia
  use Tibia, Left
  use Tibia, Right
Lateral cuneiform bone
  use Tarsal, Left
  use Tarsal, Right
Lateral epicondyle of femur
  use Femur, Lower, Left
  use Femur, Lower, Right
Lateral epicondyle of humerus
  use Humeral Shaft, Left
  use Humeral Shaft, Right
Lateral femoral cutaneous nerve
  use Nerve, Lumbar Plexus
Lateral malleolus
  use Fibula, Left
  use Fibula, Right
Lateral meniscus
  use Joint, Knee, Left
  use Joint, Knee, Right
Lateral nasal cartilage
  use Nose
Lateral plantar artery
  use Artery, Foot, Left
  use Artery, Foot, Right
Lateral plantar nerve
  use Nerve, Tibial
Lateral rectus muscle
  use Muscle, Extraocular, Left
  use Muscle, Extraocular, Right
Lateral sacral artery
  use Artery, Internal Iliac, Left
  use Artery, Internal Iliac, Right
Lateral sacral vein
  use Vein, Hypogastric, Left
  use Vein, Hypogastric, Right
Lateral sural cutaneous nerve
  use Nerve, Peroneal
Lateral tarsal artery
  use Artery, Foot, Left
  use Artery, Foot, Right
Lateral temporomandibular ligament
  use Bursa and Ligament, Head and Neck

INDEX TO PROCEDURES – 2016 ICD-10-PCS

Lateral thoracic artery
  use Artery, Axillary, Left
  use Artery, Axillary, Right
Latissimus dorsi muscle
  use Muscle, Trunk, Left
  use Muscle, Trunk, Right
Latissimus Dorsi Myocutaneous Flap
  Bilateral 0HRV075
  Left 0HRU075
  Right 0HRT075
Lavage
  see Irrigation
  bronchial alveolar, diagnostic see Drainage, Respiratory System 0B9-
Least splanchnic nerve
  use Nerve, Thoracic Sympathetic
Left ascending lumbar vein
  use Vein, Hemiazygos
Left atrioventricular valve
  use Valve, Mitral
Left auricular appendix
  use Atrium, Left
Left colic vein
  use Vein, Colic
Left coronary sulcus
  use Heart, Left
Left gastric artery
  use Artery, Gastric
Left gastroepiploic artery
  use Artery, Splenic
Left gastroepiploic vein
  use Vein, Splenic
Left inferior phrenic vein
  use Vein, Renal, Left
Left inferior pulmonary vein
  use Vein, Pulmonary, Left
Left jugular trunk
  use Lymphatic, Thoracic Duct
Left lateral ventricle
  use Cerebral Ventricle
Left ovarian vein
  use Vein, Renal, Left
Left second lumbar vein
  use Vein, Renal, Left
Left subclavian trunk
  use Lymphatic, Thoracic Duct
Left subcostal vein
  use Vein, Hemiazygos
Left superior pulmonary vein
  use Vein, Pulmonary, Left
Left suprarenal vein
  use Vein, Renal, Left
Left testicular vein
  use Vein, Renal, Left
Lengthening
  Bone, with device see Insertion of Limb Lengthening Device
  Muscle, by incision see Division, Muscles 0K8-
  Tendon, by incision see Division, Tendons 0L8-
Leptomeninges, intracranial
  use Cerebral Meninges
Leptomeninges, spinal
  use Spinal Meninges
Lesser alar cartilage
  use Nose
Lesser occipital nerve
  use Nerve, Cervical Plexus
Lesser splanchnic nerve
  use Nerve, Thoracic Sympathetic
Lesser trochanter
  use Femur, Upper, Left
  use Femur, Upper, Right
Lesser tuberosity
  use Humeral Head, Left
  use Humeral Head, Right
Lesser wing
  use Bone, Sphenoid, Left
  use Bone, Sphenoid, Right

Leukopheresis, therapeutic see Pheresis, Circulatory 6A55-
Levator anguli oris muscle
  use Muscle, Facial
Levator ani muscle
  use Muscle, Trunk, Left
  use Muscle, Trunk, Right
Levator labii superioris alaeque nasi muscle
  use Muscle, Facial
Levator labii superioris muscle
  use Muscle, Facial
Levator palpebrae superioris muscle
  use Eyelid, Upper, Left
  use Eyelid, Upper, Right
Levator scapulae muscle
  use Muscle, Neck, Left
  use Muscle, Neck, Right
Levator veli palatini muscle
  use Muscle, Tongue, Palate, Pharynx
Levatores costarum muscle
  use Muscle, Thorax, Left
  use Muscle, Thorax, Right
LifeStent® (Flexstar) (XL) Vascular Stent System
  use Intraluminal Device
Ligament of head of fibula
  use Bursa and Ligament, Knee, Left
  use Bursa and Ligament, Knee, Right
Ligament of the lateral malleolus
  use Bursa and Ligament, Ankle, Left
  use Bursa and Ligament, Ankle, Right
Ligamentum flavum
  use Bursa and Ligament, Trunk, Left
  use Bursa and Ligament, Trunk, Right
Ligation see Occlusion
Ligation, hemorrhoid see Occlusion, Lower Veins, Hemorrhoidal Plexus
Light Therapy GZJZZZZ
Liner
  Removal of device from
    Hip
      Left 0SPB09Z
      Right 0SP909Z
    Knee
      Left 0SPD09Z
      Right 0SPC09Z
  Revision of device in
    Hip
      Left 0SWB09Z
      Right 0SW909Z
    Knee
      Left 0SWD09Z
      Right 0SWC09Z
  Supplement
    Hip
      Left 0SUB09Z
        Acetabular Surface 0SUE09Z
        Femoral Surface 0SUS09Z
      Right 0SU909Z
        Acetabular Surface 0SUA09Z
        Femoral Surface 0SUR09Z
    Knee
      Left 0SUD09-
        Femoral Surface 0SUU09Z
        Tibial Surface 0SUW09Z
      Right 0SUC09-
        Femoral Surface 0SUT09Z
        Tibial Surface 0SUV09Z
Lingual artery
  use Artery, External Carotid, Left
  use Artery, External Carotid, Right
Lingual tonsil use Tongue
Lingulectomy, lung
  see Excision, Lung Lingula 0BBH-
  see Resection, Lung Lingula 0BTH-
Lithotripsy
  see Fragmentation
  With removal of fragments see Extirpation

LITT (laser interstitial thermal therapy)
  see Laser Interstitial Thermal Therapy
LIVIAN™ CRT-D
  use Cardiac Resynchronization Defibrillator Pulse Generator in 0JH-
Lobectomy
  see Excision, Central Nervous System 00B-
  see Excision, Endocrine System 0GB-
  see Excision, Hepatobiliary System and Pancreas 0FB-
  see Excision, Respiratory System 0BB-
  see Resection, Endocrine System 0GT-
  see Resection, Hepatobiliary System and Pancreas 0FT-
  see Resection, Respiratory System 0BT-
Lobotomy see Division, Brain 0080-
Localization
  see Imaging
  see Map
Locus ceruleus
  use Pons
Long thoracic nerve
  use Nerve, Brachial Plexus
Loop ileostomy see Bypass, Ileum 0D1B-
Loop recorder, implantable
  use Monitoring Device
Lower GI series see Fluoroscopy, Colon BD14-
Lumbar artery
  use Aorta, Abdominal
Lumbar facet joint
  use Joint, Lumbar Vertebral
Lumbar ganglion
  use Nerve, Lumbar Sympathetic
Lumbar lymph node
  use Lymphatic, Aortic
Lumbar lymphatic trunk
  use Cisterna Chyli
Lumbar splanchnic nerve
  use Nerve, Lumbar Sympathetic
Lumbosacral facet joint
  use Joint, Lumbosacral
Lumbosacral trunk
  use Nerve, Lumbar
Lumpectomy see Excision
Lunate bone
  use Carpal, Left
  use Carpal, Right
Lunotriquetral ligament
  use Bursa and Ligament, Hand, Left
  use Bursa and Ligament, Hand, Right
Lymphadenectomy
  see Excision, Lymphatic and Hemic Systems 07B-
  see Resection, Lymphatic and Hemic Systems 07T-
Lymphadenotomy see Drainage, Lymphatic and Hemic Systems 079-
Lymphangiectomy
  see Excision, Lymphatic and Hemic Systems 07B-
  see Resection, Lymphatic and Hemic Systems 07T-
Lymphangiogram see Plain Radiography, Lymphatic System B70-
Lymphangioplasty
  see Repair, Lymphatic and Hemic Systems 07Q-
  see Supplement, Lymphatic and Hemic Systems 07U-
Lymphangiorrhaphy see Repair, Lymphatic and Hemic Systems 07Q-
Lymphangiotomy see Drainage, Lymphatic and Hemic Systems 079-
Lysis see Release

M

Macula
  use Retina, Left
  use Retina, Right
Magnet extraction, ocular foreign body see Extirpation, Eye 08C-
Magnetic Resonance Imaging (MRI)
  Abdomen BW30-
  Ankle
    Left BQ3H-
    Right BQ3G-
  Aorta
    Abdominal B430-
    Thoracic B330-
  Arm
    Left BP3F-
    Right BP3E-
  Artery
    Celiac B431-
    Cervico-Cerebral Arch B33Q-
    Common Carotid, Bilateral B335-
    Coronary
      Bypass Graft, Multiple B233-
      Multiple B231-
    Internal Carotid, Bilateral B338-
    Intracranial B33R-
    Lower Extremity
      Bilateral B43H-
      Left B43G-
      Right B43F-
    Pelvic B43C-
    Renal, Bilateral B438-
    Spinal B33M-
    Superior Mesenteric B434-
    Upper Extremity
      Bilateral B33K-
      Left B33J-
      Right B33H-
    Vertebral, Bilateral B33G-
  Bladder BT30-
  Brachial Plexus BW3P-
  Brain B030-
  Breast
    Bilateral BH32-
    Left BH31-
    Right BH30-
  Calcaneus
    Left BQ3K-
    Right BQ3J-
  Chest BW33Y-
  Coccyx BR3F-
  Connective Tissue
    Lower Extremity BL31-
    Upper Extremity BL30-
  Corpora Cavernosa BV30-
  Disc
    Cervical BR31-
    Lumbar BR33-
    Thoracic BR32-
  Ear B930-
  Elbow
    Left BP3H-
    Right BP3G-
  Eye
    Bilateral B837-
    Left B836-
    Right B835-
  Femur
    Left BQ34-
    Right BQ33-
  Fetal Abdomen BY33-
  Fetal Extremity BY35-
  Fetal Head BY30-
  Fetal Heart BY31-
  Fetal Spine BY34-
  Fetal Thorax BY32-
  Fetus, Whole BY36-

Magnetic

INDEX TO PROCEDURES – 2016 ICD-10-PCS

Magnetic Resonance Imaging (MRI) — continued
Foot
  Left **BQ3M-**
  Right **BQ3L-**
Forearm
  Left **BP3K-**
  Right **BP3J-**
Gland
  Adrenal, Bilateral **BG32-**
  Parathyroid **BG33-**
  Parotid, Bilateral **B936-**
  Salivary, Bilateral **B93D-**
  Submandibular, Bilateral **B939-**
  Thyroid **BG34-**
Head **BW38-**
Heart, Right and Left **B236-**
Hip
  Left **BQ31-**
  Right **BQ30-**
Intracranial Sinus **B532-**
Joint
  Finger
    Left **BP3D-**
    Right **BP3C-**
  Hand
    Left **BP3D-**
    Right **BP3C-**
  Temporomandibular, Bilateral **BN39-**
Kidney
  Bilateral **BT33-**
  Left **BT32-**
  Right **BT31-**
  Transplant **BT39-**
Knee
  Left **BQ38-**
  Right **BQ37-**
Larynx **B93J-**
Leg
  Left **BQ3F-**
  Right **BQ3D-**
Liver **BF35-**
Liver and Spleen **BF36-**
Lung Apices **BB3G-**
Nasopharynx **B93F-**
Neck **BW3F-**
Nerve
  Acoustic **B03C-**
  Brachial Plexus **BW3P-**
Oropharynx **B93F-**
Ovary
  Bilateral **BU35-**
  Left **BU34-**
  Right **BU33-**
Ovary and Uterus **BU3C-**
Pancreas **BF37-**
Patella
  Left **BQ3W-**
  Right **BQ3V-**
Pelvic Region **BW3G-**
Pelvis **BR3C-**
Pituitary Gland **B039-**
Plexus, Brachial **BW3P-**
Prostate **BV33-**
Retroperitoneum **BW3H-**
Sacrum **BR3F-**
Scrotum **BV34-**
Sella Turcica **B039-**
Shoulder
  Left **BP39-**
  Right **BP38-**
Sinus
  Intracranial **B532-**
  Paranasal **B932-**
Spinal Cord **B03B-**
Spine
  Cervical **BR30-**
  Lumbar **BR39-**
  Thoracic **BR37-**
Spleen and Liver **BF36-**

Magnetic Resonance Imaging (MRI) — continued
Subcutaneous Tissue
  Abdomen **BH3H-**
  Extremity
    Lower **BH3J-**
    Upper **BH3F-**
  Head **BH3D-**
  Neck **BH3D-**
  Pelvis **BH3H-**
  Thorax **BH3G-**
Tendon
  Lower Extremity **BL33-**
  Upper Extremity **BL32-**
Testicle
  Bilateral **BV37-**
  Left **BV36-**
  Right **BV35-**
Toe
  Left **BQ3Q-**
  Right **BQ3P-**
Uterus **BU36-**
  Pregnant **BU3B-**
Uterus and Ovary **BU3C-**
Vagina **BU39-**
Vein
  Cerebellar **B531-**
  Cerebral **B531-**
  Jugular, Bilateral **B535-**
  Lower Extremity
    Bilateral **B53D-**
    Left **B53C-**
    Right **B53B-**
  Other **B53V-**
  Pelvic (Iliac) Bilateral **B53H-**
  Portal **B53T-**
  Pulmonary, Bilateral **B53S-**
  Renal, Bilateral **B53L-**
  Spanchnic **B53T-**
  Upper Extremity
    Bilateral **B53P-**
    Left **B53N-**
    Right **B53M-**
Vena Cava
  Inferior **B539-**
  Superior **B538-**
Wrist
  Left **BP3M-**
  Right **BP3L-**
Malleotomy see Drainage, Ear, Nose, Sinus **099-**

Malleus
use Auditory Ossicle, Left
use Auditory Ossicle, Right

Mammaplasty, mammoplasty
see Alteration, Skin and Breast **0H0-**
see Repair, Skin and Breast **0HQ-**
see Replacement, Skin and Breast **0HR-**
see Supplement, Skin and Breast **0HU-**

Mammary duct
use Breast, Bilateral
use Breast, Left
use Breast, Right

Mammary gland
use Breast, Bilateral
use Breast, Left
use Breast, Right

Mammectomy
see Excision, Skin and Breast **0HB-**
see Resection, Skin and Breast **0HT-**

Mammillary body
use Hypothalamus

Mammography see Plain Radiography, Skin, Subcutaneous Tissue and Breast **BH0-**

Mammotomy see Drainage, Skin and Breast **0H9-**

Mandibular nerve
use Nerve, Trigeminal

Mandibular notch
use Mandible, Left
use Mandible, Right

Mandibulectomy
see Excision, Head and Facial Bones **0NB-**
see Resection, Head and Facial Bones **0NT-**

Manipulation
Adhesions see Release
Chiropractic see Chiropractic Manipulation

Manubrium
use Sternum

Map
Basal Ganglia **00K8-**
Brain **00K0-**
Cerebellum **00KC-**
Cerebral Hemisphere **00K7-**
Conduction Mechanism **02K8-**
Hypothalamus **00KA-**
Medulla Oblongata **00KD-**
Pons **00KB-**
Thalamus **00K9-**

Mapping
Doppler ultrasound see Ultrasonography
Electrocardiogram only see Measurement, Cardiac **4A02-**

Mark IV Breathing Pacemaker System
use Stimulator Generator in Subcutaneous Tissue and Fascia

Marsupialization
see Drainage
see Excision

Massage, cardiac
External **5A12012**
Open **02QA0ZZ**

Masseter muscle
use Muscle, Head

Masseteric fascia
use Subcutaneous Tissue and Fascia, Face

Mastectomy
see Excision, Skin and Breast **0HB-**
see Resection, Skin and Breast **0HT-**

Mastoid (postauricular) lymph node
use Lymphatic, Neck, Left
use Lymphatic, Neck, Right

Mastoid air cells
use Sinus, Mastoid, Left
use Sinus, Mastoid, Right

Mastoid process
use Bone, Temporal, Left
use Bone, Temporal, Right

Mastoidectomy
see Excision, Ear, Nose, Sinus **09B-**
see Resection, Ear, Nose, Sinus **09T-**

Mastoidotomy see Drainage, Ear, Nose, Sinus **099-**

Mastopexy
see Reposition, Skin and Breast **0HS-**
see Repair, Skin and Breast **0HQ-**

Mastorrhaphy see Repair, Skin and Breast **0HQ-**

Mastotomy see Drainage, Skin and Breast **0H9-**

Maxillary artery
use Artery, External Carotid, Left
use Artery, External Carotid, Right

Maxillary nerve
use Nerve, Trigeminal

Maximo II DR (VR)
use Defibrillator, Generator in **0JH-**

Maximo II DR CRT-D
use Cardiac Resynchronization Defibrillator Pulse Generator in **0JH-**

Measurement
Arterial
  Flow
    Coronary **4A03-**
    Peripheral **4A03-**
    Pulmonary **4A03-**
  Pressure
    Coronary **4A03-**
    Peripheral **4A03-**
    Pulmonary **4A03-**
    Thoracic, Other **4A03-**
  Pulse
    Coronary **4A03-**
    Peripheral **4A03-**
    Pulmonary **4A03-**
  Saturation, Peripheral **4A03-**
  Sound, Peripheral **4A03-**
Biliary
  Flow **4A0C-**
  Pressure **4A0C-**
Cardiac
  Action Currents **4A02-**
  Defibrillator **4B02XTZ**
  Electrical Activity **4A02-**
    Guidance **4A02X4A**
    No Qualifier **4A02X4Z**
  Output **4A02-**
  Pacemaker **4B02XSZ**
  Rate **4A02-**
  Rhythm **4A02-**
  Sampling and Pressure
    Bilateral **4A02-**
    Left Heart **4A02-**
    Right Heart **4A02-**
  Sound **4A02-**
  Total Activity, Stress **4A02XM4**
Central Nervous
  Conductivity **4A00-**
  Electrical Activity **4A00-**
  Pressure **4A000BZ**
    Intracranial **4A00-**
  Saturation, Intracranial **4A00-**
  Stimulator **4B00XVZ**
  Temperature, Intracranial **4A00-**
Circulatory, Volume **4A05XLZ**
Gastrointestinal
  Motility **4A0B-**
  Pressure **4A0B-**
  Secretion **4A0B-**
Lymphatic
  Flow **4A06-**
  Pressure **4A06-**
Metabolism **4A0Z-**
Musculoskeletal
  Contractility **4A0F-**
  Stimulator **4B0FXVZ**
Olfactory, Acuity **4A08X0Z**
Peripheral Nervous
  Conductivity
    Motor **4A01-**
    Sensory **4A01-**
  Electrical Activity **4A01-**
  Stimulator **4B01XVZ**
Products of Conception
  Cardiac
    Electrical Activity **4A0H-**
    Rate **4A0H-**
    Rhythm **4A0H-**
    Sound **4A0H-**
  Nervous
    Conductivity **4A0J-**
    Electrical Activity **4A0J-**
    Pressure **4A0J-**
Respiratory
  Capacity **4A09-**
  Flow **4A09-**
  Pacemaker **4B09XSZ**
  Rate **4A09-**
  Resistance **4A09-**
  Total Activity **4A09-**
  Volume **4A09-**
Sleep **4A0ZXQZ**

Measurement — *continued*
  Temperature 4A0Z-
  Urinary
    Contractility 4A0D73Z
    Flow 4A0D75Z
    Pressure 4A0D7BZ
    Resistance 4A0D7DZ
    Volume 4A0D7LZ
  Venous
    Flow
      Central 4A04-
      Peripheral 4A04-
      Portal 4A04-
      Pulmonary 4A04-
    Pressure
      Central 4A04-
      Peripheral 4A04-
      Portal 4A04-
      Pulmonary 4A04-
    Pulse
      Central 4A04-
      Peripheral 4A04-
      Portal 4A04-
      Pulmonary 4A04-
    Saturation, Peripheral 4A04-
  Visual
    Acuity 4A07X0Z
    Mobility 4A07X7Z
    Pressure 4A07XBZ
Meatoplasty, urethra *see* Repair, Urethra 0TQD-
Meatotomy *see* Drainage, Urinary System 0T9-
Mechanical ventilation *see* Performance, Respiratory 5A19-
Medial canthus
  use Eyelid, Lower, Left
  use Eyelid, Lower, Right
Medial collateral ligament (MCL)
  use Bursa and Ligament, Knee, Left
  use Bursa and Ligament, Knee, Right
Medial condyle of femur
  use Femur, Lower, Left
  use Femur, Lower, Right
Medial condyle of tibia
  use Tibia, Left
  use Tibia, Right
Medial cuneiform bone
  use Tarsal, Left
  use Tarsal, Right
Medial epicondyle of femur
  use Femur, Lower, Left
  use Femur, Lower, Right
Medial epicondyle of humerus
  use Humeral Shaft, Left
  use Humeral Shaft, Right
Medial malleolus
  use Tibia, Left
  use Tibia, Right
Medial meniscus
  use Joint, Knee, Left
  use Joint, Knee, Right
Medial plantar artery
  use Artery, Foot, Left
  use Artery, Foot, Right
Medial plantar nerve
  use Nerve, Tibial
Medial popliteal nerve
  use Nerve, Tibial
Medial rectus muscle
  use Muscle, Extraocular, Left
  use Muscle, Extraocular, Right
Medial sural cutaneous nerve
  use Nerve, Tibial
Median antebrachial vein
  use Vein, Basilic, Left
  use Vein, Basilic, Right
Median cubital vein
  use Vein, Basilic, Left
  use Vein, Basilic, Right
Median sacral artery
  use Aorta, Abdominal

Mediastinal lymph node
  use Lymphatic, Thorax
Mediastinoscopy 0WJC4ZZ
Medication Management GZ3ZZZZ
  For substance abuse
    Antabuse HZ83ZZZ
    Bupropion HZ87ZZZ
    Clonidine HZ86ZZZ
    Levo-alpha-acetyl-methadol (LAAM) HZ82ZZZ
    Methadone Maintenance HZ81ZZZ
    Naloxone HZ85ZZZ
    Naltrexone HZ84ZZZ
    Nicotine Replacement HZ80ZZZ
    Other Replacement Medication HZ89ZZZ
    Psychiatric Medication HZ88ZZZ
Meditation 8E0ZXY5
Meissner's (submucous) plexus
  use Nerve, Abdominal Sympathetic
Melody® transcatheter pulmonary valve
  use Zooplastic Tissue in Heart and Great Vessels
Membranous urethra
  use Urethra
Meningeorrhaphy
  see Repair, Cerebral Meninges 00Q1-
  see Repair, Spinal Meninges 00QT-
Meniscectomy, knee
  see Excision, Lower Joints 0SB-
Mental foramen
  use Mandible, Left
  use Mandible, Right
Mentalis muscle
  use Muscle, Facial
Mentoplasty *see* Alteration, Jaw, Lower 0W05-
Mesenterectomy *see* Excision, Mesentery 0DBV-
Mesenteriorrhaphy, mesenterorrhaphy *see* Repair, Mesentery 0DQV-
Mesenteriplication *see* Repair, Mesentery 0DQV-
Mesoappendix
  use Mesentery
Mesocolon
  use Mesentery
Metacarpal ligament
  use Bursa and Ligament, Hand, Left
  use Bursa and Ligament, Hand, Right
Metacarpophalangeal ligament
  use Bursa and Ligament, Hand, Left
  use Bursa and Ligament, Hand, Right
Metatarsal ligament
  use Bursa and Ligament, Foot, Left
  use Bursa and Ligament, Foot, Right
Metatarsectomy
  see Excision, Lower Bones 0QB-
  see Resection, Lower Bones 0QT-
Metatarsophalangeal (MTP) joint
  use Joint, Metatarsal-Phalangeal, Left
  use Joint, Metatarsal-Phalangeal, Right
Metatarsophalangeal ligament
  use Bursa and Ligament, Foot, Left
  use Bursa and Ligament, Foot, Right
Metathalamus
  use Thalamus
Micro-Driver stent (RX) (OTW)
  use Intraluminal Device
MicroMed HeartAssist
  use Implantable Heart Assist System in Heart and Great Vessels
Micrus CERECYTE microcoil
  use Intraluminal Device, Bioactive in Upper Arteries

Midcarpal joint
  use Joint, Carpal, Left
  use Joint, Carpal, Right
Middle cardiac nerve
  use Nerve, Thoracic Sympathetic
Middle cerebral artery
  use Artery, Intracranial
Middle cerebral vein
  use Vein, Intracranial
Middle colic vein
  use Vein, Colic
Middle genicular artery
  use Artery, Popliteal, Left
  use Artery, Popliteal, Right
Middle hemorrhoidal vein
  use Vein, Hypogastric, Left
  use Vein, Hypogastric, Right
Middle rectal artery
  use Artery, Internal Iliac, Left
  use Artery, Internal Iliac, Right
Middle suprarenal artery
  use Aorta, Abdominal
Middle temporal artery
  use Artery, Temporal, Left
  use Artery, Temporal, Right
Middle turbinate
  use Turbinate, Nasal
MitraClip valve repair system
  use Synthetic Substitute
Mitral annulus
  use Valve, Mitral
Mitroflow® Aortic Pericardial Heart Valve
  use Zooplastic Tissue in Heart and Great Vessels
Mobilization, adhesions *see* Release
Molar gland
  use Buccal Mucosa
Monitoring
  Arterial
    Flow
      Coronary 4A13-
      Peripheral 4A13-
      Pulmonary 4A13-
    Pressure
      Coronary 4A13-
      Peripheral 4A13-
      Pulmonary 4A13-
    Pulse
      Coronary 4A13-
      Peripheral 4A13-
      Pulmonary 4A13-
    Saturation, Peripheral 4A13-
    Sound, Peripheral 4A13-
  Cardiac
    Electrical Activity 4A12-
      Ambulatory 4A12X45
      No Qualifier 4A12X4Z
    Output 4A12-
    Rate 4A12-
    Rhythm 4A12-
    Sound 4A12-
    Total Activity, Stress 4A12XM4
  Central Nervous
    Conductivity 4A10-
    Electrical Activity
      Intraoperative 4A10-
      No Qualifier 4A10-
    Pressure 4A100BZ
      Intracranial 4A10-
    Saturation, Intracranial 4A10-
    Temperature, Intracranial 4A10-
  Gastrointestinal
    Motility 4A1B-
    Pressure 4A1B-
    Secretion 4A1B-
  Intraoperative Knee Replacement Sensor XR2-
  Lymphatic
    Flow 4A16-
    Pressure 4A16-

Monitoring — *continued*
  Peripheral Nervous
    Conductivity
      Motor 4A11-
      Sensory 4A11-
    Electrical Activity
      Intraoperative 4A11-
      No Qualifier 4A11-
  Products of Conception
    Cardiac
      Electrical Activity 4A1H-
      Rate 4A1H-
      Rhythm 4A1H-
      Sound 4A1H-
    Nervous
      Conductivity 4A1J-
      Electrical Activity 4A1J-
      Pressure 4A1J-
  Respiratory
    Capacity 4A19-
    Flow 4A19-
    Rate 4A19-
    Resistance 4A19-
    Volume 4A19-
  Sleep 4A1ZXQZ
  Temperature 4A1Z-
  Urinary
    Contractility 4A1D73Z
    Flow 4A1D75Z
    Pressure 4A1D7BZ
    Resistance 4A1D7DZ
    Volume 4A1D7LZ
  Venous
    Flow
      Central 4A14-
      Peripheral 4A14-
      Portal 4A14-
      Pulmonary 4A14-
    Pressure
      Central 4A14-
      Peripheral 4A14-
      Portal 4A14-
      Pulmonary 4A14-
    Pulse
      Central 4A14-
      Peripheral 4A14-
      Portal 4A14-
      Pulmonary 4A14-
    Saturation
      Central 4A14-
      Portal 4A14-
      Pulmonary 4A14-
Monitoring Device, Hemodynamic
  Abdomen 0JH8-
  Chest 0JH6-
Mosaic Bioprosthesis (aortic) (mitral) valve
  use Zooplastic Tissue in Heart and Great Vessels
Motor Function Assessment F01-
Motor Treatment F07-
MR Angiography
  see Magnetic Resonance Imaging (MRI), Heart B23-
  see Magnetic Resonance Imaging (MRI), Lower Arteries B43-
  see Magnetic Resonance Imaging (MRI), Upper Arteries B33-
MULTI-LINK (VISION) (MINI-VISION) (ULTRA) Coronary Stent System
  use Intraluminal Device
Multiple sleep latency test 4A0ZXQZ
Musculocutaneous nerve
  use Nerve, Brachial Plexus
Musculopexy
  see Repair, Muscles 0KQ-
  see Reposition, Muscles 0KS-

Musculophrenic artery
  use Artery, Internal Mammary, Left
  use Artery, Internal Mammary, Right
Musculoplasty
  see Repair, Muscles 0KQ-
  see Supplement, Muscles 0KU-
Musculorrhaphy see Repair, Muscles 0KQ-
Musculospiral nerve
  use Nerve, Radial
Myectomy
  see Excision, Muscles 0KB-
  see Resection, Muscles 0KT-
Myelencephalon
  use Medulla Oblongata
Myelogram
  CT see Computerized Tomography (CT Scan), Central Nervous System B02-
  MRI see Magnetic Resonance Imaging (MRI), Central Nervous System B03-
Myenteric (Auerbach's) plexus
  use Nerve, Abdominal Sympathetic
Myomectomy see Excision, Female Reproductive System 0UB-
Myometrium
  use Uterus
Myopexy
  see Repair, Muscles 0KQ-
  see Reposition, Muscles 0KS-
Myoplasty
  see Repair, Muscles 0KQ-
  see Supplement, Muscles 0KU-
Myorrhaphy see Repair, Muscles 0KQ-
Myoscopy see Inspection, Muscles 0KJ-
Myotomy
  see Division, Muscles 0K8-
  see Drainage, Muscles 0K9-
Myringectomy
  see Excision, Ear, Nose, Sinus 09B-
  see Resection, Ear, Nose, Sinus 09T-
Myringoplasty
  see Repair, Ear, Nose, Sinus 09Q-
  see Replacement, Ear, Nose, Sinus 09R-
  see Supplement, Ear, Nose, Sinus 09U-
Myringostomy see Drainage, Ear, Nose, Sinus 099-
Myringotomy see Drainage, Ear, Nose, Sinus 099-

N

Nail bed
  use Finger Nail
  use Toe Nail
Nail plate
  use Finger Nail
  use Toe Nail
Narcosynthesis GZGZZZZ
Nasal cavity
  use Nose
Nasal concha
  use Turbinate, Nasal
Nasalis muscle
  use Muscle, Facial
Nasolacrimal duct
  use Duct, Lacrimal, Left
  use Duct, Lacrimal, Right
Nasopharyngeal airway (NPA)
  use Intraluminal Device, Airway in Ear, Nose, Sinus
Navicular bone
  use Tarsal, Left
  use Tarsal, Right
Near Infrared Spectroscopy, Circulatory System 8E023DZ
Neck of femur
  use Femur, Upper, Left
  use Femur, Upper, Right
Neck of humerus (anatomical) (surgical)
  use Humeral Head, Left
  use Humeral Head, Right
Nephrectomy
  see Excision, Urinary System 0TB-
  see Resection, Urinary System 0TT-
Nephrolithotomy see Extirpation, Urinary System 0TC-
Nephrolysis see Release, Urinary System 0TN-
Nephropexy
  see Repair, Urinary System 0TQ-
  see Reposition, Urinary System 0TS-
Nephroplasty
  see Repair, Urinary System 0TQ-
  see Supplement, Urinary System 0TU-
Nephropyeloureterostomy
  see Bypass, Urinary System 0T1-
  see Drainage, Urinary System 0T9-
Nephrorrhaphy see Repair, Urinary System 0TQ-
Nephroscopy, transurethral 0TJ58ZZ
Nephrostomy
  see Bypass, Urinary System 0T1-
  see Drainage, Urinary System 0T9-
Nephrotomography
  see Fluoroscopy, Urinary System BT1-
  see Plain Radiography, Urinary System BT0-
Nephrotomy
  see Drainage, Urinary System 0T9-
  see Division, Urinary System 0T8-
Nerve conduction study
  see Measurement, Central Nervous 4A00-
  see Measurement, Peripheral Nervous 4A01-
Nerve Function Assessment F01-
Nerve to the stapedius
  use Nerve, Facial
Nesiritide
  use Human B-type Natriuretic Peptide
Neurectomy
  see Excision, Central Nervous System 00B-
  see Excision, Peripheral Nervous System 01B-

Neurexeresis
  see Extraction, Central Nervous System 00D-
  see Extraction, Peripheral Nervous System 01D-
Neurohypophysis
  use Gland, Pituitary
Neurolysis
  see Release, Central Nervous System 00N-
  see Release, Peripheral Nervous System 01N-
Neuromuscular electrical stimulation (NEMS) lead
  use Stimulator Lead in Muscles
Neurophysiologic monitoring see Monitoring, Central Nervous 4A10-
Neuroplasty
  see Repair, Central Nervous System 00Q-
  see Repair, Peripheral Nervous System 01Q-
  see Supplement, Central Nervous System 00U-
  see Supplement, Peripheral Nervous System 01U-
Neurorrhaphy
  see Repair, Central Nervous System 00Q-
  see Repair, Peripheral Nervous System 01Q-
Neurostimulator Generator
  Insertion of device in, Skull 0NH00NZ
  Removal of device from, Skull 0NP00NZ
  Revision of device in, Skull 0NW00NZ
Neurostimulator generator, multiple channel
  use Stimulator Generator, Multiple Array in 0JH-
Neurostimulator generator, multiple channel rechargeable
  use Stimulator Generator, Multiple Array Rechargeable in 0JH-
Neurostimulator generator, single channel
  use Stimulator Generator, Single Array in 0JH-
Neurostimulator generator, single channel rechargeable
  use Stimulator Generator, Single Array Rechargeable in 0JH-
Neurostimulator Lead
  Insertion of device in
    Brain 00H0-
    Cerebral Ventricle 00H6-
    Nerve
      Cranial 00HE-
      Peripheral 01HY-
    Spinal Canal 00HU-
    Spinal Cord 00HV-
  Removal of device from
    Brain 00P0-
    Cerebral Ventricle 00P6-
    Nerve
      Cranial 00PE-
      Peripheral 01PY-
    Spinal Canal 00PU-
    Spinal Cord 00PV-
  Revision of device in
    Brain 00W0-
    Cerebral Ventricle 00W6-
    Nerve
      Cranial 00WE-
      Peripheral 01WY-
    Spinal Canal 00WU-
    Spinal Cord 00WV-

Neurotomy
  see Division, Central Nervous System 008-
  see Division, Peripheral Nervous System 018-
Neurotripsy
  see Destruction, Central Nervous System 005-
  see Destruction, Peripheral Nervous System 015-
Neutralization plate
  use Internal Fixation Device in Head and Facial Bones
  use Internal Fixation Device in Lower Bones
  use Internal Fixation Device in Upper Bones
New Technology
  Blinatumomab antineoplastic immunotherapy XW0-
  Ceftazidime-avibactam anti-infective XW0-
  Idarucizumab, Dabigatran reversal agent XW0-
  Intraoperative knee replacement sensor XR2-
  Isavuconazole anti-infective XW0-
  Orbital atherectomy technology X2C-
Ninth cranial nerve
  use Nerve, Glossopharyngeal
Nitinol framed polymer mesh
  use Synthetic Substitute
Non-tunneled central venous catheter
  use Infusion Device
Nonimaging Nuclear Medicine Assay
  Bladder, Kidneys and Ureters CT63-
  Blood C763-
  Kidneys, Ureters and Bladder CT63-
  Lymphatics and Hematologic System C76YYZZ
  Ureters, Kidneys and Bladder CT63-
  Urinary System CT6YYZZ
Nonimaging Nuclear Medicine Probe
  Abdomen CW50-
  Abdomen and Chest CW54-
  Abdomen and Pelvis CW51-
  Brain C050-
  Central Nervous System C05YYZZ
  Chest CW53-
  Chest and Abdomen CW54-
  Chest and Neck CW56-
  Extremity
    Lower CP5PZZZ
    Upper CP5NZZZ
  Head and Neck CW5B-
  Heart C25YYZZ
    Right and Left C256-
  Lymphatics
    Head C75J-
    Head and Neck C755-
    Lower Extremity C75P-
    Neck C75K-
    Pelvic C75D-
    Trunk C75M-
    Upper Chest C75L-
    Upper Extremity C75N-
  Lymphatics and Hematologic System C75YYZZ
  Musculoskeletal System, Other CP5YYZZ
  Neck and Chest CW56-
  Neck and Head CW5B-
  Pelvic Region CW5J-
  Pelvis and Abdomen CW51-
  Spine CP55ZZZ

Nonimaging Nuclear Medicine Uptake
  Endocrine System **CG4YYZZ**
  Gland, Thyroid **CG42-**
Nostril
  use Nose
Novacor Left Ventricular Assist Device
  use Implantable Heart Assist System in Heart and Great Vessels
Novation® Ceramic AHS® (Articulation Hip System)
  use Synthetic Substitute, Ceramic in 0SR-
Nuclear medicine
  see Nonimaging Nuclear Medicine Assay
  see Nonimaging Nuclear Medicine Probe
  see Nonimaging Nuclear Medicine Uptake
  see Planar Nuclear Medicine Imaging
  see Positron Emission Tomographic (PET) Imaging
  see Systemic Nuclear Medicine Therapy
  see Tomographic (Tomo) Nuclear Medicine Imaging
Nuclear scintigraphy see Nuclear Medicine
Nutrition, concentrated substances
  Enteral infusion **3E0G36Z**
  Parenteral (peripheral) infusion see Introduction of Nutritional Substance

Obliteration see Destruction
Obturator artery
  use Artery, Internal Iliac, Left
  use Artery, Internal Iliac, Right
Obturator lymph node
  use Lymphatic, Pelvis
Obturator muscle
  use Muscle, Hip, Left
  use Muscle, Hip, Right
Obturator nerve
  use Nerve, Lumbar Plexus
Obturator vein
  use Vein, Hypogastric, Left
  use Vein, Hypogastric, Right
Obtuse margin
  use Heart, Left
Occipital artery
  use Artery, External Carotid, Left
  use Artery, External Carotid, Right
Occipital lobe
  use Cerebral Hemisphere
Occipital lymph node
  use Lymphatic, Neck, Left
  use Lymphatic, Neck, Right
Occipitofrontalis muscle
  use Muscle, Facial
Occlusion
  Ampulla of Vater **0FLC-**
  Anus **0DLQ**
  Aorta, Abdominal **04L0-**
  Artery
    Anterior Tibial
      Left **04LQ-**
      Right **04LP-**
    Axillary
      Left **03L6-**
      Right **03L5-**
    Brachial
      Left **03L8-**
      Right **03L7-**
    Celiac **04L1-**
    Colic
      Left **04L7-**
      Middle **04L8-**
      Right **04L6-**
    Common Carotid
      Left **03LJ-**
      Right **03LH-**
    Common Iliac
      Left **04LD-**
      Right **04LC-**
    External Carotid
      Left **03LN-**
      Right **03LM-**
    External Iliac
      Left **04LJ-**
      Right **04LH-**
    Face **03LR-**
    Femoral
      Left **04LL-**
      Right **04LK-**
    Foot
      Left **04LW-**
      Right **04LV-**
    Gastric **04L2-**
    Hand
      Left **03LF-**
      Right **03LD-**
    Hepatic **04L3-**
    Inferior Mesenteric **04LB-**
    Innominate **03L2-**
    Internal Carotid
      Left **03LL-**
      Right **03LK-**
    Internal Iliac
      Left, **04LF-**
      Right, **04LE-**

Occlusion — continued
  Artery — continued
    Internal Mammary
      Left **03L1-**
      Right **03L0-**
    Intracranial **03LG-**
    Lower **04LY-**
    Peroneal
      Left **04LU-**
      Right **04LT-**
    Popliteal
      Left **04LN-**
      Right **04LM-**
    Posterior Tibial
      Left **04LS-**
      Right **04LR-**
    Pulmonary, Left **02LR-**
    Radial
      Left **03LC-**
      Right **03LB-**
    Renal
      Left **04LA-**
      Right **04L9-**
    Splenic **04L4-**
    Subclavian
      Left **03L4-**
      Right **03L3-**
    Superior Mesenteric **04L5-**
    Temporal
      Left **03LT-**
      Right **03LS-**
    Thyroid
      Left **03LV-**
      Right **03LU-**
    Ulnar
      Left **03LA-**
      Right **03L9-**
    Upper **03LY-**
    Vertebral
      Left **03LQ-**
      Right **03LP-**
  Atrium, Left **02L7-**
  Bladder **0TLB-**
  Bladder Neck **0TLC-**
  Bronchus
    Lingula **0BL9-**
    Lower Lobe
      Left **0BLB-**
      Right **0BL6-**
    Main
      Left **0BL7-**
      Right **0BL3-**
    Middle Lobe, Right **0BL5-**
    Upper Lobe
      Left **0BL8-**
      Right **0BL4-**
  Carina **0BL2-**
  Cecum **0DLH-**
  Cisterna Chyli **07LL-**
  Colon
    Ascending **0DLK-**
    Descending **0DLM-**
    Sigmoid **0DLN-**
    Transverse **0DLL-**
  Cord
    Bilateral **0VLH-**
    Left **0VLG-**
    Right **0VLF-**
  Cul-de-sac **0ULF-**
  Duct
    Common Bile **0FL9-**
    Cystic **0FL8-**
    Hepatic
      Left **0FL6-**
      Right **0FL5-**
    Lacrimal
      Left **08LY-**
      Right **08LX-**
    Pancreatic **0FLD-**
      Accessory **0FLF-**

Occlusion — continued
  Duct — continued
    Parotid
      Left **0CLC-**
      Right **0CLB-**
  Duodenum **0DL9-**
  Esophagogastric Junction **0DL4-**
  Esophagus **0DL5-**
    Lower **0DL3-**
    Middle **0DL2-**
    Upper **0DL1-**
  Fallopian Tube
    Left **0UL6-**
    Right **0UL5-**
  Fallopian Tubes, Bilateral **0UL7-**
  Ileocecal Valve **0DLC-**
  Ileum **0DLB-**
  Intestine
    Large **0DLE-**
      Left **0DLG-**
      Right **0DLF-**
    Small **0DL8-**
  Jejunum **0DLA-**
  Kidney Pelvis
    Left **0TL4-**
    Right **0TL3-**
  Left atrial appendage (LAA) see Occlusion, Atrium, Left **02L7-**
  Lymphatic
    Aortic **07LD-**
    Axillary
      Left **07L6-**
      Right **07L5-**
    Head **07L0-**
    Inguinal
      Left **07LJ-**
      Right **07LH-**
    Internal Mammary
      Left **07L9-**
      Right **07L8-**
    Lower Extremity
      Left **07LG-**
      Right **07LF-**
    Mesenteric **07LB-**
    Neck
      Left **07L2-**
      Right **07L1-**
    Pelvis **07LC-**
    Thoracic Duct **07LK-**
    Thorax **07L7-**
    Upper Extremity
      Left **07L4-**
      Right **07L3-**
  Rectum **0DLP-**
  Stomach **0DL6-**
  Pylorus **0DL7-**
  Trachea **0BL1-**
  Ureter
    Left **0TL7-**
    Right **0TL6-**
  Urethra **0TLD-**
  Vagina **0ULG-**
  Vas Deferens
    Bilateral **0VLQ-**
    Left **0VLP-**
    Right **0VLN-**
  Vein
    Axillary
      Left **05L8-**
      Right **05L7-**
    Azygos **05L0-**
    Basilic
      Left **05LC-**
      Right **05LB-**
    Brachial
      Left **05LA-**
      Right **05L9-**
    Cephalic
      Left **05LF-**
      Right **05LD-**

Occlusion — INDEX TO PROCEDURES – 2016 ICD-10-PCS

Occlusion — *continued*
  Vein — *continued*
    Colic 06L7-
    Common Iliac
      Left 06LD-
      Right 06LC-
    Esophageal 06L3-
    External Iliac
      Left 06LG-
      Right 06LF-
    External Jugular
      Left 05LQ-
      Right 05LP-
    Face
      Left 05LV-
      Right 05LT-
    Femoral
      Left 06LN-
      Right 06LM-
    Foot
      Left 06LV-
      Right 06LT-
    Gastric 06L2-
    Greater Saphenous
      Left 06LQ-
      Right 06LP-
    Hand
      Left 05LH-
      Right 05LG-
    Hemiazygos 05L1-
    Hepatic 06L4-
    Hypogastric
      Left 06LJ-
      Right 06LH-
    Inferior Mesenteric 06L6-
    Innominate
      Left 05L4-
      Right 05L3-
    Internal Jugular
      Left 05LN-
      Right 05LM-
    Intracranial 05LL-
    Lesser Saphenous
      Left 06LS-
      Right 06LR-
    Lower 06LY-
    Portal 06L8-
    Pulmonary
      Left 02LT-
      Right 02LS-
    Renal
      Left 06LB-
      Right 06L9-
    Splenic 06L1-
    Subclavian
      Left 05L6-
      Right 05L5-
    Superior Mesenteric 06L5-
    Upper 05LY-
    Vertebral
      Left 05LS-
      Right 05LR-
    Vena Cava
      Inferior 06L0-
      Superior 02LV-
Occupational therapy *see* Activities of Daily Living Treatment, Rehabilitation F08-
Odentectomy
  see Excision, Mouth and Throat 0CB-
  see Resection, Mouth and Throat 0CT-
Olecranon bursa
  use Bursa and Ligament, Elbow, Left
  use Bursa and Ligament, Elbow, Right
Olecranon process
  use Ulna, Left
  use Ulna, Right
Olfactory bulb
  use Nerve, Olfactory

Omentectomy, omentumectomy
  see Excision, Gastrointestinal System 0DB-
  see Resection, Gastrointestinal System 0DT-
Omentofixation *see* Repair, Gastrointestinal System 0DQ-
Omentoplasty
  see Repair, Gastrointestinal System 0DQ-
  see Replacement, Gastrointestinal System 0DR-
  see Supplement, Gastrointestinal System 0DU-
Omentorrhaphy *see* Repair, Gastrointestinal System 0DQ-
Omentotomy *see* Drainage, Gastrointestinal System 0D9-
Omnilink Elite Vascular Balloon Expandable Stent System
  use Intraluminal Device
Onychectomy
  see Excision, Skin and Breast 0HB-
  see Resection, Skin and Breast 0HT-
Onychoplasty
  see Repair, Skin and Breast 0HQ-
  see Replacement, Skin and Breast 0HR-
Onychotomy *see* Drainage, Skin and Breast 0H9-
Oophorectomy
  see Excision, Female Reproductive System 0UB-
  see Resection, Female Reproductive System 0UT-
Oophoropexy
  see Repair, Female Reproductive System 0UQ-
  see Reposition, Female Reproductive System 0US-
Oophoroplasty
  see Repair, Female Reproductive System 0UQ-
  see Supplement, Female Reproductive System 0UU-
Oophororrhaphy *see* Repair, Female Reproductive System 0UQ-
Oophorostomy *see* Drainage, Female Reproductive System 0U9-
Oophorotomy
  see Drainage, Female Reproductive System 0U9-
  see Division, Female Reproductive System 0U8-
Oophorrhaphy *see* Repair, Female Reproductive System 0UQ-
Open Pivot Aortic Valve Graft (AVG)
  use Synthetic Substitute
Open Pivot (mechanical) valve
  use Synthetic Substitute
Ophthalmic artery
  use Artery, Internal Carotid, Left
  use Artery, Internal Carotid, Right
Ophthalmic nerve
  use Nerve, Trigeminal
Ophthalmic vein
  use Vein, Intracranial
Opponensplasty
  Tendon replacement *see* Replacement, Tendons 0LR-
  Tendon transfer *see* Transfer, Tendons 0LX-
Optic chiasma
  use Nerve, Optic
Optic disc
  use Retina, Left
  use Retina, Right
Optic foramen
  use Bone, Sphenoid, Left
  use Bone, Sphenoid, Right

Optical coherence tomography, intravascular *see* Computerized Tomography (CT Scan)
Optimizer™ III implantable pulse generator
  use Contractility Modulation Device in 0JH-
Orbicularis oculi muscle
  use Eyelid, Upper, Left
  use Eyelid, Upper, Right
Orbicularis oris muscle
  use Muscle, Facial
Orbital atherectomy technology X2C-
Orbital fascia
  use Subcutaneous Tissue and Fascia, Face
Orbital portion of ethmoid bone
  use Orbit, Left
  use Orbit, Right
Orbital portion of frontal bone
  use Orbit, Left
  use Orbit, Right
Orbital portion of lacrimal bone
  use Orbit, Left
  use Orbit, Right
Orbital portion of maxilla
  use Orbit, Left
  use Orbit, Right
Orbital portion of palatine bone
  use Orbit, Left
  use Orbit, Right
Orbital portion of sphenoid bone
  use Orbit, Left
  use Orbit, Right
Orbital portion of zygomatic bone
  use Orbit, Left
Orchectomy, orchidectomy, orchiectomy
  see Excision, Male Reproductive System 0VB-
  see Resection, Male Reproductive System 0VT-
Orchidoplasty, orchioplasty
  see Repair, Male Reproductive System 0VQ-
  see Replacement, Male Reproductive System 0VR-
  see Supplement, Male Reproductive System 0VU-
Orchidorrhaphy, orchiorrhaphy
  see Repair, Male Reproductive System 0VQ-
Orchidotomy, orchiotomy, orchotomy *see* Drainage, Male Reproductive System 0V9-
Orchiopexy
  see Repair, Male Reproductive System 0VQ-
  see Reposition, Male Reproductive System 0VS-
Oropharyngeal airway (OPA)
  use Intraluminal Device, Airway in Mouth and Throat
Oropharynx
  use Pharynx
Ossicular chain
  use Auditory Ossicle, Left
  use Auditory Ossicle, Right
Ossiculectomy
  see Excision, Ear, Nose, Sinus 09B-
  see Resection, Ear, Nose, Sinus 09T-
Ossiculotomy *see* Drainage, Ear, Nose, Sinus 099-

Ostectomy
  see Excision, Head and Facial Bones 0NB-
  see Excision, Lower Bones 0QB-
  see Excision, Upper Bones 0PB-
  see Resection, Head and Facial Bones 0NT-
  see Resection, Lower Bones 0QT-
  see Resection, Upper Bones 0PT-
Osteoclasis
  see Division, Head and Facial Bones 0N8-
  see Division, Lower Bones 0Q8-
  see Division, Upper Bones 0P8-
Osteolysis
  see Release, Head and Facial Bones 0NN-
  see Release, Lower Bones 0QN-
  see Release, Upper Bones 0PN-
Osteopathic Treatment
  Abdomen 7W09X-
  Cervical 7W01X-
  Extremity
    Lower 7W06X-
    Upper 7W07X-
  Head 7W00X-
  Lumbar 7W03X-
  Pelvis 7W05X-
  Rib Cage 7W08X-
  Sacrum 7W04X-
  Thoracic 7W02X-
Osteopexy
  see Repair, Head and Facial Bones 0NQ-
  see Repair, Lower Bones 0QQ-
  see Repair, Upper Bones 0PQ-
  see Reposition, Head and Facial Bones 0NS-
  see Reposition, Lower Bones 0QS-
  see Reposition, Upper Bones 0PS-
Osteoplasty
  see Repair, Head and Facial Bones 0NQ-
  see Repair, Lower Bones 0QQ-
  see Repair, Upper Bones 0PQ-
  see Replacement, Head and Facial Bones 0NR-
  see Replacement, Lower Bones 0QR-
  see Replacement, Upper Bones 0PR-
  see Supplement, Head and Facial Bones 0NU-
  see Supplement, Lower Bones 0QU-
  see Supplement, Upper Bones 0PU-
Osteorrhaphy
  see Repair, Head and Facial Bones 0NQ-
  see Repair, Lower Bones 0QQ-
  see Repair, Upper Bones 0PQ-
Osteotomy, ostotomy
  see Division, Head and Facial Bones 0N8-
  see Division, Lower Bones 0Q8-
  see Division, Upper Bones 0P8-
  see Drainage, Head and Facial Bones 0N9-
  see Drainage, Lower Bones 0Q9-
  see Drainage, Upper Bones 0P9-
Otic ganglion
  use Nerve, Head and Neck Sympathetic
Otoplasty
  see Repair, Ear, Nose, Sinus 09Q-
  see Replacement, Ear, Nose, Sinus 09R-
  see Supplement, Ear, Nose, Sinus 09U-
Otoscopy *see* Inspection, Ear, Nose, Sinus 09J-

Oval window
 use Ear, Middle, Left
 use Ear, Middle, Right
Ovarian artery
 use Aorta, Abdominal
Ovarian ligament
 use Uterine Supporting Structure
Ovariectomy
 see Excision, Female Reproductive System 0UB-
 see Resection, Female Reproductive System 0UT-
Ovariocentesis see Drainage, Female Reproductive System 0U9-
Ovariopexy
 see Repair, Female Reproductive System 0UQ-
 see Reposition, Female Reproductive System 0US-
Ovariotomy
 see Drainage, Female Reproductive System 0U9-
 see Division, Female Reproductive System 0U8-
Ovatio™ CRT-D
 use Cardiac Resynchronization Defibrillator Pulse Generator in 0JH-
Oversewing
 Gastrointestinal ulcer see Repair, Gastrointestinal System 0DQ-
 Pleural bleb see Repair, Respiratory System 0BQ-
Oviduct
 use Fallopian Tube, Left
 use Fallopian Tube, Right
Oxidized zirconium ceramic hip bearing surface
 use Synthetic Substitute, Ceramic on Polyethylene in 0SR-
Oximetry, Fetal pulse 10H073Z
Oxygenation
 Extracorporeal membrane (ECMO) see Performance, Circulatory 5A15-
 Hyperbaric see Assistance, Circulatory 5A05-
 Supersaturated see Assistance, Circulatory 5A05-

P

Pacemaker
 Dual Chamber
  Abdomen 0JH8-
  Chest 0JH6-
 Single Chamber
  Abdomen 0JH8-
  Chest 0JH6-
 Single Chamber Rate Responsive
  Abdomen 0JH8-
  Chest 0JH6-
Packing
 Abdominal Wall 2W43X5Z
 Anorectal 2Y43X5Z
 Arm
  Lower
   Left 2W4DX5Z
   Right 2W4CX5Z
  Upper
   Left 2W4BX5Z
   Right 2W4AX5Z
 Back 2W45X5Z
 Chest Wall 2W44X5Z
 Ear 2Y42X5Z
 Extremity
  Lower
   Left 2W4MX5Z
   Right 2W4LX5Z
  Upper
   Left 2W49X5Z
   Right 2W48X5Z
 Face 2W41X5Z
 Finger
  Left 2W4KX5Z
  Right 2W4JX5Z
 Foot
  Left 2W4TX5Z
  Right 2W4SX5Z
 Genital Tract, Female 2Y44X5Z
 Hand
  Left 2W4FX5Z
  Right 2W4EX5Z
 Head 2W40X5Z
 Inguinal Region
  Left 2W47X5Z
  Right 2W46X5Z
 Leg
  Lower
   Left 2W4RX5Z
   Right 2W4QX5Z
  Upper
   Left 2W4PX5Z
   Right 2W4NX5Z
 Mouth and Pharynx 2Y40X5Z
 Nasal 2Y41X5Z
 Neck 2W42X5Z
 Thumb
  Left 2W4HX5Z
  Right 2W4GX5Z
 Toe
  Left 2W4VX5Z
  Right 2W4UX5Z
 Urethra 2Y45X5Z
Paclitaxel-eluting coronary stent
 use Intraluminal Device, Drug-eluting in Heart and Great Vessels
Paclitaxel-eluting peripheral stent
 use Intraluminal Device, Drug-eluting in Lower Arteries
 use Intraluminal Device, Drug-eluting in Upper Arteries
Palatine gland
 use Buccal Mucosa
Palatine tonsil
 use Tonsils
Palatine uvula
 use Uvula
Palatoglossal muscle
 use Muscle, Tongue, Palate, Pharynx

Palatopharyngeal muscle
 use Muscle, Tongue, Palate, Pharynx
Palatoplasty
 see Repair, Mouth and Throat 0CQ-
 see Replacement, Mouth and Throat 0CR-
 see Supplement, Mouth and Throat 0CU-
Palatorrhaphy see Repair, Mouth and Throat 0CQ-
Palmar (volar) digital vein
 use Vein, Hand, Left
 use Vein, Hand, Right
Palmar (volar) metacarpal vein
 use Vein, Hand, Left
 use Vein, Hand, Right
Palmar cutaneous nerve
 use Nerve, Median
 use Nerve, Radial
Palmar fascia (aponeurosis)
 use Subcutaneous Tissue and Fascia, Hand, Left
 use Subcutaneous Tissue and Fascia, Hand, Right
Palmar interosseous muscle
 use Muscle, Hand, Left
 use Muscle, Hand, Right
Palmar ulnocarpal ligament
 use Bursa and Ligament, Wrist, Left
 use Bursa and Ligament, Wrist, Right
Palmaris longus muscle
 use Muscle, Lower Arm and Wrist, Left
 use Muscle, Lower Arm and Wrist, Right
Pancreatectomy
 see Excision, Pancreas 0FBG-
 see Resection, Pancreas 0FTG-
Pancreatic artery
 use Artery, Splenic
Pancreatic plexus
 use Nerve, Abdominal Sympathetic
Pancreatic vein
 use Vein, Splenic
Pancreaticoduodenostomy see Bypass, Hepatobiliary System and Pancreas 0F1-
Pancreaticosplenic lymph node
 use Lymphatic, Aortic
Pancreatogram, endoscopic retrograde see Fluoroscopy, Pancreatic Duct BF18-
Pancreatolithotomy see Extirpation, Pancreas 0FCG-
Pancreatotomy
 see Drainage, Pancreas 0F9G-
 see Division, Pancreas 0F8G-
Panniculectomy
 see Excision, Abdominal Wall 0WBF-
 see Excision, Skin, Abdomen 0HB7-
Paraaortic lymph node
 use Lymphatic, Aortic
Paracentesis
 Eye see Drainage, Eye 089-
 Peritoneal Cavity see Drainage, Peritoneal Cavity 0W9G-
 Tympanum see Drainage, Ear, Nose, Sinus 099-
Pararectal lymph node
 use Lymphatic, Mesenteric
Parasternal lymph node
 use Lymphatic, Thorax
Parathyroidectomy
 see Excision, Endocrine System 0GB-
 see Resection, Endocrine System 0GT-
Paratracheal lymph node
 use Lymphatic, Thorax
Paraurethral (Skene's) gland
 use Gland, Vestibular
Parenteral nutrition, total see Introduction of Nutritional Substance

Parietal lobe
 use Cerebral Hemisphere
Parotid lymph node
 use Lymphatic, Head
Parotid plexus
 use Nerve, Facial
Parotidectomy
 see Excision, Mouth and Throat 0CB-
 see Resection, Mouth and Throat 0CT-
Pars flaccida
 use Tympanic Membrane, Left
 use Tympanic Membrane, Right
Partial joint replacement
 Hip see Replacement, Lower Joints 0SR-
 Knee see Replacement, Lower Joints 0SR-
 Shoulder see Replacement, Upper Joints 0RR-
Partially absorbable mesh
 use Synthetic Substitute
Patch, blood, spinal 3E0S3GC
Patellapexy
 see Repair, Lower Bones 0QQ-
 see Reposition, Lower Bones 0QS-
Patellaplasty
 see Repair, Lower Bones 0QQ-
 see Replacement, Lower Bones 0QR-
 see Supplement, Lower Bones 0QU-
Patellar ligament
 use Bursa and Ligament, Knee, Left
 use Bursa and Ligament, Knee, Right
Patellar tendon
 use Tendon, Knee, Left
 use Tendon, Knee, Right
Patellectomy
 see Excision, Lower Bones 0QB-
 see Resection, Lower Bones 0QT-
Patellofemoral joint
 use Joint, Knee, Left
 use Joint, Knee, Right
 use Joint, Knee, Left, Femoral Surface
 use Joint, Knee, Right, Femoral Surface
Pectineus muscle
 use Muscle, Upper Leg, Left
 use Muscle, Upper Leg, Right
Pectoral (anterior) lymph node
 use Lymphatic, Axillary, Left
 use Lymphatic, Axillary, Right
Pectoral fascia
 use Subcutaneous Tissue and Fascia, Chest
Pectoralis major muscle
 use Muscle, Thorax, Left
 use Muscle, Thorax, Right
Pectoralis minor muscle
 use Muscle, Thorax, Left
 use Muscle, Thorax, Right
Pedicle-based dynamic stabilization device
 use Spinal Stabilization Device, Pedicle-Based in 0RH-
 use Spinal Stabilization Device, Pedicle-Based in 0SH-
PEEP (positive end expiratory pressure) see Assistance, Respiratory 5A09-
PEG (percutaneous endoscopic gastrostomy) 0DH63UZ
PEJ (percutaneous endoscopic jejunostomy) 0DHA3UZ
Pelvic splanchnic nerve
 use Nerve, Abdominal Sympathetic
 use Nerve, Sacral Sympathetic
Penectomy
 see Excision, Male Reproductive System 0VB-
 see Resection, Male Reproductive System 0VT-

Penile — INDEX TO PROCEDURES – 2016 ICD-10-PCS

Penile urethra
 use Urethra
Percutaneous endoscopic gastrojejunostomy (PEG/J) tube
 use Feeding Device in Gastrointestinal System
Percutaneous endoscopic gastrostomy (PEG) tube
 use Feeding Device in Gastrointestinal System
Percutaneous nephrostomy catheter
 use Drainage Device
Percutaneous transluminal coronary angioplasty (PTCA)
 see Dilation, Heart and Great Vessels 027-
Performance
 Biliary
  Multiple, Filtration 5A1C60Z
  Single, Filtration 5A1C00Z
 Cardiac
  Continuous
   Output 5A1221Z
   Pacing 5A1223Z
  Intermittent, Pacing 5A1213Z
  Single, Output, Manual 5A12012
 Circulatory, Continuous, Oxygenation, Membrane 5A15223
 Respiratory
  24-96 Consecutive Hours, Ventilation 5A1945Z
  Greater than 96 Consecutive Hours, Ventilation 5A1955Z
  Less than 24 Consecutive Hours, Ventilation 5A1935Z
  Single, Ventilation, Nonmechanical 5A19054
 Urinary
  Multiple, Filtration 5A1D60Z
  Single, Filtration 5A1D00Z
Perfusion see Introduction of substance in or on
Pericardiectomy
 see Excision, Pericardium 02BN-
 see Resection, Pericardium 02TN-
Pericardiocentesis see Drainage, Pericardial Cavity 0W9D-
Pericardiolysis see Release, Pericardium 02NN-
Pericardiophrenic artery
 use Artery, Internal Mammary, Left
 use Artery, Internal Mammary, Right
Pericardioplasty
 see Repair, Pericardium 02QN-
 see Replacement, Pericardium 02RN-
 see Supplement, Pericardium 02UN-
Pericardiorrhaphy see Repair, Pericardium 02QN-
Pericardiostomy see Drainage, Pericardial Cavity 0W9D-
Pericardiotomy see Drainage, Pericardial Cavity 0W9D-
Perimetrium
 use Uterus
Peripheral parenteral nutrition
 see Introduction of Nutritional Substance
Peripherally inserted central catheter (PICC)
 use Infusion Device
Peritoneal dialysis 3E1M39Z
Peritoneocentesis
 see Drainage, Peritoneal Cavity 0W9G-
 see Drainage, Peritoneum 0D9W-
Peritoneoplasty
 see Repair, Peritoneum 0DQW-
 see Replacement, Peritoneum 0DRW-
 see Supplement, Peritoneum 0DUW-

Peritoneoscopy 0DJW4ZZ
Peritoneotomy see Drainage, Peritoneum 0D9W-
Peritoneumectomy see Excision, Peritoneum 0DBW-
Peroneus brevis muscle
 use Muscle, Lower Leg, Left
 use Muscle, Lower Leg, Right
Peroneus longus muscle
 use Muscle, Lower Leg, Left
 use Muscle, Lower Leg, Right
Pessary ring
 use Intraluminal Device, Pessary in Female Reproductive System
PET scan see Positron Emission Tomography (PET) Imaging
Petrous part of temporal bone
 use Bone, Temporal, Left
 use Bone, Temporal, Right
Phacoemulsification, lens
 With IOL implant see Replacement, Eye 08R-
 Without IOL implant see Extraction, Eye 08D-
Phalangectomy
 see Excision, Lower Bones 0QB-
 see Excision, Upper Bones 0PB-
 see Resection, Lower Bones 0QT-
 see Resection, Upper Bones 0PT-
Phallectomy
 see Excision, Penis 0VBS-
 see Resection, Penis 0VTS-
Phalloplasty
 see Repair, Penis 0VQS-
 see Supplement, Penis 0VUS-
Phallotomy see Drainage, Penis 0V9S-
Pharmacotherapy, for substance abuse
 Antabuse HZ93ZZZ
 Bupropion HZ97ZZZ
 Clonidine HZ96ZZZ
 Levo-alpha-acetyl-methadol (LAAM) HZ92ZZZ
 Methadone Maintenance HZ91ZZZ
 Naloxone HZ95ZZZ
 Naltrexone HZ94ZZZ
 Nicotine Replacement HZ90ZZZ
 Psychiatric Medication HZ98ZZZ
 Replacement Medication, Other HZ99ZZZ
Pharyngeal constrictor muscle
 use Muscle, Tongue, Palate, Pharynx
Pharyngeal plexus
 use Nerve, Vagus
Pharyngeal recess
 use Nasopharynx
Pharyngeal tonsil
 use Adenoids
Pharyngogram see Fluoroscopy, Pharynix B91G-
Pharyngoplasty
 see Repair, Mouth and Throat 0CQ-
 see Replacement, Mouth and Throat 0CR-
 see Supplement, Mouth and Throat 0CU-
Pharyngorrhaphy see Repair, Mouth and Throat 0CQ-
Pharyngotomy see Drainage, Mouth and Throat 0C9-
Pharyngotympanic tube
 use Eustachian Tube, Left
 use Eustachian Tube, Right
Pheresis
 Erythrocytes 6A55-
 Leukocytes 6A55-
 Plasma 6A55-
 Platelets 6A55-
 Stem Cells
  Cord Blood 6A55-
  Hematopoietic 6A55-

Phlebectomy
 see Excision, Lower Veins 06B-
 see Excision, Upper Veins 05B-
 see Extraction, Lower Veins 06D-
 see Extraction, Upper Veins 05D-
Phlebography
 see Plain Radiography, Veins B50-
 Impedance 4A04X51
Phleborrhaphy
 see Repair, Lower Veins 06Q-
 see Repair, Upper Veins 05Q-
Phlebotomy
 see Drainage, Lower Veins 069-
 see Drainage, Upper Veins 059-
Photocoagulation
 for Destruction see Destruction
 for Repair see Repair
Photopheresis, therapeutic see Phototherapy, Circulatory 6A65-
Phototherapy
 Circulatory 6A65-
 Skin 6A60-
Phrenectomy, phrenoneurectomy
 see Excision, Nerve, Phrenic 01B2-
Phrenemphraxis see Destruction, Nerve, Phrenic 0152-
Phrenic nerve stimulator generator
 use Stimulator Generator in Subcutaneous Tissue and Fascia
Phrenic nerve stimulator lead
 use Diaphragmatic Pacemaker Lead in Respiratory System
Phreniclasis see Destruction, Nerve, Phrenic 0152-
Phrenicoexeresis see Extraction, Nerve, Phrenic 01D2-
Phrenicotomy see Division, Nerve, Phrenic 0182-
Phrenicotripsy see Destruction, Nerve, Phrenic 0152-
Phrenoplasty
 see Repair, Respiratory System 0BQ-
 see Supplement, Respiratory System 0BU-
Phrenotomy see Drainage, Respiratory System 0B9-
Physiatry see Motor Treatment, Rehabilitation F07-
Physical medicine see Motor Treatment, Rehabilitation F07-
Physical therapy see Motor Treatment, Rehabilitation F07-
PHYSIOMESH™ Flexible Composite Mesh
 use Synthetic Substitute
Pia mater, intracranial
 use Cerebral Meninges
Pia mater, spinal
 use Spinal Meninges
Pinealectomy
 see Excision, Pineal Body 0GB1-
 see Resection, Pineal Body 0GT1-
Pinealoscopy 0GJ14ZZ
Pinealotomy see Drainage, Pineal Body 0G91-
Pinna
 use Ear, External, Bilateral
 use Ear, External, Left
 use Ear, External, Right
Pipeline™ Embolization device (PED)
 use Intraluminal Device
Piriform recess (sinus)
 use Pharynx
Piriformis muscle
 use Muscle, Hip, Left
 use Muscle, Hip, Right
Pisiform bone
 use Carpal, Left
 use Carpal, Right

Pisohamate ligament
 use Bursa and Ligament, Hand, Left
 use Bursa and Ligament, Hand, Right
Pisometacarpal ligament
 use Bursa and Ligament, Hand, Left
 use Bursa and Ligament, Hand, Right
Pituitectomy
 see Excision, Gland, Pituitary 0GB0-
 see Resection, Gland, Pituitary 0GT0-
Plain film radiology see Plain Radiography
Plain Radiography
 Abdomen BW00ZZZ
 Abdomen and Pelvis BW01ZZZ
 Abdominal Lymphatic
  Bilateral B701-
  Unilateral B700-
 Airway, Upper BB0DZZZ
 Ankle
  Left BQ0H-
  Right BQ0G-
 Aorta
  Abdominal B400-
  Thoracic B300-
  Thoraco-Abdominal B30P-
 Aorta and Bilateral Lower Extremity Arteries B40D-
 Arch
  Bilateral BN0DZZZ
  Left BN0CZZZ
  Right BN0BZZZ
 Arm
  Left BP0FZZZ
  Right BP0EZZZ
 Artery
  Brachiocephalic-Subclavian, Right B301-
  Bronchial B30L-
  Bypass Graft, Other B20F-
  Cervico-Cerebral Arch B30Q-
  Common Carotid
   Bilateral B305-
   Left B304-
   Right B303-
  Coronary
   Bypass Graft
    Multiple B203-
    Single B202-
   Multiple B201-
   Single B200-
  External Carotid
   Bilateral B30C-
   Left B30B-
   Right B309-
  Hepatic B402-
  Inferior Mesenteric B405-
  Intercostal B30L-
  Internal Carotid
   Bilateral B308-
   Left B307-
   Right B306-
  Internal Mammary Bypass Graft
   Left B208-
   Right B207-
  Intra-Abdominal, Other B40B-
  Intracranial B30R-
  Lower, Other B40J-
  Lower Extremity
   Bilateral and Aorta B40D-
   Left B40G-
   Right B40F-
  Lumbar B409-
  Pelvic B40C-
  Pulmonary
   Left B30T-
   Right B30S-
  Renal
   Bilateral B408-
   Left B407-
   Right B406-
   Transplant B40M-
  Spinal B30M-

Plain Radiography — continued
Artery — continued
Splenic **B403**-
Subclavian, Left **B302**-
Superior Mesenteric **B404**-
Upper, Other **B30N**-
Upper Extremity
  Bilateral **B30K**-
  Left **B30J**-
  Right **B30H**-
Vertebral
  Bilateral **B30G**-
  Left **B30F**-
  Right **B30D**-
Bile Duct **BF00**-
Bile Duct and Gallbladder **BF03**-
Bladder **BT00**-
  Kidney and Ureter **BT04**-
Bladder and Urethra **BT03**-
Bone
  Facial **BN05ZZZ**
  Nasal **BN04ZZZ**
Bones, Long, All **BW0BZZZ**
Breast
  Bilateral **BH02ZZZ**
  Left **BH01ZZZ**
  Right **BH00ZZZ**
Calcaneus
  Left **BQ0KZZZ**
  Right **BQ0JZZZ**
Chest **BW03ZZZ**
Clavicle
  Left **BP05ZZZ**
  Right **BP04ZZZ**
Coccyx **BR0FZZZ**
Corpora Cavernosa **BV00**-
Dialysis Fistula **B50W**-
Dialysis Shunt **B50W**-
Disc
  Cervical **BR01**-
  Lumbar **BR03**-
  Thoracic **BR02**-
Duct
  Lacrimal
    Bilateral **B802**-
    Left **B801**-
    Right **B800**-
  Mammary
    Multiple
      Left **BH06**-
      Right **BH05**-
    Single
      Left **BH04**-
      Right **BH03**-
Elbow
  Left **BP0H**-
  Right **BP0G**-
Epididymis
  Left **BV02**-
  Right **BV01**-
Extremity
  Lower **BW0CZZZ**
  Upper **BW0JZZZ**
Eye
  Bilateral **B807ZZZ**
  Left **B806ZZZ**
  Right **B805ZZZ**
Facet Joint
  Cervical **BR04**-
  Lumbar **BR06**-
  Thoracic **BR05**-
Fallopian Tube
  Bilateral **BU02**-
  Left **BU01**-
  Right **BU00**-
Fallopian Tube and Uterus **BU08**-
Femur
  Left, Densitometry **BQ04ZZ1**
  Right, Densitometry **BQ03ZZ1**
Finger
  Left **BP0SZZZ**
  Right **BP0RZZZ**

Plain Radiography — continued
Foot
  Left **BQ0MZZZ**
  Right **BQ0LZZZ**
Forearm
  Left **BP0KZZZ**
  Right **BP0JZZZ**
Gallbladder and Bile Duct **BF03**-
Gland
  Parotid
    Bilateral **B906**-
    Left **B905**-
    Right **B904**-
  Salivary
    Bilateral **B90D**-
    Left **B90C**-
    Right **B90B**-
  Submandibular
    Bilateral **B909**-
    Left **B908**-
    Right **B907**-
Hand
  Left **BP0PZZZ**
  Right **BP0NZZZ**
Heart
  Left **B205**-
  Right **B204**-
  Right and Left **B206**-
Hepatobiliary System, All **BF0C**-
Hip
  Left **BQ01**-
    Densitometry **BQ01ZZ1**
  Right **BQ00**-
    Densitometry **BQ00ZZ1**
Humerus
  Left **BP0BZZZ**
  Right **BP0AZZZ**
Ileal Diversion Loop **BT0C**-
Intracranial Sinus **B502**-
Joint
  Acromioclavicular, Bilateral
    BP03ZZZ
  Finger
    Left **BP0D**-
    Right **BP0C**-
  Foot
    Left **BQ0Y**-
    Right **BQ0X**-
  Hand
    Left **BP0D**-
    Right **BP0C**-
  Lumbosacral **BR0BZZZ**
  Sacroiliac **BR0D**-
  Sternoclavicular
    Bilateral **BP02ZZZ**
    Left **BP01ZZZ**
    Right **BP00ZZZ**
  Temporomandibular
    Bilateral **BN09**-
    Left **BN08**-
    Right **BN07**-
  Thoracolumbar **BR08ZZZ**
  Toe
    Left **BQ0Y**-
    Right **BQ0X**-
Kidney
  Bilateral **BT03**-
  Left **BT02**-
  Right **BT01**-
  Ureter and Bladder **BT04**-
Knee
  Left **BQ08**-
  Right **BQ07**-
Leg
  Left **BQ0FZZZ**
  Right **BQ0DZZZ**
Lymphatic
  Head **B704**-
  Lower Extremity
    Bilateral **B70B**-
    Left **B709**-
    Right **B708**-

Plain Radiography — continued
Lymphatic — continued
Neck **B704**-
Pelvic **B70C**-
Upper Extremity
  Bilateral **B707**-
  Left **B706**-
  Right **B705**-
Mandible **BN06ZZZ**
Mastoid **B90HZZZ**
Nasopharynx **B90FZZZ**
Optic Foramina
  Left **B804ZZZ**
  Right **B803ZZZ**
Orbit
  Bilateral **BN03ZZZ**
  Left **BN02ZZZ**
  Right **BN01ZZZ**
Oropharynx **B90FZZZ**
Patella
  Left **BQ0WZZZ**
  Right **BQ0VZZZ**
Pelvis **BR0CZZZ**
Pelvis and Abdomen **BW01ZZZ**
Prostate **BV03**-
Retroperitoneal Lymphatic
  Bilateral **B701**-
  Unilateral **B700**-
Ribs
  Left **BP0YZZZ**
  Right **BP0XZZZ**
Sacrum **BR0FZZZ**
Scapula
  Left **BP07ZZZ**
  Right **BP06ZZZ**
Shoulder
  Left **BP09**-
  Right **BP08**-
Sinus
  Intracranial **B502**-
  Paranasal **B902ZZZ**
Skull **BN00ZZZ**
Spinal Cord **B00B**-
Spine
  Cervical, Densitometry **BR00ZZ1**
  Lumbar, Densitometry **BR09ZZ1**
  Thoracic, Densitometry **BR07ZZ1**
  Whole, Densitometry **BR0GZZ1**
Sternum **BR0HZZZ**
Teeth
  All **BN0JZZZ**
  Multiple **BN0HZZZ**
Testicle
  Left **BV06**-
  Right **BV05**-
Toe
  Left **BQ0QZZZ**
  Right **BQ0PZZZ**
Tooth, Single **BN0GZZZ**
Tracheobronchial Tree
  Bilateral **BB09YZZ**
  Left **BB08YZZ**
  Right **BB07YZZ**
Ureter
  Bilateral **BT08**-
  Kidney and Bladder **BT04**-
  Left **BT07**-
  Right **BT06**-
Urethra **BT05**-
Urethra and Bladder **BT0B**-
Uterus **BU06**-
Uterus and Fallopian Tube **BU08**-
Vagina **BU09**-
Vasa Vasorum **BV08**-
Vein
  Cerebellar **B501**-
  Cerebral **B501**-
  Epidural **B500**-
  Jugular
    Bilateral **B505**-
    Left **B504**-
    Right **B503**-

Plain Radiography — continued
Vein — continued
Lower Extremity
  Bilateral **B50D**-
  Left **B50C**-
  Right **B50B**-
Other **B50V**-
Pelvic (Iliac)
  Bilateral **B50H**-
  Left **B50G**-
  Right **B50F**-
Portal **B50T**-
Pulmonary
  Bilateral **B50S**-
  Left **B50R**-
  Right **B50Q**-
Renal
  Bilateral **B50L**-
  Left **B50K**-
  Right **B50J**-
Spanchnic **B50T**-
Subclavian
  Left **B507**-
  Right **B506**-
Upper Extremity
  Bilateral **B50P**-
  Left **B50N**-
  Right **B50M**-
Vena Cava
  Inferior **B509**-
  Superior **B508**-
Whole Body **BW0KZZZ**
  Infant **BW0MZZZ**
Whole Skeleton **BW0LZZZ**
Wrist
  Left **BP0M**-
  Right **BP0L**-

Planar Nuclear Medicine Imaging
Abdomen **CW10**-
Abdomen and Chest **CW14**-
Abdomen and Pelvis **CW11**-
Anatomical Region, Other **CW1ZZZZ**
Anatomical Regions, Multiple
  CW1YYZZ
Bladder and Ureters **CT1H**-
Bladder, Kidneys and Ureters **CT13**-
Blood **C713**-
Bone Marrow **C710**-
Brain **C010**-
Breast **CH1YYZZ**
  Bilateral **CH12**-
  Left **CH11**-
  Right **CH10**-
Bronchi and Lungs **CB12**-
Central Nervous System **C01YYZZ**
Cerebrospinal Fluid **C015**-
Chest **CW13**-
Chest and Abdomen **CW14**-
Chest and Neck **CW16**-
Digestive System **CD1YYZZ**
Ducts, Lacrimal, Bilateral **C819**-
Ear, Nose, Mouth and Throat
  C91YYZZ
Endocrine System **CG1YYZZ**
Extremity
  Lower **CW1D**-
    Bilateral **CP1F**-
    Left **CP1D**-
    Right **CP1C**-
  Upper **CW1M**-
    Bilateral **CP1B**-
    Left **CP19**-
    Right **CP18**-
Eye **C81YYZZ**
Gallbladder **CF14**-
Gastrointestinal Tract **CD17**-
  Upper **CD15**-
Gland
  Adrenal, Bilateral **CG14**-
  Parathyroid **CG11**-
  Thyroid **CG12**-
Glands, Salivary, Bilateral **C91B**-

Planar

Planar Nuclear Medicine Imaging — continued
  Head and Neck **CW1B-**
  Heart **C21YYZZ**
    Right and Left **C216-**
  Hepatobiliary System, All **CF1C-**
  Hepatobiliary System and Pancreas **CF1YYZZ**
  Kidneys, Ureters and Bladder **CT13-**
  Liver **CF15-**
  Liver and Spleen **CF16-**
  Lungs and Bronchi **CB12-**
  Lymphatics
    Head **C71J-**
    Head and Neck **C715-**
    Lower Extremity **C71P-**
    Neck **C71K-**
    Pelvic **C71D-**
    Trunk **C71M-**
    Upper Chest **C71L-**
    Upper Extremity **C71N-**
  Lymphatics and Hematologic System **C71YYZZ**
  Musculoskeletal System
    All **CP1Z-**
    Other **CP1YYZZ-**
  Myocardium **C21G-**
  Neck and Chest **CW16-**
  Neck and Head **CW1B-**
  Pancreas and Hepatobiliary System **CF1YYZZ**
  Pelvic Region **CW1J-**
  Pelvis **CP16-**
  Pelvis and Abdomen **CW11-**
  Pelvis and Spine **CP17-**
  Reproductive System, Male **CV1YYZZ**
  Respiratory System **CB1YYZZ**
  Skin **CH1YYZZ**
  Skull **CP11-**
  Spine **CP15-**
  Spine and Pelvis **CP17-**
  Spleen **C712-**
  Spleen and Liver **CF16-**
  Subcutaneous Tissue **CH1YYZZ**
  Testicles, Bilateral **CV19-**
  Thorax **CP14-**
  Ureters, Kidneys and Bladder **CT13-**
  Ureters and Bladder **CT1H-**
  Urinary System **CT1YYZZ**
  Veins **C51YYZZ**
    Central **C51R-**
    Lower Extremity
      Bilateral **C51D-**
      Left **C51C-**
      Right **C51B-**
    Upper Extremity
      Bilateral **C51Q-**
      Left **C51P-**
      Right **C51N-**
  Whole Body **CW1N-**
Plantar digital vein
  use Vein, Foot, Left
  use Vein, Foot, Right
Plantar fascia (aponeurosis)
  use Subcutaneous Tissue and Fascia, Foot, Left
  use Subcutaneous Tissue and Fascia, Foot, Right
Plantar metatarsal vein
  use Vein, Foot, Left
  use Vein, Foot, Right
Plantar venous arch
  use Vein, Foot, Left
  use Vein, Foot, Right
Plaque Radiation
  Abdomen **DWY3FZZ**
  Adrenal Gland **DGY2FZZ**
  Anus **DDY8FZZ**
  Bile Ducts **DFY2FZZ**
  Bladder **DTY2FZZ**
  Bone, Other **DPYCFZZ**
  Bone Marrow **D7Y0FZZ**

Plaque Radiation — continued
  Brain **D0Y0FZZ**
  Brain Stem **D0Y1FZZ**
  Breast
    Left **DMY0FZZ**
    Right **DMY1FZZ**
  Bronchus **DBY1FZZ**
  Cervix **DUY1FZZ**
  Chest **DWY2FZZ**
  Chest Wall **DBY7FZZ**
  Colon **DDY5FZZ**
  Diaphragm **DBY8FZZ**
  Duodenum **DDY2FZZ**
  Ear **D9Y0FZZ**
  Esophagus **DDY0FZZ**
  Eye **D8Y0FZZ**
  Femur **DPY9FZZ**
  Fibula **DPYBFZZ**
  Gallbladder **DFY1FZZ**
  Gland
    Adrenal **DGY2FZZ**
    Parathyroid **DGY4FZZ**
    Pituitary **DGY0FZZ**
    Thyroid **DGY5FZZ**
  Glands, Salivary **D9Y6FZZ**
  Head and Neck **DWY1FZZ**
  Hemibody **DWY4FZZ**
  Humerus **DPY6FZZ**
  Ileum **DDY4FZZ**
  Jejunum **DDY3FZZ**
  Kidney **DTY0FZZ**
  Larynx **D9YBFZZ**
  Liver **DFY0FZZ**
  Lung **DBY2FZZ**
  Lymphatics
    Abdomen **D7Y6FZZ**
    Axillary **D7Y4FZZ**
    Inguinal **D7Y8FZZ**
    Neck **D7Y3FZZ**
    Pelvis **D7Y7FZZ**
    Thorax **D7Y5FZZ**
  Mandible **DPY3FZZ**
  Maxilla **DPY2FZZ**
  Mediastinum **DBY6FZZ**
  Mouth **D9Y4FZZ**
  Nasopharynx **D9YDFZZ**
  Neck and Head **DWY1FZZ**
  Nerve, Peripheral **D0Y7FZZ**
  Nose **D9Y1FZZ**
  Ovary **DUY0FZZ**
  Palate
    Hard **D9Y8FZZ**
    Soft **D9Y9FZZ**
  Pancreas **DFY3FZZ**
  Parathyroid Gland **DGY4FZZ**
  Pelvic Bones **DPY8FZZ**
  Pelvic Region **DWY6FZZ**
  Pharynx **D9YCFZZ**
  Pineal Body **DGY1FZZ**
  Pituitary Gland **DGY0FZZ**
  Pleura **DBY5FZZ**
  Prostate **DVY0FZZ**
  Radius **DPY7FZZ**
  Rectum **DDY7FZZ**
  Rib **DPY5FZZ**
  Sinuses **D9Y7FZZ**
  Skin
    Abdomen **DHY8FZZ**
    Arm **DHY4FZZ**
    Back **DHY7FZZ**
    Buttock **DHY9FZZ**
    Chest **DHY6FZZ**
    Face **DHY2FZZ**
    Foot **DHYCFZZ**
    Hand **DHY5FZZ**
    Leg **DHYBFZZ**
    Neck **DHY3FZZ**
  Skull **DPY0FZZ**
  Spinal Cord **D0Y6FZZ**
  Spleen **D7Y2FZZ**
  Sternum **DPY4FZZ**
  Stomach **DDY1FZZ**

Plaque Radiation — continued
  Testis **DVY1FZZ**
  Thymus **D7Y1FZZ**
  Thyroid Gland **DGY5FZZ**
  Tibia **DPYBFZZ**
  Tongue **D9Y5FZZ**
  Trachea **DBY0FZZ**
  Ulna **DPY7FZZ**
  Ureter **DTY1FZZ**
  Urethra **DTY3FZZ**
  Uterus **DUY2FZZ**
  Whole Body **DWY5FZZ**
Plasmapheresis, therapeutic 6A550Z3
Plateletpheresis, therapeutic 6A550Z2
Platysma muscle
  use Muscle, Neck, Left
  use Muscle, Neck, Right
Pleurectomy
  see Excision, Respiratory System **0BB-**
  see Resection, Respiratory System **0BT-**
Pleurocentesis see Drainage, Anatomical Regions, General **0W9-**
Pleurodesis, pleurosclerosis
  Chemical injection see Introduction of substance in or on, Pleural Cavity **3E0L-**
  Surgical see Destruction, Respiratory System **0B5-**
Pleurolysis see Release, Respiratory System **0BN-**
Pleuroscopy 0BJQ4ZZ
Pleurotomy see Drainage, Respiratory System **0B9-**
Plica semilunaris
  use Conjunctiva, Left
  use Conjunctiva, Right
Plication see Restriction
Pneumectomy
  see Excision, Respiratory System **0BB-**
  see Resection, Respiratory System **0BT-**
Pneumocentesis see Drainage, Respiratory System **0B9-**
Pneumogastric nerve
  use Nerve, Vagus
Pneumolysis see Release, Respiratory System **0BN-**
Pneumonectomy
  see Resection, Respiratory System **0BT-**
Pneumonolysis see Release, Respiratory System **0BN-**
Pneumonopexy
  see Repair, Respiratory System **0BQ-**
  see Reposition, Respiratory System **0BS-**
Pneumonorrhaphy see Repair, Respiratory System **0BQ-**
Pneumonotomy see Drainage, Respiratory System **0B9-**
Pneumotaxic center
  use Pons
Pneumotomy see Drainage, Respiratory System **0B9-**
Pollicization see Transfer, Anatomical Regions, Upper Extremities **0XX-**
Polyethylene socket
  use Synthetic Substitute, Polyethylene in **0SR-**
Polymethylmethacrylate (PMMA)
  use Synthetic Substitute
Polypectomy, gastrointestinal see Excision, Gastrointestinal System **0DB-**
Polypropylene mesh
  use Synthetic Substitute
Polysomnogram 4A1ZXQZ
Pontine tegmentum
  use Pons

Popliteal ligament
  use Bursa and Ligament, Knee, Left
  use Bursa and Ligament, Knee, Right
Popliteal lymph node
  use Lymphatic, Lower Extremity, Left
  use Lymphatic, Lower Extremity, Right
Popliteal vein
  use Vein, Femoral, Left
  use Vein, Femoral, Right
Popliteus muscle
  use Muscle, Lower Leg, Left
  use Muscle, Lower Leg, Right
Porcine (bioprosthetic) valve
  use Zooplastic Tissue in Heart and Great Vessels
Positive end expiratory pressure
  see Performance, Respiratory **5A19-**
Positron Emission Tomographic (PET) Imaging
  Brain **C030-**
  Bronchi and Lungs **CB32-**
  Central Nervous System **C03YYZZ**
  Heart **C23YYZZ**
  Lungs and Bronchi **CB32-**
  Myocardium **C23G-**
  Respiratory System **CB3YYZZ**
  Whole Body **CW3NYZZ**
Positron emission tomography see Positron Emission Tomographic (PET) Imaging
Postauricular (mastoid) lymph node
  use Lymphatic, Neck, Left
  use Lymphatic, Neck, Right
Postcava
  use Vena Cava, Inferior
Posterior (subscapular) lymph node
  use Lymphatic, Axillary, Left
  use Lymphatic, Axillary, Right
Posterior auricular artery
  use Artery, External Carotid, Left
  use Artery, External Carotid, Right
Posterior auricular nerve
  use Nerve, Facial
Posterior auricular vein
  use Vein, External Jugular, Left
  use Vein, External Jugular, Right
Posterior cerebral artery
  use Artery, Intracranial
Posterior chamber
  use Eye, Left
  use Eye, Right
Posterior circumflex humeral artery
  use Artery, Axillary, Left
  use Artery, Axillary, Right
Posterior communicating artery
  use Artery, Intracranial
Posterior cruciate ligament (PCL)
  use Bursa and Ligament, Knee, Left
  use Bursa and Ligament, Knee, Right
Posterior facial (retromandibular) vein
  use Vein, Face, Left
  use Vein, Face, Right
Posterior femoral cutaneous nerve
  use Nerve, Sacral Plexus
Posterior inferior cerebellar artery (PICA)
  use Artery, Intracranial
Posterior interosseous nerve
  use Nerve, Radial
Posterior labial nerve
  use Nerve, Pudendal
Posterior scrotal nerve
  use Nerve, Pudendal
Posterior spinal artery
  use Artery, Vertebral, Left
  use Artery, Vertebral, Right

INDEX TO PROCEDURES – 2016 ICD-10-PCS

Posterior tibial recurrent artery
 use Artery, Anterior Tibial, Left
 use Artery, Anterior Tibial, Right
Posterior ulnar recurrent artery
 use Artery, Ulnar, Left
 use Artery, Ulnar, Right
Posterior vagal trunk
 use Nerve, Vagus
PPN (peripheral parenteral nutrition) see Introduction of Nutritional Substance
Preauricular lymph node
 use Lymphatic, Head
Precava
 use Vena Cava, Superior
Prepatellar bursa
 use Bursa and Ligament, Knee, Left
 use Bursa and Ligament, Knee, Right
Preputiotomy see Drainage, Male Reproductive System 0V9-
Pressure support ventilation see Performance, Respiratory 5A19-
PRESTIGE® Cervical Disc
 use Synthetic Substitute
Pretracheal fascia
 use Subcutaneous Tissue and Fascia, Neck, Anterior
Prevertebral fascia
 use Subcutaneous Tissue and Fascia, Neck, Posterior
PrimeAdvanced neurostimulator (SureScan) (MRI Safe)
 use Stimulator Generator, Multiple Array in 0JH
Princeps pollicis artery
 use Artery, Hand, Left
 use Artery, Hand, Right
Probing, duct
 Diagnostic see Inspection
 Dilation see Dilation
PROCEED™ Ventral Patch
 use Synthetic Substitute
Procerus muscle
 use Muscle, Facial
Proctectomy
 see Excision, Rectum 0DBP-
 see Resection, Rectum 0DTP-
Proctoclysis see Introduction of substance in or on, Gastrointestinal Tract, Lower 3E0H-
Proctocolectomy
 see Excision, Gastrointestinal System 0DB-
 see Resection, Gastrointestinal System 0DT-
Proctocolpoplasty
 see Repair, Gastrointestinal System 0DQ-
 see Supplement, Gastrointestinal System 0DU-
Proctoperineoplasty
 see Repair, Gastrointestinal System 0DQ-
 see Supplement, Gastrointestinal System 0DU-
Proctoperineorrhaphy see Repair, Gastrointestinal System 0DQ-
Proctopexy
 see Repair, Rectum 0DQP-
 see Reposition, Rectum 0DSP-
Proctoplasty
 see Repair, Rectum 0DQP-
 see Supplement, Rectum 0DUP-
Proctorrhaphy see Repair, Rectum 0DQP-
Proctoscopy 0DJD8ZZ
Proctosigmoidectomy
 see Excision, Gastrointestinal System 0DB-
 see Resection, Gastrointestinal System 0DT-
Proctosigmoidoscopy 0DJD8ZZ

Proctostomy see Drainage, Rectum 0D9P-
Proctotomy see Drainage, Rectum 0D9P-
Prodisc-C
 use Synthetic Substitute
Prodisc-L
 use Synthetic Substitute
Production, atrial septal defect see Excision, Septum, Atrial 02B5-
Profunda brachii
 use Artery, Brachial, Left
 use Artery, Brachial, Right
Profunda femoris (deep femoral) vein
 use Vein, Femoral, Left
 use Vein, Femoral, Right
PROLENE Polypropylene Hernia System (PHS)
 use Synthetic Substitute
Pronator quadratus muscle
 use Muscle, Lower Arm and Wrist, Left
 use Muscle, Lower Arm and Wrist, Right
Pronator teres muscle
 use Muscle, Lower Arm and Wrist, Left
 use Muscle, Lower Arm and Wrist, Right
Prostatectomy
 see Excision, Prostate 0VB0-
 see Resection, Prostate 0VT0-
Prostatic urethra
 use Urethra
Prostatomy, prostatotomy see Drainage, Prostate 0V90-
Protecta XT CRT-D
 use Cardiac Resynchronization Defibrillator Pulse Generator in 0JH-
Protecta XT DR (XT VR)
 use Defibrillator Generator in 0JH-
Protégé® RX Carotid Stent System
 use Intraluminal Device
Proximal radioulnar joint
 use Joint, Elbow, Left
 use Joint, Elbow, Right
Psoas muscle
 use Muscle, Hip, Left
 use Muscle, Hip, Right
PSV (pressure support ventilation) see Performance, Respiratory 5A19-
Psychoanalysis GZ54ZZZ
Psychological Tests
 Cognitive Status GZ14ZZZ
 Developmental GZ10ZZZ
 Intellectual and Psychoeducational GZ12ZZZ
 Neurobehavioral Status GZ14ZZZ
 Neuropsychological GZ13ZZZ
 Personality and Behavioral GZ11ZZZ
Psychotherapy
 Family, Mental Health Services GZ72ZZZ
 Group GZHZZZZ
  Mental Health Services GZHZZZZ
 Individual
  see Psychotherapy, Individual, Mental Health Services
 For substance abuse
  12-Step HZ53ZZZ
  Behavioral HZ51ZZZ
  Cognitive HZ50ZZZ
  Cognitive-Behavioral HZ52ZZZ
  Confrontational HZ58ZZZ
  Interactive HZ55ZZZ
  Interpersonal HZ54ZZZ
  Motivational Enhancement HZ57ZZZ
  Psychoanalysis HZ5BZZZ

Psychotherapy — continued
 Individual — continued
  For substance abuse — continued
   Psychodynamic HZ5CZZZ
   Psychoeducation HZ56ZZZ
   Psychophysiological HZ5DZZZ
   Supportive HZ59ZZZ
 Mental Health Services
  Behavioral GZ51ZZZ
  Cognitive GZ52ZZZ
  Cognitive-Behavioral GZ58ZZZ
  Interactive GZ50ZZZ
  Interpersonal GZ53ZZZ
  Psychoanalysis GZ54ZZZ
  Psychodynamic GZ55ZZZ
  Psychophysiological GZ59ZZZ
  Supportive GZ56ZZZ
PTCA (percutaneous transluminal coronary angioplasty) see Dilation, Heart and Great Vessels 027-
Pterygoid muscle
 use Muscle, Head
Pterygoid process
 use Bone, Sphenoid, Left
 use Bone, Sphenoid, Right
Pterygopalatine (sphenopalatine) ganglion
 use Nerve, Head and Neck Sympathetic
Pubic ligament
 use Bursa and Ligament, Trunk, Left
 use Bursa and Ligament, Trunk, Right
Pubis
 use Bone, Pelvic, Left
 use Bone, Pelvic, Right
Pubofemoral ligament
 use Bursa and Ligament, Hip, Left
 use Bursa and Ligament, Hip, Right
Pudendal nerve
 use Nerve, Sacral Plexus
Pull-through, rectal see Resection, Rectum 0DTP-
Pulmoaortic canal
 use Artery, Pulmonary, Left
Pulmonary annulus
 use Valve, Pulmonary
Pulmonary artery wedge monitoring see Monitoring, Arterial 4A13-
Pulmonary plexus
 use Nerve, Thoracic Sympathetic
 use Nerve, Vagus
Pulmonic valve
 use Valve, Pulmonary
Pulpectomy see Excision, Mouth and Throat 0CB-
Pulverization see Fragmentation
Pulvinar
 use Thalamus
Pump reservoir
 use Infusion Device, Pump in Subcutaneous Tissue and Fascia
Punch biopsy see Excision with qualifier Diagnostic
Puncture see Drainage
Puncture, lumbar see Drainage, Spinal Canal 009U-
Pyelography
 see Fluoroscopy, Urinary System BT1-
 see Plain Radiography, Urinary System BT0-
Pyeloileostomy, urinary diversion
 see Bypass, Urinary System 0T1-

Pyeloplasty
 see Repair, Urinary System 0TQ-
 see Replacement, Urinary System 0TR-
 see Supplement, Urinary System 0TU-
Pyelorrhaphy see Repair, Urinary System 0TQ-
Pyeloscopy 0TJ58ZZ
Pyelostomy
 see Drainage, Urinary System 0T9-
 see Bypass, Urinary System 0T1-
Pyelotomy see Drainage, Urinary System 0T9-
Pylorectomy
 see Excision, Stomach, Pylorus 0DB7-
 see Resection, Stomach, Pylorus 0DT7-
Pyloric antrum
 use Stomach, Pylorus
Pyloric canal
 use Stomach, Pylorus
Pyloric sphincter
 use Stomach, Pylorus
Pylorodiosis see Dilation, Stomach, Pylorus 0D77-
Pylorogastrectomy
 see Excision, Gastrointestinal System 0DB-
 see Resection, Gastrointestinal System 0DT-
Pyloroplasty
 see Repair, Stomach, Pylorus 0DQ7-
 see Supplement, Stomach, Pylorus 0DU7-
Pyloroscopy 0DJ68ZZ
Pylorotomy see Drainage, Stomach, Pylorus 0D97-
Pyramidalis muscle
 use Muscle, Abdomen, Left
 use Muscle, Abdomen, Right

Q

Quadrangular cartilage
 use Septum, Nasal
Quadrant resection of breast see
 Excision, Skin and Breast 0HB-
Quadrate lobe
 use Liver
Quadratus femoris muscle
 use Muscle, Hip, Left
 use Muscle, Hip, Right
Quadratus lumborum muscle
 use Muscle, Trunk, Left
 use Muscle, Trunk, Right
Quadratus plantae muscle
 use Muscle, Foot, Left
 use Muscle, Foot, Right
Quadriceps (femoris)
 use Muscle, Upper Leg, Left
 use Muscle, Upper Leg, Right
Quarantine 8E0ZXY6

R

Radial collateral carpal ligament
 use Bursa and Ligament, Wrist, Left
 use Bursa and Ligament, Wrist, Right
Radial collateral ligament
 use Bursa and Ligament, Elbow, Left
 use Bursa and Ligament, Elbow, Right
Radial notch
 use Ulna, Left
 use Ulna, Right
Radial recurrent artery
 use Artery, Radial, Left
 use Artery, Radial, Right
Radial vein
 use Vein, Brachial, Left
 use Vein, Brachial, Right
Radialis indicis
 use Artery, Hand, Left
 use Artery, Hand, Right
Radiation Therapy
 see Beam Radiation
 see Brachytherapy
 see Stereotactic Radiosurgery
Radiation treatment see Radiation Therapy
Radiocarpal joint
 use Joint, Wrist, Left
 use Joint, Wrist, Right
Radiocarpal ligament
 use Bursa and Ligament, Wrist, Left
 use Bursa and Ligament, Wrist, Right
Radiography see Plain Radiography
Radiology, analog see Plain Radiography
Radiology, diagnostic see Imaging, Diagnostic
Radioulnar ligament
 use Bursa and Ligament, Wrist, Left
 use Bursa and Ligament, Wrist, Right
Range of motion testing see Motor Function Assessment, Rehabilitation F01-
REALIZE® Adjustable Gastric Band
 use Extraluminal Device
Reattachment
 Abdominal Wall 0WMF0ZZ
 Ampulla of Vater 0FMC-
 Ankle Region
  Left 0YML0ZZ
  Right 0YMK0ZZ
 Arm
  Lower
   Left 0XMF0ZZ
   Right 0XMD0ZZ
  Upper
   Left 0XM90ZZ
   Right 0XM80ZZ
 Axilla
  Left 0XM50ZZ
  Right 0XM40ZZ
 Back
  Lower 0WML0ZZ
  Upper 0WMK0ZZ
 Bladder 0TMB-
 Bladder Neck 0TMC-
 Breast
  Bilateral 0HMVXZZ
  Left 0HMUXZZ
  Right 0HMTXZZ
 Bronchus
  Lingula 0BM90ZZ
  Lower Lobe
   Left 0BMB0ZZ
   Right 0BM60ZZ
  Main
   Left 0BM70ZZ
   Right 0BM30ZZ
  Middle Lobe, Right 0BM50ZZ
  Upper Lobe
   Left 0BM80ZZ
   Right 0BM40ZZ

Reattachment — continued
 Bursa and Ligament
  Abdomen
   Left 0MMJ-
   Right 0MMH-
  Ankle
   Left 0MMR-
   Right 0MMQ-
  Elbow
   Left 0MM4-
   Right 0MM3-
  Foot
   Left 0MMT-
   Right 0MMS-
  Hand
   Left 0MM8-
   Right 0MM7-
  Head and Neck 0MM0-
  Hip
   Left 0MMM-
   Right 0MML-
  Knee
   Left 0MMP-
   Right 0MMN-
  Lower Extremity
   Left 0MMW-
   Right 0MMV-
  Perineum 0MMK-
  Shoulder
   Left 0MM2-
   Right 0MM1-
  Thorax
   Left 0MMG-
   Right 0MMF-
  Trunk
   Left 0MMD-
   Right 0MMC-
  Upper Extremity
   Left 0MMB-
   Right 0MM9-
  Wrist
   Left 0MM6-
   Right 0MM5-
 Buttock
  Left 0YM10ZZ
  Right 0YM00ZZ
 Carina 0BM20ZZ
 Cecum 0DMH-
 Cervix 0UMC-
 Chest Wall 0WM80ZZ
 Clitoris 0UMJXZZ
 Colon
  Ascending 0DMK-
  Descending 0DMM-
  Sigmoid 0DMN-
  Transverse 0DML-
 Cord
  Bilateral 0VMH-
  Left 0VMG-
  Right 0VMF-
 Cul-de-sac 0UMF-
 Diaphragm
  Left 0BMS0ZZ
  Right 0BMR0ZZ
 Duct
  Common Bile 0FM9-
  Cystic 0FM8-
  Hepatic
   Left 0FM6-
   Right 0FM5-
  Pancreatic 0FMD-
   Accessory 0FMF-
 Duodenum 0DM9-
 Ear
  Left 09M1XZZ
  Right 09M0XZZ
 Elbow Region
  Left 0XMC0ZZ
  Right 0XMB0ZZ
 Esophagus 0DM5-

Reattachment — continued
 Extremity
  Lower
   Left 0YMB0ZZ
   Right 0YM90ZZ
  Upper
   Left 0XM70ZZ
   Right 0XM60ZZ
 Eyelid
  Lower
   Left 08MRXZZ
   Right 08MQXZZ
  Upper
   Left 08MPXZZ
   Right 08MNXZZ
 Face 0WM20ZZ
 Fallopian Tube
  Left 0UM6-
  Right 0UM5-
 Fallopian Tubes, Bilateral 0UM7-
 Femoral Region
  Left 0YM80ZZ
  Right 0YM70ZZ
 Finger
  Index
   Left 0XMP0ZZ
   Right 0XMN0ZZ
  Little
   Left 0XMW0ZZ
   Right 0XMV0ZZ
  Middle
   Left 0XMR0ZZ
   Right 0XMQ0ZZ
  Ring
   Left 0XMT0ZZ
   Right 0XMS0ZZ
 Foot
  Left 0YMN0ZZ
  Right 0YMM0ZZ
 Forequarter
  Left 0XM10ZZ
  Right 0XM00ZZ
 Gallbladder 0FM4
 Gland
  Left 0GM2-
  Right 0GM3-
 Hand
  Left 0XMK0ZZ
  Right 0XMJ0ZZ
 Hindquarter
  Bilateral 0YM40ZZ
  Left 0YM30ZZ
  Right 0YM20ZZ
 Hymen 0UMK-
 Ileum 0DMB-
 Inguinal Region
  Left 0YM60ZZ
  Right 0YM50ZZ
 Intestine
  Large 0DME-
   Left 0DMG-
   Right 0DMF-
  Small 0DM8-
 Jaw
  Lower 0WM50ZZ
  Upper 0WM40ZZ
 Jejunum 0DMA-
 Kidney
  Left 0TM1-
  Right 0TM0-
 Kidney Pelvis
  Left 0TM4-
  Right 0TM3-
 Kidneys, Bilateral 0TM2-
 Knee Region
  Left 0YMG0ZZ
  Right 0YMF0ZZ
 Leg
  Lower
   Left 0YMJ0ZZ
   Right 0YMH0ZZ

INDEX TO PROCEDURES – 2016 ICD-10-PCS

Reattachment — *continued*
Leg — *continued*
  Upper
    Left 0YMD0ZZ
    Right 0YMC0ZZ
Lip
  Lower 0CM10ZZ
  Upper 0CM00ZZ
Liver 0FM0-
  Left Lobe 0FM2-
  Right Lobe 0FM1-
Lung
  Left 0BML0ZZ
  Lower Lobe
    Left 0BMJ0ZZ
    Right 0BMF0ZZ
  Middle Lobe, Right 0BMD0ZZ
  Right 0BMK0ZZ
  Upper Lobe
    Left 0BMG0ZZ
    Right 0BMC0ZZ
Lung Lingula 0BMH0ZZ
Muscle
  Abdomen
    Left 0KML-
    Right 0KMK-
  Facial 0KM1-
  Foot
    Left 0KMW-
    Right 0KMV-
  Hand
    Left 0KMD-
    Right 0KMC-
  Head 0KM0-
  Hip
    Left 0KMP-
    Right 0KMN-
  Lower Arm and Wrist
    Left 0KMB-
    Right 0KM9-
  Lower Leg
    Left 0KMT-
    Right 0KMS-
  Neck
    Left 0KM3-
    Right 0KM2-
  Perineum 0KMM-
  Shoulder
    Left 0KM6-
    Right 0KM5-
  Thorax
    Left 0KMJ-
    Right 0KMH-
  Tongue, Palate, Pharynx 0KM4-
  Trunk
    Left 0KMG-
    Right 0KMF-
  Upper Arm
    Left 0KM8-
    Right 0KM7-
  Upper Leg
    Left 0KMR-
    Right 0KMQ-
Neck 0WM60ZZ
Nipple
  Left 0HMXXZZ
  Right 0HMWXZZ
Nose 09MKXZZ
Ovary
  Bilateral 0UM2-
  Left 0UM1-
  Right 0UM0-
Palate, Soft 0CM30ZZ
Pancreas 0FMG-
Parathyroid Gland 0GMR-
  Inferior
    Left 0GMP-
    Right 0GMN-
  Multiple 0GMQ-
  Superior
    Left 0GMM-
    Right 0GML-

Reattachment — *continued*
Penis 0VMSXZZ
Perineum
  Female 0WMN0ZZ
  Male 0WMM0ZZ
Rectum 0DMP-
Scrotum 0VM5XZZ
Shoulder Region
  Left 0XM30ZZ
  Right 0XM20ZZ
Skin
  Abdomen 0HM7XZZ
  Back 0HM6XZZ
  Buttock 0HM8XZZ
  Chest 0HM5XZZ
  Ear
    Left 0HM3XZZ
    Right 0HM2XZZ
  Face 0HM1XZZ
  Foot
    Left 0HMNXZZ
    Right 0HMMXZZ
  Genitalia 0HMAXZZ
  Hand
    Left 0HMGXZZ
    Right 0HMFXZZ
  Lower Arm
    Left 0HMEXZZ
    Right 0HMDXZZ
  Lower Leg
    Left 0HMLXZZ
    Right 0HMKXZZ
  Neck 0HM4XZZ
  Perineum 0HM9XZZ
  Scalp 0HM0XZZ
  Upper Arm
    Left 0HMCXZZ
    Right 0HMBXZZ
  Upper Leg
    Left 0HMJXZZ
    Right 0HMHXZZ
Stomach 0DM6-
Tendon
  Abdomen
    Left 0LMG-
    Right 0LMF-
  Ankle
    Left 0LMT-
    Right 0LMS-
  Foot
    Left 0LMW-
    Right 0LMV-
  Hand
    Left 0LM8-
    Right 0LM7-
  Head and Neck 0LM0-
  Hip
    Left 0LMK-
    Right 0LMJ-
  Knee
    Left 0LMR-
    Right 0LMQ-
  Lower Arm and Wrist
    Left 0LM6-
    Right 0LM5-
  Lower Leg
    Left 0LMP-
    Right 0LMN-
  Perineum 0LMH-
  Shoulder
    Left 0LM2-
    Right 0LM1-
  Thorax
    Left 0LMD-
    Right 0LMC-
  Trunk
    Left 0LMB-
    Right 0LM9-
  Upper Arm
    Left 0LM4-
    Right 0LM3-

Reattachment — *continued*
Tendon — *continued*
  Upper Leg
    Left 0LMM-
    Right 0LML-
Testis
  Bilateral 0VMC-
  Left 0VMB-
  Right 0VM9-
Thumb
  Left 0XMM0ZZ
  Right 0XML0ZZ
Thyroid Gland
  Left Lobe 0GMG-
  Right Lobe 0GMH-
Toe
  1st
    Left 0YMQ0ZZ
    Right 0YMP0ZZ
  2nd
    Left 0YMS0ZZ
    Right 0YMR0ZZ
  3rd
    Left 0YMU0ZZ
    Right 0YMT0ZZ
  4th
    Left 0YMW0ZZ
    Right 0YMV0ZZ
  5th
    Left 0YMY0ZZ
    Right 0YMX0ZZ
Tongue 0CM70ZZ
Tooth
  Lower 0CMX-
  Upper 0CMW-
Trachea 0BM10ZZ
Tunica Vaginalis
  Left 0VM7-
  Right 0VM6-
Ureter
  Left 0TM7-
  Right 0TM6-
Ureters, Bilateral 0TM8-
Urethra 0TMD-
Uterine Supporting Structure 0UM4-
Uterus 0UM9-
Uvula 0CMN0ZZ
Vagina 0UMG-
Vulva 0UMMXZZ
Wrist Region
  Left 0XMH0ZZ
  Right 0XMG0ZZ
Rebound HRD® (Hernia Repair Device)
  use Synthetic Substitute
Recession
  see Repair
  see Reposition
Reclosure, disrupted abdominal wall 0WQFXZZ
Reconstruction
  see Repair
  see Replacement
  see Supplement
Rectectomy
  see Excision, Rectum 0DBP-
  see Resection, Rectum 0DTP-
Rectocele repair
  see Repair, Subcutaneous Tissue and Fascia, Pelvic Region 0JQC-
Rectopexy
  see Repair, Gastrointestinal System 0DQ-
  see Reposition, Gastrointestinal System 0DS-
Rectoplasty
  see Repair, Gastrointestinal System 0DQ-
  see Supplement, Gastrointestinal System 0DU-
Rectorrhaphy *see* Repair, Gastrointestinal System 0DQ -

Rectoscopy 0DJD8ZZ
Rectosigmoid junction
  use Colon, Sigmoid
Rectosigmoidectomy
  see Excision, Gastrointestinal System 0DB-
  see Resection, Gastrointestinal System 0DT-
Rectostomy *see* Drainage, Rectum 0D9P-
Rectotomy *see* Drainage, Rectum 0D9P-
Rectus abdominis muscle
  use Muscle, Abdomen, Left
  use Muscle, Abdomen, Right
Rectus femoris muscle
  use Muscle, Upper Leg, Left
  use Muscle, Upper Leg, Right
Recurrent laryngeal nerve
  use Nerve, Vagus
Reduction
  Dislocation *see* Reposition
  Fracture *see* Reposition
  Intussusception, intestinal *see* Reposition, Gastrointestinal System 0DS-
  Mammoplasty *see* Excision, Skin and Breast 0HB-
  Prolapse *see* Reposition
  Torsion *see* Reposition
  Volvulus, gastrointestinal *see* Reposition, Gastrointestinal System 0DS-
Refusion *see* Fusion
Rehabilitation
  see Activities of Daily Living Assessment, Rehabilitation F02-
  see Activities of Daily Living Treatment, Rehabilitation F08-
  see Caregiver Training, Rehabilitation F0F-
  see Cochlear Implant Treatment, Rehabilitation F0B-
  see Device Fitting, Rehabilitation F0D-
  see Hearing Treatment, Rehabilitation F09-
  see Motor Function Assessment, Rehabilitation F01-
  see Motor Treatment, Rehabilitation F07-
  see Speech Assessment, Rehabilitation F00-
  see Speech Treatment, Rehabilitation F06-
  see Vestibular Treatment, Rehabilitation F0C-
Reimplantation
  see Reattachment
  see Reposition
  see Transfer
Reinforcement
  see Repair
  see Supplement
Relaxation, scar tissue *see* Release
Release
  Acetabulum
    Left 0QN5-
    Right 0QN4-
  Adenoids 0CNQ-
  Ampulla of Vater 0FNC-
  Anal Sphincter 0DNR-
  Anterior Chamber
    Left 08N33ZZ
    Right 08N23ZZ
  Anus 0DNQ-
  Aorta
    Abdominal 04N0-
    Thoracic 02NW-
  Aortic Body 0GND-
  Appendix 0DNJ-

Release

Release — continued
- Artery
  - Anterior Tibial
    - Left 04NQ-
    - Right 04NP-
  - Axillary
    - Left 03N6-
    - Right 03N5-
  - Brachial
    - Left 03N8-
    - Right 03N7-
  - Celiac 04N1-
  - Colic
    - Left 04N7-
    - Middle 04N8-
    - Right 04N6-
  - Common Carotid
    - Left 03NJ-
    - Right 03NH-
  - Common Iliac
    - Left 04ND-
    - Right 04NC-
  - External Carotid
    - Left 03NN-
    - Right 03NM-
  - External Iliac
    - Left 04NJ-
    - Right 04NH-
  - Face 03NR-
  - Femoral
    - Left 04NL-
    - Right 04NK-
  - Foot
    - Left 04NW-
    - Right 04NV-
  - Gastric 04N2-
  - Hand
    - Left 03NF-
    - Right 03ND-
  - Hepatic 04N3-
  - Inferior Mesenteric 04NB-
  - Innominate 03N2-
  - Internal Carotid
    - Left 03NL-
    - Right 03NK-
  - Internal Iliac
    - Left 04NF-
    - Right 04NE-
  - Internal Mammary
    - Left 03N1-
    - Right 03N0-
  - Intracranial 03NG-
  - Lower 04NY-
  - Peroneal
    - Left 04NU-
    - Right 04NT-
  - Popliteal
    - Left 04NN-
    - Right 04NM-
  - Posterior Tibial
    - Left 04NS-
    - Right 04NR-
  - Pulmonary
    - Left 02NR-
    - Right 02NQ-
  - Pulmonary Trunk 02NP-
  - Radial
    - Left 03NC-
    - Right 03NB-
  - Renal
    - Left 04NA-
    - Right 04N9-
  - Splenic 04N4-
  - Subclavian
    - Left 03N4-
    - Right 03N3-
  - Superior Mesenteric 04N5-
  - Temporal
    - Left 03NT-
    - Right 03NS-

Release — continued
- Artery — continued
  - Thyroid
    - Left 03NV-
    - Right 03NU-
  - Ulnar
    - Left 03NA-
    - Right 03N9-
    - Upper 03NY-
  - Vertebral
    - Left 03NQ-
    - Right 03NP-
- Atrium
  - Left 02N7-
  - Right 02N6-
- Auditory Ossicle
  - Left 09NA0ZZ
  - Right 09N90ZZ
- Basal Ganglia 00N8-
- Bladder 0TNB-
- Bladder Neck 0TNC-
- Bone
  - Ethmoid
    - Left 0NNG-
    - Right 0NNF-
  - Frontal
    - Left 0NN2-
    - Right 0NN1-
  - Hyoid 0NNX-
  - Lacrimal
    - Left 0NNJ-
    - Right 0NNH-
  - Nasal 0NNB-
  - Occipital
    - Left 0NN8-
    - Right 0NN7-
  - Palatine
    - Left 0NNL-
    - Right 0NNK-
  - Parietal
    - Left 0NN4-
    - Right 0NN3-
  - Pelvic
    - Left 0QN3-
    - Right 0QN2-
  - Sphenoid
    - Left 0NND-
    - Right 0NNC-
  - Temporal
    - Left 0NN6-
    - Right 0NN5-
  - Zygomatic
    - Left 0NNN-
    - Right 0NNM-
- Brain 00N0-
- Breast
  - Bilateral 0HNV-
  - Left 0HNU-
  - Right 0HNT-
- Bronchus
  - Lingula 0BN9-
  - Lower Lobe
    - Left 0BNB-
    - Right 0BN6-
  - Main
    - Left 0BN7-
    - Right 0BN3-
  - Middle Lobe, Right 0BN5-
  - Upper Lobe
    - Left 0BN8-
    - Right 0BN4-
- Buccal Mucosa 0CN4-
- Bursa and Ligament
  - Abdomen
    - Left 0MNJ-
    - Right 0MNH-
  - Ankle
    - Left 0MNR-
    - Right 0MNQ-
  - Elbow
    - Left 0MN4-
    - Right 0MN3-

Release — continued
- Bursa and Ligament — continued
  - Foot
    - Left 0MNT-
    - Right 0MNS-
  - Hand
    - Left 0MN8-
    - Right 0MN7-
  - Head and Neck 0MN0-
  - Hip
    - Left 0MNM-
    - Right 0MNL-
  - Knee
    - Left 0MNP-
    - Right 0MNN-
  - Lower Extremity
    - Left 0MNW-
    - Right 0MNV-
  - Perineum 0MNK-
  - Shoulder
    - Left 0MN2-
    - Right 0MN1-
  - Thorax
    - Left 0MNG-
    - Right 0MNF-
  - Trunk
    - Left 0MND-
    - Right 0MNC-
  - Upper Extremity
    - Left 0MNB-
    - Right 0MN9-
  - Wrist
    - Left 0MN6-
    - Right 0MN5-
- Carina 0BN2-
- Carotid Bodies, Bilateral 0GN8-
- Carotid Body
  - Left 0GN6-
  - Right 0GN7-
- Carpal
  - Left 0PNN-
  - Right 0PNM-
- Cecum 0DNH-
- Cerebellum 00NC-
- Cerebral Hemisphere 00N7-
- Cerebral Meninges 00N1-
- Cerebral Ventricle 00N6-
- Cervix 0UNC-
- Chordae Tendineae 02N9-
- Choroid
  - Left 08NB-
  - Right 08NA-
- Cisterna Chyli 07NL-
- Clavicle
  - Left 0PNB-
  - Right 0PN9-
- Clitoris 0UNJ-
- Coccygeal Glomus 0GNB-
- Coccyx 0QNS-
- Colon
  - Ascending 0DNK-
  - Descending 0DNM-
  - Sigmoid 0DNN-
  - Transverse 0DNL-
- Conduction Mechanism 02N8-
- Conjunctiva
  - Left 08NTXZZ
  - Right 08NSXZZ
- Cord
  - Bilateral 0VNH-
  - Left 0VNG-
  - Right 0VNF-
- Cornea
  - Left 08N9XZZ
  - Right 08N8XZZ
- Cul-de-sac 0UNF-
- Diaphragm
  - Left 0BNS-
  - Right 0BNR-
- Disc
  - Cervical Vertebral 0RN3-
  - Cervicothoracic Vertebral 0RN5-

Release — continued
- Disc — continued
  - Lumbar Vertebral 0SN2-
  - Lumbosacral 0SN4-
  - Thoracic Vertebral 0RN9-
  - Thoracolumbar Vertebral 0RNB-
- Duct
  - Common Bile 0FN9-
  - Cystic 0FN8-
  - Hepatic
    - Left 0FN6-
    - Right 0FN5-
  - Lacrimal
    - Left 08NY-
    - Right 08NX-
  - Pancreatic 0FND-
    - Accessory 0FNF-
  - Parotid
    - Left 0CNC-
    - Right 0CNB-
- Duodenum 0DN9-
- Dura Mater 00N2-
- Ear
  - External
    - Left 09N1-
    - Right 09N0-
  - External Auditory Canal
    - Left 09N4-
    - Right 09N3-
  - Inner
    - Left 09NE0ZZ
    - Right 09ND0ZZ
  - Middle
    - Left 09N60ZZ
    - Right 09N50ZZ
- Epididymis
  - Bilateral 0VNL-
  - Left 0VNK-
  - Right 0VNJ-
- Epiglottis 0CNR-
- Esophagogastric Junction 0DN4-
- Esophagus 0DN5-
  - Lower 0DN3-
  - Middle 0DN2-
  - Upper 0DN1-
- Eustachian Tube
  - Left 09NG-
  - Right 09NF-
- Eye
  - Left 08N1XZZ
  - Right 08N0XZZ
- Eyelid
  - Lower
    - Left 08NR-
    - Right 08NQ-
  - Upper
    - Left 08NP-
    - Right 08NN-
- Fallopian Tube
  - Left 0UN6-
  - Right 0UN5-
- Fallopian Tubes, Bilateral 0UN7-
- Femoral Shaft
  - Left 0QN9-
  - Right 0QN8-
- Femur
  - Lower
    - Left 0QNC-
    - Right 0QNB-
  - Upper
    - Left 0QN7-
    - Right 0QN6-
- Fibula
  - Left 0QNK-
  - Right 0QNJ-
- Finger Nail 0HNQXZZ
- Gallbladder 0FN4-
- Gingiva
  - Lower 0CN6-
  - Upper 0CN5-

INDEX TO PROCEDURES – 2016 ICD-10-PCS

Release

Release — *continued*
Gland
　Adrenal
　　Bilateral 0GN4-
　　Left 0GN2-
　　Right 0GN3-
　Lacrimal
　　Left 08NW-
　　Right 08NV-
　Minor Salivary 0CNJ-
　Parotid
　　Left 0CN9-
　　Right 0CN8-
　Pituitary 0GN0-
　Sublingual
　　Left 0CNF-
　　Right 0CND-
　Submaxillary
　　Left 0CNH-
　　Right 0CNG-
　Vestibular 0UNL-
Glenoid Cavity
　Left 0PN8-
　Right 0PN7-
Glomus Jugulare 0GNC-
Humeral Head
　Left 0PND-
　Right 0PNC-
Humeral Shaft
　Left 0PNG-
　Right 0PNF-
Hymen 0UNK-
Hypothalamus 00NA-
Ileocecal Valve 0DNC-
Ileum 0DNB-
Intestine
　Large 0DNE-
　　Left 0DNG-
　　Right 0DNF-
　Small 0DN8-
Iris
　Left 08ND3ZZ
　Right 08NC3ZZ
Jejunum 0DNA-
Joint
　Acromioclavicular
　　Left 0RNH-
　　Right 0RNG-
　Ankle
　　Left 0SNG-
　　Right 0SNF-
　Carpal
　　Left 0RNR-
　　Right 0RNQ-
　Cervical Vertebral 0RN1-
　Cervicothoracic Vertebral 0RN4-
　Coccygeal 0SN6-
　Elbow
　　Left 0RNM-
　　Right 0RNL-
　Finger Phalangeal
　　Left 0RNX-
　　Right 0RNW-
　Hip
　　Left 0SNB-
　　Right 0SN9-
　Knee
　　Left 0SND-
　　Right 0SNC-
　Lumbar Vertebral 0SN0-
　Lumbosacral 0SN3-
　Metacarpocarpal
　　Left 0RNT-
　　Right 0RNS-
　Metacarpophalangeal
　　Left 0RNV-
　　Right 0RNU-
　Metatarsal-Phalangeal
　　Left 0SNN-
　　Right 0SNM-

Release — *continued*
Joint — *continued*
　Metatarsal-Tarsal
　　Left 0SNL-
　　Right 0SNK-
　Occipital-cervical 0RN0-
　Sacrococcygeal 0SN5-
　Sacroiliac
　　Left 0SN8-
　　Right 0SN7-
　Shoulder
　　Left 0RNK-
　　Right 0RNJ-
　Sternoclavicular
　　Left 0RNF-
　　Right 0RNE-
　Tarsal
　　Left 0SNJ-
　　Right 0SNH-
　Temporomandibular
　　Left 0RND-
　　Right 0RNC-
　Thoracic Vertebral 0RN6-
　Thoracolumbar Vertebral 0RNA-
　Toe Phalangeal
　　Left 0SNQ-
　　Right 0SNP-
　Wrist
　　Left 0RNP-
　　Right 0RNN-
Kidney
　Left 0TN1-
　Right 0TN0-
Kidney Pelvis
　Left 0TN4-
　Right 0TN3-
Larynx 0CNS-
Lens
　Left 08NK3ZZ
　Right 08NJ3ZZ
Lip
　Lower 0CN1-
　Upper 0CN0-
Liver 0FN0-
　Left Lobe 0FN2-
　Right Lobe 0FN1-
Lung
　Bilateral 0BNM-
　Left 0BNL-
　Lower Lobe
　　Left 0BNJ-
　　Right 0BNF-
　Middle Lobe, Right 0BND-
　Right 0BNK-
　Upper Lobe
　　Left 0BNG-
　　Right 0BNC-
Lung Lingula 0BNH-
Lymphatic
　Aortic 07ND-
　Axillary
　　Left 07N6-
　　Right 07N5-
　Head 07N0-
　Inguinal
　　Left 07NJ-
　　Right 07NH-
　Internal Mammary
　　Left 07N9-
　　Right 07N8-
　Lower Extremity
　　Left 07NG-
　　Right 07NF-
　Mesenteric 07NB-
　Neck
　　Left 07N2-
　　Right 07N1-
　Pelvis 07NC-
　Thoracic Duct 07NK-
　Thorax 07N7-

Release — *continued*
Lymphatic — *continued*
　Upper Extremity
　　Left 07N4-
　　Right 07N3-
Mandible
　Left 0NNV-
　Right 0NNT-
Maxilla
　Left 0NNS-
　Right 0NNR-
Medulla Oblongata 00ND-
Mesentery 0DNV-
Metacarpal
　Left 0PNQ-
　Right 0PNP-
Metatarsal
　Left 0QNP-
　Right 0QNN-
Muscle
　Abdomen
　　Left 0KNL-
　　Right 0KNK-
　Extraocular
　　Left 08NM-
　　Right 08NL-
　Facial 0KN1-
　Foot
　　Left 0KNW-
　　Right 0KNV-
　Hand
　　Left 0KND-
　　Right 0KNC-
　Head 0KN0-
　Hip
　　Left 0KNP-
　　Right 0KNN-
　Lower Arm and Wrist
　　Left 0KNB-
　　Right 0KN9-
　Lower Leg
　　Left 0KNT-
　　Right 0KNS-
　Neck
　　Left 0KN3-
　　Right 0KN2-
　Papillary 02ND-
　Perineum 0KNM-
　Shoulder
　　Left 0KN6-
　　Right 0KN5-
　Thorax
　　Left 0KNJ-
　　Right 0KNH-
　Tongue, Palate, Pharynx 0KN4-
　Trunk
　　Left 0KNG-
　　Right 0KNF-
　Upper Arm
　　Left 0KN8-
　　Right 0KN7-
　Upper Leg
　　Left 0KNR-
　　Right 0KNQ-
Nasopharynx 09NN-
Nerve
　Abdominal Sympathetic 01NM-
　Abducens 00NL-
　Accessory 00NR-
　Acoustic 00NN-
　Brachial Plexus 01N3-
　Cervical 01N1-
　Cervical Plexus 01N0-
　Facial 00NM-
　Femoral 01ND-
　Glossopharyngeal 00NP-
　Head and Neck Sympathetic 01NK-
　Hypoglossal 00NS-

Release — *continued*
Nerve — *continued*
　Lumbar 01NB-
　Lumbar Plexus 01N9-
　Lumbar Sympathetic 01NN-
　Lumbosacral Plexus 01NA-
　Median 01N5-
　Oculomotor 00NH-
　Olfactory 00NF-
　Optic 00NG-
　Peroneal 01NH-
　Phrenic 01N2-
　Pudendal 01NC-
　Radial 01N6-
　Sacral 01NR-
　Sacral Plexus 01NQ-
　Sacral Sympathetic 01NP-
　Sciatic 01NF-
　Thoracic 01N8-
　Thoracic Sympathetic 01NL-
　Tibial 01NG-
　Trigeminal 00NK-
　Trochlear 00NJ-
　Ulnar 01N4-
　Vagus 00NQ-
Nipple
　Left 0HNX-
　Right 0HNW-
Nose 09NK-
Omentum
　Greater 0DNS-
　Lesser 0DNT-
Orbit
　Left 0NNQ-
　Right 0NNP-
Ovary
　Bilateral 0UN2-
　Left 0UN1-
　Right 0UN0-
Palate
　Hard 0CN2-
　Soft 0CN3-
Pancreas 0FNG-
Para-aortic Body 0GN9-
Paraganglion Extremity 0GNF-
Parathyroid Gland 0GNR-
　Inferior
　　Left 0GNP-
　　Right 0GNN-
　Multiple 0GNQ-
　Superior
　　Left 0GNM-
　　Right 0GNL-
Patella
　Left 0QNF-
　Right 0QND-
Penis 0VNS-
Pericardium 02NN-
Peritoneum 0DNW-
Phalanx
　Finger
　　Left 0PNV-
　　Right 0PNT-
　Thumb
　　Left 0PNS-
　　Right 0PNR-
　Toe
　　Left 0QNR-
　　Right 0QNQ-
Pharynx 0CNM-
Pineal Body 0GN1-
Pleura
　Left 0BNP-
　Right 0BNN-
Pons 00NB-
Prepuce 0VNT-
Prostate 0VN0-
Radius
　Left 0PNJ-
　Right 0PNH-
Rectum 0DNP-

Release

Release — continued
Retina
  Left 08NF3ZZ
  Right 08NE3ZZ
Retinal Vessel
  Left 08NH3ZZ
  Right 08NG3ZZ
Rib
  Left 0PN2-
  Right 0PN1-
Sacrum 0QN1-
Scapula
  Left 0PN6-
  Right 0PN5-
Sclera
  Left 08N7XZZ
  Right 08N6XZZ
Scrotum 0VN5-
Septum
  Atrial 02N5-
  Nasal 09NM-
  Ventricular 02NM-
Sinus
  Accessory 09NP-
  Ethmoid
    Left 09NV-
    Right 09NU-
  Frontal
    Left 09NT-
    Right 09NS-
  Mastoid
    Left 09NC-
    Right 09NB-
  Maxillary
    Left 09NR-
    Right 09NQ-
  Sphenoid
    Left 09NX-
    Right 09NW-
Skin
  Abdomen 0HN7XZZ
  Back 0HN6XZZ
  Buttock 0HN8XZZ
  Chest 0HN5XZZ
  Ear
    Left 0HN3XZZ
    Right 0HN2XZZ
  Face 0HN1XZZ
  Foot
    Left 0HNNXZZ
    Right 0HNMXZZ
  Genitalia 0HNAXZZ
  Hand
    Left 0HNGXZZ
    Right 0HNFXZZ
  Lower Arm
    Left 0HNEXZZ
    Right 0HNDXZZ
  Lower Leg
    Left 0HNLXZZ
    Right 0HNKXZZ
  Neck 0HN4XZZ
  Perineum 0HN9XZZ
  Scalp 0HN0XZZ
  Upper Arm
    Left 0HNCXZZ
    Right 0HNBXZZ
  Upper Leg
    Left 0HNJXZZ
    Right 0HNHXZZ
Spinal Cord
  Cervical 00NW-
  Lumbar 00NY-
  Thoracic 00NX-
Spinal Meninges 00NT-
Spleen 07NP-
Sternum 0PN0-
Stomach 0DN6-
  Pylorus 0DN7-

Release — continued
Subcutaneous Tissue and Fascia
  Abdomen 0JN8-
  Back 0JN7-
  Buttock 0JN9-
  Chest 0JN6-
  Face 0JN1-
  Foot
    Left 0JNR-
    Right 0JNQ-
  Hand
    Left 0JNK-
    Right 0JNJ-
  Lower Arm
    Left 0JNH-
    Right 0JNG-
  Lower Leg
    Left 0JNP-
    Right 0JNN-
  Neck
    Anterior 0JN4-
    Posterior 0JN5-
  Pelvic Region 0JNC-
  Perineum 0JNB-
  Scalp 0JN0-
  Upper Arm
    Left 0JNF-
    Right 0JND-
  Upper Leg
    Left 0JNM-
    Right 0JNL-
Tarsal
  Left 0QNM-
  Right 0QNL-
Tendon
  Abdomen
    Left 0LNG-
    Right 0LNF-
  Ankle
    Left 0LNT-
    Right 0LNS-
  Foot
    Left 0LNW-
    Right 0LNV-
  Hand
    Left 0LN8-
    Right 0LN7-
  Head and Neck 0LN0-
  Hip
    Left 0LNK-
    Right 0LNJ-
  Knee
    Left 0LNR-
    Right 0LNQ-
  Lower Arm and Wrist
    Left 0LN6-
    Right 0LN5-
  Lower Leg
    Left 0LNP-
    Right 0LNN-
  Perineum 0LNH-
  Shoulder
    Left 0LN2-
    Right 0LN1-
  Thorax
    Left 0LND-
    Right 0LNC-
  Trunk
    Left 0LNB-
    Right 0LN9-
  Upper Arm
    Left 0LN4-
    Right 0LN3-
  Upper Leg
    Left 0LNM-
    Right 0LNL-
Testis
  Bilateral 0VNC-
  Left 0VNB-
  Right 0VN9-

Release — continued
Thalamus 00N9-
Thymus 07NM-
Thyroid Gland 0GNK-
  Left Lobe 0GNG-
  Right Lobe 0GNH-
Tibia
  Left 0QNH-
  Right 0QNG-
Toe Nail 0HNRXZZ
Tongue 0CN7-
Tonsils 0CNP-
Tooth
  Lower 0CNX-
  Upper 0CNW-
Trachea 0BN1-
Tunica Vaginalis
  Left 0VN7-
  Right 0VN6-
Turbinate, Nasal 09NL-
Tympanic Membrane
  Left 09N8-
  Right 09N7-
Ulna
  Left 0PNL-
  Right 0PNK-
Ureter
  Left 0TN7-
  Right 0TN6-
Urethra 0TND-
Uterine Supporting Structure 0UN4-
Uterus 0UN9-
Uvula 0CNN-
Vagina 0UNG-
Valve
  Aortic 02NF-
  Mitral 02NG-
  Pulmonary 02NH-
  Tricuspid 02NJ-
Vas Deferens
  Bilateral 0VNQ-
  Left 0VNP-
  Right 0VNN-
Vein
  Axillary
    Left 05N8-
    Right 05N7-
  Azygos 05N0-
  Basilic
    Left 05NC-
    Right 05NB-
  Brachial
    Left 05NA-
    Right 05N9-
  Cephalic
    Left 05NF-
    Right 05ND-
  Colic 06N7-
  Common Iliac
    Left 06ND-
    Right 06NC-
  Coronary 02N4-
  Esophageal 06N3-
  External Iliac
    Left 06NG-
    Right 06NF-
  External Jugular
    Left 05NQ-
    Right 05NP-
  Face
    Left 05NV-
    Right 05NT-
  Femoral
    Left 06NN-
    Right 06NM-
  Foot
    Left 06NV-
    Right 06NT-
  Gastric 06N2-

Release — continued
Vein — continued
  Greater Saphenous
    Left 06NQ-
    Right 06NP-
  Hand
    Left 05NH-
    Right 05NG-
  Hemiazygos 05N1-
  Hepatic 06N4-
  Hypogastric
    Left 06NJ-
    Right 06NH-
  Inferior Mesenteric 06N6-
  Innominate
    Left 05N4-
    Right 05N3-
  Internal Jugular
    Left 05NN-
    Right 05NM-
  Intracranial 05NL-
  Lesser Saphenous
    Left 06NS-
    Right 06NR-
  Lower 06NY-
  Portal 06N8-
  Pulmonary
    Left 02NT-
    Right 02NS-
  Renal
    Left 06NB-
    Right 06N9-
  Splenic 06N1-
  Subclavian
    Left 05N6-
    Right 05N5-
  Superior Mesenteric 06N5-
  Upper 05NY-
  Vertebral
    Left 05NS-
    Right 05NR-
Vena Cava
  Inferior 06N0-
  Superior 02NV-
Ventricle
  Left 02NL-
  Right 02NK-
Vertebra
  Cervical 0PN3-
  Lumbar 0QN0-
  Thoracic 0PN4-
Vesicle
  Bilateral 0VN3-
  Left 0VN2-
  Right 0VN1-
Vitreous
  Left 08N53ZZ
  Right 08N43ZZ
Vocal Cord
  Left 0CNV-
  Right 0CNT-
Vulva 0UNM-
Relocation see Reposition
Removal
  Abdominal Wall 2W53X-
  Anorectal 2Y53X5Z
  Arm
    Lower
      Left 2W5DX-
      Right 2W5CX-
    Upper
      Left 2W5BX-
      Right 2W5AX-
  Back 2W55X-
  Chest Wall 2W54X-
  Ear 2Y52X5Z

INDEX TO PROCEDURES – 2016 ICD-10-PCS

Removal — continued
Extremity
　Lower
　　Left 2W5MX-
　　Right 2W5LX-
　Upper
　　Left 2W59X-
　　Right 2W58X-
Face 2W51X-
Finger
　Left 2W5KX-
　Right 2W5JX-
Foot
　Left 2W5TX-
　Right 2W5SX-
Genital Tract, Female 2Y54X5Z
Hand
　Left 2W5FX-
　Right 2W5EX-
Head 2W50X-
Inguinal Region
　Left 2W57X-
　Right 2W56X-
Leg
　Lower
　　Left 2W5RX-
　　Right 2W5QX-
　Upper
　　Left 2W5PX-
　　Right 2W5NX-
Mouth and Pharynx 2Y50X5Z
Nasal 2Y51X5Z
Neck 2W52X-
Thumb
　Left 2W5HX-
　Right 2W5GX-
Toe
　Left 2W5VX-
　Right 2W5UX-
Urethra 2Y55X5Z

Removal of device from
Abdominal Wall 0WPF-
Acetabulum
　Left 0QP5-
　Right 0QP4-
Anal Sphincter 0DPR-
Anus 0DPQ-
Artery
　Lower 04PY-
　Upper 03PY-
Back
　Lower 0WPL-
　Upper 0WPK-
Bladder 0TPB-
Bone
　Facial 0NPW-
　Lower 0QPY-
　Nasal 0NPB-
　Pelvic
　　Left 0QP3-
　　Right 0QP2-
　Upper 0PPY-
Bone Marrow 07PT-
Brain 00P0-
Breast
　Left 0HPU-
　Right 0HPT-
Bursa and Ligament
　Lower 0MPY-
　Upper 0MPX-
Carpal
　Left 0PPN-
　Right 0PPM-
Cavity, Cranial 0WP1-
Cerebral Ventricle 00P6-
Chest Wall 0WP8-
Cisterna Chyli 07PL-
Clavicle
　Left 0PPB-
　Right 0PP9-
Coccyx 0QPS-

Removal of device from — continued
Diaphragm 0BPT-
Disc
　Cervical Vertebral 0RP3-
　Cervicothoracic Vertebral 0RP5-
　Lumbar Vertebral 0SP2-
　Lumbosacral 0SP4-
　Thoracic Vertebral 0RP9-
　Thoracolumbar Vertebral 0RPB-
Duct
　Hepatobiliary 0FPB-
　Pancreatic 0FPD-
Ear
　Inner
　　Left 09PE-
　　Right 09PD-
　Left 09PJ-
　Right 09PH-
Epididymis and Spermatic Cord 0VPM-
Esophagus 0DP5-
Extremity
　Lower
　　Left 0YPB-
　　Right 0YP9-
　Upper
　　Left 0XP7-
　　Right 0XP6-
Eye
　Left 08P1-
　Right 08P0-
Face 0WP2-
Fallopian Tube 0UP8-
Femoral Shaft
　Left 0QP9-
　Right 0QP8-
Femur
　Lower
　　Left 0QPC-
　　Right 0QPB-
　Upper
　　Left 0QP7-
　　Right 0QP6-
Fibula
　Left 0QPK-
　Right 0QPJ-
Finger Nail 0HPQX-
Gallbladder 0FP4-
Gastrointestinal Tract 0WPP-
Genitourinary Tract 0WPR-
Gland
　Adrenal 0GP5-
　Endocrine 0GPS-
　Pituitary 0GP0-
　Salivary 0CPA-
Glenoid Cavity
　Left 0PP8-
　Right 0PP7-
Great Vessel 02PY-
Hair 0HPSX-
Head 0WP0-
Heart 02PA-
Humeral Head
　Left 0PPD-
　Right 0PPC-
Humeral Shaft
　Left 0PPG-
　Right 0PPF-
Intestinal Tract
　Lower 0DPD-
　Upper 0DP0-
Jaw
　Lower 0WP5-
　Upper 0WP4-

Removal of device from — continued
Joint
　Acromioclavicular
　　Left 0RPH-
　　Right 0RPG-
　Ankle
　　Left 0SPG-
　　Right 0SPF-
　Carpal
　　Left 0RPR-
　　Right 0RPQ-
　Cervical Vertebral 0RP1-
　Cervicothoracic Vertebral 0RP4-
　Coccygeal 0SP6-
　Elbow
　　Left 0RPM-
　　Right 0RPL-
　Finger Phalangeal
　　Left 0RPX-
　　Right 0RPW-
　Hip
　　Left 0SPB-
　　Right 0SP9-
　Knee
　　Left 0SPD-
　　Right 0SPC-
　Lumbar Vertebral 0SP0-
　Lumbosacral 0SP3-
　Metacarpocarpal
　　Left 0RPT-
　　Right 0RPS-
　Metacarpophalangeal
　　Left 0RPV-
　　Right 0RPU-
　Metatarsal-Phalangeal
　　Left 0SPN-
　　Right 0SPM-
　Metatarsal-Tarsal
　　Left 0SPL-
　　Right 0SPK-
　Occipital-cervical 0RP0-
　Sacrococcygeal 0SP5-
　Sacroiliac
　　Left 0SP8-
　　Right 0SP7-
　Shoulder
　　Left 0RPK-
　　Right 0RPJ-
　Sternoclavicular
　　Left 0RPF-
　　Right 0RPE-
　Tarsal
　　Left 0SPJ-
　　Right 0SPH-
　Temporomandibular
　　Left 0RPD-
　　Right 0RPC-
　Thoracic Vertebral 0RP6-
　Thoracolumbar Vertebral 0RPA-
　Toe Phalangeal
　　Left 0SPQ-
　　Right 0SPP-
　Wrist
　　Left 0RPP-
　　Right 0RPN-
Kidney 0TP5-
Larynx 0CPS-
Lens
　Left 08PK3JZ
　Right 08PJ3JZ
Liver 0FP0-
Lung
　Left 0BPL-
　Right 0BPK-
Lymphatic 07PN-
　Thoracic Duct 07PK-
Mediastinum 0WPC-
Mesentery 0DPV-

Removal of device from — continued
Metacarpal
　Left 0PPQ-
　Right 0PPP-
Metatarsal
　Left 0QPP-
　Right 0QPN-
Mouth and Throat 0CPY-
Muscle
　Extraocular
　　Left 08PM-
　　Right 08PL-
　Lower 0KPY-
　Upper 0KPX-
Neck 0WP6-
Nerve
　Cranial 00PE-
　Peripheral 01PY-
Nose 09PK-
Omentum 0DPU-
Ovary 0UP3-
Pancreas 0FPG-
Parathyroid Gland 0GPR-
Patella
　Left 0QPF-
　Right 0QPD-
Pelvic Cavity 0WPJ-
Penis 0VPS-
Pericardial Cavity 0WPD-
Perineum
　Female 0WPN-
　Male 0WPM-
Peritoneal Cavity 0WPG-
Peritoneum 0DPW-
Phalanx
　Finger
　　Left 0PPV-
　　Right 0PPT-
　Thumb
　　Left 0PPS-
　　Right 0PPR-
　Toe
　　Left 0QPR-
　　Right 0QPQ-
Pineal Body 0GP1-
Pleura 0BPQ-
Pleural Cavity
　Left 0WPB-
　Right 0WP9-
Products of Conception 10P0-
Prostate and Seminal Vesicles 0VP4-
Radius
　Left 0PPJ-
　Right 0PPH-
Rectum 0DPP-
Respiratory Tract 0WPQ-
Retroperitoneum 0WPH-
Rib
　Left 0PP2-
　Right 0PP1-
Sacrum 0QP1-
Scapula
　Left 0PP6-
　Right 0PP5-
Scrotum and Tunica Vaginalis 0VP8-
Sinus 09PY-
Skin 0HPPX-
Skull 0NP0-
Spinal Canal 00PU-
Spinal Cord 00PV-
Spleen 07PP-
Sternum 0PP0-
Stomach 0DP6-
Subcutaneous Tissue and Fascia
　Head and Neck 0JPS-
　Lower Extremity 0JPW-
　Trunk 0JPT-
　Upper Extremity 0JPV-

57

Removal of — INDEX TO PROCEDURES – 2016 ICD-10-PCS

Removal of device from — *continued*
  Tarsal
    Left 0QPM-
    Right 0QPL-
  Tendon
    Lower 0LPY-
    Upper 0LPX-
  Testis 0VPD-
  Thymus 07PM-
  Thyroid Gland 0GPK-
  Tibia
    Left 0QPH-
    Right 0QPG-
  Toe Nail 0HPRX-
  Trachea 0BP1-
  Tracheobronchial Tree 0BP0-
  Tympanic Membrane
    Left 09P8-
    Right 09P7-
  Ulna
    Left 0PPL-
    Right 0PPK-
  Ureter 0TP9-
  Urethra 0TPD-
  Uterus and Cervix 0UPD-
  Vagina and Cul-de-sac 0UPH-
  Vas Deferens 0VPR-
  Vein
    Lower 06PY-
    Upper 05PY-
  Vertebra
    Cervical 0PP3-
    Lumbar 0QP0-
    Thoracic 0PP4-
  Vulva 0UPM-

Renal calyx
  use Kidney
  use Kidneys, Bilateral
  use Kidney, Left
  use Kidney, Right

Renal capsule
  use Kidney
  use Kidneys, Bilateral
  use Kidney, Left
  use Kidney, Right

Renal cortex
  use Kidney
  use Kidneys, Bilateral
  use Kidney, Left
  use Kidney, Right

Renal dialysis *see* Performance, Urinary 5A1D-

Renal plexus
  use Nerve, Abdominal Sympathetic

Renal segment
  use Kidney
  use Kidney, Left
  use Kidney, Right
  use Kidneys, Bilateral

Renal segmental artery
  use Artery, Renal, Left
  use Artery, Renal, Right

Reopening, operative site
  Control of bleeding *see* Control postprocedural bleeding in
  Inspection only *see* Inspection

Repair
  Abdominal Wall 0WQF-
  Acetabulum
    Left 0QQ5-
    Right 0QQ4-
  Adenoids 0CQQ-
  Ampulla of Vater 0FQC-
  Anal Sphincter 0DQR-
  Ankle Region
    Left 0YQL-
    Right 0YQK-

Repair — *continued*
  Anterior Chamber
    Left 08Q33ZZ
    Right 08Q23ZZ
  Anus 0DQQ-
  Aorta
    Abdominal 04Q0-
    Thoracic 02QW-
  Aortic Body 0GQD-
  Appendix 0DQJ-
  Arm
    Lower
      Left 0XQF-
      Right 0XQD-
    Upper
      Left 0XQ9-
      Right 0XQ8-
  Artery
    Anterior Tibial
      Left 04QQ-
      Right 04QP-
    Axillary
      Left 03Q6-
      Right 03Q5-
    Brachial
      Left 03Q8-
      Right 03Q7-
    Celiac 04Q1-
    Colic
      Left 04Q7-
      Middle 04Q8-
      Right 04Q6-
    Common Carotid
      Left 03QJ-
      Right 03QH-
    Common Iliac
      Left 04QD-
      Right 04QC-
    Coronary
      One Site 02Q0-
      Two Sites 02Q1-
      Three Sites 02Q2-
      Four or More Sites 02Q3-
    External Carotid
      Left 03QN-
      Right 03QM-
    External Iliac
      Left 04QJ-
      Right 04QH-
    Face 03QR-
    Femoral
      Left 04QL-
      Right 04QK-
    Foot
      Left 04QW-
      Right 04QV-
    Gastric 04Q2-
    Hand
      Left 03QF-
      Right 03QD-
    Hepatic 04Q3-
    Inferior Mesenteric 04QB-
    Innominate 03Q2-
    Internal Carotid
      Left 03QL-
      Right 03QK-
    Internal Iliac
      Left 04QF-
      Right 04QE-
    Internal Mammary
      Left 03Q1-
      Right 03Q0-
    Intracranial 03QG-
    Lower 04QY-
    Peroneal
      Left 04QU-
      Right 04QT-
    Popliteal
      Left 04QN-
      Right 04QM-

Repair — *continued*
  Artery — *continued*
    Posterior Tibial
      Left 04QS-
      Right 04QR-
    Pulmonary
      Left 02QR-
      Right 02QQ-
    Pulmonary Trunk 02QP-
    Radial
      Left 03QC-
      Right 03QB-
    Renal
      Left 04QA-
      Right 04Q9-
    Splenic 04Q4-
    Subclavian
      Left 03Q4-
      Right 03Q3-
    Superior Mesenteric 04Q5-
    Temporal
      Left 03QT-
      Right 03QS-
    Thyroid
      Left 03QV-
      Right 03QU-
    Ulnar
      Left 03QA-
      Right 03Q9-
    Upper 03QY-
    Vertebral
      Left 03QQ-
      Right 03QP-
  Atrium
    Left 02Q7-
    Right 02Q6-
  Auditory Ossicle
    Left 09QA0ZZ
    Right 09Q90ZZ
  Axilla
    Left 0XQ5-
    Right 0XQ4-
  Back
    Lower 0WQL-
    Upper 0WQK-
  Basal Ganglia 00Q8-
  Bladder 0TQB-
  Bladder Neck 0TQC-
  Bone
    Ethmoid
      Left 0NQG-
      Right 0NQF-
    Frontal
      Left 0NQ2-
      Right 0NQ1-
    Hyoid 0NQX-
    Lacrimal
      Left 0NQJ-
      Right 0NQH-
    Nasal 0NQB-
    Occipital
      Left 0NQ8-
      Right 0NQ7-
    Palatine
      Left 0NQL-
      Right 0NQK-
    Parietal
      Left 0NQ4-
      Right 0NQ3-
    Pelvic
      Left 0QQ3-
      Right 0QQ2-
    Sphenoid
      Left 0NQD-
      Right 0NQC-
    Temporal
      Left 0NQ6-
      Right 0NQ5-
    Zygomatic
      Left 0NQN-
      Right 0NQM-

Repair — *continued*
  Brain 00Q0-
  Breast
    Bilateral 0HQV-
    Left 0HQU-
    Right 0HQT-
    Supernumerary 0HQY-
  Bronchus
    Lingula 0BQ9-
    Lower Lobe
      Left 0BQB-
      Right 0BQ6-
    Main
      Left 0BQ7-
      Right 0BQ3-
    Middle Lobe, Right 0BQ5-
    Upper Lobe
      Left 0BQ8-
      Right 0BQ4-
  Buccal Mucosa 0CQ4-
  Bursa and Ligament
    Abdomen
      Left 0MQJ-
      Right 0MQH-
    Ankle
      Left 0MQR-
      Right 0MQQ-
    Elbow
      Left 0MQ4-
      Right 0MQ3-
    Foot
      Left 0MQT-
      Right 0MQS-
    Hand
      Left 0MQ8-
      Right 0MQ7-
    Head and Neck 0MQ0-
    Hip
      Left 0MQM-
      Right 0MQL-
    Knee
      Left 0MQP-
      Right 0MQN-
    Lower Extremity
      Left 0MQW-
      Right 0MQV-
    Perineum 0MQK-
    Shoulder
      Left 0MQ2-
      Right 0MQ1-
    Thorax
      Left 0MQG-
      Right 0MQF-
    Trunk
      Left 0MQD-
      Right 0MQC-
    Upper Extremity
      Left 0MQB-
      Right 0MQ9-
    Wrist
      Left 0MQ6-
      Right 0MQ5-
  Buttock
    Left 0YQ1-
    Right 0YQ0-
  Carina 0BQ2
  Carotid Bodies, Bilateral 0GQ8-
  Carotid Body
    Left 0GQ6-
    Right 0GQ7-
  Carpal
    Left 0PQN-
    Right 0PQM-
  Cecum 0DQH-
  Cerebellum 00QC-
  Cerebral Hemisphere 00Q7-
  Cerebral Meninges 00Q1-
  Cerebral Ventricle 00Q6-
  Cervix 0UQC-
  Chest Wall 0WQ8-
  Chordae Tendineae 02Q9-

Repair — *continued*
  Choroid
    Left 08QB-
    Right 08QA-
  Cisterna Chyli 07QL-
  Clavicle
    Left 0PQB-
    Right 0PQ9-
  Clitoris 0UQJ-
  Coccygeal Glomus 0GQB-
  Coccyx 0QQS-
  Colon
    Ascending 0DQK-
    Descending 0DQM-
    Sigmoid 0DQN-
    Transverse 0DQL-
  Conduction Mechanism 02Q8-
  Conjunctiva
    Left 08QTXZZ
    Right 08QSXZZ
  Cord
    Bilateral 0VQH-
    Left 0VQG-
    Right 0VQF-
  Cornea
    Left 08Q9XZZ
    Right 08Q8XZZ
  Cul-de-sac 0UQF-
  Diaphragm
    Left 0BQS-
    Right 0BQR-
  Disc
    Cervical Vertebral 0RQ3-
    Cervicothoracic Vertebral 0RQ5-
    Lumbar Vertebral 0SQ2-
    Lumbosacral 0SQ4-
    Thoracic Vertebral 0RQ9-
    Thoracolumbar Vertebral 0RQB-
  Duct
    Common Bile 0FQ9-
    Cystic 0FQ8-
    Hepatic
      Left 0FQ6-
      Right 0FQ5-
    Lacrimal
      Left 08QY-
      Right 08QX-
    Pancreatic 0FQD-
      Accessory 0FQF-
    Parotid
      Left 0CQC-
      Right 0CQB-
  Duodenum 0DQ9-
  Dura Mater 00Q2-
  Ear
    External
      Bilateral 09Q2-
      Left 09Q1-
      Right 09Q0-
    External Auditory Canal
      Left 09Q4-
      Right 09Q3-
    Inner
      Left 09QE0ZZ
      Right 09QD0ZZ
    Middle
      Left 09Q60ZZ
      Right 09Q50ZZ
  Elbow Region
    Left 0XQC-
    Right 0XQB-
  Epididymis
    Bilateral 0VQL-
    Left 0VQK-
    Right 0VQJ-
  Epiglottis 0CQR-
  Esophagogastric Junction 0DQ4-
  Esophagus 0DQ5-
    Lower 0DQ3-
    Middle 0DQ2-
    Upper 0DQ1-

Repair — *continued*
  Eustachian Tube
    Left 09QG-
    Right 09QF-
  Extremity
    Lower
      Left 0YQB-
      Right 0YQ9-
    Upper
      Left 0XQ7-
      Right 0XQ6-
  Eye
    Left 08Q1XZZ
    Right 08Q0XZZ
  Eyelid
    Lower
      Left 08QR-
      Right 08QQ-
    Upper
      Left 08QP-
      Right 08QN-
  Face 0WQ2-
  Fallopian Tube
    Left 0UQ6-
    Right 0UQ5-
  Fallopian Tubes, Bilateral 0UQ7-
  Femoral Region
    Bilateral 0YQE-
    Left 0YQ8-
    Right 0YQ7-
  Femoral Shaft
    Left 0QQ9-
    Right 0QQ8-
  Femur
    Lower
      Left 0QQC-
      Right 0QQB-
    Upper
      Left 0QQ7-
      Right 0QQ6-
  Fibula
    Left 0QQK-
    Right 0QQJ-
  Finger
    Index
      Left 0XQP-
      Right 0XQN-
    Little
      Left 0XQW-
      Right 0XQV-
    Middle
      Left 0XQR-
      Right 0XQQ-
    Ring
      Left 0XQT-
      Right 0XQS-
  Finger Nail 0HQQXZZ
  Foot
    Left 0YQN-
    Right 0YQM-
  Gallbladder 0FQ4-
  Gingiva
    Lower 0CQ6-
    Upper 0CQ5-
  Gland
    Adrenal
      Bilateral 0GQ4-
      Left 0GQ2-
      Right 0GQ3-
    Lacrimal
      Left 08QW-
      Right 08QV-
    Minor Salivary 0CQJ-
    Parotid
      Left 0CQ9-
      Right 0CQ8-
    Pituitary 0GQ0-
    Sublingual
      Left 0CQF-
      Right 0CQD-

Repair — *continued*
  Gland — *continued*
    Submaxillary
      Left 0CQH-
      Right 0CQG-
    Vestibular 0UQL-
  Glenoid Cavity
    Left 0PQ8-
    Right 0PQ7-
  Glomus Jugulare 0GQC-
  Hand
    Left 0XQK-
    Right 0XQJ-
  Head 0WQ0-
  Heart 02QA-
    Left 02QC-
    Right 02QB-
  Humeral Head
    Left 0PQD-
    Right 0PQC-
  Humeral Shaft
    Left 0PQG-
    Right 0PQF-
  Hymen 0UQK-
  Hypothalamus 00QA-
  Ileocecal Valve 0DQC-
  Ileum 0DQB-
  Inguinal Region
    Bilateral 0YQA-
    Left 0YQ6-
    Right 0YQ5-
  Intestine
    Large 0DQE-
      Left 0DQG-
      Right 0DQF-
    Small 0DQ8-
  Iris
    Left 08QD3ZZ
    Right 08QC3ZZ
  Jaw
    Lower 0WQ5-
    Upper 0WQ4-
  Jejunum 0DQA-
  Joint
    Acromioclavicular
      Left 0RQH-
      Right 0RQG-
    Ankle
      Left 0SQG-
      Right 0SQF-
    Carpal
      Left 0RQR-
      Right 0RQQ-
    Cervical Vertebral 0RQ1-
    Cervicothoracic Vertebral 0RQ4-
    Coccygeal 0SQ6-
    Elbow
      Left 0RQM-
      Right 0RQL-
    Finger Phalangeal
      Left 0RQX-
      Right 0RQW-
    Hip
      Left 0SQB-
      Right 0SQ9-
    Knee
      Left 0SQD-
      Right 0SQC-
    Lumbar Vertebral 0SQ0-
    Lumbosacral 0SQ3-
    Metacarpocarpal
      Left 0RQT-
      Right 0RQS-
    Metacarpophalangeal
      Left 0RQV-
      Right 0RQU-
    Metatarsal-Phalangeal
      Left 0SQN-
      Right 0SQM-

Repair — *continued*
  Joint — *continued*
    Metatarsal-Tarsal
      Left 0SQL-
      Right 0SQK-
    Occipital-cervical 0RQ0-
    Sacrococcygeal 0SQ5-
    Sacroiliac
      Left 0SQ8-
      Right 0SQ7-
    Shoulder
      Left 0RQK-
      Right 0RQJ-
    Sternoclavicular
      Left 0RQF-
      Right 0RQE-
    Tarsal
      Left 0SQJ-
      Right 0SQH-
    Temporomandibular
      Left 0RQD-
      Right 0RQC-
    Thoracic Vertebral 0RQ6-
    Thoracolumbar Vertebral 0RQA-
    Toe Phalangeal
      Left 0SQQ-
      Right 0SQP
    Wrist
      Left 0RQP-
      Right 0RQN-
  Kidney
    Left 0TQ1-
    Right 0TQ0-
  Kidney Pelvis
    Left 0TQ4-
    Right 0TQ3-
  Knee Region
    Left 0YQG-
    Right 0YQF-
  Larynx 0CQS-
  Leg
    Lower
      Left 0YQJ-
      Right 0YQH-
    Upper
      Left 0YQD-
      Right 0YQC-
  Lens
    Left 08QK3ZZ
    Right 08QJ3ZZ
  Lip
    Lower 0CQ1-
    Upper 0CQ0-
  Liver 0FQ0-
    Left Lobe 0FQ2-
    Right Lobe 0FQ1-
  Lung
    Bilateral 0BQM-
    Left 0BQL-
    Lower Lobe
      Left 0BQJ-
      Right 0BQF-
    Middle Lobe, Right 0BQD-
    Right 0BQK-
    Upper Lobe
      Left 0BQG-
      Right 0BQC-
  Lung Lingula 0BQH-
  Lymphatic
    Aortic 07QD-
    Axillary
      Left 07Q6-
      Right 07Q5-
    Head 07Q0-
    Inguinal
      Left 07QJ-
      Right 07QH-
    Internal Mammary
      Left 07Q9-
      Right 07Q8-

Repair — continued
 Lymphatic — continued
  Lower Extremity
   Left 07QG-
   Right 07QF-
  Mesenteric 07QB-
  Neck
   Left 07Q2-
   Right 07Q1-
  Pelvis 07QC-
  Thoracic Duct 07QK-
  Thorax 07Q7-
  Upper Extremity
   Left 07Q4-
   Right 07Q3-
 Mandible
  Left 0NQV-
  Right 0NQT-
 Maxilla
  Left 0NQS-
  Right 0NQR-
 Mediastinum 0WQC-
 Medulla Oblongata 00QD-
 Mesentery 0DQV-
 Metacarpal
  Left 0PQQ-
  Right 0PQP-
 Metatarsal
  Left 0QQP-
  Right 0QQN-
 Muscle
  Abdomen
   Left 0KQL-
   Right 0KQK-
  Extraocular
   Left 08QM-
   Right 08QL-
  Facial 0KQ1-
  Foot
   Left 0KQW-
   Right 0KQV-
  Hand
   Left 0KQD-
   Right 0KQC-
  Head 0KQ0-
  Hip
   Left 0KQP-
   Right 0KQN-
  Lower Arm and Wrist
   Left 0KQB-
   Right 0KQ9-
  Lower Leg
   Left 0KQT-
   Right 0KQS-
  Neck
   Left 0KQ3-
   Right 0KQ2-
  Papillary 02QD-
  Perineum 0KQM-
  Shoulder
   Left 0KQ6-
   Right 0KQ5-
  Thorax
   Left 0KQJ-
   Right 0KQH-
  Tongue, Palate, Pharynx 0KQ4-
  Trunk
   Left 0KQG-
   Right 0KQF-
  Upper Arm
   Left 0KQ8-
   Right 0KQ7-
  Upper Leg
   Left 0KQR-
   Right 0KQQ-
 Nasopharynx 09QN-
 Neck 0WQ6-

Repair — continued
 Nerve
  Abdominal Sympathetic 01QM-
  Abducens 00QL-
  Accessory 00QR-
  Acoustic 00QN-
  Brachial Plexus 01Q3-
  Cervical 01Q1-
  Cervical Plexus 01Q0-
  Facial 00QM-
  Femoral 01QD-
  Glossopharyngeal 00QP-
  Head and Neck Sympathetic 01QK-
  Hypoglossal 00QS-
  Lumbar 01QB-
  Lumbar Plexus 01Q9-
  Lumbar Sympathetic 01QN-
  Lumbosacral Plexus 01QA-
  Median 01Q5-
  Oculomotor 00QH-
  Olfactory 00QF-
  Optic 00QG-
  Peroneal 01QH-
  Phrenic 01Q2-
  Pudendal 01QC-
  Radial 01Q6-
  Sacral 01QR-
  Sacral Plexus 01QQ-
  Sacral Sympathetic 01QP-
  Sciatic 01QF-
  Thoracic 01Q8-
  Thoracic Sympathetic 01QL-
  Tibial 01QG-
  Trigeminal 00QK-
  Trochlear 00QJ-
  Ulnar 01Q4-
  Vagus 00QQ-
 Nipple
  Left 0HQX-
  Right 0HQW-
 Nose 09QK-
 Omentum
  Greater 0DQS-
  Lesser 0DQT-
 Orbit
  Left 0NQQ-
  Right 0NQP-
 Ovary
  Bilateral 0UQ2-
  Left 0UQ1-
  Right 0UQ0-
 Palate
  Hard 0CQ2-
  Soft 0CQ3-
 Pancreas 0FQG-
 Para-aortic Body 0GQ9-
 Paraganglion Extremity 0GQF-
 Parathyroid Gland 0GQR-
  Inferior
   Left 0GQP-
   Right 0GQN-
  Multiple 0GQQ-
  Superior
   Left 0GQM-
   Right 0GQL-
 Patella
  Left 0QQF-
  Right 0QQD-
 Penis 0VQS-
 Pericardium 02QN-
 Perineum
  Female 0WQN-
  Male 0WQM-
 Peritoneum 0DQW-

Repair — continued
 Phalanx
  Finger
   Left 0PQV-
   Right 0PQT-
  Thumb
   Left 0PQS-
   Right 0PQR-
  Toe
   Left 0QQR-
   Right 0QQQ-
 Pharynx 0CQM-
 Pineal Body 0GQ1-
 Pleura
  Left 0BQP-
  Right 0BQN-
 Pons 00QB-
 Prepuce 0VQT-
 Products of Conception 10Q0-
 Prostate 0VQ0-
 Radius
  Left 0PQJ-
  Right 0PQH-
 Rectum 0DQP-
 Retina
  Left 08QF3ZZ
  Right 08QE3ZZ
 Retinal Vessel
  Left 08QH3ZZ
  Right 08QG3ZZ
 Rib
  Left 0PQ2-
  Right 0PQ1-
 Sacrum 0QQ1-
 Scapula
  Left 0PQ6-
  Right 0PQ5-
 Sclera
  Left 08Q7XZZ
  Right 08Q6XZZ
 Scrotum 0VQ5-
 Septum
  Atrial 02Q5-
  Nasal 09QM-
  Ventricular 02QM-
 Shoulder Region
  Left 0XQ3-
  Right 0XQ2-
 Sinus
  Accessory 09QP-
  Ethmoid
   Left 09QV-
   Right 09QU-
  Frontal
   Left 09QT-
   Right 09QS-
  Mastoid
   Left 09QC-
   Right 09QB-
  Maxillary
   Left 09QR-
   Right 09QQ-
  Sphenoid
   Left 09QX-
   Right 09QW-
 Skin
  Abdomen 0HQ7XZZ
  Back 0HQ6XZZ
  Buttock 0HQ8XZZ
  Chest 0HQ5XZZ
  Ear
   Left 0HQ3XZZ
   Right 0HQ2XZZ
  Face 0HQ1XZZ
  Foot
   Left 0HQNXZZ
   Right 0HQMXZZ
  Genitalia 0HQAXZZ
  Hand
   Left 0HQGXZZ
   Right 0HQFXZZ

Repair — continued
 Skin — continued
  Lower Arm
   Left 0HQEXZZ
   Right 0HQDXZZ
  Lower Leg
   Left 0HQLXZZ
   Right 0HQKXZZ
  Neck 0HQ4XZZ
  Perineum 0HQ9XZZ
  Scalp 0HQ0XZZ
  Upper Arm
   Left 0HQCXZZ
   Right 0HQBXZZ
  Upper Leg
   Left 0HQJXZZ
   Right 0HQHXZZ
 Skull 0NQ0-
 Spinal Cord
  Cervical 00QW-
  Lumbar 00QY-
  Thoracic 00QX-
 Spinal Meninges 00QT-
 Spleen 07QP-
 Sternum 0PQ0-
 Stomach 0DQ6-
  Pylorus 0DQ7-
 Subcutaneous Tissue and Fascia
  Abdomen 0JQ8-
  Back 0JQ7-
  Buttock 0JQ9-
  Chest 0JQ6-
  Face 0JQ1-
  Foot
   Left 0JQR-
   Right 0JQQ-
  Hand
   Left 0JQK-
   Right 0JQJ-
  Lower Arm
   Left 0JQH-
   Right 0JQG-
  Lower Leg
   Left 0JQP-
   Right 0JQN-
  Neck
   Anterior 0JQ4-
   Posterior 0JQ5-
  Pelvic Region 0JQC-
  Perineum 0JQB-
  Scalp 0JQ0-
  Upper Arm
   Left 0JQF-
   Right 0JQD-
  Upper Leg
   Left 0JQM-
   Right 0JQL-
 Tarsal
  Left 0QQM-
  Right 0QQL-
 Tendon
  Abdomen
   Left 0LQG-
   Right 0LQF-
  Ankle
   Left 0LQT-
   Right 0LQS-
  Foot
   Left 0LQW-
   Right 0LQV-
  Hand
   Left 0LQ8-
   Right 0LQ7-
  Head and Neck 0LQ0-
  Hip
   Left 0LQK-
   Right 0LQJ-
  Knee
   Left 0LQR-
   Right 0LQQ-

INDEX TO PROCEDURES – 2016 ICD-10-PCS

Repair — *continued*
Tendon — *continued*
  Lower Arm and Wrist
    Left 0LQ6-
    Right 0LQ5-
  Lower Leg
    Left 0LQP-
    Right 0LQN-
  Perineum 0LQH-
  Shoulder
    Left 0LQ2-
    Right 0LQ1-
  Thorax
    Left 0LQD-
    Right 0LQC-
  Trunk
    Left 0LQB-
    Right 0LQ9-
  Upper Arm
    Left 0LQ4-
    Right 0LQ3-
  Upper Leg
    Left 0LQM-
    Right 0LQL-
Testis
  Bilateral 0VQC-
  Left 0VQB-
  Right 0VQ9-
Thalamus 00Q9-
Thumb
  Left 0XQM-
  Right 0XQL-
Thymus 07QM-
Thyroid Gland 0GQK-
  Left Lobe 0GQG-
  Right Lobe 0GQH-
Thyroid Gland Isthmus 0GQJ-
Tibia
  Left 0QQH-
  Right 0QQG-
Toe
  1st
    Left 0YQQ-
    Right 0YQP-
  2nd
    Left 0YQS-
    Right 0YQR-
  3rd
    Left 0YQU-
    Right 0YQT-
  4th
    Left 0YQW-
    Right 0YQV-
  5th
    Left 0YQY-
    Right 0YQX-
Toe Nail 0HQRXZZ
Tongue 0CQ7-
Tonsils 0CQP-
Tooth
  Lower 0CQX-
  Upper 0CQW-
Trachea 0BQ1-
Tunica Vaginalis
  Left 0VQ7-
  Right 0VQ6-
Turbinate, Nasal 09QL-
Tympanic Membrane
  Left 09Q8-
  Right 09Q7-
Ulna
  Left 0PQL-
  Right 0PQK-
Ureter
  Left 0TQ7-
  Right 0TQ6-
Urethra 0TQD-
Uterine Supporting Structure 0UQ4-
Uterus 0UQ9-
Uvula 0CQN-
Vagina 0UQG-

Repair — *continued*
Valve
  Aortic 02QF-
  Mitral 02QG-
  Pulmonary 02QH-
  Tricuspid 02QJ-
Vas Deferens
  Bilateral 0VQQ-
  Left 0VQP-
  Right 0VQN-
Vein
  Axillary
    Left 05Q8-
    Right 05Q7-
  Azygos 05Q0-
  Basilic
    Left 05QC-
    Right 05QB-
  Brachial
    Left 05QA-
    Right 05Q9-
  Cephalic
    Left 05QF-
    Right 05QD-
  Colic 06Q7-
  Common Iliac
    Left 06QD-
    Right 06QC-
  Coronary 02Q4-
  Esophageal 06Q3-
  External Iliac
    Left 06QG-
    Right 06QF-
  External Jugular
    Left 05QQ-
    Right 05QP-
  Face
    Left 05QV-
    Right 05QT-
  Femoral
    Left 06QN-
    Right 06QM-
  Foot
    Left 06QV-
    Right 06QT-
  Gastric 06Q2-
  Greater Saphenous
    Left 06QQ-
    Right 06QP-
  Hand
    Left 05QH-
    Right 05QG-
  Hemiazygos 05Q1-
  Hepatic 06Q4-
  Hypogastric
    Left 06QJ-
    Right 06QH-
  Inferior Mesenteric 06Q6-
  Innominate
    Left 05Q4-
    Right 05Q3-
  Internal Jugular
    Left 05QN-
    Right 05QM-
  Intracranial 05QL-
  Lesser Saphenous
    Left 06QS-
    Right 06QR-
  Lower 06QY-
  Portal 06Q8-
  Pulmonary
    Left 02QT-
    Right 02QS-
  Renal
    Left 06QB-
    Right 06Q9-
  Splenic 06Q1-
  Subclavian
    Left 05Q6-
    Right 05Q5-
  Superior Mesenteric 06Q5-

Repair — *continued*
Vein — *continued*
  Upper 05QY-
  Vertebral
    Left 05QS-
    Right 05QR-
Vena Cava
  Inferior 06Q0-
  Superior 02QV-
Ventricle
  Left 02QL-
  Right 02QK-
Vertebra
  Cervical 0PQ3-
  Lumbar 0QQ0-
  Thoracic 0PQ4-
Vesicle
  Bilateral 0VQ3-
  Left 0VQ2-
  Right 0VQ1-
Vitreous
  Left 08Q53ZZ
  Right 08Q43ZZ
Vocal Cord
  Left 0CQV-
  Right 0CQT-
Vulva 0UQM-
Wrist Region
  Left 0XQH-
  Right 0XQG-
Repair, obstetric laceration, periurethral 0UQMXZZ
Replacement
Acetabulum
  Left 0QR5-
  Right 0QR4
Ampulla of Vater 0FRC-
Anal Sphincter 0DRR-
Aorta
  Abdominal 04R0-
  Thoracic 02RW-
Artery
  Anterior Tibial
    Left 04RQ-
    Right 04RP-
  Axillary
    Left 03R6-
    Right 03R5-
  Brachial
    Left 03R8-
    Right 03R7-
  Celiac 04R1-
  Colic
    Left 04R7-
    Middle 04R8-
    Right 04R6-
  Common Carotid
    Left 03RJ-
    Right 03RH-
  Common Iliac
    Left 04RD-
    Right 04RC-
  External Carotid
    Left 03RN-
    Right 03RM-
  External Iliac
    Left 04RJ-
    Right 04RH-
  Face 03RR-
  Femoral
    Left 04RL-
    Right 04RK-
  Foot
    Left 04RW-
    Right 04RV-
  Gastric 04R2-
  Hand
    Left 03RF-
    Right 03RD-
  Hepatic 04R3-
  Inferior Mesenteric 04RB-
  Innominate 03R2-

Replacement — *continued*
Artery — *continued*
  Internal Carotid
    Left 03RL-
    Right 03RK-
  Internal Iliac
    Left 04RF-
    Right 04RE-
  Internal Mammary
    Left 03R1-
    Right 03R0-
  Intracranial 03RG-
  Lower 04RY-
  Peroneal
    Left 04RU-
    Right 04RT-
  Popliteal
    Left 04RN-
    Right 04RM-
  Posterior Tibial
    Left 04RS-
    Right 04RR-
  Pulmonary
    Left 02RR-
    Right 02RQ-
  Pulmonary Trunk 02RP-
  Radial
    Left 03RC-
    Right 03RB-
  Renal
    Left 04RA-
    Right 04R9-
  Splenic 04R4-
  Subclavian
    Left 03R4-
    Right 03R3-
  Superior Mesenteric 04R5-
  Temporal
    Left 03RT-
    Right 03RS-
  Thyroid
    Left 03RV-
    Right 03RU-
  Ulnar
    Left 03RA-
    Right 03R9-
  Upper 03RY-
  Vertebral
    Left 03RQ-
    Right 03RP-
Atrium
  Left 02R7-
  Right 02R6-
Auditory Ossicle
  Left 09RA0-
  Right 09R90-
Bladder 0TRB-
Bladder Neck 0TRC-
Bone
  Ethmoid
    Left 0NRG-
    Right 0NRF-
  Frontal
    Left 0NR2-
    Right 0NR1-
  Hyoid 0NRX-
  Lacrimal
    Left 0NRJ-
    Right 0NRH-
  Nasal 0NRB-
  Occipital
    Left 0NR8-
    Right 0NR7-
  Palatine
    Left 0NRL-
    Right 0NRK-
  Parietal
    Left 0NR4-
    Right 0NR3-

Replacement — *continued*
  Bone — *continued*
    Pelvic
      Left 0QR3-
      Right 0QR2-
    Sphenoid
      Left 0NRD-
      Right 0NRC-
    Temporal
      Left 0NR6-
      Right 0NR5-
    Zygomatic
      Left 0NRN-
      Right 0NRM-
  Breast
    Bilateral 0HRV-
    Left 0HRU-
    Right 0HRT-
  Buccal Mucosa 0CR4-
  Carpal
    Left 0PRN-
    Right 0PRM-
  Chordae Tendineae 02R9-
  Choroid
    Left 08RB-
    Right 08RA-
  Clavicle
    Left 0PRB-
    Right 0PR9-
  Coccyx 0QRS-
  Conjunctiva
    Left 08RTX-
    Right 08RSX-
  Cornea
    Left 08R9-
    Right 08R8-
  Disc
    Cervical Vertebral 0RR30-
    Cervicothoracic Vertebral 0RR50-
    Lumbar Vertebral 0SR20-
    Lumbosacral 0SR40-
    Thoracic Vertebral 0RR90-
    Thoracolumbar Vertebral 0RRB0-
  Duct
    Common Bile 0FR9-
    Cystic 0FR8-
    Hepatic
      Left 0FR6-
      Right 0FR5-
    Lacrimal
      Left 08RY-
      Right 08RX-
    Pancreatic 0FRD-
      Accessory 0FRF-
    Parotid
      Left 0CRC-
      Right 0CRB-
  Ear
    External
      Bilateral 09R2-
      Left 09R1-
      Right 09R0-
    Inner
      Left 09RE0-
      Right 09RD0-
    Middle
      Left 09R60-
      Right 09R50-
  Epiglottis 0CRR-
  Esophagus 0DR5-
  Eye
    Left 08R1-
    Right 08R0-
  Eyelid
    Lower
      Left 08RR-
      Right 08RQ-
    Upper
      Left 08RP-
      Right 08RN-

Replacement — *continued*
  Femoral Shaft
    Left 0QR9-
    Right 0QR8-
  Femur
    Lower
      Left 0QRC-
      Right 0QRB-
    Upper
      Left 0QR7-
      Right 0QR6-
  Fibula
    Left 0QRK-
    Right 0QRJ-
  Finger Nail 0HRQX-
  Gingiva
    Lower 0CR6-
    Upper 0CR5-
  Glenoid Cavity
    Left 0PR8-
    Right 0PR7-
  Hair 0HRSX-
  Humeral Head
    Left 0PRD-
    Right 0PRC-
  Humeral Shaft
    Left 0PRG-
    Right 0PRF-
  Iris
    Left 08RD3-
    Right 08RC3-
  Joint
    Acromioclavicular
      Left 0RRH0-
      Right 0RRG0-
    Ankle
      Left 0SRG-
      Right 0SRF-
    Carpal
      Left 0RRR0-
      Right 0RRQ0-
    Cervical Vertebral 0RR10-
    Cervicothoracic Vertebral 0RR40-
    Coccygeal 0SR60-
    Elbow
      Left 0RRM0-
      Right 0RRL0-
    Finger Phalangeal
      Left 0RRX0-
      Right 0RRW0-
    Hip
      Left 0SRB-
        Acetabular Surface 0SRE-
        Femoral Surface 0SRS-
      Right 0SR9-
        Acetabular Surface 0SRA-
        Femoral Surface 0SRR-
    Knee
      Left 0SRD-
        Femoral Surface 0SRU-
        Tibial Surface 0SRW-
      Right 0SRC-
        Femoral Surface 0SRT-
        Tibial Surface 0SRV-
    Lumbar Vertebral 0SR00-
    Lumbosacral 0SR30-
    Metacarpocarpal
      Left 0RRT0-
      Right 0RRS0-
    Metacarpophalangeal
      Left 0RRV0-
      Right 0RRU0-
    Metatarsal-Phalangeal
      Left 0SRN0-
      Right 0SRM0-
    Metatarsal-Tarsal
      Left 0SRL0-
      Right 0SRK0-
    Occipital-cervical 0RR00-
    Sacrococcygeal 0SR50-

Replacement — *continued*
  Joint — *continued*
    Sacroiliac
      Left 0SR80-
      Right 0SR70-
    Shoulder
      Left 0RRK-
      Right 0RRJ-
    Sternoclavicular
      Left 0RRF0-
      Right 0RRE0-
    Tarsal
      Left 0SRJ0-
      Right 0SRH0-
    Temporomandibular
      Left 0RRD0-
      Right 0RRC0-
    Thoracic Vertebral 0RR60-
    Thoracolumbar Vertebral 0RRA0-
    Toe Phalangeal
      Left 0SRQ0-
      Right 0SRP0-
    Wrist
      Left 0RRP0-
      Right 0RRN0-
  Kidney Pelvis
    Left 0TR4-
    Right 0TR3-
  Larynx 0CRS-
  Lens
    Left 08RK30Z
    Right 08RJ30Z
  Lip
    Lower 0CR1-
    Upper 0CR0-
  Mandible
    Left 0NRV-
    Right 0NRT-
  Maxilla
    Left 0NRS-
    Right 0NRR-
  Mesentery 0DRV-
  Metacarpal
    Left 0PRQ-
    Right 0PRP-
  Metatarsal
    Left 0QRP-
    Right 0QRN-
  Muscle, Papillary 02RD-
  Nasopharynx 09RN-
  Nipple
    Left 0HRX-
    Right 0HRW-
  Nose 09RK-
  Omentum
    Greater 0DRS-
    Lesser 0DRT-
  Orbit
    Left 0NRQ-
    Right 0NRP-
  Palate
    Hard 0CR2-
    Soft 0CR3-
  Patella
    Left 0QRF-
    Right 0QRD-
  Pericardium 02RN-
  Peritoneum 0DRW-
  Phalanx
    Finger
      Left 0PRV-
      Right 0PRT-
    Thumb
      Left 0PRS-
      Right 0PRR-
    Toe
      Left 0QRR-
      Right 0QRQ-
  Pharynx 0CRM-

Replacement — *continued*
  Radius
    Left 0PRJ-
    Right 0PRH-
  Retinal Vessel
    Left 08RH3-
    Right 08RG3-
  Rib
    Left 0PR2-
    Right 0PR1-
  Sacrum 0QR1-
  Scapula
    Left 0PR6-
    Right 0PR5-
  Sclera
    Left 08R7X-
    Right 08R6X-
  Septum
    Atrial 02R5-
    Nasal 09RM-
    Ventricular 02RM-
  Skin
    Abdomen 0HR7-
    Back 0HR6-
    Buttock 0HR8-
    Chest 0HR5-
    Ear
      Left 0HR3-
      Right 0HR2-
    Face 0HR1-
    Foot
      Left 0HRN-
      Right 0HRM-
    Genitalia 0HRA-
    Hand
      Left 0HRG-
      Right 0HRF-
    Lower Arm
      Left 0HRE-
      Right 0HRD-
    Lower Leg
      Left 0HRL-
      Right 0HRK-
    Neck 0HR4-
    Perineum 0HR9-
    Scalp 0HR0-
    Upper Arm
      Left 0HRC-
      Right 0HRB-
    Upper Leg
      Left 0HRJ-
      Right 0HRH-
  Skull 0NR0-
  Sternum 0PR0-
  Subcutaneous Tissue and Fascia
    Abdomen 0JR8-
    Back 0JR7-
    Buttock 0JR9-
    Chest 0JR6-
    Face 0JR1-
    Foot
      Left 0JRR-
      Right 0JRQ-
    Hand
      Left 0JRK-
      Right 0JRJ-
    Lower Arm
      Left 0JRH-
      Right 0JRG-
    Lower Leg
      Left 0JRP-
      Right 0JRN-
    Neck
      Anterior 0JR4-
      Posterior 0JR5-
    Pelvic Region 0JRC-
    Perineum 0JRB-
    Scalp 0JR0-
    Upper Arm
      Left 0JRF-
      Right 0JRD-

Replacement — *continued*
Subcutaneous Tissue and Fascia — *continued*
Upper Leg
Left 0JRM-
Right 0JRL-
Tarsal
Left 0QRM-
Right 0QRL-
Tendon
Abdomen
Left 0LRG-
Right 0LRF-
Ankle
Left 0LRT-
Right 0LRS-
Foot
Left 0LRW-
Right 0LRV-
Hand
Left 0LR8-
Right 0LR7-
Head and Neck 0LR0-
Hip
Left 0LRK-
Right 0LRJ-
Knee
Left 0LRR-
Right 0LRQ-
Lower Arm and Wrist
Left 0LR6-
Right 0LR5-
Lower Leg
Left 0LRP-
Right 0LRN-
Perineum 0LRH-
Shoulder
Left 0LR2-
Right 0LR1-
Thorax
Left 0LRD-
Right 0LRC-
Trunk
Left 0LRB-
Right 0LR9-
Upper Arm
Left 0LR4-
Right 0LR3-
Upper Leg
Left 0LRM-
Right 0LRL-
Testis
Bilateral 0VRC0JZ
Left 0VRB0JZ
Right 0VR90JZ
Thumb
Left 0XRM-
Right 0XRL-
Tibia
Left 0QRH-
Right 0QRG-
Toe Nail 0HRRX-
Tongue 0CR7-
Tooth
Lower 0CRX-
Upper 0CRW-
Turbinate, Nasal 09RL-
Tympanic Membrane
Left 09R8-
Right 09R7-
Ulna
Left 0PRL-
Right 0PRK-
Ureter
Left 0TR7-
Right 0TR6-
Urethra 0TRD-
Uvula 0CRN-

Replacement — *continued*
Valve
Aortic 02RF-
Mitral 02RG-
Pulmonary 02RH-
Tricuspid 02RJ-
Vein
Axillary
Left 05R8-
Right 05R7-
Azygos 05R0-
Basilic
Left 05RC-
Right 05RB-
Brachial
Left 05RA-
Right 05R9-
Cephalic
Left 05RF-
Right 05RD-
Colic 06R7-
Common Iliac
Left 06RD-
Right 06RC-
Esophageal 06R3-
External Iliac
Left 06RG-
Right 06RF-
External Jugular
Left 05RQ-
Right 05RP-
Face
Left 05RV-
Right 05RT-
Femoral
Left 06RN-
Right 06RM-
Foot
Left 06RV-
Right 06RT-
Gastric 06R2-
Greater Saphenous
Left 06RQ-
Right 06RP-
Hand
Left 05RH-
Right 05RG-
Hemiazygos 05R1-
Hepatic 06R4-
Hypogastric
Left 06RJ-
Right 06RH-
Inferior Mesenteric 06R6-
Innominate
Left 05R4-
Right 05R3-
Internal Jugular
Left 05RN-
Right 05RM-
Intracranial 05RL-
Lesser Saphenous
Left 06RS-
Right 06RR-
Lower 06RY-
Portal 06R8-
Pulmonary
Left 02RT-
Right 02RS-
Renal
Left 06RB-
Right 06R9-
Splenic 06R1-
Subclavian
Left 05R6-
Right 05R5-
Superior Mesenteric 06R5-
Upper 05RY-
Vertebral
Left 05RS-
Right 05RR-

Replacement — *continued*
Vena Cava
Inferior 06R0-
Superior 02RV-
Ventricle
Left 02RL-
Right 02RK-
Vertebra
Cervical 0PR3-
Lumbar 0QR0-
Thoracic 0PR4-
Vitreous
Left 08R53-
Right 08R43-
Vocal Cord
Left 0CRV-
Right 0CRT-
Replacement, hip
Partial or total *see* Replacement, Lower Joints 0SR-
Resurfacing only *see* Supplement, Lower Joints 0SU-
Replantation *see* Reposition
Replantation, scalp *see* Reattachment, Skin, Scalp 0HM0-
Reposition
Acetabulum
Left 0QS5-
Right 0QS4-
Ampulla of Vater 0FSC-
Anus 0DSQ-
Aorta
Abdominal 04S0-
Thoracic 02SW0ZZ
Artery
Anterior Tibial
Left 04SQ-
Right 04SP-
Axillary
Left 03S6-
Right 03S5-
Brachial
Left 03S8-
Right 03S7-
Celiac 04S1-
Colic
Left 04S7-
Middle 04S8-
Right 04S6-
Common Carotid
Left 03SJ-
Right 03SH-
Common Iliac
Left 04SD-
Right 04SC-
External Carotid
Left 03SN-
Right 03SM-
External Iliac
Left 04SJ-
Right 04SH-
Face 03SR-
Femoral
Left 04SL-
Right 04SK-
Foot
Left 04SW-
Right 04SV-
Gastric 04S2-
Hand
Left 03SF-
Right 03SD-
Hepatic 04S3-
Inferior Mesenteric 04SB-
Innominate 03S2-
Internal Carotid
Left 03SL-
Right 03SK-
Internal Iliac
Left 04SF-
Right 04SE-

Reposition — *continued*
Artery — *continued*
Internal Mammary
Left 03S1-
Right 03S0-
Intracranial 03SG-
Lower 04SY-
Peroneal
Left 04SU-
Right 04ST-
Popliteal
Left 04SN-
Right 04SM-
Posterior Tibial
Left 04SS-
Right 04SR-
Pulmonary
Left 02SR0ZZ
Right 02SQ0ZZ
Pulmonary Trunk 02SP0ZZ
Radial
Left 03SC-
Right 03SB-
Renal
Left 04SA-
Right 04S9-
Splenic 04S4-
Subclavian
Left 03S4-
Right 03S3-
Superior Mesenteric 04S5-
Temporal
Left 03ST-
Right 03SS-
Thyroid
Left 03SV-
Right 03SU-
Ulnar
Left 03SA-
Right 03S9-
Upper 03SY-
Vertebral
Left 03SQ-
Right 03SP-
Auditory Ossicle
Left 09SA-
Right 09S9-
Bladder 0TSB
Bladder Neck 0TSC-
Bone
Ethmoid
Left 0NSG-
Right 0NSF-
Frontal
Left 0NS2-
Right 0NS1-
Hyoid 0NSX-
Lacrimal
Left 0NSJ-
Right 0NSH-
Nasal 0NSB-
Occipital
Left 0NS8-
Right 0NS7-
Palatine
Left 0NSL-
Right 0NSK-
Parietal
Left 0NS4-
Right 0NS3-
Pelvic
Left 0QS3-
Right 0QS2-
Sphenoid
Left 0NSD-
Right 0NSC-
Temporal
Left 0NS6-
Right 0NS5-
Zygomatic
Left 0NSN-
Right 0NSM-

Reposition — continued
Breast
  Bilateral 0HSV0ZZ
  Left 0HSU0ZZ
  Right 0HST0ZZ
Bronchus
  Lingula 0BS90ZZ
  Lower Lobe
    Left 0BSB0ZZ
    Right 0BS60ZZ
  Main
    Left 0BS70ZZ
    Right 0BS30ZZ
  Middle Lobe, Right 0BS50ZZ
  Upper Lobe
    Left 0BS80ZZ
    Right 0BS40ZZ
Bursa and Ligament
  Abdomen
    Left 0MSJ-
    Right 0MSH-
  Ankle
    Left 0MSR-
    Right 0MSQ-
  Elbow
    Left 0MS4-
    Right 0MS3-
  Foot
    Left 0MST-
    Right 0MSS-
  Hand
    Left 0MS8-
    Right 0MS7-
  Head and Neck 0MS0-
  Hip
    Left 0MSM-
    Right 0MSL-
  Knee
    Left 0MSP-
    Right 0MSN-
  Lower Extremity
    Left 0MSW-
    Right 0MSV-
  Perineum 0MSK-
  Shoulder
    Left 0MS2-
    Right 0MS1-
  Thorax
    Left 0MSG-
    Right 0MSF-
  Trunk
    Left 0MSD-
    Right 0MSC-
  Upper Extremity
    Left 0MSB-
    Right 0MS9-
  Wrist
    Left 0MS6-
    Right 0MS5-
Carina 0BS20ZZ
Carpal
  Left 0PSN-
  Right 0PSM-
Cecum 0DSH-
Cervix 0USC-
Clavicle
  Left 0PSB-
  Right 0PS9-
Coccyx 0QSS-
Colon
  Ascending 0DSK-
  Descending 0DSM-
  Sigmoid 0DSN-
  Transverse 0DSL-
Cord
  Bilateral 0VSH-
  Left 0VSG-
  Right 0VSF-
Cul-de-sac 0USF-

Reposition — continued
Diaphragm
  Left 0BSS0ZZ
  Right 0BSR0ZZ
Duct
  Common Bile 0FS9-
  Cystic 0FS8-
  Hepatic
    Left 0FS6-
    Right 0FS5-
  Lacrimal
    Left 08SY-
    Right 08SX-
  Pancreatic 0FSD-
    Accessory 0FSF-
  Parotid
    Left 0CSC-
    Right 0CSB-
Duodenum 0DS9-
Ear
  Bilateral 09S2-
  Left 09S1-
  Right 09S0-
Epiglottis 0CSR-
Esophagus 0DS5-
Eustachian Tube
  Left 09SG-
  Right 09SF-
Eyelid
  Lower
    Left 08SR-
    Right 08SQ-
  Upper
    Left 08SP-
    Right 08SN-
Fallopian Tube
  Left 0US6-
  Right 0US5-
Fallopian Tubes, Bilateral 0US7-
Femoral Shaft
  Left 0QS9-
  Right 0QS8-
Femur
  Lower
    Left 0QSC-
    Right 0QSB-
  Upper
    Left 0QS7-
    Right 0QS6-
Fibula
  Left 0QSK-
  Right 0QSJ-
Gallbladder 0FS4-
Gland
  Adrenal
    Left 0GS2-
    Right 0GS3-
  Lacrimal
    Left 08SW-
    Right 08SV-
Glenoid Cavity
  Left 0PS8-
  Right 0PS7-
Hair 0HSSXZZ
Humeral Head
  Left 0PSD-
  Right 0PSC-
Humeral Shaft
  Left 0PSG-
  Right 0PSF-
Ileum 0DSB-
Iris
  Left 08SD3ZZ
  Right 08SC3ZZ
Jejunum 0DSA-

Reposition — continued
Joint
  Acromioclavicular
    Left 0RSH-
    Right 0RSG-
  Ankle
    Left 0SSG-
    Right 0SSF-
  Carpal
    Left 0RSR-
    Right 0RSQ-
  Cervical Vertebral 0RS1-
  Cervicothoracic Vertebral 0RS4-
  Coccygeal 0SS6-
  Elbow
    Left 0RSM-
    Right 0RSL-
  Finger Phalangeal
    Left 0RSX-
    Right 0RSW-
  Hip
    Left 0SSB-
    Right 0SS9-
  Knee
    Left 0SSD-
    Right 0SSC-
  Lumbar Vertebral 0SS0-
  Lumbosacral 0SS3-
  Metacarpocarpal
    Left 0RST-
    Right 0RSS-
  Metacarpophalangeal
    Left 0RSV-
    Right 0RSU-
  Metatarsal-Phalangeal
    Left 0SSN-
    Right 0SSM-
  Metatarsal-Tarsal
    Left 0SSL-
    Right 0SSK-
  Occipital-cervical 0RS0-
  Sacrococcygeal 0SS5-
  Sacroiliac
    Left 0SS8-
    Right 0SS7-
  Shoulder
    Left 0RSK-
    Right 0RSJ-
  Sternoclavicular
    Left 0RSF-
    Right 0RSE-
  Tarsal
    Left 0SSJ-
    Right 0SSH-
  Temporomandibular
    Left 0RSD-
    Right 0RSC-
  Thoracic Vertebral 0RS6-
  Thoracolumbar Vertebral 0RSA-
  Toe Phalangeal
    Left 0SSQ-
    Right 0SSP-
  Wrist
    Left 0RSP-
    Right 0RSN-
Kidney
  Left 0TS1-
  Right 0TS0-
Kidney Pelvis
  Left 0TS4-
  Right 0TS3-
Kidneys, Bilateral 0TS2-
Lens
  Left 08SK3ZZ
  Right 08SJ3ZZ
Lip
  Lower 0CS1-
  Upper 0CS0-
Liver 0FS0-

Reposition — continued
Lung
  Left 0BSL0ZZ
  Lower Lobe
    Left 0BSJ0ZZ
    Right 0BSF0ZZ
  Middle Lobe, Right 0BSD0ZZ
  Right 0BSK0ZZ
  Upper Lobe
    Left 0BSG0ZZ
    Right 0BSC0ZZ
Lung Lingula 0BSH0ZZ
Mandible
  Left 0NSV-
  Right 0NST-
Maxilla
  Left 0NSS-
  Right 0NSR-
Metacarpal
  Left 0PSQ-
  Right 0PSP-
Metatarsal
  Left 0QSP-
  Right 0QSN-
Muscle
  Abdomen
    Left 0KSL-
    Right 0KSK-
  Extraocular
    Left 08SM-
    Right 08SL-
  Facial 0KS1-
  Foot
    Left 0KSW-
    Right 0KSV-
  Hand
    Left 0KSD-
    Right 0KSC-
  Head 0KS0-
  Hip
    Left 0KSP-
    Right 0KSN-
  Lower Arm and Wrist
    Left 0KSB-
    Right 0KS9-
  Lower Leg
    Left 0KST-
    Right 0KSS-
  Neck
    Left 0KS3-
    Right 0KS2-
  Perineum 0KSM-
  Shoulder
    Left 0KS6-
    Right 0KS5-
  Thorax
    Left 0KSJ-
    Right 0KSH-
  Tongue, Palate, Pharynx 0KS4-
  Trunk
    Left 0KSG-
    Right 0KSF-
  Upper Arm
    Left 0KS8-
    Right 0KS7-
  Upper Leg
    Left 0KSR-
    Right 0KSQ-
Nerve
  Abducens 00SL-
  Accessory 00SR-
  Acoustic 00SN-
  Brachial Plexus 01S3-
  Cervical 01S1-
  Cervical Plexus 01S0-
  Facial 00SM-
  Femoral 01SD-
  Glossopharyngeal 00SP-
  Hypoglossal 00SS-

Reposition — continued
Nerve — continued
Lumbar 01SB-
Lumbar Plexus 01S9-
Lumbosacral Plexus 01SA-
Median 01S5-
Oculomotor 00SH-
Olfactory 00SF-
Optic 00SG-
Peroneal 01SH-
Phrenic 01S2-
Pudendal 01SC-
Radial 01S6-
Sacral 01SR-
Sacral Plexus 01SQ-
Sciatic 01SF-
Thoracic 01S8-
Tibial 01SG-
Trigeminal 00SK-
Trochlear 00SJ-
Ulnar 01S4-
Vagus 00SQ-
Nipple
Left 0HSXXZZ
Right 0HSWXZZ
Nose 09SK-
Orbit
Left 0NSQ-
Right 0NSP-
Ovary
Bilateral 0US2-
Left 0US1-
Right 0US0-
Palate
Hard 0CS2-
Soft 0CS3-
Pancreas 0FSG-
Parathyroid Gland 0GSR-
Inferior
Left 0GSP-
Right 0GSN-
Multiple 0GSQ-
Superior
Left 0GSM-
Right 0GSL-
Patella
Left 0QSF-
Right 0QSD-
Phalanx
Finger
Left 0PSV-
Right 0PST-
Thumb
Left 0PSS-
Right 0PSR-
Toe
Left 0QSR-
Right 0QSQ-
Products of Conception 10S0-
Ectopic 10S2-
Radius
Left 0PSJ-
Right 0PSH-
Rectum 0DSP-
Retinal Vessel
Left 08SH3ZZ
Right 08SG3ZZ
Rib
Left 0PS2-
Right 0PS1-
Sacrum 0QS1-
Scapula
Left 0PS6-
Right 0PS5-
Septum, Nasal 09SM-
Skull 0NS0-
Spinal Cord
Cervical 00SW-
Lumbar 00SY-
Thoracic 00SX-
Spleen 07SP0ZZ

Reposition — continued
Sternum 0PS0-
Stomach 0DS6-
Tarsal
Left 0QSM-
Right 0QSL-
Tendon
Abdomen
Left 0LSG-
Right 0LSF-
Ankle
Left 0LST-
Right 0LSS-
Foot
Left 0LSW-
Right 0LSV-
Hand
Left 0LS8-
Right 0LS7-
Head and Neck 0LS0-
Hip
Left 0LSK-
Right 0LSJ-
Knee
Left 0LSR-
Right 0LSQ-
Lower Arm and Wrist
Left 0LS6-
Right 0LS5-
Lower Leg
Left 0LSP-
Right 0LSN-
Perineum 0LSH-
Shoulder
Left 0LS2-
Right 0LS1-
Thorax
Left 0LSD-
Right 0LSC-
Trunk
Left 0LSB-
Right 0LS9-
Upper Arm
Left 0LS4-
Right 0LS3-
Upper Leg
Left 0LSM-
Right 0LSL-
Testis
Bilateral 0VSC-
Left 0VSB-
Right 0VS9-
Thymus 07SM0ZZ
Thyroid Gland
Left Lobe 0GSG-
Right Lobe 0GSH-
Tibia
Left 0QSH-
Right 0QSG-
Tongue 0CS7-
Tooth
Lower 0CSX-
Upper 0CSW-
Trachea 0BS10ZZ
Turbinate, Nasal 09SL-
Tympanic Membrane
Left 09S8-
Right 09S7-
Ulna
Left 0PSL-
Right 0PSK-
Ureter
Left 0TS7-
Right 0TS6-
Ureters, Bilateral 0TS8-
Urethra 0TSD-
Uterine Supporting Structure 0US4-
Uterus 0US9-
Uvula 0CSN-
Vagina 0USG-

Reposition — continued
Vein
Axillary
Left 05S8-
Right 05S7-
Azygos 05S0-
Basilic
Left 05SC-
Right 05SB-
Brachial
Left 05SA-
Right 05S9-
Cephalic
Left 05SF-
Right 05SD-
Colic 06S7-
Common Iliac
Left 06SD-
Right 06SC-
Esophageal 06S3-
External Iliac
Left 06SG-
Right 06SF-
External Jugular
Left 05SQ-
Right 05SP-
Face
Left 05SV-
Right 05ST-
Femoral
Left 06SN-
Right 06SM-
Foot
Left 06SV-
Right 06ST-
Gastric 06S2-
Greater Saphenous
Left 06SQ-
Right 06SP-
Hand
Left 05SH-
Right 05SG-
Hemiazygos 05S1-
Hepatic 06S4-
Hypogastric
Left 06SJ-
Right 06SH-
Inferior Mesenteric 06S6-
Innominate
Left 05S4-
Right 05S3-
Internal Jugular
Left 05SN-
Right 05SM-
Intracranial 05SL-
Lesser Saphenous
Left 06SS-
Right 06SR-
Lower 06SY-
Portal 06S8-
Pulmonary
Left 02ST0ZZ
Right 02SS0ZZ
Renal
Left 06SB-
Right 06S9-
Splenic 06S1-
Subclavian
Left 05S6-
Right 05S5-
Superior Mesenteric 06S5-
Upper 05SY-
Vertebral
Left 05SS-
Right 05SR-
Vena Cava
Inferior 06S0-
Superior 02SV0ZZ
Vertebra
Cervical 0PS3-
Lumbar 0QS0-
Thoracic 0PS4-

Reposition — continued
Vocal Cord
Left 0CSV-
Right 0CST-
Resection
Acetabulum
Left 0QT50ZZ
Right 0QT40ZZ
Adenoids 0CTQ-
Ampulla of Vater 0FTC-
Anal Sphincter 0DTR-
Anus 0DTQ-
Aortic Body 0GTD-
Appendix 0DTJ-
Auditory Ossicle
Left 09TA0ZZ
Right 09T90ZZ
Bladder 0TTB-
Bladder Neck 0TTC-
Bone
Ethmoid
Left 0NTG0ZZ
Right 0NTF0ZZ
Frontal
Left 0NT20ZZ
Right 0NT10ZZ
Hyoid 0NTX0ZZ
Lacrimal
Left 0NTJ0ZZ
Right 0NTH0ZZ
Nasal 0NTB0ZZ
Occipital
Left 0NT80ZZ
Right 0NT70ZZ
Palatine
Left 0NTL0ZZ
Right 0NTK0ZZ
Parietal
Left 0NT40ZZ
Right 0NT30ZZ
Pelvic
Left 0QT30ZZ
Right 0QT20ZZ
Sphenoid
Left 0NTD0ZZ
Right 0NTC0ZZ
Temporal
Left 0NT60ZZ
Right 0NT50ZZ
Zygomatic
Left 0NTN0ZZ
Right 0NTM0ZZ
Breast
Bilateral 0HTV0ZZ
Left 0HTU0ZZ
Right 0HTT0ZZ
Supernumerary 0HTY0ZZ
Bronchus
Lingula 0BT9-
Lower Lobe
Left 0BTB-
Right 0BT6-
Main
Left 0BT7-
Right 0BT3-
Middle Lobe, Right 0BT5-
Upper Lobe
Left 0BT8-
Right 0BT4-
Bursa and Ligament
Abdomen
Left 0MTJ-
Right 0MTH-
Ankle
Left 0MTR-
Right 0MTQ-
Elbow
Left 0MT4-
Right 0MT3-

Resection — *continued*
  Bursa and Ligament — *continued*
    Foot
      Left 0MTT-
      Right 0MTS-
    Hand
      Left 0MT8-
      Right 0MT7-
    Head and Neck 0MT0-
    Hip
      Left 0MTM-
      Right 0MTL-
    Knee
      Left 0MTP-
      Right 0MTN-
    Lower Extremity
      Left 0MTW-
      Right 0MTV-
    Perineum 0MTK-
    Shoulder
      Left 0MT2-
      Right 0MT1-
    Thorax
      Left 0MTG-
      Right 0MTF-
    Trunk
      Left 0MTD-
      Right 0MTC-
    Upper Extremity
      Left 0MTB-
      Right 0MT9-
    Wrist
      Left 0MT6-
      Right 0MT5-
  Carina 0BT2-
  Carotid Bodies, Bilateral 0GT8-
  Carotid Body
    Left 0GT6-
    Right 0GT7-
  Carpal
    Left 0PTN0ZZ
    Right 0PTM0ZZ
  Cecum 0DTH-
  Cerebral Hemisphere 00T7-
  Cervix 0UTC-
  Chordae Tendineae 02T9-
  Cisterna Chyli 07TL-
  Clavicle
    Left 0PTB0ZZ
    Right 0PT90ZZ
  Clitoris 0UTJ-
  Coccygeal Glomus 0GTB-
  Coccyx 0QTS0ZZ
  Colon
    Ascending 0DTK-
    Descending 0DTM-
    Sigmoid 0DTN-
    Transverse 0DTL-
  Conduction Mechanism 02T8-
  Cord
    Bilateral 0VTH-
    Left 0VTG-
    Right 0VTF-
  Cornea
    Left 08T9XZZ
    Right 08T8XZZ
  Cul-de-sac 0UTF-
  Diaphragm
    Left 0BTS-
    Right 0BTR-
  Disc
    Cervical Vertebral 0RT30ZZ
    Cervicothoracic Vertebral 0RT50ZZ
    Lumbar Vertebral 0ST20ZZ
    Lumbosacral 0ST40ZZ
    Thoracic Vertebral 0RT90ZZ
    Thoracolumbar Vertebral 0RTB0ZZ

Resection — *continued*
  Duct
    Common Bile 0FT9-
    Cystic 0FT8-
    Hepatic
      Left 0FT6-
      Right 0FT5-
    Lacrimal
      Left 08TY-
      Right 08TX-
    Pancreatic 0FTD-
      Accessory 0FTF-
    Parotid
      Left 0CTC0ZZ
      Right 0CTB0ZZ
  Duodenum 0DT9-
  Ear
    External
      Left 09T1-
      Right 09T0-
    Inner
      Left 09TE0ZZ
      Right 09TD0ZZ
    Middle
      Left 09T60ZZ
      Right 09T50ZZ
  Epididymis
    Bilateral 0VTL-
    Left 0VTK-
    Right 0VTJ-
  Epiglottis 0CTR-
  Esophagogastric Junction 0DT4-
  Esophagus 0DT5-
    Lower 0DT3-
    Middle 0DT2-
    Upper 0DT1-
  Eustachian Tube
    Left 09TG-
    Right 09TF-
  Eye
    Left 08T1XZZ
    Right 08T0XZZ
  Eyelid
    Lower
      Left 08TR-
      Right 08TQ-
    Upper
      Left 08TP-
      Right 08TN-
  Fallopian Tube
    Left 0UT6-
    Right 0UT5-
  Fallopian Tubes, Bilateral 0UT7-
  Femoral Shaft
    Left 0QT90ZZ
    Right 0QT80ZZ
  Femur
    Lower
      Left 0QTC0ZZ
      Right 0QTB0ZZ
    Upper
      Left 0QT70ZZ
      Right 0QT60ZZ
  Fibula
    Left 0QTK0ZZ
    Right 0QTJ0ZZ
  Finger Nail 0HTQXZZ
  Gallbladder 0FT4-
  Gland
    Adrenal
      Bilateral 0GT4-
      Left 0GT2-
      Right 0GT3-
    Lacrimal
      Left 08TW-
      Right 08TV-
    Minor Salivary 0CTJ0ZZ
    Parotid
      Left 0CT90ZZ
      Right 0CT80ZZ
    Pituitary 0GT0-

Resection — *continued*
  Gland — *continued*
    Sublingual
      Left 0CTF0ZZ
      Right 0CTD0ZZ
    Submaxillary
      Left 0CTH0ZZ
      Right 0CTG0ZZ
    Vestibular 0UTL-
  Glenoid Cavity
    Left 0PT80ZZ
    Right 0PT70ZZ
  Glomus Jugulare 0GTC-
  Humeral Head
    Left 0PTD0ZZ
    Right 0PTC0ZZ
  Humeral Shaft
    Left 0PTG0ZZ
    Right 0PTF0ZZ
  Hymen 0UTK-
  Ileocecal Valve 0DTC-
  Ileum 0DTB-
  Intestine
    Large 0DTE-
      Left 0DTG-
      Right 0DTF-
    Small 0DT8-
  Iris
    Left 08TD3ZZ
    Right 08TC3ZZ
  Jejunum 0DTA-
  Joint
    Acromioclavicular
      Left 0RTH0ZZ
      Right 0RTG0ZZ
    Ankle
      Left 0STG0ZZ
      Right 0STF0ZZ
    Carpal
      Left 0RTR0ZZ
      Right 0RTQ0ZZ
    Cervicothoracic Vertebral 0RT40ZZ
    Coccygeal 0ST60ZZ
    Elbow
      Left 0RTM0ZZ
      Right 0RTL0ZZ
    Finger Phalangeal
      Left 0RTX0ZZ
      Right 0RTW0ZZ
    Hip
      Left 0STB0ZZ
      Right 0ST90ZZ
    Knee
      Left 0STD0ZZ
      Right 0STC0ZZ
    Metacarpocarpal
      Left 0RTT0ZZ
      Right 0RTS0ZZ
    Metacarpophalangeal
      Left 0RTV0ZZ
      Right 0RTU0ZZ
    Metatarsal-Phalangeal
      Left 0STN0ZZ
      Right 0STM0ZZ
    Metatarsal-Tarsal
      Left 0STL0ZZ
      Right 0STK0ZZ
    Sacrococcygeal 0ST50ZZ
    Sacroiliac
      Left 0ST80ZZ
      Right 0ST70ZZ
    Shoulder
      Left 0RTK0ZZ
      Right 0RTJ0ZZ
    Sternoclavicular
      Left 0RTF0ZZ
      Right 0RTE0ZZ
    Tarsal
      Left 0STJ0ZZ
      Right 0STH0ZZ

Resection — *continued*
  Joint — *continued*
    Temporomandibular
      Left 0RTD0ZZ
      Right 0RTC0ZZ
    Toe Phalangeal
      Left 0STQ0ZZ
      Right 0STP0ZZ
    Wrist
      Left 0RTP0ZZ
      Right 0RTN0ZZ
  Kidney
    Left 0TT1-
    Right 0TT0-
  Kidney Pelvis
    Left 0TT4-
    Right 0TT3-
  Kidneys, Bilateral 0TT2-
  Larynx 0CTS-
  Lens
    Left 08TK3ZZ
    Right 08TJ3ZZ
  Lip
    Lower 0CT1-
    Upper 0CT0-
  Liver 0FT0-
    Left Lobe 0FT2-
    Right Lobe 0FT1-
  Lung
    Bilateral 0BTM-
    Left 0BTL-
    Lower Lobe
      Left 0BTJ-
      Right 0BTF-
    Middle Lobe, Right 0BTD-
    Right 0BTK-
    Upper Lobe
      Left 0BTG-
      Right 0BTC-
  Lung Lingula 0BTH-
  Lymphatic
    Aortic 07TD-
    Axillary
      Left 07T6-
      Right 07T5-
    Head 07T0-
    Inguinal
      Left 07TJ-
      Right 07TH-
    Internal Mammary
      Left 07T9-
      Right 07T8-
    Lower Extremity
      Left 07TG-
      Right 07TF-
    Mesenteric 07TB-
    Neck
      Left 07T2-
      Right 07T1-
    Pelvis 07TC-
    Thoracic Duct 07TK-
    Thorax 07T7-
    Upper Extremity
      Left 07T4-
      Right 07T3-
  Mandible
    Left 0NTV0ZZ
    Right 0NTT0ZZ
  Maxilla
    Left 0NTS0ZZ
    Right 0NTR0ZZ
  Metacarpal
    Left 0PTQ0ZZ
    Right 0PTP0ZZ
  Metatarsal
    Left 0QTP0ZZ
    Right 0QTN0ZZ

Resection — *continued*
Muscle
　Abdomen
　　Left 0KTL-
　　Right 0KTK-
　Extraocular
　　Left 08TM-
　　Right 08TL-
　Facial 0KT1-
　Foot
　　Left 0KTW-
　　Right 0KTV-
　Hand
　　Left 0KTD-
　　Right 0KTC-
　Head 0KT0-
　Hip
　　Left 0KTP-
　　Right 0KTN-
　Lower Arm and Wrist
　　Left 0KTB-
　　Right 0KT9-
　Lower Leg
　　Left 0KTT-
　　Right 0KTS-
　Neck
　　Left 0KT3-
　　Right 0KT2-
　Papillary 02TD-
　Perineum 0KTM-
　Shoulder
　　Left 0KT6-
　　Right 0KT5-
　Thorax
　　Left 0KTJ-
　　Right 0KTH-
　Tongue, Palate, Pharynx 0KT4-
　Trunk
　　Left 0KTG-
　　Right 0KTF-
　Upper Arm
　　Left 0KT8-
　　Right 0KT7-
　Upper Leg
　　Left 0KTR-
　　Right 0KTQ-
Nasopharynx 09TN-
Nipple
　Left 0HTXXZZ
　Right 0HTWXZZ
Nose 09TK-
Omentum
　Greater 0DTS-
　Lesser 0DTT-
Orbit
　Left 0NTQ0ZZ
　Right 0NTP0ZZ
Ovary
　Bilateral 0UT2-
　Left 0UT1-
　Right 0UT0-
Palate
　Hard 0CT2-
　Soft 0CT3-
Pancreas 0FTG-
Para-aortic Body 0GT9-
Paraganglion Extremity 0GTF-
Parathyroid Gland 0GTR-
　Inferior
　　Left 0GTP-
　　Right 0GTN-
　Multiple 0GTQ-
　Superior
　　Left 0GTM-
　　Right 0GTL-
Patella
　Left 0QTF0ZZ
　Right 0QTD0ZZ
Penis 0VTS-
Pericardium 02TN-

Resection — *continued*
Phalanx
　Finger
　　Left 0PTV0ZZ
　　Right 0PTT0ZZ
　Thumb
　　Left 0PTS0ZZ
　　Right 0PTR0ZZ
　Toe
　　Left 0QTR0ZZ
　　Right 0QTQ0ZZ
Pharynx 0CTM-
Pineal Body 0GT1-
Prepuce 0VTT-
Products of Conception, Ectopic 10T2-
Prostate 0VT0-
Radius
　Left 0PTJ0ZZ
　Right 0PTH0ZZ
Rectum 0DTP-
Rib
　Left 0PT20ZZ
　Right 0PT10ZZ
Scapula
　Left 0PT60ZZ
　Right 0PT50ZZ
Scrotum 0VT5-
Septum
　Atrial 02T5-
　Nasal 09TM-
　Ventricular 02TM-
Sinus
　Accessory 09TP-
　Ethmoid
　　Left 09TV-
　　Right 09TU-
　Frontal
　　Left 09TT-
　　Right 09TS-
　Mastoid
　　Left 09TC-
　　Right 09TB-
　Maxillary
　　Left 09TR-
　　Right 09TQ-
　Sphenoid
　　Left 09TX-
　　Right 09TW-
Spleen 07TP-
Sternum 0PT00ZZ
Stomach 0DT6-
　Pylorus 0DT7-
Tarsal
　Left 0QTM0ZZ
　Right 0QTL0ZZ
Tendon
　Abdomen
　　Left 0LTG-
　　Right 0LTF-
　Ankle
　　Left 0LTT-
　　Right 0LTS-
　Foot
　　Left 0LTW-
　　Right 0LTV-
　Hand
　　Left 0LT8-
　　Right 0LT7-
　Head and Neck 0LT0-
　Hip
　　Left 0LTK-
　　Right 0LTJ-
　Knee
　　Left 0LTR-
　　Right 0LTQ-
　Lower Arm and Wrist
　　Left 0LT6-
　　Right 0LT5-
　Lower Leg
　　Left 0LTP-
　　Right 0LTN-

Resection — *continued*
Tendon — *continued*
　Perineum 0LTH-
　Shoulder
　　Left 0LT2-
　　Right 0LT1-
　Thorax
　　Left 0LTD-
　　Right 0LTC-
　Trunk
　　Left 0LTB-
　　Right 0LT9-
　Upper Arm
　　Left 0LT4-
　　Right 0LT3-
　Upper Leg
　　Left 0LTM-
　　Right 0LTL-
Testis
　Bilateral 0VTC-
　Left 0VTB-
　Right 0VT9-
Thymus 07TM-
Thyroid Gland 0GTK-
　Left Lobe 0GTG-
　Right Lobe 0GTH-
Tibia
　Left 0QTH0ZZ
　Right 0QTG0ZZ
Toe Nail 0HTRXZZ
Tongue 0CT7-
Tonsils 0CTP-
Tooth
　Lower 0CTX0Z-
　Upper 0CTW0Z-
Trachea 0BT1-
Tunica Vaginalis
　Left 0VT7-
　Right 0VT6-
Turbinate, Nasal 09TL-
Tympanic Membrane
　Left 09T8-
　Right 09T7-
Ulna
　Left 0PTL0ZZ
　Right 0PTK0ZZ
Ureter
　Left 0TT7-
　Right 0TT6-
Urethra 0TTD-
Uterine Supporting Structure 0UT4-
Uterus 0UT9-
Uvula 0CTN-
Vagina 0UTG-
Valve, Pulmonary 02TH-
Vas Deferens
　Bilateral 0VTQ-
　Left 0VTP-
　Right 0VTN-
Vesicle
　Bilateral 0VT3-
　Left 0VT2-
　Right 0VT1-
Vitreous
　Left 08T53ZZ
　Right 08T43ZZ
Vocal Cord
　Left 0CTV-
　Right 0CTT-
Vulva 0UTM-
Restoration, Cardiac, Single, Rhythm 5A2204Z
RestoreAdvanced neurostimulator (SureScan) (MRI Safe)
　use Stimulator Generator, Multiple Array Rechargeable in 0JH-
RestoreSensor neurostimulator (SureScan) (MRI Safe)
　use Stimulator Generator, Multiple Array Rechargeable in 0JH-

RestoreUltra neurostimulator (SureScan) (MRI Safe)
　use Stimulator Generator, Multiple Array Rechargeable in 0JH-
Restriction
Ampulla of Vater 0FVC-
Anus 0DVQ-
Aorta
　Abdominal 04V0-
　Thoracic 02VW-
Artery
　Anterior Tibial
　　Left 04VQ-
　　Right 04VP-
　Axillary
　　Left 03V6-
　　Right 03V5-
　Brachial
　　Left 03V8-
　　Right 03V7-
　Celiac 04V1-
　Colic
　　Left 04V7-
　　Middle 04V8-
　　Right 04V6-
　Common Carotid
　　Left 03VJ-
　　Right 03VH-
　Common Iliac
　　Left 04VD-
　　Right 04VC-
　External Carotid
　　Left 03VN-
　　Right 03VM-
　External Iliac
　　Left 04VJ-
　　Right 04VH-
　Face 03VR-
　Femoral
　　Left 04VL-
　　Right 04VK-
　Foot
　　Left 04VW-
　　Right 04VV-
　Gastric 04V2-
　Hand
　　Left 03VF-
　　Right 03VD-
　Hepatic 04V3-
　Inferior Mesenteric 04VB-
　Innominate 03V2-
　Internal Carotid
　　Left 03VL-
　　Right 03VK-
　Internal Iliac
　　Left 04VF-
　　Right 04VE-
　Internal Mammary
　　Left 03V1-
　　Right 03V0-
　Intracranial 03VG-
　Lower 04VY-
　Peroneal
　　Left 04VU-
　　Right 04VT-
　Popliteal
　　Left 04VN-
　　Right 04VM-
　Posterior Tibial
　　Left 04VS-
　　Right 04VR-
　Pulmonary
　　Left 02VR-
　　Right 02VQ-
　Pulmonary Trunk 02VP-
　Radial
　　Left 03VC-
　　Right 03VB-
　Renal
　　Left 04VA-
　　Right 04V9-
　Splenic 04V4-

Restriction — continued
Artery — continued
Subclavian
Left 03V4-
Right 03V3-
Superior Mesenteric 04V5-
Temporal
Left 03VT-
Right 03VS-
Thyroid
Left 03VV-
Right 03VU-
Ulnar
Left 03VA-
Right 03V9-
Upper 03VY-
Vertebral
Left 03VQ-
Right 03VP-
Bladder 0TVB-
Bladder Neck 0TVC-
Bronchus
Lingula 0BV9-
Lower Lobe
Left 0BVB-
Right 0BV6-
Main
Left 0BV7-
Right 0BV3-
Middle Lobe, Right 0BV5-
Upper Lobe
Left 0BV8-
Right 0BV4-
Carina 0BV2-
Cecum 0DVH-
Cervix 0UVC-
Cisterna Chyli 07VL-
Colon
Ascending 0DVK-
Descending 0DVM-
Sigmoid 0DVN-
Transverse 0DVL-
Duct
Common Bile 0FV9-
Cystic 0FV8-
Hepatic
Left 0FV6-
Right 0FV5-
Lacrimal
Left 08VY-
Right 08VX-
Pancreatic 0FVD-
Accessory 0FVF-
Parotid
Left 0CVC-
Right 0CVB-
Duodenum 0DV9-
Esophagogastric Junction 0DV4-
Esophagus 0DV5-
Lower 0DV3-
Middle 0DV2-
Upper 0DV1-
Heart 02VA-
Ileocecal Valve 0DVC-
Ileum 0DVB-
Intestine
Large 0DVE-
Left 0DVG-
Right 0DVF-
Small 0DV8-
Jejunum 0DVA-
Kidney Pelvis
Left 0TV4-
Right 0TV3-
Lymphatic
Aortic 07VD-
Axillary
Left 07V6-
Right 07V5-
Head 07V0-

Restriction — continued
Lymphatic — continued
Inguinal
Left 07VJ-
Right 07VH-
Internal Mammary
Left 07V9-
Right 07V8-
Lower Extremity
Left 07VG-
Right 07VF-
Mesenteric 07VB-
Neck
Left 07V2-
Right 07V1-
Pelvis 07VC-
Thoracic Duct 07VK-
Thorax 07V7-
Upper Extremity
Left 07V4-
Right 07V3-
Rectum 0DVP-
Stomach 0DV6-
Pylorus 0DV7-
Trachea 0BV1-
Ureter
Left 0TV7-
Right 0TV6-
Urethra 0TVD-
Vein
Axillary
Left 05V8-
Right 05V7-
Azygos 05V0-
Basilic
Left 05VC-
Right 05VB-
Brachial
Left 05VA-
Right 05V9-
Cephalic
Left 05VF-
Right 05VD-
Colic 06V7-
Common Iliac
Left 06VD-
Right 06VC-
Esophageal 06V3-
External Iliac
Left 06VG-
Right 06VF-
External Jugular
Left 05VQ-
Right 05VP-
Face
Left 05VV-
Right 05VT-
Femoral
Left 06VN-
Right 06VM-
Foot
Left 06VV-
Right 06VT-
Gastric 06V2-
Greater Saphenous
Left 06VQ-
Right 06VP-
Hand
Left 05VH-
Right 05VG-
Hemiazygos 05V1-
Hepatic 06V4-
Hypogastric
Left 06VJ-
Right 06VH-
Inferior Mesenteric 06V6-
Innominate
Left 05V4-
Right 05V3-
Internal Jugular
Left 05VN-
Right 05VM-

Restriction — continued
Vein — continued
Intracranial 05VL-
Lesser Saphenous
Left 06VS-
Right 06VR-
Lower 06V8-
Portal 06V8-
Pulmonary
Left 02VT-
Right 02VS-
Renal
Left 06VB-
Right 06V9-
Splenic 06V1-
Subclavian
Left 05V6-
Right 05V5-
Superior Mesenteric 06V5-
Upper 05VY-
Vertebral
Left 05VS-
Right 05VR-
Vena Cava
Inferior 06V0-
Superior 02VV-
Resurfacing Device
Removal of device from
Hip joint
Left 0SPB0BZ
Right 0SP90BZ
Revision of device in
Hip joint
Left 0SWB0BZ
Right 0SW90BZ
Supplement
Hip joint
Left 0SUB0BZ
Acetabular Surface 0SUE0BZ
Femoral Surface 0SUS0BZ
Right 0SU90BZ
Acetabular Surface 0SUA0BZ
Femoral Surface 0SUR0BZ
Resuscitation
Cardiopulmonary see Assistance, Cardiac 5A02-
Cardioversion 5A2204Z
Defibrillation 5A2204Z
Endotracheal intubation see Insertion of device in, Trachea 0BH1-
External chest compression 5A12012
Pulmonary 5A19054
Resuture, Heart valve prosthesis see Revision of device in, Heart and Great Vessels 02W-
Retraining
Cardiac see Motor Treatment, Rehabilitation F07-
Vocational see Activities of Daily Living Treatment, Rehabilitation F08-
Retrogasserian rhizotomy see Division, Nerve, Trigeminal 008K-
Retroperitoneal lymph node use Lymphatic, Aortic
Retroperitoneal space use Retroperitoneum
Retropharyngeal lymph node
use Lymphatic, Neck, Left
use Lymphatic, Neck, Right
Retropubic space use Pelvic Cavity
Reveal (DX) (XT) use Monitoring Device
Reverse total shoulder replacement see Replacement, Upper Joints 0RR-
Reverse® Shoulder Prosthesis use Synthetic Substitute, Reverse Ball and Socket in 0RR-

Revision
Correcting a portion of existing device
see Revision of device in
Removal of device without replacement
see Removal of device from
Replacement of existing device
see Removal of device from
see Root operation to place new device, e.g., Insertion, Replacement, Supplement
Revision of device in
Abdominal Wall 0WWF-
Acetabulum
Left 0QW5-
Right 0QW4-
Anal Sphincter 0DWR-
Anus 0DWQ-
Artery
Lower 04WY-
Upper 03WY-
Auditory Ossicle
Left 09WA-
Right 09W9-
Back
Lower 0WWL-
Upper 0WWK-
Bladder 0TWB-
Bone
Facial 0NWW-
Lower 0QWY-
Nasal 0NWB-
Pelvic
Left 0QW3-
Right 0QW2-
Upper 0PWY-
Bone Marrow 07WT-
Brain 00W0-
Breast
Left 0HWU-
Right 0HWT-
Bursa and Ligament
Lower 0MWY-
Upper 0MWX-
Carpal
Left 0PWN-
Right 0PWM-
Cavity, Cranial 0WW1-
Cerebral Ventricle 00W6-
Chest Wall 0WW8-
Cisterna Chyli 07WL-
Clavicle
Left 0PWB-
Right 0PW9-
Coccyx 0QWS-
Diaphragm 0BWT-
Disc
Cervical Vertebral 0RW3-
Cervicothoracic Vertebral 0RW5-
Lumbar Vertebral 0SW2-
Lumbosacral 0SW4-
Thoracic Vertebral 0RW9-
Thoracolumbar Vertebral 0RWB-
Duct
Hepatobiliary 0FWB-
Pancreatic 0FWD-
Ear
Inner
Left 09WE-
Right 09WD-
Left 09WJ-
Right 09WH-
Epididymis and Spermatic Cord 0VWM-
Esophagus 0DW5-
Extremity
Lower
Left 0YWB-
Right 0YW9-
Upper
Left 0XW7-
Right 0XW6-

INDEX TO PROCEDURES – 2016 ICD-10-PCS

Revision of device in — *continued*
Eye
  Left 08W1-
  Right 08W0-
Face 0WW2-
Fallopian Tube 0UW8-
Femoral Shaft
  Left 0QW9-
  Right 0QW8-
Femur
  Lower
    Left 0QWC-
    Right 0QWB-
  Upper
    Left 0QW7-
    Right 0QW6-
Fibula
  Left 0QWK-
  Right 0QWJ-
Finger Nail 0HWQX-
Gallbladder 0FW4-
Gastrointestinal Tract 0WWP-
Genitourinary Tract 0WWR-
Gland
  Adrenal 0GW5-
  Endocrine 0GWS-
  Pituitary 0GW0-
  Salivary 0CWA-
Glenoid Cavity
  Left 0PW8-
  Right 0PW7-
Great Vessel 02WY-
Hair 0HWSX-
Head 0WW0-
Heart 02WA-
Humeral Head
  Left 0PWD-
  Right 0PWC-
Humeral Shaft
  Left 0PWG-
  Right 0PWF-
Intestinal Tract
  Lower 0DWD-
  Upper 0DW0-
Intestine
  Large 0DWE-
  Small 0DW8-
Jaw
  Lower 0WW5-
  Upper 0WW4-
Joint
  Acromioclavicular
    Left 0RWH-
    Right 0RWG-
  Ankle
    Left 0SWG-
    Right 0SWF-
  Carpal
    Left 0RWR-
    Right 0RWQ-
  Cervical Vertebral 0RW1-
  Cervicothoracic Vertebral 0RW4-
  Coccygeal 0SW6-
  Elbow
    Left 0RWM-
    Right 0RWL-
  Finger Phalangeal
    Left 0RWX-
    Right 0RWW-
  Hip
    Left 0SWB-
    Right 0SW9-
  Knee
    Left 0SWD-
    Right 0SWC-
  Lumbar Vertebral 0SW0-
  Lumbosacral 0SW3-
  Metacarpocarpal
    Left 0RWT-
    Right 0RWS-

Revision of device in — *continued*
Joint — *continued*
  Metacarpophalangeal
    Left 0RWV-
    Right 0RWU-
  Metatarsal-Phalangeal
    Left 0SWN-
    Right 0SWM-
  Metatarsal-Tarsal
    Left 0SWL-
    Right 0SWK-
  Occipital-cervical 0RW0-
  Sacrococcygeal 0SW5-
  Sacroiliac
    Left 0SW8-
    Right 0SW7-
  Shoulder
    Left 0RWK-
    Right 0RWJ-
  Sternoclavicular
    Left 0RWF-
    Right 0RWE-
  Tarsal
    Left 0SWJ-
    Right 0SWH-
  Temporomandibular
    Left 0RWD-
    Right 0RWC-
  Thoracic Vertebral 0RW6-
  Thoracolumbar Vertebral 0RWA-
  Toe Phalangeal
    Left 0SWQ-
    Right 0SWP-
  Wrist
    Left 0RWP-
    Right 0RWN-
Kidney 0TW5-
Larynx 0CWS-
Lens
  Left 08WK-
  Right 08WJ-
Liver 0FW0-
Lung
  Left 0BWL-
  Right 0BWK-
Lymphatic 07WN-
  Thoracic Duct 07WK-
Mediastinum 0WWC-
Mesentery 0DWV-
Metacarpal
  Left 0PWQ-
  Right 0PWP-
Metatarsal
  Left 0QWP-
  Right 0QWN-
Mouth and Throat 0CWY-
Muscle
  Extraocular
    Left 08WM-
    Right 08WL-
  Lower 0KWY-
  Upper 0KWX-
Neck 0WW6-
Nerve
  Cranial 00WE-
  Peripheral 01WY-
Nose 09WK-
Omentum 0DWU-
Ovary 0UW3-
Pancreas 0FWG-
Parathyroid Gland 0GWR-
Patella
  Left 0QWF-
  Right 0QWD-
Pelvic Cavity 0WWJ-
Penis 0VWS-
Pericardial Cavity 0WWD-
Perineum
  Female 0WWN-
  Male 0WWM-
Peritoneal Cavity 0WWG-
Peritoneum 0DWW-

Revision of device in — *continued*
Phalanx
  Finger
    Left 0PWV-
    Right 0PWT-
  Thumb
    Left 0PWS-
    Right 0PWR-
  Toe
    Left 0QWR-
    Right 0QWQ-
Pineal Body 0GW1-
Pleura 0BWQ-
Pleural Cavity
  Left 0WWB-
  Right 0WW9-
Prostate and Seminal Vesicles 0VW4-
Radius
  Left 0PWJ-
  Right 0PWH-
Respiratory Tract 0WWQ-
Retroperitoneum 0WWH-
Rib
  Left 0PW2-
  Right 0PW1-
Sacrum 0QW1-
Scapula
  Left 0PW6-
  Right 0PW5-
Scrotum and Tunica Vaginalis 0VW8-
Septum
  Atrial 02W5-
  Ventricular 02WM-
Sinus 09WY-
Skin 0HWPX-
Skull 0NW0-
Spinal Canal 00WU-
Spinal Cord 00WV-
Spleen 07WP-
Sternum 0PW0-
Stomach 0DW6-
Subcutaneous Tissue and Fascia
  Head and Neck 0JWS-
  Lower Extremity 0JWW-
  Trunk 0JWT-
  Upper Extremity 0JWV-
Tarsal
  Left 0QWM-
  Right 0QWL-
Tendon
  Lower 0LWY-
  Upper 0LWX-
Testis 0VWD-
Thymus 07WM-
Thyroid Gland 0GWK-
Tibia
  Left 0QWH-
  Right 0QWG-
Toe Nail 0HWRX-
Trachea 0BW1-
Tracheobronchial Tree 0BW0-
Tympanic Membrane
  Left 09W8-
  Right 09W7-
Ulna
  Left 0PWL-
  Right 0PWK-
Ureter 0TW9-
Urethra 0TWD-
Uterus and Cervix 0UWD-
Vagina and Cul-de-sac 0UWH-
Valve
  Aortic 02WF-
  Mitral 02WG-
  Pulmonary 02WH-
  Tricuspid 02WJ-
Vas Deferens 0VWR-
Vein
  Lower 06WY-
  Upper 05WY-

Revision of device in — *continued*
Vertebra
  Cervical 0PW3-
  Lumbar 0QW0-
  Thoracic 0PW4-
Vulva 0UWM-
Revo MRI™ SureScan® pacemaker
  use Pacemaker, Dual Chamber in **0JH**
rhBMP-2 *use* Recombinant Bone Morphogenetic Protein
Rheos® System device
  use Stimulator Generator in Subcutaneous Tissue and Fascia
Rheos® System lead
  use Stimulator Lead in Upper Arteries
Rhinopharynx
  use Nasopharynx
Rhinoplasty
  see Alteration, Nose 090K-
  see Repair, Nose 09QK-
  see Replacement, Nose 09RK-
  see Supplement, Nose 09UK-
Rhinorrhaphy *see* Repair, Nose 09QK-
Rhinoscopy 09JKXZZ
Rhizotomy
  see Division, Central Nervous System 008-
  see Division, Peripheral Nervous System 018-
Rhomboid major muscle
  use Muscle, Trunk, Left
  use Muscle, Trunk, Right
Rhomboid minor muscle
  use Muscle, Trunk, Left
  use Muscle, Trunk, Right
Rhythm electrocardiogram *see* Measurement, Cardiac 4A02-
Rhytidectomy *see* Face lift
Right ascending lumbar vein
  use Vein, Azygos
Right atrioventricular valve
  use Valve, Tricuspid
Right auricular appendix
  use Atrium, Right
Right colic vein
  use Vein, Colic
Right coronary sulcus
  use Heart, Right
Right gastric artery
  use Artery, Gastric
Right gastroepiploic vein
  use Vein, Superior Mesenteric
Right inferior phrenic vein
  use Vena Cava, Inferior
Right inferior pulmonary vein
  use Vein, Pulmonary, Right
Right jugular trunk
  use Lymphatic, Neck, Right
Right lateral ventricle
  use Cerebral Ventricle
Right lymphatic duct
  use Lymphatic, Neck, Right
Right ovarian vein
  use Vena Cava, Inferior
Right second lumbar vein
  use Vena Cava, Inferior
Right subclavian trunk
  use Lymphatic, Neck, Right
Right subcostal vein
  use Vein, Azygos
Right superior pulmonary vein
  use Vein, Pulmonary, Right
Right suprarenal vein
  use Vena Cava, Inferior
Right testicular vein
  use Vena Cava, Inferior
Rima glottidis
  use Larynx

Risorius muscle
 use Muscle, Facial
RNS System lead
 use Neurostimulator Lead in Central Nervous System
RNS system neurostimulator generator
 use Neurostimulator Generator in Head and Facial Bones
Robotic Assisted Procedure
 Extremity
  Lower 8E0Y
  Upper 8E0X
 Head and Neck Region 8E09-
 Trunk Region 8E0W-
Rotation of fetal head
 Forceps 10S07ZZ
 Manual 10S0XZZ
Round ligament of uterus
 use Uterine Supporting Structure
Round window
 use Ear, Inner, Left
 use Ear, Inner, Right
Roux-en-Y operation
 see Bypass, Gastrointestinal System 0D1-
 see Bypass, Hepatobiliary System and Pancreas 0F1-
Rupture
 Adhesions see Release
 Fluid collection see Drainage

S

Sacral ganglion
 use Nerve, Sacral Sympathetic
Sacral lymph node
 use Lymphatic, Pelvis
Sacral nerve modulation (SNM) lead
 use Stimulator Lead in Urinary System
Sacral neuromodulation lead
 use Stimulator Lead in Urinary System
Sacral splanchnic nerve
 use Nerve, Sacral Sympathetic
Sacrectomy see Excision, Lower Bones 0QB-
Sacrococcygeal ligament
 use Bursa and Ligament, Trunk, Left
 use Bursa and Ligament, Trunk, Right
Sacrococcygeal symphysis
 use Joint, Sacrococcygeal
Sacroiliac ligament
 use Bursa and Ligament, Trunk, Left
 use Bursa and Ligament, Trunk, Right
Sacrospinous ligament
 use Bursa and Ligament, Trunk, Left
 use Bursa and Ligament, Trunk, Right
Sacrotuberous ligament
 use Bursa and Ligament, Trunk, Left
 use Bursa and Ligament, Trunk, Right
Salpingectomy
 see Excision, Female Reproductive System 0UB-
 see Resection, Female Reproductive System 0UT-
Salpingolysis see Release, Female Reproductive System 0UN-
Salpingopexy
 see Repair, Female Reproductive System 0UQ-
 see Reposition, Female Reproductive System 0US-
Salpingopharyngeus muscle
 use Muscle, Tongue, Palate, Pharynx
Salpingoplasty
 see Repair, Female Reproductive System 0UQ-
 see Supplement, Female Reproductive System 0UU-
Salpingorrhaphy see Repair, Female Reproductive System 0UQ-
Salpingoscopy 0UJ88ZZ
Salpingostomy see Drainage, Female Reproductive System 0U9-
Salpingotomy see Drainage, Female Reproductive System 0U9-
Salpinx
 use Fallopian Tube, Left
 use Fallopian Tube, Right
Saphenous nerve
 use Nerve, Femoral
SAPIEN transcatheter aortic valve
 use Zooplastic Tissue in Heart and Great Vessels
Sartorius muscle
 use Muscle, Upper Leg, Left
 use Muscle, Upper Leg, Right
Scalene muscle
 use Muscle, Neck, Left
 use Muscle, Neck, Right
Scan
 Computerized Tomography (CT) see Computerized Tomography (CT Scan)
 Radioisotope see Planar Nuclear Medicine Imaging
Scaphoid bone
 use Carpal, Left
 use Carpal, Right

Scapholunate ligament
 use Bursa and Ligament, Hand, Left
 use Bursa and Ligament, Hand, Right
Scaphotrapezium ligament
 use Bursa and Ligament, Hand, Left
 use Bursa and Ligament, Hand, Right
Scapulectomy
 see Excision, Upper Bones 0PB-
 see Resection, Upper Bones 0PT-
Scapulopexy
 see Repair, Upper Bones 0PQ-
 see Reposition, Upper Bones 0PS-
Scarpa's (vestibular) ganglion
 use Nerve, Acoustic
Sclerectomy see Excision, Eye 08B-
Sclerotherapy, mechanical see Destruction
Sclerotomy see Drainage, Eye 089-
Scrotectomy
 see Excision, Male Reproductive System 0VB-
 see Resection, Male Reproductive System 0VT-
Scrotoplasty
 see Repair, Male Reproductive System 0VQ-
 see Supplement, Male Reproductive System 0VU-
Scrotorrhaphy see Repair, Male Reproductive System 0VQ-
Scrototomy see Drainage, Male Reproductive System 0V9-
Sebaceous gland
 use Skin
Second cranial nerve
 use Nerve, Optic
Section, cesarean see Extraction, Pregnancy 10D-
Secura (DR) (VR)
 use Defibrillator Generator in 0JH-
Sella Turcica
 use Bone, Sphenoid, Left
 use Bone, Sphenoid, Right
Semicircular canal
 use Ear, Inner, Left
 use Ear, Inner, Right
Semimembranosus muscle
 use Muscle, Upper Leg, Left
 use Muscle, Upper Leg, Right
Semitendinosus muscle
 use Muscle, Upper Leg, Left
 use Muscle, Upper Leg, Right
Seprafilm
 use Adhesion Barrier
Septal cartilage
 use Septum, Nasal
Septectomy
 see Excision, Ear, Nose, Sinus 09B-
 see Excision, Heart and Great Vessels 02B-
 see Resection, Ear, Nose, Sinus 09T-
 see Resection, Heart and Great Vessels 02T-
Septoplasty
 see Repair, Ear, Nose, Sinus 09Q-
 see Repair, Heart and Great Vessels 02Q-
 see Replacement, Ear, Nose, Sinus 09R-
 see Replacement, Heart and Great Vessels 02R-
 see Reposition, Ear, Nose, Sinus 09S-
 see Supplement, Ear, Nose, Sinus 09U-
 see Supplement, Heart and Great Vessels 02U-
Septotomy see Drainage, Ear, Nose, Sinus 099-
Sequestrectomy, bone see Extirpation

Serratus anterior muscle
 use Muscle, Thorax, Left
 use Muscle, Thorax, Right
Serratus posterior muscle
 use Muscle, Trunk, Left
 use Muscle, Trunk, Right
Seventh cranial nerve
 use Nerve, Facial
Sheffield hybrid external fixator
 use External Fixation Device, Hybrid in 0PH-
 use External Fixation Device, Hybrid in 0PS-
 use External Fixation Device, Hybrid in 0QH-
 use External Fixation Device, Hybrid in 0QS-
Sheffield ring external fixator
 use External Fixation Device, Ring in 0PH-
 use External Fixation Device, Ring in 0PS-
 use External Fixation Device, Ring in 0QH-
 use External Fixation Device, Ring in 0QS-
Shirodkar cervical cerclage 0UVC7ZZ
Shock Wave Therapy, Musculoskeletal 6A93-
Short gastric artery
 use Artery, Splenic
Shortening
 see Excision
 see Repair
 see Reposition
Shunt creation see Bypass
Sialoadenectomy
 Complete see Resection, Mouth and Throat 0CT-
 Partial see Excision, Mouth and Throat 0CB-
Sialodochoplasty
 see Repair, Mouth and Throat 0CQ-
 see Replacement, Mouth and Throat 0CR-
 see Supplement, Mouth and Throat 0CU-
Sialoectomy
 see Excision, Mouth and Throat 0CB-
 see Resection, Mouth and Throat 0CT-
Sialography see Plain Radiography, Ear, Nose, Mouth and Throat B90-
Sialolithotomy see Extirpation, Mouth and Throat 0CC-
Sigmoid artery
 use Artery, Inferior Mesenteric
Sigmoid flexure
 use Colon, Sigmoid
Sigmoid vein
 use Vein, Inferior Mesenteric
Sigmoidectomy
 see Excision, Gastrointestinal System 0DB-
 see Resection, Gastrointestinal System 0DT-
Sigmoidorrhaphy see Repair, Gastrointestinal System 0DQ-
Sigmoidoscopy 0DJD8ZZ
Sigmoidotomy see Drainage, Gastrointestinal System 0D9-
Single lead pacemaker (atrium) (ventricle)
 use Pacemaker, Single Chamber in 0JH-
Single lead rate responsive pacemaker (atrium) (ventricle)
 use Pacemaker, Single Chamber Rate Responsive in 0JH-
Sinoatrial node
 use Conduction Mechanism

INDEX TO PROCEDURES – 2016 ICD-10-PCS

Spinal

Sinogram
Abdominal Wall see Fluoroscopy, Abdomen and Pelvis BW11-
Chest Wall see Plain Radiography, Chest BW03-
Retroperitoneum see Fluoroscopy, Abdomen and Pelvis BW11-

Sinus venosus
use Atrium, Right

Sinusectomy
see Excision, Ear, Nose, Sinus 09B-
see Resection, Ear, Nose, Sinus 09T-

Sinusoscopy 09JY4ZZ

Sinusotomy see Drainage, Ear, Nose, Sinus 099-

Sirolimus-eluting coronary stent
use Intraluminal Device, Drug-eluting in Heart and Great Vessels

Sixth cranial nerve
use Nerve, Abducens

Size reduction, breast see Excision, Skin and Breast 0HB-

SJM Biocor® Stented Valve System
use Zooplastic Tissue in Heart and Great Vessels

Skene's (paraurethral) gland
use Gland, Vestibular

Sling
Fascial, orbicularis muscle (mouth) see Supplement, Muscle, Facial 0KU1-
Levator muscle, for urethral suspension see Reposition, Bladder Neck 0TSC-
Pubococcygeal, for urethral suspension see Reposition, Bladder Neck 0TSC-
Rectum see Reposition, Rectum 0DSP-

Small bowel series see Fluoroscopy, Bowel, Small BD13-

Small saphenous vein
use Vein, Lesser Saphenous, Left
use Vein, Lesser Saphenous, Right

Snaring, polyp, colon see Excision, Gastrointestinal System 0DB-

Solar (celiac) plexus
use Nerve, Abdominal Sympathetic

Soleus muscle
use Muscle, Lower Leg, Left
use Muscle, Lower Leg, Right

Spacer
Insertion of device in
  Disc
    Lumbar Vertebral 0SH2-
    Lumbosacral 0SH4-
  Joint
    Acromioclavicular
      Left 0RHH-
      Right 0RHG-
    Ankle
      Left 0SHG-
      Right 0SHF-
    Carpal
      Left 0RHR-
      Right 0RHQ-
    Cervical Vertebral 0RH1-
    Cervicothoracic Vertebral 0RH4-
    Coccygeal 0SH6-
    Elbow
      Left 0RHM-
      Right 0RHL-
    Finger Phalangeal
      Left 0RHX-
      Right 0RHW-
    Hip
      Left 0SHB-
      Right 0SH9-

Spacer — *continued*
Insertion of device in — *continued*
  Joint — *continued*
    Knee
      Left 0SHD-
      Right 0SHC-
    Lumbar Vertebral 0SH0-
    Lumbosacral 0SH3-
    Metacarpocarpal
      Left 0RHT-
      Right 0RHS-
    Metacarpophalangeal
      Left 0RHV-
      Right 0RHU-
    Metatarsal-Phalangeal
      Left 0SHN-
      Right 0SHM-
    Metatarsal-Tarsal
      Left 0SHL-
      Right 0SHK-
    Occipital-cervical 0RH0-
    Sacrococcygeal 0SH5-
    Sacroiliac
      Left 0SH8-
      Right 0SH7-
    Shoulder
      Left 0RHK-
      Right 0RHJ-
    Sternoclavicular
      Left 0RHF-
      Right 0RHE-
    Tarsal
      Left 0SHJ-
      Right 0SHH-
    Temporomandibular
      Left 0RHD-
      Right 0RHC-
    Thoracic Vertebral 0RH6-
    Thoracolumbar Vertebral 0RHA-
    Toe Phalangeal
      Left 0SHQ-
      Right 0SHP-
    Wrist
      Left 0RHP-
      Right 0RHN-
Removal of device from
  Acromioclavicular
    Left 0RPH-
    Right 0RPG-
  Ankle
    Left 0SPG-
    Right 0SPF-
  Carpal
    Left 0RPR-
    Right 0RPQ-
  Cervical Vertebral 0RP1-
  Cervicothoracic Vertebral 0RP4-
  Coccygeal 0SP6-
  Elbow
    Left 0RPM-
    Right 0RPL-
  Finger Phalangeal
    Left 0RPX-
    Right 0RPW-
  Hip
    Left 0SPB-
    Right 0SP9-
  Knee
    Left 0SPD-
    Right 0SPC-
  Lumbar Vertebral 0SP0-
  Lumbosacral 0SP3-
  Metacarpocarpal
    Left 0RPT-
    Right 0RPS-
  Metacarpophalangeal
    Left 0RPV-
    Right 0RPU-
  Metatarsal-Phalangeal
    Left 0SPN-
    Right 0SPM-

Spacer — *continued*
Removal of device from — *continued*
  Metatarsal-Tarsal
    Left 0SPL-
    Right 0SPK-
  Occipital-cervical 0RP0-
  Sacrococcygeal 0SP5-
  Sacroiliac
    Left 0SP8-
    Right 0SP7-
  Shoulder
    Left 0RPK-
    Right 0RPJ-
  Sternoclavicular
    Left 0RPF-
    Right 0RPE-
  Tarsal
    Left 0SPJ-
    Right 0SPH-
  Temporomandibular
    Left 0RPD-
    Right 0RPC-
  Thoracic Vertebral 0RP6-
  Thoracolumbar Vertebral 0RPA-
  Toe Phalangeal
    Left 0SPQ-
    Right 0SPP-
  Wrist
    Left 0RPP-
    Right 0RPN-
Revision of device in
  Acromioclavicular
    Left 0RWH-
    Right 0RWG-
  Ankle
    Left 0SWG-
    Right 0SWF-
  Carpal
    Left 0RWR-
    Right 0RWQ-
  Cervical Vertebral 0RW1-
  Cervicothoracic Vertebral 0RW4-
  Coccygeal 0SW6-
  Elbow
    Left 0RWM-
    Right 0RWL-
  Finger Phalangeal
    Left 0RWX-
    Right 0RWW-
  Hip
    Left 0SWB-
    Right 0SW9-
  Knee
    Left 0SWD-
    Right 0SWC-
  Lumbar Vertebral 0SW0-
  Lumbosacral 0SW3-
  Metacarpocarpal
    Left 0RWT-
    Right 0RWS-
  Metacarpophalangeal
    Left 0RWV-
    Right 0RWU-
  Metatarsal-Phalangeal
    Left 0SWN-
    Right 0SWM-
  Metatarsal-Tarsal
    Left 0SWL-
    Right 0SWK-
  Occipital-cervical 0RW0-
  Sacrococcygeal 0SW5-
  Sacroiliac
    Left 0SW8-
    Right 0SW7-
  Shoulder
    Left 0RWK-
    Right 0RWJ-
  Sternoclavicular
    Left 0RWF-
    Right 0RWE-

Spacer — *continued*
Revision of device in — *continued*
  Tarsal
    Left 0SWJ-
    Right 0SWH-
  Temporomandibular
    Left 0RWD-
    Right 0RWC-
  Thoracic Vertebral 0RW6-
  Thoracolumbar Vertebral 0RWA-
  Toe Phalangeal
    Left 0SWQ-
    Right 0SWP-
  Wrist
    Left 0RWP-
    Right 0RWN-

Spectroscopy
Intravascular 8E023DZ
Near infrared 8E023DZ

Speech Assessment F00

Speech therapy see Speech Treatment, Rehabilitation F06-

Speech Treatment F06-

Sphenoidectomy
see Excision, Ear, Nose, Sinus 09B-
see Excision, Head and Facial Bones 0NB-
see Resection, Ear, Nose, Sinus 09T-
see Resection, Head and Facial Bones 0NT-

Sphenoidotomy see Drainage, Ear, Nose, Sinus 099-

Sphenomandibular ligament
use Bursa and Ligament, Head and Neck

Sphenopalatine (pterygopalatine) ganglion
use Nerve, Head and Neck Sympathetic

Sphincterorrhaphy, anal see Repair, Anal Sphincter 0DQR-

Sphincterotomy, anal
see Division, Anal Sphincter 0D8R-
see Drainage, Anal Sphincter 0D9R-

Spinal cord neurostimulator lead
use Neurostimulator Lead in Central Nervous System

Spinal nerve, cervical
use Nerve, Cervical

Spinal nerve, lumbar
use Nerve, Lumbar

Spinal nerve, sacral
use Nerve, Sacral

Spinal nerve, thoracic
use Nerve, Thoracic

Spinal Stabilization Device
Facet Replacement
  Cervical Vertebral 0RH1-
  Cervicothoracic Vertebral 0RH4-
  Lumbar Vertebral 0SH0-
  Lumbosacral 0SH3-
  Occipital-cervical 0RH0-
  Thoracic Vertebral 0RH6-
  Thoracolumbar Vertebral 0RHA-
Interspinous Process
  Cervical Vertebral 0RH1-
  Cervicothoracic Vertebral 0RH4-
  Lumbar Vertebral 0SH0-
  Lumbosacral 0SH3-
  Occipital-cervical 0RH0-
  Thoracic Vertebral 0RH6-
  Thoracolumbar Vertebral 0RHA-
Pedicle-Based
  Cervical Vertebral 0RH1-
  Cervicothoracic Vertebral 0RH4-
  Lumbar Vertebral 0SH0-
  Lumbosacral 0SH3-
  Occipital-cervical 0RH0-
  Thoracic Vertebral 0RH6-
  Thoracolumbar Vertebral 0RHA-

Spinous

INDEX TO PROCEDURES – 2016 ICD-10-PCS

Spinous process
 use Vertebra, Cervical
 use Vertebra, Lumbar
 use Vertebra, Thoracic

Spiral ganglion
 use Nerve, Acoustic

Spiration IBV™ Valve System
 use Intraluminal Device, Endobronchial Valve in Respiratory System

Splenectomy
 see Excision, Lymphatic and Hemic Systems 07B-
 see Resection, Lymphatic and Hemic Systems 07T-

Splenic flexure
 use Colon, Transverse

Splenic plexus
 use Nerve, Abdominal Sympathetic

Splenius capitis muscle
 use Muscle, Head

Splenius cervicis muscle
 use Muscle, Neck, Left
 use Muscle, Neck, Right

Splenolysis see Release, Lymphatic and Hemic Systems 07N-

Splenopexy
 see Repair, Lymphatic and Hemic Systems 07Q-
 see Reposition, Lymphatic and Hemic Systems 07S-

Splenoplasty see Repair, Lymphatic and Hemic Systems 07Q-

Splenorrhaphy see Repair, Lymphatic and Hemic Systems 07Q-

Splenotomy see Drainage, Lymphatic and Hemic Systems 079-

Splinting, musculoskeletal see Immobilization, Anatomical Regions 2W3-

Stapedectomy
 see Excision, Ear, Nose, Sinus 09B-
 see Resection, Ear, Nose, Sinus 09T-

Stapediolysis see Release, Ear, Nose, Sinus 09N-

Stapedioplasty
 see Repair, Ear, Nose, Sinus 09Q-
 see Replacement, Ear, Nose, Sinus 09R-
 see Supplement, Ear, Nose, Sinus 09U-

Stapedotomy see Drainage, Ear, Nose, Sinus 099-

Stapes
 use Auditory Ossicle, Left
 use Auditory Ossicle, Right

Stellate ganglion
 use Nerve, Head and Neck Sympathetic

Stensen's duct
 use Duct, Parotid, Left
 use Duct, Parotid, Right

Stent, intraluminal (cardiovascular) (gastrointestinal) (hepatobiliary) (urinary)
 use Intraluminal Device

Stented tissue valve
 use Zooplastic Tissue in Heart and Great Vessels

Stereotactic Radiosurgery
 Abdomen DW23-
 Adrenal Gland DG22-
 Bile Ducts DF22-
 Bladder DT22-
 Bone Marrow D720-
 Brain D020-
 Brain Stem D021-
 Breast
  Left DM20-
  Right DM21-
 Bronchus DB21-

Stereotactic Radiosurgery — continued
 Cervix DU21-
 Chest DW22-
 Chest Wall DB27-
 Colon DD25-
 Diaphragm DB28-
 Duodenum DD22-
 Ear D920-
 Esophagus DD20-
 Eye D820-
 Gallbladder DF21-
 Gamma Beam
  Abdomen DW23JZZ
  Adrenal Gland DG22JZZ
  Bile Ducts DF22JZZ
  Bladder DT22JZZ
  Bone Marrow D720JZZ
  Brain D020JZZ
  Brain Stem D021JZZ
  Breast
   Left DM20JZZ
   Right DM21JZZ
  Bronchus DB21JZZ
  Cervix DU21JZZ
  Chest DW22JZZ
  Chest Wall DB27JZZ
  Colon DD25JZZ
  Diaphragm DB28JZZ
  Duodenum DD22JZZ
  Ear D920JZZ
  Esophagus DD20JZZ
  Eye D820JZZ
  Gallbladder DF21JZZ
  Gland
   Adrenal DG22JZZ
   Parathyroid DG24JZZ
   Pituitary DG20JZZ
   Thyroid DG25JZZ
  Glands, Salivary D926JZZ
  Head and Neck DW21JZZ
  Ileum DD24JZZ
  Jejunum DD23JZZ
  Kidney DT20JZZ
  Larynx D92BJZZ
  Liver DF20JZZ
  Lung DB22JZZ
  Lymphatics
   Abdomen D726JZZ
   Axillary D724JZZ
   Inguinal D728JZZ
   Neck D723JZZ
   Pelvis D727JZZ
   Thorax D725JZZ
  Mediastinum DB26JZZ
  Mouth D924JZZ
  Nasopharynx D92DJZZ
  Neck and Head DW21JZZ
  Nerve, Peripheral D027JZZ
  Nose D921JZZ
  Ovary DU20JZZ
  Palate
   Hard D928JZZ
   Soft D929JZZ
  Pancreas DF23JZZ
  Parathyroid Gland DG24JZZ
  Pelvic Region DW26JZZ
  Pharynx D92CJZZ
  Pineal Body DG21JZZ
  Pituitary Gland DG20JZZ
  Pleura DB25JZZ
  Prostate DV20JZZ
  Rectum DD27JZZ
  Sinuses D927JZZ
  Spinal Cord D026JZZ
  Spleen D722JZZ
  Stomach DD21JZZ
  Testis DV21JZZ
  Thymus D721JZZ
  Thyroid Gland DG25JZZ
  Tongue D925JZZ
  Trachea DB20JZZ

Stereotactic Radiosurgery — continued
 Gamma Beam — continued
  Ureter DT21JZZ
  Urethra DT23JZZ
  Uterus DU22JZZ
 Gland
  Adrenal DG22-
  Parathyroid DG24-
  Pituitary DG20-
  Thyroid DG25-
 Glands, Salivary D926-
 Head and Neck DW21-
 Ileum DD24-
 Jejunum DD23-
 Kidney DT20-
 Larynx D92B-
 Liver DF20-
 Lung DB22-
 Lymphatics
  Abdomen D726-
  Axillary D724-
  Inguinal D728-
  Neck D723-
  Pelvis D727-
  Thorax D725-
 Mediastinum DB26-
 Mouth D924-
 Nasopharynx D92D-
 Neck and Head DW21-
 Nerve, Peripheral D027-
 Nose D921-
 Other Photon
  Abdomen DW23DZZ
  Adrenal Gland DG22DZZ
  Bile Ducts DF22DZZ
  Bladder DT22DZZ
  Bone Marrow D720DZZ
  Brain D020DZZ
  Brain Stem D021DZZ
  Breast
   Left DM20DZZ
   Right DM21DZZ
  Bronchus DB21DZZ
  Cervix DU21DZZ
  Chest DW22DZZ
  Chest Wall DB27DZZ
  Colon DD25DZZ
  Diaphragm DB28DZZ
  Duodenum DD22DZZ
  Ear D920DZZ
  Esophagus DD20DZZ
  Eye D820DZZ
  Gallbladder DF21DZZ
  Gland
   Adrenal DG22DZZ
   Parathyroid DG24DZZ
   Pituitary DG20DZZ
   Thyroid DG25DZZ
  Glands, Salivary D926DZZ
  Head and Neck DW21DZZ
  Ileum DD24DZZ
  Jejunum DD23DZZ
  Kidney DT20DZZ
  Larynx D92BDZZ
  Liver DF20DZZ
  Lung DB22DZZ
  Lymphatics
   Abdomen D726DZZ
   Axillary D724DZZ
   Inguinal D728DZZ
   Neck D723DZZ
   Pelvis D727DZZ
   Thorax D725DZZ
  Mediastinum DB26DZZ
  Mouth D924DZZ
  Nasopharynx D92DDZZ
  Neck and Head DW21DZZ
  Nerve, Peripheral D027DZZ
  Nose D921DZZ
  Ovary DU20DZZ

Stereotactic Radiosurgery — continued
 Other Photon — continued
  Palate
   Hard D928DZZ
   Soft D929DZZ
  Pancreas DF23DZZ
  Parathyroid Gland DG24DZZ
  Pelvic Region DW26DZZ
  Pharynx D92CDZZ
  Pineal Body DG21DZZ
  Pituitary Gland DG20DZZ
  Pleura DB25DZZ
  Prostate DV20DZZ
  Rectum DD27DZZ
  Sinuses D927DZZ
  Spinal Cord D026DZZ
  Spleen D722DZZ
  Stomach DD21DZZ
  Testis DV21DZZ
  Thymus D721DZZ
  Thyroid Gland DG25DZZ
  Tongue D925DZZ
  Trachea DB20DZZ
  Ureter DT21DZZ
  Urethra DT23DZZ
  Uterus DU22DZZ
 Ovary DU20-
 Palate
  Hard D928-
  Soft D929-
 Pancreas DF23-
 Parathyroid Gland DG24-
 Particulate
  Abdomen DW23HZZ
  Adrenal Gland DG22HZZ
  Bile Ducts DF22HZZ
  Bladder DT22HZZ
  Bone Marrow D720HZZ
  Brain D020HZZ
  Brain Stem D021HZZ
  Breast
   Left DM20HZZ
   Right DM21HZZ
  Bronchus DB21HZZ
  Cervix DU21HZZ
  Chest DW22HZZ
  Chest Wall DB27HZZ
  Colon DD25HZZ
  Diaphragm DB28HZZ
  Duodenum DD22HZZ
  Ear D920HZZ
  Esophagus DD20HZZ
  Eye D820HZZ
  Gallbladder DF21HZZ
  Gland
   Adrenal DG22HZZ
   Parathyroid DG24HZZ
   Pituitary DG20HZZ
   Thyroid DG25HZZ
  Glands, Salivary D926HZZ
  Head and Neck DW21HZZ
  Ileum DD24HZZ
  Jejunum DD23HZZ
  Kidney DT20HZZ
  Larynx D92BHZZ
  Liver DF20HZZ
  Lung DB22HZZ
  Lymphatics
   Abdomen D726HZZ
   Axillary D724HZZ
   Inguinal D728HZZ
   Neck D723HZZ
   Pelvis D727HZZ
   Thorax D725HZZ
  Mediastinum DB26HZZ
  Mouth D924HZZ
  Nasopharynx D92DHZZ
  Neck and Head DW21HZZ
  Nerve, Peripheral D027HZZ
  Nose D921HZZ
  Ovary DU20HZZ

INDEX TO PROCEDURES – 2016 ICD-10-PCS

Stereotactic Radiosurgery — continued
Particulate — continued
  Palate
    Hard **D92**8HZZ
    Soft **D92**9HZZ
  Pancreas **DF2**3HZZ
  Parathyroid Gland **DG2**4HZZ
  Pelvic Region **DW2**6HZZ
  Pharynx **D92**CHZZ
  Pineal Body **DG2**1HZZ
  Pituitary Gland **DG2**0HZZ
  Pleura **DB2**5HZZ
  Prostate **DV2**0HZZ
  Rectum **DD2**7HZZ
  Sinuses **D92**7HZZ
  Spinal Cord **D02**6HZZ
  Spleen **D72**2HZZ
  Stomach **DD2**1HZZ
  Testis **DV2**1HZZ
  Thymus **D72**1HZZ
  Thyroid Gland **DG2**5HZZ
  Tongue **D92**5HZZ
  Trachea **DB2**0HZZ
  Ureter **DT2**1HZZ
  Urethra **DT2**3HZZ
  Uterus **DU2**2HZZ
Pelvic Region **DW2**6-
Pharynx **D92**C-
Pineal Body **DG2**1-
Pituitary Gland **DG2**0-
Pleura **DB2**5-
Prostate **DV2**0-
Rectum **DD2**7-
Sinuses **D92**7-
Spinal Cord **D02**6-
Spleen **D72**2-
Stomach **DD2**1-
Testis **DV2**1-
Thymus **D72**1-
Thyroid Gland **DG2**5-
Tongue **D92**5-
Trachea **DB2**0-
Ureter **DT2**1-
Urethra **DT2**3-
Uterus **DU2**2-

Sternoclavicular ligament
  use Bursa and Ligament, Shoulder, Left
  use Bursa and Ligament, Shoulder, Right

Sternocleidomastoid artery
  use Artery, Thyroid, Left
  use Artery, Thyroid, Right

Sternocleidomastoid muscle
  use Muscle, Neck, Left
  use Muscle, Neck, Right

Sternocostal ligament
  use Bursa and Ligament, Thorax, Left
  use Bursa and Ligament, Thorax, Right

Sternotomy
  see Division, Sternum **0P8**0-
  see Drainage, Sternum **0P9**0-

Stimulation, cardiac
  Cardioversion **5A2**204Z
  Electrophysiologic testing *see* Measurement, Cardiac **4A0**2-

Stimulator Generator
Insertion of device in
  Abdomen **0JH**8-
  Back **0JH**7-
  Chest **0JH**6-
Multiple Array
  Abdomen **0JH**8-
  Back **0JH**7-
  Chest **0JH**6-
Multiple Array Rechargeable
  Abdomen **0JH**8-
  Back **0JH**7-
  Chest **0JH**6-
Removal of device from, Subcutaneous Tissue and Fascia, Trunk **0JPT**-

Stimulator Generator — continued
Revision of device in, Subcutaneous Tissue and Fascia, Trunk **0JWT**-
Single Array
  Abdomen **0JH**8-
  Back **0JH**7-
  Chest **0JH**6-
Single Array Rechargeable
  Abdomen **0JH**8-
  Back **0JH**7-
  Chest **0JH**6-

Stimulator Lead
Insertion of device in
  Anal Sphincter **0DH**R-
  Artery
    Left **03H**L-
    Right **03H**K-
  Bladder **0TH**B-
  Muscle
    Lower **0KH**Y-
    Upper **0KH**X-
  Stomach **0DH**6-
  Ureter **0TH**9-
Removal of device from
  Anal Sphincter **0DP**R-
  Artery, Upper **03P**Y-
  Bladder **0TP**B-
  Muscle
    Lower **0KP**Y-
    Upper **0KP**X-
  Stomach **0DP**6-
  Ureter **0TP**9-
Revision of device in
  Anal Sphincter **0DW**R-
  Artery, Upper **03W**Y-
  Bladder **0TW**B-
  Muscle
    Lower **0KW**Y-
    Upper **0KW**X-
  Stomach **0DW**6-
  Ureter **0TW**9-

Stoma
Excision
  Abdominal Wall **0WB**FXZ2
  Neck **0WB**6XZ2
Repair
  Abdominal Wall **0WQ**FXZ2
  Neck **0WQ**6XZ2

Stomatoplasty
  see Repair, Mouth and Throat **0CQ**-
  see Replacement, Mouth and Throat **0CR**-
  see Supplement, Mouth and Throat **0CU**-

Stomatorrhaphy *see* Repair, Mouth and Throat **0CQ**-

Stratos LV
  use Cardiac Resynchronization Pacemaker Pulse Generator in **0JH**-

Stress test
  4A02XM4
  4A12XM4

Stripping *see* Extraction

Study
Electrophysiologic stimulation, cardiac *see* Measurement, Cardiac **4A0**2-
Ocular motility **4A0**7X7Z
Pulmonary airway flow measurement *see* Measurement, Respiratory **4A0**9-
Visual acuity **4A0**7X0Z

Styloglossus muscle
  use Muscle, Tongue, Palate, Pharynx

Stylomandibular ligament
  use Bursa and Ligament, Head and Neck

Stylopharyngeus muscle
  use Muscle, Tongue, Palate, Pharynx

Subacromial bursa
  use Bursa and Ligament, Shoulder, Left
  use Bursa and Ligament, Shoulder, Right

Subaortic (common iliac) lymph node
  use Lymphatic, Pelvis

Subarachnoid space, intracranial
  use Subarachnoid Space

Subarachnoid space, spinal
  use Spinal Canal

Subclavicular (apical) lymph node
  use Lymphatic, Axillary, Left
  use Lymphatic, Axillary, Right

Subclavius muscle
  use Muscle, Thorax, Left
  use Muscle, Thorax, Right

Subclavius nerve
  use Nerve, Brachial Plexus

Subcostal artery
  use Aorta, Thoracic

Subcostal muscle
  use Muscle, Thorax, Left
  use Muscle, Thorax, Right

Subcostal nerve
  use Nerve, Thoracic

Subcutaneous injection reservoir, port
  use Vascular Access Device, Reservoir in Subcutaneous Tissue and Fascia

Subcutaneous injection reservoir, pump
  use Infusion Device, Pump in Subcutaneous Tissue and Fascia

Subdermal progesterone implant
  use Contraceptive Device in Subcutaneous Tissue and Fascia

Subdural space, intracranial
  use Subdural Space

Subdural space, spinal
  use Spinal Canal

Submandibular ganglion
  use Nerve, Facial
  use Nerve, Head and Neck Sympathetic

Submandibular gland
  use Gland, Submaxillary, Left
  use Gland, Submaxillary, Right

Submandibular lymph node
  use Lymphatic, Head

Submaxillary ganglion
  use Nerve, Head and Neck Sympathetic

Submaxillary lymph node
  use Lymphatic, Head

Submental artery
  use Artery, Face

Submental lymph node
  use Lymphatic, Head

Submucous (Meissner's) plexus
  use Nerve, Abdominal Sympathetic

Suboccipital nerve
  use Nerve, Cervical

Suboccipital venous plexus
  use Vein, Vertebral, Left
  use Vein, Vertebral, Right

Subparotid lymph node
  use Lymphatic, Head

Subscapular (posterior) lymph node
  use Lymphatic, Axillary, Left
  use Lymphatic, Axillary, Right

Subscapular aponeurosis
  use Subcutaneous Tissue and Fascia, Upper Arm, Left
  use Subcutaneous Tissue and Fascia, Upper Arm, Right

Subscapular artery
  use Artery, Axillary, Left
  use Artery, Axillary, Right

Subscapularis muscle
  use Muscle, Shoulder, Left
  use Muscle, Shoulder, Right

Substance Abuse Treatment
Counseling
  Family, for substance abuse, Other Family Counseling **HZ6**3ZZZ
  Group
    12-Step **HZ4**3ZZZ
    Behavioral **HZ4**1ZZZ
    Cognitive **HZ4**0ZZZ
    Cognitive-Behavioral **HZ4**2ZZZ
    Confrontational **HZ4**8ZZZ
    Continuing Care **HZ4**9ZZZ
    Infectious Disease
      Post-Test **HZ4**CZZZ
      Pre-Test **HZ4**CZZZ
    Interpersonal **HZ4**4ZZZ
    Motivational Enhancement **HZ4**7ZZZ
    Psychoeducation **HZ4**6ZZZ
    Spiritual **HZ4**BZZZ
    Vocational **HZ4**5ZZZ
  Individual
    12-Step **HZ3**3ZZZ
    Behavioral **HZ3**1ZZZ
    Cognitive **HZ3**0ZZZ
    Cognitive-Behavioral **HZ3**2ZZZ
    Confrontational **HZ3**8ZZZ
    Continuing Care **HZ3**9ZZZ
    Infectious Disease
      Post-Test **HZ3**CZZZ
      Pre-Test **HZ3**CZZZ
    Interpersonal **HZ3**4ZZZ
    Motivational Enhancement **HZ3**7ZZZ
    Psychoeducation **HZ3**6ZZZ
    Spiritual **HZ3**BZZZ
    Vocational **HZ3**5ZZZ
Detoxification Services, for substance abuse **HZ2**ZZZZ
Medication Management
  Antabuse **HZ8**3ZZZ
  Bupropion **HZ8**7ZZZ
  Clonidine **HZ8**6ZZZ
  Levo-alpha-acetyl-methadol (LAAM) **HZ8**2ZZZ
  Methadone Maintenance **HZ8**1ZZZ
  Naloxone **HZ8**5ZZZ
  Naltrexone **HZ8**4ZZZ
  Nicotine Replacement **HZ8**0ZZZ
  Other Replacement Medication **HZ8**9ZZZ
  Psychiatric Medication **HZ8**8ZZZ
Pharmacotherapy
  Antabuse **HZ9**3ZZZ
  Bupropion **HZ9**7ZZZ
  Clonidine **HZ9**6ZZZ
  Levo-alpha-acetyl-methadol (LAAM) **HZ9**2ZZZ
  Methadone Maintenance **HZ9**1ZZZ
  Naloxone **HZ9**5ZZZ
  Naltrexone **HZ9**4ZZZ
  Nicotine Replacement **HZ9**0ZZZ
  Psychiatric Medication **HZ9**8ZZZ
  Replacement Medication, Other **HZ9**9ZZZ
Psychotherapy
  12-Step **HZ5**3ZZZ
  Behavioral **HZ5**1ZZZ
  Cognitive **HZ5**0ZZZ
  Cognitive-Behavioral **HZ5**2ZZZ
  Confrontational **HZ5**8ZZZ
  Interactive **HZ5**5ZZZ
  Interpersonal **HZ5**4ZZZ
  Motivational Enhancement **HZ5**7ZZZ
  Psychoanalysis **HZ5**BZZZ
  Psychodynamic **HZ5**CZZZ
  Psychoeducation **HZ5**6ZZZ
  Psychophysiological **HZ5**DZZZ
  Supportive **HZ5**9ZZZ

Substantia | INDEX TO PROCEDURES – 2016 ICD-10-PCS | [2016.PCS]

Substantia nigra
  use Basal Ganglia
Subtalar (talocalcaneal) joint
  use Joint, Tarsal, Left
  use Joint, Tarsal, Right
Subtalar ligament
  use Bursa and Ligament, Foot, Left
  use Bursa and Ligament, Foot, Right
Subthalamic nucleus
  use Basal Ganglia
Suction curettage (D&C), nonobstetric see Extraction, Endometrium 0UDB-
Suction curettage, obstetric post-delivery see Extraction, Products of Conception, Retained 10D1-
Superficial circumflex iliac vein
  use Vein, Greater Saphenous, Left
  use Vein, Greater Saphenous, Right
Superficial epigastric artery
  use Artery, Femoral, Left
  use Artery, Femoral, Right
Superficial epigastric vein
  use Vein, Greater Saphenous, Left
  use Vein, Greater Saphenous, Right
Superficial Inferior Epigastric Artery Flap
  Bilateral 0HRV078
  Left 0HRU078
  Right 0HRT078
Superficial palmar arch
  use Artery, Hand, Left
  use Artery, Hand, Right
Superficial palmar venous arch
  use Vein, Hand, Left
  use Vein, Hand, Right
Superficial temporal artery
  use Artery, Temporal, Left
  use Artery, Temporal, Right
Superficial transverse perineal muscle
  use Muscle, Perineum
Superior cardiac nerve
  use Nerve, Thoracic Sympathetic
Superior cerebellar vein
  use Vein, Intracranial
Superior cerebral vein
  use Vein, Intracranial
Superior clunic (cluneal) nerve
  use Nerve, Lumbar
Superior epigastric artery
  use Artery, Internal Mammary, Left
  use Artery, Internal Mammary, Right
Superior genicular artery
  use Artery, Popliteal, Left
  use Artery, Popliteal, Right
Superior gluteal artery
  use Artery, Internal Iliac, Left
  use Artery, Internal Iliac, Right
Superior gluteal nerve
  use Nerve, Lumbar Plexus
Superior hypogastric plexus
  use Nerve, Abdominal Sympathetic
Superior labial artery
  use Artery, Face
Superior laryngeal artery
  use Artery, Thyroid, Left
  use Artery, Thyroid, Right
Superior laryngeal nerve
  use Nerve, Vagus
Superior longitudinal muscle
  use Muscle, Tongue, Palate, Pharynx
Superior mesenteric ganglion
  use Nerve, Abdominal Sympathetic
Superior mesenteric lymph node
  use Lymphatic, Mesenteric
Superior mesenteric plexus
  use Nerve, Abdominal Sympathetic
Superior oblique muscle
  use Muscle, Extraocular, Left
  use Muscle, Extraocular, Right

Superior olivary nucleus
  use Pons
Superior rectal artery
  use Artery, Inferior Mesenteric
Superior rectal vein
  use Vein, Inferior Mesenteric
Superior rectus muscle
  use Muscle, Extraocular, Left
  use Muscle, Extraocular, Right
Superior tarsal plate
  use Eyelid, Upper, Left
  use Eyelid, Upper, Right
Superior thoracic artery
  use Artery, Axillary, Left
  use Artery, Axillary, Right
Superior thyroid artery
  use Artery, External Carotid, Left
  use Artery, External Carotid, Right
  use Artery, Thyroid, Left
  use Artery, Thyroid, Right
Superior turbinate
  use Turbinate, Nasal
Superior ulnar collateral artery
  use Artery, Brachial, Left
  use Artery, Brachial, Right
Supplement
  Abdominal Wall 0WUF-
  Acetabulum
    Left 0QU5-
    Right 0QU4-
  Ampulla of Vater 0FUC-
  Anal Sphincter 0DUR-
  Ankle Region
    Left 0YUL-
    Right 0YUK-
  Anus 0DUQ-
  Aorta
    Abdominal 04U0-
    Thoracic 02UW-
  Arm
    Lower
      Left 0XUF-
      Right 0XUD-
    Upper
      Left 0XU9-
      Right 0XU8-
  Artery
    Anterior Tibial
      Left 04UQ-
      Right 04UP-
    Axillary
      Left 03U6-
      Right 03U5-
    Brachial
      Left 03U8-
      Right 03U7-
    Celiac 04U1-
    Colic
      Left 04U7-
      Middle 04U8-
      Right 04U6-
    Common Carotid
      Left 03UJ-
      Right 03UH-
    Common Iliac
      Left 04UD-
      Right 04UC-
    External Carotid
      Left 03UN-
      Right 03UM-
    External Iliac
      Left 04UJ-
      Right 04UH-
    Face 03UR-
    Femoral
      Left 04UL-
      Right 04UK-
    Foot
      Left 04UW-
      Right 04UV-
    Gastric 04U2-

Supplement — continued
  Artery — continued
    Hand
      Left 03UF-
      Right 03UD-
    Hepatic 04U3-
    Inferior Mesenteric 04UB-
    Innominate 03U2-
    Internal Carotid
      Left 03UL-
      Right 03UK-
    Internal Iliac
      Left 04UF-
      Right 04UE-
    Internal Mammary
      Left 03U1-
      Right 03U0-
    Intracranial 03UG-
    Lower 04UY-
    Peroneal
      Left 04UU-
      Right 04UT-
    Popliteal
      Left 04UN-
      Right 04UM-
    Posterior Tibial
      Left 04US-
      Right 04UR-
    Pulmonary
      Left 02UR-
      Right 02UQ-
    Pulmonary Trunk 02UP-
    Radial
      Left 03UC-
      Right 03UB-
    Renal
      Left 04UA-
      Right 04U9-
    Splenic 04U4-
    Subclavian
      Left 03U4-
      Right 03U3-
    Superior Mesenteric 04U5-
    Temporal
      Left 03UT-
      Right 03US-
    Thyroid
      Left 03UV-
      Right 03UU-
    Ulnar
      Left 03UA-
      Right 03U9-
    Upper 03UY-
    Vertebral
      Left 03UQ-
      Right 03UP-
  Atrium
    Left 02U7-
    Right 02U6-
  Auditory Ossicle
    Left 09UA0-
    Right 09U90-
  Axilla
    Left 0XU5-
    Right 0XU4-
  Back
    Lower 0WUL-
    Upper 0WUK-
  Bladder 0TUB-
  Bladder Neck 0TUC-
  Bone
    Ethmoid
      Left 0NUG-
      Right 0NUF-
    Frontal
      Left 0NU2-
      Right 0NU1-
    Hyoid 0NUX-
    Lacrimal
      Left 0NUJ-
      Right 0NUH-
    Nasal 0NUB-

Supplement — continued
  Bone — continued
    Occipital
      Left 0NU8-
      Right 0NU7-
    Palatine
      Left 0NUL-
      Right 0NUK-
    Parietal
      Left 0NU4-
      Right 0NU3-
    Pelvic
      Left 0QU3-
      Right 0QU2-
    Sphenoid
      Left 0NUD-
      Right 0NUC-
    Temporal
      Left 0NU6-
      Right 0NU5-
    Zygomatic
      Left 0NUN-
      Right 0NUM-
  Breast
    Bilateral 0HUV-
    Left 0HUU-
    Right 0HUT-
  Bronchus
    Lingula 0BU9-
    Lower Lobe
      Left 0BUB-
      Right 0BU6-
    Main
      Left 0BU7-
      Right 0BU3-
    Middle Lobe, Right 0BU5-
    Upper Lobe
      Left 0BU8-
      Right 0BU4-
  Buccal Mucosa 0CU4-
  Bursa and Ligament
    Abdomen
      Left 0MUJ-
      Right 0MUH-
    Ankle
      Left 0MUR-
      Right 0MUQ-
    Elbow
      Left 0MU4-
      Right 0MU3-
    Foot
      Left 0MUT-
      Right 0MUS-
    Hand
      Left 0MU8-
      Right 0MU7-
    Head and Neck 0MU0-
    Hip
      Left 0MUM-
      Right 0MUL-
    Knee
      Left 0MUP-
      Right 0MUN-
    Lower Extremity
      Left 0MUW-
      Right 0MUV-
    Perineum 0MUK-
    Shoulder
      Left 0MU2-
      Right 0MU1-
    Thorax
      Left 0MUG-
      Right 0MUF-
    Trunk
      Left 0MUD-
      Right 0MUC-
    Upper Extremity
      Left 0MUB-
      Right 0MU9-
    Wrist
      Left 0MU6-
      Right 0MU5-

Supplement — *continued*
Buttock
 Left 0YU1-
 Right 0YU0-
Carina 0BU2-
Carpal
 Left 0PUN-
 Right 0PUM-
Cecum 0DUH-
Cerebral Meninges 00U1-
Chest Wall 0WU8-
Chordae Tendineae 02U9-
Cisterna Chyli 07UL-
Clavicle
 Left 0PUB-
 Right 0PU9-
Clitoris 0UUJ-
Coccyx 0QUS-
Colon
 Ascending 0DUK-
 Descending 0DUM-
 Sigmoid 0DUN-
 Transverse 0DUL-
Cord
 Bilateral 0VUH-
 Left 0VUG-
 Right 0VUF-
Cornea
 Left 08U9-
 Right 08U8-
Cul-de-sac 0UUF-
Diaphragm
 Left 0BUS-
 Right 0BUR-
Disc
 Cervical Vertebral 0RU3-
 Cervicothoracic Vertebral 0RU5-
 Lumbar Vertebral 0SU2-
 Lumbosacral 0SU4-
 Thoracic Vertebral 0RU9-
 Thoracolumbar Vertebral 0RUB-
Duct
 Common Bile 0FU9-
 Cystic 0FU8-
 Hepatic
  Left 0FU6-
  Right 0FU5-
 Lacrimal
  Left 08UY-
  Right 08UX-
 Pancreatic 0FUD-
  Accessory 0FUF-
Duodenum 0DU9-
Dura Mater 00U2-
Ear
 External
  Bilateral 09U2-
  Left 09U1-
  Right 09U0-
 Inner
  Left 09UE0-
  Right 09UD0-
 Middle
  Left 09U60-
  Right 09U50-
Elbow Region
 Left 0XUC-
 Right 0XUB-
Epididymis
 Bilateral 0VUL-
 Left 0VUK-
 Right 0VUJ-
Epiglottis 0CUR-
Esophagogastric Junction 0DU4-
Esophagus 0DU5-
 Lower 0DU3-
 Middle 0DU2-
 Upper 0DU1-
Extremity
 Lower
  Left 0YUB-
  Right 0YU9-

Supplement — *continued*
Extremity — *continued*
 Upper
  Left 0XU7-
  Right 0XU6-
Eye
 Left 08U1-
 Right 08U0-
Eyelid
 Lower
  Left 08UR-
  Right 08UQ-
 Upper
  Left 08UP-
  Right 08UN-
Face 0WU2-
Fallopian Tube
 Left 0UU6-
 Right 0UU5-
Fallopian Tubes, Bilateral 0UU/-
Femoral Region
 Bilateral 0YUE-
 Left 0YU8-
 Right 0YU7-
Femoral Shaft
 Left 0QU9-
 Right 0QU8-
Femur
 Lower
  Left 0QUC-
  Right 0QUB-
 Upper
  Left 0QU7-
  Right 0QU6-
Fibula
 Left 0QUK-
 Right 0QUJ-
Finger
 Index
  Left 0XUP-
  Right 0XUN-
 Little
  Left 0XUW-
  Right 0XUV-
 Middle
  Left 0XUR-
  Right 0XUQ-
 Ring
  Left 0XUT-
  Right 0XUS-
Foot
 Left 0YUN-
 Right 0YUM-
Gingiva
 Lower 0CU6-
 Upper 0CU5-
Glenoid Cavity
 Left 0PU8-
 Right 0PU7-
Hand
 Left 0XUK-
 Right 0XUJ-
Head 0WU0-
Heart 02UA-
Humeral Head
 Left 0PUD-
 Right 0PUC-
Humeral Shaft
 Left 0PUG-
 Right 0PUF-
Hymen 0UUK-
Ileocecal Valve 0DUC-
Ileum 0DUB-
Inguinal Region
 Bilateral 0YUA-
 Left 0YU6-
 Right 0YU5-
Intestine
 Large 0DUE-
  Left 0DUG-
  Right 0DUF-
 Small 0DU8-

Supplement — *continued*
Iris
 Left 08UD-
 Right 08UC-
Jaw
 Lower 0WU5-
 Upper 0WU4-
Jejunum 0DUA-
Joint
 Acromioclavicular
  Left 0RUH-
  Right 0RUG-
 Ankle
  Left 0SUG-
  Right 0SUF-
 Carpal
  Left 0RUR-
  Right 0RUQ-
 Cervical Vertebral 0RU1-
 Cervicothoracic Vertebral 0RU4-
 Coccygeal 0SU6-
 Elbow
  Left 0RUM-
  Right 0RUL-
 Finger Phalangeal
  Left 0RUX-
  Right 0RUW-
 Hip
  Left 0SUB-
   Acetabular Surface 0SUE-
   Femoral Surface 0SUS-
  Right 0SU9-
   Acetabular Surface 0SUA-
   Femoral Surface 0SUR-
 Knee
  Left 0SUD-
   Femoral Surface 0SUU09Z
   Tibial Surface 0SUW09Z
  Right 0SUC-
   Femoral Surface 0SUT09Z
   Tibial Surface 0SUV09Z
 Lumbar Vertebral 0SU0-
 Lumbosacral 0SU3-
 Metacarpocarpal
  Left 0RUT-
  Right 0RUS-
 Metacarpophalangeal
  Left 0RUV-
  Right 0RUU-
 Metatarsal-Phalangeal
  Left 0SUN-
  Right 0SUM-
 Metatarsal-Tarsal
  Left 0SUL-
  Right 0SUK-
 Occipital-cervical 0RU0-
 Sacrococcygeal 0SU5-
 Sacroiliac
  Left 0SU8-
  Right 0SU7-
 Shoulder
  Left 0RUK-
  Right 0RUJ-
 Sternoclavicular
  Left 0RUF-
  Right 0RUE-
 Tarsal
  Left 0SUJ-
  Right 0SUH-
 Temporomandibular
  Left 0RUD-
  Right 0RUC-
 Thoracic Vertebral 0RU6-
 Thoracolumbar Vertebral 0RUA-
 Toe Phalangeal
  Left 0SUQ-
  Right 0SUP-
 Wrist
  Left 0RUP-
  Right 0RUN-

Supplement — *continued*
Kidney Pelvis
 Left 0TU4-
 Right 0TU3-
Knee Region
 Left 0YUG-
 Right 0YUF-
Larynx 0CUS-
Leg
 Lower
  Left 0YUJ-
  Right 0YUH-
 Upper
  Left 0YUD-
  Right 0YUC-
Lip
 Lower 0CU1-
 Upper 0CU0-
Lymphatic
 Aortic 07UD-
 Axillary
  Left 07U6-
  Right 07U5-
 Head 07U0-
 Inguinal
  Left 07UJ-
  Right 07UH-
 Internal Mammary
  Left 07U9-
  Right 07U8-
 Lower Extremity
  Left 07UG-
  Right 07UF-
 Mesenteric 07UB-
 Neck
  Left 07U2-
  Right 07U1-
 Pelvis 07UC-
 Thoracic Duct 07UK-
 Thorax 07U7-
 Upper Extremity
  Left 07U4-
  Right 07U3-
Mandible
 Left 0NUV-
 Right 0NUT-
Maxilla
 Left 0NUS-
 Right 0NUR-
Mediastinum 0WUC-
Mesentery 0DUV-
Metacarpal
 Left 0PUQ-
 Right 0PUP-
Metatarsal
 Left 0QUP-
 Right 0QUN-
Muscle
 Abdomen
  Left 0KUL-
  Right 0KUK-
 Extraocular
  Left 08UM-
  Right 08UL-
 Facial 0KU1-
 Foot
  Left 0KUW-
  Right 0KUV-
 Hand
  Left 0KUD-
  Right 0KUC-
 Head 0KU0-
 Hip
  Left 0KUP-
  Right 0KUN-
 Lower Arm and Wrist
  Left 0KUB-
  Right 0KU9-
 Lower Leg
  Left 0KUT-
  Right 0KUS-

75

Supplement — *continued*
  Muscle — *continued*
    Neck
      Left 0KU3-
      Right 0KU2-
    Papillary 02UD-
    Perineum 0KUM-
    Shoulder
      Left 0KU6-
      Right 0KU5-
    Thorax
      Left 0KUJ-
      Right 0KUH-
    Tongue, Palate, Pharynx 0KU4-
    Trunk
      Left 0KUG-
      Right 0KUF-
    Upper Arm
      Left 0KU8-
      Right 0KU7-
    Upper Leg
      Left 0KUR-
      Right 0KUQ-
  Nasopharynx 09UN-
  Neck 0WU6-
  Nerve
    Abducens 00UL-
    Accessory 00UR-
    Acoustic 00UN-
    Cervical 01U1-
    Facial 00UM-
    Femoral 01UD-
    Glossopharyngeal 00UP-
    Hypoglossal 00US-
    Lumbar 01UB-
    Median 01U5-
    Oculomotor 00UH-
    Olfactory 00UF-
    Optic 00UG-
    Peroneal 01UH-
    Phrenic 01U2-
    Pudendal 01UC-
    Radial 01U6-
    Sacral 01UR-
    Sciatic 01UF-
    Thoracic 01U8-
    Tibial 01UG-
    Trigeminal 00UK-
    Trochlear 00UJ-
    Ulnar 01U4-
    Vagus 00UQ-
  Nipple
    Left 0HUX-
    Right 0HUW-
  Nose 09UK-
  Omentum
    Greater 0DUS-
    Lesser 0DUT-
  Orbit
    Left 0NUQ-
    Right 0NUP-
  Palate
    Hard 0CU2-
    Soft 0CU3-
  Patella
    Left 0QUF-
    Right 0QUD-
  Penis 0VUS-
  Pericardium 02UN-
  Perineum
    Female 0WUN-
    Male 0WUM-
  Peritoneum 0DUW-
  Phalanx
    Finger
      Left 0PUV-
      Right 0PUT-
    Thumb
      Left 0PUS-
      Right 0PUR-

Supplement — *continued*
  Phalanx — *continued*
    Toe
      Left 0QUR-
      Right 0QUQ-
  Pharynx 0CUM-
  Prepuce 0VUT-
  Radius
    Left 0PUJ-
    Right 0PUH-
  Rectum 0DUP-
  Retina
    Left 08UF-
    Right 08UE-
  Retinal Vessel
    Left 08UH-
    Right 08UG-
  Rib
    Left 0PU2-
    Right 0PU1-
  Sacrum 0QU1-
  Scapula
    Left 0PU6-
    Right 0PU5-
  Scrotum 0VU5-
  Septum
    Atrial 02U5-
    Nasal 09UM-
    Ventricular 02UM-
  Shoulder Region
    Left 0XU3-
    Right 0XU2-
  Skull 0NU0-
  Spinal Meninges 00UT-
  Sternum 0PU0-
  Stomach 0DU6-
    Pylorus 0DU7-
  Subcutaneous Tissue and Fascia
    Abdomen 0JU8-
    Back 0JU7-
    Buttock 0JU9-
    Chest 0JU6-
    Face 0JU1-
    Foot
      Left 0JUR-
      Right 0JUQ-
    Hand
      Left 0JUK-
      Right 0JUJ-
    Lower Arm
      Left 0JUH-
      Right 0JUG-
    Lower Leg
      Left 0JUP-
      Right 0JUN-
    Neck
      Anterior 0JU4-
      Posterior 0JU5-
    Pelvic Region 0JUC-
    Perineum 0JUB-
    Scalp 0JU0-
    Upper Arm
      Left 0JUF-
      Right 0JUD-
    Upper Leg
      Left 0JUM-
      Right 0JUL-
  Tarsal
    Left 0QUM-
    Right 0QUL-
  Tendon
    Abdomen
      Left 0LUG-
      Right 0LUF-
    Ankle
      Left 0LUT-
      Right 0LUS-
    Foot
      Left 0LUW-
      Right 0LUV-

Supplement — *continued*
  Tendon — *continued*
    Hand
      Left 0LU8-
      Right 0LU7-
    Head and Neck 0LU0-
    Hip
      Left 0LUK-
      Right 0LUJ-
    Knee
      Left 0LUR-
      Right 0LUQ-
    Lower Arm and Wrist
      Left 0LU6-
      Right 0LU5-
    Lower Leg
      Left 0LUP-
      Right 0LUN-
    Perineum 0LUH-
    Shoulder
      Left 0LU2-
      Right 0LU1-
    Thorax
      Left 0LUD-
      Right 0LUC-
    Trunk
      Left 0LUB-
      Right 0LU9-
    Upper Arm
      Left 0LU4-
      Right 0LU3-
    Upper Leg
      Left 0LUM-
      Right 0LUL-
  Testis
    Bilateral 0VUC0-
    Left 0VUB0-
    Right 0VU90-
  Thumb
    Left 0XUM-
    Right 0XUL-
  Tibia
    Left 0QUH-
    Right 0QUG-
  Toe
    1st
      Left 0YUQ-
      Right 0YUP-
    2nd
      Left 0YUS-
      Right 0YUR-
    3rd
      Left 0YUU-
      Right 0YUT-
    4th
      Left 0YUW-
      Right 0YUV-
    5th
      Left 0YUY-
      Right 0YUX-
  Tongue 0CU7-
  Trachea 0BU1-
  Tunica Vaginalis
    Left 0VU7-
    Right 0VU6-
  Turbinate, Nasal 09UL-
  Tympanic Membrane
    Left 09U8-
    Right 09U7-
  Ulna
    Left 0PUL-
    Right 0PUK-
  Ureter
    Left 0TU7-
    Right 0TU6-
  Urethra 0TUD-
  Uterine Supporting Structure 0UU4-
  Uvula 0CUN-
  Vagina 0UUG-

Supplement — *continued*
  Valve
    Aortic 02UF-
    Mitral 02UG-
    Pulmonary 02UH-
    Tricuspid 02UJ-
  Vas Deferens
    Bilateral 0VUQ-
    Left 0VUP-
    Right 0VUN-
  Vein
    Axillary
      Left 05U8-
      Right 05U7-
    Azygos 05U0-
    Basilic
      Left 05UC-
      Right 05UB-
    Brachial
      Left 05UA-
      Right 05U9-
    Cephalic
      Left 05UF-
      Right 05UD-
    Colic 06U7-
    Common Iliac
      Left 06UD-
      Right 06UC-
    Esophageal 06U3-
    External Iliac
      Left 06UG-
      Right 06UF-
    External Jugular
      Left 05UQ-
      Right 05UP-
    Face
      Left 05UV-
      Right 05UT-
    Femoral
      Left 06UN-
      Right 06UM-
    Foot
      Left 06UV-
      Right 06UT-
    Gastric 06U2-
    Greater Saphenous
      Left 06UQ-
      Right 06UP-
    Hand
      Left 05UH-
      Right 05UG-
    Hemiazygos 05U1-
    Hepatic 06U4-
    Hypogastric
      Left 06UJ-
      Right 06UH-
    Inferior Mesenteric 06U6-
    Innominate
      Left 05U4-
      Right 05U3-
    Internal Jugular
      Left 05UN-
      Right 05UM-
    Intracranial 05UL-
    Lesser Saphenous
      Left 06US-
      Right 06UR-
    Lower 06UY-
    Portal 06U8-
    Pulmonary
      Left 02UT-
      Right 02US-
    Renal
      Left 06UB-
      Right 06U9-
    Splenic 06U1-
    Subclavian
      Left 05U6-
      Right 05U5-
    Superior Mesenteric 06U5-
    Upper 05UY-

Supplement — continued
Vein — continued
  Vertebral
    Left 05US-
    Right 05UR-
  Vena Cava
    Inferior 06U0-
    Superior 02UV-
  Ventricle
    Left 02UL-
    Right 02UK-
  Vertebra
    Cervical 0PU3-
    Lumbar 0QU0-
    Thoracic 0PU4-
  Vesicle
    Bilateral 0VU3-
    Left 0VU2-
    Right 0VU1-
  Vocal Cord
    Left 0CUV-
    Right 0CUT-
  Vulva 0UUM-
  Wrist Region
    Left 0XUH-
    Right 0XUG-
Supraclavicular (Virchow's) lymph node
  use Lymphatic, Neck, Left
  use Lymphatic, Neck, Right
Supraclavicular nerve
  use Nerve, Cervical Plexus
Suprahyoid lymph node
  use Lymphatic, Head
Suprahyoid muscle
  use Muscle, Neck, Left
  use Muscle, Neck, Right
Suprainguinal lymph node
  use Lymphatic, Pelvis
Supraorbital vein
  use Vein, Face, Left
  use Vein, Face, Right
Suprarenal gland
  use Gland, Adrenal
  use Gland, Adrenal, Bilateral
  use Gland, Adrenal, Left
  use Gland, Adrenal, Right
Suprarenal plexus
  use Nerve, Abdominal Sympathetic
Suprascapular nerve
  use Nerve, Brachial Plexus
Supraspinatus fascia
  use Subcutaneous Tissue and Fascia, Upper Arm, Left
  use Subcutaneous Tissue and Fascia, Upper Arm, Right
Supraspinatus muscle
  use Muscle, Shoulder, Left
  use Muscle, Shoulder, Right
Supraspinous ligament
  use Bursa and Ligament, Trunk, Left
  use Bursa and Ligament, Trunk, Right
Suprasternal notch
  use Sternum
Supratrochlear lymph node
  use Lymphatic, Upper Extremity, Left
  use Lymphatic, Upper Extremity, Right
Sural artery
  use Artery, Popliteal, Left
  use Artery, Popliteal, Right
Suspension
  Bladder Neck *see* Reposition, Bladder Neck 0TSC-
  Kidney *see* Reposition, Urinary System 0TS-
  Urethra *see* Reposition, Urinary System 0TS-
  Urethrovesical *see* Reposition, Bladder Neck 0TSC-
  Uterus *see* Reposition, Uterus 0US9-
  Vagina *see* Reposition, Vagina 0USG-

Suture
  Laceration repair *see* Repair
  Ligation *see* Occlusion
Suture Removal
  Extremity
    Lower 8E0YXY8
    Upper 8E0XXY8
  Head and Neck Region 8E09XY8
  Trunk Region 8E0WXY8
Sweat gland
  use Skin
Sympathectomy *see* Excision, Peripheral Nervous System 01B-
SynCardia Total Artificial Heart
  use Synthetic Substitute
Synchra CRT-P
  use Cardiac Resynchronization Pacemaker Pulse Generator in 0JH-
SynchroMed pump
  use Infusion Device, Pump in Subcutaneous Tissue and Fascia
Synechiotomy, iris *see* Release, Eye 08N-
Synovectomy
  Lower joint *see* Excision, Lower Joints 0SB-
  Upper joint *see* Excision, Upper Joints 0RB-
Systemic Nuclear Medicine Therapy
  Abdomen CW70-
  Anatomical Regions, Multiple CW7YYZZ
  Chest CW73-
  Thyroid CW7G-
  Whole Body CW7N-

T

Takedown
  Arteriovenous shunt *see* Removal of device from, Upper Arteries 03P-
  Arteriovenous shunt, with creation of new shunt *see* Bypass, Upper Arteries 031-
  Stoma *see* Repair
Talent® Converter
  use Intraluminal Device
Talent® Occluder
  use Intraluminal Device
Talent® Stent Graft (abdominal) (thoracic)
  use Intraluminal Device
Talocalcaneal (subtalar) joint
  use Joint, Tarsal, Left
  use Joint, Tarsal, Right
Talocalcaneal ligament
  use Bursa and Ligament, Foot, Left
  use Bursa and Ligament, Foot, Right
Talocalcaneonavicular joint
  use Joint, Tarsal, Left
  use Joint, Tarsal, Right
Talocalcaneonavicular ligament
  use Bursa and Ligament, Foot, Left
  use Bursa and Ligament, Foot, Right
Talocrural joint
  use Joint, Ankle, Left
  use Joint, Ankle, Right
Talofibular ligament
  use Bursa and Ligament, Ankle, Left
  use Bursa and Ligament, Ankle, Right
Talus bone
  use Tarsal, Left
  use Tarsal, Right
TandemHeart® System
  use External Heart Assist System in Heart and Great Vessels
Tarsectomy
  see Excision, Lower Bones 0QB-
  see Resection, Lower Bones 0QT-
Tarsometatarsal joint
  use Joint, Metatarsal-Tarsal, Left
  use Joint, Metatarsal-Tarsal, Right
Tarsometatarsal ligament
  use Bursa and Ligament, Foot, Left
  use Bursa and Ligament, Foot, Right
Tarsorrhaphy *see* Repair, Eye 08Q-
Tattooing
  Cornea 3E0CXMZ
  Skin *see* Introduction of substance in or on, Skin 3E00-
TAXUS® Liberté® Paclitaxel-eluting Coronary Stent System
  use Intraluminal Device, Drug-eluting in Heart and Great Vessels
TBNA (transbronchial needle aspiration) *see* Drainage, Respiratory System 0B9-
Telemetry 4A12X4Z
  Ambulatory 4A12X45
Temperature gradient study 4A0ZXKZ
Temporal lobe
  use Cerebral Hemisphere
Temporalis muscle
  use Muscle, Head
Temporoparietalis muscle
  use Muscle, Head
Tendolysis *see* Release, Tendons 0LN-
Tendonectomy
  see Excision, Tendons 0LB-
  see Resection, Tendons 0LT-
Tendonoplasty, tenoplasty
  see Repair, Tendons 0LQ-
  see Replacement, Tendons 0LR-
  see Supplement, Tendons 0LU-
Tendorrhaphy *see* Repair, Tendons 0LQ-

Tendototomy
  see Division, Tendons 0L8-
  see Drainage, Tendons 0L9-
Tenectomy, tenonectomy
  see Excision, Tendons 0LB-
  see Resection, Tendons 0LT-
Tenolysis *see* Release, Tendons 0LN-
Tenontorrhaphy *see* Repair, Tendons 0LQ-
Tenontotomy
  see Division, Tendons 0L8-
  see Drainage, Tendons 0L9-
Tenorrhaphy *see* Repair, Tendons 0LQ-
Tenosynovectomy
  see Excision, Tendons 0LB-
  see Resection, Tendons 0LT-
Tenotomy
  see Division, Tendons 0L8-
  see Drainage, Tendons 0L9-
Tensor fasciae latae muscle
  use Muscle, Hip, Left
  use Muscle, Hip, Right
Tensor veli palatini muscle
  use Muscle, Tongue, Palate, Pharynx
Tenth cranial nerve
  use Nerve, Vagus
Tentorium cerebelli
  use Dura Mater
Teres major muscle
  use Muscle, Shoulder, Left
  use Muscle, Shoulder, Right
Teres minor muscle
  use Muscle, Shoulder, Left
  use Muscle, Shoulder, Right
Termination of pregnancy
  Aspiration curettage 10A07ZZ
  Dilation and curettage 10A07ZZ
  Hysterotomy 10A00ZZ
  Intra-amniotic injection 10A03ZZ
  Laminaria 10A07ZW
  Vacuum 10A07Z6
Testectomy
  see Excision, Male Reproductive System 0VB-
  see Resection, Male Reproductive System 0VT-
Testicular artery
  use Aorta, Abdominal
Testing
  Glaucoma 4A07XBZ
  Hearing *see* Hearing Assessment, Diagnostic Audiology F13-
  Mental health *see* Psychological Tests
  Muscle function, electromyography (EMG) *see* Measurement, Musculoskeletal 4A0F-
  Muscle function, manual *see* Motor Function Assessment, Rehabilitation F01-
  Neurophysiologic monitoring, intra-operative *see* Monitoring, Physiological Systems 4A1-
  Range of motion *see* Motor Function Assessment, Rehabilitation F01-
  Vestibular function *see* Vestibular Assessment, Diagnostic Audiology F15-
Thalamectomy *see* Excision, Thalamus 00B9-
Thalamotomy *see* Drainage, Thalamus 0099-
Thenar muscle
  use Muscle, Hand, Left
  use Muscle, Hand, Right
Therapeutic Massage
  Musculoskeletal System 8E0KX1Z
  Reproductive System
    Prostate 8E0VX1C
    Rectum 8E0VX1D

Therapeutic occlusion — INDEX TO PROCEDURES – 2016 ICD-10-PCS [2016.PCS]

Therapeutic occlusion coil(s)
use Intraluminal Device
Thermography 4A0ZXKZ
Thermotherapy, prostate see Destruction, Prostate 0V50-
Third cranial nerve
use Nerve, Oculomotor
Third occipital nerve
use Nerve, Cervical
Third ventricle
use Cerebral Ventricle
Thoracectomy see Excision, Anatomical Regions, General 0WB-
Thoracentesis see Drainage, Anatomical Regions, General 0W9-
Thoracic aortic plexus
use Nerve, Thoracic Sympathetic
Thoracic esophagus
use Esophagus, Middle
Thoracic facet joint
use Joint, Thoracic Vertebral
Thoracic ganglion
use Nerve, Thoracic Sympathetic
Thoracoacromial artery
use Artery, Axillary, Left
use Artery, Axillary, Right
Thoracocentesis see Drainage, Anatomical Regions, General 0W9-
Thoracolumbar facet joint
use Joint, Thoracolumbar Vertebral
Thoracoplasty
see Repair, Anatomical Regions, General 0WQ-
see Supplement, Anatomical Regions, General 0WU-
Thoracostomy tube
use Drainage Device
Thoracostomy, for lung collapse
see Drainage, Respiratory System 0B9-
Thoracotomy see Drainage, Anatomical Regions, General 0W9-
Thoratec IVAD (Implantable Ventricular Assist Device)
use Implantable Heart Assist System in Heart and Great Vessels
Thoratec Paracorporeal Ventricular Assist Device
use External Heart Assist System in Heart and Great Vessels
Thrombectomy see Extirpation
Thymectomy
see Excision, Lymphatic and Hemic Systems 07B-
see Resection, Lymphatic and Hemic Systems 07T-
Thymopexy
see Repair, Lymphatic and Hemic Systems 07Q-
see Reposition, Lymphatic and Hemic Systems 07S-
Thymus gland
use Thymus
Thyroarytenoid muscle
use Muscle, Neck, Left
use Muscle, Neck, Right
Thyrocervical trunk
use Artery, Thyroid, Left
use Artery, Thyroid, Right
Thyroid cartilage
use Larynx
Thyroidectomy
see Excision, Endocrine System 0GB-
see Resection, Endocrine System 0GT-
Thyroidorrhaphy see Repair, Endocrine System 0GQ-
Thyroidoscopy 0GJK4ZZ
Thyroidotomy see Drainage, Endocrine System 0G9-

Tibial insert
use Liner in Lower Joints
Tibialis anterior muscle
use Muscle, Lower Leg, Left
use Muscle, Lower Leg, Right
Tibialis posterior muscle
use Muscle, Lower Leg, Left
use Muscle, Lower Leg, Right
Tibiofemoral joint
use Joint, Knee, Left
use Joint, Knee, Right
use Joint, Knee, Left, Tibial Surface
use Joint, Knee, Right, Tibial Surface
TigerPaw® system for closure of left atrial appendage
use Extraluminal Device
Tissue bank graft
use Nonautologous Tissue Substitute
Tissue Expander
Insertion of device in
  Breast
    Bilateral 0HHV-
    Left 0HHU-
    Right 0HHT-
  Nipple
    Left 0HHX-
    Right 0HHW-
  Subcutaneous Tissue and Fascia
    Abdomen 0JH8-
    Back 0JH7-
    Buttock 0JH9-
    Chest 0JH6-
    Face 0JH1-
    Foot
      Left 0JHR-
      Right 0JHQ-
    Hand
      Left 0JHK-
      Right 0JHJ-
    Lower Arm
      Left 0JHH-
      Right 0JHG-
    Lower Leg
      Left 0JHP-
      Right 0JHN-
    Neck
      Anterior 0JH4-
      Posterior 0JH5-
    Pelvic Region 0JHC-
    Perineum 0JHB-
    Scalp 0JH0-
    Upper Arm
      Left 0JHF-
      Right 0JHD-
    Upper Leg
      Left 0JHM-
      Right 0JHL-
Removal of device from
  Breast
    Left 0HPU-
    Right 0HPT-
  Subcutaneous Tissue and Fascia
    Head and Neck 0JPS-
    Lower Extremity 0JPW-
    Trunk 0JPT-
    Upper Extremity 0JPV-
Revision of device in
  Breast
    Left 0HWU-
    Right 0HWT-
  Subcutaneous Tissue and Fascia
    Head and Neck 0JWS-
    Lower Extremity 0JWW-
    Trunk 0JWT-
    Upper Extremity 0JWV-
Tissue expander (inflatable) (injectable)
use Tissue Expander in Skin and Breast
use Tissue Expander in Subcutaneous Tissue and Fascia

Tissue Plasminogen Activator (tPA) (r-tPA)
use Thrombolytic, Other
Titanium Sternal Fixation System (TSFS)
use Internal Fixation Device, Rigid Plate in 0PS-
use Internal Fixation Device, Rigid Plate in 0PH-
Tomographic (Tomo) Nuclear Medicine Imaging
Abdomen CW20-
Abdomen and Chest CW24-
Abdomen and Pelvis CW21-
Anatomical Regions, Multiple CW2YYZZ
Bladder, Kidneys and Ureters CT23-
Brain C020-
Breast CH2YYZZ
  Bilateral CH22-
  Left CH21-
  Right CH20-
Bronchi and Lungs CB22-
Central Nervous System C02YYZZ
Cerebrospinal Fluid C025-
Chest CW23-
Chest and Abdomen CW24-
Chest and Neck CW26-
Digestive System CD2YYZZ
Endocrine System CG2YYZZ
Extremity
  Lower CW2D-
    Bilateral CP2F-
    Left CP2D-
    Right CP2C-
  Upper CW2M-
    Bilateral CP2B-
    Left CP29-
    Right CP28-
Gallbladder CF24-
Gastrointestinal Tract CD27-
Gland, Parathyroid CG21-
Head and Neck CW2B-
Heart C22YYZZ
  Right and Left C226-
Hepatobiliary System and Pancreas CF2YYZZ
Kidneys, Ureters and Bladder CT23-
Liver CF25-
Liver and Spleen CF26-
Lungs and Bronchi CB22-
Lymphatics and Hematologic System C72YYZZ
Musculoskeletal System, Other CP2YYZZ
Myocardium C22G-
Neck and Chest CW26-
Neck and Head CW2B-
Pancreas and Hepatobiliary System CF2YYZZ
Pelvic Region CW2J-
Pelvis CP26-
Pelvis and Abdomen CW21-
Pelvis and Spine CP27-
Respiratory System CB2YYZZ
Skin CH2YYZZ
Skull CP21-
Skull and Cervical Spine CP23-
Spine
  Cervical CP22-
  Cervical and Skull CP23-
  Lumbar CP2H-
  Thoracic CP2G-
  Thoracolumbar CP2J-
Spine and Pelvis CP27-
Spleen C722-
Spleen and Liver CF26-
Subcutaneous Tissue CH2YYZZ
Thorax CP24-
Ureters, Kidneys and Bladder CT23-
Urinary System CT2YYZZ

Tomography, computerized see Computerized Tomography (CT Scan)
Tonometry 4A07XBZ
Tonsillectomy
see Excision, Mouth and Throat 0CB-
see Resection, Mouth and Throat 0CT-
Tonsillotomy see Drainage, Mouth and Throat 0C9-
Total artificial (replacement) heart
use Synthetic Substitute
Total parenteral nutrition (TPN)
see Introduction of Nutritional Substance
Trachectomy
see Excision, Trachea 0BB1-
see Resection, Trachea 0BT1-
Trachelectomy
see Excision, Cervix 0UBC-
see Resection, Cervix 0UTC-
Trachelopexy
see Repair, Cervix 0UQC-
see Reposition, Cervix 0USC-
Tracheloplasty see Repair, Cervix 0UQC-
Trachelorrhaphy see Repair, Cervix 0UQC-
Trachelotomy see Drainage, Cervix 0U9C-
Tracheobronchial lymph node
use Lymphatic, Thorax
Tracheoesophageal fistulization 0B110D6
Tracheolysis see Release, Respiratory System 0BN-
Tracheoplasty
see Repair, Respiratory System 0BQ-
see Supplement, Respiratory System 0BU-
Tracheorrhaphy see Repair, Respiratory System 0BQ-
Tracheoscopy 0BJ18ZZ
Tracheostomy see Bypass, Respiratory System 0B1-
Tracheostomy Device
Bypass, Trachea 0B11-
Change device in, Trachea 0B21XFZ
Removal of device from, Trachea 0BP1-
Revision of device in, Trachea 0BW1-
Tracheostomy tube
use Tracheostomy Device in Respiratory System
Tracheotomy see Drainage, Respiratory System 0B9-
Traction
Abdominal Wall 2W63X-
Arm
  Lower
    Left 2W6DX-
    Right 2W6CX-
  Upper
    Left 2W6BX-
    Right 2W6AX-
Back 2W65X-
Chest Wall 2W64X-
Extremity
  Lower
    Left 2W6MX-
    Right 2W6LX-
  Upper
    Left 2W69X-
    Right 2W68X-
Face 2W61X-
Finger
  Left 2W6KX-
  Right 2W6JX-
Foot
  Left 2W6TX-
  Right 2W6SX-

INDEX TO PROCEDURES – 2016 ICD-10-PCS

Traction — *continued*
  Hand
    Left 2W6FX-
    Right 2W6EX-
  Head 2W60X-
  Inguinal Region
    Left 2W67X-
    Right 2W66X-
  Leg
    Lower
      Left 2W6RX-
      Right 2W6QX-
    Upper
      Left 2W6PX-
      Right 2W6NX-
  Neck 2W62X-
  Thumb
    Left 2W6HX-
    Right 2W6GX-
  Toe
    Left 2W6VX-
    Right 2W6UX-
Tractotomy *see* Division, Central Nervous System 008-
Tragus
  use Ear, External, Bilateral
  use Ear, External, Left
  use Ear, External, Right
Training, caregiver *see* Caregiver Training
TRAM (transverse rectus abdominis myocutaneous) flap reconstruction
  Free *see* Replacement, Skin and Breast 0HR-
  Pedicled *see* Transfer, Muscles 0KX-
Transection *see* Division
Transfer
  Buccal Mucosa 0CX4-
  Bursa and Ligament
    Abdomen
      Left 0MXJ-
      Right 0MXH-
    Ankle
      Left 0MXR-
      Right 0MXQ-
    Elbow
      Left 0MX4-
      Right 0MX3-
    Foot
      Left 0MXT-
      Right 0MXS-
    Hand
      Left 0MX8-
      Right 0MX7-
    Head and Neck 0MX0-
    Hip
      Left 0MXM-
      Right 0MXL-
    Knee
      Left 0MXP-
      Right 0MXN-
    Lower Extremity
      Left 0MXW-
      Right 0MXV-
    Perineum 0MXK-
    Shoulder
      Left 0MX2-
      Right 0MX1-
    Thorax
      Left 0MXG-
      Right 0MXF-
    Trunk
      Left 0MXD-
      Right 0MXC-
    Upper Extremity
      Left 0MXB-
      Right 0MX9-
    Wrist
      Left 0MX6-
      Right 0MX5-

Transfer — *continued*
  Finger
    Left 0XXP0ZM
    Right 0XXN0ZL
  Gingiva
    Lower 0CX6-
    Upper 0CX5-
  Intestine
    Large 0DXE-
    Small 0DX8-
  Lip
    Lower 0CX1-
    Upper 0CX0-
  Muscle
    Abdomen
      Left 0KXL-
      Right 0KXK-
    Extraocular
      Left 08XM-
      Right 08XL-
    Facial 0KX1-
    Foot
      Left 0KXW-
      Right 0KXV-
    Hand
      Left 0KXD-
      Right 0KXC-
    Head 0KX0-
    Hip
      Left 0KXP-
      Right 0KXN-
    Lower Arm and Wrist
      Left 0KXB-
      Right 0KX9-
    Lower Leg
      Left 0KXT-
      Right 0KXS-
    Neck
      Left 0KX3-
      Right 0KX2-
    Perineum 0KXM-
    Shoulder
      Left 0KX6-
      Right 0KX5-
    Thorax
      Left 0KXJ-
      Right 0KXH-
    Tongue, Palate, Pharynx 0KX4-
    Trunk
      Left 0KXG-
      Right 0KXF-
    Upper Arm
      Left 0KX8-
      Right 0KX7-
    Upper Leg
      Left 0KXR-
      Right 0KXQ-
  Nerve
    Abducens 00XL-
    Accessory 00XR-
    Acoustic 00XN-
    Cervical 01X1-
    Facial 00XM-
    Femoral 01XD-
    Glossopharyngeal 00XP-
    Hypoglossal 00XS-
    Lumbar 01XB-
    Median 01X5-
    Oculomotor 00XH-
    Olfactory 00XF-
    Optic 00XG-
    Peroneal 01XH-
    Phrenic 01X2-
    Pudendal 01XC-
    Radial 01X6-
    Sciatic 01XF-
    Thoracic 01X8-
    Tibial 01XG-
    Trigeminal 00XK-
    Trochlear 00XJ-
    Ulnar 01X4-
    Vagus 00XQ-

Transfer — *continued*
  Palate, Soft 0CX3-
  Skin
    Abdomen 0HX7XZZ
    Back 0HX6XZZ
    Buttock 0HX8XZZ
    Chest 0HX5XZZ
    Ear
      Left 0HX3XZZ
      Right 0HX2XZZ
    Face 0HX1XZZ
    Foot
      Left 0HXNXZZ
      Right 0HXMXZZ
    Genitalia 0HXAXZZ
    Hand
      Left 0HXGXZZ
      Right 0HXFXZZ
    Lower Arm
      Left 0HXEXZZ
      Right 0HXDXZZ
    Lower Leg
      Left 0HXLXZZ
      Right 0HXKXZZ
    Neck 0HX4XZZ
    Perineum 0HX9XZZ
    Scalp 0HX0XZZ
    Upper Arm
      Left 0HXCXZZ
      Right 0HXBXZZ
    Upper Leg
      Left 0HXJXZZ
      Right 0HXHXZZ
  Stomach 0DX6-
  Subcutaneous Tissue and Fascia
    Abdomen 0JX8-
    Back 0JX7-
    Buttock 0JX9-
    Chest 0JX6-
    Face 0JX1-
    Foot
      Left 0JXR-
      Right 0JXQ-
    Hand
      Left 0JXK-
      Right 0JXJ-
    Lower Arm
      Left 0JXH-
      Right 0JXG-
    Lower Leg
      Left 0JXP-
      Right 0JXN-
    Neck
      Anterior 0JX4-
      Posterior 0JX5-
    Pelvic Region 0JXC-
    Perineum 0JXB-
    Scalp 0JX0-
    Upper Arm
      Left 0JXF-
      Right 0JXD-
    Upper Leg
      Left 0JXM-
      Right 0JXL-
  Tendon
    Abdomen
      Left 0LXG-
      Right 0LXF-
    Ankle
      Left 0LXT-
      Right 0LXS-
    Foot
      Left 0LXW-
      Right 0LXV-
    Hand
      Left 0LX8-
      Right 0LX7-
    Head and Neck 0LX0-
    Hip
      Left 0LXK-
      Right 0LXJ-

Transfer — *continued*
  Tendon — *continued*
    Knee
      Left 0LXR-
      Right 0LXQ-
    Lower Arm and Wrist
      Left 0LX6-
      Right 0LX5-
    Lower Leg
      Left 0LXP-
      Right 0LXN-
    Perineum 0LXH-
    Shoulder
      Left 0LX2-
      Right 0LX1-
    Thorax
      Left 0LXD-
      Right 0LXC-
    Trunk
      Left 0LXB-
      Right 0LX9-
    Upper Arm
      Left 0LX4-
      Right 0LX3-
    Upper Leg
      Left 0LXM-
      Right 0LXL-
  Tongue 0CX7-
Transfusion
  Artery
    Central
      Antihemophilic Factors 3026-
      Blood
        Platelets 3026-
        Red Cells 3026-
          Frozen 3026-
        White Cells 3026-
        Whole 3026-
      Bone Marrow 3026-
      Factor IX 3026-
      Fibrinogen 3026-
      Globulin 3026-
      Plasma
        Fresh 3026-
        Frozen 3026-
      Plasma Cryoprecipitate 3026-
      Serum Albumin 3026-
      Stem Cells
        Cord Blood 3026-
        Hematopoietic 3026-
    Peripheral
      Antihemophilic Factors 3025-
      Blood
        Platelets 3025-
        Red Cells 3025-
          Frozen 3025-
        White Cells 3025-
        Whole 3025-
      Bone Marrow 3025-
      Factor IX 3025-
      Fibrinogen 3025-
      Globulin 3025-
      Plasma
        Fresh 3025-
        Frozen 3025-
      Plasma Cryoprecipitate 3025-
      Serum Albumin 3025-
      Stem Cells
        Cord Blood 3025-
        Hematopoietic 3025-
  Products of Conception
    Antihemophilic Factors 3027-
    Blood
      Platelets 3027-
      Red Cells 3027-
        Frozen 3027-
      White Cells 3027-
      Whole 3027-
    Factor IX 3027-
    Fibrinogen 3027-
    Globulin 3027-

Transfusion

INDEX TO PROCEDURES – 2016 ICD-10-PCS [2016.PCS]

Transfusion — *continued*
Products of Conception — *continued*
  Plasma
   Fresh 3027-
   Frozen 3027-
   Plasma Cryoprecipitate 3027-
   Serum Albumin 3027-
  Vein
   4-Factor Prothrombin Complex Concentrate 3028-
   Central
    Antihemophilic Factors 3024-
    Blood
     Platelets 3024-
     Red Cells 3024-
      Frozen 3024-
     White Cells 3024-
     Whole 3024-
    Bone Marrow 3024-
    Factor IX 3024-
    Fibrinogen 3024-
    Globulin 3024-
    Plasma
     Fresh 3024-
     Frozen 3024-
    Plasma Cryoprecipitate 3024-
    Serum Albumin 3024-
    Stem Cells
     Cord Blood 3024-
     Embryonic 3024-
     Hematopoietic 3024-
   Peripheral
    Antihemophilic Factors 3023-
    Blood
     Platelets 3023-
     Red Cells 3023-
      Frozen 3023-
     White Cells 3023-
     Whole 3023-
    Bone Marrow 3023-
    Factor IX 3023-
    Fibrinogen 3023-
    Globulin 3023-
    Plasma
     Fresh 3023-
     Frozen 3023-
    Plasma Cryoprecipitate 3023-
    Serum Albumin 3023-
    Stem Cells
     Cord Blood 3023-
     Embryonic 3023-
     Hematopoietic 3023-
Transplantation
 Esophagus 0DY50Z-
 Heart 02YA0Z-
 Intestine
  Large 0DYE0Z-
  Small 0DY80Z-
 Kidney
  Left 0TY10Z-
  Right 0TY00Z-
 Liver 0FY00Z-
 Lung
  Bilateral 0BYM0Z-
  Left 0BYL0Z-
  Lower Lobe
   Left 0BYJ0Z-
   Right 0BYF0Z-
  Middle Lobe, Right 0BYD0Z-
  Right 0BYK0Z-
  Upper Lobe
   Left 0BYG0Z-
   Right 0BYC0Z-
 Lung Lingula 0BYH0Z-
 Ovary
  Left 0UY10Z-
  Right 0UY00Z-
 Pancreas 0FYG0Z-
 Products of Conception 10Y0-
 Spleen 07YP0Z-
 Stomach 0DY60Z-
 Thymus 07YM0Z-

Transposition
 see Reposition
 see Transfer
Transversalis fascia
 use Subcutaneous Tissue and Fascia, Trunk
Transverse (cutaneous) cervical nerve
 use Nerve, Cervical Plexus
Transverse acetabular ligament
 use Bursa and Ligament, Hip, Left
 use Bursa and Ligament, Hip, Right
Transverse facial artery
 use Artery, Temporal, Left
 use Artery, Temporal, Right
Transverse humeral ligament
 use Bursa and Ligament, Shoulder, Left
 use Bursa and Ligament, Shoulder, Right
Transverse ligament of atlas
 use Bursa and Ligament, Head and Neck
Transverse Rectus Abdominis Myocutaneous Flap
 Replacement
  Bilateral 0HRV076
  Left 0HRU076
  Right 0HRT076
 Transfer
  Left 0KXL-
  Right 0KXK-
Transverse scapular ligament
 use Bursa and Ligament, Shoulder, Left
 use Bursa and Ligament, Shoulder, Right
Transverse thoracis muscle
 use Muscle, Thorax, Left
 use Muscle, Thorax, Right
Transversospinalis muscle
 use Muscle, Trunk, Left
 use Muscle, Trunk, Right
Transversus abdominis muscle
 use Muscle, Abdomen, Left
 use Muscle, Abdomen, Right
Trapezium bone
 use Carpal, Left
 use Carpal, Right
Trapezius muscle
 use Muscle, Trunk, Left
 use Muscle, Trunk, Right
Trapezoid bone
 use Carpal, Left
 use Carpal, Right
Triceps brachii muscle
 use Muscle, Upper Arm, Left
 use Muscle, Upper Arm, Right
Tricuspid annulus
 use Valve, Tricuspid
Trifacial nerve
 use Nerve, Trigeminal
Trifecta™ Valve (aortic)
 use Zooplastic Tissue in Heart and Great Vessels
Trigone of bladder
 use Bladder
Trimming, excisional *see* Excision
Triquetral bone
 use Carpal, Left
 use Carpal, Right
Trochanteric bursa
 use Bursa and Ligament, Hip, Left
 use Bursa and Ligament, Hip, Right
TUMT (Transurethral microwave thermotherapy of prostate) 0V507ZZ
TUNA (transurethral needle ablation of prostate) 0V507ZZ
Tunneled central venous catheter
 use Vascular Access Device in Subcutaneous Tissue and Fascia

Tunneled spinal (intrathecal) catheter
 use Infusion Device
Turbinectomy
 see Excision, Ear, Nose, Sinus 09B-
 see Resection, Ear, Nose, Sinus 09T-
Turbinoplasty
 see Repair, Ear, Nose, Sinus 09Q-
 see Replacement, Ear, Nose, Sinus 09R-
 see Supplement, Ear, Nose, Sinus 09U-
Turbinotomy
 see Drainage, Ear, Nose, Sinus 099-
 see Division, Ear, Nose, Sinus 098-
TURP (transurethral resection of prostate)
 see Excision, Prostate 0VB0-
 see Resection, Prostate 0VT0-
Twelfth cranial nerve
 use Nerve, Hypoglossal
Two lead pacemaker
 use Pacemaker, Dual Chamber in 0JH-
Tympanic cavity
 use Ear, Middle, Left
 use Ear, Middle, Right
Tympanic nerve
 use Nerve, Glossopharyngeal
Tympanic part of temporal bone
 use Bone, Temporal, Left
 use Bone, Temporal, Right
Tympanogram *see* Hearing Assessment, Diagnostic Audiology F13-
Tympanoplasty
 see Repair, Ear, Nose, Sinus 09Q-
 see Replacement, Ear, Nose, Sinus 09R-
 see Supplement, Ear, Nose, Sinus 09U-
Tympanosympathectomy *see* Excision, Nerve, Head and Neck Sympathetic 01BK-
Tympanotomy *see* Drainage, Ear, Nose, Sinus 099-

U

Ulnar collateral carpal ligament
 use Bursa and Ligament, Wrist, Left
 use Bursa and Ligament, Wrist, Right
Ulnar collateral ligament
 use Bursa and Ligament, Elbow, Left
 use Bursa and Ligament, Elbow, Right
Ulnar notch
 use Radius, Left
 use Radius, Right
Ulnar vein
 use Vein, Brachial, Left
 use Vein, Brachial, Right
Ultrafiltration
 Hemodialysis *see* Performance, Urinary 5A1D-
 Therapeutic plasmapheresis *see* Pheresis, Circulatory 6A55-
Ultraflex™ Precision Colonic Stent System
 use Intraluminal Device
ULTRAPRO Hernia System (UHS)
 use Synthetic Substitute
ULTRAPRO Partially Absorbable Lightweight Mesh
 use Synthetic Substitute
ULTRAPRO Plug
 use Synthetic Substitute
Ultrasonic osteogenic stimulator
 use Bone Growth Stimulator in Head and Facial Bones
 use Bone Growth Stimulator in Lower Bones
 use Bone Growth Stimulator in Upper Bones
Ultrasonography
 Abdomen BW40ZZZ
 Abdomen and Pelvis BW41ZZZ
 Abdominal Wall BH49ZZZ
 Aorta
  Abdominal, Intravascular B440ZZ3
  Thoracic, Intravascular B340ZZ3
 Appendix BD48ZZZ
 Artery
  Brachiocephalic-Subclavian, Right, Intravascular B341ZZ3
  Celiac and Mesenteric, Intravascular B44KZZ3
  Common Carotid
   Bilateral, Intravascular B345ZZ3
   Left, Intravascular B344ZZ3
   Right, Intravascular B343ZZ3
  Coronary
   Multiple B241YZZ
    Intravascular B241ZZ3
    Transesophageal B241ZZ4
   Single B240YZZ
    Intravascular B240ZZ3
    Transesophageal B240ZZ4
  Femoral, Intravascular B44LZZ3
  Inferior Mesenteric, Intravascular B445ZZ3
  Internal Carotid
   Bilateral, Intravascular B348ZZ3
   Left, Intravascular B347ZZ3
   Right, Intravascular B346ZZ3
  Intra-Abdominal, Other, Intravascular B44BZZ3
  Intracranial, Intravascular B34RZZ3
  Lower Extremity
   Bilateral, Intravascular B44HZZ3
   Left, Intravascular B44GZZ3
   Right, Intravascular B44FZZ3
  Mesenteric and Celiac, Intravascular B44KZZ3
  Ophthalmic, Intravascular B34VZZ3
  Penile, Intravascular B44NZZ3

INDEX TO PROCEDURES – 2016 ICD-10-PCS

Ultrasonography — continued
Artery — continued
  Pulmonary
    Left, Intravascular **B34TZZ3**
    Right, Intravascular **B34SZZ3**
  Renal
    Bilateral, Intravascular **B448ZZ3**
    Left, Intravascular **B447ZZ3**
    Right, Intravascular **B446ZZ3**
  Subclavian, Left, Intravascular **B342ZZ3**
  Superior Mesenteric, Intravascular **B444ZZ3**
  Upper Extremity
    Bilateral, Intravascular **B34KZZ3**
    Left, Intravascular **B34JZZ3**
    Right, Intravascular **B34HZZ3**
Bile Duct **BF40ZZZ**
Bile Duct and Gallbladder **BF43ZZZ**
Bladder **BT40ZZZ**
  and Kidney **BT4JZZZ**
Brain **B040ZZZ**
Breast
  Bilateral **BH42ZZZ**
  Left **BH41ZZZ**
  Right **BH40ZZZ**
Chest Wall **BH4BZZZ**
Coccyx **BR4FZZZ**
Connective Tissue
  Lower Extremity **BL41ZZZ**
  Upper Extremity **BL40ZZZ**
Duodenum **BD49ZZZ**
Elbow
  Left, Densitometry **BP4HZZ1**
  Right, Densitometry **BP4GZZ1**
Esophagus **BD41ZZZ**
Extremity
  Lower **BH48ZZZ**
  Upper **BH47ZZZ**
Eye
  Bilateral **B847ZZZ**
  Left **B846ZZZ**
  Right **B845ZZZ**
Fallopian Tube
  Bilateral **BU42-**
  Left **BU41-**
  Right **BU40-**
Fetal Umbilical Cord **BY47ZZZ**
Fetus
  First Trimester, Multiple Gestation **BY4BZZZ**
  Second Trimester, Multiple Gestation **BY4DZZZ**
  Single
    First Trimester **BY49ZZZ**
    Second Trimester **BY4CZZZ**
    Third Trimester **BY4FZZZ**
  Third Trimester, Multiple Gestation **BY4GZZZ**
Gallbladder **BF42ZZZ**
Gallbladder and Bile Duct **BF43ZZZ**
Gastrointestinal Tract **BD47ZZZ**
Gland
  Adrenal
    Bilateral **BG42ZZZ**
    Left **BG41ZZZ**
    Right **BG40ZZZ**
  Parathyroid **BG43ZZZ**
  Thyroid **BG44ZZZ**
Hand
  Left, Densitometry **BP4PZZ1**
  Right, Densitometry **BP4NZZ1**
Head and Neck **BH4CZZZ**

Ultrasonography — continued
Heart
  Left **B245YZZ**
    Intravascular **B245ZZ3**
    Transesophageal **B245ZZ4**
  Pediatric **B24DYZZ**
    Intravascular **B24DZZ3**
    Transesophageal **B24DZZ4**
  Right **B244YZZ**
    Intravascular **B244ZZ3**
    Transesophageal **B244ZZ4**
  Right and Left **B246YZZ**
    Intravascular **B246ZZ3**
    Transesophageal **B246ZZ4**
Heart with Aorta **B24BYZZ**
    Intravascular **B24BZZ3**
    Transesophageal **B24BZZ4**
Hepatobiliary System, All **BF4CZZZ**
Hip
  Bilateral **BQ42ZZZ**
  Left **BQ41ZZZ**
  Right **BQ40ZZZ**
Kidney
  and Bladder **BT4JZZZ**
  Bilateral **BT43ZZZ**
  Left **BT42ZZZ**
  Right **BT41ZZZ**
  Transplant **BT49ZZZ**
Knee
  Bilateral **BQ49ZZZ**
  Left **BQ48ZZZ**
  Right **BQ47ZZZ**
Liver **BF45ZZZ**
Liver and Spleen **BF46ZZZ**
Mediastinum **BB4CZZZ**
Neck **BW4FZZZ**
Ovary
  Bilateral **BU45-**
  Left **BU44-**
  Right **BU43-**
Ovary and Uterus **BU4C-**
Pancreas **BF47ZZZ**
Pelvic Region **BW4GZZZ**
Pelvis and Abdomen **BW41ZZZ**
Penis **BV4BZZZ**
Pericardium **B24CYZZ**
    Intravascular **B24CZZ3**
    Transesophageal **B24CZZ4**
Placenta **BY48ZZZ**
Pleura **BB4BZZZ**
Prostate and Seminal Vesicle **BV49ZZZ**
Rectum **BD4CZZZ**
Sacrum **BR4FZZZ**
Scrotum **BV44ZZZ**
Seminal Vesicle and Prostate **BV49ZZZ**
Shoulder
  Left, Densitometry **BP49ZZ1**
  Right, Densitometry **BP48ZZ1**
Spinal Cord **B04BZZZ**
Spine
  Cervical **BR40ZZZ**
  Lumbar **BR49ZZZ**
  Thoracic **BR47ZZZ**
Spleen and Liver **BF46ZZZ**
Stomach **BD42ZZZ**
Tendon
  Lower Extremity **BL43ZZZ**
  Upper Extremity **BL42ZZZ**
Ureter
  Bilateral **BT48ZZZ**
  Left **BT47ZZZ**
  Right **BT46ZZZ**
Urethra **BT45ZZZ**
Uterus **BU46-**
Uterus and Ovary **BU4C-**

Ultrasonography — continued
Vein
  Jugular
    Left, Intravascular **B544ZZ3**
    Right, Intravascular **B543ZZ3**
  Lower Extremity
    Bilateral, Intravascular **B54DZZ3**
    Left, Intravascular **B54CZZ3**
    Right, Intravascular **B54BZZ3**
  Portal, Intravascular **B54TZZ3**
  Renal
    Bilateral, Intravascular **B54LZZ3**
    Left, Intravascular **B54KZZ3**
    Right, Intravascular **B54JZZ3**
  Spanchnic, Intravascular **B54TZZ3**
  Subclavian
    Left, Intravascular **B547ZZ3**
    Right, Intravascular **B546ZZ3**
  Upper Extremity
    Bilateral, Intravascular **B54PZZ3**
    Left, Intravascular **B54NZZ3**
    Right, Intravascular **B54MZZ3**
  Vena Cava
    Inferior, Intravascular **B549ZZ3**
    Superior, Intravascular **B548ZZ3**
  Wrist
    Left, Densitometry **BP4MZZ1**
    Right, Densitometry **BP4LZZ1**
Ultrasound bone healing system
  use Bone Growth Stimulator in Head and Facial Bones
  use Bone Growth Stimulator in Lower Bones
  use Bone Growth Stimulator in Upper Bones
Ultrasound Therapy
  Heart **6A75-**
  No Qualifier **6A75-**
  Vessels
    Head and Neck **6A75-**
    Other **6A75-**
    Peripheral **6A75-**
Ultraviolet Light Therapy, Skin 6A80-
Umbilical artery
  use Artery, Internal Iliac, Left
  use Artery, Internal Iliac, Right
Uniplanar external fixator
  use External Fixation Device, Monoplanar in **0PH-**
  use External Fixation Device, Monoplanar in **0PS-**
  use External Fixation Device, Monoplanar in **0QH-**
  use External Fixation Device, Monoplanar in **0QS-**
Upper GI series see Fluoroscopy, Gastrointestinal, Upper **BD15-**
Ureteral orifice
  use Ureter
  use Ureter, Left
  use Ureter, Right
  use Ureters, Bilateral
Ureterectomy
  see Excision, Urinary System **0TB-**
  see Resection, Urinary System **0TT-**
Ureterocolostomy see Bypass, Urinary System **0T1-**
Ureterocystostomy see Bypass, Urinary System **0T1-**
Ureteroenterostomy see Bypass, Urinary System **0T1-**
Ureteroileostomy see Bypass, Urinary System **0T1-**
Ureterolithotomy see Extirpation, Urinary System **0TC-**
Ureterolysis see Release, Urinary System **0TN-**
Ureteroneocystostomy
  see Bypass, Urinary System **0T1-**
  see Reposition, Urinary System **0TS-**

Ureteropelvic junction (UPJ)
  use Kidney Pelvis, Left
  use Kidney Pelvis, Right
Ureteropexy
  see Repair, Urinary System **0TQ-**
  see Reposition, Urinary System **0TS-**
Ureteroplasty
  see Repair, Urinary System **0TQ-**
  see Replacement, Urinary System **0TR-**
  see Supplement, Urinary System **0TU-**
Ureteroplication see Restriction, Urinary System **0TV-**
Ureteropyelography see Fluoroscopy, Urinary System **BT1-**
Ureterorrhaphy see Repair, Urinary System **0TQ-**
Ureteroscopy 0TJ98ZZ
Ureterostomy
  see Bypass, Urinary System **0T1**
  see Drainage, Urinary System **0T9-**
Ureterotomy see Drainage, Urinary System **0T9-**
Ureteroureterostomy see Bypass, Urinary System **0T1-**
Ureterovesical orifice
  use Ureter
  use Ureter, Left
  use Ureter, Right
  use Ureters, Bilateral
Urethral catheterization, indwelling 0T9B70Z
Urethrectomy
  see Excision, Urethra **0TBD-**
  see Resection, Urethra **0TTD-**
Urethrolithotomy see Extirpation, Urethra **0TCD-**
Urethrolysis see Release, Urethra **0TND-**
Urethropexy
  see Repair, Urethra **0TQD-**
  see Reposition, Urethra **0TSD-**
Urethroplasty
  see Repair, Urethra **0TQD-**
  see Replacement, Urethra **0TRD-**
  see Supplement, Urethra **0TUD-**
Urethrorrhaphy see Repair, Urethra **0TQD-**
Urethroscopy 0TJD8ZZ
Urethrotomy see Drainage, Urethra **0T9D-**
Urinary incontinence stimulator lead
  use Stimulator Lead in Urinary System
Urography see Fluoroscopy, Urinary System **BT1-**
Uterine Artery
  use Artery, Internal Iliac, Left
  use Artery, Internal Iliac, Right
Uterine artery embolization (UAE) see Occlusion, Lower Arteries **04L-**
Uterine cornu
  use Uterus
Uterine tube
  use Fallopian Tube, Left
  use Fallopian Tube, Right
Uterine vein
  use Vein, Hypogastric, Left
  use Vein, Hypogastric, Right
Uvulectomy
  see Excision, Uvula **0CBN-**
  see Resection, Uvula **0CTN-**
Uvulorrhaphy see Repair, Uvula **0CQN-**
Uvulotomy see Drainage, Uvula **0C9N-**

V

Vaccination see Introduction of Serum, Toxoid, and Vaccine
Vacuum extraction, obstetric 10D07Z6
Vaginal artery
 use Artery, Internal Iliac, Left
 use Artery, Internal Iliac, Right
Vaginal pessary
 use Intraluminal Device, Pessary in Female Reproductive System
Vaginal vein
 use Vein, Hypogastric, Left
 use Vein, Hypogastric, Right
Vaginectomy
 see Excision, Vagina 0UBG-
 see Resection, Vagina 0UTG-
Vaginofixation
 see Repair, Vagina 0UQG-
 see Reposition, Vagina 0USG-
Vaginoplasty
 see Repair, Vagina 0UQG-
 see Supplement, Vagina 0UUG-
Vaginorrhaphy see Repair, Vagina 0UQG-
Vaginoscopy 0UJH8ZZ
Vaginotomy see Drainage, Female Reproductive System 0U9-
Vagotomy see Division, Nerve, Vagus 008Q-
Valiant Thoracic Stent Graft
 use Intraluminal Device
Valvotomy, valvulotomy
 see Division, Heart and Great Vessels 028-
 see Release, Heart and Great Vessels 02N-
Valvuloplasty
 see Repair, Heart and Great Vessels 02Q-
 see Replacement, Heart and Great Vessels 02R-
 see Supplement, Heart and Great Vessels 02U-
Vascular Access Device
 Insertion of device in
  Abdomen 0JH8-
  Chest 0JH6-
  Lower Arm
   Left 0JHH-
   Right 0JHG-
  Lower Leg
   Left 0JHP-
   Right 0JHN-
  Upper Arm
   Left 0JHF-
   Right 0JHD-
  Upper Leg
   Left 0JHM-
   Right 0JHL-
 Removal of device from
  Lower Extremity 0JPW-
  Trunk 0JPT-
  Upper Extremity 0JPV-
 Reservoir
  Insertion of device in
   Abdomen 0JH8-
   Chest 0JH6-
   Lower Arm
    Left 0JHH-
    Right 0JHG-
   Lower Leg
    Left 0JHP-
    Right 0JHN-
   Upper Arm
    Left 0JHF-
    Right 0JHD-
   Upper Leg
    Left 0JHM-
    Right 0JHL-

Vascular Access Device — continued
 Reservoir — continued
  Removal of device from
   Lower Extremity 0JPW-
   Trunk 0JPT-
   Upper Extremity 0JPV-
  Revision of device in
   Lower Extremity 0JWW-
   Trunk 0JWT-
   Upper Extremity 0JWV-
 Revision of device in
  Lower Extremity 0JWW-
  Trunk 0JWT-
  Upper Extremity 0JWV
Vasectomy see Excision, Male Reproductive System 0VB-
Vasography
 see Fluoroscopy, Male Reproductive System BV1-
 see Plain Radiography, Male Reproductive System BV0-
Vasoligation see Occlusion, Male Reproductive System 0VL-
Vasorrhaphy see Repair, Male Reproductive System 0VQ-
Vasostomy see Bypass, Male Reproductive System 0V1-
Vasotomy
 Drainage see Drainage, Male Reproductive System 0V9-
 With ligation see Occlusion, Male Reproductive System 0VL-
Vasovasostomy see Repair, Male Reproductive System 0VQ-
Vastus intermedius muscle
 use Muscle, Upper Leg, Left
 use Muscle, Upper Leg, Right
Vastus lateralis muscle
 use Muscle, Upper Leg, Left
 use Muscle, Upper Leg, Right
Vastus medialis muscle
 use Muscle, Upper Leg, Left
 use Muscle, Upper Leg, Right
VCG (vectorcardiogram) see Measurement, Cardiac 4A02-
Vectra® Vascular Access Graft
 use Vascular Access Device in Subcutaneous Tissue and Fascia
Venectomy
 see Excision, Lower Veins 06B-
 see Excision, Upper Veins 05B-
Venography
 see Fluoroscopy, Veins B51-
 see Plain Radiography, Veins B50-
Venorrhaphy
 see Repair, Lower Veins 06Q-
 see Repair, Upper Veins 05Q-
Venotripsy
 see Occlusion, Lower Veins 06L-
 see Occlusion, Upper Veins 05L-
Ventricular fold
 use Larynx
Ventriculoatriostomy see Bypass, Central Nervous System 001-
Ventriculocisternostomy see Bypass, Central Nervous System 001-
Ventriculogram, cardiac
 Combined left and right heart see Fluoroscopy, Heart, Right and Left B216-
 Left ventricle see Fluoroscopy, Heart, Left B215-
 Right ventricle see Fluoroscopy, Heart, Right B214-
Ventriculopuncture, through previously implanted catheter 8C01X6J
Ventriculoscopy 00J04ZZ

Ventriculostomy
 External drainage see Drainage, Cerebral Ventricle 0096-
 Internal shunt see Bypass, Cerebral Ventricle 0016-
Ventriculovenostomy see Bypass, Cerebral Ventricle 0016-
Ventrio™ Hernia Patch
 use Synthetic Substitute
VEP (visual evoked potential) 4A07X0Z
Vermiform appendix
 use Appendix
Vermilion border
 use Lip, Lower
 use Lip, Upper
Versa
 use Pacemaker, Dual chamber in 0JH-
Version, obstetric
 External 10S0XZZ
 Internal 10S07ZZ
Vertebral arch
 use Vertebra, Cervical
 use Vertebra, Lumbar
 use Vertebra, Thoracic
Vertebral canal
 use Spinal Canal
Vertebral foramen
 use Vertebra, Cervical
 use Vertebra, Lumbar
 use Vertebra, Thoracic
Vertebral lamina
 use Vertebra, Cervical
 use Vertebra, Lumbar
 use Vertebra, Thoracic
Vertebral pedicle
 use Vertebra, Cervical
 use Vertebra, Lumbar
 use Vertebra, Thoracic
Vesical vein
 use Vein, Hypogastric, Left
 use Vein, Hypogastric, Right
Vesicotomy see Drainage, Urinary System 0T9-
Vesiculectomy
 see Excision, Male Reproductive System 0VB-
 see Resection, Male Reproductive System 0VT-
Vesiculogram, seminal see Plain Radiography, Male Reproductive System BV0-
Vesiculotomy see Drainage, Male Reproductive System 0V9-
Vestibular (Scarpa's) ganglion
 use Nerve, Acoustic
Vestibular Assessment F15Z-
Vestibular nerve
 use Nerve, Acoustic
Vestibular Treatment F0C-
Vestibulocochlear nerve
 use Nerve, Acoustic
VH-IVUS (virtual histology intravascular ultrasound)
 see Ultrasonography, Heart B24-
Virchow's (supraclavicular) lymph node
 use Lymphatic, Neck, Left
 use Lymphatic, Neck, Right
Virtuoso (II) (DR) (VR)
 use Defibrillator Generator in 0JH-
Vitrectomy
 see Excision, Eye 08B-
 see Resection, Eye 08T-
Vitreous body
 use Vitreous, Left
 use Vitreous, Right
Viva (XT) (S)
 use Cardiac Resynchronization Defibrillator Pulse Generator in 0JH-

Vocal fold
 use Vocal Cord, Left
 use Vocal Cord, Right
Vocational
 Assessment see Activities of Daily Living Assessment, Rehabilitation F02-
 Retraining see Activities of Daily Living Treatment, Rehabilitation F08-
Volar (palmar) digital vein
 use Vein, Hand, Left
 use Vein, Hand, Right
Volar (palmar) metacarpal vein
 use Vein, Hand, Left
 use Vein, Hand, Right
Vomer bone
 use Septum, Nasal
Vomer of nasal septum
 use Bone, Nasal
Voraxaze
 use Glucarpidase
Vulvectomy
 see Excision, Female Reproductive System 0UB-
 see Resection, Female Reproductive System 0UT-

W

WALLSTENT® Endoprosthesis
 use Intraluminal Device
Washing see Irrigation
Wedge resection, pulmonary see Excision, Respiratory System 0BB-
Window see Drainage
Wiring, dental 2W31X9Z

X

Xact Carotid Stent System
 use Intraluminal Device
X-ray see Plain Radiography
X-STOP® Spacer
 use Spinal Stabilization Device, Interspinous Process in 0RH-
 use Spinal Stabilization Device, Interspinous Process in 0SH-
Xenograft
 use Zooplastic Tissue in Heart and Great Vessels
XIENCE Everolimus Eluting Coronary Stent System
 use Intraluminal Device, Drug-eluting in Heart and Great Vessels
Xiphoid process
 use Sternum
XLIF® System
 use Interbody Fusion Device in Lower Joints

Y

Yoga Therapy 8E0ZXY4

Z

Z-plasty, skin for scar contracture
 see Release, Skin and Breast 0HN-
Zenith Flex® AAA Endovascular Graft
 use Intraluminal Device
Zenith TX2® TAA Endovascular Graft
 use Intraluminal Device
Zenith® Renu™ AAA Ancillary Graft
 use Intraluminal Device
Zilver® PTX® (paclitaxel) Drug-Eluting Peripheral Stent
 use Intraluminal Device, Drug-eluting in Lower Arteries
 use Intraluminal Device, Drug-eluting in Upper Arteries
Zimmer® NexGen® LPS Mobile Bearing Knee
 use Synthetic Substitute
Zimmer® NexGen® LPS-Flex Mobile Knee
 use Synthetic Substitute
Zonule of Zinn
 use Lens, Left
 use Lens, Right
Zotarolimus-eluting coronary stent
 use Intraluminal Device, Drug-eluting in Heart and Great Vessels
Zygomatic process of frontal bone
 use Bone, Frontal, Left
 use Bone, Frontal, Right
Zygomatic process of temporal bone
 use Bone, Temporal, Left
 use Bone, Temporal, Right
Zygomaticus muscle
 use Muscle, Facial
Zyvox
 use Oxazolidinones

NOTES

Educational Annotations | 0 – Central Nervous System

Body System Specific Educational Annotations for the Central Nervous System include:
- Anatomy and Physiology Review
- Anatomical Illustrations
- Definitions of Common Procedures
- AHA Coding Clinic® Reference Notations
- Body Part Key Listings
- Device Key Listings
- Device Aggregation Table Listings
- Coding Notes

Anatomy and Physiology Review of Central Nervous System

BODY PART VALUES – 0 - CENTRAL NERVOUS SYSTEM

Abducens Nerve – The sixth (VI) cranial nerve that innervates the lateral rectus muscles of the eye.

Accessory Nerve – The eleventh (XI) cranial nerve that innervates the sternocleidomastoideus and trapezius muscles.

Acoustic Nerve – The cochlear (hearing) portion of the eighth (VIII) cranial nerve (also known as the vestibulocochlear or auditory nerve).

Basal Ganglia – ANATOMY – The basal ganglia are masses of gray matter located deep within the cerebral hemispheres, including the globus pallidus. The corpus striatum consists of 2 of the basal ganglia, the caudate and lentiform nuclei. PHYSIOLOGY – The basal ganglia function as relay stations for motor impulses.

Brain – ANATOMY – The brain is the largest and most complex part of the nervous system, and is located in the cranial cavity. The cerebrum is the largest part of the brain, and is divided sagittally (front and back through the center) into 2 hemispheres. The corpus callosum lies below and connects the 2 hemispheres. The frontal lobe forms the anterior portion of each cerebral hemisphere. The temporal lobes lie below the frontal lobe on the lateral side of each cerebral hemisphere. The parietal lobe forms the superior portion of the cerebrum, lying posterior to the frontal lobe. The occipital lobe forms the posterior portion of each cerebral hemisphere. The brain stem connects the upper end of the spinal cord with the cerebrum. It contains the pons, cerebral peduncle, medulla oblongata, and midbrain. The tapetum is a layer of fibers from the corpus callosum forming the roof and lateral walls of the lateral ventricles. PHYSIOLOGY – The cerebrum, including its lobes and cerebral cortex, is concerned with the higher brain functions, such as memory, learning, thought, reasoning, hearing, vision, speech, language, and voluntary muscle control.

Cerebellum – ANATOMY – The cerebellum is the second largest portion of the brain, located below the occipital lobe and behind the brain stem. PHYSIOLOGY – The cerebellum functions primarily as a reflex center in the coordination of skeletal muscle movements and the maintenance of equilibrium.

Cerebral Hemisphere – ANATOMY – The cerebrum is the largest portion of the brain and is symmetrically divided into left and right cerebral hemispheres that are linked by the corpus callosum. PHYSIOLOGY – Although both hemispheres are involved in most brain functions, the left hemisphere generally controls the right half of the body, and the right hemisphere generally controls the left half of the body.

Cerebral Meninges – ANATOMY – The cerebral meninges are continuous with the spinal meninges, completely enclosing the brain (and spinal cord), and consist of three layers: Dura mater, arachnoid mater, and pia mater. The dura mater is the outermost tough, fibroelastic tissue layer. The arachnoid mater is the thin, transparent middle layer. The pia mater is the thin, delicate layer that adheres to the brain and spinal cord tissues. PHYSIOLOGY – The spinal meninges function to protect the spinal cord and contain the cerebrospinal fluid. The subarachnoid space is the cerebrospinal fluid-filled space between the arachnoid and the pia mater.

Cerebral Ventricle – ANATOMY – The ventricles are a series of four interconnected cavities of the brain and are continuous with the central canal of the spinal cord, which are filled with the cerebrospinal fluid. The tapetum is a layer of fibers from the corpus callosum forming the roof and lateral walls of the lateral ventricles. PHYSIOLOGY – The ventricles produce and are filled by continuously replaced cerebrospinal fluid which serves to protect the brain by absorbing shocks and removing any waste substances. It also provides a stable ionic concentration in the central nervous system, which is important for maximum nerve impulse transfers.

Cervical Spinal Cord – That portion within the cervical vertebral column.

Cranial Nerve – ANATOMY – The 12 pairs of nerves arising from the brain stem and cerebrum. PHYSIOLOGY – The cranial nerves serve the various specific organs of the head and neck, with some being mostly sensory (olfactory, optic), others being mostly motor (abducens), and most being of mixed sensory and motor nerve fibers and function.

Continued on next page

Educational Annotations

0 – Central Nervous System

Anatomy and Physiology Review of Central Nervous System

BODY PART VALUES – 0 - CENTRAL NERVOUS SYSTEM
Continued from previous page

Dura Mater – ANATOMY – The dura mater is the outermost cerebral and spinal cord layer comprised of tough, fibroelastic tissue. PHYSIOLOGY – The dura mater protects the brain and spinal cord from injury, pathogens, and any contaminates.

Epidural Space – The space inside the vertebral column and outside of the dura mater spinal meninges layer.

Facial Nerve – The seventh (VII) cranial nerve that innervates a significant number of structures both motor and sensory including facial expression and sensation, salivary glands, taste sense from the anterior portion of the tongue, and the oral and nasal cavities.

Glossopharyngeal Nerve – The ninth (IX) cranial nerve that innervates most of the motor and sensory structures of the tongue and pharynx.

Hypoglossal Nerve – The twelfth (XII) cranial nerve that innervates the musculature of the tongue and pharynx.

Hypothalamus – ANATOMY – The hypothalamus lies above the brain stem and forms the floor of the third ventricle. PHYSIOLOGY – The hypothalamus functions to control homeostasis by regulation of the heart rate, arterial blood pressure, body temperature, body weight, sleep, and controls the anterior pituitary gland.

Lumbar Spinal Cord – That portion within the lumbar vertebral column.

Medulla Oblongata – ANATOMY – The cone-shaped part of the brainstem that is situated between the pons and the spinal cord. PHYSIOLOGY – The medulla oblongata connects the higher levels of the cerebrum to the spinal cord and transmits ascending and descending impulses. The medulla oblongata helps regulate breathing, heart rate, blood pressure, digestion, sneezing, and swallowing.

Oculomotor Nerve – The third (III) cranial nerve that innervates most of the motor function of the eye, both somatic and autonomic.

Olfactory Nerve – The first (I) cranial nerve that innervates the olfactory epithelium (sense of smell).

Optic Nerve – The second (II) cranial nerve that innervates the retina.

Pons – ANATOMY – The pons is part of the brainstem that is situated between the below midbrain and above the medulla oblongata. PHYSIOLOGY – The pons transmits impulses between the cerebrum and cerebellum and other parts of the nervous system.

Spinal Canal – The spinal canal is the round space in the vertebrae through which the spinal cord passes.

Spinal Cord – ANATOMY – The spinal cord is a long cylindrical structure of nervous tissue that runs the length of the vertebral column from the medulla oblongata to the lumbar vertebral column. There are two consecutive rows of nerve roots that form 31 pairs of spinal nerves that emerge on each side. PHYSIOLOGY – The spinal cord is the nervous system link between the brain and most of the body through sensory, autonomic, and motor pathways.

Spinal Meninges – ANATOMY – The spinal meninges are continuous with the cerebral meninges, completely enclosing the spinal cord (and brain), and consist of three layers: Dura mater, arachnoid mater, and pia mater. The dura mater is the outermost tough, fibroelastic tissue layer. The arachnoid mater is the thin, transparent middle layer. The pia mater is the thin, delicate layer that adheres to the brain and spinal cord tissues. PHYSIOLOGY – The spinal meninges function to protect the spinal cord and contain the cerebrospinal fluid. The subarachnoid space is the cerebrospinal fluid-filled space between the arachnoid and the pia mater.

Subarachnoid Space – The subarachnoid space is the cerebrospinal fluid-filled space between the arachnoid and the pia mater.

Subdural Space – The potential space between the dura mater and the subarachnoid mater. Any actual space may develop due to illness or trauma.

Thalamus – ANATOMY – The thalamus lies below the corpus callosum on either side of the third ventricle. PHYSIOLOGY – The thalamus functions as a central relay station for sensory impulses and regulation of motor functions. It also functions to regulate the states of sleep and consciousness.

Continued on next page

Educational Annotations | 0 – Central Nervous System

Anatomy and Physiology Review of Central Nervous System – *continued*

BODY PART VALUES – 0 - CENTRAL NERVOUS SYSTEM
Continued from previous page

Thoracic Spinal Cord – That portion within the thoracic vertebral column.

Trigeminal Nerve – The fifth (V) cranial nerve that innervates a large number of structures, both motor and sensory, including touch, pain, and temperature of the face, nose, and mouth.

Trochlear Nerve – The fourth (IV) cranial nerve that innervates the superior oblique muscle of the orbit.

Vagus Nerve – The tenth (X) cranial nerve that innervates a large number of parasympathetic nerves of the heart, lungs, and digestive tract and controls the muscles of swallowing.

Anatomical Illustrations of Central Nervous System

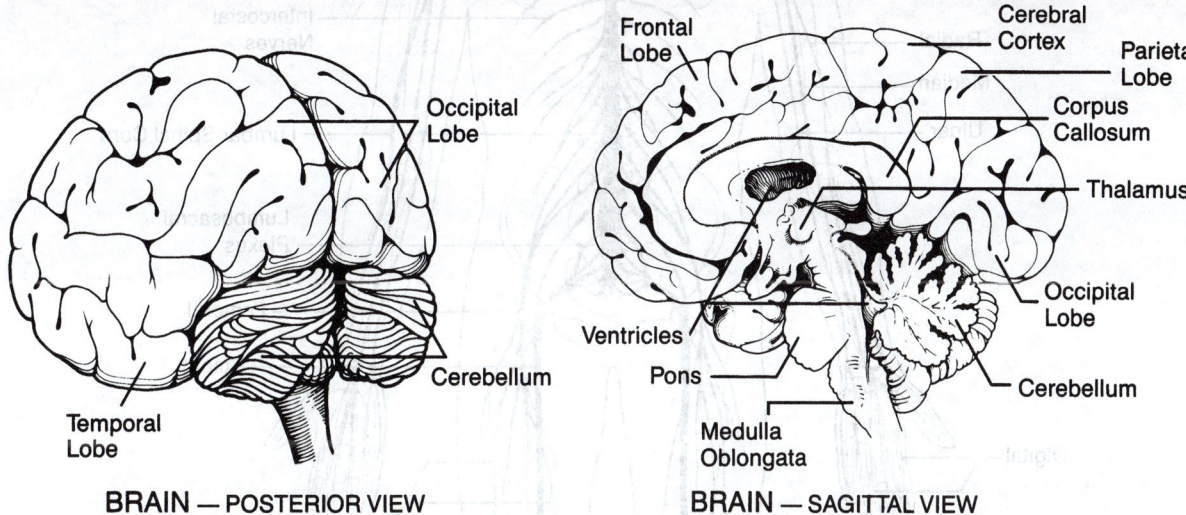

BRAIN — POSTERIOR VIEW

BRAIN — SAGITTAL VIEW

CRANIAL NERVES

Continued on next page

Educational Annotations
0 – Central Nervous System

Continued from previous page

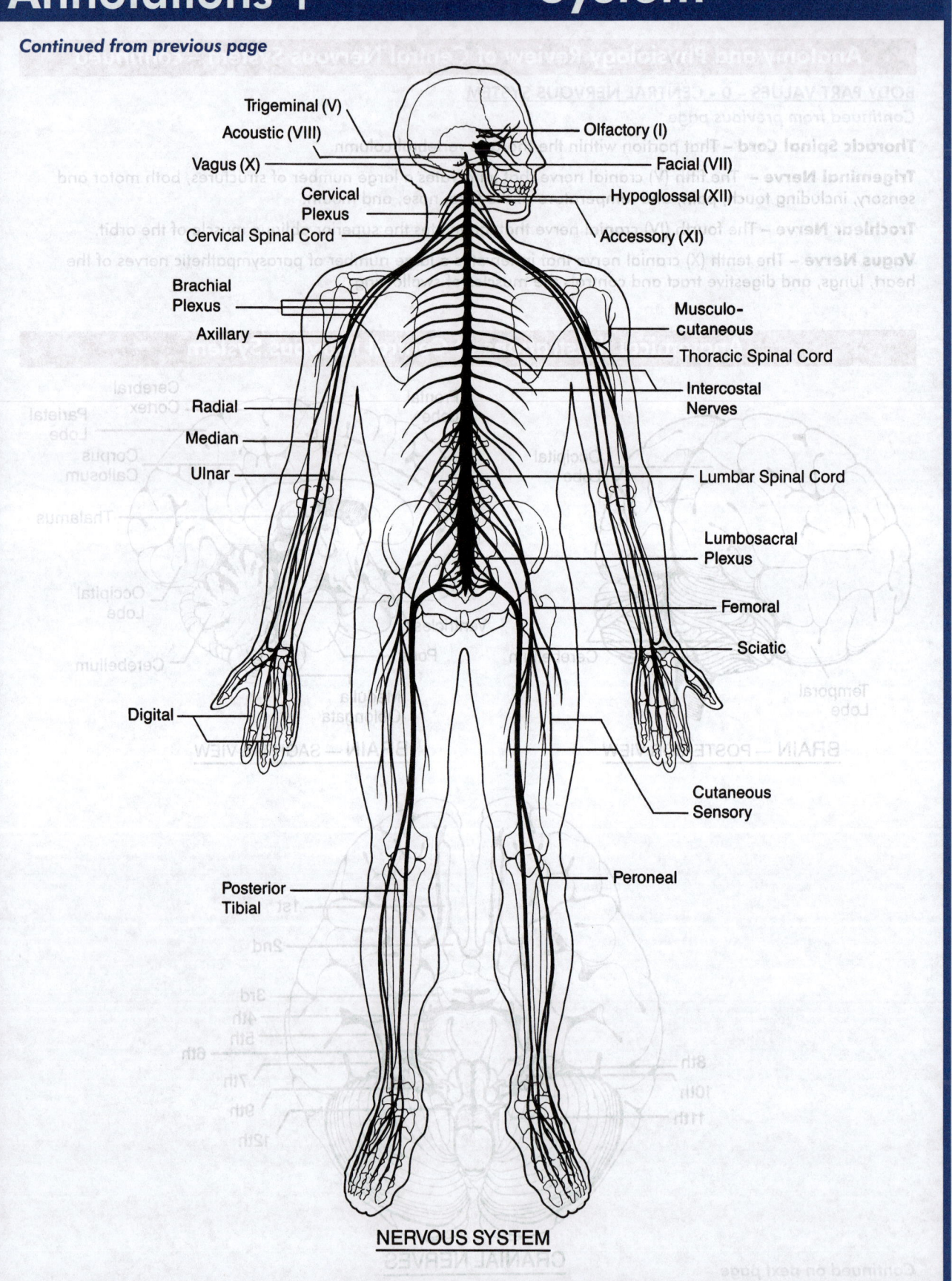

NERVOUS SYSTEM

Educational Annotations | 0 – Central Nervous System

Definitions of Common Procedures of Central Nervous System

Anterior temporal lobectomy – The surgical removal of a portion of the temporal lobe of the brain to treat medically intractable temporal lobe epilepsy.

Brain biopsy – The removal of brain tissue for microscopic examination that is performed through a small hole (burr hole) drilled into the skull, often using the stereotactic navigation system.

Chiari decompression – The surgical procedure to reduce or eliminate the pressure on the spinal cord by removal of a portion of the base of the skull that creates space at the level of the foramen magnum and is often accompanied by durotomy/duraplasty.

Gasserian ganglionectomy – The surgical removal of gasserian ganglion of the trigeminal nerve.

Lumbar puncture (spinal tap) – The insertion of a needle into the lumbar subarachnoid space to withdraw cerebrospinal fluid, usually for diagnostic reasons.

Ventriculoperitoneal shunt – The shunting redirection of excessive cerebrospinal fluid (hydrocephalus) by placing a catheter into a cerebral ventricle and tunneling it under the skin and into the peritoneal cavity.

AHA Coding Clinic® Reference Notations of Central Nervous System

ROOT OPERATION SPECIFIC - 0 - CENTRAL NERVOUS SYSTEM

BYPASS - 1
    Ventriculoperitoneal shunt (VP) with laparoscopic assistance .... AHA 13:2Q:p36

CHANGE - 2

DESTRUCTION - 5

DIVISION - 8

DRAINAGE - 9
    Aspiration via a lumbar drain port .... AHA 14:1Q:p8
    Diagnostic lumbar tap .... AHA 14:1Q:p8
    Shunting (drainage) of spinal syrinx .... AHA 15:2Q:p30

EXCISION - B
    Brain biopsy .... AHA 15:1Q:p12
    Excision of spinal cord lipoma .... AHA 14:3Q:p24
    Resection of brain tumor .... AHA 14:4Q:p34

EXTIRPATION - C
    Evacuation of brain hematoma .... AHA 15:1Q:p12

EXTRACTION - D

FRAGMENTATION - F

INSERTION - H
    Replacement of Baclofen medication pump/spinal canal catheter .... AHA 14:3Q:p19

INSPECTION - J

MAP - K

RELEASE - N
    Decompressive cervical laminectomy at multiple sites .... AHA 15:2Q:p21
    Laminoplasty to expand spinal canal space .... AHA 15:2Q:p20
    Release of tethered spinal cord .... AHA 14:3Q:p24

REMOVAL - P
    Replacement of Baclofen medication pump/spinal canal catheter .... AHA 14:3Q:p19

REPAIR - Q
    Dural rent repair .... AHA 13:3Q:p25
    .... AHA 14:3Q:p7

REPOSITION - S
    Reimplantation of transected facial nerve into muscle .... AHA 14:4Q:p35

RESECTION - T

SUPPLEMENT - U
    Dural patch graft with Durepair® .... AHA 14:3Q:p24

REVISION - W

TRANSFER - X

0 – Central Nervous System

Educational Annotations

Body Part Key Listings of Central Nervous System

See also Body Part Key in Appendix C

Anterior vagal trunk	*use* Vagus Nerve
Apneustic center	*use* Pons
Aqueduct of Sylvius	*use* Cerebral Ventricle
Arachnoid mater, intracranial	*use* Cerebral Meninges
Arachnoid mater, spinal	*use* Spinal Meninges
Basal nuclei	*use* Basal Ganglia
Basis pontis	*use* Pons
Carotid sinus nerve	*use* Glossopharyngeal Nerve
Cauda equina	*use* Lumbar Spinal Cord
Cerebral aqueduct (Sylvius)	*use* Cerebral Ventricle
Cerebrum	*use* Brain
Chorda tympani	*use* Facial Nerve
Choroid plexus	*use* Cerebral Ventricle
Claustrum	*use* Basal Ganglia
Cochlear nerve	*use* Acoustic Nerve
Conus medullaris	*use* Lumbar Spinal Cord
Corpus callosum	*use* Brain
Corpus striatum	*use* Basal Ganglia
Culmen	*use* Cerebellum
Denticulate (dentate) ligament	*use* Spinal Meninges
Diaphragma sellae	*use* Dura Mater
Dura mater, intracranial	*use* Dura Mater
Dura mater, spinal	*use* Spinal Meninges
Eighth cranial nerve	*use* Acoustic Nerve
Eleventh cranial nerve	*use* Accessory Nerve
Encephalon	*use* Brain
Ependyma	*use* Cerebral Ventricle
Epidural space, intracranial	*use* Epidural Space
Epidural space, spinal	*use* Spinal Canal
Epithalamus	*use* Thalamus
Extradural space, intracranial	*use* Epidural Space
Extradural space, spinal	*use* Spinal Canal
Extradural space	*use* Epidural Space
Falx cerebri	*use* Dura Mater
Fifth cranial nerve	*use* Trigeminal Nerve
First cranial nerve	*use* Olfactory Nerve
Foramen of Monro (intraventricular)	*use* Cerebral Ventricle
Fourth cranial nerve	*use* Trochlear Nerve
Fourth ventricle	*use* Cerebral Ventricle
Frontal lobe	*use* Cerebral Hemisphere
Gasserian ganglion	*use* Trigeminal Nerve
Geniculate ganglion	*use* Facial Nerve
Geniculate nucleus	*use* Thalamus
Globus pallidus	*use* Basal Ganglia
Greater superficial petrosal nerve	*use* Facial Nerve
Interventricular foramen (Monro)	*use* Cerebral Ventricle
Left lateral ventricle	*use* Cerebral Ventricle

Continued on next page

Educational Annotations | 0 – Central Nervous System

Body Part Key Listings of Central Nervous System

Continued from previous page

Leptomeninges, intracranial	*use* Cerebral Meninges
Leptomeninges, spinal	*use* Spinal Meninges
Locus ceruleus	*use* Pons
Mammillary body	*use* Hypothalamus
Mandibular nerve	*use* Trigeminal Nerve
Maxillary nerve	*use* Trigeminal Nerve
Metathalamus	*use* Thalamus
Myelencephalon	*use* Medulla Oblongata
Nerve to the stapedius	*use* Facial Nerve
Ninth cranial nerve	*use* Glossopharyngeal Nerve
Occipital lobe	*use* Cerebral Hemisphere
Olfactory bulb	*use* Olfactory Nerve
Ophthalmic nerve	*use* Trigeminal Nerve
Optic chiasma	*use* Optic Nerve
Parietal lobe	*use* Cerebral Hemisphere
Parotid plexus	*use* Facial Nerve
Pharyngeal plexus	*use* Vagus Nerve
Pia mater, intracranial	*use* Cerebral Meninges
Pia mater, spinal	*use* Spinal Meninges
Pneumogastric nerve	*use* Vagus Nerve
Pneumotaxic center	*use* Pons
Pontine tegmentum	*use* Pons
Posterior auricular nerve	*use* Facial Nerve
Posterior vagal trunk	*use* Vagus Nerve
Pulmonary plexus	*use* Vagus Nerve/Thoracic Sympathetic Nerve
Pulvinar	*use* Thalamus
Recurrent laryngeal nerve	*use* Vagus Nerve
Right lateral ventricle	*use* Cerebral Ventricle
Scarpa's (vestibular) ganglion	*use* Acoustic Nerve
Second cranial nerve	*use* Optic Nerve
Seventh cranial nerve	*use* Facial Nerve
Sixth cranial nerve	*use* Abducens Nerve
Spiral ganglion	*use* Acoustic Nerve
Subarachnoid space, intracranial	*use* Subarchnoid Space
Subarachnoid space, spinal	*use* Spinal Canal
Subdural space, intracranial	*use* Subdural Space
Subdural space, spinal	*use* Spinal Canal
Submandibular ganglion	*use* Facial Nerve
Substantia nigra	*use* Basal Ganglia
Subthalamic nucleus	*use* Basal Ganglia
Superior laryngeal nerve	*use* Vagus Nerve
Superior olivary nucleus	*use* Pons
Temporal lobe	*use* Cerebral Hemisphere
Tenth cranial nerve	*use* Vagus Nerve
Tentorium cerebelli	*use* Dura Mater
Third cranial nerve	*use* Oculomotor Nerve
Third ventricle	*use* Cerebral Ventricle
Trifacial nerve	*use* Trigeminal Nerve

Continued on next page

Educational Annotations

0 – Central Nervous System

Body Part Key Listings of Central Nervous System

Continued from previous page

Twelfth cranial nerve	use Hypoglossal Nerve
Tympanic nerve	use Glossopharyngeal Nerve
Vertebral canal	use Spinal Canal
Vestibular (Scarpa's) ganglion	use Acoustic Nerve
Vestibular nerve	use Acoustic Nerve
Vestibulocochlear nerve	use Acoustic Nerve

Device Key Listings of Central Nervous System

See also Device Key in Appendix D

Ascenda Intrathecal Catheter	use Infusion Device
Autograft	use Autologous Tissue Substitute
Cortical strip neurostimulator lead	use Neurostimulator Lead in Central Nervous System
DBS lead	use Neurostimulator Lead in Central Nervous System
Deep brain neurostimulator lead	use Neurostimulator Lead in Central Nervous System
Holter valve ventricular shunt	use Synthetic Substitute
InDura, intrathecal catheter (1P) (spinal)	use Infusion Device
RNS System lead	use Neurostimulator Lead in Central Nervous System
Spinal cord neurostimulator lead	use Neurostimulator Lead in Central Nervous System
Tissue bank graft	use Nonautologous Tissue Substitute
Tunneled spinal (intrathecal) catheter	use Infusion Device

Device Aggregation Table Listings of Central Nervous System

See also Device Aggregation Table in Appendix E

Specific Device	For Operation	In Body System	General Device
None Listed in Device Aggregation Table for this Body System			

Coding Notes of Central Nervous System

Body System Specific PCS Reference Manual Exercises

PCS CODE	0 – CENTRAL NERVOUS SYSTEM EXERCISES
00160J6	Shunting of intrathecal cerebrospinal fluid to peritoneal cavity using synthetic shunt.
00163J6	Percutaneous placement of ventriculoperitoneal shunt for treatment of hydrocephalus.
0020X0Z	Exchange of cerebral ventriculostomy drainage tube.
009630Z	External ventricular CSF drainage catheter placement via burr hole.
00K00ZZ	Intraoperative whole brain mapping via craniotomy.
00K74ZZ	Mapping of left cerebral hemisphere, percutaneous endoscopic.
00K83ZZ	Percutaneous mapping of basal ganglia.
00XK4ZM	Trigeminal to facial nerve transfer, percutaneous endoscopic.

0 – CENTRAL NERVOUS SYSTEM

TUBULAR GROUP: Bypass, (Dilation), (Occlusion), (Restriction)
Root Operations that alter the diameter/route of a tubular body part.

1ST – **0** Medical and Surgical
2ND – **0** Central Nervous System
3RD – **1 BYPASS**

EXAMPLE: Ventriculoperitoneal shunt | CMS Ex: Coronary artery bypass

BYPASS: Altering the route of passage of the contents of a tubular body part.

EXPLANATION: Rerouting contents to a downstream part ...

Body Part – 4TH	Approach – 5TH	Device – 6TH	Qualifier – 7TH
6 Cerebral Ventricle	0 Open 3 Percutaneous	7 Autologous tissue substitute J Synthetic substitute K Nonautologous tissue substitute	0 Nasopharynx 1 Mastoid sinus 2 Atrium 3 Blood vessel 4 Pleural cavity 5 Intestine 6 Peritoneal cavity 7 Urinary tract 8 Bone marrow B Cerebral cisterns
U Spinal Canal	0 Open 3 Percutaneous	7 Autologous tissue substitute J Synthetic substitute K Nonautologous tissue substitute	4 Pleural cavity 6 Peritoneal cavity 7 Urinary tract 9 Fallopian tube

DEVICE GROUP: Change, Insertion, Removal, (Replacement), Revision, Supplement
Root Operations that always involve a device.

1ST – **0** Medical and Surgical
2ND – **0** Central Nervous System
3RD – **2 CHANGE**

EXAMPLE: Exchange ventriculostomy tube | CMS Ex: Change urinary cath

CHANGE: Taking out or off a device from a body part and putting back an identical or similar device in or on the same body part without cutting or puncturing the skin or a mucous membrane.

EXPLANATION: ALL Changes use EXTERNAL approach only...

Body Part – 4TH	Approach – 5TH	Device – 6TH	Qualifier – 7TH
0 Brain E Cranial Nerve U Spinal Canal	X External	0 Drainage device Y Other device	Z No qualifier

005 MEDICAL AND SURGICAL SECTION – 2016 ICD-10-PCS [2016.PCS]

EXCISION GROUP: Excision, Resection, Destruction, Extraction, (Detachment)
Root Operations that take out some or all of a body part.

- 1ST – **0** Medical and Surgical
- 2ND – **0** Central Nervous System
- 3RD – **5 DESTRUCTION**

EXAMPLE: Ablation trigeminal nerve   CMS Ex: Fulguration polyp

DESTRUCTION: Physical eradication of all or a portion of a body part by the direct use of energy, force, or a destructive agent.

EXPLANATION: None of the body part is physically taken out

Body Part – 4TH		Approach – 5TH	Device – 6TH	Qualifier – 7TH
0 Brain	J Trochlear Nerve	0 Open	Z No device	Z No qualifier
1 Cerebral Meninges	K Trigeminal Nerve	3 Percutaneous		
2 Dura Mater	L Abducens Nerve	4 Percutaneous endoscopic		
6 Cerebral Ventricle	M Facial Nerve			
7 Cerebral Hemisphere	N Acoustic Nerve			
8 Basal Ganglia	P Glossopharyngeal Nerve			
9 Thalamus	Q Vagus Nerve			
A Hypothalamus	R Accessory Nerve			
B Pons	S Hypoglossal Nerve			
C Cerebellum	T Spinal Meninges			
D Medulla Oblongata	W Cervical Spinal Cord			
F Olfactory Nerve	X Thoracic Spinal Cord			
G Optic Nerve	Y Lumbar Spinal Cord			
H Oculomotor Nerve				

DIVISION GROUP: Division, Release
Root Operations involving cutting or separation only.

- 1ST – **0** Medical and Surgical
- 2ND – **0** Central Nervous System
- 3RD – **8 DIVISION**

EXAMPLE: Bisection facial nerve   CMS Ex: Osteotomy

DIVISION: Cutting into a body part without draining fluids and/or gases from the body part in order to separate or transect a body part.

EXPLANATION: Separated into two or more portions ...

Body Part – 4TH	Approach – 5TH	Device – 6TH	Qualifier – 7TH
0 Brain	0 Open	Z No device	Z No qualifier
7 Cerebral Hemisphere	3 Percutaneous		
8 Basal Ganglia	4 Percutaneous endoscopic		
F Olfactory Nerve			
G Optic Nerve			
H Oculomotor Nerve			
J Trochlear Nerve			
K Trigeminal Nerve			
L Abducens Nerve			
M Facial Nerve			
N Acoustic Nerve			
P Glossopharyngeal Nerve			
Q Vagus Nerve			
R Accessory Nerve			
S Hypoglossal Nerve			
W Cervical Spinal Cord			
X Thoracic Spinal Cord			
Y Lumbar Spinal Cord			

0 – CENTRAL NERVOUS SYSTEM 009

DRAINAGE GROUP: Drainage, Extirpation, Fragmentation
Root Operations that take out solids/fluids/gases from a body part.

1ST - **0** Medical and Surgical

2ND - **0** Central Nervous System

3RD - **9 DRAINAGE**

EXAMPLE: Lumbar puncture   CMS Ex: Thoracentesis

DRAINAGE: Taking or letting out fluids and/or gases from a body part.

EXPLANATION: Qualifier "X Diagnostic" indicates biopsy ...

Body Part – 4TH		Approach – 5TH	Device – 6TH	Qualifier – 7TH
0 Brain 1 Cerebral Meninges 2 Dura Mater 3 Epidural Space 4 Subdural Space 5 Subarachnoid Space 6 Cerebral Ventricle 7 Cerebral Hemisphere 8 Basal Ganglia 9 Thalamus A Hypothalamus B Pons C Cerebellum D Medulla Oblongata F Olfactory Nerve G Optic Nerve	H Oculomotor Nerve J Trochlear Nerve K Trigeminal Nerve L Abducens Nerve M Facial Nerve N Acoustic Nerve P Glossopharyngeal Nerve Q Vagus Nerve R Accessory Nerve S Hypoglossal Nerve T Spinal Meninges U Spinal Canal W Cervical Spinal Cord X Thoracic Spinal Cord Y Lumbar Spinal Cord	0 Open 3 Percutaneous 4 Percutaneous endoscopic	0 Drainage device	Z No qualifier
0 Brain 1 Cerebral Meninges 2 Dura Mater 3 Epidural Space 4 Subdural Space 5 Subarachnoid Space 6 Cerebral Ventricle 7 Cerebral Hemisphere 8 Basal Ganglia 9 Thalamus A Hypothalamus B Pons C Cerebellum D Medulla Oblongata F Olfactory Nerve G Optic Nerve	H Oculomotor Nerve J Trochlear Nerve K Trigeminal Nerve L Abducens Nerve M Facial Nerve N Acoustic Nerve P Glossopharyngeal Nerve Q Vagus Nerve R Accessory Nerve S Hypoglossal Nerve T Spinal Meninges U Spinal Canal W Cervical Spinal Cord X Thoracic Spinal Cord Y Lumbar Spinal Cord	0 Open 3 Percutaneous 4 Percutaneous endoscopic	Z No device	X Diagnostic Z No qualifier

0 0 B — MEDICAL AND SURGICAL SECTION – 2016 ICD-10-PCS

[2016.PCS]

EXCISION GROUP: Excision, Resection, Destruction, Extraction, (Detachment)
Root Operations that take out some or all of a body part.

- 1ST – **0** Medical and Surgical
- 2ND – **0** Central Nervous System
- 3RD – **B** EXCISION

EXAMPLE: Stereotactic thalamic biopsy CMS Ex: Liver biopsy

EXCISION: Cutting out or off, without replacement, a portion of a body part.

EXPLANATION: Qualifier "X Diagnostic" indicates biopsy …

Body Part – 4TH		Approach – 5TH	Device – 6TH	Qualifier – 7TH
0 Brain	J Trochlear Nerve	0 Open	Z No device	X Diagnostic
1 Cerebral Meninges	K Trigeminal Nerve	3 Percutaneous		Z No qualifier
2 Dura Mater	L Abducens Nerve	4 Percutaneous endoscopic		
6 Cerebral Ventricle	M Facial Nerve			
7 Cerebral Hemisphere	N Acoustic Nerve			
8 Basal Ganglia	P Glossopharyngeal Nerve			
9 Thalamus	Q Vagus Nerve			
A Hypothalamus	R Accessory Nerve			
B Pons	S Hypoglossal Nerve			
C Cerebellum	T Spinal Meninges			
D Medulla Oblongata	W Cervical Spinal Cord			
F Olfactory Nerve	X Thoracic Spinal Cord			
G Optic Nerve	Y Lumbar Spinal Cord			
H Oculomotor Nerve				

DRAINAGE GROUP: Drainage, Extirpation, Fragmentation
Root Operations that take out solids/fluids/gases from a body part.

- 1ST – **0** Medical and Surgical
- 2ND – **0** Central Nervous System
- 3RD – **C** EXTIRPATION

EXAMPLE: Removal FB lumbar spinal cord CMS Ex: Choledocholithotomy

EXTIRPATION: Taking or cutting out solid matter from a body part.

EXPLANATION: Abnormal byproduct or foreign body …

Body Part – 4TH		Approach – 5TH	Device – 6TH	Qualifier – 7TH
0 Brain	H Oculomotor Nerve	0 Open	Z No device	Z No qualifier
1 Cerebral Meninges	J Trochlear Nerve	3 Percutaneous		
2 Dura Mater	K Trigeminal Nerve	4 Percutaneous endoscopic		
3 Epidural Space	L Abducens Nerve			
4 Subdural Space	M Facial Nerve			
5 Subarachnoid Space	N Acoustic Nerve			
6 Cerebral Ventricle	P Glossopharyngeal Nerve			
7 Cerebral Hemisphere	Q Vagus Nerve			
8 Basal Ganglia	R Accessory Nerve			
9 Thalamus	S Hypoglossal Nerve			
A Hypothalamus	T Spinal Meninges			
B Pons	W Cervical Spinal Cord			
C Cerebellum	X Thoracic Spinal Cord			
D Medulla Oblongata	Y Lumbar Spinal Cord			
F Olfactory Nerve				
G Optic Nerve				

0 – CENTRAL NERVOUS SYSTEM — 00H

EXCISION GROUP: Excision, Resection, Destruction, Extraction, (Detachment)
Root Operations that take out some or all of a body part.

- 1ST – **0** Medical and Surgical
- 2ND – **0** Central Nervous System
- 3RD – **D** EXTRACTION

EXAMPLE: Extraction vagus nerve segment
CMS Ex: D&C

EXTRACTION: Pulling or stripping out or off all or a portion of a body part by the use of force.

EXPLANATION: None for this Body System

Body Part – 4TH		Approach – 5TH	Device – 6TH	Qualifier – 7TH
1 Cerebral Meninges	M Facial Nerve	0 Open	Z No device	Z No qualifier
2 Dura Mater	N Acoustic Nerve	3 Percutaneous		
F Olfactory Nerve	P Glossopharyngeal Nerve	4 Percutaneous endoscopic		
G Optic Nerve	Q Vagus Nerve			
H Oculomotor Nerve	R Accessory Nerve			
J Trochlear Nerve	S Hypoglossal Nerve			
K Trigeminal Nerve	T Spinal Meninges			
L Abducens Nerve				

DRAINAGE GROUP: Drainage, Extirpation, Fragmentation
Root Operations that take out solids/fluids/gases from a body part.

- 1ST – **0** Medical and Surgical
- 2ND – **0** Central Nervous System
- 3RD – **F** FRAGMENTATION

EXAMPLE: Fragmentation foreign body
CMS Ex: ESWL

FRAGMENTATION: Breaking solid matter in a body part into pieces.

EXPLANATION: Pieces are not taken out during procedure …

Body Part – 4TH	Approach – 5TH	Device – 6TH	Qualifier – 7TH
3 Epidural Space	0 Open	Z No device	Z No qualifier
4 Subdural Space	3 Percutaneous		
5 Subarachnoid Space	4 Percutaneous endoscopic		
6 Cerebral Ventricle	X External NC*		
U Spinal Canal			

NC* – Some procedures are considered non-covered by Medicare. See current Medicare Code Editor for details.

DEVICE GROUP: Change, Insertion, Removal, (Replacement), Revision, Supplement
Root Operations that always involve a device.

- 1ST – **0** Medical and Surgical
- 2ND – **0** Central Nervous System
- 3RD – **H** INSERTION

EXAMPLE: Intrathecal spinal cord cath
CMS Ex: Central venous catheter

INSERTION: Putting in a nonbiological appliance that monitors, assists, performs, or prevents a physiological function but does not physically take the place of a body part.

EXPLANATION: None

Body Part – 4TH	Approach – 5TH	Device – 6TH	Qualifier – 7TH
0 Brain	0 Open	2 Monitoring device	Z No qualifier
6 Cerebral Ventricle	3 Percutaneous	3 Infusion device	
E Cranial Nerve	4 Percutaneous endoscopic	M Neurostimulator lead	
U Spinal Canal			
V Spinal Cord			

0 0 J

MEDICAL AND SURGICAL SECTION – 2016 ICD-10-PCS

EXAMINATION GROUP: Inspection, Map
Root Operations involving examination only.

- 1ST – **0** Medical and Surgical
- 2ND – **0** Central Nervous System
- 3RD – **J** INSPECTION

EXAMPLE: Examination cranial nerve
CMS Ex: Colonoscopy

INSPECTION: Visually and/or manually exploring a body part.

EXPLANATION: Direct or instrumental visualization …

Body Part – 4TH	Approach – 5TH	Device – 6TH	Qualifier – 7TH
0 Brain	0 Open	Z No device	Z No qualifier
E Cranial Nerve	3 Percutaneous		
U Spinal Canal	4 Percutaneous endoscopic		
V Spinal Cord			

EXAMINATION GROUP: Inspection, Map
Root Operations involving examination only.

- 1ST – **0** Medical and Surgical
- 2ND – **0** Central Nervous System
- 3RD – **K** MAP

EXAMPLE: Mapping of basal ganglia
CMS Ex: Cardiac mapping

MAP: Locating the route of passage of electrical impulses and/or locating functional areas in a body part.

EXPLANATION: Limited to cardiac and nervous systems…

Body Part – 4TH	Approach – 5TH	Device – 6TH	Qualifier – 7TH
0 Brain	0 Open	Z No device	Z No qualifier
7 Cerebral Hemisphere	3 Percutaneous		
8 Basal Ganglia	4 Percutaneous endoscopic		
9 Thalamus			
A Hypothalamus			
B Pons			
C Cerebellum			
D Medulla Oblongata			

CENTRAL NERVOUS 0 0 J

0 – CENTRAL NERVOUS SYSTEM — 0 0 N

DIVISION GROUP: Division, Release
Root Operations involving cutting or separation only.

1ST - **0** Medical and Surgical
2ND - **0** Central Nervous System
3RD - **N RELEASE**

EXAMPLE: Lysis acoustic nerve scar tissue | **CMS Ex:** Carpal tunnel release

RELEASE: Freeing a body part from an abnormal physical constraint by cutting or by the use of force.

EXPLANATION: None of the body part is taken out ...

Body Part – 4TH		Approach – 5TH	Device – 6TH	Qualifier – 7TH
0 Brain	J Trochlear Nerve	0 Open	Z No device	Z No qualifier
1 Cerebral Meninges	K Trigeminal Nerve	3 Percutaneous		
2 Dura Mater	L Abducens Nerve	4 Percutaneous endoscopic		
6 Cerebral Ventricle	M Facial Nerve			
7 Cerebral Hemisphere	N Acoustic Nerve			
8 Basal Ganglia	P Glossopharyngeal Nerve			
9 Thalamus	Q Vagus Nerve			
A Hypothalamus	R Accessory Nerve			
B Pons	S Hypoglossal Nerve			
C Cerebellum	T Spinal Meninges			
D Medulla Oblongata	W Cervical Spinal Cord			
F Olfactory Nerve	X Thoracic Spinal Cord			
G Optic Nerve	Y Lumbar Spinal Cord			
H Oculomotor Nerve				

0 0 P — MEDICAL AND SURGICAL SECTION – 2016 ICD-10-PCS

DEVICE GROUP: Change, Insertion, Removal, (Replacement), Revision, Supplement
Root Operations that always involve a device.

1ST - 0 Medical and Surgical
2ND - 0 Central Nervous System
3RD - P REMOVAL

EXAMPLE: Removal neurostimulator lead | CMS Ex: Chest tube removal

REMOVAL: Taking out or off a device from a body part.

EXPLANATION: Removal device without reinsertion ...

Body Part – 4TH	Approach – 5TH	Device – 6TH	Qualifier – 7TH
0 Brain V Spinal Cord	0 Open 3 Percutaneous 4 Percutaneous endoscopic	0 Drainage device 2 Monitoring device 3 Infusion device 7 Autologous tissue substitute J Synthetic substitute K Nonautologous tissue substitute M Neurostimulator lead	Z No qualifier
0 Brain V Spinal Cord	X External	0 Drainage device 2 Monitoring device 3 Infusion device M Neurostimulator lead	Z No qualifier
6 Cerebral Ventricle U Spinal Canal	0 Open 3 Percutaneous 4 Percutaneous endoscopic	0 Drainage device 2 Monitoring device 3 Infusion device J Synthetic substitute M Neurostimulator lead	Z No qualifier
6 Cerebral Ventricle U Spinal Canal	X External	0 Drainage device 2 Monitoring device 3 Infusion device M Neurostimulator lead	Z No qualifier
E Cranial Nerve	0 Open 3 Percutaneous 4 Percutaneous endoscopic	0 Drainage device 2 Monitoring device 3 Infusion device 7 Autologous tissue substitute M Neurostimulator lead	Z No qualifier
E Cranial Nerve	X External	0 Drainage device 2 Monitoring device 3 Infusion device M Neurostimulator lead	Z No qualifier

0 – CENTRAL NERVOUS SYSTEM   0 0 S

OTHER REPAIRS GROUP: (Control), Repair
Root Operations that define other repairs.

1ST - 0 Medical and Surgical
2ND - 0 Central Nervous System
3RD - Q REPAIR

EXAMPLE: Cerebral meningeorrhaphy   CMS Ex: Suture laceration

REPAIR: Restoring, to the extent possible, a body part to its normal anatomic structure and function.

EXPLANATION: Only when no other root operation applies ...

Body Part – 4TH		Approach – 5TH	Device – 6TH	Qualifier – 7TH
0 Brain	J Trochlear Nerve	0 Open	Z No device	Z No qualifier
1 Cerebral Meninges	K Trigeminal Nerve	3 Percutaneous		
2 Dura Mater	L Abducens Nerve	4 Percutaneous endoscopic		
6 Cerebral Ventricle	M Facial Nerve			
7 Cerebral Hemisphere	N Acoustic Nerve			
8 Basal Ganglia	P Glossopharyngeal Nerve			
9 Thalamus	Q Vagus Nerve			
A Hypothalamus	R Accessory Nerve			
B Pons	S Hypoglossal Nerve			
C Cerebellum	T Spinal Meninges			
D Medulla Oblongata	W Cervical Spinal Cord			
F Olfactory Nerve	X Thoracic Spinal Cord			
G Optic Nerve	Y Lumbar Spinal Cord			
H Oculomotor Nerve				

MOVE GROUP: (Reattachment), Reposition, Transfer, (Transplantation)
Root Operations that put in/put back or move some/all of a body part.

1ST - 0 Medical and Surgical
2ND - 0 Central Nervous System
3RD - S REPOSITION

EXAMPLE: Relocation hypoglossal nerve   CMS Ex: Fracture reduction

REPOSITION: Moving to its normal location, or other suitable location, all or a portion of a body part.

EXPLANATION: May or may not be cut to be moved ...

Body Part – 4TH		Approach – 5TH	Device – 6TH	Qualifier – 7TH
F Olfactory Nerve	P Glossopharyngeal Nerve	0 Open	Z No device	Z No qualifier
G Optic Nerve	Q Vagus Nerve	3 Percutaneous		
H Oculomotor Nerve	R Accessory Nerve	4 Percutaneous endoscopic		
J Trochlear Nerve	S Hypoglossal Nerve			
K Trigeminal Nerve	W Cervical Spinal Cord			
L Abducens Nerve	X Thoracic Spinal Cord			
M Facial Nerve	Y Lumbar Spinal Cord			
N Acoustic Nerve				

0 0 T — MEDICAL AND SURGICAL SECTION – 2016 ICD-10-PCS

EXCISION GROUP: Excision, Resection, Destruction, Extraction, (Detachment)
Root Operations that take out some or all of a body part.

- 1ST – **0** Medical and Surgical
- 2ND – **0** Central Nervous System
- 3RD – **T** RESECTION

EXAMPLE: Cerebral hemispherectomy   CMS Ex: Cholecystectomy

RESECTION: Cutting out or off, without replacement, all of a body part.

EXPLANATION: None

Body Part – 4TH	Approach – 5TH	Device – 6TH	Qualifier – 7TH
7 Cerebral Hemisphere	0 Open 3 Percutaneous 4 Percutaneous endoscopic	Z No device	Z No qualifier

DEVICE GROUP: Change, Insertion, Removal, (Replacement), Revision, Supplement
Root Operations that always involve a device.

- 1ST – **0** Medical and Surgical
- 2ND – **0** Central Nervous System
- 3RD – **U** SUPPLEMENT

EXAMPLE: Dural patch graft   CMS Ex: Hernia repair with mesh

SUPPLEMENT: Putting in or on biological or synthetic material that physically reinforces and/or augments the function of a portion of a body part.

EXPLANATION: Biological material from same individual ...

Body Part – 4TH	Approach – 5TH	Device – 6TH	Qualifier – 7TH
1 Cerebral Meninges 2 Dura Mater T Spinal Meninges	0 Open 3 Percutaneous 4 Percutaneous endoscopic	7 Autologous tissue substitute J Synthetic substitute K Nonautologous tissue substitute	Z No qualifier
F Olfactory Nerve M Facial Nerve G Optic Nerve N Acoustic Nerve H Oculomotor Nerve P Glossopharyngeal Nerve J Trochlear Nerve Q Vagus Nerve K Trigeminal Nerve R Accessory Nerve L Abducens Nerve S Hypoglossal Nerve	0 Open 3 Percutaneous 4 Percutaneous endoscopic	7 Autologous tissue substitute	Z No qualifier

CENTRAL NERVOUS 0 0 T

0 – CENTRAL NERVOUS SYSTEM — 00W

DEVICE GROUP: Change, Insertion, Removal, (Replacement), Revision, Supplement
Root Operations that always involve a device.

- 1ST – **0** Medical and Surgical
- 2ND – **0** Central Nervous System
- 3RD – **W** REVISION

EXAMPLE: Reposition neurostimulator lead | **CMS Ex:** Adjust pacemaker lead

REVISION: Correcting, to the extent possible, a portion of a malfunctioning device or the position of a displaced device.

EXPLANATION: May replace components of a device ...

Body Part – 4TH	Approach – 5TH	Device – 6TH	Qualifier – 7TH
0 Brain V Spinal Cord	0 Open 3 Percutaneous 4 Percutaneous endoscopic X External	0 Drainage device 2 Monitoring device 3 Infusion device 7 Autologous tissue substitute J Synthetic substitute K Nonautologous tissue substitute M Neurostimulator lead	Z No qualifier
6 Cerebral Ventricle U Spinal Canal	0 Open 3 Percutaneous 4 Percutaneous endoscopic X External	0 Drainage device 2 Monitoring device 3 Infusion device J Synthetic substitute M Neurostimulator lead	Z No qualifier
E Cranial Nerve	0 Open 3 Percutaneous 4 Percutaneous endoscopic X External	0 Drainage device 2 Monitoring device 3 Infusion device 7 Autologous tissue substitute M Neurostimulator lead	Z No qualifier

0 0 X

MEDICAL AND SURGICAL SECTION – 2016 ICD-10-PCS

MOVE GROUP: (Reattachment), Reposition, Transfer, (Transplantation)
Root Operations that put in/put back or move some/all of a body part.

- 1ST – **0** Medical and Surgical
- 2ND – **0** Central Nervous System
- 3RD – **X** TRANSFER

EXAMPLE: Transfer trigeminal to facial nerve | **CMS Ex:** Tendon transfer

TRANSFER: Moving, without taking out, all or a portion of a body part to another location to take over the function of all or a portion of a body part.

EXPLANATION: The body part remains connected ...

Body Part – 4TH	Approach – 5TH	Device – 6TH	Qualifier – 7TH
F Olfactory Nerve	0 Open	Z No device	F Olfactory Nerve
G Optic Nerve	4 Percutaneous endoscopic		G Optic Nerve
H Oculomotor Nerve			H Oculomotor Nerve
J Trochlear Nerve			J Trochlear Nerve
K Trigeminal Nerve			K Trigeminal Nerve
L Abducens Nerve			L Abducens Nerve
M Facial Nerve			M Facial Nerve
N Acoustic Nerve			N Acoustic Nerve
P Glossopharyngeal Nerve			P Glossopharyngeal Nerve
Q Vagus Nerve			Q Vagus Nerve
R Accessory Nerve			R Accessory Nerve
S Hypoglossal Nerve			S Hypoglossal Nerve

Educational Annotations | 1 – Peripheral Nervous System

Body System Specific Educational Annotations for the Peripheral Nervous System include:
- Anatomy and Physiology Review
- Anatomical Illustrations
- Definitions of Common Procedures
- AHA Coding Clinic® Reference Notations
- Body Part Key Listings
- Device Key Listings
- Device Aggregation Table Listings
- Coding Notes

Anatomy and Physiology Review of Peripheral Nervous System

BODY PART VALUES – 1 - PERIPHERAL NERVOUS SYSTEM

Abdominal Sympathetic Nerve – The autonomic nervous system sympathetic nerve trunk portion that innervates the smooth muscles, glands, and organs of the abdominal region.

Brachial Plexus – A branching network of the last four cervical spinal nerves and the first thoracic spinal nerve (C5-C8, T1) that primarily innervates the skin and muscles of the upper limbs.

Cervical Nerve – One of eight pairs of spinal nerves emerging from the cervical vertebrae.

Cervical Plexus – A branching network of the first four cervical spinal nerves (C1-C4) that primarily innervates the skin and muscles of the head and neck.

Femoral Nerve – The femoral nerve is the major nerve that innervates the muscles and skin of the thigh and leg.

Head and Neck Sympathetic Nerve – The autonomic nervous system sympathetic nerve trunk portion that innervates the smooth muscles, glands, and organs of the head and neck region.

Lumbar Nerve – One of five pairs of spinal nerves emerging from the lumbar vertebrae.

Lumbar Plexus – A branching network of the first four lumbar spinal nerves and the last thoracic spinal nerve (L1-L4, T12) that primarily innervates the skin and muscles of the lower abdomen and upper legs.

Lumbar Sympathetic Nerve – The autonomic nervous system sympathetic nerve trunk portion that innervates the smooth muscles, glands, and organs of the lower abdominal and pelvic regions.

Lumbosacral Plexus – A branching network of the lumbar spinal nerves, the last thoracic spinal nerve (L1-L5, T12), the sacral plexus (S1-S3) and pudendal plexus (S4-S5 and coccygeal nerve) that primarily innervates the skin and muscles of the lower abdomen and legs.

Median Nerve – The median nerve is one of the three major upper limb nerves that innervates the muscles and skin of the forearm and hand.

Peripheral Nerve – ANATOMY – A nerve outside of the brain and spinal cord. PHYSIOLOGY – The peripheral nervous system consists of a network of nerves that coordinates its voluntary and involuntary actions and communication among its parts.

Peroneal Nerve – The peroneal nerve is a division of the sciatic nerve that innervates the muscles and skin of the lower leg.

Phrenic Nerve – The phrenic nerve is the major nerve that innervates the muscles of the diaphragm and is the nerve responsible for the hiccough reflex.

Pudendal Nerve – The pudendal nerve is the major nerve that innervates the perineum, external genitalia, and anus.

Radial Nerve – The radial nerve is one of the three major upper limb nerves that innervates the muscles and skin of the arm (specifically the triceps muscle), wrist, and hand.

Sacral Nerve – One of five pairs of spinal nerves emerging from the sacrum.

Sacral Plexus – A branching network of the sacral nerves (S1-S5) and coccygeal nerve that primarily innervates the skin and muscles of the legs.

Sacral Sympathetic Nerve – The autonomic nervous system sympathetic nerve trunk portion that innervates the smooth muscles, glands, and organs of the pelvic region.

Sciatic Nerve – The sciatic nerve is the major nerve that innervates the muscles and skin of the thighs, lower legs and feet.

Thoracic Nerve – One of twelve pairs of spinal nerves emerging from the thoracic vertebrae.

Continued on next page

01 MEDICAL AND SURGICAL SECTION – 2016 ICD-10-PCS

Educational Annotations | 1 – Peripheral Nervous System

Anatomy and Physiology Review of Peripheral Nervous System

BODY PART VALUES – 1 - PERIPHERAL NERVOUS SYSTEM
Continued from previous page

Thoracic Sympathetic Nerve – The autonomic nervous system sympathetic nerve trunk portion that innervates the smooth muscles, glands, and organs of the thoracic region.

Tibial Nerve – The tibial nerve is a division of the sciatic nerve that innervates the muscles and skin of the lower legs and feet.

Ulnar Nerve – The ulnar nerve is one of the three major upper limb nerves that innervates the muscles and skin of the arm, hand, little finger, and half of the ring finger.

Anatomical Illustrations of Peripheral Nervous System

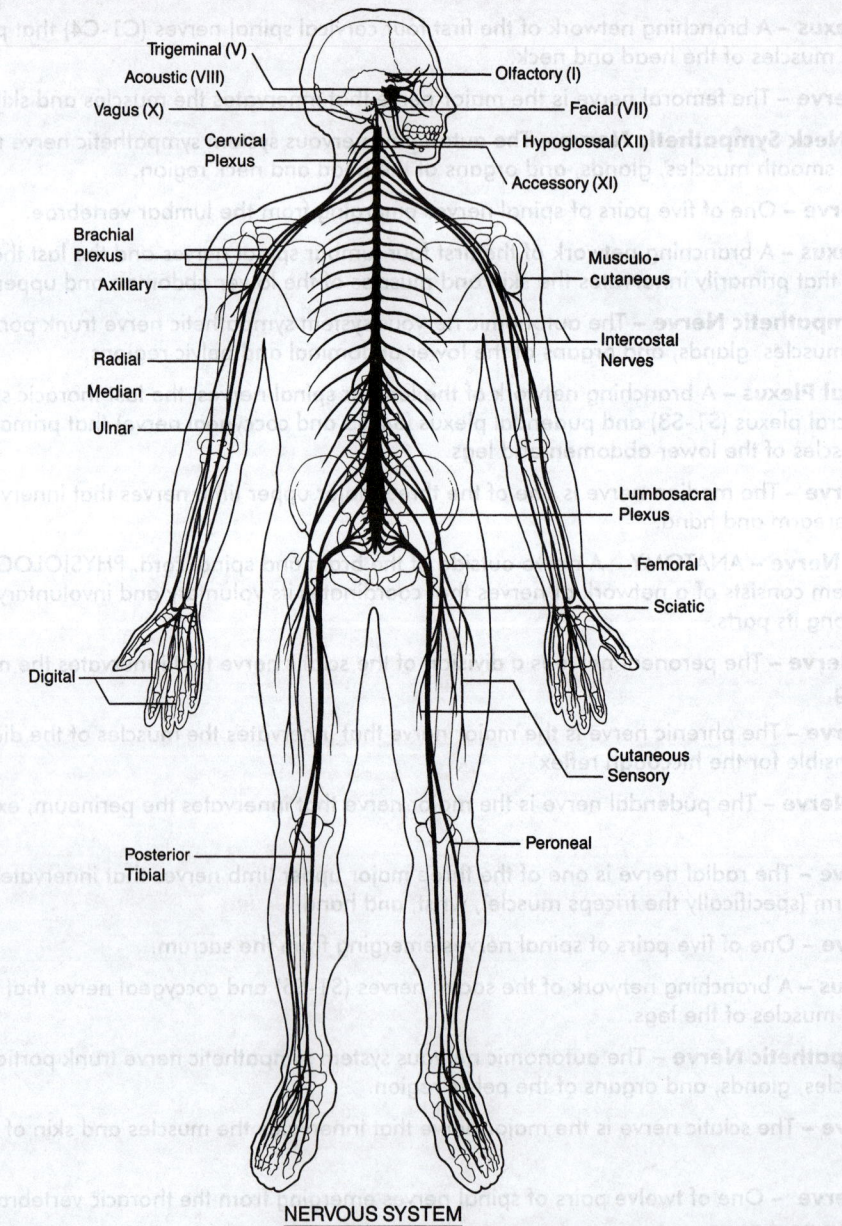

NERVOUS SYSTEM

Educational Annotations | 1 – Peripheral Nervous System

Definitions of Common Procedures of Peripheral Nervous System

Carpal tunnel release – The surgical relief from pain and weakness of the hand due to compression of the median nerve at the wrist by dividing the transverse carpal ligament causing the compression.

Free nerve graft – The surgical repair of a damaged nerve to restore nerve function using a harvested nerve section to connect both ends of the damaged nerve.

Nerve transfer – The surgical dissection to free a viable redundant nerve branch to connect to the damaged nerve in order to restore movement or sensory function.

Thoracic sympathectomy – The surgical excision or destruction of the thoracic sympathetic nerve chain ganglia to alleviate the symptoms of hyperhidrosis, sweaty palms, or Raynaud's disease.

AHA Coding Clinic® Reference Notations of Peripheral Nervous System

ROOT OPERATION SPECIFIC - 1 - PERIPHERAL NERVOUS SYSTEM
CHANGE - 2
DESTRUCTION - 5
DIVISION - 8
DRAINAGE - 9
EXCISION - B
EXTIRPATION - C
EXTRACTION - D
INSERTION - H
INSPECTION - J
RELEASE - N
    Carpal tunnel release ....AHA 14:3Q:p33
REMOVAL - P
REPAIR - Q
REPOSITION - S
SUPPLEMENT - U
REVISION - W
TRANSFER - X

Body Part Key Listings of Peripheral Nervous System

See also Body Part Key in Appendix C
Abdominal aortic plexus ....*use* Abdominal Sympathetic Nerve
Accessory obturator nerve ....*use* Lumbar Plexus
Accessory phrenic nerve ....*use* Phrenic Nerve
Ansa cervicalis ....*use* Cervical Plexus
Anterior crural nerve ....*use* Femoral Nerve
Anterior interosseous nerve ....*use* Median Nerve
Auerbach's (myenteric) plexus ....*use* Abdominal Sympathetic Nerve
Axillary nerve ....*use* Brachial Plexus
Cardiac plexus ....*use* Thoracic Sympathetic Nerve
Cavernous plexus ....*use* Head and Neck Sympathetic Nerve
Celiac (solar) plexus ....*use* Abdominal Sympathetic Nerve
Celiac ganglion ....*use* Abdominal Sympathetic Nerve
Cervical ganglion ....*use* Head and Neck Sympathetic Nerve
Ciliary ganglion ....*use* Head and Neck Sympathetic Nerve

Continued on next page

Educational Annotations | 1 – Peripheral Nervous System

Body Part Key Listings of Peripheral Nervous System

Continued from previous page

Common fibular nerve	*use* Peroneal Nerve
Common peroneal nerve	*use* Peroneal Nerve
Cubital nerve	*use* Ulnar Nerve
Cutaneous (transverse) cervical nerve	*use* Cervical Plexus
Dorsal digital nerve	*use* Radial Nerve
Dorsal scapular nerve	*use* Brachial Plexus
Esophageal plexus	*use* Thoracic Sympathetic Nerve
External popliteal nerve	*use* Peroneal Nerve
First intercostal nerve	*use* Brachial Plexus
Ganglion impar (ganglion of Walther)	*use* Sacral Sympathetic Nerve
Gastric plexus	*use* Abdominal Sympathetic Nerve
Genitofemoral nerve	*use* Lumbar Plexus
Great auricular nerve	*use* Cervical Plexus
Greater occipital nerve	*use* Cervical Nerve
Greater splanchnic nerve	*use* Thoracic Sympathetic Nerve
Hepatic plexus	*use* Abdominal Sympathetic Nerve
Iliohypogastric nerve	*use* Lumbar Plexus
Ilioinguinal nerve	*use* Lumbar Plexus
Inferior cardiac nerve	*use* Thoracic Sympathetic Nerve
Inferior gluteal nerve	*use* Sacral Plexus
Inferior hypogastric plexus	*use* Abdominal Sympathetic Nerve
Inferior mesenteric ganglion	*use* Abdominal Sympathetic Nerve
Inferior mesenteric plexus	*use* Abdominal Sympathetic Nerve
Intercostal nerve	*use* Thoracic Nerve
Intercostobrachial nerve	*use* Thoracic Nerve
Internal carotid plexus	*use* Head and Neck Sympathetic Nerve
Ischiatic nerve	*use* Sciatic Nerve
Lateral femoral cutaneous nerve	*use* Lumbar Plexus
Lateral plantar nerve	*use* Tibial Nerve
Lateral sural cutaneous nerve	*use* Peroneal Nerve
Least splanchnic nerve	*use* Thoracic Sympathetic Nerve
Lesser occipital nerve	*use* Cervical Plexus
Lesser splanchnic nerve	*use* Thoracic Sympathetic Nerve
Long thoracic nerve	*use* Brachial Plexus
Lumbar ganglion	*use* Lumbar Sympathetic Nerve
Lumbar splanchnic nerve	*use* Lumbar Sympathetic Nerve
Lumbosacral trunk	*use* Lumbar Nerve
Medial plantar nerve	*use* Tibial Nerve
Medial popliteal nerve	*use* Tibial Nerve
Medial sural cutaneous nerve	*use* Tibial Nerve
Meissner's (submucous) plexus	*use* Abdominal Sympathetic Nerve
Middle cardiac nerve	*use* Thoracic Sympathetic Nerve
Musculocutaneous nerve	*use* Brachial Plexus
Musculospiral nerve	*use* Radial Nerve
Myenteric (Auerbach's) plexus	*use* Abdominal Sympathetic Nerve
Obturator nerve	*use* Lumbar Plexus
Otic ganglion	*use* Head and Neck Sympathetic Nerve

Continued on next page

Educational Annotations | 1 – Peripheral Nervous System

Body Part Key Listings of Peripheral Nervous System

Continued from previous page

Palmar cutaneous nerve	*use* Median Nerve, Radial Nerve
Pancreatic plexus	*use* Abdominal Sympathetic Nerve
Pelvic splanchnic nerve	*use* Abdominal Sympathetic Nerve
	use Sacral Sympathetic Nerve
Posterior femoral cutaneous nerve	*use* Sacral Plexus
Posterior interosseous nerve	*use* Radial Nerve
Posterior labial nerve	*use* Pudendal Nerve
Posterior scrotal nerve	*use* Pudendal Nerve
Pterygopalatine (sphenopalatine) ganglion	*use* Head and Neck Sympathetic Nerve
Pudendal nerve	*use* Sacral Plexus
Pulmonary plexus	*use* Vagus Nerve/Thoracic Sympathetic Nerve
Renal plexus	*use* Abdominal Sympathetic Nerve
Sacral ganglion	*use* Sacral Sympathetic Nerve
Sacral splanchnic nerve	*use* Sacral Sympathetic Nerve
Saphenous nerve	*use* Femoral Nerve
Solar (celiac) plexus	*use* Abdominal Sympathetic Nerve
Sphenopalatine (pterygopalatine) ganglion	*use* Head and Neck Sympathetic Nerve
Spinal nerve, cervical	*use* Cervical Nerve
Spinal nerve, lumbar	*use* Lumbar Nerve
Spinal nerve, sacral	*use* Sacral Nerve
Spinal nerve, thoracic	*use* Thoracic Nerve
Splenic plexus	*use* Abdominal Sympathetic Nerve
Stellate ganglion	*use* Head and Neck Sympathetic Nerve
Subclavius nerve	*use* Brachial Plexus
Subcostal nerve	*use* Thoracic Nerve
Submandibular ganglion	*use* Head and Neck Sympathetic Nerve
Submaxillary ganglion	*use* Head and Neck Sympathetic Nerve
Submucous (Meissner's) plexus	*use* Abdominal Sympathetic Nerve
Suboccipital nerve	*use* Cervical Nerve
Superior cardiac nerve	*use* Thoracic Sympathetic Nerve
Superior clunic (cluneal) nerve	*use* Lumbar Nerve
Superior gluteal nerve	*use* Lumbar Plexus
Superior hypogastric plexus	*use* Abdominal Sympathetic Nerve
Superior mesenteric ganglion	*use* Abdominal Sympathetic Nerve
Superior mesenteric plexus	*use* Abdominal Sympathetic Nerve
Supraclavicular nerve	*use* Cervical Plexus
Suprascapular nerve	*use* Brachial Plexus
Suprarenal plexus	*use* Abdominal Sympathetic Nerve
Third occipital nerve	*use* Cervical Nerve
Thoracic aortic plexus	*use* Thoracic Sympathetic Nerve
Thoracic ganglion	*use* Thoracic Sympathetic Nerve
Transverse (cutaneous) cervical nerve	*use* Cervical Plexus

01 MEDICAL AND SURGICAL SECTION – 2016 ICD-10-PCS

Educational Annotations | 1 – Peripheral Nervous System

Device Key Listings of Peripheral Nervous System

See also Device Key in Appendix D
Autograft .... *use* Autologous Tissue Substitute
InterStim® Therapy lead .... *use* Neurostimulator Lead in Peripheral Nervous System

Device Aggregation Table Listings of Peripheral Nervous System

See also Device Aggregation Table in Appendix E

Specific Device	For Operation	In Body System	General Device
None Listed in Device Aggregation Table for this Body System			

Coding Notes of Peripheral Nervous System

Body System Relevant Coding Guidelines

Branches of body parts
B4.2
Where a specific branch of a body part does not have its own body part value in PCS, the body part is coded to the closest proximal branch that has a specific body part value.
Example: A procedure performed on the mandibular branch of the trigeminal nerve is coded to the trigeminal nerve body part value.

Body System Specific PCS Reference Manual Exercises

PCS CODE	1 – PERIPHERAL NERVOUS SYSTEM EXERCISES
018R3ZZ	Sacral rhizotomy for pain control, percutaneous.
01N0ZZ	Open posterior tarsal tunnel release. (The nerve released in the posterior tarsal tunnel is the tibial nerve.)
01PY0MZ	Open removal of lumbar sympathetic neurostimulator.
01Q60ZZ	Suture repair of left radial nerve laceration. (The approach value is Open, though the surgical exposure may have been created by the wound itself.)
01S40ZZ	Open transposition of ulnar nerve.
01U547Z	Autograft nerve graft to right median nerve, percutaneous endoscopic (graft harvest not coded for this exercise example).
01X64Z5	Endoscopic radial to median nerve transfer.

1 – PERIPHERAL NERVOUS SYSTEM   015

DEVICE GROUP: Change, Insertion, Removal, (Replacement), Revision, Supplement
Root Operations that always involve a device.

1ST - **0** Medical and Surgical
2ND - **1** Peripheral Nervous System
3RD - **2 CHANGE**

EXAMPLE: Exchange ulnar nerve drain tube | CMS Ex: Change urinary cath

CHANGE: Taking out or off a device from a body part and putting back an identical or similar device in or on the same body part without cutting or puncturing the skin or a mucous membrane.

EXPLANATION: ALL Changes use EXTERNAL approach only...

Body Part – 4TH	Approach – 5TH	Device – 6TH	Qualifier – 7TH
Y Peripheral Nerve	X External	0 Drainage device Y Other device	Z No qualifier

EXCISION GROUP: Excision, Resection, Destruction, Extraction, (Detachment)
Root Operations that take out some or all of a body part.

1ST - **0** Medical and Surgical
2ND - **1** Peripheral Nervous System
3RD - **5 DESTRUCTION**

EXAMPLE: Cryoablation nerve lesion | CMS Ex: Fulguration polyp

DESTRUCTION: Physical eradication of all or a portion of a body part by the direct use of energy, force, or a destructive agent.

EXPLANATION: None of the body part is physically taken out

Body Part – 4TH		Approach – 5TH	Device – 6TH	Qualifier – 7TH
0 Cervical Plexus	F Sciatic Nerve	0 Open	Z No device	Z No qualifier
1 Cervical Nerve	G Tibial Nerve	3 Percutaneous		
2 Phrenic Nerve	H Peroneal Nerve	4 Percutaneous endoscopic		
3 Brachial Plexus	K Head and Neck Sympathetic Nerve			
4 Ulnar Nerve				
5 Median Nerve	L Thoracic Sympathetic Nerve			
6 Radial Nerve	M Abdominal Sympathetic Nerve			
8 Thoracic Nerve				
9 Lumbar Plexus	N Lumbar Sympathetic Nerve			
A Lumbosacral Plexus	P Sacral Sympathetic Nerve			
B Lumbar Nerve	Q Sacral Plexus			
C Pudendal Nerve	R Sacral Nerve			
D Femoral Nerve				

018 MEDICAL AND SURGICAL SECTION – 2016 ICD-10-PCS

DIVISION GROUP: Division, Release
Root Operations involving cutting or separation only.

- 1ST – **0** Medical and Surgical
- 2ND – **1** Peripheral Nervous System
- 3RD – **8 DIVISION**

EXAMPLE: Sacral nerve rhizotomy **CMS Ex:** Osteotomy

DIVISION: Cutting into a body part without draining fluids and/or gases from the body part in order to separate or transect a body part.

EXPLANATION: Separated into two or more portions …

Body Part – 4TH		Approach – 5TH	Device – 6TH	Qualifier – 7TH
0 Cervical Plexus	F Sciatic Nerve	0 Open	Z No device	Z No qualifier
1 Cervical Nerve	G Tibial Nerve	3 Percutaneous		
2 Phrenic Nerve	H Peroneal Nerve	4 Percutaneous endoscopic		
3 Brachial Plexus	K Head and Neck Sympathetic Nerve			
4 Ulnar Nerve				
5 Median Nerve	L Thoracic Sympathetic Nerve			
6 Radial Nerve	M Abdominal Sympathetic Nerve			
8 Thoracic Nerve				
9 Lumbar Plexus	N Lumbar Sympathetic Nerve			
A Lumbosacral Plexus	P Sacral Sympathetic Nerve			
B Lumbar Nerve	Q Sacral Plexus			
C Pudendal Nerve	R Sacral Nerve			
D Femoral Nerve				

1 – PERIPHERAL NERVOUS SYSTEM

DRAINAGE GROUP: Drainage, Extirpation, (Fragmentation)
Root Operations that take out solids/fluids/gases from a body part.

1ST - **0** Medical and Surgical
2ND - **1** Peripheral Nervous System
3RD - **9 DRAINAGE**

EXAMPLE: Aspiration nerve abscess   CMS Ex: Thoracentesis

DRAINAGE: Taking or letting out fluids and/or gases from a body part.

EXPLANATION: Qualifier "X Diagnostic" indicates biopsy ...

Body Part – 4TH		Approach – 5TH	Device – 6TH	Qualifier – 7TH
0 Cervical Plexus	F Sciatic Nerve	0 Open	0 Drainage device	Z No qualifier
1 Cervical Nerve	G Tibial Nerve	3 Percutaneous		
2 Phrenic Nerve	H Peroneal Nerve	4 Percutaneous endoscopic		
3 Brachial Plexus	K Head and Neck Sympathetic Nerve			
4 Ulnar Nerve				
5 Median Nerve	L Thoracic Sympathetic Nerve			
6 Radial Nerve	M Abdominal Sympathetic Nerve			
8 Thoracic Nerve				
9 Lumbar Plexus	N Lumbar Sympathetic Nerve			
A Lumbosacral Plexus	P Sacral Sympathetic Nerve			
B Lumbar Nerve	Q Sacral Plexus			
C Pudendal Nerve	R Sacral Nerve			
D Femoral Nerve				
0 Cervical Plexus	F Sciatic Nerve	0 Open	Z No device	X Diagnostic
1 Cervical Nerve	G Tibial Nerve	3 Percutaneous		Z No qualifier
2 Phrenic Nerve	H Peroneal Nerve	4 Percutaneous endoscopic		
3 Brachial Plexus	K Head and Neck Sympathetic Nerve			
4 Ulnar Nerve				
5 Median Nerve	L Thoracic Sympathetic Nerve			
6 Radial Nerve	M Abdominal Sympathetic Nerve			
8 Thoracic Nerve				
9 Lumbar Plexus	N Lumbar Sympathetic Nerve			
A Lumbosacral Plexus	P Sacral Sympathetic Nerve			
B Lumbar Nerve	Q Sacral Plexus			
C Pudendal Nerve	R Sacral Nerve			
D Femoral Nerve				

01B MEDICAL AND SURGICAL SECTION – 2016 ICD-10-PCS [2016.PCS]

EXCISION GROUP: Excision, Resection, Destruction, Extraction, (Detachment)
Root Operations that take out some or all of a body part.

- 1ST – **0** Medical and Surgical
- 2ND – **1** Peripheral Nervous System
- 3RD – **B** EXCISION

EXAMPLE: Biopsy of lumbosacral plexus   CMS Ex: Liver biopsy

EXCISION: Cutting out or off, without replacement, a portion of a body part.

EXPLANATION: Qualifier "X Diagnostic" indicates biopsy …

Body Part – 4TH		Approach – 5TH	Device – 6TH	Qualifier – 7TH
0 Cervical Plexus	F Sciatic Nerve	0 Open	Z No device	X Diagnostic
1 Cervical Nerve	G Tibial Nerve	3 Percutaneous		Z No qualifier
2 Phrenic Nerve	H Peroneal Nerve	4 Percutaneous endoscopic		
3 Brachial Plexus	K Head and Neck Sympathetic Nerve			
4 Ulnar Nerve				
5 Median Nerve	L Thoracic Sympathetic Nerve			
6 Radial Nerve	M Abdominal Sympathetic Nerve			
8 Thoracic Nerve				
9 Lumbar Plexus	N Lumbar Sympathetic Nerve			
A Lumbosacral Plexus	P Sacral Sympathetic Nerve			
B Lumbar Nerve	Q Sacral Plexus			
C Pudendal Nerve	R Sacral Nerve			
D Femoral Nerve				

DRAINAGE GROUP: Drainage, Extirpation, (Fragmentation)
Root Operations that take out solids/fluids/gases from a body part.

- 1ST – **0** Medical and Surgical
- 2ND – **1** Peripheral Nervous System
- 3RD – **C** EXTIRPATION

EXAMPLE: Removal FB cervical plexus   CMS Ex: Choledocholithotomy

EXTIRPATION: Taking or cutting out solid matter from a body part.

EXPLANATION: Abnormal byproduct or foreign body …

Body Part – 4TH		Approach – 5TH	Device – 6TH	Qualifier – 7TH
0 Cervical Plexus	F Sciatic Nerve	0 Open	Z No device	Z No qualifier
1 Cervical Nerve	G Tibial Nerve	3 Percutaneous		
2 Phrenic Nerve	H Peroneal Nerve	4 Percutaneous endoscopic		
3 Brachial Plexus	K Head and Neck Sympathetic Nerve			
4 Ulnar Nerve				
5 Median Nerve	L Thoracic Sympathetic Nerve			
6 Radial Nerve	M Abdominal Sympathetic Nerve			
8 Thoracic Nerve				
9 Lumbar Plexus	N Lumbar Sympathetic Nerve			
A Lumbosacral Plexus	P Sacral Sympathetic Nerve			
B Lumbar Nerve	Q Sacral Plexus			
C Pudendal Nerve	R Sacral Nerve			
D Femoral Nerve				

PERIPHERAL NERVOUS 01B

1 – PERIPHERAL NERVOUS SYSTEM — 01H

EXCISION GROUP: Excision, Resection, Destruction, Extraction, (Detachment)
Root Operations that take out some or all of a body part.

1ST - 0 Medical and Surgical
2ND - 1 Peripheral Nervous System
3RD - D EXTRACTION

EXAMPLE: Neurexeresis radial nerve CMS Ex: D&C

EXTRACTION: Pulling or stripping out or off all or a portion of a body part by the use of force.

EXPLANATION: None for this Body System

Body Part – 4TH		Approach – 5TH	Device – 6TH	Qualifier – 7TH
0 Cervical Plexus	F Sciatic Nerve	0 Open	Z No device	Z No qualifier
1 Cervical Nerve	G Tibial Nerve	3 Percutaneous		
2 Phrenic Nerve	H Peroneal Nerve	4 Percutaneous endoscopic		
3 Brachial Plexus	K Head and Neck Sympathetic Nerve			
4 Ulnar Nerve				
5 Median Nerve	L Thoracic Sympathetic Nerve			
6 Radial Nerve	M Abdominal Sympathetic Nerve			
8 Thoracic Nerve				
9 Lumbar Plexus	N Lumbar Sympathetic Nerve			
A Lumbosacral Plexus	P Sacral Sympathetic Nerve			
B Lumbar Nerve	Q Sacral Plexus			
C Pudendal Nerve	R Sacral Nerve			
D Femoral Nerve				

DEVICE GROUP: Change, Insertion, Removal, (Replacement), Revision, Supplement
Root Operations that always involve a device.

1ST - 0 Medical and Surgical
2ND - 1 Peripheral Nervous System
3RD - H INSERTION

EXAMPLE: Insertion neurostimulator lead CMS Ex: Central venous catheter

INSERTION: Putting in a nonbiological appliance that monitors, assists, performs, or prevents a physiological function but does not physically take the place of a body part.

EXPLANATION: None

Body Part – 4TH	Approach – 5TH	Device – 6TH	Qualifier – 7TH
Y Peripheral Nerve	0 Open 3 Percutaneous 4 Percutaneous endoscopic	2 Monitoring device M Neurostimulator lead	Z No qualifier

01J MEDICAL AND SURGICAL SECTION – 2016 ICD-10-PCS [2016.PCS]

EXAMINATION GROUP: Inspection, (Map)
Root Operations involving examination only.

- 1ST – **0** Medical and Surgical
- 2ND – **1** Peripheral Nervous System
- 3RD – **J** INSPECTION

EXAMPLE: Examination injured nerve CMS Ex: Colonoscopy

INSPECTION: Visually and/or manually exploring a body part.

EXPLANATION: Direct or instrumental visualization …

Body Part – 4TH	Approach – 5TH	Device – 6TH	Qualifier – 7TH
Y Peripheral Nerve	0 Open 3 Percutaneous 4 Percutaneous endoscopic	Z No device	Z No qualifier

DIVISION GROUP: Division, Release
Root Operations involving cutting or separation only.

- 1ST – **0** Medical and Surgical
- 2ND – **1** Peripheral Nervous System
- 3RD – **N** RELEASE

EXAMPLE: Carpal tunnel release CMS Ex: Carpal tunnel release

RELEASE: Freeing a body part from an abnormal physical constraint by cutting or by the use of force.

EXPLANATION: None of the body part is taken out …

Body Part – 4TH		Approach – 5TH	Device – 6TH	Qualifier – 7TH
0 Cervical Plexus 1 Cervical Nerve 2 Phrenic Nerve 3 Brachial Plexus 4 Ulnar Nerve 5 Median Nerve 6 Radial Nerve 8 Thoracic Nerve 9 Lumbar Plexus A Lumbosacral Plexus B Lumbar Nerve C Pudendal Nerve D Femoral Nerve	F Sciatic Nerve G Tibial Nerve H Peroneal Nerve K Head and Neck Sympathetic Nerve L Thoracic Sympathetic Nerve M Abdominal Sympathetic Nerve N Lumbar Sympathetic Nerve P Sacral Sympathetic Nerve Q Sacral Plexus R Sacral Nerve	0 Open 3 Percutaneous 4 Percutaneous endoscopic	Z No device	Z No qualifier

1 – PERIPHERAL NERVOUS SYSTEM — 01Q

DEVICE GROUP: Change, Insertion, Removal, (Replacement), Revision, Supplement
Root Operations that always involve a device.

- 1ST – **0** Medical and Surgical
- 2ND – **1** Peripheral Nervous System
- 3RD – **P REMOVAL**

EXAMPLE: Removal neurostimulator lead | CMS Ex: Chest tube removal

REMOVAL: Taking out or off a device from a body part.

EXPLANATION: Removal device without reinsertion ...

Body Part – 4TH	Approach – 5TH	Device – 6TH	Qualifier – 7TH
Y Peripheral Nerve	0 Open 3 Percutaneous 4 Percutaneous endoscopic	0 Drainage device 2 Monitoring device 7 Autologous tissue substitute M Neurostimulator lead	Z No qualifier
Y Peripheral Nerve	X External	0 Drainage device 2 Monitoring device M Neurostimulator lead	Z No qualifier

OTHER REPAIRS GROUP: (Control), Repair
Root Operations that define other repairs.

- 1ST – **0** Medical and Surgical
- 2ND – **1** Peripheral Nervous System
- 3RD – **Q REPAIR**

EXAMPLE: Microsurgical repair nerve | CMS Ex: Suture laceration

REPAIR: Restoring, to the extent possible, a body part to its normal anatomic structure and function.

EXPLANATION: Only when no other root operation applies ...

Body Part – 4TH	Approach – 5TH	Device – 6TH	Qualifier – 7TH
0 Cervical Plexus 1 Cervical Nerve 2 Phrenic Nerve 3 Brachial Plexus 4 Ulnar Nerve 5 Median Nerve 6 Radial Nerve 8 Thoracic Nerve 9 Lumbar Plexus A Lumbosacral Plexus B Lumbar Nerve C Pudendal Nerve D Femoral Nerve F Sciatic Nerve G Tibial Nerve H Peroneal Nerve K Head and Neck Sympathetic Nerve L Thoracic Sympathetic Nerve M Abdominal Sympathetic Nerve N Lumbar Sympathetic Nerve P Sacral Sympathetic Nerve Q Sacral Plexus R Sacral Nerve	0 Open 3 Percutaneous 4 Percutaneous endoscopic	Z No device	Z No qualifier

01S MEDICAL AND SURGICAL SECTION – 2016 ICD-10-PCS

MOVE GROUP: (Reattachment), Reposition, Transfer, (Transplantation)
Root Operations that put in/put back or move some/all of a body part.

- 1ST – **0** Medical and Surgical
- 2ND – **1** Peripheral Nervous System
- 3RD – **S REPOSITION**

EXAMPLE: Relocation femoral nerve   **CMS Ex:** Fracture reduction

REPOSITION: Moving to its normal location, or other suitable location, all or a portion of a body part.

EXPLANATION: May or may not be cut to be moved …

Body Part – 4TH		Approach – 5TH	Device – 6TH	Qualifier – 7TH
0 Cervical Plexus	A Lumbosacral Plexus	0 Open	Z No device	Z No qualifier
1 Cervical Nerve	B Lumbar Nerve	3 Percutaneous		
2 Phrenic Nerve	C Pudendal Nerve	4 Percutaneous endoscopic		
3 Brachial Plexus	D Femoral Nerve			
4 Ulnar Nerve	F Sciatic Nerve			
5 Median Nerve	G Tibial Nerve			
6 Radial Nerve	H Peroneal Nerve			
8 Thoracic Nerve	Q Sacral Plexus			
9 Lumbar Plexus	R Sacral Nerve			

DEVICE GROUP: Change, Insertion, Removal, (Replacement), Revision, Supplement
Root Operations that always involve a device.

- 1ST – **0** Medical and Surgical
- 2ND – **1** Peripheral Nervous System
- 3RD – **U SUPPLEMENT**

EXAMPLE: Free nerve autograft   **CMS Ex:** Hernia repair with mesh

SUPPLEMENT: Putting in or on biological or synthetic material that physically reinforces and/or augments the function of a portion of a body part.

EXPLANATION: Biological material from same individual …

Body Part – 4TH		Approach – 5TH	Device – 6TH	Qualifier – 7TH
1 Cervical Nerve	C Pudendal Nerve	0 Open	7 Autologous tissue substitute	Z No qualifier
2 Phrenic Nerve	D Femoral Nerve	3 Percutaneous		
4 Ulnar Nerve	F Sciatic Nerve	4 Percutaneous endoscopic		
5 Median Nerve	G Tibial Nerve			
6 Radial Nerve	H Peroneal Nerve			
8 Thoracic Nerve	R Sacral Nerve			
B Lumbar Nerve				

1 – PERIPHERAL NERVOUS SYSTEM — 01X

DEVICE GROUP: Change, Insertion, Removal, (Replacement), Revision, Supplement
Root Operations that always involve a device.

- 1ST – **0** Medical and Surgical
- 2ND – **1** Peripheral Nervous System
- 3RD – **W** REVISION

EXAMPLE: Reposition neurostimulator lead | CMS Ex: Adjust pacemaker lead

REVISION: Correcting, to the extent possible, a portion of a malfunctioning device or the position of a displaced device.

EXPLANATION: May replace components of a device ...

Body Part – 4TH	Approach – 5TH	Device – 6TH	Qualifier – 7TH
Y Peripheral Nerve	0 Open 3 Percutaneous 4 Percutaneous endoscopic X External	0 Drainage device 2 Monitoring device 7 Autologous tissue substitute M Neurostimulator lead	Z No qualifier

MOVE GROUP: (Reattachment), Reposition, Transfer, (Transplantation)
Root Operations that put in/put back or move some/all of a body part.

- 1ST – **0** Medical and Surgical
- 2ND – **1** Peripheral Nervous System
- 3RD – **X** TRANSFER

EXAMPLE: Radial to median nerve transfer | CMS Ex: Tendon transfer

TRANSFER: Moving, without taking out, all or a portion of a body part to another location to take over the function of all or a portion of a body part.

EXPLANATION: The body part remains connected ...

Body Part – 4TH	Approach – 5TH	Device – 6TH	Qualifier – 7TH
1 Cervical Nerve 2 Phrenic Nerve	0 Open 4 Percutaneous endoscopic	Z No device	1 Cervical Nerve 2 Phrenic Nerve
4 Ulnar Nerve 5 Median Nerve 6 Radial Nerve	0 Open 4 Percutaneous endoscopic	Z No device	4 Ulnar Nerve 5 Median Nerve 6 Radial Nerve
8 Thoracic Nerve	0 Open 4 Percutaneous endoscopic	Z No device	8 Thoracic Nerve
B Lumbar Nerve C Pudendal Nerve	0 Open 4 Percutaneous endoscopic	Z No device	B Lumbar Nerve C Perineal Nerve
D Femoral Nerve F Sciatic Nerve G Tibial Nerve H Peroneal Nerve	0 Open 4 Percutaneous endoscopic	Z No device	D Femoral Nerve F Sciatic Nerve G Tibial Nerve H Peroneal Nerve

MEDICAL AND SURGICAL SECTION – 2016 ICD-10-PCS

NOTES

PERIPHERAL NERVOUS 01

0 Medical and Surgical
1 Peripheral Nervous System
W REVISION

DEVICE GROUP: Change, Insertion, Removal, Revision, Supplement
Root Operations that always involve a device.

REVISION: Correcting, to the extent possible, a portion of a malfunctioning device or the position of a displaced device.

EXPLANATION: May replace components of a device.

EXAMPLE: Reposition neurostimulator lead. (CMS Ex. Adjust pacemaker lead)

Body Part – 4th	Approach – 5th	Device – 6th	Qualifier – 7th
Y Peripheral Nerve	0 Open 3 Percutaneous 4 Percutaneous endoscopic X External	0 Drainage device 2 Monitoring device 7 Autologous tissue substitute M Neurostimulator lead	Z No qualifier

---

0 Medical and Surgical
1 Peripheral Nervous System
X TRANSFER

MOVE GROUP: Map, Reattach, Reposition, Transfer, Transplant
Root Operations that put back or move something of a body part.

TRANSFER: Moving, without taking out, all or a portion of a body part to another location to take over the function of all or a portion of a body part.

EXPLANATION: The body part remains connected...

EXAMPLE: Radial to median nerve transfer. (CMS Ex. linear transfer)

Body Part – 4th	Approach – 5th	Device – 6th	Qualifier – 7th
1 Cervical Nerve 2 Phrenic Nerve	0 Open 4 Percutaneous endoscopic	Z No device	1 Cervical Nerve 2 Phrenic Nerve
4 Ulnar Nerve 5 Median Nerve 6 Radial Nerve	0 Open 4 Percutaneous endoscopic	Z No device	4 Ulnar Nerve 5 Median Nerve 6 Radial Nerve
8 Thoracic Nerve	0 Open 4 Percutaneous endoscopic	Z No device	8 Thoracic Nerve
B Lumbar Nerve C Pudendal Nerve	0 Open 4 Percutaneous endoscopic	Z No device	B Lumbar Nerve C Perineal Nerve
D Femoral Nerve F Sciatic Nerve G Tibial Nerve H Peroneal Nerve	0 Open 4 Percutaneous endoscopic	Z No device	D Femoral Nerve F Sciatic Nerve G Tibial Nerve H Peroneal Nerve

Educational Annotations | 2 – Heart and Great Vessels

Body System Specific Educational Annotations for the Heart and Great Vessels include:
- Anatomy and Physiology Review
- Anatomical Illustrations
- Definitions of Common Procedures
- AHA Coding Clinic® Reference Notations
- Body Part Key Listings
- Device Key Listings
- Device Aggregation Table Listings
- Coding Notes

Anatomy and Physiology Review of Heart and Great Vessels

BODY PART VALUES – 2 - HEART AND GREAT VESSELS

Aortic Valve – ANATOMY – The aortic valve has three cusps and is located between the outlet of the left ventricle and the base of the aorta. PHYSIOLOGY – The aortic valve prevents backflow of blood into the left ventricle from the aorta via its one-way valve function.

Atrial Septum – The strong tissue wall that separates the left and right atria.

Atrium, Left – ANATOMY – One of the two smaller chambers of the heart's four chambers. PHYSIOLOGY – The left atrium receives and pools the oxygenated blood from the lungs briefly before the tricuspid valve opens and the blood flows into the left ventricle.

Atrium, Right – ANATOMY – One of the two smaller chambers of the heart's four chambers. PHYSIOLOGY – The right atrium receives and pools the de-oxygenated blood from the inferior vena cava and the superior vena cava briefly before the pulmonary valve opens and the blood flows into the right ventricle.

Chordae Tendineae – The very strong tendinous cord attaching a papillary muscle to a valve leaflet.

Conduction Mechanism – The electrical signal transmission system that controls the rhythmical heart beat through various structures and fibers including the sinoatrial node (the heart's pacemaker), the atrioventricular node, and the Bundle of HIS.

Coronary Artery – Coronary arteries supply oxygenated blood to the heart.

Coronary Vein – Coronary veins remove the deoxygenated blood from the heart muscle and return it to the right atrium.

Great Vessel – The major vessels associated with the heart that lie within the thoracic cavity including: Thoracic aorta, pulmonary arteries, pulmonary veins, and the superior vena cava and thoracic portion of the inferior vena cava.

Heart – ANATOMY – The heart is the 4 chambered, muscular, blood pumping organ behind the mediastinum in the thorax, and is approximately 5.5 inches (14 cm) long and 3.5 inches (9 cm) wide. The heart has 3 layers: The endocardium, myocardium, and pericardium. The endocardium is the interior lining of endothelium. The myocardium is the thick muscular layer. The pericardium is the double-layered serous membrane protecting the heart from friction as it beats. The heart has 4 valves and 4 chambers: The tricuspid valve, mitral valve, aortic valve, the pulmonary valve, right and left atria, and right and left ventricles. The mediastinum is the mass of tissue between the sternum and vertebral column which divides the thoracic cavity. PHYSIOLOGY – The heart functions to pump and maintain sufficient pressure of the blood to constantly meet the needs of the body cells. The venous blood is returned from the body via the inferior and superior vena cava to the right atrium where it is pooled momentarily before the tricuspid valve opens and allows the venous blood to enter the right ventricle. The right ventricle then contracts forcing the blood through the pulmonary valve to the lungs. The lungs return the reoxygenated blood to the left atrium where it is pooled momentarily before the mitral valve opens and allows the venous blood to enter the left ventricle. The left ventricle then contracts, forcing the blood through the aortic valve to all the tissues of the body.

Heart, Left – ANATOMY – The portion of the heart that includes the left atria and left ventricle.
PHYSIOLOGY – The left heart receives the re-oxygenated blood from the lungs and pumps it out to the body.

Heart, Right – ANATOMY – The portion of the heart that includes the right atria and right ventricle.
PHYSIOLOGY – The right heart receives the venous blood and pumps it to the lungs for re-oxygenation.

Mitral Valve – ANATOMY – The mitral valve (also known as the bicuspid valve) has two cusps and is located between the left atrium and the left ventricle. PHYSIOLOGY – The mitral valve prevents backflow of blood from the left ventricle back into the left atrium via its one-way valve function. The mitral valve's closure is strengthened by the papillary muscles and their chordae tendineae during the left ventricle's forceful contraction.

Continued on next page

Educational Annotations

2 – Heart and Great Vessels

Anatomy and Physiology Review of Heart and Great Vessels

BODY PART VALUES – 2 - HEART AND GREAT VESSELS
Continued from previous page

Papillary Muscle – ANATOMY – The intraventricular muscles that connect with the mitral and tricuspid valves via a chordae tendineae. PHYSIOLOGY – The papillary muscles contract at the same time as the ventricle, thus reinforcing the closure of the atrial inlet valve.

Pericardium – The pericardium is the double-layered serous membrane protecting the heart from friction as it beats.

Pulmonary Artery, Left – The major blood vessel transporting de-oxygenated blood from the right ventricle to the left lobes of the lungs. Blood vessels with blood flow going away from the heart are termed arteries. Pulmonary arteries carry venous blood, the opposite of the rest of the arteries.

Pulmonary Artery, Right – The major blood vessel transporting de-oxygenated blood from the right ventricle to the right lobes of the lungs. Blood vessels with blood flow going away from the heart are termed arteries. Pulmonary arteries carry venous blood, the opposite of the rest of the arteries.

Pulmonary Trunk – The short, large blood vessel connecting the right ventricle to the right and left pulmonary arteries.

Pulmonary Valve – ANATOMY – The pulmonary valve has three cusps and is located between the outlet of the right ventricle and the base of the pulmonary artery. PHYSIOLOGY – The pulmonary valve prevents backflow of blood into the right ventricle from the pulmonary artery via its one-way valve function.

Pulmonary Vein, Left – The major blood vessel transporting oxygenated blood from the left lobes of the lungs to the left atrium. Blood vessels with blood flow going to the heart are termed veins. Pulmonary veins carry arterial blood, the opposite of the rest of the veins.

Pulmonary Vein, Right – The major blood vessel transporting oxygenated blood from the right lobes of the lungs to the left atrium. Blood vessels with blood flow going to the heart are termed veins. Pulmonary veins carry arterial blood, the opposite of the rest of the veins.

Superior Vena Cava – The major vein transporting de-oxygenated blood from the upper body and head that empties into the right atrium.

Thoracic Aorta – The upper most portion of the aorta that lies within the thoracic cavity.

Tricuspid Valve – ANATOMY – The tricuspid valve has three cusps and is located between the right atrium and the right ventricle. PHYSIOLOGY – The tricuspid valve prevents backflow of blood from the right ventricle back into the right atrium via its one-way valve function. The tricuspid valve's closure is strengthened by the papillary muscles and their chordae tendineae during the right ventricle's forceful contraction.

Ventricle, Left – ANATOMY – One of the two large chambers of the heart's four chambers. PHYSIOLOGY – The left ventricle pumps oxygenated blood from the heart into the aorta to be carried throughout the body.

Ventricle, Right – ANATOMY – One of the two large chambers of the heart's four chambers. PHYSIOLOGY – The right ventricle pumps de-oxygenated blood from the heart to the lungs through the pulmonary arteries.

Ventricular Septum – The strong tissue wall that separates the left and right ventricles.

Educational Annotations | 2 – Heart and Great Vessels

Anatomical Illustrations of Heart and Great Vessels

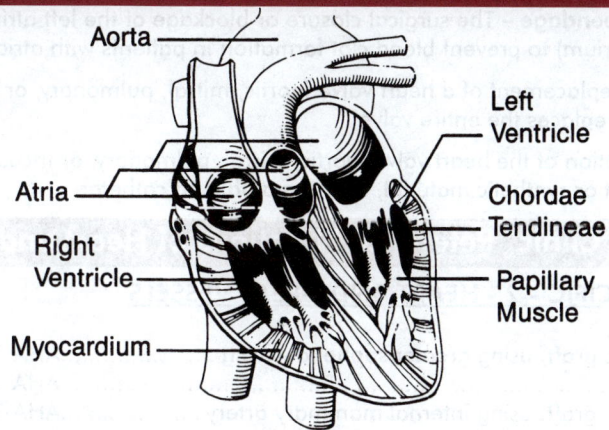

HEART — ANTERIOR (CUT-AWAY) VIEW

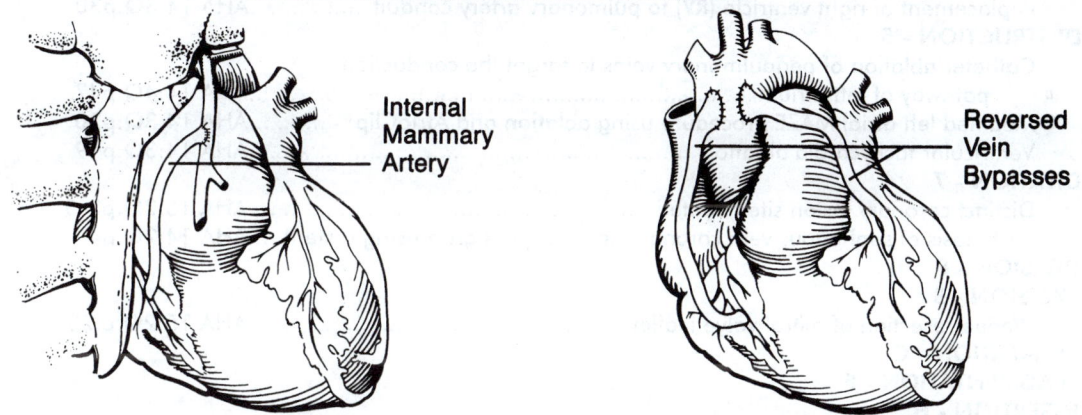

INTERNAL MAMMARY-CORONARY BYPASS   DOUBLE AORTOCORONARY BYPASS

Definitions of Common Procedures of Heart and Great Vessels

Aortocoronary artery bypass – The restoration of coronary artery blood flow by using a tubular graft (usually a saphenous vein) to bring blood from the aorta to the coronary artery that is distal to the blocked site.

Coronary artery stent – The widening of the coronary artery lumen by placing a stent (tubular supporting device) in the narrowed arterial site. The stent may or may not be coated in a drug-eluting substance.

Heart transplant – The removal of the end-staged diseased heart and replacement with a donor heart.

Internal mammary artery coronary artery bypass – The restoration of coronary artery blood flow by using the direct connection of an internal mammary artery to the coronary artery that is distal to the blocked site.

Intra-aortic balloon pump (IABP) – The computer-controlled inflatable circulatory assist device that is placed in the descending thoracic aorta. The balloon is inflated during diastole (heart not contracting and filling with blood) to increase cardiac output pressure and increase coronary blood flow.

MAZE procedure (Cox-MAZE) – The surgical cutting or destruction of atrial tissue to disrupt the electrical pathways and re-direct them through a maze-like pattern that creates only one path that the electrical impulse can take from the SA node to the AV node, which prevents the irregular electrical impulses of atrial fibrillation.

Continued on next page

Educational Annotations | 2 – Heart and Great Vessels

Definitions of Common Procedures of Heart and Great Vessels

Occlusion of left atrial appendage – The surgical closure or blockage of the left atrial appendage (small pouch in muscle wall of the left atrium) to prevent blood clot formation in patients with atrial fibrillation.

Valve replacement – The replacement of a heart valve (aortic, mitral, pulmonary, or tricuspid) using a mechanical or bioprosthetic valve that replaces the entire valve.

Valvuloplasty – The restoration of the heart valve (aortic, mitral, pulmonary, or tricuspid) anatomy and/or function using a tissue graft or synthetic material, or using a balloon catheter.

AHA Coding Clinic® Reference Notations of Heart and Great Vessels

ROOT OPERATION SPECIFIC - 2 - HEART AND GREAT VESSELS

BYPASS - 1
- Coronary artery bypass graft, using greater saphenous vein ....AHA 14:3Q:p20
  ....AHA 14:1Q:p10
- Coronary artery bypass graft, using internal mammary artery ....AHA 14:3Q:p8,20
- Fontan completion stage II procedure..AHA 14:3Q:p29
- Modified Blalock-Taussig shunt procedure..AHA 14:3Q:p3
- Replacement of right ventricle (RV) to pulmonary artery conduit ....AHA 14:3Q:p30

DESTRUCTION - 5
- Catheter ablation of peripulmonary veins to target the conduction
  pathway of left atrium ....AHA 14:4Q:p47
- Modified left atrial MAZE procedure using ablation and AtrioClip® ....AHA 14:3Q:p20
- Ventricular tachycardia ablation ....AHA 14:3Q:p19

DILATION - 7
- Distinct coronary lesion sites treated...AHA 15:2Q:p3-5
- Restenosis of saphenous vein coronary artery bypass graft using a stent ....AHA 14:2Q:p4

DIVISION - 8

EXCISION - B
- Wedge resection of mitral valve leaflet ....AHA 15:2Q:p.23

EXTIRPATION - C

FRAGMENTATION - F

INSERTION - H
- Insertion of infusion device into superior vena cava ....AHA 15:2Q:p.33
- Insertion of leadless pacemaker ....AHA 15:2Q:p.31
- Placement of peripherally inserted central catheter (PICC line) into
  superior vena cava ....AHA 13:3Q:p18

INSPECTION - J

MAP - K

OCCLUSION - L
- Modified left atrial MAZE procedure using ablation and AtrioClip® ....AHA 14:3Q:p20

RELEASE - N
- Widening of right ventricular outflow tract ....AHA 14:3Q:p16

REMOVAL - P

REPAIR - Q
- Thoracic aortic valve repair (TAVR) ....AHA 13:3Q:p26

REPLACEMENT - R
- Graft repair of thoracic aortic arch aneurysm ....AHA 14:1Q:p10

REPOSITION - S

RESECTION - T

SUPPLEMENT - U
- Closure of ventricular septal defect with Goretex® patch ....AHA 14:3Q:p16
- Mitral valve ring annuloplasty ....AHA 15:2Q:p.23

RESTRICTION - V

REVISION - W
- Closure of paravalvular leak ....AHA 14:3Q:p31

TRANSPLANTATION - Y
- Heart transplant..AHA 13:3Q:p18

Educational Annotations | 2 – Heart and Great Vessels

Body Part Key Listings of Heart and Great Vessels

See also Body Part Key in Appendix C

Aortic annulus	*use* Aortic Valve
Aortic arch	*use* Thoracic Aorta
Aortic intercostal artery	*use* Thoracic Aorta
Arterial canal (duct)	*use* Pulmonary Artery, Left
Ascending aorta	*use* Thoracic Aorta
Atrioventricular node	*use* Conduction Mechanism
Atrium dextrum cordis	*use* Atrium, Right
Atrium pulmonale	*use* Atrium, Left
Bicuspid valve	*use* Mitral Valve
Botallo's duct	*use* Pulmonary Artery, Left
Bronchial artery	*use* Thoracic Aorta
Bundle of His	*use* Conduction Mechanism
Bundle of Kent	*use* Conduction Mechanism
Conus arteriosus	*use* Ventricle, Right
Esophageal artery	*use* Thoracic Aorta
Interatrial septum	*use* Atrial Septum
Interventricular septum	*use* Ventricular Septum
Left atrioventricular valve	*use* Mitral Valve
Left auricular appendix	*use* Atrium, Left
Left coronary sulcus	*use* Heart, Left
Left inferior pulmonary vein	*use* Pulmonary Vein, Left
Left superior pulmonary vein	*use* Pulmonary Vein, Left
Mitral annulus	*use* Mitral Valve
Obtuse margin	*use* Heart, Left
Precava	*use* Superior Vena Cava
Pulmoaortic canal	*use* Pulmonary Artery, Left
Pulmonary annulus	*use* Pulmonary Valve
Pulmonic valve	*use* Pulmonary Valve
Right atrioventricular valve	*use* Tricuspid Valve
Right auricular appendix	*use* Atrium, Right
Right coronary sulcus	*use* Heart, Right
Right inferior pulmonary vein	*use* Pulmonary Vein, Right
Right superior pulmonary vein	*use* Pulmonary Vein, Right
Sinoatrial node	*use* Conduction Mechanism
Sinus venosus	*use* Atrium, Right
Subcostal artery	*use* Thoracic Aorta
Tricuspid annulus	*use* Tricuspid Valve

Device Key Listings of Heart and Great Vessels

See also Device Key in Appendix D

3f (Aortic) Bioprosthesis valve	*use* Zooplastic Tissue in Heart and Great Vessels
AbioCor® Total Replacement Heart	*use* Synthetic Substitute
ACUITY™ Steerable Lead	*use* Cardiac Lead, Pacemaker for Insertion in Heart and Great Vessels
	use Cardiac Lead, Defibrillator for Insertion in Heart and Great Vessels
AMPLATZER® Muscular VSD Occluder	*use* Synthetic Substitute
Annuloplasty ring	*use* Synthetic Substitute

Continued on next page

Educational Annotations | 2 – Heart and Great Vessels

Device Key Listings of Heart and Great Vessels

Continued from previous page

Attain Ability® lead	*use* Cardiac Lead, Pacemaker for Insertion in Heart and Great Vessels
	use Cardiac Lead, Defibrillator for Insertion in Heart and Great Vessels
Attain StarFix® (OTW) lead	*use* Cardiac Lead, Pacemaker for Insertion in Heart and Great Vessels
	use Cardiac Lead, Defibrillator for Insertion in Heart and Great Vessels
Autograft	*use* Autologous Tissue Substitute
Autologous artery graft	*use* Autologous Arterial Tissue in Heart and Great Vessels
Autologous vein graft	*use* Autologous Venous Tissue in Heart and Great Vessels
Berlin Heart Ventricular Assist Device	*use* Implantable Heart Assist System in Heart and Great Vessels
Biventricular external heart assist system	*use* External Heart Assist System in Heart and Great Vessels
Bovine pericardial valve	*use* Zooplastic Tissue in Heart and Great Vessels
Bovine pericardium graft	*use* Zooplastic Tissue in Heart and Great Vessels
BVS 5000 Ventricular Assist Device	*use* External Heart Assist System in Heart and Great Vessels
Cardiac contractility modulation lead	*use* Cardiac Lead in Heart and Great Vessels
Cardiac event recorder	*use* Monitoring Device
Cardiac resynchronization therapy (CRT) lead	*use* Cardiac Lead, Pacemaker for Insertion in Heart and Great Vessels
	use Cardiac Lead, Defibrillator for Insertion in Heart and Great Vessels
CardioMEMS® pressure sensor	*use* Monitoring Device, Pressure Sensor for Insertion in Heart and Great Vessels
Centrimag® Blood Pump	*use* External Heart Assist System in Heart and Great Vessels
CoAxia NeuroFlo catheter	*use* Intraluminal Device
Contegra Pulmonary Valved Conduit	*use* Zooplastic Tissue in Heart and Great Vessels
CoreValve transcatheter aortic valve	*use* Zooplastic Tissue in Heart and Great Vessels
Corox OTW (Bipolar) Lead	*use* Cardiac Lead, Pacemaker for Insertion in Heart and Great Vessels
	use Cardiac Lead, Defibrillator for Insertion in Heart and Great Vessels
CYPHER® Stent	*use* Intraluminal Device, Drug-eluting in Heart and Great Vessels
DeBakey Left Ventricular Assist Device	*use* Implantable Heart Assist System in Heart and Great Vessels
Driver stent (RX) (OTW)	*use* Intraluminal Device
DuraHeart Left Ventricular Assist System	*use* Implantable Heart Assist System in Heart and Great Vessels
Durata® Defibrillation Lead	*use* Cardiac Lead, Defibrillator for Insertion in Heart and Great Vessels
Endeavor® (III) (IV) (Sprint) Zotarolimus-eluting Coronary Stent System	*use* Intraluminal Device, Drug-eluting in Heart and Great Vessels
EndoSure® sensor	*use* Monitoring Device, Pressure Sensor for Insertion in Heart and Great Vessels
ENDOTAK RELIANCE® (G) Defibrillation Lead	*use* Cardiac Lead, Defibrillator for Insertion in Heart and Great Vessels
Epic™ Stented Tissue Valve (aortic)	*use* Zooplastic Tissue in Heart and Great Vessels
Everolimus-eluting coronary stent	*use* Intraluminal Device, Drug-eluting in Heart and Great Vessels
Freestyle (Stentless) Aortic Root Bioprosthesis	*use* Zooplastic Tissue in Heart and Great Vessels
Hancock Bioprosthesis (aortic) (mitral) valve	*use* Zooplastic Tissue in Heart and Great Vessels
Hancock Bioprosthetic Valved Conduit	*use* Zooplastic Tissue in Heart and Great Vessels
HeartMate II® Left Ventricular Assist Device (LVAD)	*use* Implantable Heart Assist System in Heart and Great Vessels
HeartMate XVE® Left Ventricular Assist Device (LVAD)	*use* Implantable Heart Assist System in Heart and Great Vessels
Melody® transcatheter pulmonary valve	*use* Zooplastic Tissue in Heart and Great Vessels
Micro-Driver stent (RX) (OTW)	*use* Intraluminal Device
MicroMed HeartAssist	*use* Implantable Heart Assist System in Heart and Great Vessels
MitraClip valve repair system	*use* Synthetic Substitute
Mitroflow® Aortic Pericardial Heart Valve	*use* Zooplastic Tissue in Heart and Great Vessels
Mosaic Bioprosthesis (aortic) (mitral) valve	*use* Zooplastic Tissue in Heart and Great Vessels
MULTI-LINK (VISION) (MINI-VISION) (ULTRA) Coronary Stent System	*use* Intraluminal Device

Continued on next page

Educational Annotations | 2 – Heart and Great Vessels

Device Key Listings of Heart and Great Vessels

Continued from previous page

Novacor Left Ventricular Assist Device	*use* Implantable Heart Assist System in Heart and Great Vessels
Open Pivot Aortic Valve Graft (AVG)	*use* Synthetic Substitute
Open Pivot (mechanical) valve	*use* Synthetic Substitute
Paclitaxel-eluting coronary stent	*use* Intraluminal Device, Drug-eluting in Heart and Great Vessels
Peripherally inserted central catheter (PICC)	*use* Infusion Device
Porcine (bioprosthetic) valve	*use* Zooplastic Tissue in Heart and Great Vessels
SAPIEN transcatheter aortic valve	*use* Zooplastic Tissue in Heart and Great Vessels
Sirolimus-eluting coronary stent	*use* Intraluminal Device, Drug-eluting in Heart and Great Vessels
SJM Biocor® Stented Valve System	*use* Zooplastic Tissue in Heart and Great Vessels
Stent, intraluminal (cardiovascular) (gastrointestinal) (hepatobiliary) (urinary)	*use* Intraluminal Device
Stented tissue valve	*use* Zooplastic Tissue in Heart and Great Vessels
SynCardia Total Artificial Heart	*use* Synthetic Substitute
TandemHeart® System	*use* External Heart Assist System in Heart and Great Vessels
TAXUS® Liberté® Paclitaxel-eluting Coronary Stent System	*use* Intraluminal Device, Drug-eluting in Heart and Great Vessels
Thoratec IVAD (Implantable Ventricular Assist Device)	*use* Implantable Heart Assist System in Heart and Great Vessels
Thoratec Paracorporeal Ventricular Assist Device	*use* External Heart Assist System in Heart and Great Vessels
TigerPaw® system for closure of left atrial appendage	*use* Extraluminal Device
Tissue bank graft	*use* Nonautologous Tissue Substitute
Total artificial (replacement) heart	*use* Synthetic Substitute
Trifecta™ Valve (aortic)	*use* Zooplastic Tissue in Heart and Great Vessels
Valiant Thoracic Stent Graft	*use* Intraluminal Device
Xenograft	*use* Zooplastic Tissue in Heart and Great Vessels
XIENCE Everolimus Eluting Coronary Stent System	*use* Intraluminal Device, Drug-eluting in Heart and Great Vessels
Zenith TX2® TAA Endovascular Graft	*use* Intraluminal Device
Zotarolimus-eluting coronary stent	*use* Intraluminal Device, Drug-eluting in Heart and Great Vessels

Device Aggregation Table Listings of Heart and Great Vessels

See also Device Aggregation Table in Appendix E

Specific Device	For Operation	In Body System	General Device
Autologous Arterial Tissue	All applicable	Heart and Great Vessels	7 Autologous Tissue Substitute
Autologous Venous Tissue	All applicable	Heart and Great Vessels	7 Autologous Tissue Substitute
Cardiac Lead, Defibrillator	Insertion	Heart and Great Vessels	M Cardiac Lead
Cardiac Lead, Pacemaker	Insertion	Heart and Great Vessels	M Cardiac Lead
Intraluminal Device, Drug-eluting	All applicable	Heart and Great Vessels	D Intraluminal Device
Intraluminal Device, Radioactive	All applicable	Heart and Great Vessels	D Intraluminal Device
Monitoring Device, Pressure Sensor	Insertion	Heart and Great Vessels	2 Monitoring Device

02 — MEDICAL AND SURGICAL SECTION – 2016 ICD-10-PCS

Educational Annotations | 2 – Heart and Great Vessels

Coding Notes of Heart and Great Vessels

Body System Relevant Coding Guidelines

Bypass procedures

B3.6b
Coronary arteries are classified by number of distinct sites treated, rather than number of coronary arteries or anatomic name of a coronary artery (e.g., left anterior descending). Coronary artery bypass procedures are coded differently than other bypass procedures as described in the previous guideline. Rather than identifying the body part bypassed from, the body part identifies the number of coronary artery sites bypassed to, and the qualifier specifies the vessel bypassed from.
Example: Aortocoronary artery bypass of one site on the left anterior descending coronary artery and one site on the obtuse marginal coronary artery is classified in the body part axis of classification as two coronary artery sites and the qualifier specifies the aorta as the body part bypassed from.

B3.6c
If multiple coronary artery sites are bypassed, a separate procedure is coded for each coronary artery site that uses a different device and/or qualifier.
Example: Aortocoronary artery bypass and internal mammary coronary artery bypass are coded separately.

Coronary arteries

B4.4
The coronary arteries are classified as a single body part that is further specified by number of sites treated and not by name or number of arteries. Separate body part values are used to specify the number of sites treated when the same procedure is performed on multiple sites in the coronary arteries.
Examples: Angioplasty of two distinct sites in the left anterior descending coronary artery with placement of two stents is coded as Dilation of Coronary Arteries, Two Sites, with Intraluminal Device. Angioplasty of two distinct sites in the left anterior descending coronary artery, one with stent placed and one without, is coded separately as Dilation of Coronary Arteries, One Site with Intraluminal Device, and Dilation of Coronary Artery, One Site with no device.

Body System Specific PCS Reference Manual Exercises

PCS CODE	2 – HEART AND GREAT VESSELS EXERCISES
02100Z9	CABG of LAD using left internal mammary artery, open off-bypass.
02103D4	PICVA (Percutaneous in-situ coronary venous arterialization) of single coronary artery.
02583ZZ	Left heart catheterization with laser destruction of arrhythmogenic focus, A-V node.
02703DZ	PTCA of two coronary arteries, LAD with stent placement, RCA with no stent.
02703ZZ	(A separate procedure is coded for each artery dilated, since the device value differs for each artery.)
02883ZZ	Left heart catheterization with division of bundle of HIS.
02FN0ZZ	Thoracotomy with crushing of pericardial calcifications.
02H73JZ	Percutaneous replacement of broken pacemaker lead in left atrium. (Taking out the broken pacemaker lead is coded separately to the root operation Removal.)
02HP32Z	Percutaneous placement of Swan-Ganz catheter in pulmonary trunk. The Swan-Ganz catheter is coded to the device value Monitoring Device because it monitors pulmonary artery output.)
02K80ZZ	Intraoperative cardiac mapping during open heart surgery.
02K83ZZ	Heart catheterization with cardiac mapping.
02L70CK	Open occlusion of left atrial appendage, using extraluminal pressure clips.
02L73ZK	Percutaneous suture exclusion of left atrial appendage, via femoral artery access.
02NG0ZZ	Mitral valvulotomy for release of fused leaflets, open approach.
02PYX2Z	Non-incisional removal of Swan-Ganz catheter from right pulmonary artery.
02RG08Z	Mitral valve replacement using porcine valve, open.
02RH38Z	Transcatheter replacement of pulmonary valve using a bovine jugular vein valve.
02TD0ZZ	Open resection of papillary muscle. (The papillary muscle refers to the heart and is found in the Heart and Great Vessels body system.)
02UA0JZ	Implantation of CorCap cardiac support device, open approach.

Continued on next page

Educational Annotations | 2 – Heart and Great Vessels

Coding Notes of Heart and Great Vessels

Continued from previous page

0 2 U F 0 J Z	Aortic valve annuloplasty using ring, open.
0 2 H V 3 3 Z	Percutaneous placement of venous central line in right internal jugular, with tip in superior vena cava.
0 2 V R 0 C Z	Thoracotomy with banding of left pulmonary artery using extraluminal device.
0 2 V W 3 D J	Catheter-based temporary restriction of blood flow in descending aorta for treatment of cerebral ischemia.
0 2 W A 3 M Z	Adjustment of position, pacemaker lead in left ventricle, percutaneous.
0 2 Y A 0 Z 2	Orthotopic heart transplant using porcine heart. (The donor heart comes from an animal (pig), so the qualifier value is Zooplastic.)

Educational Annotations

2 – Heart and Great Vessels

NOTES

2 – HEART AND GREAT VESSELS

TUBULAR GROUP: Bypass, Dilation, Occlusion, Restriction
Root Operations that alter the diameter/route of a tubular body part.

1ST - **0** Medical and Surgical
2ND - **2** Heart and Great Vessels
3RD - **1** BYPASS

EXAMPLE: Coronary artery bypass   CMS Ex: Coronary artery bypass

BYPASS: Altering the route of passage of the contents of a tubular body part.

EXPLANATION: Rerouting contents to a downstream part ...

Body Part – 4TH	Approach – 5TH	Device – 6TH	Qualifier – 7TH
0 Coronary Artery, One Site 1 Coronary Artery, Two Sites 2 Coronary Artery, Three Sites 3 Coronary Artery, Four or More Sites	0 Open	9 Autologous venous tissue A Autologous arterial tissue J Synthetic substitute K Nonautologous tissue substitute	3 Coronary Artery 8 Internal Mammary, Right 9 Internal Mammary, Left C Thoracic Artery F Abdominal Artery W Aorta
0 Coronary Artery, One Site 1 Coronary Artery, Two Sites 2 Coronary Artery, Three Sites 3 Coronary Artery, Four or More Sites	0 Open	Z No device	3 Coronary Artery 8 Internal Mammary, Right 9 Internal Mammary, Left C Thoracic Artery F Abdominal Artery
0 Coronary Artery, One Site 1 Coronary Artery, Two Sites 2 Coronary Artery, Three Sites 3 Coronary Artery, Four or More Sites	3 Percutaneous	4 Drug-eluting intraluminal device D Intraluminal device	4 Coronary Vein
0 Coronary Artery, One Site 1 Coronary Artery, Two Sites 2 Coronary Artery, Three Sites 3 Coronary Artery, Four or More Sites	4 Percutaneous endoscopic	4 Drug-eluting intraluminal device D Intraluminal device	4 Coronary Vein

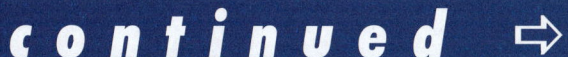

continued ➪

021 BYPASS – continued

0 **2** **1**

Body Part – 4ᵀᴴ	Approach – 5ᵀᴴ	Device – 6ᵀᴴ	Qualifier – 7ᵀᴴ
0 Coronary Artery, One Site 1 Coronary Artery, Two Sites 2 Coronary Artery, Three Sites 3 Coronary Artery, Four or More Sites	4 Percutaneous endoscopic	9 Autologous venous tissue A Autologous arterial tissue J Synthetic substitute K Nonautologous tissue substitute	3 Coronary Artery 8 Internal Mammary, Right 9 Internal Mammary, Left C Thoracic Artery F Abdominal Artery W Aorta
0 Coronary Artery, One Site 1 Coronary Artery, Two Sites 2 Coronary Artery, Three Sites 3 Coronary Artery, Four or More Sites	4 Percutaneous endoscopic	Z No device	3 Coronary Artery 8 Internal Mammary, Right 9 Internal Mammary, Left C Thoracic Artery F Abdominal Artery
6 Atrium, Right	0 Open 4 Percutaneous endoscopic	9 Autologous venous tissue A Autologous arterial tissue J Synthetic substitute K Nonautologous tissue substitute	P Pulmonary Trunk Q Pulmonary Artery, Right R Pulmonary Artery, Left
6 Atrium, Right	0 Open 4 Percutaneous endoscopic	Z No device	7 Atrium, Left P Pulmonary Trunk Q Pulmonary Artery, Right R Pulmonary Artery, Left
7 Atrium, Left V Superior Vena Cava	0 Open 4 Percutaneous endoscopic	9 Autologous venous tissue A Autologous arterial tissue J Synthetic substitute K Nonautologous tissue substitute Z No device	P Pulmonary Trunk Q Pulmonary Artery, Right R Pulmonary Artery, Left
K Ventricle, Right L Ventricle, Left	0 Open 4 Percutaneous endoscopic	9 Autologous venous tissue A Autologous arterial tissue J Synthetic substitute K Nonautologous tissue substitute	P Pulmonary Trunk Q Pulmonary Artery, Right R Pulmonary Artery, Left

continued

021 BYPASS – continued

Body Part – 4TH	Approach – 5TH	Device – 6TH	Qualifier – 7TH
K Ventricle, Right L Ventricle, Left	0 Open 4 Percutaneous endoscopic	Z No device	5 Coronary Circulation 8 Internal Mammary, Right 9 Internal Mammary, Left C Thoracic Artery F Abdominal Artery P Pulmonary Trunk Q Pulmonary Artery, Right R Pulmonary Artery, Left W Aorta
W Thoracic Aorta	0 Open 4 Percutaneous endoscopic	9 Autologous venous tissue A Autologous arterial tissue J Synthetic substitute K Nonautologous tissue substitute Z No device	B Subclavian D Carotid P Pulmonary Trunk Q Pulmonary Artery, Right R Pulmonary Artery, Left

---

EXCISION GROUP: Excision, Resection, Destruction, (Extraction), (Detachment)
Root Operations that take out some or all of a body part.

1ST - 0 Medical and Surgical
2ND - 2 Heart and Great Vessels
3RD - 5 DESTRUCTION

EXAMPLE: Atrioventricular node ablation CMS Ex: Fulguration polyp

DESTRUCTION: Physical eradication of all or a portion of a body part by the direct use of energy, force, or a destructive agent.

EXPLANATION: None of the body part is physically taken out

Body Part – 4TH	Approach – 5TH	Device – 6TH	Qualifier – 7TH
4 Coronary Vein 5 Atrial Septum 6 Atrium, Right 8 Conduction Mechanism 9 Chordae Tendineae D Papillary Muscle F Aortic Valve G Mitral Valve H Pulmonary Valve J Tricuspid Valve K Ventricle, Right L Ventricle, Left M Ventricular Septum N Pericardium P Pulmonary Trunk Q Pulmonary Artery, Right R Pulmonary Artery, Left S Pulmonary Vein, Right T Pulmonary Vein, Left V Superior Vena Cava W Thoracic Aorta	0 Open 3 Percutaneous 4 Percutaneous endoscopic	Z No device	Z No qualifier
7 Atrium, Left	0 Open 3 Percutaneous 4 Percutaneous endoscopic	Z No device	K Left Atrial Appendage Z No qualifier

TUBULAR GROUP: Bypass, Dilation, Occlusion, Restriction
Root Operations that alter the diameter/route of a tubular body part.

1ST - 0 Medical and Surgical
2ND - 2 Heart and Great Vessels
3RD - 7 DILATION

EXAMPLE: PTCA coronary artery   CMS Ex: Transluminal angioplasty

DILATION: Expanding an orifice or the lumen of a tubular body part.

EXPLANATION: By force (stretching) or cutting ...

Body Part – 4TH	Approach – 5TH	Device – 6TH	Qualifier – 7TH
0 Coronary Artery, One Site 1 Coronary Artery, Two Sites 2 Coronary Artery, Three Sites 3 Coronary Artery, Four or More Sites	0 Open 3 Percutaneous 4 Percutaneous endoscopic	4 Drug-eluting intraluminal device D Intraluminal device T Intraluminal device, radioactive Z No device	6 Bifurcation Z No qualifier
F Aortic Valve Q Pulmonary Artery, Right G Mitral Valve S Pulmonary Vein, Right H Pulmonary Valve T Pulmonary Vein, Left J Tricuspid Valve V Superior Vena Cava K Ventricle, Right W Thoracic Aorta P Pulmonary Trunk	0 Open 3 Percutaneous 4 Percutaneous endoscopic	4 Drug-eluting intraluminal device D Intraluminal device Z No device	Z No qualifier
R Pulmonary Artery, Left	0 Open 3 Percutaneous 4 Percutaneous endoscopic	4 Drug-eluting intraluminal device D Intraluminal device Z No device	T Ductus Arteriosus Z No qualifier

DIVISION GROUP: Division, Release
Root Operations involving cutting or separation only.

1ST - 0 Medical and Surgical
2ND - 2 Heart and Great Vessels
3RD - 8 DIVISION

EXAMPLE: Division bundle of HIS   CMS Ex: Osteotomy

DIVISION: Cutting into a body part without draining fluids and/or gases from the body part in order to separate or transect a body part.

EXPLANATION: Separated into two or more portions ...

Body Part – 4TH	Approach – 5TH	Device – 6TH	Qualifier – 7TH
8 Conduction Mechanism 9 Chordae Tendineae D Papillary Muscle	0 Open 3 Percutaneous 4 Percutaneous endoscopic	Z No device	Z No qualifier

2 – HEART AND GREAT VESSELS — 02B

EXCISION GROUP: Excision, Resection, Destruction, (Extraction), (Detachment)
Root Operations that take out some or all of a body part.

- 1ST – **0** Medical and Surgical
- 2ND – **2** Heart and Great Vessels
- 3RD – **B** EXCISION

EXAMPLE: Pericardial biopsy   **CMS Ex:** Liver biopsy

EXCISION: Cutting out or off, without replacement, a portion of a body part.

EXPLANATION: Qualifier "X Diagnostic" indicates biopsy …

Body Part – 4TH		Approach – 5TH	Device – 6TH	Qualifier – 7TH
4 Coronary Vein 5 Atrial Septum 6 Atrium, Right 8 Conduction Mechanism 9 Chordae Tendineae D Papillary Muscle F Aortic Valve G Mitral Valve H Pulmonary Valve J Tricuspid Valve K Ventricle, Right NC*	L Ventricle, Left NC* M Ventricular Septum N Pericardium P Pulmonary Trunk Q Pulmonary Artery, Right R Pulmonary Artery, Left S Pulmonary Vein, Right T Pulmonary Vein, Left V Superior Vena Cava W Thoracic Aorta	0 Open 3 Percutaneous 4 Percutaneous endoscopic	Z No device	X Diagnostic Z No qualifier
7 Atrium, Left		0 Open 3 Percutaneous 4 Percutaneous endoscopic	Z No device	K Left Atrial Appendage X Diagnostic Z No qualifier

NC* – Some procedures are considered non-covered by Medicare. See current Medicare Code Editor for details.

02C — MEDICAL AND SURGICAL SECTION – 2016 ICD-10-PCS

DRAINAGE GROUP: (Drainage), Extirpation, Fragmentation
Root Operations that take out solids/fluids/gases from a body part.

- 1ST – **0** Medical and Surgical
- 2ND – **2** Heart and Great Vessels
- 3RD – **C** EXTIRPATION

EXAMPLE: Pulmonary artery thrombectomy | CMS Ex: Choledocholithotomy

EXTIRPATION: Taking or cutting out solid matter from a body part.

EXPLANATION: Abnormal byproduct or foreign body ...

Body Part – 4TH	Approach – 5TH	Device – 6TH	Qualifier – 7TH
0 Coronary Artery, One Site 1 Coronary Artery, Two Sites 2 Coronary Artery, Three Sites 3 Coronary Artery, Four or More Sites 4 Coronary Vein 5 Atrial Septum 6 Atrium, Right 7 Atrium, Left 8 Conduction Mechanism 9 Chordae Tendineae D Papillary Muscle F Aortic Valve G Mitral Valve H Pulmonary Valve J Tricuspid Valve K Ventricle, Right L Ventricle, Left M Ventricular Septum N Pericardium P Pulmonary Trunk Q Pulmonary Artery, Right R Pulmonary Artery, Left S Pulmonary Vein, Right T Pulmonary Vein, Left V Superior Vena Cava W Thoracic Aorta	0 Open 3 Percutaneous 4 Percutaneous endoscopic	Z No device	Z No qualifier

DRAINAGE GROUP: (Drainage), Extirpation, Fragmentation
Root Operations that take out solids/fluids/gases from a body part.

- 1ST – **0** Medical and Surgical
- 2ND – **2** Heart and Great Vessels
- 3RD – **F** FRAGMENTATION

EXAMPLE: Pulverization pericardial calcifications | CMS Ex: ESWL

FRAGMENTATION: Breaking solid matter in a body part into pieces.

EXPLANATION: Pieces are not taken out during procedure ...

Body Part – 4TH	Approach – 5TH	Device – 6TH	Qualifier – 7TH
N Pericardium	0 Open 3 Percutaneous 4 Percutaneous endoscopic X External NC*	Z No device	Z No qualifier

NC* – Non-covered by Medicare. See current Medicare Code Editor for details.

2 – HEART AND GREAT VESSELS — 02H

DEVICE GROUP: (Change), Insertion, Removal, Replacement, Revision, Supplement
Root Operations that always involve a device.

1ST - 0 Medical and Surgical
2ND - 2 Heart and Great Vessels
3RD - H INSERTION

EXAMPLE: Insertion pacemaker lead
CMS Ex: Central venous catheter

INSERTION: Putting in a nonbiological appliance that monitors, assists, performs, or prevents a physiological function but does not physically take the place of a body part.

EXPLANATION: None

Body Part – 4TH	Approach – 5TH	Device – 6TH	Qualifier – 7TH
4 Coronary Vein 6 Atrium, Right 7 Atrium, Left K Ventricle, Right L Ventricle, Left	0 Open 3 Percutaneous 4 Percutaneous endoscopic	0 Monitoring device, pressure sensor 2 Monitoring device 3 Infusion device D Intraluminal device J Cardiac lead, pacemaker K Cardiac lead, defibrillator M Cardiac lead	Z No qualifier
A Heart NC*	0 Open 3 Percutaneous 4 Percutaneous endoscopic	Q Implantable heart assist system	Z No qualifier
A Heart	0 Open 3 Percutaneous 4 Percutaneous endoscopic	R External heart assist system	S Biventricular Z No qualifier
N Pericardium	0 Open 3 Percutaneous 4 Percutaneous endoscopic	0 Monitoring device, pressure sensor 2 Monitoring device J Cardiac lead, pacemaker K Cardiac lead, defibrillator M Cardiac lead	Z No qualifier
P Pulmonary Trunk Q Pulmonary Artery, Right R Pulmonary Artery, Left S Pulmonary Vein, Right T Pulmonary Vein, Left V Superior Vena Cava W Thoracic Aorta	0 Open 3 Percutaneous 4 Percutaneous endoscopic	0 Monitoring device, pressure sensor 2 Monitoring device 3 Infusion device D Intraluminal device	Z No qualifier

NC* – Some procedures are considered non-covered by Medicare. See current Medicare Code Editor for details.

0 2 J — MEDICAL AND SURGICAL SECTION – 2016 ICD-10-PCS [2016.PCS]

EXAMINATION GROUP: Inspection, Map
Root Operations involving examination only.

1ST – 0 Medical and Surgical
2ND – 2 Heart and Great Vessels
3RD – J INSPECTION

EXAMPLE: Thoracoscopic visualization heart CMS Ex: Colonoscopy

INSPECTION: Visually and/or manually exploring a body part.

EXPLANATION: Direct or instrumental visualization ...

Body Part – 4TH	Approach – 5TH	Device – 6TH	Qualifier – 7TH
A Heart Y Great Vessel	0 Open 3 Percutaneous 4 Percutaneous endoscopic	Z No device	Z No qualifier

EXAMINATION GROUP: Inspection, Map
Root Operations involving examination only.

1ST – 0 Medical and Surgical
2ND – 2 Heart and Great Vessels
3RD – K MAP

EXAMPLE: Cardiac mapping CMS Ex: Cardiac mapping

MAP: Locating the route of passage of electrical impulses and/or locating functional areas in a body part.

EXPLANATION: Limited to cardiac and nervous systems...

Body Part – 4TH	Approach – 5TH	Device – 6TH	Qualifier – 7TH
8 Conduction Mechanism	0 Open 3 Percutaneous 4 Percutaneous endoscopic	Z No device	Z No qualifier

2 – HEART AND GREAT VESSELS — 02N

TUBULAR GROUP: Bypass, Dilation, Occlusion, Restriction
Root Operations that alter the diameter/route of a tubular body part.

- 1ST – **0** Medical and Surgical
- 2ND – **2** Heart and Great Vessels
- 3RD – **L** OCCLUSION

EXAMPLE: Suture closure of LAA   CMS Ex: Fallopian tube ligation

OCCLUSION: Completely closing an orifice or lumen of a tubular body part.

EXPLANATION: Natural or artificially created orifice ...

Body Part – 4TH	Approach – 5TH	Device – 6TH	Qualifier – 7TH
7 Atrium, Left	0 Open 3 Percutaneous 4 Percutaneous endoscopic	C Extraluminal device D Intraluminal device Z No device	K Left Atrial Appendage
R Pulmonary Artery, Left	0 Open 3 Percutaneous 4 Percutaneous endoscopic	C Extraluminal device D Intraluminal device Z No device	T Ductus Arteriosus
S Pulmonary Vein, Right T Pulmonary Vein, Left V Superior Vena Cava	0 Open 3 Percutaneous 4 Percutaneous endoscopic	C Extraluminal device D Intraluminal device Z No device	Z No qualifier

DIVISION GROUP: Division, Release
Root Operations involving cutting or separation only.

- 1ST – **0** Medical and Surgical
- 2ND – **2** Heart and Great Vessels
- 3RD – **N** RELEASE

EXAMPLE: Mitral valvulotomy of fused leaflets   CMS Ex: Carpal tunnel

RELEASE: Freeing a body part from an abnormal physical constraint by cutting or by the use of force.

EXPLANATION: None of the body part is taken out ...

Body Part – 4TH	Approach – 5TH	Device – 6TH	Qualifier – 7TH
4 Coronary Vein 5 Atrial Septum 6 Atrium, Right 7 Atrium, Left 8 Conduction Mechanism 9 Chordae Tendineae D Papillary Muscle F Aortic Valve G Mitral Valve H Pulmonary Valve J Tricuspid Valve K Ventricle, Right L Ventricle, Left M Ventricular Septum N Pericardium P Pulmonary Trunk Q Pulmonary Artery, Right R Pulmonary Artery, Left S Pulmonary Vein, Right T Pulmonary Vein, Left V Superior Vena Cava W Thoracic Aorta	0 Open 3 Percutaneous 4 Percutaneous endoscopic	Z No device	Z No qualifier

0 2 P

MEDICAL AND SURGICAL SECTION – 2016 ICD-10-PCS

DEVICE GROUP: (Change), Insertion, Removal, Replacement, Revision, Supplement
Root Operations that always involve a device.

1ST - 0 Medical and Surgical
2ND - 2 Heart and Great Vessels
3RD - P REMOVAL

EXAMPLE: Removal of Swan Ganz catheter | **CMS Ex:** Chest tube removal

REMOVAL: Taking out or off a device from a body part.

EXPLANATION: Removal device without reinsertion ...

Body Part – 4TH	Approach – 5TH	Device – 6TH	Qualifier – 7TH
A Heart	0 Open 3 Percutaneous 4 Percutaneous endoscopic	2 Monitoring device 3 Infusion device 7 Autologous tissue substitute 8 Zooplastic tissue C Extraluminal device D Intraluminal device J Synthetic substitute K Nonautologous tissue substitute M Cardiac lead Q Implantable heart assist system R External heart assist system	Z No qualifier
A Heart	X External	2 Monitoring device 3 Infusion device D Intraluminal device M Cardiac lead	Z No qualifier
Y Great Vessel	0 Open 3 Percutaneous 4 Percutaneous endoscopic	2 Monitoring device 3 Infusion device 7 Autologous tissue substitute 8 Zooplastic tissue C Extraluminal device D Intraluminal device J Synthetic substitute K Nonautologous tissue substitute	Z No qualifier
Y Great Vessel	X External	2 Monitoring device 3 Infusion device D Intraluminal device	Z No qualifier

HEART & GREAT V. 02P

2 – HEART AND GREAT VESSELS 02Q

OTHER REPAIRS GROUP: (Control), **Repair**
Root Operations that define other repairs.

1ST - **0** Medical and Surgical
2ND - **2** Heart and Great Vessels
3RD - **Q REPAIR**

EXAMPLE: Suture pericardial injury **CMS Ex:** Suture laceration

REPAIR: Restoring, to the extent possible, a body part to its normal anatomic structure and function.

EXPLANATION: Only when no other root operation applies ...

Body Part – 4TH		Approach – 5TH	Device – 6TH	Qualifier – 7TH
0 Coronary Artery, One Site	D Papillary Muscle	0 Open	Z No device	Z No qualifier
1 Coronary Artery, Two Sites	F Aortic Valve	3 Percutaneous		
2 Coronary Artery, Three Sites	G Mitral Valve	4 Percutaneous endoscopic		
3 Coronary Artery, Four or More Sites	H Pulmonary Valve			
4 Coronary Vein	J Tricuspid Valve			
5 Atrial Septum	K Ventricle, Right			
6 Atrium, Right	L Ventricle, Left			
7 Atrium, Left	M Ventricular Septum			
8 Conduction Mechanism	N Pericardium			
9 Chordae Tendineae	P Pulmonary Trunk			
A Heart	Q Pulmonary Artery, Right			
B Heart, Right	R Pulmonary Artery, Left			
C Heart, Left	S Pulmonary Vein, Right			
	T Pulmonary Vein, Left			
	V Superior Vena Cava			
	W Thoracic Aorta			

141

0 2 R

MEDICAL AND SURGICAL SECTION – 2016 ICD-10-PCS

[2016.PCS]

DEVICE GROUP: (Change), Insertion, Removal, Replacement, Revision, Supplement
Root Operations that always involve a device.

- 1ST – **0** Medical and Surgical
- 2ND – **2** Heart and Great Vessels
- 3RD – **R REPLACEMENT**

EXAMPLE: Mitral valve replacement   CMS Ex: Total hip

REPLACEMENT: Putting in or on a biological or synthetic material that physically takes the place and/or function of all or a portion of a body part.

EXPLANATION: Includes taking out body part, or eradication...

Body Part – 4TH		Approach – 5TH	Device – 6TH	Qualifier – 7TH
5 Atrial Septum 6 Atrium, Right 7 Atrium, Left 9 Chordae Tendineae D Papillary Muscle J Tricuspid Valve K Ventricle, Right NC*LC* L Ventricle, Left NC*LC* M Ventricular Septum	N Pericardium P Pulmonary Trunk Q Pulmonary Artery, Right R Pulmonary Artery, Left S Pulmonary Vein, Right T Pulmonary Vein, Left V Superior Vena Cava W Thoracic Aorta	0 Open 4 Percutaneous endoscopic	7 Autologous tissue substitute 8 Zooplastic tissue J Synthetic substitute K Nonautologous tissue substitute	Z No qualifier
F Aortic Valve G Mitral Valve H Pulmonary Valve		0 Open 4 Percutaneous endoscopic	7 Autologous tissue substitute 8 Zooplastic tissue J Synthetic substitute K Nonautologous tissue substitute	Z No qualifier
F Aortic Valve G Mitral Valve H Pulmonary Valve		3 Percutaneous	7 Autologous tissue substitute 8 Zooplastic tissue J Synthetic substitute K Nonautologous tissue substitute	H Transapical Z No qualifier

NC*LC* – Some procedures are considered non-covered or limited coverage by Medicare. See current Medicare Code Editor for details.

MOVE GROUP: (Reattachment), Reposition, (Transfer), Transplantation
Root Operations that put in/put back or move some/all of a body part.

- 1ST – **0** Medical and Surgical
- 2ND – **2** Heart and Great Vessels
- 3RD – **S REPOSITION**

EXAMPLE: Relocation pulmonary vein   CMS Ex: Fracture reduction

REPOSITION: Moving to its normal location, or other suitable location, all or a portion of a body part.

EXPLANATION: May or may not be cut to be moved ...

Body Part – 4TH	Approach – 5TH	Device – 6TH	Qualifier – 7TH
P Pulmonary Trunk Q Pulmonary Artery, Right R Pulmonary Artery, Left S Pulmonary Vein, Right T Pulmonary Vein, Left V Superior Vena Cava W Thoracic Aorta	0 Open	Z No device	Z No qualifier

2 – HEART AND GREAT VESSELS 02U

EXCISION GROUP: Excision, Resection, Destruction, (Extraction), (Detachment)
Root Operations that take out some or all of a body part.

- 1ST – **0** Medical and Surgical
- 2ND – **2** Heart and Great Vessels
- 3RD – **T** RESECTION

EXAMPLE: Atrial septectomy **CMS Ex:** Cholecystectomy

RESECTION: Cutting out or off, without replacement, all of a body part.

EXPLANATION: None

Body Part – 4TH	Approach – 5TH	Device – 6TH	Qualifier – 7TH
5 Atrial Septum 8 Conduction Mechanism 9 Chordae Tendineae D Papillary Muscle H Pulmonary Valve M Ventricular Septum N Pericardium	0 Open 3 Percutaneous 4 Percutaneous endoscopic	Z No device	Z No qualifier

DEVICE GROUP: (Change), Insertion, Removal, Replacement, Revision, Supplement
Root Operations that always involve a device.

- 1ST – **0** Medical and Surgical
- 2ND – **2** Heart and Great Vessels
- 3RD – **U** SUPPLEMENT

EXAMPLE: Valve graft annuloplasty **CMS Ex:** Hernia repair with mesh

SUPPLEMENT: Putting in or on biological or synthetic material that physically reinforces and/or augments the function of a portion of a body part.

EXPLANATION: Biological material from same individual ...

Body Part – 4TH	Approach – 5TH	Device – 6TH	Qualifier – 7TH
5 Atrial Septum 6 Atrium, Right 7 Atrium, Left 9 Chordae Tendineae A Heart D Papillary Muscle F Aortic Valve G Mitral Valve H Pulmonary Valve J Tricuspid Valve K Ventricle, Right L Ventricle, Left M Ventricular Septum N Pericardium P Pulmonary Trunk Q Pulmonary Artery, Right R Pulmonary Artery, Left S Pulmonary Vein, Right T Pulmonary Vein, Left V Superior Vena Cava W Thoracic Aorta	0 Open 3 Percutaneous 4 Percutaneous endoscopic	7 Autologous tissue substitute 8 Zooplastic tissue J Synthetic substitute K Nonautologous tissue substitute	Z No qualifier

0 2 V — MEDICAL AND SURGICAL SECTION – 2016 ICD-10-PCS

TUBULAR GROUP: Bypass, Dilation, Occlusion, Restriction
Root Operations that alter the diameter/route of a tubular body part.

- 1ST – **0** Medical and Surgical
- 2ND – **2** Heart and Great Vessels
- 3RD – **V** RESTRICTION

EXAMPLE: Banding left pulmonary artery
CMS Ex: Cervical cerclage

RESTRICTION: Partially closing an orifice or the lumen of a tubular body part.

EXPLANATION: Natural or artificially created orifice ...

Body Part – 4TH	Approach – 5TH	Device – 6TH	Qualifier – 7TH
A Heart	0 Open 3 Percutaneous 4 Percutaneous endoscopic	C Extraluminal device Z No device	Z No qualifier
P Pulmonary Trunk Q Pulmonary Artery, Right S Pulmonary Vein, Right T Pulmonary Vein, Left V Superior Vena Cava W Thoracic aorta	0 Open 3 Percutaneous 4 Percutaneous endoscopic	C Extraluminal device D Intraluminal device Z No device	Z No qualifier
R Pulmonary Artery, Left	0 Open 3 Percutaneous 4 Percutaneous endoscopic	C Extraluminal device D Intraluminal device Z No device	T Ductus Arteriosus Z No qualifier

02W

2 – HEART AND GREAT VESSELS

DEVICE GROUP: (Change), Insertion, Removal, Replacement, **Revision**, Supplement
Root Operations that always involve a device.

1ST – 0	Medical and Surgical
2ND – 2	Heart and Great Vessels
3RD – W	**REVISION**

EXAMPLE: Reposition cardiac lead **CMS Ex:** Adjustment pacemaker lead

REVISION: Correcting, to the extent possible, a portion of a malfunctioning device or the position of a displaced device.

EXPLANATION: May replace components of a device ...

Body Part – 4TH	Approach – 5TH	Device – 6TH	Qualifier – 7TH
5 Atrial Septum M Ventricular Septum	0 Open 4 Percutaneous endoscopic	J Synthetic substitute	Z No qualifier
A Heart	0 Open 3 Percutaneous 4 Percutaneous endoscopic X External	2 Monitoring device 3 Infusion device 7 Autologous tissue substitute 8 Zooplastic tissue C Extraluminal device D Intraluminal device J Synthetic substitute LC* K Nonautologous tissue substitute M Cardiac lead Q Implantable heart assist system LC* R External heart assist system	Z No qualifier
F Aortic Valve G Mitral Valve H Pulmonary Valve J Tricuspid Valve	0 Open 4 Percutaneous endoscopic	7 Autologous tissue substitute 8 Zooplastic tissue J Synthetic substitute K Nonautologous tissue substitute	Z No qualifier
Y Great Vessel	0 Open 3 Percutaneous 4 Percutaneous endoscopic X External	2 Monitoring device 3 Infusion device 7 Autologous tissue substitute 8 Zooplastic tissue C Extraluminal device D Intraluminal device J Synthetic substitute K Nonautologous tissue substitute	Z No qualifier

LC* – Some procedures are considered limited coverage by Medicare. See current Medicare Code Editor for details.

0 2 Y — MEDICAL AND SURGICAL SECTION – 2016 ICD-10-PCS

MOVE GROUP: (Reattachment), Reposition, (Transfer), **Transplantation**
Root Operations that put in/put back or move some/all of a body part.

- 1ST – **0** Medical and Surgical
- 2ND – **2** Heart and Great Vessels
- 3RD – **Y** TRANSPLANTATION

EXAMPLE: Heart transplant **CMS Ex:** Kidney transplant

TRANSPLANTATION: Putting in or on all or a portion of a living body part taken from another individual or animal to physically take the place and/or function of all or a portion of a similar body part.

EXPLANATION: May take over all or part of its function …

Body Part – 4TH	Approach – 5TH	Device – 6TH	Qualifier – 7TH
A Heart LC*	0 Open	Z No device	0 Allogenic 1 Syngeneic 2 Zooplastic

LC* – Some procedures are considered limited coverage by Medicare. See current Medicare Code Editor for details.

Educational Annotations | 3 – Upper Arteries

Body System Specific Educational Annotations for the Upper Arteries include:
- Anatomy and Physiology Review
- Anatomical Illustrations
- Definitions of Common Procedures
- AHA Coding Clinic® Reference Notations
- Body Part Key Listings
- Device Key Listings
- Device Aggregation Table Listings
- Coding Notes

Anatomy and Physiology Review of Upper Arteries

BODY PART VALUES – 3 - UPPER ARTERIES

Artery – Blood vessels that carry oxygenated (arterial) blood away from the heart and to the organs and tissues of the body. Arteries have a higher blood pressure than other parts of the circulatory system in order to adequately perfuse all the tissues with oxygenated red blood cells.

Axillary Artery – The axillary artery branches from the subclavian artery and serves the lateral thorax and upper limb.

Brachial Artery – The brachial artery branches from the axillary artery and serves the upper limb.

Common Carotid Artery – The left common carotid artery branches from the aortic arch and serves the head and brain. The right common carotid artery branches from the innominate artery (also known as the brachiocephalic artery) and serves the head and brain.

External Carotid Artery – The external carotid artery branches from the common carotid artery and serves the head.

Face Artery – Any of the smaller arterial branches that serves the face.

Hand Artery – Any of the smaller arterial branches that serves the hand.

Innominate Artery – The innominate artery (also known as the brachiocephalic artery) branches from the aortic arch and branches to the right common carotid artery, the internal mammary artery, and the subclavian artery.

Internal Carotid Artery – The internal carotid artery branches from the common carotid artery and serves primarily the brain.

Internal Mammary Artery – The internal mammary artery branches from the innominate artery and serves the anterior chest wall and breasts.

Intracranial Artery – Any of the smaller arterial branches that lies within the skull.

Radial Artery – The radial artery branches from the brachial artery and serves the forearm, wrist, and hand.

Subclavian Artery – The left subclavian artery branches from the aortic arch and serves the thorax, head, and left upper limb. The right subclavian artery branches from the innominate artery (also known as the brachiocephalic artery) and serves the thorax, head, and right upper limb.

Temporal Artery – The temporal artery branches from the external carotid artery and serves the head.

Thyroid Artery – The thyroid artery branches from the thyrocervical trunk of the subclavian artery and serves the thyroid gland.

Ulnar Artery – The ulnar artery branches from the brachial artery and serves the forearm and wrist.

Upper Artery – The arteries located above the diaphragm (see Coding Guideline B2.1b).

Vertebral Artery – The vertebral artery branches from the subclavian artery and serves the brain.

Educational Annotations | 3 – Upper Arteries

MEDICAL AND SURGICAL SECTION – 2016 ICD-10-PCS

Anatomical Illustrations of Upper Arteries

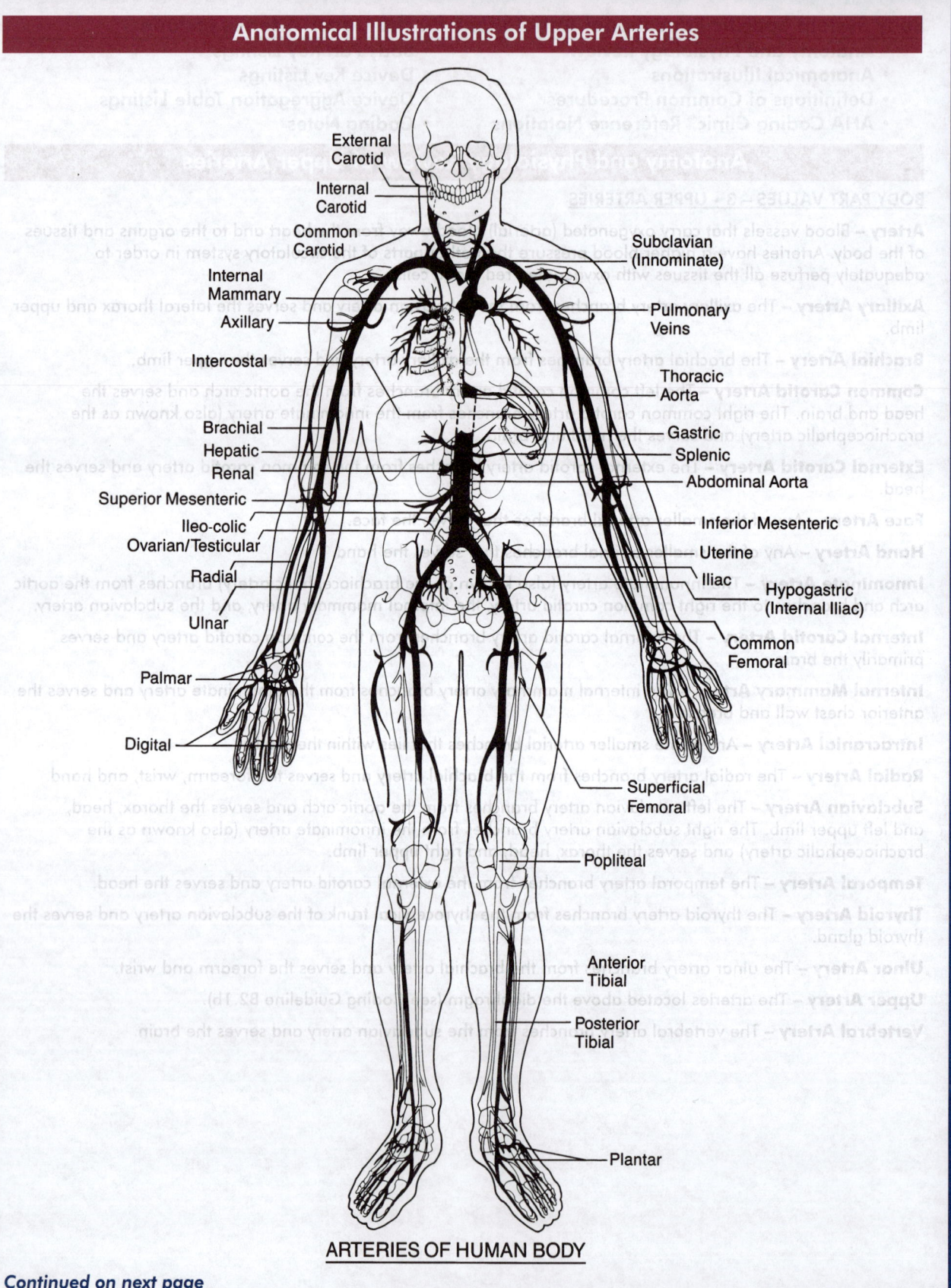

ARTERIES OF HUMAN BODY

Continued on next page

Educational Annotations | 3 – Upper Arteries

Anatomical Illustrations of Upper Arteries

Continued from previous page

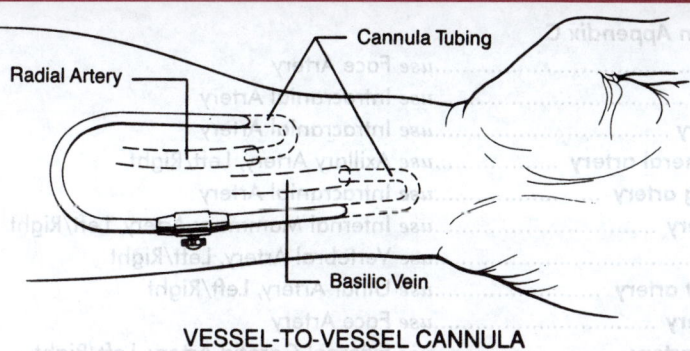

VESSEL-TO-VESSEL CANNULA

Definitions of Common Procedures of Upper Arteries

Balloon angioplasty – The surgical restoration of a narrowed arterial lumen using a balloon-dilating catheter.

Carotid artery to vertebral artery bypass – The restoration of vertebral artery blood flow by using a tubular graft (tissue or synthetic) from a carotid artery to bypass the diseased section of a vertebral artery.

Carotid endarterectomy – The surgical removal of lumen-reducing plaque from a carotid artery to increase the blood flow to the head and reduce the risk of stroke.

Creation of arteriovenous (AV) fistula – The surgical re-routing of an artery in the forearm directly into a vein in the forearm to create an easy and reliable access for repeated hemodialysis.

AHA Coding Clinic® Reference Notations of Upper Arteries

ROOT OPERATION SPECIFIC - 3 - UPPER ARTERIES
BYPASS - 1
    Anastomosis between an artery and a vein for hemodialysis access ....AHA 13:1Q:p27
    Arteriovenous anastomosis of brachial artery ....AHA 13:4Q:p125
DESTRUCTION - 5
DILATION - 7
DRAINAGE - 9
EXCISION - B
EXTIRPATION - C
INSERTION - H
INSPECTION - J
    Discontinued carotid artery procedure ....AHA 15:1Q:p29
OCCLUSION - L
    Endovascular Onyx-18 liquid embolization ....AHA 14:4Q:p37
RELEASE - N
REMOVAL - P
REPAIR - Q
    Epistaxis control using sutures ....AHA 14:4Q:p20
REPLACEMENT - R
REPOSITION - S
SUPPLEMENT - U
RESTRICTION - V
REVISION - W
    Stent to trap herniated/migrated coil in basilar artery ....AHA 15:1Q:p32

Educational Annotations

3 – Upper Arteries

Body Part Key Listings of Upper Arteries

See also Body Part Key in Appendix C

Angular artery	*use* Face Artery
Anterior cerebral artery	*use* Intracranial Artery
Anterior choroidal artery	*use* Intracranial Artery
Anterior circumflex humeral artery	*use* Axillary Artery, Left/Right
Anterior communicating artery	*use* Intracranial Artery
Anterior intercostal artery	*use* Internal Mammary Artery, Left/Right
Anterior spinal artery	*use* Vertebral Artery, Left/Right
Anterior ulnar recurrent artery	*use* Ulnar Artery, Left/Right
Ascending palatine artery	*use* Face Artery
Ascending pharyngeal artery	*use* External Carotid Artery, Left/Right
Basilar artery	*use* Intracranial Artery
Brachiocephalic artery	*use* Innominate Artery
Brachiocephalic trunk	*use* Innominate Artery
Caroticotympanic artery	*use* Internal Carotid Artery, Left/Right
Carotid sinus	*use* Internal Carotid Artery, Left/Right
Circle of Willis	*use* Intracranial Artery
Common interosseous artery	*use* Ulnar Artery, Left/Right
Costocervical trunk	*use* Subclavian Artery, Left/Right
Cricothyroid artery	*use* Thyroid Artery, Left/Right
Deep palmar arch	*use* Hand Artery, Left/Right
Dorsal scapular artery	*use* Subclavian Artery, Left/Right
External maxillary artery	*use* Face Artery
Facial artery	*use* Face Artery
Hyoid artery	*use* Thyroid Artery, Left/Right
Inferior labial artery	*use* Face Artery
Inferior ulnar collateral artery	*use* Brachial Artery, Left/Right
Internal maxillary artery	*use* External Carotid Artery, Left/Right
Internal thoracic artery	*use* Internal Mammary Artery, Left/Right
	use Subclavian Artery, Left/Right
Lateral thoracic artery	*use* Axillary Artery, Left/Right
Lingual artery	*use* External Carotid Artery, Left/Right
Maxillary artery	*use* External Carotid Artery, Left/Right
Middle cerebral artery	*use* Intracranial Artery
Middle temporal artery	*use* Temporal Artery, Left/Right
Musculophrenic artery	*use* Internal Mammary Artery, Left/Right
Occipital artery	*use* External Carotid Artery, Left/Right
Ophthalmic artery	*use* Internal Carotid Artery, Left/Right
Pericardiophrenic artery	*use* Internal Mammary Artery, Left/Right
Posterior auricular artery	*use* External Carotid Artery, Left/Right
Posterior cerebral artery	*use* Intracranial Artery
Posterior circumflex humeral artery	*use* Axillary Artery, Left/Right
Posterior communicating artery	*use* Intracranial Artery
Posterior inferior cerebellar artery (PICA)	*use* Intracranial Artery
Posterior spinal artery	*use* Vertebral Artery, Left/Right
Posterior ulnar recurrent artery	*use* Ulnar Artery, Left/Right
Princeps pollicis artery	*use* Hand Artery, Left/Right
Profunda brachii	*use* Brachial Artery, Left/Right
Radial recurrent artery	*use* Radial Artery, Left/Right

Continued on next page

3 – Upper Arteries

Body Part Key Listings of Upper Arteries

Continued from previous page

Radialis indicis	*use* Hand Artery, Left/Right
Sternocleidomastoid artery	*use* Thyroid Artery, Left/Right
Submental artery	*use* Face Artery
Subscapular artery	*use* Axillary Artery, Left/Right
Superficial palmar arch	*use* Hand Artery, Left/Right
Superficial temporal artery	*use* Temporal Artery, Left/Right
Superior epigastric artery	*use* Internal Mammary Artery, Left/Right
Superior labial artery	*use* Face Artery
Superior laryngeal artery	*use* Thyroid Artery, Left/Right
Superior thoracic artery	*use* Axillary Artery, Left/Right
Superior thyroid artery	*use* External Carotid Artery, Left/Right
	use Thyroid Artery, Left/Right
Superior ulnar collateral artery	*use* Brachial Artery, Left/Right
Thoracoacromial artery	*use* Axillary Artery, Left/Right
Thyrocervical trunk	*use* Thyroid Artery, Left/Right
Transverse facial artery	*use* Temporal Artery, Left/Right

Device Key Listings of Upper Arteries

See also Device Key in Appendix D

Absolute Pro Vascular (OTW) Self-Expanding Stent System	*use* Intraluminal Device
Acculink (RX) Carotid Stent System	*use* Intraluminal Device
AneuRx® AAA Advantage®	*use* Intraluminal Device
Autograft	*use* Autologous Tissue Substitute
Autologous artery graft	*use* Autologous Arterial Tissue in Upper Arteries
Autologous vein graft	*use* Autologous Venous Tissue in Upper Arteries
Baroreflex Activation Therapy® (BAT®)	*use* Stimulator Lead in Upper Arteries
Bioactive embolization coil(s)	*use* Intraluminal Device, Bioactive in Upper Arteries
Carotid (artery) sinus (baroreceptor) lead	*use* Stimulator Lead in Upper Arteries
Carotid WALLSTENT® Monorail® Endoprosthesis	*use* Intraluminal Device
Embolization coil(s)	*use* Intraluminal Device
FLAIR® Endovascular Stent Graft	*use* Intraluminal Device
Micrus CERECYTE microcoil	*use* Intraluminal Device, Bioactive in Upper Arteries
Paclitaxel-eluting peripheral stent	*use* Intraluminal Device, Drug-eluting in Upper Arteries, Lower Arteries
Pipeline™ Embolization device (PED)	*use* Intraluminal Device
Protégé® RX Carotid Stent System	*use* Intraluminal Device
Rheos® System lead	*use* Stimulator Lead in Upper Arteries
Stent, intraluminal (cardiovascular) (gastrointestinal) (hepatobiliary) (urinary)	*use* Intraluminal Device
Talent® Converter	*use* Intraluminal Device
Talent® Occluder	*use* Intraluminal Device
Talent® Stent Graft (abdominal) (thoracic)	*use* Intraluminal Device
Therapeutic occlusion coil(s)	*use* Intraluminal Device
Tissue bank graft	*use* Nonautologous Tissue Substitute
WALLSTENT® Endoprosthesis	*use* Intraluminal Device
Xact Carotid Stent System	*use* Intraluminal Device
Zilver® PTX® (paclitaxel) Drug-Eluting Peripheral Stent	*use* Intraluminal Device, Drug-eluting in Upper Arteries, Lower Arteries

Educational Annotations | 3 – Upper Arteries

Device Aggregation Table Listings of Upper Arteries

See also Device Aggregation Table in Appendix E

Specific Device	For Operation	In Body System		General Device
Autologous Arterial Tissue	All applicable	Upper Arteries	7	Autologous Tissue Substitute
Autologous Venous Tissue	All applicable	Upper Arteries	7	Autologous Tissue Substitute
Intraluminal Device, Bioactive	All applicable	Upper Arteries	D	Intraluminal Device
Intraluminal Device, Drug-eluting	All applicable	Upper Arteries	D	Intraluminal Device

Coding Notes of Upper Arteries

Body System Relevant Coding Guidelines

General Guidelines

B2.1b

Where the general body part values "upper" and "lower" are provided as an option in the Upper Arteries, Lower Arteries, Upper Veins, Lower Veins, Muscles and Tendons body systems, "upper" and "lower" specifies body parts located above or below the diaphragm respectively.

Example: Vein body parts above the diaphragm are found in the Upper Veins body system; vein body parts below the diaphragm are found in the Lower Veins body system.

Branches of body parts

B4.2

Where a specific branch of a body part does not have its own body part value in PCS, the body part is coded to the closest proximal branch that has a specific body part value.

Example: A procedure performed on the mandibular branch of the trigeminal nerve is coded to the trigeminal nerve body part value.

Body System Specific PCS Reference Manual Exercises

PCS CODE	3 – UPPER ARTERIES EXERCISES
031S0JG	Right temporal artery to intracranial artery bypass using goretex graft, open.
03773ZZ	PTA of right brachial artery stenosis.
03C83ZZ	Percutaneous mechanical thrombectomy, left brachial artery.
03CH0ZZ	Right common carotid endarterectomy, open.
03L80ZZ	Open suture ligation of failed AV graft, left brachial artery.
03LG3DZ	Percutaneous embolization of vascular supply, intracranial meningioma.
03LL3DZ	Percutaneous embolization of left internal carotid-cavernous fistula.
03VG0CZ	Craniotomy with clipping of cerebral aneurysm. (A clip is placed lengthwise on the outside wall of the widened portion of the vessel.)

3 – UPPER ARTERIES 031

TUBULAR GROUP: Bypass, Dilation, Occlusion, Restriction
Root Operations that alter the diameter/route of a tubular body part.

1ST - **0** Medical and Surgical
2ND - **3** Upper Arteries
3RD - **1 BYPASS**

EXAMPLE: Arteriovenous hemodialysis fistula | CMS Ex: Coronary bypass

BYPASS: Altering the route of passage of the contents of a tubular body part.

EXPLANATION: Rerouting contents to a downstream part …

Body Part – 4TH	Approach – 5TH	Device – 6TH	Qualifier – 7TH
2 Innominate Artery 5 Axillary Artery, Right 6 Axillary Artery, Left	0 Open	9 Autologous venous tissue A Autologous arterial tissue J Synthetic substitute K Nonautologous tissue substitute Z No device	0 Upper Arm Artery, Right 1 Upper Arm Artery, Left 2 Upper Arm Artery, Bilateral 3 Lower Arm Artery, Right 4 Lower Arm Artery, Left 5 Lower Arm Artery, Bilateral 6 Upper Leg Artery, Right 7 Upper Leg Artery, Left 8 Upper Leg Artery, Bilateral 9 Lower Leg Artery, Right B Lower Leg Artery, Left C Lower Leg Artery, Bilateral D Upper Arm Vein F Lower Arm Vein J Extracranial Artery, Right K Extracranial Artery, Left
3 Subclavian Artery, Right 4 Subclavian Artery, Left	0 Open	9 Autologous venous tissue A Autologous arterial tissue J Synthetic substitute K Nonautologous tissue substitute Z No device	0 Upper Arm Artery, Right 1 Upper Arm Artery, Left 2 Upper Arm Artery, Bilateral 3 Lower Arm Artery, Right 4 Lower Arm Artery, Left 5 Lower Arm Artery, Bilateral 6 Upper Leg Artery, Right 7 Upper Leg Artery, Left 8 Upper Leg Artery, Bilateral 9 Lower Leg Artery, Right B Lower Leg Artery, Left C Lower Leg Artery, Bilateral D Upper Arm Vein F Lower Arm Vein J Extracranial Artery, Right K Extracranial Artery, Left M Pulmonary Artery, Right N Pulmonary Artery, Left

continued ➡

031 BYPASS – continued

Body Part – 4ᵀᴴ	Approach – 5ᵀᴴ	Device – 6ᵀᴴ	Qualifier – 7ᵀᴴ
7 Brachial Artery, Right	0 Open	9 Autologous venous tissue A Autologous arterial tissue J Synthetic substitute K Nonautologous tissue substitute Z No device	0 Upper Arm Artery, Right 3 Lower Arm Artery, Right D Upper Arm Vein F Lower Arm Vein
8 Brachial Artery, Left	0 Open	9 Autologous venous tissue A Autologous arterial tissue J Synthetic substitute K Nonautologous tissue substitute Z No device	1 Upper Arm Artery, Left 4 Lower Arm Artery, Left D Upper Arm Vein F Lower Arm Vein
9 Ulnar Artery, Right B Radial Artery, Right	0 Open	9 Autologous venous tissue A Autologous arterial tissue J Synthetic substitute K Nonautologous tissue substitute Z No device	3 Lower Arm Artery, Right F Lower Arm Vein
A Ulnar Artery, Left C Radial Artery, Left	0 Open	9 Autologous venous tissue A Autologous arterial tissue J Synthetic substitute K Nonautologous tissue substitute Z No device	4 Lower Arm Artery, Left F Lower Arm Vein
G Intracranial Artery S Temporal Artery, Right NC* T Temporal Artery, Left NC*	0 Open	9 Autologous venous tissue A Autologous arterial tissue J Synthetic substitute K Nonautologous tissue substitute Z No device	G Intracranial Artery

continued ⇨

0 3 1 BYPASS – continued

Body Part – 4TH	Approach – 5TH	Device – 6TH	Qualifier – 7TH
H Common Carotid Artery, Right	0 Open	9 Autologous venous tissue A Autologous arterial tissue J Synthetic substitute K Nonautologous tissue substitute Z No device	G Intracranial Artery NC* J Extracranial Artery, Right
J Common Carotid Artery, Left	0 Open	9 Autologous venous tissue A Autologous arterial tissue J Synthetic substitute K Nonautologous tissue substitute Z No device	G Intracranial Artery NC* K Extracranial Artery, Left
K Internal Carotid Artery, Right M External Carotid Artery, Right	0 Open	9 Autologous venous tissue A Autologous arterial tissue J Synthetic substitute K Nonautologous tissue substitute Z No device	J Extracranial Artery, Right
L Internal Carotid Artery, Left N External Carotid Artery, Left	0 Open	9 Autologous venous tissue A Autologous arterial tissue J Synthetic substitute K Nonautologous tissue substitute Z No device	K Extracranial Artery, Left

NC* – Non-covered by Medicare. See current Medicare Code Editor for details.

0 3 5 — MEDICAL AND SURGICAL SECTION – 2016 ICD-10-PCS

EXCISION GROUP: Excision, (Resection), **Destruction**, (Extraction), (Detachment)
Root Operations that take out some or all of a body part.

- 1ST – **0** Medical and Surgical
- 2ND – **3** Upper Arteries
- 3RD – **5 DESTRUCTION**

EXAMPLE: Fulguration arterial lesion **CMS Ex:** Fulguration polyp

DESTRUCTION: Physical eradication of all or a portion of a body part by the direct use of energy, force, or a destructive agent.

EXPLANATION: None of the body part is physically taken out

Body Part – 4TH		Approach – 5TH	Device – 6TH	Qualifier – 7TH
0 Internal Mammary Artery, Right	J Common Carotid Artery, Left	0 Open	Z No device	Z No qualifier
1 Internal Mammary Artery, Left	K Internal Carotid Artery, Right	3 Percutaneous		
2 Innominate Artery	L Internal Carotid Artery, Left	4 Percutaneous endoscopic		
3 Subclavian Artery, Right	M External Carotid Artery, Right			
4 Subclavian Artery, Left	N External Carotid Artery, Left			
5 Axillary Artery, Right	P Vertebral Artery, Right			
6 Axillary Artery, Left	Q Vertebral Artery, Left			
7 Brachial Artery, Right	R Face Artery			
8 Brachial Artery, Left	S Temporal Artery, Right			
9 Ulnar Artery, Right	T Temporal Artery, Left			
A Ulnar Artery, Left	U Thyroid Artery, Right			
B Radial Artery, Right	V Thyroid Artery, Left			
C Radial Artery, Left	Y Upper Artery			
D Hand Artery, Right				
F Hand Artery, Left				
G Intracranial Artery				
H Common Carotid Artery, Right				

3 – UPPER ARTERIES

037

TUBULAR GROUP: Bypass, Dilation, Occlusion, Restriction
Root Operations that alter the diameter/route of a tubular body part.

1ST - **0** Medical and Surgical
2ND - **3** Upper Arteries
3RD - **7 DILATION**

EXAMPLE: PTA common carotid   CMS Ex: Transluminal angioplasty

DILATION: Expanding an orifice or the lumen of a tubular body part.

EXPLANATION: By force (stretching) or cutting ...

Body Part – 4TH		Approach – 5TH	Device – 6TH	Qualifier – 7TH
0 Internal Mammary Artery, Right	J Common Carotid Artery, Left	0 Open	4 Drug-eluting intraluminal device	Z No qualifier
1 Internal Mammary Artery, Left	K Internal Carotid Artery, Right	3 Percutaneous	D Intraluminal device	
2 Innominate Artery	L Internal Carotid Artery, Left	4 Percutaneous endoscopic	Z No device	
3 Subclavian Artery, Right	M External Carotid Artery, Right			
4 Subclavian Artery, Left	N External Carotid Artery, Left			
5 Axillary Artery, Right	P Vertebral Artery, Right			
6 Axillary Artery, Left	Q Vertebral Artery, Left			
7 Brachial Artery, Right	R Face Artery			
8 Brachial Artery, Left	S Temporal Artery, Right			
9 Ulnar Artery, Right	T Temporal Artery, Left			
A Ulnar Artery, Left	U Thyroid Artery, Right			
B Radial Artery, Right	V Thyroid Artery, Left			
C Radial Artery, Left	Y Upper Artery			
D Hand Artery, Right				
F Hand Artery, Left				
G Intracranial Artery NC*				
H Common Carotid Artery, Right				

NC* – Some procedures are considered non-covered by Medicare. See current Medicare Code Editor for details.

039

MEDICAL AND SURGICAL SECTION – 2016 ICD-10-PCS

DRAINAGE GROUP: Drainage, Extirpation, (Fragmentation)
Root Operations that take out solids/fluids/gases from a body part.

- 1ST - **0** Medical and Surgical
- 2ND - **3** Upper Arteries
- 3RD - **9 DRAINAGE**

EXAMPLE: Aspiration arterial abscess CMS Ex: Thoracentesis

DRAINAGE: Taking or letting out fluids and/or gases from a body part.

EXPLANATION: Qualifier "X Diagnostic" indicates biopsy ...

UPPER ARTERIES 039

Body Part – 4TH	Approach – 5TH	Device – 6TH	Qualifier – 7TH
0 Internal Mammary Artery, Right 1 Internal Mammary Artery, Left 2 Innominate Artery 3 Subclavian Artery, Right 4 Subclavian Artery, Left 5 Axillary Artery, Right 6 Axillary Artery, Left 7 Brachial Artery, Right 8 Brachial Artery, Left 9 Ulnar Artery, Right A Ulnar Artery, Left B Radial Artery, Right C Radial Artery, Left D Hand Artery, Right F Hand Artery, Left G Intracranial Artery H Common Carotid Artery, Right J Common Carotid Artery, Left K Internal Carotid Artery, Right L Internal Carotid Artery, Left M External Carotid Artery, Right N External Carotid Artery, Left P Vertebral Artery, Right Q Vertebral Artery, Left R Face Artery S Temporal Artery, Right T Temporal Artery, Left U Thyroid Artery, Right V Thyroid Artery, Left Y Upper Artery	0 Open 3 Percutaneous 4 Percutaneous endoscopic	0 Drainage device	Z No qualifier
0 Internal Mammary Artery, Right 1 Internal Mammary Artery, Left 2 Innominate Artery 3 Subclavian Artery, Right 4 Subclavian Artery, Left 5 Axillary Artery, Right 6 Axillary Artery, Left 7 Brachial Artery, Right 8 Brachial Artery, Left 9 Ulnar Artery, Right A Ulnar Artery, Left B Radial Artery, Right C Radial Artery, Left D Hand Artery, Right F Hand Artery, Left G Intracranial Artery H Common Carotid Artery, Right J Common Carotid Artery, Left K Internal Carotid Artery, Right L Internal Carotid Artery, Left M External Carotid Artery, Right N External Carotid Artery, Left P Vertebral Artery, Right Q Vertebral Artery, Left R Face Artery S Temporal Artery, Right T Temporal Artery, Left U Thyroid Artery, Right V Thyroid Artery, Left Y Upper Artery	0 Open 3 Percutaneous 4 Percutaneous endoscopic	Z No device	X Diagnostic Z No qualifier

3 – UPPER ARTERIES 03B

EXCISION GROUP: Excision, (Resection), **Destruction,** (Extraction), (Detachment)
Root Operations that take out some or all of a body part.

1ST – **0** Medical and Surgical

2ND – **3** Upper Arteries

3RD – **B EXCISION**

EXAMPLE: Temporal artery biopsy   CMS Ex: Liver biopsy

EXCISION: Cutting out or off, without replacement, a portion of a body part.

EXPLANATION: Qualifier "X Diagnostic" indicates biopsy …

Body Part – 4TH		Approach – 5TH	Device – 6TH	Qualifier – 7TH
0 Internal Mammary Artery, Right	J Common Carotid Artery, Left	0 Open	Z No device	X Diagnostic
1 Internal Mammary Artery, Left	K Internal Carotid Artery, Right	3 Percutaneous		Z No qualifier
2 Innominate Artery	L Internal Carotid Artery, Left	4 Percutaneous endoscopic		
3 Subclavian Artery, Right	M External Carotid Artery, Right			
4 Subclavian Artery, Left	N External Carotid Artery, Left			
5 Axillary Artery, Right				
6 Axillary Artery, Left	P Vertebral Artery, Right			
7 Brachial Artery, Right	Q Vertebral Artery, Left			
8 Brachial Artery, Left	R Face Artery			
9 Ulnar Artery, Right	S Temporal Artery, Right			
A Ulnar Artery, Left	T Temporal Artery, Left			
B Radial Artery, Right	U Thyroid Artery, Right			
C Radial Artery, Left	V Thyroid Artery, Left			
D Hand Artery, Right	Y Upper Artery			
F Hand Artery, Left				
G Intracranial Artery				
H Common Carotid Artery, Right				

03C

MEDICAL AND SURGICAL SECTION – 2016 ICD-10-PCS

DRAINAGE GROUP: Drainage, Extirpation, (Fragmentation)
Root Operations that take out solids/fluids/gases from a body part.

1ST - **0** Medical and Surgical
2ND - **3** Upper Arteries
3RD - **C EXTIRPATION**

EXAMPLE: Carotid artery endarterectomy **CMS Ex:** Choledocholithotomy

EXTIRPATION: Taking or cutting out solid matter from a body part.

EXPLANATION: Abnormal byproduct or foreign body ...

Body Part – 4TH		Approach – 5TH	Device – 6TH	Qualifier – 7TH
0 Internal Mammary Artery, Right	J Common Carotid Artery, Left	0 Open	Z No device	Z No qualifier
1 Internal Mammary Artery, Left	K Internal Carotid Artery, Right	3 Percutaneous		
2 Innominate Artery	L Internal Carotid Artery, Left	4 Percutaneous endoscopic		
3 Subclavian Artery, Right	M External Carotid Artery, Right			
4 Subclavian Artery, Left	N External Carotid Artery, Left			
5 Axillary Artery, Right	P Vertebral Artery, Right			
6 Axillary Artery, Left	Q Vertebral Artery, Left			
7 Brachial Artery, Right	R Face Artery			
8 Brachial Artery, Left	S Temporal Artery, Right			
9 Ulnar Artery, Right	T Temporal Artery, Left			
A Ulnar Artery, Left	U Thyroid Artery, Right			
B Radial Artery, Right	V Thyroid Artery, Left			
C Radial Artery, Left	Y Upper Artery			
D Hand Artery, Right				
F Hand Artery, Left				
G Intracranial Artery NC*				
H Common Carotid Artery, Right				

NC* – Some procedures are considered non-covered by Medicare. See current Medicare Code Editor for details.

3 – UPPER ARTERIES
03J

DEVICE GROUP: (Change), Insertion, Removal, Replacement, Revision, Supplement
Root Operations that always involve a device.

1ST - 0	Medical and Surgical
2ND - 3	Upper Arteries
3RD - H	INSERTION

EXAMPLE: Carotid artery stimulator lead | **CMS Ex:** Central venous cath

INSERTION: Putting in a nonbiological appliance that monitors, assists, performs, or prevents a physiological function but does not physically take the place of a body part.

EXPLANATION: None

Body Part – 4TH		Approach – 5TH	Device – 6TH	Qualifier – 7TH
0 Internal Mammary Artery, Right	G Intracranial Artery	0 Open	3 Infusion device	Z No qualifier
1 Internal Mammary Artery, Left	H Common Carotid Artery, Right	3 Percutaneous	D Intraluminal device	
2 Innominate Artery	J Common Carotid Artery, Left	4 Percutaneous endoscopic		
3 Subclavian Artery, Right	M External Carotid Artery, Right			
4 Subclavian Artery, Left	N External Carotid Artery, Left			
5 Axillary Artery, Right	P Vertebral Artery, Right			
6 Axillary Artery, Left	Q Vertebral Artery, Left			
7 Brachial Artery, Right	R Face Artery			
8 Brachial Artery, Left	S Temporal Artery, Right			
9 Ulnar Artery, Right	T Temporal Artery, Left			
A Ulnar Artery, Left	U Thyroid Artery, Right			
B Radial Artery, Right	V Thyroid Artery, Left			
C Radial Artery, Left				
D Hand Artery, Right				
F Hand Artery, Left				
K Internal Carotid Artery, Right		0 Open	3 Infusion device	Z No qualifier
L Internal Carotid Artery, Left		3 Percutaneous	D Intraluminal device	
		4 Percutaneous endoscopic	M Stimulator lead	
Y Upper Artery		0 Open	2 Monitoring device	Z No qualifier
		3 Percutaneous	3 Infusion device	
		4 Percutaneous endoscopic	D Intraluminal device	

EXAMINATION GROUP: Inspection, (Map)
Root Operations involving examination only.

1ST - 0	Medical and Surgical
2ND - 3	Upper Arteries
3RD - J	INSPECTION

EXAMPLE: Exploration arterial cath removal site | **CMS Ex:** Colonoscopy

INSPECTION: Visually and/or manually exploring a body part.

EXPLANATION: Direct or instrumental visualization ...

Body Part – 4TH	Approach – 5TH	Device – 6TH	Qualifier – 7TH
Y Upper Artery	0 Open	Z No device	Z No qualifier
	3 Percutaneous		
	4 Percutaneous endoscopic		
	X External		

03L

MEDICAL AND SURGICAL SECTION – 2016 ICD-10-PCS

TUBULAR GROUP: Bypass, Dilation, Occlusion, Restriction
Root Operations that alter the diameter/route of a tubular body part.

1ST - **0** Medical and Surgical	EXAMPLE: Embolization carotid fistula	CMS Ex: Fallopian tube ligation
2ND - **3** Upper Arteries	**OCCLUSION:** Completely closing an orifice or lumen of a tubular body part.	
3RD - **L** OCCLUSION	EXPLANATION: Natural or artificially created orifice ...	

Body Part – 4TH		Approach – 5TH	Device – 6TH	Qualifier – 7TH
0 Internal Mammary Artery, Right	A Ulnar Artery, Left	0 Open	C Extraluminal device	Z No qualifier
1 Internal Mammary Artery, Left	B Radial Artery, Right	3 Percutaneous	D Intraluminal device	
2 Innominate Artery	C Radial Artery, Left	4 Percutaneous endoscopic	Z No device	
3 Subclavian Artery, Right	D Hand Artery, Right			
4 Subclavian Artery, Left	F Hand Artery, Left			
5 Axillary Artery, Right	R Face Artery			
6 Axillary Artery, Left	S Temporal Artery, Right			
7 Brachial Artery, Right	T Temporal Artery, Left			
8 Brachial Artery, Left	U Thyroid Artery, Right			
9 Ulnar Artery, Right	V Thyroid Artery, Left			
	Y Upper Artery			
G Intracranial Artery		0 Open	B Bioactive intraluminal device	Z No qualifier
H Common Carotid Artery, Right		3 Percutaneous	C Extraluminal device	
J Common Carotid Artery, Left		4 Percutaneous endoscopic	D Intraluminal device	
K Internal Carotid Artery, Right			Z No device	
L Internal Carotid Artery, Left				
M External Carotid Artery, Right				
N External Carotid Artery, Left				
P Vertebral Artery, Right				
Q Vertebral Artery, Left				

3 – UPPER ARTERIES 03N

DIVISION GROUP: (Division), **Release**
Root Operations involving cutting or separation only.

1ST - **0** Medical and Surgical
2ND - **3** Upper Arteries
3RD - **N RELEASE**

EXAMPLE: Arterial adhesiolysis **CMS Ex:** Carpal tunnel release

RELEASE: Freeing a body part from an abnormal physical constraint by cutting or by the use of force.

EXPLANATION: None of the body part is taken out ...

Body Part – 4TH		Approach – 5TH	Device – 6TH	Qualifier – 7TH
0 Internal Mammary Artery, Right	J Common Carotid Artery, Left	0 Open	Z No device	Z No qualifier
1 Internal Mammary Artery, Left	K Internal Carotid Artery, Right	3 Percutaneous		
2 Innominate Artery	L Internal Carotid Artery, Left	4 Percutaneous endoscopic		
3 Subclavian Artery, Right				
4 Subclavian Artery, Left	M External Carotid Artery, Right			
5 Axillary Artery, Right				
6 Axillary Artery, Left	N External Carotid Artery, Left			
7 Brachial Artery, Right				
8 Brachial Artery, Left	P Vertebral Artery, Right			
9 Ulnar Artery, Right	Q Vertebral Artery, Left			
A Ulnar Artery, Left	R Face Artery			
B Radial Artery, Right	S Temporal Artery, Right			
C Radial Artery, Left	T Temporal Artery, Left			
D Hand Artery, Right	U Thyroid Artery, Right			
F Hand Artery, Left	V Thyroid Artery, Left			
G Intracranial Artery	Y Upper Artery			
H Common Carotid Artery, Right				

0 3 P

MEDICAL AND SURGICAL SECTION – 2016 ICD-10-PCS

DEVICE GROUP: (Change), Insertion, Removal, Replacement, Revision, Supplement
Root Operations that always involve a device.

- 1ST – **0** Medical and Surgical
- 2ND – **3** Upper Arteries
- 3RD – **P** REMOVAL

EXAMPLE: Removal vascular clip
CMS Ex: Chest tube removal

REMOVAL: Taking out or off a device from a body part.

EXPLANATION: Removal device without reinsertion ...

Body Part – 4TH	Approach – 5TH	Device – 6TH	Qualifier – 7TH
Y Upper Artery	0 Open 3 Percutaneous 4 Percutaneous endoscopic	0 Drainage device 2 Monitoring device 3 Infusion device 7 Autologous tissue substitute C Extraluminal device D Intraluminal device J Synthetic substitute K Nonautologous tissue substitute M Stimulator lead	Z No qualifier
Y Upper Artery	X External	0 Drainage device 2 Monitoring device 3 Infusion device D Intraluminal device M Stimulator lead	Z No qualifier

OTHER REPAIRS GROUP: (Control), Repair
Root Operations that define other repairs.

1ST - **0** Medical and Surgical

2ND - **3** Upper Arteries

3RD - **Q REPAIR**

EXAMPLE: Suture arterial laceration   CMS Ex: Suture laceration

REPAIR: Restoring, to the extent possible, a body part to its normal anatomic structure and function.

EXPLANATION: Only when no other root operation applies ...

Body Part – 4TH		Approach – 5TH	Device – 6TH	Qualifier – 7TH
0 Internal Mammary Artery, Right	J Common Carotid Artery, Left	0 Open	Z No device	Z No qualifier
1 Internal Mammary Artery, Left	K Internal Carotid Artery, Right	3 Percutaneous		
2 Innominate Artery	L Internal Carotid Artery, Left	4 Percutaneous endoscopic		
3 Subclavian Artery, Right				
4 Subclavian Artery, Left	M External Carotid Artery, Right			
5 Axillary Artery, Right	N External Carotid Artery, Left			
6 Axillary Artery, Left				
7 Brachial Artery, Right	P Vertebral Artery, Right			
8 Brachial Artery, Left	Q Vertebral Artery, Left			
9 Ulnar Artery, Right	R Face Artery			
A Ulnar Artery, Left	S Temporal Artery, Right			
B Radial Artery, Right	T Temporal Artery, Left			
C Radial Artery, Left	U Thyroid Artery, Right			
D Hand Artery, Right	V Thyroid Artery, Left			
F Hand Artery, Left	Y Upper Artery			
G Intracranial Artery				
H Common Carotid Artery, Right				

03R

MEDICAL AND SURGICAL SECTION – 2016 ICD-10-PCS

DEVICE GROUP: (Change), Insertion, Removal, Replacement, Revision, Supplement
Root Operations that always involve a device.

1ST – **0** Medical and Surgical
2ND – **3** Upper Arteries
3RD – **R** REPLACEMENT

EXAMPLE: Reconstruction artery using graft | **CMS Ex:** Total hip

REPLACEMENT: Putting in or on a biological or synthetic material that physically takes the place and/or function of all or a portion of a body part.

EXPLANATION: Includes taking out body part, or eradication...

Body Part – 4TH		Approach – 5TH	Device – 6TH	Qualifier – 7TH
0 Internal Mammary Artery, Right	J Common Carotid Artery, Left	0 Open	7 Autologous tissue substitute	Z No qualifier
1 Internal Mammary Artery, Left	K Internal Carotid Artery, Right	4 Percutaneous endoscopic	J Synthetic substitute	
2 Innominate Artery	L Internal Carotid Artery, Left		K Nonautologous tissue substitute	
3 Subclavian Artery, Right	M External Carotid Artery, Right			
4 Subclavian Artery, Left	N External Carotid Artery, Left			
5 Axillary Artery, Right	P Vertebral Artery, Right			
6 Axillary Artery, Left	Q Vertebral Artery, Left			
7 Brachial Artery, Right	R Face Artery			
8 Brachial Artery, Left	S Temporal Artery, Right			
9 Ulnar Artery, Right	T Temporal Artery, Left			
A Ulnar Artery, Left	U Thyroid Artery, Right			
B Radial Artery, Right	V Thyroid Artery, Left			
C Radial Artery, Left	Y Upper Artery			
D Hand Artery, Right				
F Hand Artery, Left				
G Intracranial Artery				
H Common Carotid Artery, Right				

3 – UPPER ARTERIES 03S

MOVE GROUP: (Reattachment), **Reposition**, (Transfer), (Transplantation)
Root Operations that put in/put back or move some/all of a body part.

- 1ST – **0** Medical and Surgical
- 2ND – **3** Upper Arteries
- 3RD – **S** REPOSITION

EXAMPLE: Relocation ulnar artery

CMS Ex: Fracture reduction

REPOSITION: Moving to its normal location, or other suitable location, all or a portion of a body part.

EXPLANATION: May or may not be cut to be moved ...

Body Part – 4TH		Approach – 5TH	Device – 6TH	Qualifier – 7TH
0 Internal Mammary Artery, Right	J Common Carotid Artery, Left	0 Open	Z No device	Z No qualifier
1 Internal Mammary Artery, Left	K Internal Carotid Artery, Right	3 Percutaneous		
2 Innominate Artery	L Internal Carotid Artery, Left	4 Percutaneous endoscopic		
3 Subclavian Artery, Right	M External Carotid Artery, Right			
4 Subclavian Artery, Left	N External Carotid Artery, Left			
5 Axillary Artery, Right	P Vertebral Artery, Right			
6 Axillary Artery, Left	Q Vertebral Artery, Left			
7 Brachial Artery, Right	R Face Artery			
8 Brachial Artery, Left	S Temporal Artery, Right			
9 Ulnar Artery, Right	T Temporal Artery, Left			
A Ulnar Artery, Left	U Thyroid Artery, Right			
B Radial Artery, Right	V Thyroid Artery, Left			
C Radial Artery, Left	Y Upper Artery			
D Hand Artery, Right				
F Hand Artery, Left				
G Intracranial Artery				
H Common Carotid Artery, Right				

0 3 U

MEDICAL AND SURGICAL SECTION – 2016 ICD-10-PCS

DEVICE GROUP: (Change), Insertion, Removal, Replacement, Revision, Supplement
Root Operations that always involve a device.

1ST – **0** Medical and Surgical
2ND – **3** Upper Arteries
3RD – **U SUPPLEMENT**

EXAMPLE: Bovine patch angioplasty   CMS Ex: Hernia repair with mesh

SUPPLEMENT: Putting in or on biological or synthetic material that physically reinforces and/or augments the function of a portion of a body part.

EXPLANATION: Biological material from same individual ...

Body Part – 4TH		Approach – 5TH	Device – 6TH	Qualifier – 7TH
0 Internal Mammary Artery, Right	J Common Carotid Artery, Left	0 Open	7 Autologous tissue substitute	Z No qualifier
1 Internal Mammary Artery, Left	K Internal Carotid Artery, Right	3 Percutaneous	J Synthetic substitute	
2 Innominate Artery	L Internal Carotid Artery, Left	4 Percutaneous endoscopic	K Nonautologous tissue substitute	
3 Subclavian Artery, Right	M External Carotid Artery, Right			
4 Subclavian Artery, Left	N External Carotid Artery, Left			
5 Axillary Artery, Right	P Vertebral Artery, Right			
6 Axillary Artery, Left	Q Vertebral Artery, Left			
7 Brachial Artery, Right	R Face Artery			
8 Brachial Artery, Left	S Temporal Artery, Right			
9 Ulnar Artery, Right	T Temporal Artery, Left			
A Ulnar Artery, Left	U Thyroid Artery, Right			
B Radial Artery, Right	V Thyroid Artery, Left			
C Radial Artery, Left	Y Upper Artery			
D Hand Artery, Right				
F Hand Artery, Left				
G Intracranial Artery				
H Common Carotid Artery, Right				

3 – UPPER ARTERIES 03V

TUBULAR GROUP: Bypass, Dilation, Occlusion, Restriction
Root Operations that alter the diameter/route of a tubular body part.

1ST - **0** Medical and Surgical
2ND - **3** Upper Arteries
3RD - **V** RESTRICTION

EXAMPLE: Clipping cerebral aneurysm | CMS Ex: Cervical cerclage

RESTRICTION: Partially closing an orifice or the lumen of a tubular body part.

EXPLANATION: Natural or artificially created orifice ...

Body Part – 4TH		Approach – 5TH	Device – 6TH	Qualifier – 7TH
0 Internal Mammary Artery, Right 1 Internal Mammary Artery, Left 2 Innominate Artery 3 Subclavian Artery, Right 4 Subclavian Artery, Left 5 Axillary Artery, Right 6 Axillary Artery, Left 7 Brachial Artery, Right 8 Brachial Artery, Left 9 Ulnar Artery, Right	A Ulnar Artery, Left B Radial Artery, Right C Radial Artery, Left D Hand Artery, Right F Hand Artery, Left R Face Artery S Temporal Artery, Right T Temporal Artery, Left U Thyroid Artery, Right V Thyroid Artery, Left Y Upper Artery	0 Open 3 Percutaneous 4 Percutaneous endoscopic	C Extraluminal device D Intraluminal device Z No device	Z No qualifier
G Intracranial Artery H Common Carotid Artery, Right J Common Carotid Artery, Left K Internal Carotid Artery, Right L Internal Carotid Artery, Left M External Carotid Artery, Right N External Carotid Artery, Left P Vertebral Artery, Right Q Vertebral Artery, Left		0 Open 3 Percutaneous 4 Percutaneous endoscopic	B Bioactive intraluminal device C Extraluminal device D Intraluminal device Z No device	Z No qualifier

0 3 W — MEDICAL AND SURGICAL SECTION – 2016 ICD-10-PCS

DEVICE GROUP: (Change), Insertion, Removal, Replacement, Revision, Supplement
Root Operations that always involve a device.

- 1ST – **0** Medical and Surgical
- 2ND – **3** Upper Arteries
- 3RD – **W** REVISION

EXAMPLE: Repair ruptured graft   **CMS Ex:** Adjustment pacemaker lead

REVISION: Correcting, to the extent possible, a portion of a malfunctioning device or the position of a displaced device.

EXPLANATION: May replace components of a device ...

Body Part – 4TH	Approach – 5TH	Device – 6TH	Qualifier – 7TH
Y Upper Artery	0 Open 3 Percutaneous 4 Percutaneous endoscopic X External	0 Drainage device 2 Monitoring device 3 Infusion device 7 Autologous tissue substitute C Extraluminal device D Intraluminal device J Synthetic substitute K Nonautologous tissue substitute M Stimulator lead	Z No qualifier

Educational Annotations | 4 – Lower Arteries

Body System Specific Educational Annotations for the Lower Arteries include:
- Anatomy and Physiology Review
- Anatomical Illustrations
- Definitions of Common Procedures
- AHA Coding Clinic® Reference Notations
- Body Part Key Listings
- Device Key Listings
- Device Aggregation Table Listings
- Coding Notes

Anatomy and Physiology Review of Lower Arteries

BODY PART VALUES – 4 - LOWER ARTERIES

Abdominal Aorta – The abdominal aorta is continuous from the thoracic aorta artery and ends by branching into the right and left common iliac arteries. Many abdominal arteries branch off from the abdominal aorta.

Anterior Tibial Artery – The anterior tibial artery branches from the popliteal artery and serves the anterior portion of the lower leg and dorsal portion of the foot.

Artery – Blood vessels that carry oxygenated (arterial) blood away from the heart and to the organs and tissues of the body. Arteries have a higher blood pressure than other parts of the circulatory system in order to adequately perfuse all the tissues with oxygenated red blood cells.

Celiac Artery – The celiac artery (also known as the celiac trunk) branches from the abdominal aorta and then almost immediately (1-2cm) branches into the common hepatic artery, the splenic artery, and left gastric artery.

Colic Artery – The colic artery branches from the superior mesenteric artery and serves the colon, ileum, appendix.

Common Iliac Artery – The common iliac artery branches from the aortic bifurcation of the abdominal aorta and branch almost immediately (4 cm in length) into the internal and external iliac arteries.

External Iliac Artery – The external iliac artery branches from the common iliac artery and serves the legs.

Femoral Artery – The femoral artery branches from the external iliac artery and serves the legs.

Foot Artery – Any of the smaller arterial branches that serve the foot.

Gastric Artery – The gastric artery branches from the celiac artery and serves the stomach and esophagus.

Hepatic Artery – The hepatic artery branches from the celiac artery and serves the gallbladder, liver, duodenum, pylorus, and pancreas.

Inferior Mesenteric Artery – The inferior mesenteric artery branches from the abdominal aorta and serves the descending colon, part of the transverse colon, sigmoid colon, and the upper part of the rectum.

Internal Iliac Artery – The internal iliac artery branches from the common iliac artery and serves the pelvic viscera, buttocks, and reproductive organs.

Lower Artery – The arteries located below the diaphragm (see Coding Guideline B2.1b).

Peroneal Artery – The peroneal artery (also known as the fibular artery) branches from the posterior tibial artery and serves the lateral portion of the leg.

Popliteal Artery – The popliteal artery branches from the femoral artery and serves the knee and lower leg.

Posterior Tibial Artery – The posterior tibial artery branches from the popliteal artery and serves the posterior portion of the lower leg and the plantar portion of the foot.

Renal Artery – The renal artery branches from the abdominal aorta and serves the kidney.

Splenic Artery – The splenic artery branches from the celiac artery and serves the spleen.

Superior Mesenteric Artery – The superior mesenteric artery branches from the abdominal aorta and serves the duodenum, ascending colon, part of the transverse colon, and pancreas.

Uterine Artery – The uterine artery branches from the internal iliac artery and serves the uterus.

Educational Annotations | 4 – Lower Arteries

Anatomical Illustrations of Lower Arteries

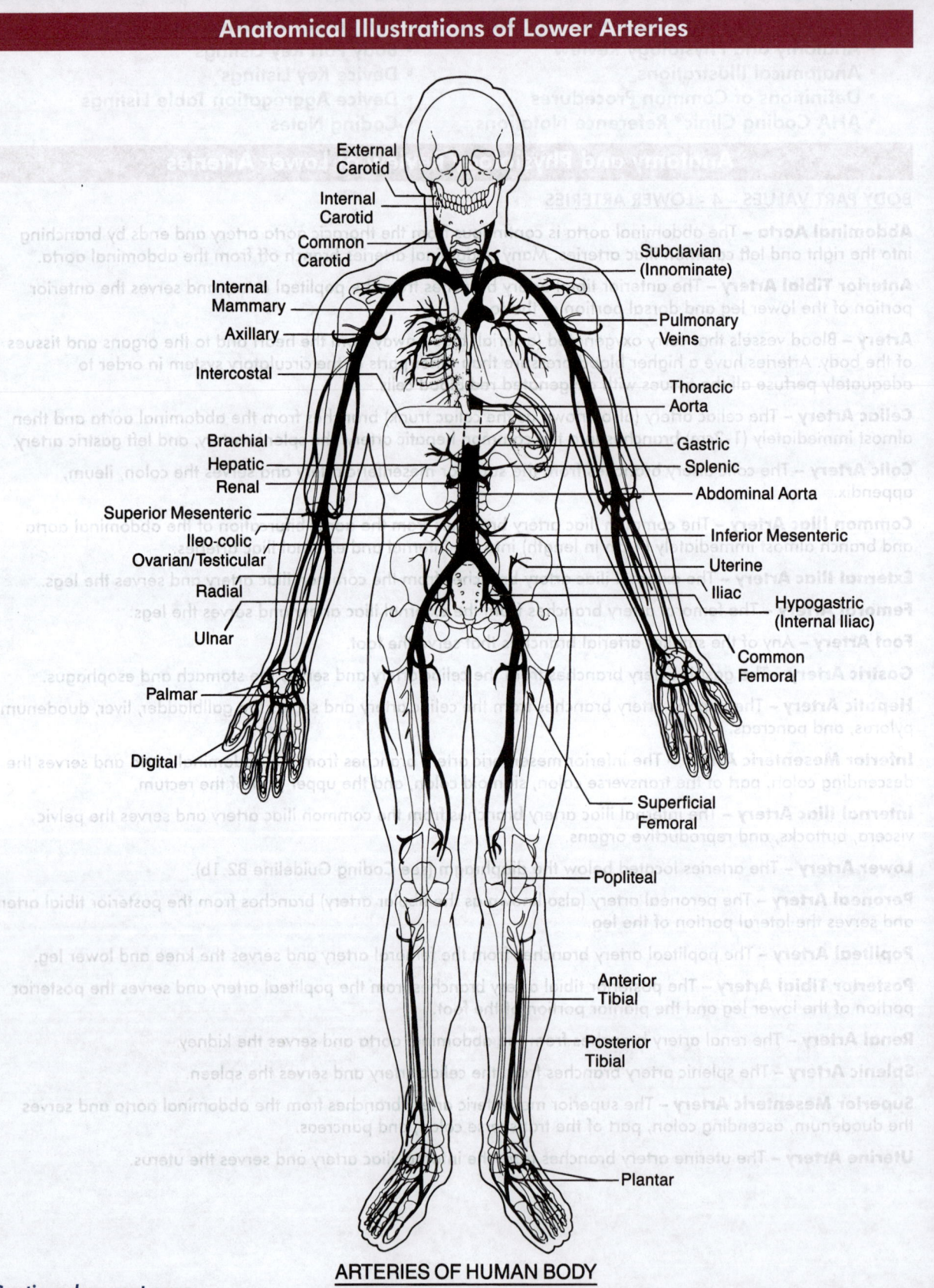

ARTERIES OF HUMAN BODY

Continued on next page

Educational Annotations | 4 – Lower Arteries

Anatomical Illustrations of Lower Arteries

Continued from previous page

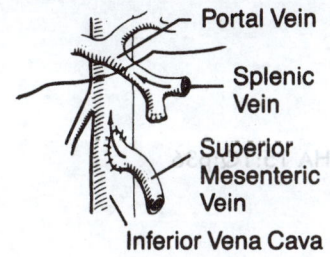
MESOCAVAL SHUNT

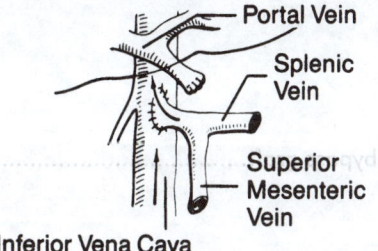
PORTACAVAL ANASTOMOSIS

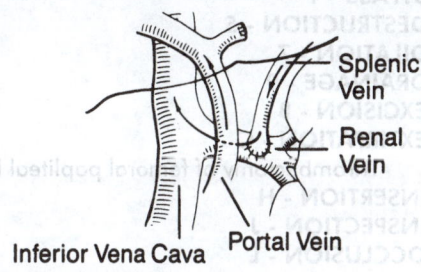
SPLENORENAL SHUNT

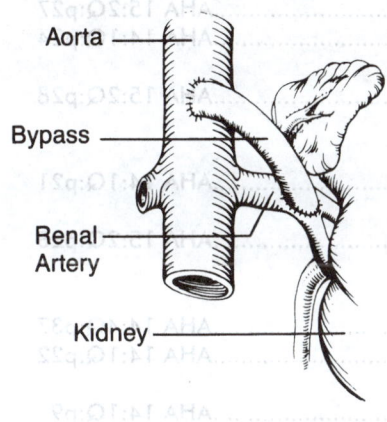
AORTA-RENAL BYPASS

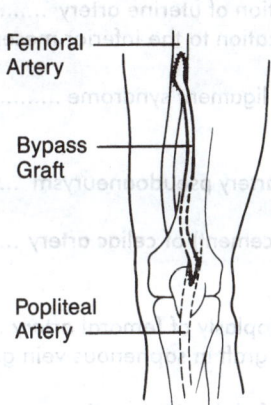
FEMORAL-POPLITEAL BYPASS

Definitions of Common Procedures of Lower Arteries

Aorto-bifemoral bypass – The restoration of blood flow to the legs by replacing the aortic-femoral bifurcation with a replacement graft that is usually synthetic, or the addition of a bypass graft sewn to the distal aorta and to the femoral arteries distal to the blockage site(s).

Abdominal aortic aneurysmectomy – The resection of an enlarged abdominal aortic wall protrusion and replacement with a graft that is usually synthetic. An endovascular version inserts a synthetic graft intravascularly to reinforce the weakened section without resecting any of the native aorta.

Femoral-popliteal bypass – The restoration of blood flow to the popliteal artery by using a bypass graft from the femoral artery.

Percutaneous mechanical thrombectomy – A minimally invasive approach to remove an acute thrombus in a lower extremity artery or graft by an endovascular approach using attachments to break up and remove the clot.

04 — 4 – Lower Arteries

Educational Annotations

AHA Coding Clinic® Reference Notations of Lower Arteries

ROOT OPERATION SPECIFIC - 4 - LOWER ARTERIES

BYPASS - 1
DESTRUCTION - 5
DILATION - 7
DRAINAGE - 9
EXCISION - B
EXTIRPATION - C
   Thrombectomy of femoral popliteal bypass graft ....AHA 15:1Q:p36
INSERTION - H
INSPECTION - J
OCCLUSION - L
   Coil embolization of gastroduodenal artery, and chemoembolization of
      hepatic artery ....AHA 14:3Q:p26
   Endovascular embolization using microcoils of colic artery ....AHA 14:1Q:p24
   Gelfoam embolization of uterine artery ....AHA 15:2Q:p27
   Microbead embolization to the inferior mesenteric artery ....AHA 14:1Q:p24
RELEASE - N
   Release of arcuate ligament syndrome ....AHA 15:2Q:p28
REMOVAL - P
REPAIR - Q
   Repair of femoral artery pseudoaneurysm ....AHA 14:1Q:p21
REPLACEMENT - R
   Bypass graft (replacement) of celiac artery ....AHA 15:2Q:p28
REPOSITION - S
SUPPLEMENT - U
   Bovine patch arterioplasty of femoral artery ....AHA 14:4Q:p37
   Placement of stent graft in saphenous vein graft ....AHA 14:1Q:p22
RESTRICTION - V
   Stent graft repair of abdominal aortic aneurysm ....AHA 14:1Q:p9
REVISION - W
   Reanastomosed femoral popliteal bypass graft ....AHA 15:1Q:p36
   Reattachment of abdominal aortic stent graft ....AHA 14:1Q:p9
   Repair of ruptured femoral-popliteal bypass graft ....AHA 14:1Q:p22

Body Part Key Listings of Lower Arteries

See also Body Part Key in Appendix C

Anterior lateral malleolar artery	*use* Anterior Tibial Artery, Left/Right
Anterior medial malleolar artery	*use* Anterior Tibial Artery, Left/Right
Anterior tibial recurrent artery	*use* Anterior Tibial Artery, Left/Right
Arcuate artery	*use* Foot Artery, Left/Right
Celiac trunk	*use* Celiac Artery
Circumflex iliac artery	*use* Femoral Artery, Left/Right
Common hepatic artery	*use* Hepatic Artery
Deep circumflex iliac artery	*use* External Iliac Artery, Left/Right
Deep femoral artery	*use* Femoral Artery, Left/Right
Deferential artery	*use* Internal Iliac Artery, Left/Right
Descending genicular artery	*use* Femoral Artery, Left/Right
Dorsal metatarsal artery	*use* Foot Artery, Left/Right
Dorsalis pedis artery	*use* Anterior Tibial Artery, Left/Right
External pudendal artery	*use* Femoral Artery, Left/Right
Fibular artery	*use* Peroneal Artery, Left/Right

Continued on next page

Educational Annotations | 4 – Lower Arteries

Body Part Key Listings of Lower Arteries

Continued from previous page

Gastroduodenal artery	*use* Hepatic Artery
Hepatic artery proper	*use* Hepatic Artery
Hypogastric artery	*use* Internal Iliac Artery, Left/Right
Ileal artery	*use* Superior Mesenteric Artery
Ileocolic artery	*use* Superior Mesenteric Artery
Iliolumbar artery	*use* Internal Iliac Artery, Left/Right
Inferior epigastric artery	*use* External Iliac Artery, Left/Right
Inferior genicular artery	*use* Popliteal Artery, Left/Right
Inferior gluteal artery	*use* Internal Iliac Artery, Left/Right
Inferior pancreaticoduodenal artery	*use* Superior Mesenteric Artery
Inferior phrenic artery	*use* Abdominal Aorta
Inferior suprarenal artery	*use* Renal Artery, Left/Right
Inferior vesical artery	*use* Internal Iliac Artery, Left/Right
Internal pudendal artery	*use* Internal Iliac Artery, Left/Right
Internal thoracic artery	*use* Internal Mammary Artery, Left/Right
	use Subclavian Artery, Left/Right
Jejunal artery	*use* Superior Mesenteric Artery
Lateral plantar artery	*use* Foot Artery, Left/Right
Lateral sacral artery	*use* Internal Iliac Artery, Left/Right
Lateral tarsal artery	*use* Foot Artery, Left/Right
Left gastric artery	*use* Gastric Artery
Left gastroepiploic artery	*use* Splenic Artery
Lumbar artery	*use* Abdominal Aorta
Medial plantar artery	*use* Foot Artery, Left/Right
Median sacral artery	*use* Abdominal Aorta
Middle genicular artery	*use* Popliteal Artery, Left/Right
Middle rectal artery	*use* Internal Iliac Artery, Left/Right
Middle suprarenal artery	*use* Abdominal Aorta
Obturator artery	*use* Internal Iliac Artery, Left/Right
Ovarian artery	*use* Abdominal Aorta
Pancreatic artery	*use* Splenic Artery
Posterior tibial recurrent artery	*use* Anterior Tibial Artery, Left/Right
Renal segmental artery	*use* Renal Artery, Left/Right
Right gastric artery	*use* Gastric Artery
Short gastric artery	*use* Splenic Artery
Sigmoid artery	*use* Inferior Mesenteric Artery
Superficial epigastric artery	*use* Femoral Artery, Left/Right
Superior genicular artery	*use* Popliteal Artery, Left/Right
Superior gluteal artery	*use* Internal Iliac Artery, Left/Right
Superior rectal artery	*use* Inferior Mesenteric Artery
Sural artery	*use* Popliteal Artery, Left/Right
Testicular artery	*use* Abdominal Aorta
Umbilical artery	*use* Internal Iliac Artery, Left/Right
Uterine artery	*use* Internal Iliac Artery, Left/Right
Vaginal artery	*use* Internal Iliac Artery, Left/Right

Educational Annotations | 4 – Lower Arteries

Device Key Listings of Lower Arteries

See also Device Key in Appendix D

Absolute Pro Vascular (OTW) Self-Expanding Stent System	*use* Intraluminal Device
AneuRx® AAA Advantage®	*use* Intraluminal Device
Assurant (Cobalt) stent	*use* Intraluminal Device
Autograft	*use* Autologous Tissue Substitute
Autologous artery graft	*use* Autologous Arterial Tissue in Lower Arteries
Autologous vein graft	*use* Autologous Venous Tissue in Lower Arteries
Brachytherapy seeds	*use* Radioactive Element
CoAxia NeuroFlo catheter	*use* Intraluminal Device
Complete (SE) stent	*use* Intraluminal Device
E-Luminexx™ (Biliary) (Vascular) Stent	*use* Intraluminal Device
Embolization coil(s)	*use* Intraluminal Device
Endurant® Endovascular Stent Graft	*use* Intraluminal Device
Express® (LD) Premounted Stent System	*use* Intraluminal Device
Express® Biliary SD Monorail® Premounted Stent System	*use* Intraluminal Device
Express® SD Renal Monorail® Premounted Stent System	*use* Intraluminal Device
Formula™ Balloon-Expandable Renal Stent System	*use* Intraluminal Device
Herculink (RX) Elite Renal Stent System	*use* Intraluminal Device
LifeStent® (Flexstar) (XL) Vascular Stent System	*use* Intraluminal Device
Omnilink Elite Vascular Balloon Expandable Stent System	*use* Intraluminal Device
Paclitaxel-eluting peripheral stent	*use* Intraluminal Device, Drug-eluting in Upper Arteries, Lower Arteries
Stent, intraluminal (cardiovascular) (gastrointestinal) (hepatobiliary) (urinary)	*use* Intraluminal Device
Talent® Converter	*use* Intraluminal Device
Talent® Occluder	*use* Intraluminal Device
Talent® Stent Graft (abdominal) (thoracic)	*use* Intraluminal Device
Tissue bank graft	*use* Nonautologous Tissue Substitute
Zenith Flex® AAA Endovascular Graft	*use* Intraluminal Device
Zenith® Renu™ AAA Ancillary Graft	*use* Intraluminal Device
Zilver® PTX® (paclitaxel) Drug-Eluting Peripheral Stent	*use* Intraluminal Device, Drug-eluting in Upper Arteries, Lower Arteries

Device Aggregation Table Listings of Lower Arteries

See also Device Aggregation Table in Appendix E

Specific Device	For Operation	In Body System	General Device
Autologous Arterial Tissue	All applicable	Lower Arteries	7 Autologous Tissue Substitute
Autologous Venous Tissue	All applicable	Lower Arteries	7 Autologous Tissue Substitute
Intraluminal Device, Drug-eluting	All applicable	Lower Arteries	D Intraluminal Device

Educational Annotations | 4 – Lower Arteries

Coding Notes of Lower Arteries

Body System Relevant Coding Guidelines

General Guidelines
  B2.1b
   Where the general body part values "upper" and "lower" are provided as an option in the Upper Arteries, Lower Arteries, Upper Veins, Lower Veins, Muscles and Tendons body systems, "upper" and "lower" specifies body parts located above or below the diaphragm respectively.
   Example: Vein body parts above the diaphragm are found in the Upper Veins body system; vein body parts below the diaphragm are found in the Lower Veins body system.

Branches of body parts
  B4.2
   Where a specific branch of a body part does not have its own body part value in PCS, the body part is coded to the closest proximal branch that has a specific body part value.
   Example: A procedure performed on the mandibular branch of the trigeminal nerve is coded to the trigeminal nerve body part value.

Body System Specific PCS Reference Manual Exercises

PCS CODE	4 – LOWER ARTERIES EXERCISES
041L0KL	Open left femoral-popliteal artery bypass using cadaver vein graft.
047L0ZZ	Open dilation of old anastomosis, left femoral artery.
04LE3DT	Percutaneous embolization of right uterine artery, using coils.
04R00JZ	Excision of abdominal aorta with goretex graft replacement, open.
04WY0JZ	Trimming and reanastomosis of stenosed femorofemoral synthetic bypass graft, open.

Educational Annotations

4 – Lower Arteries

NOTES

4 – LOWER ARTERIES

TUBULAR GROUP: Bypass, Dilation, Occlusion, Restriction
Root Operations that alter the diameter/route of a tubular body part.

1ST - 0 Medical and Surgical
2ND - 4 Lower Arteries
3RD - 1 BYPASS

EXAMPLE: Aorto-bifemoral bypass   **CMS Ex:** Coronary artery bypass

BYPASS: Altering the route of passage of the contents of a tubular body part.

EXPLANATION: Rerouting contents to a downstream part ...

Body Part – 4TH	Approach – 5TH	Device – 6TH	Qualifier – 7TH
0 Abdominal Aorta C Common Iliac Artery, Right D Common Iliac Artery, Left	0 Open 4 Percutaneous endoscopic	9 Autologous venous tissue A Autologous arterial tissue J Synthetic substitute K Nonautologous tissue substitute Z No device	0 Abdominal Aorta 1 Celiac Artery 2 Mesenteric Artery 3 Renal Artery, Right 4 Renal Artery, Left 5 Renal Artery, Bilateral 6 Common Iliac Artery, Right 7 Common Iliac Artery, Left 8 Common Iliac Arteries, Bilateral 9 Internal Iliac Artery, Right B Internal Iliac Artery, Left C Internal Iliac Arteries, Bilateral D External Iliac Artery, Right F External Iliac Artery, Left G External Iliac Arteries, Bilateral H Femoral Artery, Right J Femoral Artery, Left K Femoral Arteries, Bilateral Q Lower Extremity Artery R Lower Artery
4 Splenic Artery	0 Open 4 Percutaneous endoscopic	9 Autologous venous tissue A Autologous arterial tissue J Synthetic substitute K Nonautologous tissue substitute Z No device	3 Renal Artery, Right 4 Renal Artery, Left 5 Renal Artery, Bilateral
E Internal Iliac Artery, Right F Internal Iliac Artery, Left H External Iliac Artery, Right J External Iliac Artery, Left	0 Open 4 Percutaneous endoscopic	9 Autologous venous tissue A Autologous arterial tissue J Synthetic substitute K Nonautologous tissue substitute Z No device	9 Internal Iliac Artery, Right B Internal Iliac Artery, Left C Internal Iliac Arteries, Bilateral D External Iliac Artery, Right F External Iliac Artery, Left G External Iliac Arteries, Bilateral H Femoral Artery, Right J Femoral Artery, Left K Femoral Arteries, Bilateral P Foot Artery Q Lower Extremity Artery

continued ⇨

041 MEDICAL AND SURGICAL SECTION – 2016 ICD-10-PCS [2016.PCS]

0 4 1 BYPASS – continued

Body Part – 4ᵗʰ	Approach – 5ᵗʰ	Device – 6ᵗʰ	Qualifier – 7ᵗʰ
K Femoral Artery, Right L Femoral Artery, Left	0 Open 4 Percutaneous endoscopic	9 Autologous venous tissue A Autologous arterial tissue J Synthetic substitute K Nonautologous tissue substitute Z No device	H Femoral Artery, Right J Femoral Artery, Left K Femoral Arteries, Bilateral L Popliteal Artery M Peroneal Artery N Posterior Tibial Artery P Foot Artery Q Lower Extremity Artery S Lower Extremity Vein
M Popliteal Artery, Right N Popliteal Artery, Left	0 Open 4 Percutaneous endoscopic	9 Autologous venous tissue A Autologous arterial tissue J Synthetic substitute K Nonautologous tissue substitute Z No device	L Popliteal Artery M Peroneal Artery P Foot Artery Q Lower Extremity Artery S Lower Extremity Vein

LOWER ARTERIES

EXCISION GROUP: Excision, (Resection), Destruction, (Extraction), (Detachment)
Root Operations that take out some or all of a body part.

0 4 1

- 1ˢᵀ – **0** Medical and Surgical
- 2ᴺᴰ – **4** Lower Arteries
- 3ᴿᴰ – **5 DESTRUCTION**

EXAMPLE: Fulguration arterial lesion **CMS Ex:** Fulguration polyp

DESTRUCTION: Physical eradication of all or a portion of a body part by the direct use of energy, force, or a destructive agent.

EXPLANATION: None of the body part is physically taken out

Body Part – 4ᵗʰ	Approach – 5ᵗʰ	Device – 6ᵗʰ	Qualifier – 7ᵗʰ
0 Abdominal Aorta 1 Celiac Artery 2 Gastric Artery 3 Hepatic Artery 4 Splenic Artery 5 Superior Mesenteric Artery 6 Colic Artery, Right 7 Colic Artery, Left 8 Colic Artery, Middle 9 Renal Artery, Right A Renal Artery, Left B Inferior Mesenteric Artery C Common Iliac Artery, Right D Common Iliac Artery, Left E Internal Iliac Artery, Right F Internal Iliac Artery, Left H External Iliac Artery, Right J External Iliac Artery, Left K Femoral Artery, Right L Femoral Artery, Left M Popliteal Artery, Right N Popliteal Artery, Left P Anterior Tibial Artery, Right Q Anterior Tibial Artery, Left R Posterior Tibial Artery, Right S Posterior Tibial Artery, Left T Peroneal Artery, Right U Peroneal Artery, Left V Foot Artery, Right W Foot Artery, Left Y Lower Artery	0 Open 3 Percutaneous 4 Percutaneous endoscopic	Z No device	Z No qualifier

4 – LOWER ARTERIES   047

TUBULAR GROUP: Bypass, Dilation, Occlusion, Restriction
Root Operations that alter the diameter/route of a tubular body part.

1ST - **0** Medical and Surgical
2ND - **4** Lower Arteries
3RD - **7 DILATION**

EXAMPLE: PTA femoral artery   **CMS Ex:** Transluminal angioplasty

DILATION: Expanding an orifice or the lumen of a tubular body part.

EXPLANATION: By force (stretching) or cutting …

Body Part – 4TH		Approach – 5TH	Device – 6TH	Qualifier – 7TH
0 Abdominal Aorta	E Internal Iliac Artery, Right	0 Open	4 Drug-eluting intraluminal device	Z No qualifier
1 Celiac Artery	F Internal Iliac Artery, Left	3 Percutaneous	D Intraluminal device	
2 Gastric Artery	H External Iliac Artery, Right	4 Percutaneous endoscopic	Z No device	
3 Hepatic Artery	J External Iliac Artery, Left			
4 Splenic Artery	P Anterior Tibial Artery, Right			
5 Superior Mesenteric Artery	Q Anterior Tibial Artery, Left			
6 Colic Artery, Right	R Posterior Tibial Artery, Right			
7 Colic Artery, Left	S Posterior Tibial Artery, Left			
8 Colic Artery, Middle	T Peroneal Artery, Right			
9 Renal Artery, Right	U Peroneal Artery, Left			
A Renal Artery, Left	V Foot Artery, Right			
B Inferior Mesenteric Artery	W Foot Artery, Left			
C Common Iliac Artery, Right	Y Lower Artery			
D Common Iliac Artery, Left				
K Femoral Artery, Right		0 Open	4 Drug-eluting intraluminal device	1 Drug-coated balloon
L Femoral Artery, Left		3 Percutaneous	D Intraluminal device	Z No qualifier
M Popliteal Artery, Right		4 Percutaneous endoscopic	Z No device	
N Popliteal Artery, Left				

0 4 9

MEDICAL AND SURGICAL SECTION – 2016 ICD-10-PCS

DRAINAGE GROUP: Drainage, Extirpation, (Fragmentation)
Root Operations that take out solids/fluids/gases from a body part.

- 1ST - **0** Medical and Surgical
- 2ND - **4** Lower Arteries
- 3RD - **9 DRAINAGE**

EXAMPLE: Aspiration arterial abscess   **CMS Ex:** Thoracentesis

DRAINAGE: Taking or letting out fluids and/or gases from a body part.

EXPLANATION: Qualifier "X Diagnostic" indicates biopsy ...

Body Part – 4TH		Approach – 5TH	Device – 6TH	Qualifier – 7TH
0 Abdominal Aorta 1 Celiac Artery 2 Gastric Artery 3 Hepatic Artery 4 Splenic Artery 5 Superior Mesenteric Artery 6 Colic Artery, Right 7 Colic Artery, Left 8 Colic Artery, Middle 9 Renal Artery, Right A Renal Artery, Left B Inferior Mesenteric Artery C Common Iliac Artery, Right D Common Iliac Artery, Left E Internal Iliac Artery, Right F Internal Iliac Artery, Left	H External Iliac Artery, Right J External Iliac Artery, Left K Femoral Artery, Right L Femoral Artery, Left M Popliteal Artery, Right N Popliteal Artery, Left P Anterior Tibial Artery, Right Q Anterior Tibial Artery, Left R Posterior Tibial Artery, Right S Posterior Tibial Artery, Left T Peroneal Artery, Right U Peroneal Artery, Left V Foot Artery, Right W Foot Artery, Left Y Lower Artery	0 Open 3 Percutaneous 4 Percutaneous endoscopic	0 Drainage device	Z No qualifier
0 Abdominal Aorta 1 Celiac Artery 2 Gastric Artery 3 Hepatic Artery 4 Splenic Artery 5 Superior Mesenteric Artery 6 Colic Artery, Right 7 Colic Artery, Left 8 Colic Artery, Middle 9 Renal Artery, Right A Renal Artery, Left B Inferior Mesenteric Artery C Common Iliac Artery, Right D Common Iliac Artery, Left E Internal Iliac Artery, Right F Internal Iliac Artery, Left	H External Iliac Artery, Right J External Iliac Artery, Left K Femoral Artery, Right L Femoral Artery, Left M Popliteal Artery, Right N Popliteal Artery, Left P Anterior Tibial Artery, Right Q Anterior Tibial Artery, Left R Posterior Tibial Artery, Right S Posterior Tibial Artery, Left T Peroneal Artery, Right U Peroneal Artery, Left V Foot Artery, Right W Foot Artery, Left Y Lower Artery	0 Open 3 Percutaneous 4 Percutaneous endoscopic	Z No device	X Diagnostic Z No qualifier

LOWER ARTERIES 049

4 – LOWER ARTERIES   0 4 B

EXCISION GROUP: Excision, (Resection), **Destruction,** (Extraction), (Detachment)
Root Operations that take out some or all of a body part.

1ST - **0** Medical and Surgical

2ND - **4** Lower Arteries

3RD - **B EXCISION**

EXAMPLE: Femoral artery biopsy

CMS Ex: Liver biopsy

EXCISION: Cutting out or off, without replacement, a portion of a body part.

EXPLANATION: Qualifier "X Diagnostic" indicates biopsy ...

Body Part – 4TH		Approach – 5TH	Device – 6TH	Qualifier – 7TH
0 Abdominal Aorta	H External Iliac Artery, Right	0 Open	Z No device	X Diagnostic
1 Celiac Artery	J External Iliac Artery, Left	3 Percutaneous		Z No qualifier
2 Gastric Artery	K Femoral Artery, Right	4 Percutaneous endoscopic		
3 Hepatic Artery	L Femoral Artery, Left			
4 Splenic Artery	M Popliteal Artery, Right			
5 Superior Mesenteric Artery	N Popliteal Artery, Left			
6 Colic Artery, Right	P Anterior Tibial Artery, Right			
7 Colic Artery, Left	Q Anterior Tibial Artery, Left			
8 Colic Artery, Middle	R Posterior Tibial Artery, Right			
9 Renal Artery, Right	S Posterior Tibial Artery, Left			
A Renal Artery, Left	T Peroneal Artery, Right			
B Inferior Mesenteric Artery	U Peroneal Artery, Left			
C Common Iliac Artery, Right	V Foot Artery, Right			
D Common Iliac Artery, Left	W Foot Artery, Left			
E Internal Iliac Artery, Right	Y Lower Artery			
F Internal Iliac Artery, Left				

183

04C MEDICAL AND SURGICAL SECTION – 2016 ICD-10-PCS

DRAINAGE GROUP: Drainage, Extirpation, (Fragmentation)
Root Operations that take out solids/fluids/gases from a body part.

1ST - **0** Medical and Surgical
2ND - **4** Lower Arteries
3RD - **C EXTIRPATION**

EXAMPLE: Iliac artery thrombectomy CMS Ex: Choledocholithotomy

EXTIRPATION: Taking or cutting out solid matter from a body part.

EXPLANATION: Abnormal byproduct or foreign body ...

Body Part – 4TH		Approach – 5TH	Device – 6TH	Qualifier – 7TH
0 Abdominal Aorta	H External Iliac Artery, Right	0 Open	Z No device	Z No qualifier
1 Celiac Artery	J External Iliac Artery, Left	3 Percutaneous		
2 Gastric Artery	K Femoral Artery, Right	4 Percutaneous endoscopic		
3 Hepatic Artery	L Femoral Artery, Left			
4 Splenic Artery	M Popliteal Artery, Right			
5 Superior Mesenteric Artery	N Popliteal Artery, Left			
	P Anterior Tibial Artery, Right			
6 Colic Artery, Right	Q Anterior Tibial Artery, Left			
7 Colic Artery, Left				
8 Colic Artery, Middle	R Posterior Tibial Artery, Right			
9 Renal Artery, Right				
A Renal Artery, Left	S Posterior Tibial Artery, Left			
B Inferior Mesenteric Artery				
C Common Iliac Artery, Right	T Peroneal Artery, Right			
	U Peroneal Artery, Left			
D Common Iliac Artery, Left	V Foot Artery, Right			
	W Foot Artery, Left			
E Internal Iliac Artery, Right	Y Lower Artery			
F Internal Iliac Artery, Left				

4 – LOWER ARTERIES

0 4 H

DEVICE GROUP: (Change), Insertion, Removal, Replacement, Revision, Supplement
Root Operations that always involve a device.

- 1ST – **0** Medical and Surgical
- 2ND – **4** Lower Arteries
- 3RD – **H** INSERTION

EXAMPLE: Arterial infusion catheter   **CMS Ex:** Central venous catheter

INSERTION: Putting in a nonbiological appliance that monitors, assists, performs, or prevents a physiological function but does not physically take the place of a body part.

EXPLANATION: None

Body Part – 4TH		Approach – 5TH	Device – 6TH	Qualifier – 7TH
0 Abdominal Aorta Y Lower Artery		0 Open 3 Percutaneous 4 Percutaneous endoscopic	2 Monitoring device 3 Infusion device D Intraluminal device	Z No qualifier
1 Celiac Artery 2 Gastric Artery 3 Hepatic Artery 4 Splenic Artery 5 Superior Mesenteric Artery 6 Colic Artery, Right 7 Colic Artery, Left 8 Colic Artery, Middle 9 Renal Artery, Right A Renal Artery, Left B Inferior Mesenteric Artery C Common Iliac Artery, Right D Common Iliac Artery, Left E Internal Iliac Artery, Right F Internal Iliac Artery, Left	H External Iliac Artery, Right J External Iliac Artery, Left K Femoral Artery, Right L Femoral Artery, Left M Popliteal Artery, Right N Popliteal Artery, Left P Anterior Tibial Artery, Right Q Anterior Tibial Artery, Left R Posterior Tibial Artery, Right S Posterior Tibial Artery, Left T Peroneal Artery, Right U Peroneal Artery, Left V Foot Artery, Right W Foot Artery, Left	0 Open 3 Percutaneous 4 Percutaneous endoscopic	3 Infusion device D Intraluminal device	Z No qualifier

04J MEDICAL AND SURGICAL SECTION – 2016 ICD-10-PCS [2016.PCS]

EXAMINATION GROUP: Inspection, (Map)
Root Operations involving examination only.

1ST - **0** Medical and Surgical
2ND - **4** Lower Arteries
3RD - **J** INSPECTION

EXAMPLE: Exploration arterial cath removal site | CMS Ex: Colonoscopy

INSPECTION: Visually and/or manually exploring a body part.

EXPLANATION: Direct or instrumental visualization ...

Body Part – 4TH	Approach – 5TH	Device – 6TH	Qualifier – 7TH
Y Lower Artery	0 Open 3 Percutaneous 4 Percutaneous endoscopic X External	Z No device	Z No qualifier

---

TUBULAR GROUP: Bypass, Dilation, Occlusion, Restriction
Root Operations that alter the diameter/route of a tubular body part.

1ST - **0** Medical and Surgical
2ND - **4** Lower Arteries
3RD - **L** OCCLUSION

EXAMPLE: Renal artery embolization | CMS Ex: Fallopian tube ligation

OCCLUSION: Completely closing an orifice or lumen of a tubular body part.

EXPLANATION: Natural or artificially created orifice ...

Body Part – 4TH		Approach – 5TH	Device – 6TH	Qualifier – 7TH
0 Abdominal Aorta 1 Celiac Artery 2 Gastric Artery 3 Hepatic Artery 4 Splenic Artery 5 Superior Mesenteric Artery 6 Colic Artery, Right 7 Colic Artery, Left 8 Colic Artery, Middle 9 Renal Artery, Right A Renal Artery, Left B Inferior Mesenteric Artery C Common Iliac Artery, Right D Common Iliac Artery, Left	H External Iliac Artery, Right J External Iliac Artery, Left K Femoral Artery, Right L Femoral Artery, Left M Poplical Artery, Right N Popliteal Artery, Left P Anterior Tibial Artery, Right Q Anterior Tibial Artery, Left R Posterior Tibial Artery, Right S Posterior Tibial Artery, Left T Peroneal Artery, Right U Peroneal Artery, Left V Foot Artery, Right W Foot Artery, Left Y Lower Artery	0 Open 3 Percutaneous 4 Percutaneous endoscopic	C Extraluminal device D Intraluminal device Z No device	Z No qualifier
E Internal Iliac Artery, Right		0 Open 3 Percutaneous 4 Percutaneous endoscopic	C Extraluminal device D Intraluminal device Z No device	T Uterine artery, right ♀ Z No qualifier
F Internal Iliac Artery, Left		0 Open 3 Percutaneous 4 Percutaneous endoscopic	C Extraluminal device D Intraluminal device Z No device	U Uterine artery, left ♀ Z No qualifier

4 – LOWER ARTERIES

0 4 N

DIVISION GROUP: (Division), **Release**
Root Operations involving cutting or separation only.

- 1ST – **0** Medical and Surgical
- 2ND – **4** Lower Arteries
- 3RD – **N** RELEASE

EXAMPLE: Arterial adhesiolysis
CMS Ex: Carpal tunnel release

RELEASE: Freeing a body part from an abnormal physical constraint by cutting or by the use of force.

EXPLANATION: None of the body part is taken out ...

Body Part – 4TH	Approach – 5TH	Device – 6TH	Qualifier – 7TH
0 Abdominal Aorta	0 Open	Z No device	Z No qualifier
1 Celiac Artery	3 Percutaneous		
2 Gastric Artery	4 Percutaneous endoscopic		
3 Hepatic Artery			
4 Splenic Artery			
5 Superior Mesenteric Artery			
6 Colic Artery, Right			
7 Colic Artery, Left			
8 Colic Artery, Middle			
9 Renal Artery, Right			
A Renal Artery, Left			
B Inferior Mesenteric Artery			
C Common Iliac Artery, Right			
D Common Iliac Artery, Left			
E Internal Iliac Artery, Right			
F Internal Iliac Artery, Left			
H External Iliac Artery, Right			
J External Iliac Artery, Left			
K Femoral Artery, Right			
L Femoral Artery, Left			
M Popliteal Artery, Right			
N Popliteal Artery, Left			
P Anterior Tibial Artery, Right			
Q Anterior Tibial Artery, Left			
R Posterior Tibial Artery, Right			
S Posterior Tibial Artery, Left			
T Peroneal Artery, Right			
U Peroneal Artery, Left			
V Foot Artery, Right			
W Foot Artery, Left			
Y Lower Artery			

04P

MEDICAL AND SURGICAL SECTION – 2016 ICD-10-PCS

DEVICE GROUP: (Change), Insertion, Removal, Replacement, Revision, Supplement
Root Operations that always involve a device.

1ST - **0** Medical and Surgical

2ND - **4** Lower Arteries

3RD - **P REMOVAL**

EXAMPLE: Removal arterial catheter   CMS Ex: Chest tube removal

REMOVAL: Taking out or off a device from a body part.

EXPLANATION: Removal device without reinsertion ...

Body Part – 4TH	Approach – 5TH	Device – 6TH	Qualifier – 7TH
Y Lower Artery	0 Open 3 Percutaneous 4 Percutaneous endoscopic	0 Drainage device 2 Monitoring device 3 Infusion device 7 Autologous tissue substitute C Extraluminal device D Intraluminal device J Synthetic substitute K Nonautologous tissue substitute	Z No qualifier
Y Lower Artery	X External	0 Drainage device 1 Radioactive element 2 Monitoring device 3 Infusion device D Intraluminal device	Z No qualifier

4 – LOWER ARTERIES 04Q

OTHER REPAIRS GROUP: (Control), Repair
Root Operations that define other repairs.

1ST – **0** Medical and Surgical
2ND – **4** Lower Arteries
3RD – **Q REPAIR**

EXAMPLE: Repair arterial injury
CMS Ex: Suture laceration

REPAIR: Restoring, to the extent possible, a body part to its normal anatomic structure and function.

EXPLANATION: Only when no other root operation applies ...

Body Part – 4TH		Approach – 5TH	Device – 6TH	Qualifier – 7TH
0 Abdominal Aorta	H External Iliac Artery, Right	0 Open	Z No device	Z No qualifier
1 Celiac Artery	J External Iliac Artery, Left	3 Percutaneous		
2 Gastric Artery	K Femoral Artery, Right	4 Percutaneous endoscopic		
3 Hepatic Artery	L Femoral Artery, Left			
4 Splenic Artery	M Popliteal Artery, Right			
5 Superior Mesenteric Artery	N Popliteal Artery, Left			
6 Colic Artery, Right	P Anterior Tibial Artery, Right			
7 Colic Artery, Left	Q Anterior Tibial Artery, Left			
8 Colic Artery, Middle	R Posterior Tibial Artery, Right			
9 Renal Artery, Right	S Posterior Tibial Artery, Left			
A Renal Artery, Left	T Peroneal Artery, Right			
B Inferior Mesenteric Artery	U Peroneal Artery, Left			
C Common Iliac Artery, Right	V Foot Artery, Right			
D Common Iliac Artery, Left	W Foot Artery, Left			
E Internal Iliac Artery, Right	Y Lower Artery			
F Internal Iliac Artery, Left				

04R

MEDICAL AND SURGICAL SECTION – 2016 ICD-10-PCS

[2016.PCS]

DEVICE GROUP: (Change), Insertion, Removal, Replacement, Revision, Supplement
Root Operations that always involve a device.

1ST - **0** Medical and Surgical

2ND - **4** Lower Arteries

3RD - **R REPLACEMENT**

EXAMPLE: Reconstruction artery using graft **CMS Ex:** Total hip

REPLACEMENT: Putting in or on a biological or synthetic material that physically takes the place and/or function of all or a portion of a body part.

EXPLANATION: Includes taking out body part, or eradication...

Body Part – 4TH		Approach – 5TH	Device – 6TH	Qualifier – 7TH
0 Abdominal Aorta	H External Iliac Artery, Right	0 Open	7 Autologous tissue substitute	Z No qualifier
1 Celiac Artery	J External Iliac Artery, Left	4 Percutaneous endoscopic	J Synthetic substitute	
2 Gastric Artery	K Femoral Artery, Right		K Nonautologous tissue substitute	
3 Hepatic Artery	L Femoral Artery, Left			
4 Splenic Artery	M Popliteal Artery, Right			
5 Superior Mesenteric Artery	N Popliteal Artery, Left			
6 Colic Artery, Right	P Anterior Tibial Artery, Right			
7 Colic Artery, Left	Q Anterior Tibial Artery, Left			
8 Colic Artery, Middle	R Posterior Tibial Artery, Right			
9 Renal Artery, Right	S Posterior Tibial Artery, Left			
A Renal Artery, Left	T Peroneal Artery, Right			
B Inferior Mesenteric Artery	U Peroneal Artery, Left			
C Common Iliac Artery, Right	V Foot Artery, Right			
D Common Iliac Artery, Left	W Foot Artery, Left			
E Internal Iliac Artery, Right	Y Lower Artery			
F Internal Iliac Artery, Left				

LOWER ARTERIES 04R

4 – LOWER ARTERIES — 0 4 S

MOVE GROUP: (Reattachment), **Reposition**, (Transfer), (Transplantation)
Root Operations that put in/put back or move some/all of a body part.

- 1ST - **0** Medical and Surgical
- 2ND - **4** Lower Arteries
- 3RD - **S** REPOSITION

EXAMPLE: Relocation peroneal artery **CMS Ex:** Fracture reduction

REPOSITION: Moving to its normal location, or other suitable location, all or a portion of a body part.

EXPLANATION: May or may not be cut to be moved ...

Body Part – 4TH		Approach – 5TH	Device – 6TH	Qualifier – 7TH
0 Abdominal Aorta	H External Iliac Artery, Right	0 Open	Z No device	Z No qualifier
1 Celiac Artery	J External Iliac Artery, Left	3 Percutaneous		
2 Gastric Artery	K Femoral Artery, Right	4 Percutaneous endoscopic		
3 Hepatic Artery	L Femoral Artery, Left			
4 Splenic Artery	M Popliteal Artery, Right			
5 Superior Mesenteric Artery	N Popliteal Artery, Left			
6 Colic Artery, Right	P Anterior Tibial Artery, Right			
7 Colic Artery, Left	Q Anterior Tibial Artery, Left			
8 Colic Artery, Middle				
9 Renal Artery, Right	R Posterior Tibial Artery, Right			
A Renal Artery, Left	S Posterior Tibial Artery, Left			
B Inferior Mesenteric Artery				
C Common Iliac Artery, Right	T Peroneal Artery, Right			
D Common Iliac Artery, Left	U Peroneal Artery, Left			
	V Foot Artery, Right			
	W Foot Artery, Left			
E Internal Iliac Artery, Right	Y Lower Artery			
F Internal Iliac Artery, Left				

04U

DEVICE GROUP: (Change), Insertion, Removal, Replacement, Revision, Supplement
Root Operations that always involve a device.

1ST – 0 Medical and Surgical
2ND – 4 Lower Arteries
3RD – U SUPPLEMENT

EXAMPLE: Bovine patch angioplasty   **CMS Ex:** Hernia repair with mesh

SUPPLEMENT: Putting in or on biological or synthetic material that physically reinforces and/or augments the function of a portion of a body part.

EXPLANATION: Biological material from same individual ...

Body Part – 4TH		Approach – 5TH	Device – 6TH	Qualifier – 7TH
0 Abdominal Aorta	H External Iliac Artery, Right	0 Open	7 Autologous tissue substitute	Z No qualifier
1 Celiac Artery	J External Iliac Artery, Left	3 Percutaneous	J Synthetic substitute	
2 Gastric Artery	K Femoral Artery, Right	4 Percutaneous endoscopic	K Nonautologous tissue substitute	
3 Hepatic Artery	L Femoral Artery, Left			
4 Splenic Artery	M Popliteal Artery, Right			
5 Superior Mesenteric Artery	N Popliteal Artery, Left			
	P Anterior Tibial Artery, Right			
6 Colic Artery, Right	Q Anterior Tibial Artery, Left			
7 Colic Artery, Left				
8 Colic Artery, Middle	R Posterior Tibial Artery, Right			
9 Renal Artery, Right				
A Renal Artery, Left	S Posterior Tibial Artery, Left			
B Inferior Mesenteric Artery	T Peroneal Artery, Right			
C Common Iliac Artery, Right	U Peroneal Artery, Left			
D Common Iliac Artery, Left	V Foot Artery, Right			
	W Foot Artery, Left			
E Internal Iliac Artery, Right	Y Lower Artery			
F Internal Iliac Artery, Left				

4 – LOWER ARTERIES 04V

TUBULAR GROUP: Bypass, Dilation, Occlusion, Restriction
Root Operations that alter the diameter/route of a tubular body part.

1ST - 0 Medical and Surgical
2ND - 4 Lower Arteries
3RD - V RESTRICTION

EXAMPLE: Stent graft repair aneurysm — CMS Ex: Cervical cerclage

RESTRICTION: Partially closing an orifice or the lumen of a tubular body part.

EXPLANATION: Natural or artificially created orifice ...

Body Part – 4TH		Approach – 5TH	Device – 6TH	Qualifier – 7TH
0 Abdominal Aorta		0 Open 3 Percutaneous 4 Percutaneous endoscopic	C Extraluminal device Z No device	Z No qualifier
0 Abdominal Aorta		0 Open 3 Percutaneous 4 Percutaneous endoscopic	D Intraluminal device	J Temporary Z No qualifier
1 Celiac Artery 2 Gastric Artery 3 Hepatic Artery 4 Splenic Artery 5 Superior Mesenteric Artery 6 Colic Artery, Right 7 Colic Artery, Left 8 Colic Artery, Middle 9 Renal Artery, Right A Renal Artery, Left B Inferior Mesenteric Artery C Common Iliac Artery, Right D Common Iliac Artery, Left E Internal Iliac Artery, Right F Internal Iliac Artery, Left	H External Iliac Artery, Right J External Iliac Artery, Left K Femoral Artery, Right L Femoral Artery, Left M Popliteal Artery, Right N Popliteal Artery, Left P Anterior Tibial Artery, Right Q Anterior Tibial Artery, Left R Posterior Tibial Artery, Right S Posterior Tibial Artery, Left T Peroneal Artery, Right U Peroneal Artery, Left V Foot Artery, Right W Foot Artery, Left Y Lower Artery	0 Open 3 Percutaneous 4 Percutaneous endoscopic	C Extraluminal device D Intraluminal device Z No device	Z No qualifier

04W

MEDICAL AND SURGICAL SECTION – 2016 ICD-10-PCS

DEVICE GROUP: (Change), Insertion, Removal, Replacement, Revision, Supplement
Root Operations that always involve a device.

1ST - **0** Medical and Surgical
2ND - **4** Lower Arteries
3RD - **W REVISION**

EXAMPLE: Repair ruptured graft **CMS Ex:** Adjustment pacemaker lead

REVISION: Correcting, to the extent possible, a portion of a malfunctioning device or the position of a displaced device.

EXPLANATION: May replace components of a device ...

Body Part – 4TH	Approach – 5TH	Device – 6TH	Qualifier – 7TH
Y Lower Artery	0 Open 3 Percutaneous 4 Percutaneous endoscopic X External	0 Drainage device 2 Monitoring device 3 Infusion device 7 Autologous tissue substitute C Extraluminal device D Intraluminal device J Synthetic substitute K Nonautologous tissue substitute	Z No qualifier

Educational Annotations | 5 – Upper Veins

Body System Specific Educational Annotations for the Upper Veins include:
- Anatomy and Physiology Review
- Anatomical Illustrations
- Definitions of Common Procedures
- AHA Coding Clinic® Reference Notations
- Body Part Key Listings
- Device Key Listings
- Device Aggregation Table Listings
- Coding Notes

Anatomy and Physiology Review of Upper Veins

BODY PART VALUES – 5 - UPPER VEINS

Axillary Vein – The axillary vein drains to the subclavian vein and drains blood from the axilla, lateral thorax, and upper limb.

Azygos Vein – The azygos vein drains to the superior vena cava and drains blood from the right side of the posterior thorax.

Basilic Vein – The basilic vein drains to the axillary vein and drains blood from the hand and forearm.

Brachial Vein – The brachial vein drains to the axillary vein and drains blood from the upper limb.

Cephalic Vein – The cephalic vein drains to the axillary vein and drains blood from the hand.

External Jugular Vein – The external jugular vein drains to the subclavian vein and drains blood from the head and face.

Face Vein – Any of the smaller vein branches that drains the blood from the face.

Hand Vein – Any of the smaller vein branches that drains the blood from the hand.

Hemiazygos Vein – The hemiazygos vein drains to the azygos vein and drains blood from the left side of the posterior thorax.

Innominate Vein – The innominate vein drains to the superior vena cava and drains blood from the internal jugular vein and subclavian vein.

Internal Jugular Vein – The internal jugular vein drains to the subclavian vein and drains blood from the brain and face.

Intracranial Vein – Any of the smaller vein branches that drains the blood from within the skull.

Subclavian Vein – The subclavian vein drains to the innominate vein and drains blood from the axillary vein and external jugular vein.

Upper Vein – The veins located above the diaphragm (see Coding Guideline B2.1b).

Vein – Blood vessels that carry de-oxygenated (venous) blood away from the organs and tissues of the body and to the heart. Most veins have one-way valves to prevent backflow of venous blood and to assist the lower-pressure venous blood back to the heart.

Vertebral Vein – The vertebral vein drains to the innominate vein and drains blood from the neck.

Educational Annotations

5 – Upper Veins

Anatomical Illustrations of Upper Veins

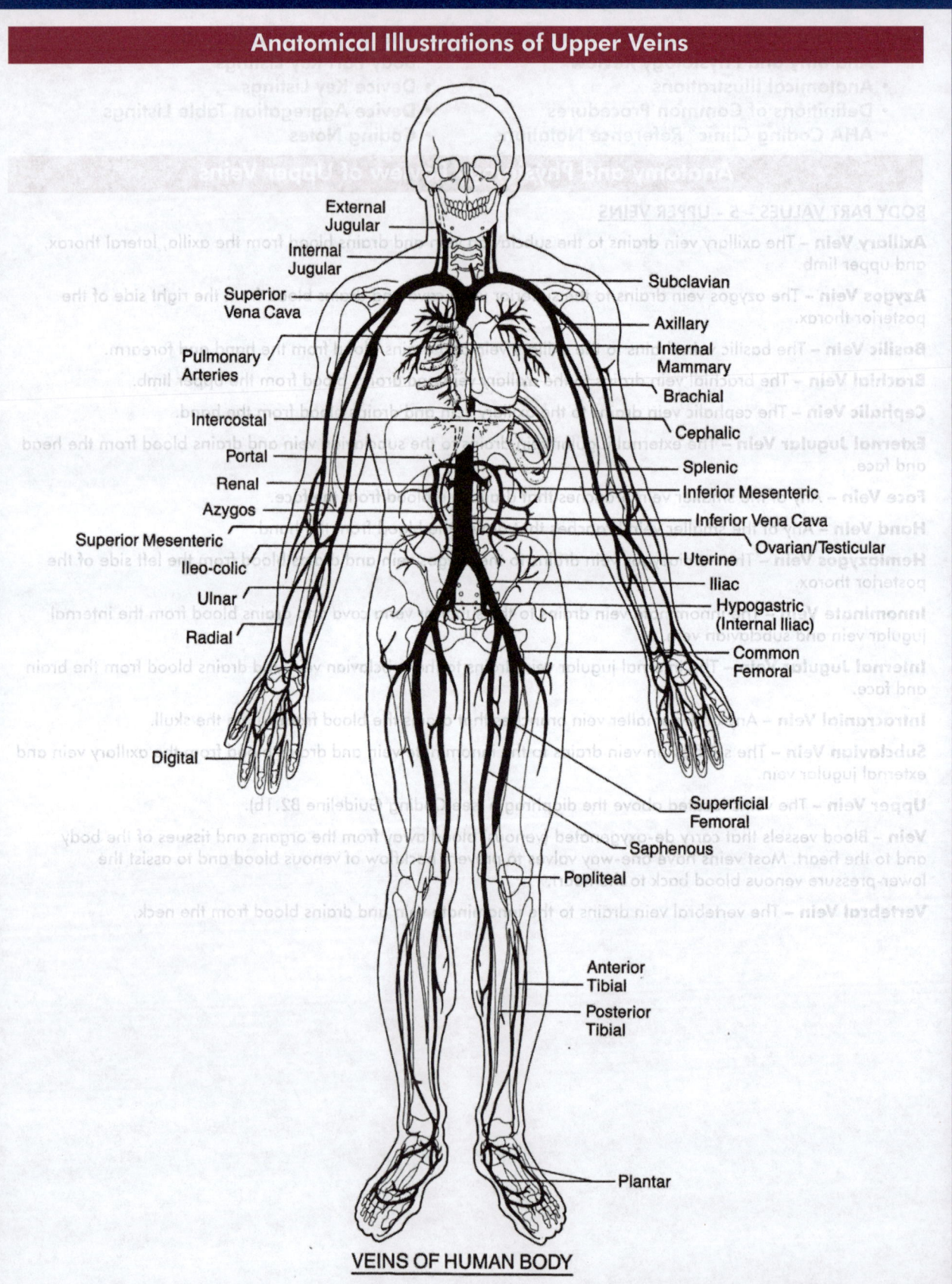

VEINS OF HUMAN BODY

Educational Annotations

5 – Upper Veins

Definitions of Common Procedures of Upper Veins

Excision of damaged vein – The surgical removal of a damaged vein segment.

Mobilization/superficialization of vein – The surgical elevation of a vein to a location just under the skin from a deeper tissue location for easier and safer cannulation access.

Superior vena cava filter – The placement of a wire filter device in the superior vena cava to prevent pulmonary emboli (PE) from upper-extremity deep vein thrombosis.

AHA Coding Clinic® Reference Notations of Upper Veins

ROOT OPERATION SPECIFIC - 5 - UPPER VEINS
BYPASS - 1
DESTRUCTION - 5
DILATION - 7
DRAINAGE - 9
EXCISION - B
EXTIRPATION - C
EXTRACTION - D
INSERTION - H
INSPECTION - J
OCCLUSION - L
RELEASE - N
REMOVAL - P
REPAIR - Q
REPLACEMENT - R
REPOSITION - S
    Superficialization of cephalic vein...AHA 13:4Q:p125
SUPPLEMENT - U
RESTRICTION - V
REVISION - W

Educational Annotations | 5 – Upper Veins

Body Part Key Listings of Upper Veins

See also Body Part Key in Appendix C

Accessory cephalic vein	*use* Cephalic Vein, Left/Right
Angular vein	*use* Face Vein, Left/Right
Anterior cerebral vein	*use* Intracranial Vein
Anterior facial vein	*use* Face Vein, Left/Right
Basal (internal) cerebral vein	*use* Intracranial Vein
Brachiocephalic vein	*use* Innominate Vein, Left/Right
Common facial vein	*use* Face Vein, Left/Right
Deep cervical vein	*use* Vertebral Vein, Left/Right
Deep facial vein	*use* Face Vein, Left/Right
Dorsal metacarpal vein	*use* Hand Vein, Left/Right
Dural venous sinus	*use* Intracranial Vein
Frontal vein	*use* Face Vein, Left/Right
Great cerebral vein	*use* Intracranial Vein
Inferior cerebellar vein	*use* Intracranial Vein
Inferior cerebral vein	*use* Intracranial Vein
Inferior thyroid vein	*use* Innominate Vein, Left/Right
Internal (basal) cerebral vein	*use* Intracranial Vein
Left ascending lumbar vein	*use* Hemiazygos Vein
Left subcostal vein	*use* Hemiazygos Vein
Median antebrachial vein	*use* Basilic Vein, Left/Right
Median cubital vein	*use* Basilic Vein, Left/Right
Middle cerebral vein	*use* Intracranial Vein
Ophthalmic vein	*use* Intracranial Vein
Palmar (volar) digital vein	*use* Hand Vein, Left/Right
Palmar (volar) metacarpal vein	*use* Hand Vein, Left/Right
Posterior auricular vein	*use* External Jugular Vein, Left/Right
Posterior facial (retromandibular) vein	*use* Face Vein, Left/Right
Radial vein	*use* Brachial Vein, Left/Right
Right ascending lumbar vein	*use* Azygos Vein
Right subcostal vein	*use* Azygos Vein
Suboccipital venous plexus	*use* Vertebral Vein, Left/Right
Superficial palmar venous arch	*use* Hand Vein, Left/Right
Superior cerebellar vein	*use* Intracranial Vein
Superior cerebral vein	*use* Intracranial Vein
Supraorbital vein	*use* Face Vein, Left/Right
Ulnar vein	*use* Brachial Vein, Left/Right
Volar (palmar) digital vein	*use* Hand Vein, Left/Right
Volar (palmar) metacarpal vein	*use* Hand Vein, Left/Right

Device Key Listings of Upper Veins

See also Device Key in Appendix D

Autograft	*use* Autologous Tissue Substitute
Autologous artery graft	*use* Autologous Arterial Tissue in Upper Veins
Autologous vein graft	*use* Autologous Venous Tissue in Upper Veins
Non-tunneled central venous catheter	*use* Infusion Device
Peripherally inserted central catheter (PICC)	*use* Infusion Device
Tissue bank graft	*use* Nonautologous Tissue Substitute

Educational Annotations | 5 – Upper Veins

Device Aggregation Table Listings of Upper Veins

See also Device Aggregation Table in Appendix E

Specific Device	For Operation	In Body System		General Device
Autologous Arterial Tissue	All applicable	Upper Veins	7	Autologous Tissue Substitute
Autologous Venous Tissue	All applicable	Upper Veins	7	Autologous Tissue Substitute

Coding Notes of Upper Veins

Body System Relevant Coding Guidelines

General Guidelines

B2.1b
Where the general body part values "upper" and "lower" are provided as an option in the Upper Arteries, Lower Arteries, Upper Veins, Lower Veins, Muscles and Tendons body systems, "upper" and "lower" specifies body parts located above or below the diaphragm respectively.
Example: Vein body parts above the diaphragm are found in the Upper Veins body system; vein body parts below the diaphragm are found in the Lower Veins body system.

Branches of body parts

B4.2
Where a specific branch of a body part does not have its own body part value in PCS, the body part is coded to the closest proximal branch that has a specific body part value.
Example: A procedure performed on the mandibular branch of the trigeminal nerve is coded to the trigeminal nerve body part value.

Body System Specific PCS Reference Manual Exercises

PCS CODE	5 – UPPER VEINS EXERCISES
059C3ZZ	Phlebotomy of left median cubital vein for polycythemia vera. (The median cubital vein is a branch of the basilic vein.)

5 – Upper Veins

Educational Annotations

NOTES

Device Aggregation Table Findings of Upper Veins

Specific Device	for Operation	in Body System	General Device
Autologous Arterial Tissue	All applicable	Upper Veins	Z Autologous Tissue Substitute
Autologous Venous Tissue	All applicable	Upper Veins	Z Autologous Tissue Substitute

See also Device Aggregation Table in Appendix E

Coding Notes of Upper Veins

Body System Relevant Coding Guidelines

General Guidelines
B2.1b
Where the general body part values "upper" and "lower" are provided as an option in the Upper Arteries, Lower Arteries, Upper Veins, Lower Veins, Muscles and Tendons body systems, "upper" and "lower" specifies body parts located above or below the diaphragm respectively.
Example: Vein body parts above the diaphragm are found in the Upper Veins body system; vein body parts below the diaphragm are found in the Lower Veins body system.

Branches of body parts
B4.2
Where a specific branch of a body part does not have its own body part value in PCS, the body part is coded to the closest proximal branch that has a specific body part value
Example: A procedure performed on the mandibular branch of the trigeminal nerve is coded to the trigeminal nerve body part value

Body System Specific PCS Reference Manual Exercises

5 – UPPER VEINS EXERCISES

PCS CODE	
0 5 9 C 3 Z Z	Phlebotomy of left median cubital vein for polycythemia vera. (The median cubital vein is a branch of the basilic vein.)

5 – UPPER VEINS

TUBULAR GROUP: Bypass, Dilation, Occlusion, Restriction
Root Operations that alter the diameter/route of a tubular body part.

1ST - 0 Medical and Surgical
2ND - 5 Upper Veins
3RD - 1 BYPASS

EXAMPLE: Bypass damaged subclavian | CMS Ex: Coronary artery bypass

BYPASS: Altering the route of passage of the contents of a tubular body part.

EXPLANATION: Rerouting contents to a downstream part ...

Body Part – 4TH		Approach – 5TH	Device – 6TH	Qualifier – 7TH
0 Azygos Vein	H Hand Vein, Left	0 Open	7 Autologous tissue substitute	Y Upper Vein
1 Hemiazygos Vein	L Intracranial Vein	4 Percutaneous endoscopic	9 Autologous venous tissue	
3 Innominate Vein, Right	M Internal Jugular Vein, Right		A Autologous arterial tissue	
4 Innominate Vein, Left	N Internal Jugular Vein, Left		J Synthetic substitute	
5 Subclavian Vein, Right			K Nonautologous tissue substitute	
6 Subclavian Vein, Left	P External Jugular Vein, Right		Z No device	
7 Axillary Vein, Right	Q External Jugular Vein, Left			
8 Axillary Vein, Left	R Vertebral Vein, Right			
9 Brachial Vein, Right	S Vertebral Vein, Left			
A Brachial Vein, Left	T Face Vein, Right			
B Basilic Vein, Right	V Face Vein, Left			
C Basilic Vein, Left				
D Cephalic Vein, Right				
F Cephalic Vein, Left				
G Hand Vein, Right				

EXCISION GROUP: Excision, (Resection), Destruction, Extraction, (Detachment)
Root Operations that take out some or all of a body part.

1ST - 0 Medical and Surgical
2ND - 5 Upper Veins
3RD - 5 DESTRUCTION

EXAMPLE: Fulguration venous lesion | CMS Ex: Fulguration polyp

DESTRUCTION: Physical eradication of all or a portion of a body part by the direct use of energy, force, or a destructive agent.

EXPLANATION: None of the body part is physically taken out

Body Part – 4TH		Approach – 5TH	Device – 6TH	Qualifier – 7TH
0 Azygos Vein	H Hand Vein, Left	0 Open	Z No device	Z No qualifier
1 Hemiazygos Vein	L Intracranial Vein	3 Percutaneous		
3 Innominate Vein, Right	M Internal Jugular Vein, Right	4 Percutaneous endoscopic		
4 Innominate Vein, Left	N Internal Jugular Vein, Left			
5 Subclavian Vein, Right				
6 Subclavian Vein, Left	P External Jugular Vein, Right			
7 Axillary Vein, Right	Q External Jugular Vein, Left			
8 Axillary Vein, Left	R Vertebral Vein, Right			
9 Brachial Vein, Right	S Vertebral Vein, Left			
A Brachial Vein, Left	T Face Vein, Right			
B Basilic Vein, Right	V Face Vein, Left			
C Basilic Vein, Left	Y Upper Vein			
D Cephalic Vein, Right				
F Cephalic Vein, Left				
G Hand Vein, Right				

057

MEDICAL AND SURGICAL SECTION – 2016 ICD-10-PCS [2016.PCS]

TUBULAR GROUP: Bypass, Dilation, Occlusion, Restriction
Root Operations that alter the diameter/route of a tubular body part.

1ST - **0** Medical and Surgical	EXAMPLE: Balloon dilation axillary vein — CMS Ex: Transluminal angioplasty
2ND - **5** Upper Veins	**DILATION:** Expanding an orifice or the lumen of a tubular body part.
3RD - **7 DILATION**	EXPLANATION: By force (stretching) or cutting ...

Body Part – 4TH		Approach – 5TH	Device – 6TH	Qualifier – 7TH
0 Azygos Vein	H Hand Vein, Left	0 Open	D Intraluminal device	Z No qualifier
1 Hemiazygos Vein	L Intracranial Vein NC*	3 Percutaneous	Z No device	
3 Innominate Vein, Right	M Internal Jugular Vein, Right	4 Percutaneous endoscopic		
4 Innominate Vein, Left				
5 Subclavian Vein, Right	N Internal Jugular Vein, Left			
6 Subclavian Vein, Left				
7 Axillary Vein, Right	P External Jugular Vein, Right			
8 Axillary Vein, Left				
9 Brachial Vein, Right	Q External Jugular Vein, Left			
A Brachial Vein, Left				
B Basilic Vein, Right	R Vertebral Vein, Right			
C Basilic Vein, Left	S Vertebral Vein, Left			
D Cephalic Vein, Right	T Face Vein, Right			
F Cephalic Vein, Left	V Face Vein, Left			
G Hand Vein, Right	Y Upper Vein			

NC* – Some procedures are considered non-covered by Medicare. See current Medicare Code Editor for details.

UPPER VEINS

057

5 – UPPER VEINS

DRAINAGE GROUP: Drainage, Extirpation, (Fragmentation)
Root Operations that take out solids/fluids/gases from a body part.

1ST - 0 Medical and Surgical
2ND - 5 Upper Veins
3RD - 9 DRAINAGE

EXAMPLE: Phlebotomy basilic vein   **CMS Ex:** Thoracentesis

DRAINAGE: Taking or letting out fluids and/or gases from a body part.

EXPLANATION: Qualifier "X Diagnostic" indicates biopsy …

Body Part – 4TH		Approach – 5TH	Device – 6TH	Qualifier – 7TH
0 Azygos Vein	H Hand Vein, Left	0 Open	0 Drainage device	Z No qualifier
1 Hemiazygos Vein	L Intracranial Vein	3 Percutaneous		
3 Innominate Vein, Right	M Internal Jugular Vein, Right	4 Percutaneous endoscopic		
4 Innominate Vein, Left				
5 Subclavian Vein, Right	N Internal Jugular Vein, Left			
6 Subclavian Vein, Left				
7 Axillary Vein, Right	P External Jugular Vein, Right			
8 Axillary Vein, Left				
9 Brachial Vein, Right	Q External Jugular Vein, Left			
A Brachial Vein, Left				
B Basilic Vein, Right	R Vertebral Vein, Right			
C Basilic Vein, Left	S Vertebral Vein, Left			
D Cephalic Vein, Right	T Face Vein, Right			
F Cephalic Vein, Left	V Face Vein, Left			
G Hand Vein, Right	Y Upper Vein			

Body Part – 4TH		Approach – 5TH	Device – 6TH	Qualifier – 7TH
0 Azygos Vein	H Hand Vein, Left	0 Open	Z No device	X Diagnostic
1 Hemiazygos Vein	L Intracranial Vein	3 Percutaneous		Z No qualifier
3 Innominate Vein, Right	M Internal Jugular Vein, Right	4 Percutaneous endoscopic		
4 Innominate Vein, Left				
5 Subclavian Vein, Right	N Internal Jugular Vein, Left			
6 Subclavian Vein, Left				
7 Axillary Vein, Right	P External Jugular Vein, Right			
8 Axillary Vein, Left				
9 Brachial Vein, Right	Q External Jugular Vein, Left			
A Brachial Vein, Left				
B Basilic Vein, Right	R Vertebral Vein, Right			
C Basilic Vein, Left	S Vertebral Vein, Left			
D Cephalic Vein, Right	T Face Vein, Right			
F Cephalic Vein, Left	V Face Vein, Left			
G Hand Vein, Right	Y Upper Vein			

05B

MEDICAL AND SURGICAL SECTION – 2016 ICD-10-PCS

EXCISION GROUP: Excision, (Resection), Destruction, Extraction, (Detachment)
Root Operations that take out some or all of a body part.

1ST – **0** Medical and Surgical	EXAMPLE: Harvest brachial vein — CMS Ex: Liver biopsy
2ND – **5** Upper Veins	**EXCISION:** Cutting out or off, without replacement, a portion of a body part.
3RD – **B** EXCISION	EXPLANATION: Qualifier "X Diagnostic" indicates biopsy ...

Body Part – 4TH		Approach – 5TH	Device – 6TH	Qualifier – 7TH
0 Azygos Vein	H Hand Vein, Left	0 Open	Z No device	X Diagnostic
1 Hemiazygos Vein	L Intracranial Vein	3 Percutaneous		Z No qualifier
3 Innominate Vein, Right	M Internal Jugular Vein, Right	4 Percutaneous endoscopic		
4 Innominate Vein, Left				
5 Subclavian Vein, Right	N Internal Jugular Vein, Left			
6 Subclavian Vein, Left				
7 Axillary Vein, Right	P External Jugular Vein, Right			
8 Axillary Vein, Left				
9 Brachial Vein, Right	Q External Jugular Vein, Left			
A Brachial Vein, Left				
B Basilic Vein, Right	R Vertebral Vein, Right			
C Basilic Vein, Left	S Vertebral Vein, Left			
D Cephalic Vein, Right	T Face Vein, Right			
F Cephalic Vein, Left	V Face Vein, Left			
G Hand Vein, Right	Y Upper Vein			

DRAINAGE GROUP: Drainage, Extirpation, (Fragmentation)
Root Operations that take out solids/fluids/gases from a body part.

1ST – **0** Medical and Surgical	EXAMPLE: Mechanical thrombectomy — CMS Ex: Choledocholithotomy
2ND – **5** Upper Veins	**EXTIRPATION:** Taking or cutting out solid matter from a body part.
3RD – **C** EXTIRPATION	EXPLANATION: Abnormal byproduct or foreign body ...

Body Part – 4TH		Approach – 5TH	Device – 6TH	Qualifier – 7TH
0 Azygos Vein	H Hand Vein, Left	0 Open	Z No device	Z No qualifier
1 Hemiazygos Vein	L Intracranial Vein NC*	3 Percutaneous		
3 Innominate Vein, Right	M Internal Jugular Vein, Right	4 Percutaneous endoscopic		
4 Innominate Vein, Left				
5 Subclavian Vein, Right	N Internal Jugular Vein, Left			
6 Subclavian Vein, Left				
7 Axillary Vein, Right	P External Jugular Vein, Right			
8 Axillary Vein, Left				
9 Brachial Vein, Right	Q External Jugular Vein, Left			
A Brachial Vein, Left				
B Basilic Vein, Right	R Vertebral Vein, Right			
C Basilic Vein, Left	S Vertebral Vein, Left			
D Cephalic Vein, Right	T Face Vein, Right			
F Cephalic Vein, Left	V Face Vein, Left			
G Hand Vein, Right	Y Upper Vein			

NC* – Some procedures are considered non-covered by Medicare. See current Medicare Code Editor for details.

5 – UPPER VEINS 0 5 H

EXCISION GROUP: Excision, (Resection), Destruction, Extraction, (Detachment)
Root Operations that take out some or all of a body part.

- 1ST – **0** Medical and Surgical
- 2ND – **5** Upper Veins
- 3RD – **D** EXTRACTION

EXAMPLE: Vein ligation and stripping CMS Ex: D&C

EXTRACTION: Pulling or stripping out or off all or a portion of a body part by the use of force.

EXPLANATION: None for this Body System

Body Part – 4TH		Approach – 5TH	Device – 6TH	Qualifier – 7TH
9 Brachial Vein, Right	D Cephalic Vein, Right	0 Open	Z No device	Z No qualifier
A Brachial Vein, Left	F Cephalic Vein, Left	3 Percutaneous		
B Basilic Vein, Right	G Hand Vein, Right			
C Basilic Vein, Left	H Hand Vein, Left			
	Y Upper Vein			

DEVICE GROUP: (Change), Insertion, Removal, Replacement, Revision, Supplement
Root Operations that always involve a device.

- 1ST – **0** Medical and Surgical
- 2ND – **5** Upper Veins
- 3RD – **H** INSERTION

EXAMPLE: Insertion central venous line CMS Ex: Insertion CVP cath

INSERTION: Putting in a nonbiological appliance that monitors, assists, performs, or prevents a physiological function but does not physically take the place of a body part.

EXPLANATION: None

Body Part – 4TH		Approach – 5TH	Device – 6TH	Qualifier – 7TH
0 Azygos Vein	H Hand Vein, Left	0 Open	3 Infusion device	Z No qualifier
1 Hemiazygos Vein	L Intracranial Vein	3 Percutaneous	D Intraluminal device	
3 Innominate Vein, Right	M Internal Jugular Vein, Right	4 Percutaneous endoscopic		
4 Innominate Vein, Left	N Internal Jugular Vein, Left			
5 Subclavian Vein, Right	P External Jugular Vein, Right			
6 Subclavian Vein, Left	Q External Jugular Vein, Left			
7 Axillary Vein, Right	R Vertebral Vein, Right			
8 Axillary Vein, Left	S Vertebral Vein, Left			
9 Brachial Vein, Right	T Face Vein, Right			
A Brachial Vein, Left	V Face Vein, Left			
B Basilic Vein, Right				
C Basilic Vein, Left				
D Cephalic Vein, Right				
F Cephalic Vein, Left				
G Hand Vein, Right				
Y Upper Vein		0 Open	2 Monitoring device	Z No qualifier
		3 Percutaneous	3 Infusion device	
		4 Percutaneous endoscopic	D Intraluminal device	

05J MEDICAL AND SURGICAL SECTION – 2016 ICD-10-PCS

EXAMINATION GROUP: Inspection, (Map)
Root Operations involving examination only.

- 1ST – **0** Medical and Surgical
- 2ND – **5** Upper Veins
- 3RD – **J** INSPECTION

EXAMPLE: Open intracranial vein examination
CMS Ex: Colonoscopy

INSPECTION: Visually and/or manually exploring a body part.

EXPLANATION: Direct or instrumental visualization ...

Body Part – 4TH	Approach – 5TH	Device – 6TH	Qualifier – 7TH
Y Upper Vein	0 Open 3 Percutaneous 4 Percutaneous endoscopic X External	Z No device	Z No qualifier

TUBULAR GROUP: Bypass, Dilation, Occlusion, Restriction
Root Operations that alter the diameter/route of a tubular body part.

- 1ST – **0** Medical and Surgical
- 2ND – **5** Upper Veins
- 3RD – **L** OCCLUSION

EXAMPLE: Ligation jugular vein
CMS Ex: Fallopian tube ligation

OCCLUSION: Completely closing an orifice or lumen of a tubular body part.

EXPLANATION: Natural or artificially created orifice ...

Body Part – 4TH	Approach – 5TH	Device – 6TH	Qualifier – 7TH
0 Azygos Vein 1 Hemiazygos Vein 3 Innominate Vein, Right 4 Innominate Vein, Left 5 Subclavian Vein, Right 6 Subclavian Vein, Left 7 Axillary Vein, Right 8 Axillary Vein, Left 9 Brachial Vein, Right A Brachial Vein, Left B Basilic Vein, Right C Basilic Vein, Left D Cephalic Vein, Right F Cephalic Vein, Left G Hand Vein, Right H Hand Vein, Left L Intracranial Vein M Internal Jugular Vein, Right N Internal Jugular Vein, Left P External Jugular Vein, Right Q External Jugular Vein, Left R Vertebral Vein, Right S Vertebral Vein, Left T Face Vein, Right V Face Vein, Left Y Upper Vein	0 Open 3 Percutaneous 4 Percutaneous endoscopic	C Extraluminal device D Intraluminal device Z No device	Z No qualifier

5 – UPPER VEINS   05P

DIVISION GROUP: (Division), Release
Root Operations involving cutting or separation only.

1ST - 0	Medical and Surgical
2ND - 5	Upper Veins
3RD - N	RELEASE

EXAMPLE: Adhesiolysis brachial vein   **CMS Ex:** Carpal tunnel release

RELEASE: Freeing a body part from an abnormal physical constraint by cutting or by the use of force.

EXPLANATION: None of the body part is taken out ...

Body Part – 4TH		Approach – 5TH	Device – 6TH	Qualifier – 7TH
0 Azygos Vein	H Hand Vein, Left	0 Open	Z No device	Z No qualifier
1 Hemiazygos Vein	L Intracranial Vein	3 Percutaneous		
3 Innominate Vein, Right	M Internal Jugular Vein, Right	4 Percutaneous endoscopic		
4 Innominate Vein, Left				
5 Subclavian Vein, Right	N Internal Jugular Vein, Left			
6 Subclavian Vein, Left				
7 Axillary Vein, Right	P External Jugular Vein, Right			
8 Axillary Vein, Left				
9 Brachial Vein, Right	Q External Jugular Vein, Left			
A Brachial Vein, Left				
B Basilic Vein, Right	R Vertebral Vein, Right			
C Basilic Vein, Left	S Vertebral Vein, Left			
D Cephalic Vein, Right	T Face Vein, Right			
F Cephalic Vein, Left	V Face Vein, Left			
G Hand Vein, Right	Y Upper Vein			

DEVICE GROUP: (Change), Insertion, Removal, Replacement, Revision, Supplement
Root Operations that always involve a device.

1ST - 0	Medical and Surgical
2ND - 5	Upper Veins
3RD - P	REMOVAL

EXAMPLE: Removal central venous line   **CMS Ex:** Chest tube removal

REMOVAL: Taking out or off a device from a body part.

EXPLANATION: Removal device without reinsertion ...

Body Part – 4TH	Approach – 5TH	Device – 6TH	Qualifier – 7TH
Y Upper Vein	0 Open 3 Percutaneous 4 Percutaneous endoscopic	0 Drainage device 2 Monitoring device 3 Infusion device 7 Autologous tissue substitute C Extraluminal device D Intraluminal device J Synthetic substitute K Nonautologous tissue substitute	Z No qualifier
Y Upper Vein	X External	0 Drainage device 2 Monitoring device 3 Infusion device D Intraluminal device	Z No qualifier

05Q — MEDICAL AND SURGICAL SECTION – 2016 ICD-10-PCS

OTHER REPAIRS GROUP: (Control), Repair
Root Operations that define other repairs.

1ST - 0 Medical and Surgical
2ND - 5 Upper Veins
3RD - Q REPAIR

EXAMPLE: Suture lacerated cephalic vein | CMS Ex: Suture laceration

REPAIR: Restoring, to the extent possible, a body part to its normal anatomic structure and function.

EXPLANATION: Only when no other root operation applies ...

Body Part – 4TH		Approach – 5TH	Device – 6TH	Qualifier – 7TH
0 Azygos Vein	H Hand Vein, Left	0 Open	Z No device	Z No qualifier
1 Hemiazygos Vein	L Intracranial Vein	3 Percutaneous		
3 Innominate Vein, Right	M Internal Jugular Vein, Right	4 Percutaneous endoscopic		
4 Innominate Vein, Left				
5 Subclavian Vein, Right	N Internal Jugular Vein, Left			
6 Subclavian Vein, Left				
7 Axillary Vein, Right	P External Jugular Vein, Right			
8 Axillary Vein, Left				
9 Brachial Vein, Right	Q External Jugular Vein, Left			
A Brachial Vein, Left				
B Basilic Vein, Right	R Vertebral Vein, Right			
C Basilic Vein, Left	S Vertebral Vein, Left			
D Cephalic Vein, Right	T Face Vein, Right			
F Cephalic Vein, Left	V Face Vein, Left			
G Hand Vein, Right	Y Upper Vein			

DEVICE GROUP: (Change), Insertion, Removal, Replacement, Revision, Supplement
Root Operations that always involve a device.

1ST - 0 Medical and Surgical
2ND - 5 Upper Veins
3RD - R REPLACEMENT

EXAMPLE: Spiral jugular vein replacement graft | CMS Ex: Total hip

REPLACEMENT: Putting in or on a biological or synthetic material that physically takes the place and/or function of all or a portion of a body part.

EXPLANATION: Includes taking out body part, or eradication...

Body Part – 4TH		Approach – 5TH	Device – 6TH	Qualifier – 7TH
0 Azygos Vein	H Hand Vein, Left	0 Open	7 Autologous tissue substitute	Z No qualifier
1 Hemiazygos Vein	L Intracranial Vein	4 Percutaneous endoscopic	J Synthetic substitute	
3 Innominate Vein, Right	M Internal Jugular Vein, Right		K Nonautologous tissue substitute	
4 Innominate Vein, Left				
5 Subclavian Vein, Right	N Internal Jugular Vein, Left			
6 Subclavian Vein, Left				
7 Axillary Vein, Right	P External Jugular Vein, Right			
8 Axillary Vein, Left				
9 Brachial Vein, Right	Q External Jugular Vein, Left			
A Brachial Vein, Left				
B Basilic Vein, Right	R Vertebral Vein, Right			
C Basilic Vein, Left	S Vertebral Vein, Left			
D Cephalic Vein, Right	T Face Vein, Right			
F Cephalic Vein, Left	V Face Vein, Left			
G Hand Vein, Right	Y Upper Vein			

5 – UPPER VEINS 05U

MOVE GROUP: (Reattachment), Reposition, (Transfer), (Transplantation)
Root Operations that put in/put back or move some/all of a body part.

1ST - 0 Medical and Surgical
2ND - 5 Upper Veins
3RD - S REPOSITION

EXAMPLE: Superficialization cephalic vein | CMS Ex: Fracture reduction

REPOSITION: Moving to its normal location, or other suitable location, all or a portion of a body part.

EXPLANATION: May or may not be cut to be moved ...

Body Part – 4TH		Approach – 5TH	Device – 6TH	Qualifier – 7TH
0 Azygos Vein	H Hand Vein, Left	0 Open	Z No device	Z No qualifier
1 Hemiazygos Vein	L Intracranial Vein	3 Percutaneous		
3 Innominate Vein, Right	M Internal Jugular Vein, Right	4 Percutaneous endoscopic		
4 Innominate Vein, Left	N Internal Jugular Vein, Left			
5 Subclavian Vein, Right				
6 Subclavian Vein, Left	P External Jugular Vein, Right			
7 Axillary Vein, Right	Q External Jugular Vein, Left			
8 Axillary Vein, Left				
9 Brachial Vein, Right	R Vertebral Vein, Right			
A Brachial Vein, Left	S Vertebral Vein, Left			
B Basilic Vein, Right	T Face Vein, Right			
C Basilic Vein, Left	V Face Vein, Left			
D Cephalic Vein, Right	Y Upper Vein			
F Cephalic Vein, Left				
G Hand Vein, Right				

DEVICE GROUP: (Change), Insertion, Removal, Replacement, Revision, Supplement
Root Operations that always involve a device.

1ST - 0 Medical and Surgical
2ND - 5 Upper Veins
3RD - U SUPPLEMENT

EXAMPLE: Patch graft venoplasty | CMS Ex: Hernia repair with mesh

SUPPLEMENT: Putting in or on biological or synthetic material that physically reinforces and/or augments the function of a portion of a body part.

EXPLANATION: Biological material from same individual ...

Body Part – 4TH		Approach – 5TH	Device – 6TH	Qualifier – 7TH
0 Azygos Vein	H Hand Vein, Left	0 Open	7 Autologous tissue substitute	Z No qualifier
1 Hemiazygos Vein	L Intracranial Vein	3 Percutaneous	J Synthetic substitute	
3 Innominate Vein, Right	M Internal Jugular Vein, Right	4 Percutaneous endoscopic	K Nonautologous tissue substitute	
4 Innominate Vein, Left	N Internal Jugular Vein, Left			
5 Subclavian Vein, Right				
6 Subclavian Vein, Left	P External Jugular Vein, Right			
7 Axillary Vein, Right	Q External Jugular Vein, Left			
8 Axillary Vein, Left				
9 Brachial Vein, Right	R Vertebral Vein, Right			
A Brachial Vein, Left	S Vertebral Vein, Left			
B Basilic Vein, Right	T Face Vein, Right			
C Basilic Vein, Left	V Face Vein, Left			
D Cephalic Vein, Right	Y Upper Vein			
F Cephalic Vein, Left				
G Hand Vein, Right				

05V — MEDICAL AND SURGICAL SECTION – 2016 ICD-10-PCS

TUBULAR GROUP: Bypass, Dilation, Occlusion, Restriction
Root Operations that alter the diameter/route of a tubular body part.

EXAMPLE: Restrictive venous stent **CMS Ex:** Cervical cerclage

- 1ST – **0** Medical and Surgical
- 2ND – **5** Upper Veins
- 3RD – **V** RESTRICTION

RESTRICTION: Partially closing an orifice or the lumen of a tubular body part.

EXPLANATION: Natural or artificially created orifice …

Body Part – 4TH		Approach – 5TH	Device – 6TH	Qualifier – 7TH
0 Azygos Vein	H Hand Vein, Left	0 Open	C Extraluminal device	Z No qualifier
1 Hemiazygos Vein	L Intracranial Vein	3 Percutaneous	D Intraluminal device	
3 Innominate Vein, Right	M Internal Jugular Vein, Right	4 Percutaneous endoscopic	Z No device	
4 Innominate Vein, Left	N Internal Jugular Vein, Left			
5 Subclavian Vein, Right	P External Jugular Vein, Right			
6 Subclavian Vein, Left	Q External Jugular Vein, Left			
7 Axillary Vein, Right	R Vertebral Vein, Right			
8 Axillary Vein, Left	S Vertebral Vein, Left			
9 Brachial Vein, Right	T Face Vein, Right			
A Brachial Vein, Left	V Face Vein, Left			
B Basilic Vein, Right	Y Upper Vein			
C Basilic Vein, Left				
D Cephalic Vein, Right				
F Cephalic Vein, Left				
G Hand Vein, Right				

DEVICE GROUP: (Change), Insertion, Removal, Replacement, Revision, Supplement
Root Operations that always involve a device.

EXAMPLE: Reposition central line line **CMS Ex:** Adjust pacemaker lead

- 1ST – **0** Medical and Surgical
- 2ND – **5** Upper Veins
- 3RD – **W** REVISION

REVISION: Correcting, to the extent possible, a portion of a malfunctioning device or the position of a displaced device.

EXPLANATION: May replace components of a device …

Body Part – 4TH	Approach – 5TH	Device – 6TH	Qualifier – 7TH
Y Upper Vein	0 Open	0 Drainage device	Z No qualifier
	3 Percutaneous	2 Monitoring device	
	4 Percutaneous endoscopic	3 Infusion device	
	X External	7 Autologous tissue substitute	
		C Extraluminal device	
		D Intraluminal device	
		J Synthetic substitute	
		K Nonautologous tissue substitute	

Educational Annotations | 6 – Lower Veins

Body System Specific Educational Annotations for the Lower Veins include:
- Anatomy and Physiology Review
- Anatomical Illustrations
- Definitions of Common Procedures
- AHA Coding Clinic® Reference Notations
- Body Part Key Listings
- Device Key Listings
- Device Aggregation Table Listings
- Coding Notes

Anatomy and Physiology Review of Lower Veins

BODY PART VALUES – 6 - LOWER VEINS

Colic Vein – The colic vein drains to the superior mesenteric vein and drains blood from the colon.

Common Iliac Vein – The common iliac vein drains to the inferior vena cava and drains blood from the external and hypogastric (also known as the internal iliac vein) veins.

Esophageal Vein – The esophageal vein drains to the azygos vein and drains blood from the esophagus.

External Iliac Vein – The external iliac vein drains to the common iliac vein and drains blood from the femoral veins.

Femoral Vein – The femoral vein drains to the external iliac vein and drains blood from the lower limb.

Foot Vein – Any of the smaller vein branches that drains the blood from the foot.

Gastric Vein – The gastric vein drains to the portal vein and drains blood from the stomach.

Greater Saphenous Vein – The greater saphenous vein drains to the femoral vein and drains blood from the lower limb including the plantar portion of the foot.

Hepatic Vein – The hepatic vein drains to the inferior vena cava and drains blood from the liver, pancreas, and small intestine.

Hypogastric Vein – The hypogastric vein (also known as the internal iliac vein) drains to the common iliac vein and drains blood from the pelvic viscera and reproductive organs.

Inferior Mesenteric Vein – The inferior mesenteric vein drains to the splenic vein and drains blood from the large intestine.

Inferior Vena Cava – The inferior vena cava drains to the right atrium of the heart and drains blood from the common iliac veins.

Lesser Saphenous Vein – The lesser saphenous vein drains to the popliteal vein and drains blood from the dorsal portion of the foot.

Lower Vein – The veins located below the diaphragm (see Coding Guideline B2.1b).

Portal Vein – The portal vein drains to the hepatic vein and drains blood from the gastrointestinal tract and liver.

Renal Vein – The renal vein drains to the inferior vena cava and drains blood from the kidney.

Splenic Vein – The splenic vein drains to the portal vein and drains blood from the spleen and pancreas.

Superior Mesenteric Vein – The superior mesenteric vein drains to the portal vein and drains blood from the small intestine.

Vein – Blood vessels that carry de-oxygenated (venous) blood away from the organs and tissues of the body and to the heart. Most veins have one-way valves to prevent backflow of venous blood and to assist the lower-pressure venous blood back to the heart.

Educational Annotations

6 – Lower Veins

Anatomical Illustrations of Lower Veins

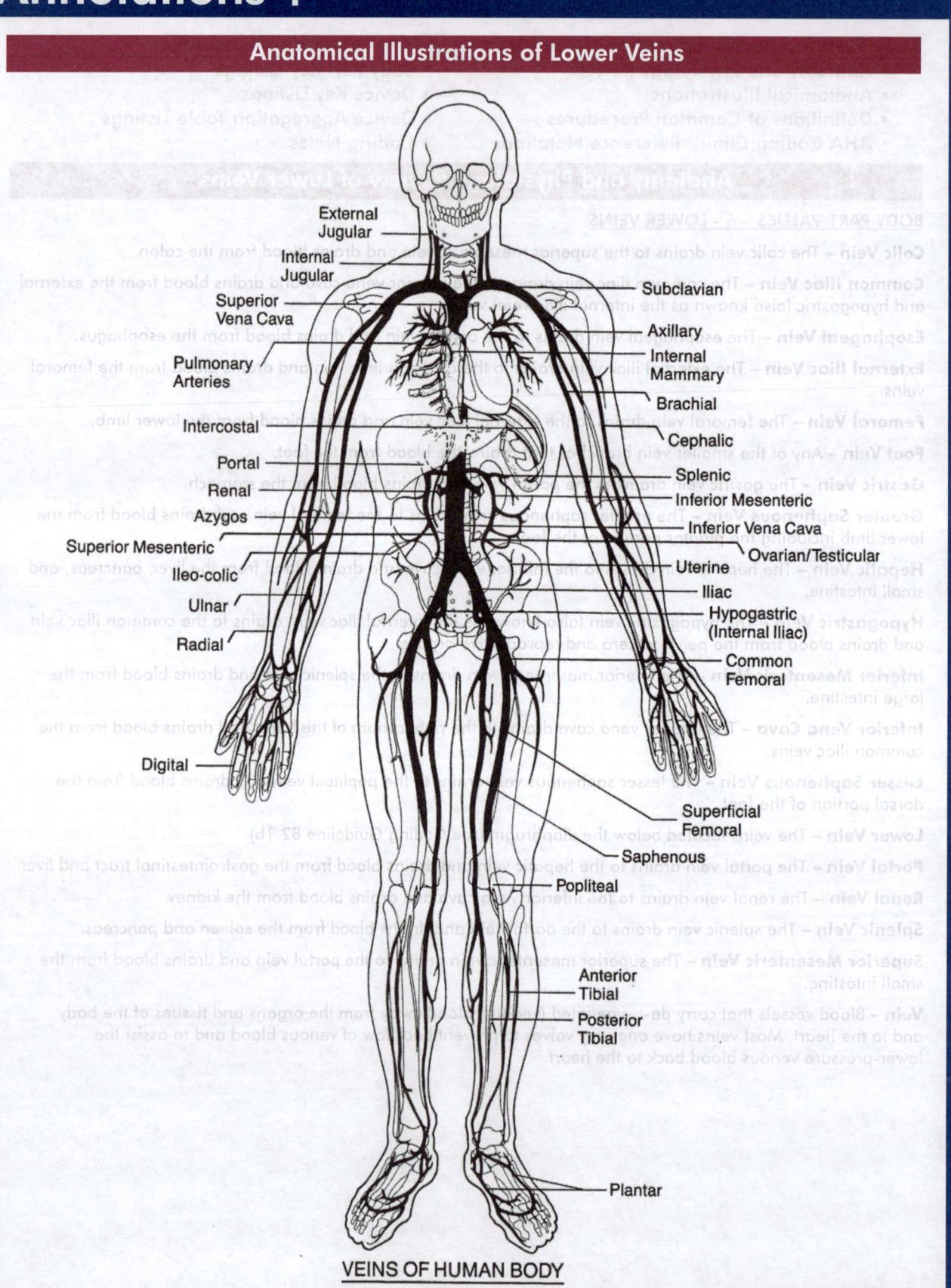

VEINS OF HUMAN BODY

Educational Annotations | 6 – Lower Veins

Definitions of Common Procedures of Lower Veins

Endovenous laser vein ablation – The placement of a laser-tipped catheter into the targeted vein, using the laser energy to destroy the vein by causing it to collapse and seal shut without removing it.

External light laser treatment of varicose veins – The use of an external laser to send strong bursts of light to small, superficial varicose veins and spider veins that make the veins slowly fade away.

Harvesting of saphenous vein – The surgical removal of a segment of a saphenous vein to be used as a vessel graft (e.g., coronary artery bypass, femoral-popliteal bypass).

Inferior vena cava filter – The placement of a wire filter device in the inferior vena cava to prevent pulmonary emboli (PE) from lower-extremity deep vein thrombosis.

Ligation and stripping of varicose veins – The surgical removal of enlarged, painful lower leg veins that is performed by making small incisions at the distal and proximal locations and using an attached endovenous wire to pull the vein out of the leg.

AHA Coding Clinic® Reference Notations of Lower Veins

ROOT OPERATION SPECIFIC - 6 - LOWER VEINS
BYPASS - 1
DESTRUCTION - 5
DILATION - 7
DIVISION - 8
EXCISION - B
    Coronary artery bypass graft, using greater saphenous vein ....AHA 14:3Q:p20
    ....AHA 14:1Q:p10
    Unspecified saphenous vein harvested ....AHA 14:3Q:p8
EXTIRPATION - C
    Pharmacomechanical thrombolysis of femoral venous thrombus ....AHA 13:4Q:p115
EXTRACTION - D
INSERTION - H
    Insertion of a Mahurkar catheter into inferior vena cava (IVC)...............AHA 13:3Q:p18
INSPECTION - J
OCCLUSION - L
    Endoscopic ligation of esophageal varices using bands ....AHA 13:4Q:p112
RELEASE - N
REMOVAL - P
REPAIR - Q
REPLACEMENT - R
REPOSITION - S
SUPPLEMENT - U
RESTRICTION - T
REVISION - W
    Removal of clots from transjugular intrahepatic portosystemic shunt (TIPS) AHA 14:3Q:p25

Educational Annotations

6 – Lower Veins

Body Part Key Listings of Lower Veins

See also Body Part Key in Appendix C

Common digital vein	*use* Foot Vein, Left/Right
Deep femoral (profunda femoris) vein	*use* Femoral Vein, Left/Right
Dorsal metatarsal vein	*use* Foot Vein, Left/Right
Dorsal venous arch	*use* Foot Vein, Left/Right
External pudendal vein	*use* Greater Saphenous Vein, Left/Right
Gluteal vein	*use* Hypogastric Vein, Left/Right
Great saphenous vein	*use* Greater Saphenous Vein, Left/Right
Hepatic portal vein	*use* Portal Vein
Ileocolic vein	*use* Colic Vein
Internal iliac vein	*use* Hypogastric Vein, Left/Right
Internal pudendal vein	*use* Hypogastric Vein, Left/Right
Lateral sacral vein	*use* Hypogastric Vein, Left/Right
Left colic vein	*use* Colic Vein
Left gastroepiploic vein	*use* Splenic Vein
Left inferior phrenic vein	*use* Renal Vein, Left
Left ovarian vein	*use* Renal Vein, Left
Left second lumbar vein	*use* Renal Vein, Left
Left suprarenal vein	*use* Renal Vein, Left
Left testicular vein	*use* Renal Vein, Left
Middle colic vein	*use* Colic Vein
Middle hemorrhoidal vein	*use* Hypogastric Vein, Left/Right
Obturator vein	*use* Hypogastric Vein, Left/Right
Pancreatic vein	*use* Splenic Vein
Plantar digital vein	*use* Foot Vein, Left/Right
Plantar metatarsal vein	*use* Foot Vein, Left/Right
Plantar venous arch	*use* Foot Vein, Left/Right
Popliteal vein	*use* Femoral Vein, Left/Right
Postcava	*use* Inferior Vena Cava
Profunda femoris (deep femoral) vein	*use* Femoral Vein, Left/Right
Right colic vein	*use* Colic Vein
Right gastroepiploic vein	*use* Superior Mesenteric Vein
Right inferior phrenic vein	*use* Inferior Vena Cava
Right ovarian vein	*use* Inferior Vena Cava
Right second lumbar vein	*use* Inferior Vena Cava
Right suprarenal vein	*use* Inferior Vena Cava
Right testicular vein	*use* Inferior Vena Cava
Sigmoid vein	*use* Inferior Mesenteric Vein
Small saphenous vein	*use* Lesser Saphenous Vein, Left/Right
Superficial circumflex iliac vein	*use* Greater Saphenous Vein, Left/Right
Superficial epigastric vein	*use* Greater Saphenous Vein, Left/Right
Superior rectal vein	*use* Inferior Mesenteric Vein
Uterine vein	*use* Hypogastric Vein, Left/Right
Vaginal vein	*use* Hypogastric Vein, Left/Right
Vesical vein	*use* Hypogastric Vein, Left/Right

Educational Annotations | 6 – Lower Veins

Device Key Listings of Lower Veins

See also Device Key in Appendix D

Autograft	*use* Autologous Tissue Substitute
Autologous artery graft	*use* Autologous Arterial Tissue in Lower Veins
Autologous vein graft	*use* Autologous Venous Tissue in Lower Veins
Non-tunneled central venous catheter	*use* Infusion Device
Tissue bank graft	*use* Nonautologous Tissue Substitute

Device Aggregation Table Listings of Lower Veins

See also Device Aggregation Table in Appendix E

Specific Device	For Operation	In Body System		General Device
Autologous Arterial Tissue	All applicable	Lower Veins	7	Autologous Tissue Substitute
Autologous Venous Tissue	All applicable	Lower Veins	7	Autologous Tissue Substitute

Coding Notes of Lower Veins

Body System Relevant Coding Guidelines

General Guidelines

B2.1b
Where the general body part values "upper" and "lower" are provided as an option in the Upper Arteries, Lower Arteries, Upper Veins, Lower Veins, Muscles and Tendons body systems, "upper" and "lower" specifies body parts located above or below the diaphragm respectively.
Example: Vein body parts above the diaphragm are found in the Upper Veins body system; vein body parts below the diaphragm are found in the Lower Veins body system.

Branches of body parts

B4.2
Where a specific branch of a body part does not have its own body part value in PCS, the body part is coded to the closest proximal branch that has a specific body part value.
Example: A procedure performed on the mandibular branch of the trigeminal nerve is coded to the trigeminal nerve body part value.

Body System Specific PCS Reference Manual Exercises

PCS CODE	6 – LOWER VEINS EXERCISES
0 6 5 Y 3 Z Z	Cautery of oozing varicose vein, left calf. (The approach is coded "Percutaneous" because that is the normal route to a vein. No mention is made of approach, because likely the skin has eroded at that spot.)
0 6 D Y 3 Z Z	Microincisional phlebectomy of spider veins, right lower leg.
0 6 H 0 3 D Z	Percutaneous insertion of Greenfield IVC filter.
0 6 L 3 3 Z Z	Percutaneous ligation of esophageal vein.

6 – Lower Veins

Educational Annotations

NOTES

TUBULAR GROUP: Bypass, Dilation, Occlusion, Restriction
Root Operations that alter the diameter/route of a tubular body part.

1ST - **0** Medical and Surgical
2ND - **6** Lower Veins
3RD - **1** BYPASS

EXAMPLE: Bypass damaged splenic vein | CMS Ex: Coronary artery bypass

BYPASS: Altering the route of passage of the contents of a tubular body part.

EXPLANATION: Rerouting contents to a downstream part ...

Body Part – 4TH	Approach – 5TH	Device – 6TH	Qualifier – 7TH
0 Inferior Vena Cava	0 Open 4 Percutaneous endoscopic	7 Autologous tissue substitute 9 Autologous venous tissue A Autologous arterial tissue J Synthetic substitute K Nonautologous tissue substitute Z No device	5 Superior Mesenteric Vein 6 Inferior Mesenteric Vein Y Lower Vein
1 Splenic Vein	0 Open 4 Percutaneous endoscopic	7 Autologous tissue substitute 9 Autologous venous tissue A Autologous arterial tissue J Synthetic substitute K Nonautologous tissue substitute Z No device	9 Renal Vein, Right B Renal Vein, Left Y Lower Vein
2 Gastric Vein 3 Esophageal Vein 4 Hepatic Vein 5 Superior Mesenteric Vein 6 Inferior Mesenteric Vein 7 Colic Vein 9 Renal Vein, Right B Renal Vein, Left C Common Iliac Vein, Right D Common Iliac Vein, Left F External Iliac Vein, Right G External Iliac Vein, Left H Hypogastric Vein, Right J Hypogastric Vein, Left M Femoral Vein, Right N Femoral Vein, Left P Greater Saphenous Vein, Right Q Greater Saphenous Vein, Left R Lesser Saphenous Vein, Right S Lesser Saphenous Vein, Left T Foot Vein, Right V Foot Vein, Left	0 Open 4 Percutaneous endoscopic	7 Autologous tissue substitute 9 Autologous venous tissue A Autologous arterial tissue J Synthetic substitute K Nonautologous tissue substitute Z No device	Y Lower Vein

continued ⇨

0 6 1 BYPASS – *continued*

Body Part – 4ᵀᴴ	Approach – 5ᵀᴴ	Device – 6ᵀᴴ	Qualifier – 7ᵀᴴ
8 Portal Vein	0 Open	7 Autologous tissue substitute 9 Autologous venous tissue A Autologous arterial tissue J Synthetic substitute K Nonautologous tissue substitute Z No device	9 Renal Vein, Right B Renal Vein, Left Y Lower Vein
8 Portal Vein	3 Percutaneous	D Intraluminal device	Y Lower Vein
8 Portal Vein	4 Percutaneous endoscopic	7 Autologous tissue substitute 9 Autologous venous tissue A Autologous arterial tissue J Synthetic substitute K Nonautologous tissue substitute Z No device	9 Renal Vein, Right B Renal Vein, Left Y Lower Vein
8 Portal Vein	4 Percutaneous endoscopic	D Intraluminal device	Y Lower Vein

6 – LOWER VEINS

EXCISION GROUP: Excision, (Resection), Destruction, Extraction, (Detachment)
Root Operations that take out some or all of a body part.

1ST - 0 Medical and Surgical
2ND - 6 Lower Veins
3RD - 5 DESTRUCTION

EXAMPLE: Fulguration venous lesion   CMS Ex: Fulguration polyp

DESTRUCTION: Physical eradication of all or a portion of a body part by the direct use of energy, force, or a destructive agent.

EXPLANATION: None of the body part is physically taken out

Body Part – 4TH		Approach – 5TH	Device – 6TH	Qualifier – 7TH
0 Inferior Vena Cava	H Hypogastric Vein, Right	0 Open	Z No device	Z No qualifier
1 Splenic Vein	J Hypogastric Vein, Left	3 Percutaneous		
2 Gastric Vein	M Femoral Vein, Right	4 Percutaneous endoscopic		
3 Esophageal Vein	N Femoral Vein, Left			
4 Hepatic Vein	P Greater Saphenous Vein, Right			
5 Superior Mesenteric Vein	Q Greater Saphenous Vein, Left			
6 Inferior Mesenteric Vein	R Lesser Saphenous Vein, Right			
7 Colic Vein	S Lesser Saphenous Vein, Left			
8 Portal Vein	T Foot Vein, Right			
9 Renal Vein, Right	V Foot Vein, Left			
B Renal Vein, Left				
C Common Iliac Vein, Right				
D Common Iliac Vein, Left				
F External Iliac Vein, Right				
G External Iliac Vein, Left				
Y Lower Vein		0 Open	Z No device	C Hemorrhoidal Plexus
		3 Percutaneous		Z No qualifier
		4 Percutaneous endoscopic		

TUBULAR GROUP: Bypass, Dilation, Occlusion, Restriction
Root Operations that alter the diameter/route of a tubular body part.

1ST - 0 Medical and Surgical
2ND - 6 Lower Veins
3RD - 7 DILATION

EXAMPLE: Balloon dilation hepatic vein   CMS Ex: Transluminal angioplasty

DILATION: Expanding an orifice or the lumen of a tubular body part.

EXPLANATION: By force (stretching) or cutting ...

Body Part – 4TH		Approach – 5TH	Device – 6TH	Qualifier – 7TH
0 Inferior Vena Cava	H Hypogastric Vein, Right	0 Open	D Intraluminal device	Z No qualifier
1 Splenic Vein	J Hypogastric Vein, Left	3 Percutaneous	Z No device	
2 Gastric Vein	M Femoral Vein, Right	4 Percutaneous endoscopic		
3 Esophageal Vein	N Femoral Vein, Left			
4 Hepatic Vein	P Greater Saphenous Vein, Right			
5 Superior Mesenteric Vein	Q Greater Saphenous Vein, Left			
6 Inferior Mesenteric Vein	R Lesser Saphenous Vein, Right			
7 Colic Vein	S Lesser Saphenous Vein, Left			
8 Portal Vein	T Foot Vein, Right			
9 Renal Vein, Right	V Foot Vein, Left			
B Renal Vein, Left	Y Lower Vein			
C Common Iliac Vein, Right				
D Common Iliac Vein, Left				
F External Iliac Vein, Right				
G External Iliac Vein, Left				

069 MEDICAL AND SURGICAL SECTION – 2016 ICD-10-PCS [2016.PCS]

DRAINAGE GROUP: Drainage, Extirpation, (Fragmentation)
Root Operations that take out solids/fluids/gases from a body part.

1ST - **0** Medical and Surgical
2ND - **6** Lower Veins
3RD - **9** DRAINAGE

EXAMPLE: Phlebotomy iliac vein   CMS Ex: Thoracentesis

DRAINAGE: Taking or letting out fluids and/or gases from a body part.

EXPLANATION: Qualifier "X Diagnostic" indicates biopsy ...

Body Part – 4TH		Approach – 5TH	Device – 6TH	Qualifier – 7TH
0 Inferior Vena Cava	H Hypogastric Vein, Right	0 Open	0 Drainage device	Z No qualifier
1 Splenic Vein	J Hypogastric Vein, Left	3 Percutaneous		
2 Gastric Vein	M Femoral Vein, Right	4 Percutaneous endoscopic		
3 Esophageal Vein	N Femoral Vein, Left			
4 Hepatic Vein	P Greater Saphenous Vein, Right			
5 Superior Mesenteric Vein				
6 Inferior Mesenteric Vein	Q Greater Saphenous Vein, Left			
7 Colic Vein				
8 Portal Vein	R Lesser Saphenous Vein, Right			
9 Renal Vein, Right				
B Renal Vein, Left	S Lesser Saphenous Vein, Left			
C Common Iliac Vein, Right				
D Common Iliac Vein, Left	T Foot Vein, Right			
F External Iliac Vein, Right	V Foot Vein, Left			
G External Iliac Vein, Left	Y Lower Vein			

Body Part		Approach	Device	Qualifier
0 Inferior Vena Cava	H Hypogastric Vein, Right	0 Open	Z No device	X Diagnostic
1 Splenic Vein	J Hypogastric Vein, Left	3 Percutaneous		Z No qualifier
2 Gastric Vein	M Femoral Vein, Right	4 Percutaneous endoscopic		
3 Esophageal Vein	N Femoral Vein, Left			
4 Hepatic Vein	P Greater Saphenous Vein, Right			
5 Superior Mesenteric Vein				
6 Inferior Mesenteric Vein	Q Greater Saphenous Vein, Left			
7 Colic Vein				
8 Portal Vein	R Lesser Saphenous Vein, Right			
9 Renal Vein, Right				
B Renal Vein, Left	S Lesser Saphenous Vein, Left			
C Common Iliac Vein, Right				
D Common Iliac Vein, Left	T Foot Vein, Right			
F External Iliac Vein, Right	V Foot Vein, Left			
G External Iliac Vein, Left	Y Lower Vein			

LOWER VEINS 069

6 – LOWER VEINS

06B

EXCISION GROUP: Excision, (Resection), Destruction, Extraction, (Detachment)
Root Operations that take out some or all of a body part.

| EXAMPLE: Harvest saphenous vein | CMS Ex: Liver biopsy |

- 1ST - **0** Medical and Surgical
- 2ND - **6** Lower Veins
- 3RD - **B** EXCISION

EXCISION: Cutting out or off, without replacement, a portion of a body part.

EXPLANATION: Qualifier "X Diagnostic" indicates biopsy ...

Body Part – 4TH		Approach – 5TH	Device – 6TH	Qualifier – 7TH
0 Inferior Vena Cava	H Hypogastric Vein, Right	0 Open	Z No device	X Diagnostic
1 Splenic Vein	J Hypogastric Vein, Left	3 Percutaneous		Z No qualifier
2 Gastric Vein	M Femoral Vein, Right	4 Percutaneous endoscopic		
3 Esophageal Vein	N Femoral Vein, Left			
4 Hepatic Vein	P Greater Saphenous Vein, Right			
5 Superior Mesenteric Vein	Q Greater Saphenous Vein, Left			
6 Inferior Mesenteric Vein	R Lesser Saphenous Vein, Right			
7 Colic Vein	S Lesser Saphenous Vein, Left			
8 Portal Vein	T Foot Vein, Right			
9 Renal Vein, Right	V Foot Vein, Left			
B Renal Vein, Left				
C Common Iliac Vein, Right				
D Common Iliac Vein, Left				
F External Iliac Vein, Right				
G External Iliac Vein, Left				
Y Lower Vein		0 Open	Z No device	C Hemorrhoidal Plexus
		3 Percutaneous		X Diagnostic
		4 Percutaneous endoscopic		Z No qualifier

06C

MEDICAL AND SURGICAL SECTION – 2016 ICD-10-PCS

[2016.PCS]

DRAINAGE GROUP: Drainage, Extirpation, (Fragmentation)
Root Operations that take out solids/fluids/gases from a body part.

- 1ST – **0** Medical and Surgical
- 2ND – **6** Lower Veins
- 3RD – **C EXTIRPATION**

EXAMPLE: Mechanical thrombectomy CMS Ex: Choledocholithotomy

EXTIRPATION: Taking or cutting out solid matter from a body part.

EXPLANATION: Abnormal byproduct or foreign body …

Body Part – 4TH		Approach – 5TH	Device – 6TH	Qualifier – 7TH
0 Inferior Vena Cava	H Hypogastric Vein, Right	0 Open	Z No device	Z No qualifier
1 Splenic Vein	J Hypogastric Vein, Left	3 Percutaneous		
2 Gastric Vein	M Femoral Vein, Right	4 Percutaneous endoscopic		
3 Esophageal Vein	N Femoral Vein, Left			
4 Hepatic Vein	P Greater Saphenous Vein, Right			
5 Superior Mesenteric Vein	Q Greater Saphenous Vein, Left			
6 Inferior Mesenteric Vein				
7 Colic Vein	R Lesser Saphenous Vein, Right			
8 Portal Vein				
9 Renal Vein, Right	S Lesser Saphenous Vein, Left			
B Renal Vein, Left				
C Common Iliac Vein, Right	T Foot Vein, Right			
D Common Iliac Vein, Left	V Foot Vein, Left			
F External Iliac Vein, Right	Y Lower Vein			
G External Iliac Vein, Left				

EXCISION GROUP: Excision, (Resection), Destruction, Extraction, (Detachment)
Root Operations that take out some or all of a body part.

- 1ST – **0** Medical and Surgical
- 2ND – **6** Lower Veins
- 3RD – **D EXTRACTION**

EXAMPLE: Vein ligation and stripping CMS Ex: D&C

EXTRACTION: Pulling or stripping out or off all or a portion of a body part by the use of force.

EXPLANATION: None for this Body System

Body Part – 4TH	Approach – 5TH	Device – 6TH	Qualifier – 7TH
M Femoral Vein, Right	0 Open	Z No device	Z No qualifier
N Femoral Vein, Left	3 Percutaneous		
P Greater Saphenous Vein, Right	4 Percutaneous endoscopic		
Q Greater Saphenous Vein, Left			
R Lesser Saphenous Vein, Right			
S Lesser Saphenous Vein, Left			
T Foot Vein, Right			
V Foot Vein, Left			
Y Lower Vein			

6 – LOWER VEINS 06J

DEVICE GROUP: (Change), Insertion, Removal, Replacement, Revision, Supplement
Root Operations that always involve a device.

1ST - 0 Medical and Surgical
2ND - 6 Lower Veins
3RD - H INSERTION

EXAMPLE: Insertion IVC filter   CMS Ex: Insertion central venous catheter

INSERTION: Putting in a nonbiological appliance that monitors, assists, performs, or prevents a physiological function but does not physically take the place of a body part.

EXPLANATION: None

Body Part – 4TH	Approach – 5TH	Device – 6TH	Qualifier – 7TH
0 Inferior Vena Cava	0 Open 3 Percutaneous	3 Infusion device	T Via Umbilical Vein Z No qualifier
0 Inferior Vena Cava	0 Open 3 Percutaneous	D Intraluminal device	Z No qualifier
0 Inferior Vena Cava	4 Percutaneous endoscopic	3 Infusion device D Intraluminal device	Z No qualifier
1 Splenic Vein 2 Gastric Vein 3 Esophageal Vein 4 Hepatic Vein 5 Superior Mesenteric Vein 6 Inferior Mesenteric Vein 7 Colic Vein 8 Portal Vein 9 Renal Vein, Right B Renal Vein, Left C Common Iliac Vein, Right D Common Iliac Vein, Left F External Iliac Vein, Right G External Iliac Vein, Left H Hypogastric Vein, Right J Hypogastric Vein, Left M Femoral Vein, Right N Femoral Vein, Left P Greater Saphenous Vein, Right Q Greater Saphenous Vein, Left R Lesser Saphenous Vein, Right S Lesser Saphenous Vein, Left T Foot Vein, Right V Foot Vein, Left	0 Open 3 Percutaneous 4 Percutaneous endoscopic	3 Infusion device D Intraluminal device	Z No qualifier
Y Lower Vein	0 Open 3 Percutaneous 4 Percutaneous endoscopic	2 Monitoring device 3 Infusion device D Intraluminal device	Z No qualifier

EXAMINATION GROUP: Inspection, (Map)
Root Operations involving examination only.

1ST - 0 Medical and Surgical
2ND - 6 Lower Veins
3RD - J INSPECTION

EXAMPLE: Open iliac vein examination   CMS Ex: Colonoscopy

INSPECTION: Visually and/or manually exploring a body part.

EXPLANATION: Direct or instrumental visualization ...

Body Part – 4TH	Approach – 5TH	Device – 6TH	Qualifier – 7TH
Y Lower Vein	0 Open 3 Percutaneous 4 Percutaneous endoscopic X External	Z No device	Z No qualifier

06L MEDICAL AND SURGICAL SECTION – 2016 ICD-10-PCS [2016.PCS]

TUBULAR GROUP: Bypass, Dilation, Occlusion, Restriction
Root Operations that alter the diameter/route of a tubular body part.

- 1ST - **0** Medical and Surgical
- 2ND - **6** Lower Veins
- 3RD - **L OCCLUSION**

EXAMPLE: Ligation esophageal varices | CMS Ex: Fallopian tube ligation

OCCLUSION: Completely closing an orifice or lumen of a tubular body part.

EXPLANATION: Natural or artificially created orifice ...

Body Part – 4TH		Approach – 5TH	Device – 6TH	Qualifier – 7TH
0 Inferior Vena Cava	H Hypogastric Vein, Right	0 Open	C Extraluminal device	Z No qualifier
1 Splenic Vein	J Hypogastric Vein, Left	3 Percutaneous	D Intraluminal device	
2 Gastric Vein	M Femoral Vein, Right	4 Percutaneous endoscopic	Z No device	
3 Esophageal Vein	N Femoral Vein, Left			
4 Hepatic Vein	P Greater Saphenous Vein, Right			
5 Superior Mesenteric Vein				
6 Inferior Mesenteric Vein	Q Greater Saphenous Vein, Left			
7 Colic Vein				
8 Portal Vein	R Lesser Saphenous Vein, Right			
9 Renal Vein, Right				
B Renal Vein, Left	S Lesser Saphenous Vein, Left			
C Common Iliac Vein, Right				
D Common Iliac Vein, Left	T Foot Vein, Right			
F External Iliac Vein, Right	V Foot Vein, Left			
G External Iliac Vein, Left				
Y Lower Vein		0 Open	C Extraluminal device	C Hemorrhoidal Plexus
		3 Percutaneous	D Intraluminal device	Z No qualifier
		4 Percutaneous endoscopic	Z No device	

DIVISION GROUP: (Division), Release
Root Operations involving cutting or separation only.

- 1ST - **0** Medical and Surgical
- 2ND - **6** Lower Veins
- 3RD - **N RELEASE**

EXAMPLE: Adhesiolysis hepatic vein | CMS Ex: Carpal tunnel release

RELEASE: Freeing a body part from an abnormal physical constraint by cutting or by the use of force.

EXPLANATION: None of the body part is taken out ...

Body Part – 4TH		Approach – 5TH	Device – 6TH	Qualifier – 7TH
0 Inferior Vena Cava	H Hypogastric Vein, Right	0 Open	Z No device	Z No qualifier
1 Splenic Vein	J Hypogastric Vein, Left	3 Percutaneous		
2 Gastric Vein	M Femoral Vein, Right	4 Percutaneous endoscopic		
3 Esophageal Vein	N Femoral Vein, Left			
4 Hepatic Vein	P Greater Saphenous Vein, Right			
5 Superior Mesenteric Vein				
6 Inferior Mesenteric Vein	Q Greater Saphenous Vein, Left			
7 Colic Vein				
8 Portal Vein	R Lesser Saphenous Vein, Right			
9 Renal Vein, Right				
B Renal Vein, Left	S Lesser Saphenous Vein, Left			
C Common Iliac Vein, Right				
D Common Iliac Vein, Left	T Foot Vein, Right			
F External Iliac Vein, Right	V Foot Vein, Left			
G External Iliac Vein, Left	Y Lower Vein			

6 – LOWER VEINS — 06Q

DEVICE GROUP: (Change), Insertion, Removal, Replacement, Revision, Supplement
Root Operations that always involve a device.

- 1ST – **0** Medical and Surgical
- 2ND – **6** Lower Veins
- 3RD – **P REMOVAL**

EXAMPLE: Removal IVC filter
CMS Ex: Chest tube removal

REMOVAL: Taking out or off a device from a body part.

EXPLANATION: Removal device without reinsertion …

Body Part – 4TH	Approach – 5TH	Device – 6TH	Qualifier – 7TH
Y Lower Vein	0 Open 3 Percutaneous 4 Percutaneous endoscopic	0 Drainage device 2 Monitoring device 3 Infusion device 7 Autologous tissue substitute C Extraluminal device D Intraluminal device J Synthetic substitute K Nonautologous tissue substitute	Z No qualifier
Y Lower Vein	X External	0 Drainage device 2 Monitoring device 3 Infusion device D Intraluminal device	Z No qualifier

OTHER REPAIRS GROUP: (Control), Repair
Root Operations that define other repairs.

- 1ST – **0** Medical and Surgical
- 2ND – **6** Lower Veins
- 3RD – **Q REPAIR**

EXAMPLE: Suture varicose vein
CMS Ex: Suture laceration

REPAIR: Restoring, to the extent possible, a body part to its normal anatomic structure and function.

EXPLANATION: Only when no other root operation applies …

Body Part – 4TH	Approach – 5TH	Device – 6TH	Qualifier – 7TH
0 Inferior Vena Cava 1 Splenic Vein 2 Gastric Vein 3 Esophageal Vein 4 Hepatic Vein 5 Superior Mesenteric Vein 6 Inferior Mesenteric Vein 7 Colic Vein 8 Portal Vein 9 Renal Vein, Right B Renal Vein, Left C Common Iliac Vein, Right D Common Iliac Vein, Left F External Iliac Vein, Right G External Iliac Vein, Left H Hypogastric Vein, Right J Hypogastric Vein, Left M Femoral Vein, Right N Femoral Vein, Left P Greater Saphenous Vein, Right Q Greater Saphenous Vein, Left R Lesser Saphenous Vein, Right S Lesser Saphenous Vein, Left T Foot Vein, Right V Foot Vein, Left Y Lower Vein	0 Open 3 Percutaneous 4 Percutaneous endoscopic	Z No device	Z No qualifier

06R — MEDICAL AND SURGICAL SECTION – 2016 ICD-10-PCS

DEVICE GROUP: (Change), Insertion, Removal, **Replacement**, Revision, Supplement
Root Operations that always involve a device.

- 1ST – **0** Medical and Surgical
- 2ND – **6** Lower Veins
- 3RD – **R** REPLACEMENT

EXAMPLE: Portal vein reconstruction graft   CMS Ex: Total hip

REPLACEMENT: Putting in or on a biological or synthetic material that physically takes the place and/or function of all or a portion of a body part.

EXPLANATION: Includes taking out body part, or eradication…

Body Part – 4TH		Approach – 5TH	Device – 6TH	Qualifier – 7TH
0 Inferior Vena Cava	H Hypogastric Vein, Right	0 Open	7 Autologous tissue substitute	Z No qualifier
1 Splenic Vein	J Hypogastric Vein, Left	4 Percutaneous endoscopic	J Synthetic substitute	
2 Gastric Vein	M Femoral Vein, Right		K Nonautologous tissue substitute	
3 Esophageal Vein	N Femoral Vein, Left			
4 Hepatic Vein	P Greater Saphenous Vein, Right			
5 Superior Mesenteric Vein	Q Greater Saphenous Vein, Left			
6 Inferior Mesenteric Vein	R Lesser Saphenous Vein, Right			
7 Colic Vein	S Lesser Saphenous Vein, Left			
8 Portal Vein	T Foot Vein, Right			
9 Renal Vein, Right	V Foot Vein, Left			
B Renal Vein, Left	Y Lower Vein			
C Common Iliac Vein, Right				
D Common Iliac Vein, Left				
F External Iliac Vein, Right				
G External Iliac Vein, Left				

MOVE GROUP: (Reattachment), **Reposition**, (Transfer), (Transplantation)
Root Operations that put in/put back or move some/all of a body part.

- 1ST – **0** Medical and Surgical
- 2ND – **6** Lower Veins
- 3RD – **S** REPOSITION

EXAMPLE: Relocate hypogastric vein   CMS Ex: Fracture reduction

REPOSITION: Moving to its normal location, or other suitable location, all or a portion of a body part.

EXPLANATION: May or may not be cut to be moved …

Body Part – 4TH		Approach – 5TH	Device – 6TH	Qualifier – 7TH
0 Inferior Vena Cava	H Hypogastric Vein, Right	0 Open	Z No device	Z No qualifier
1 Splenic Vein	J Hypogastric Vein, Left	3 Percutaneous		
2 Gastric Vein	M Femoral Vein, Right	4 Percutaneous endoscopic		
3 Esophageal Vein	N Femoral Vein, Left			
4 Hepatic Vein	P Greater Saphenous Vein, Right			
5 Superior Mesenteric Vein	Q Greater Saphenous Vein, Left			
6 Inferior Mesenteric Vein	R Lesser Saphenous Vein, Right			
7 Colic Vein	S Lesser Saphenous Vein, Left			
8 Portal Vein	T Foot Vein, Right			
9 Renal Vein, Right	V Foot Vein, Left			
B Renal Vein, Left	Y Lower Vein			
C Common Iliac Vein, Right				
D Common Iliac Vein, Left				
F External Iliac Vein, Right				
G External Iliac Vein, Left				

6 – LOWER VEINS — 0 6 V

DEVICE GROUP: (Change), Insertion, Removal, Replacement, Revision, Supplement
Root Operations that always involve a device.

1ST - 0 Medical and Surgical
2ND - 6 Lower Veins
3RD - U SUPPLEMENT

EXAMPLE: Patch graft venoplasty
CMS Ex: Hernia repair with mesh

SUPPLEMENT: Putting in or on biological or synthetic material that physically reinforces and/or augments the function of a portion of a body part.

EXPLANATION: Biological material from same individual ...

Body Part – 4TH		Approach – 5TH	Device – 6TH	Qualifier – 7TH
0 Inferior Vena Cava	H Hypogastric Vein, Right	0 Open	7 Autologous tissue substitute	Z No qualifier
1 Splenic Vein	J Hypogastric Vein, Left	3 Percutaneous	J Synthetic substitute	
2 Gastric Vein	M Femoral Vein, Right	4 Percutaneous endoscopic	K Nonautologous tissue substitute	
3 Esophageal Vein	N Femoral Vein, Left			
4 Hepatic Vein	P Greater Saphenous Vein, Right			
5 Superior Mesenteric Vein	Q Greater Saphenous Vein, Left			
6 Inferior Mesenteric Vein	R Lesser Saphenous Vein, Right			
7 Colic Vein	S Lesser Saphenous Vein, Left			
8 Portal Vein	T Foot Vein, Right			
9 Renal Vein, Right	V Foot Vein, Left			
B Renal Vein, Left	Y Lower Vein			
C Common Iliac Vein, Right				
D Common Iliac Vein, Left				
F External Iliac Vein, Right				
G External Iliac Vein, Left				

TUBULAR GROUP: Bypass, Dilation, Occlusion, Restriction
Root Operations that alter the diameter/route of a tubular body part.

1ST - 0 Medical and Surgical
2ND - 6 Lower Veins
3RD - V RESTRICTION

EXAMPLE: Restrictive venous stent
CMS Ex: Cervical cerclage

RESTRICTION: Partially closing an orifice or the lumen of a tubular body part.

EXPLANATION: Natural or artificially created orifice ...

Body Part – 4TH		Approach – 5TH	Device – 6TH	Qualifier – 7TH
0 Inferior Vena Cava	H Hypogastric Vein, Right	0 Open	C Extraluminal device	Z No qualifier
1 Splenic Vein	J Hypogastric Vein, Left	3 Percutaneous	D Intraluminal device	
2 Gastric Vein	M Femoral Vein, Right	4 Percutaneous endoscopic	Z No device	
3 Esophageal Vein	N Femoral Vein, Left			
4 Hepatic Vein	P Greater Saphenous Vein, Right			
5 Superior Mesenteric Vein	Q Greater Saphenous Vein, Left			
6 Inferior Mesenteric Vein	R Lesser Saphenous Vein, Right			
7 Colic Vein	S Lesser Saphenous Vein, Left			
8 Portal Vein	T Foot Vein, Right			
9 Renal Vein, Right	V Foot Vein, Left			
B Renal Vein, Left	Y Lower Vein			
C Common Iliac Vein, Right				
D Common Iliac Vein, Left				
F External Iliac Vein, Right				
G External Iliac Vein, Left				

0 6 W MEDICAL AND SURGICAL SECTION – 2016 ICD-10-PCS

DEVICE GROUP: (Change), Insertion, Removal, Replacement, Revision, Supplement
Root Operations that always involve a device.

1ST - 0 Medical and Surgical
2ND - 6 Lower Veins
3RD - W REVISION

EXAMPLE: Reposition IVC filter **CMS Ex:** Adjustment pacemaker lead

REVISION: Correcting, to the extent possible, a portion of a malfunctioning device or the position of a displaced device.

EXPLANATION: May replace components of a device ...

Body Part – 4TH	Approach – 5TH	Device – 6TH	Qualifier – 7TH
Y Lower Vein	0 Open 3 Percutaneous 4 Percutaneous endoscopic X External	0 Drainage device 2 Monitoring device 3 Infusion device 7 Autologous tissue substitute C Extraluminal device D Intraluminal device J Synthetic substitute K Nonautologous tissue substitute	Z No qualifier

Educational Annotations | 7 – Lymphatic and Hemic Systems

Body System Specific Educational Annotations for the Lymphatic and Hemic Systems include:

- Anatomy and Physiology Review
- Anatomical Illustrations
- Definitions of Common Procedures
- AHA Coding Clinic® Reference Notations
- Body Part Key Listings
- Device Key Listings
- Device Aggregation Table Listings
- Coding Notes

Anatomy and Physiology Review of Lymphatic and Hemic Systems

BODY PART VALUES – 7 - LYMPHATIC AND HEMIC SYSTEMS

Bone Marrow – ANATOMY – The soft tissue on the inside of bones that is comprised of red and yellow bone marrow tissue. PHYSIOLOGY – Red bone marrow produces red blood cells, platelets, and most white blood cells. Yellow bone marrow has a minor role in cell production and consists primarily of fat cells.

Cisterna Chyli – ANATOMY – The cisterna chyli is a sac-like structure formed by the junction of the lumbar, intestinal, and descending intercostal lymphatic trunks that empties into the thoracic duct. PHYSIOLOGY – The cisterna chyli collects the lymph from the lower body and chyle from the intestines.

Lymphatic – ANATOMY – The general term for structures and tissues of the lymphatic system. The lymphatic system is part of the circulatory system and its major components include: Thymus, spleen, bone marrow, cisterna chyli, thoracic duct, lymph vessels, lymph nodes, and lymph node chains. PHYSIOLOGY – The lymphatic system serves multiple functions including: Immune system defense, draining the interstitial fluid, removing waste products and cellular debris, and maintaining the balance of body fluids.

Spleen – ANATOMY – The spleen is a gland-like organ, located in the upper abdomen behind the stomach and at the tail of the pancreas, and is about 5 inches (13 cm) in length. The spleen contains both white pulp and red pulp. PHYSIOLOGY – The spleen functions as both a large lymph node (white pulp) that filters the blood and produces lymphocytes and monocytes, and as a red blood cell reservoir (red pulp) and disintegrator of worn-out red blood cells. It also plays a role in producing antibodies. Although important, the spleen is not essential to life.

Thoracic Duct – ANATOMY – The largest of the lymphatic vessels extending from the middle lumbar region to the base of the neck. PHYSIOLOGY – The thoracic duct collects most of the body's the lymphatic fluid from the chest down and drains it into the left subclavian vein.

Thymus – ANATOMY – The thymus is the small, flat bi-lobed organ lying behind the sternum, and is composed of lymphoid material. PHYSIOLOGY – The thymus functions substantially during childhood by producing lymphocytes and aids in the development of the individual's immunity.

Anatomical Illustrations of Lymphatic and Hemic Systems

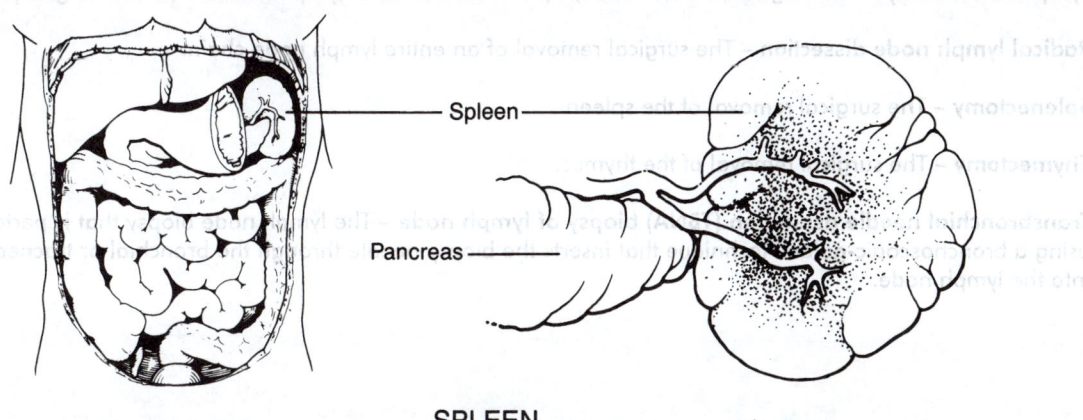

SPLEEN

Continued on next page

Educational Annotations | 7 – Lymphatic and Hemic Systems

Anatomical Illustrations of Lymphatic and Hemic Systems

Continued from previous page

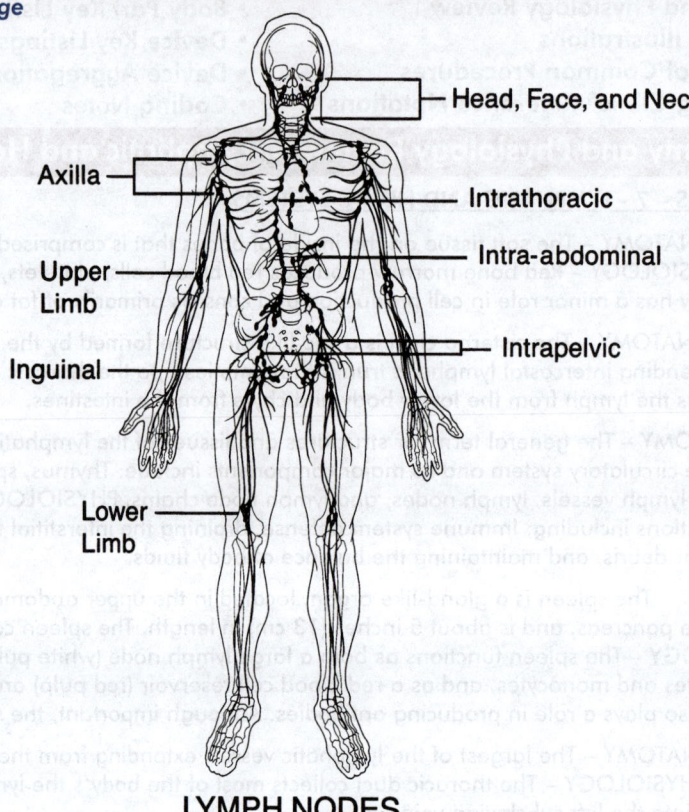

LYMPH NODES

- Head, Face, and Neck
- Axilla
- Intrathoracic
- Intra-abdominal
- Upper Limb
- Intrapelvic
- Inguinal
- Lower Limb

Definitions of Common Procedures of Lymphatic and Hemic Systems

Bone marrow biopsy – The removal of living bone marrow tissue for microscopic examination using a special needle that extracts a core (cylindrical sample) of tissue.

Lymphadenectomy – The surgical removal of a lymph node or several lymph nodes in the same group.

Radical lymph node dissection – The surgical removal of an entire lymph node chain.

Splenectomy – The surgical removal of the spleen.

Thymectomy – The surgical removal of the thymus.

Transbronchial needle aspiration (TBNA) biopsy of lymph node – The lymph node biopsy that is performed using a bronchoscopic-guided technique that inserts the biopsy needle through the bronchial or tracheal wall and into the lymph node.

Educational Annotations | 7 – Lymphatic and Hemic Systems

AHA Coding Clinic® Reference Notations of Lymphatic and Hemic Systems

ROOT OPERATION SPECIFIC - 7 - LYMPHATIC AND HEMIC SYSTEMS
CHANGE - 2
DESTRUCTION - 5
DRAINAGE - 9
EXCISION - B
    Removal of some paratracheal lymph nodes...AHA 14:3Q:p10
    Transbronchial endoscopic needle aspiration biopsy of right lung
        lymph nodes ....AHA 14:1Q:p20
    Transbronchial endoscopic lymph node aspiration biopsy
        (see also AHA 13:4Q:p111)..AHA 14:1Q:p26
EXTIRPATION - C
EXTRACTION - D
    Bone marrow biopsy ....AHA 13:4Q:p111
INSERTION - H
INSPECTION - J
OCCLUSION - L
RELEASE - N
REMOVAL - P
REPAIR - Q
REPOSITION - S
RESECTION - T
    Radical resection of level I lymph nodes, bilateral ....AHA 14:3Q:p9
    Resection of thymus ....AHA 14:3Q:p16
SUPPLEMENT - U
RESTRICTION - V
REVISION - W
TRANSPLANTATION - Y

Body Part Key Listings of Lymphatic and Hemic Systems

See also Body Part Key in Appendix C
Accessory spleen	*use* Spleen
Anterior (pectoral) lymph node	*use* Lymphatic, Axillary, Left/Right
Apical (subclavicular) lymph node	*use* Lymphatic, Axillary, Left/Right
Brachial (lateral) lymph node	*use* Lymphatic, Axillary, Left/Right
Buccinator lymph node	*use* Lymphatic, Head
Celiac lymph node	*use* Lymphatic, Aortic
Central axillary lymph node	*use* Lymphatic, Axillary, Left/Right
Cervical lymph node	*use* Lymphatic, Neck, Left/Right
Common iliac (subaortic) lymph node	*use* Lymphatic, Pelvis
Cubital lymph node	*use* Lymphatic, Upper Extremity, Left/Right
Deltopectoral (infraclavicular) lymph node	*use* Lymphatic, Upper Extremity, Left/Right
Epitrochlear lymph node	*use* Lymphatic, Upper Extremity, Left/Right
Femoral lymph node	*use* Lymphatic, Lower Extremity, Left/Right
Gastric lymph node	*use* Lymphatic, Aortic
Gluteal lymph node	*use* Lymphatic, Pelvis
Hepatic lymph node	*use* Lymphatic, Aortic
Iliac lymph node	*use* Lymphatic, Pelvis
Inferior epigastric lymph node	*use* Lymphatic, Pelvis
Inferior mesenteric lymph node	*use* Lymphatic, Mesenteric
Infraauricular lymph node	*use* Lymphatic, Head
Infraclavicular (deltopectoral) lymph node	*use* Lymphatic, Upper Extremity, Left/Right

Continued on next page

Educational Annotations | 7 – Lymphatic and Hemic Systems

Body Part Key Listings of Lymphatic and Hemic Systems

Continued from previous page

Infraparotid lymph node	*use* Lymphatic, Head
Intercostal lymph node	*use* Lymphatic, Thorax
Intestinal lymphatic trunk	*use* Cisterna Chyli
Jugular lymph node	*use* Lymphatic, Neck, Left/Right
Lateral (brachial) lymph node	*use* Lymphatic, Axillary, Left/Right
Left jugular trunk	*use* Thoracic Duct
Left subclavian trunk	*use* Thoracic Duct
Lumbar lymph node	*use* Lymphatic, Aortic
Lumbar lymphatic trunk	*use* Cisterna Chyli
Mastoid (postauricular) lymph node	*use* Lymphatic, Neck, Left/Right
Mediastinal lymph node	*use* Lymphatic, Thorax
Obturator lymph node	*use* Lymphatic, Pelvis
Occipital lymph node	*use* Lymphatic, Neck, Left/Right
Pancreaticosplenic lymph node	*use* Lymphatic, Aortic
Paraaortic lymph node	*use* Lymphatic, Aortic
Pararectal lymph node	*use* Lymphatic, Mesenteric
Parasternal lymph node	*use* Lymphatic, Thorax
Paratracheal lymph node	*use* Lymphatic, Thorax
Parotid lymph node	*use* Lymphatic, Head
Pectoral (anterior) lymph node	*use* Lymphatic, Axillary, Left/Right
Popliteal lymph node	*use* Lymphatic, Lower Extremity, Left/Right
Postauricular (mastoid) lymph node	*use* Lymphatic, Neck, Left/Right
Posterior (subscapular) lymph node	*use* Lymphatic, Axillary, Left/Right
Preauricular lymph node	*use* Lymphatic, Head
Retroperitoneal lymph node	*use* Lymphatic, Aortic
Retropharyngeal lymph node	*use* Lymphatic, Neck, Left/Right
Right jugular trunk	*use* Lymphatic, Right Neck
Right lymphatic duct	*use* Lymphatic, Right Neck
Right subclavian trunk	*use* Lymphatic, Right Neck
Sacral lymph node	*use* Lymphatic, Pelvis
Subaortic (common iliac) lymph node	*use* Lymphatic, Pelvis
Subclavicular (apical) lymph node	*use* Lymphatic, Axillary, Left/Right
Submandibular lymph node	*use* Lymphatic, Head
Submaxillary lymph node	*use* Lymphatic, Head
Submental lymph node	*use* Lymphatic, Head
Subparotid lymph node	*use* Lymphatic, Head
Subscapular (posterior) lymph node	*use* Lymphatic, Axillary, Left/Right
Superior mesenteric lymph node	*use* Lymphatic, Mesenteric
Supraclavicular (Virchow's) lymph node	*use* Lymphatic, Neck, Left/Right
Suprahyoid lymph node	*use* Lymphatic, Head
Suprainguinal lymph node	*use* Lymphatic, Pelvis
Supratrochlear lymph node	*use* Lymphatic, Upper Extremity, Left/Right
Thymus gland	*use* Thymus
Tracheobronchial lymph node	*use* Lymphatic, Thorax
Virchow's (supraclavicular) lymph node	*use* Lymphatic, Neck, Left/Right

Educational Annotations | 7 – Lymphatic and Hemic Systems

Device Key Listings of Lymphatic and Hemic Systems

See also Device Key in Appendix D
Autograft ....*use* Autologous Tissue Substitute
Tissue bank graft ....*use* Nonautologous Tissue Substitute

Device Aggregation Table Listings of Lymphatic and Hemic Systems

See also Device Aggregation Table in Appendix E

Specific Device	For Operation	In Body System	General Device
None Listed in Device Aggregation Table for this Body System			

Coding Notes of Lymphatic and Hemic Systems

Body System Specific PCS Reference Manual Exercises

PCS CODE	7 – LYMPHATIC AND HEMIC SYSTEMS EXERCISES
0 7 T 6 0 Z Z	Open left axillary total lymphadenectomy. (Resection is coded for cutting out a chain of lymph nodes.)
0 7 V K 3 D Z	Restriction of thoracic duct with intraluminal stent, percutaneous.

Educational Annotations | 7 – Lymphatic and Hemic Systems

NOTES

7 – LYMPHATIC AND HEMIC SYSTEMS

DEVICE GROUP: Change, Insertion, Removal, (Replacement), Revision, Supplement
Root Operations that always involve a device.

- 1ST – **0** Medical and Surgical
- 2ND – **7** Lymphatic and Hemic Systems
- 3RD – **2 CHANGE**

EXAMPLE: Exchange drain tube   CMS Ex: Changing urinary catheter

CHANGE: Taking out or off a device from a body part and putting back an identical or similar device in or on the same body part without cutting or puncturing the skin or a mucous membrane.

EXPLANATION: ALL Changes use EXTERNAL approach only...

Body Part – 4TH	Approach – 5TH	Device – 6TH	Qualifier – 7TH
K Thoracic Duct L Cisterna Chyli M Thymus N Lymphatic P Spleen T Bone Marrow	X External	0 Drainage device Y Other device	Z No qualifier

---

EXCISION GROUP: Excision, Resection, Destruction, Extraction, (Detachment)
Root Operations that take out some or all of a body part.

- 1ST – **0** Medical and Surgical
- 2ND – **7** Lymphatic and Hemic Systems
- 3RD – **5 DESTRUCTION**

EXAMPLE: Radiofrequency node ablation   CMS Ex: Fulguration polyp

DESTRUCTION: Physical eradication of all or a portion of a body part by the direct use of energy, force, or a destructive agent.

EXPLANATION: None of the body part is physically taken out

Body Part – 4TH	Approach – 5TH	Device – 6TH	Qualifier – 7TH
0 Lymphatic, Head 1 Lymphatic, Right Neck 2 Lymphatic, Left Neck 3 Lymphatic, Right Upper Extremity 4 Lymphatic, Left Upper Extremity 5 Lymphatic, Right Axillary 6 Lymphatic, Left Axillary 7 Lymphatic, Thorax 8 Lymphatic, Internal Mammary, Right 9 Lymphatic, Internal Mammary, Left B Lymphatic, Mesenteric C Lymphatic, Pelvis D Lymphatic, Aortic F Lymphatic, Right Lower Extremity G Lymphatic, Left Lower Extremity H Lymphatic, Right Inguinal J Lymphatic, Left Inguinal K Thoracic Duct L Cisterna Chyli M Thymus P Spleen	0 Open 3 Percutaneous 4 Percutaneous endoscopic	Z No device	Z No qualifier

079 — MEDICAL AND SURGICAL SECTION – 2016 ICD-10-PCS

DRAINAGE GROUP: Drainage, Extirpation, (Fragmentation)
Root Operations that take out solids/fluids/gases from a body part.

- 1ST – **0** Medical and Surgical
- 2ND – **7** Lymphatic and Hemic Systems
- 3RD – **9** DRAINAGE

EXAMPLE: Drainage Cisterna Chyli   **CMS Ex:** Thoracentesis

DRAINAGE: Taking or letting out fluids and/or gases from a body part.

EXPLANATION: Qualifier "X Diagnostic" indicates biopsy …

Body Part – 4TH		Approach – 5TH	Device – 6TH	Qualifier – 7TH
0 Lymphatic, Head	B Lymphatic, Mesenteric	0 Open	0 Drainage device	Z No qualifier
1 Lymphatic, Right Neck	C Lymphatic, Pelvis	3 Percutaneous		
2 Lymphatic, Left Neck	D Lymphatic, Aortic	4 Percutaneous endoscopic		
3 Lymphatic, Right Upper Extremity	F Lymphatic, Right Lower Extremity			
4 Lymphatic, Left Upper Extremity	G Lymphatic, Left Lower Extremity			
5 Lymphatic, Right Axillary	H Lymphatic, Right Inguinal			
6 Lymphatic, Left Axillary	J Lymphatic, Left Inguinal			
7 Lymphatic, Thorax	K Thoracic Duct			
8 Lymphatic, Internal Mammary, Right	L Cisterna Chyli			
	M Thymus			
9 Lymphatic, Internal Mammary, Left	P Spleen			
	T Bone Marrow			
0 Lymphatic, Head	B Lymphatic, Mesenteric	0 Open	Z No device	X Diagnostic
1 Lymphatic, Right Neck	C Lymphatic, Pelvis	3 Percutaneous		Z No qualifier
2 Lymphatic, Left Neck	D Lymphatic, Aortic	4 Percutaneous endoscopic		
3 Lymphatic, Right Upper Extremity	F Lymphatic, Right Lower Extremity			
4 Lymphatic, Left Upper Extremity	G Lymphatic, Left Lower Extremity			
5 Lymphatic, Right Axillary	H Lymphatic, Right Inguinal			
6 Lymphatic, Left Axillary	J Lymphatic, Left Inguinal			
7 Lymphatic, Thorax	K Thoracic Duct			
8 Lymphatic, Internal Mammary, Right	L Cisterna Chyli			
	M Thymus			
9 Lymphatic, Internal Mammary, Left	P Spleen			
	T Bone Marrow			

LYMPHATIC & HEMIC 079

7 – LYMPHATIC AND HEMIC SYSTEMS — 07C

EXCISION GROUP: Excision, Resection, Destruction, Extraction, (Detachment)
Root Operations that take out some or all of a body part.

- 1ST – **0** Medical and Surgical
- 2ND – **7** Lymphatic and Hemic Systems
- 3RD – **B EXCISION**

EXAMPLE: Removal single lymph node **CMS Ex:** Liver biopsy

EXCISION: Cutting out or off, without replacement, a portion of a body part.

EXPLANATION: Qualifier "X Diagnostic" indicates biopsy …

Body Part – 4TH		Approach – 5TH	Device – 6TH	Qualifier – 7TH
0 Lymphatic, Head	B Lymphatic, Mesenteric	0 Open	Z No device	X Diagnostic
1 Lymphatic, Right Neck	C Lymphatic, Pelvis	3 Percutaneous		Z No qualifier
2 Lymphatic, Left Neck	D Lymphatic, Aortic	4 Percutaneous endoscopic		
3 Lymphatic, Right Upper Extremity	F Lymphatic, Right Lower Extremity			
4 Lymphatic, Left Upper Extremity	G Lymphatic, Left Lower Extremity			
5 Lymphatic, Right Axillary	H Lymphatic, Right Inguinal			
6 Lymphatic, Left Axillary	J Lymphatic, Left Inguinal			
7 Lymphatic, Thorax	K Thoracic Duct			
8 Lymphatic, Internal Mammary, Right	L Cisterna Chyli			
9 Lymphatic, Internal Mammary, Left	M Thymus			
	P Spleen			

DRAINAGE GROUP: Drainage, Extirpation, (Fragmentation)
Root Operations that take out solids/fluids/gases from a body part.

- 1ST – **0** Medical and Surgical
- 2ND – **7** Lymphatic and Hemic Systems
- 3RD – **C EXTIRPATION**

EXAMPLE: Removal foreign body spleen **CMS Ex:** Choledocholithotomy

EXTIRPATION: Taking or cutting out solid matter from a body part.

EXPLANATION: Abnormal byproduct or foreign body …

Body Part – 4TH		Approach – 5TH	Device – 6TH	Qualifier – 7TH
0 Lymphatic, Head	B Lymphatic, Mesenteric	0 Open	Z No device	Z No qualifier
1 Lymphatic, Right Neck	C Lymphatic, Pelvis	3 Percutaneous		
2 Lymphatic, Left Neck	D Lymphatic, Aortic	4 Percutaneous endoscopic		
3 Lymphatic, Right Upper Extremity	F Lymphatic, Right Lower Extremity			
4 Lymphatic, Left Upper Extremity	G Lymphatic, Left Lower Extremity			
5 Lymphatic, Right Axillary	H Lymphatic, Right Inguinal			
6 Lymphatic, Left Axillary	J Lymphatic, Left Inguinal			
7 Lymphatic, Thorax	K Thoracic Duct			
8 Lymphatic, Internal Mammary, Right	L Cisterna Chyli			
9 Lymphatic, Internal Mammary, Left	M Thymus			
	P Spleen			

07D   MEDICAL AND SURGICAL SECTION – 2016 ICD-10-PCS   [2016.PCS]

EXCISION GROUP: Excision, Resection, Destruction, Extraction, (Detachment)
Root Operations that take out some or all of a body part.

- 1ST – **0** Medical and Surgical
- 2ND – **7** Lymphatic and Hemic Systems
- 3RD – **D EXTRACTION**

EXAMPLE: Bone marrow biopsy   CMS Ex: D&C

EXTRACTION: Pulling or stripping out or off all or a portion of a body part by the use of force.

EXPLANATION: Qualifier "X Diagnostic" indicates biopsy ...

Body Part – 4TH	Approach – 5TH	Device – 6TH	Qualifier – 7TH
Q Bone Marrow, Sternum R Bone Marrow, Iliac S Bone Marrow, Vertebral	0 Open 3 Percutaneous	Z No device	X Diagnostic Z No qualifier

DEVICE GROUP: Change, Insertion, Removal, (Replacement), Revision, Supplement
Root Operations that always involve a device.

- 1ST – **0** Medical and Surgical
- 2ND – **7** Lymphatic and Hemic Systems
- 3RD – **H INSERTION**

EXAMPLE: Insertion infusion device   CMS Ex: Central venous catheter

INSERTION: Putting in a nonbiological appliance that monitors, assists, performs, or prevents a physiological function but does not physically take the place of a body part.

EXPLANATION: None

Body Part – 4TH	Approach – 5TH	Device – 6TH	Qualifier – 7TH
K Thoracic Duct L Cisterna Chyli M Thymus N Lymphatic P Spleen	0 Open 3 Percutaneous 4 Percutaneous endoscopic	3 Infusion device	Z No qualifier

EXAMINATION GROUP: Inspection, (Map)
Root Operations involving examination only.

- 1ST – **0** Medical and Surgical
- 2ND – **7** Lymphatic and Hemic Systems
- 3RD – **J INSPECTION**

EXAMPLE: Examination of spleen   CMS Ex: Colonoscopy

INSPECTION: Visually and/or manually exploring a body part.

EXPLANATION: Direct or instrumental visualization ...

Body Part – 4TH	Approach – 5TH	Device – 6TH	Qualifier – 7TH
K Thoracic Duct L Cisterna Chyli M Thymus T Bone Marrow	0 Open 3 Percutaneous 4 Percutaneous endoscopic	Z No device	Z No qualifier
N Lymphatic P Spleen	0 Open 3 Percutaneous 4 Percutaneous endoscopic X External	Z No device	Z No qualifier

7 – LYMPHATIC AND HEMIC SYSTEMS — 07N

TUBULAR GROUP: (Bypass), (Dilation), Occlusion, Restriction
Root Operations that alter the diameter/route of a tubular body part.

- 1ST – **0** Medical and Surgical
- 2ND – **7** Lymphatic and Hemic Systems
- 3RD – **L** OCCLUSION

EXAMPLE: Occlusion para-aortic lymph | CMS Ex: Fallopian tube ligation

OCCLUSION: Completely closing an orifice or lumen of a tubular body part.

EXPLANATION: Natural or artificially created orifice ...

Body Part – 4TH		Approach – 5TH	Device – 6TH	Qualifier – 7TH
0 Lymphatic, Head	B Lymphatic, Mesenteric	0 Open	C Extraluminal device	Z No qualifier
1 Lymphatic, Right Neck	C Lymphatic, Pelvis	3 Percutaneous	D Intraluminal device	
2 Lymphatic, Left Neck	D Lymphatic, Aortic	4 Percutaneous endoscopic	Z No device	
3 Lymphatic, Right Upper Extremity	F Lymphatic, Right Lower Extremity			
4 Lymphatic, Left Upper Extremity	G Lymphatic, Left Lower Extremity			
5 Lymphatic, Right Axillary	H Lymphatic, Right Inguinal			
6 Lymphatic, Left Axillary	J Lymphatic, Left Inguinal			
7 Lymphatic, Thorax	K Thoracic Duct			
8 Lymphatic, Internal Mammary, Right	L Cisterna Chyli			
9 Lymphatic, Internal Mammary, Left				

DIVISION GROUP: (Division), Release
Root Operations involving cutting or separation only.

- 1ST – **0** Medical and Surgical
- 2ND – **7** Lymphatic and Hemic Systems
- 3RD – **N** RELEASE

EXAMPLE: Lysis of splenic adhesions | CMS Ex: Carpal tunnel release

RELEASE: Freeing a body part from an abnormal physical constraint by cutting or by the use of force.

EXPLANATION: None of the body part is taken out ...

Body Part – 4TH		Approach – 5TH	Device – 6TH	Qualifier – 7TH
0 Lymphatic, Head	B Lymphatic, Mesenteric	0 Open	Z No device	Z No qualifier
1 Lymphatic, Right Neck	C Lymphatic, Pelvis	3 Percutaneous		
2 Lymphatic, Left Neck	D Lymphatic, Aortic	4 Percutaneous endoscopic		
3 Lymphatic, Right Upper Extremity	F Lymphatic, Right Lower Extremity			
4 Lymphatic, Left Upper Extremity	G Lymphatic, Left Lower Extremity			
5 Lymphatic, Right Axillary	H Lymphatic, Right Inguinal			
6 Lymphatic, Left Axillary	J Lymphatic, Left Inguinal			
7 Lymphatic, Thorax	K Thoracic Duct			
8 Lymphatic, Internal Mammary, Right	L Cisterna Chyli			
	M Thymus			
9 Lymphatic, Internal Mammary, Left	P Spleen			

07P MEDICAL AND SURGICAL SECTION – 2016 ICD-10-PCS

DEVICE GROUP: Change, Insertion, Removal, (Replacement), Revision, Supplement
Root Operations that always involve a device.

1ST - 0 Medical and Surgical
2ND - 7 Lymphatic and Hemic Systems
3RD - P REMOVAL

EXAMPLE: Removal drain tube   CMS Ex: Chest tube removal

REMOVAL: Taking out or off a device from a body part.

EXPLANATION: Removal device without reinsertion ...

Body Part – 4TH	Approach – 5TH	Device – 6TH	Qualifier – 7TH
K Thoracic Duct L Cisterna Chyli N Lymphatic	0 Open 3 Percutaneous 4 Percutaneous endoscopic	0 Drainage device 3 Infusion device 7 Autologous tissue substitute C Extraluminal device D Intraluminal device J Synthetic substitute K Nonautologous tissue substitute	Z No qualifier
K Thoracic Duct L Cisterna Chyli N Lymphatic	X External	0 Drainage device 3 Infusion device D Intraluminal device	Z No qualifier
M Thymus P Spleen	0 Open 3 Percutaneous 4 Percutaneous endoscopic X External	0 Drainage device 3 Infusion device	Z No qualifier
T Bone Marrow	0 Open 3 Percutaneous 4 Percutaneous endoscopic X External	0 Drainage device	Z No qualifier

7 – LYMPHATIC AND HEMIC SYSTEMS — 07S

OTHER REPAIRS GROUP: (Control), Repair
Root Operations that define other repairs.

- 1ST – **0** Medical and Surgical
- 2ND – **7** Lymphatic and Hemic Systems
- 3RD – **Q REPAIR**

EXAMPLE: Splenorrhaphy
CMS Ex: Suture laceration

REPAIR: Restoring, to the extent possible, a body part to its normal anatomic structure and function.

EXPLANATION: Only when no other root operation applies …

Body Part – 4TH		Approach – 5TH	Device – 6TH	Qualifier – 7TH
0 Lymphatic, Head	B Lymphatic, Mesenteric	0 Open	Z No device	Z No qualifier
1 Lymphatic, Right Neck	C Lymphatic, Pelvis	3 Percutaneous		
2 Lymphatic, Left Neck	D Lymphatic, Aortic	4 Percutaneous endoscopic		
3 Lymphatic, Right Upper Extremity	F Lymphatic, Right Lower Extremity			
4 Lymphatic, Left Upper Extremity	G Lymphatic, Left Lower Extremity			
5 Lymphatic, Right Axillary	H Lymphatic, Right Inguinal			
6 Lymphatic, Left Axillary	J Lymphatic, Left Inguinal			
7 Lymphatic, Thorax	K Thoracic Duct			
8 Lymphatic, Internal Mammary, Right	L Cisterna Chyli			
9 Lymphatic, Internal Mammary, Left	M Thymus			
	P Spleen			

MOVE GROUP: (Reattachment), Reposition, (Transfer), Transplantation
Root Operations that put in/put back or move some/all of a body part.

- 1ST – **0** Medical and Surgical
- 2ND – **7** Lymphatic and Hemic Systems
- 3RD – **S REPOSITION**

EXAMPLE: Relocation spleen
CMS Ex: Fracture reduction

REPOSITION: Moving to its normal location, or other suitable location, all or a portion of a body part.

EXPLANATION: May or may not be cut to be moved …

Body Part – 4TH	Approach – 5TH	Device – 6TH	Qualifier – 7TH
M Thymus	0 Open	Z No device	Z No qualifier
P Spleen			

07T — MEDICAL AND SURGICAL SECTION – 2016 ICD-10-PCS

EXCISION GROUP: Excision, Resection, Destruction, Extraction, (Detachment)
Root Operations that take out some or all of a body part.

- 1ST – **0** Medical and Surgical
- 2ND – **7** Lymphatic and Hemic Systems
- 3RD – **T RESECTION**

EXAMPLE: Excision lymph node chain
CMS Ex: Cholecystectomy

RESECTION: Cutting out or off, without replacement, all of a body part.

EXPLANATION: None

Body Part – 4TH		Approach – 5TH	Device – 6TH	Qualifier – 7TH
0 Lymphatic, Head	B Lymphatic, Mesenteric	0 Open	Z No device	Z No qualifier
1 Lymphatic, Right Neck	C Lymphatic, Pelvis	4 Percutaneous endoscopic		
2 Lymphatic, Left Neck	D Lymphatic, Aortic			
3 Lymphatic, Right Upper Extremity	F Lymphatic, Right Lower Extremity			
4 Lymphatic, Left Upper Extremity	G Lymphatic, Left Lower Extremity			
5 Lymphatic, Right Axillary	H Lymphatic, Right Inguinal			
6 Lymphatic, Left Axillary	J Lymphatic, Left Inguinal			
7 Lymphatic, Thorax	K Thoracic Duct			
8 Lymphatic, Internal Mammary, Right	L Cisterna Chyli			
9 Lymphatic, Internal Mammary, Left	M Thymus			
	P Spleen			

DEVICE GROUP: Change, Insertion, Removal, (Replacement), Revision, Supplement
Root Operations that always involve a device.

- 1ST – **0** Medical and Surgical
- 2ND – **7** Lymphatic and Hemic Systems
- 3RD – **U SUPPLEMENT**

EXAMPLE: Overlay splenic graft
CMS Ex: Hernia repair with mesh

SUPPLEMENT: Putting in or on biological or synthetic material that physically reinforces and/or augments the function of a portion of a body part.

EXPLANATION: Biological material from same individual …

Body Part – 4TH		Approach – 5TH	Device – 6TH	Qualifier – 7TH
0 Lymphatic, Head	B Lymphatic, Mesenteric	0 Open	7 Autologous tissue substitute	Z No qualifier
1 Lymphatic, Right Neck	C Lymphatic, Pelvis	4 Percutaneous endoscopic	J Synthetic substitute	
2 Lymphatic, Left Neck	D Lymphatic, Aortic		K Nonautologous tissue substitute	
3 Lymphatic, Right Upper Extremity	F Lymphatic, Right Lower Extremity			
4 Lymphatic, Left Upper Extremity	G Lymphatic, Left Lower Extremity			
5 Lymphatic, Right Axillary	H Lymphatic, Right Inguinal			
6 Lymphatic, Left Axillary	J Lymphatic, Left Inguinal			
7 Lymphatic, Thorax	K Thoracic Duct			
8 Lymphatic, Internal Mammary, Right	L Cisterna Chyli			
9 Lymphatic, Internal Mammary, Left				

7 – LYMPHATIC AND HEMIC SYSTEMS   07V

TUBULAR GROUP: (Bypass), (Dilation), **Occlusion, Restriction**
Root Operations that alter the diameter/route of a tubular body part.

1ST - **0** Medical and Surgical

2ND - **7** Lymphatic and Hemic Systems

3RD - **V RESTRICTION**

EXAMPLE: Thoracic duct restrictive stent | **CMS Ex:** Cervical cerclage

RESTRICTION: Partially closing an orifice or the lumen of a tubular body part.

EXPLANATION: Natural or artificially created orifice ...

Body Part – 4TH		Approach – 5TH	Device – 6TH	Qualifier – 7TH
0 Lymphatic, Head	B Lymphatic, Mesenteric	0 Open	C Extraluminal device	Z No qualifier
1 Lymphatic, Right Neck	C Lymphatic, Pelvis	3 Percutaneous	D Intraluminal device	
2 Lymphatic, Left Neck	D Lymphatic, Aortic	4 Percutaneous endoscopic	Z No device	
3 Lymphatic, Right Upper Extremity	F Lymphatic, Right Lower Extremity			
4 Lymphatic, Left Upper Extremity	G Lymphatic, Left Lower Extremity			
5 Lymphatic, Right Axillary	H Lymphatic, Right Inguinal			
6 Lymphatic, Left Axillary	J Lymphatic, Left Inguinal			
7 Lymphatic, Thorax	K Thoracic Duct			
8 Lymphatic, Internal Mammary, Right	L Cisterna Chyli			
9 Lymphatic, Internal Mammary, Left				

07W

DEVICE GROUP: Change, Insertion, Removal, (Replacement), Revision, Supplement
Root Operations that always involve a device.

- 1ST – **0** Medical and Surgical
- 2ND – **7** Lymphatic and Hemic Systems
- 3RD – **W** REVISION

EXAMPLE: Reposition drainage tube | CMS Ex: Adjustment pacemaker lead

REVISION: Correcting, to the extent possible, a portion of a malfunctioning device or the position of a displaced device.

EXPLANATION: May replace components of a device ...

Body Part – 4TH	Approach – 5TH	Device – 6TH	Qualifier – 7TH
K Thoracic Duct L Cisterna Chyli N Lymphatic	0 Open 3 Percutaneous 4 Percutaneous endoscopic X External	0 Drainage device 3 Infusion device 7 Autologous tissue substitute C Extraluminal device D Intraluminal device J Synthetic substitute K Nonautologous tissue substitute	Z No qualifier
M Thymus P Spleen	0 Open 3 Percutaneous 4 Percutaneous endoscopic X External	0 Drainage device 3 Infusion device	Z No qualifier
T Bone Marrow	0 Open 3 Percutaneous 4 Percutaneous endoscopic X External	0 Drainage device	Z No qualifier

MOVE GROUP: (Reattachment), Reposition, (Transfer), Transplantation
Root Operations that put in/put back or move some/all of a body part.

- 1ST – **0** Medical and Surgical
- 2ND – **7** Lymphatic and Hemic Systems
- 3RD – **Y** TRANSPLANTATION

EXAMPLE: Spleen transplant | CMS Ex: Kidney transplant

TRANSPLANTATION: Putting in or on all or a portion of a living body part taken from another individual or animal to physically take the place and/or function of all or a portion of a similar body part.

EXPLANATION: May take over all or part of its function ...

Body Part – 4TH	Approach – 5TH	Device – 6TH	Qualifier – 7TH
M Thymus P Spleen	0 Open	Z No device	0 Allogenic 1 Syngeneic 2 Zooplastic

Educational Annotations | 8 – Eye

Body System Specific Educational Annotations for the Eye include:
- Anatomy and Physiology Review
- Anatomical Illustrations
- Definitions of Common Procedures
- AHA Coding Clinic® Reference Notations
- Body Part Key Listings
- Device Key Listings
- Device Aggregation Table Listings
- Coding Notes

Anatomy and Physiology Review of Eye

BODY PART VALUES – 8 - EYE

Anterior Chamber – The anterior chamber contains the watery fluid between the iris and cornea.

Choroid – ANATOMY – The choroid is the vascular layer lying between the retina and the sclera that contains the dark brown pigment. PHYSIOLOGY – The choroid functions as a vascular blood supply to most eye structures and absorbs excess light through its dark pigment.

Ciliary Body – The ciliary body consists of smooth muscle with suspensory ligaments which holds the lens in place and adjusts the focus of the lens.

Conjunctiva – ANATOMY – The conjunctiva is the delicate mucous membrane that lines the eyelids and covers the exposed surface of the sclera. PHYSIOLOGY – The conjunctiva is the protective mucous-producing membrane covering the eyelids and exposed portion of the sclera. In addition to providing lubrication, it helps prevent the entry of microorganisms.

Cornea – ANATOMY – The transparent tissue layer that covers the front part of the eye including the iris, pupil, and anterior chamber. PHYSIOLOGY – The cornea refracts and focuses most of the light entering the eye.

Extraocular Muscle – ANATOMY – The extraocular muscles attach the eyeball to the orbit by 6 different muscles. PHYSIOLOGY – The extraocular muscles function to rotate the eyeballs to look at desired objects. Four muscles move the eyeball up, down, right, and left. The other two muscles control the adjustments involved in counteracting head movement while maintaining the target.

Eye – ANATOMY – The eyes are hollow spherical structures about 1 inch (2.5 cm) in diameter, located in and protected by the orbital socket in the skull. PHYSIOLOGY – The eyes are the primary organ of sight, and are directly connected to the brain through the retina and optic nerve.

Eyelid – ANATOMY – The thin folds of skin that cover the eye when muscles draw the eyelids together. PHYSIOLOGY – The eyelids protect the eye from injury and foreign objects and aid in tear flow and distribution.

Iris – ANATOMY – The iris is a muscular diaphragm that controls the dilation of the pupil. PHYSIOLOGY – The iris contracts or dilates, allowing for varying amounts of light to enter the eye and retina.

Lacrimal Duct – ANATOMY – The lacrimal duct is located at the inner lower corner of each eye and connects the lacrimal sac with the nasal cavity. PHYSIOLOGY – The lacrimal duct drains the tears from the eyes into the nasal cavities.

Lacrimal Gland – ANATOMY – The lacrimal glands are almond-shaped glands located in the upper outer corner of each orbit. PHYSIOLOGY – The lacrimal glands produce the tears that function to keep protective fluid on the conjunctiva and cornea.

Lens – ANATOMY – The crystalline lens is a transparent elastic, biconvex structure whose shape is controlled by the action of ciliary muscles. PHYSIOLOGY – The lens and cornea refract light waves to focus them on the retina.

Retina – ANATOMY – The retina is the inner layer of the eye and is continuous with the optic nerve. It contains the visual receptor cells including the rods and cones. PHYSIOLOGY – The rods are responsible for colorless vision, like in dim light, and the cones are responsible for color vision through their light-sensitive pigment sets.

Retinal Vessels – The small arteries and veins that circulate the blood to the retina. The retinal arteries are branches of the ophthalmic artery.

Sclera – ANATOMY – The protective, outer layer of the eye (white of the eye). PHYSIOLOGY – The sclera maintains the shape of the globe and serves as the attachment insertions for the extraocular muscles. Its anterior portion, the cornea, is transparent so that it can refract light entering the eye.

Vitreous – ANATOMY – The clear, gelatinous substance filling the globe of the eye between the lens and retina. PHYSIOLOGY – The thick, gel-like substance maintains the shape of the eye globe.

Educational Annotations | 8 – Eye

Anatomical Illustrations of Eye

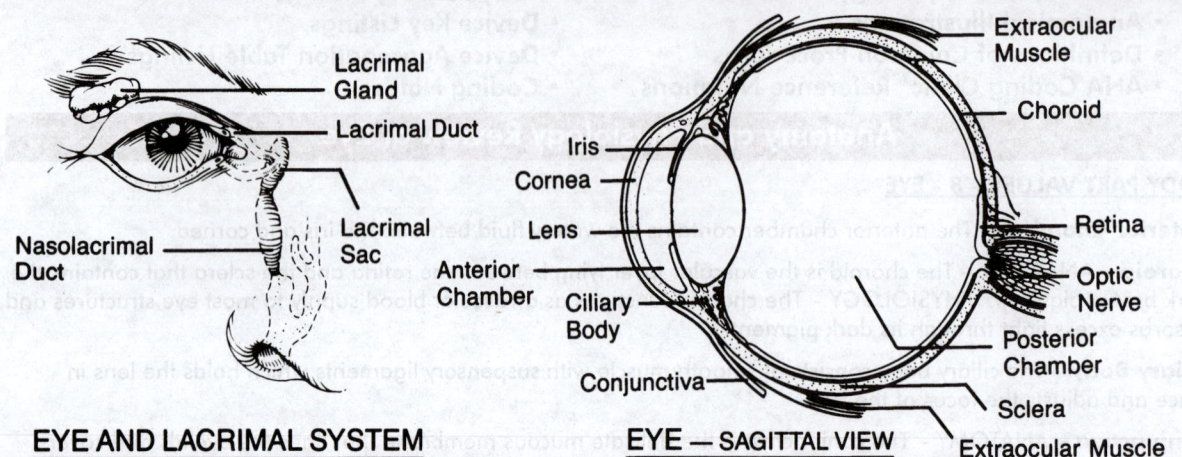

EYE AND LACRIMAL SYSTEM   EYE — SAGITTAL VIEW

Definitions of Common Procedures – Body System Specific

Blepharoplasty – The plastic surgical correction of eyelid defects and deformities. It may also be done for cosmetic reasons.

Cataract extraction – The surgical removal of a cloudy lens (normally clear) that is most often immediately replaced with an artificial lens substitute.

Conjunctivoplasty – The surgical procedure to correct a conjunctival defect or conjunctivochalasis.

Corneal transplant – The replacement of the cornea with a donor cornea graft. Also referred to as a keratoplasty.

Dacryocystorhinostomy – The surgical creation of a communicating passage between the lacrimal sac and the nasal cavity to restore the flow of tears.

Enucleation of eyeball – The surgical removal of the entire eyeball (globe) that leaves the eyelids and eye socket structures intact.

Evisceration of eyeball – The surgical removal of the iris, cornea, lens, retina, and vitreous while leaving the sclera, optic nerve, and extraocular eye muscles intact so that an artificial eye prosthesis (integrated orbital implant) moves naturally with the other eye.

Exenteration of eyeball – The surgical removal of all of the contents of the eye socket including the extraocular muscles and often including the eyelids.

Scleral buckling – The surgical placement of synthetic material around the eyeball to create an inward indentation of the sclera from the exterior creating a ridge (or buckle) that corrects the effects of retinal detachment.

Strabismus surgery – The surgical correction of strabismus by repositioning, shortening, or lengthening of one or more of the extraocular eye muscles.

Educational Annotations

8 – Eye

AHA Coding Clinic® Reference Notations of Eye

ROOT OPERATION SPECIFIC - 8 - EYE
ALTERATION - 0
BYPASS - 1
CHANGE - 2
DESTRUCTION - 5
DILATION - 7
DRAINAGE - 9
EXCISION - B
    Core vitrectomy with gas replacement ....AHA 14:4Q:p35
    Posterior pars plana vitrectomy..AHA 14:4Q:p36
EXTIRPATION - C
EXTRACTION - D
FRAGMENTATION - F
INSERTION - H
INSPECTION - J
    Unsuccessful removal of foreign body of eye ....AHA 15:1Q:p35
OCCLUSION - L
REATTACHMENT - M
RELEASE - N
    Lysis of iris adhesions...AHA 15:2Q:p24
REMOVAL - P
REPAIR - Q
REPLACEMENT - R
    Penetrating keratoplasty with anterior segment reconstruction ....AHA 15:2Q:p24
    Penetrating keratoplasty with viscoelastic filling ....AHA 15:2Q:p25
REPOSITION - S
RESECTION - T
    Radical resection of eyelid and orbital tumor ....AHA 15:2Q:p12
SUPPLEMENT - U
    Amniotic membrane corneal transplantation ....AHA 14:3Q:p31
RESTRICTION - V
REVISION - W
TRANSFER - X

Body Part Key Listings of Eye

See also Body Part Key in Appendix C

Aqueous humour	*use* Anterior Chamber, Left/Right
Ciliary body	*use* Eye, Left/Right
Fovea	*use* Retina, Left/Right
Inferior oblique muscle	*use* Extraocular Muscle, Left/Right
Inferior rectus muscle..	*use* Extraocular Muscle, Left/Right
Inferior tarsal plate	*use* Lower Eyelid, Left/Right
Lacrimal canaliculus...	*use* Lacrimal Duct, Left/Right
Lacrimal punctum	*use* Lacrimal Duct, Left/Right
Lacrimal sac	*use* Lacrimal Duct, Left/Right
Lateral canthus..	*use* Upper Eyelid, Left/Right
Lateral rectus muscle	*use* Extraocular Muscle, Left/Right
Levator palpebrae superioris muscle	*use* Upper Eyelid, Left/Right
Macula	*use* Retina, Left/Right
Medial canthus...	*use* Lower Eyelid, Left/Right
Medial rectus muscle	*use* Extraocular Muscle, Left/Right

Continued on next page

Educational Annotations | 8 – Eye

Body Part Key Listings of Eye

Continued from previous page

Nasolacrimal duct	use Lacrimal Duct, Left/Right
Optic disc	use Retina, Left/Right
Orbicularis oculi muscle	use Upper Eyelid, Left/Right
Plica semilunaris	use Conjunctiva, Left/Right
Posterior chamber	use Eye, Left/Right
Superior oblique muscle	use Extraocular Muscle, Left/Right
Superior rectus muscle	use Extraocular Muscle, Left/Right
Superior tarsal plate	use Upper Eyelid, Left/Right
Vitreous body	use Vitreous, Left/Right
Zonule of Zinn	use Lens, Left/Right

Device Key Listings of Eye

See also Device Key in Appendix D

Autograft	use Autologous Tissue Substitute
Brachytherapy seeds	use Radioactive Element
Ex-PRESS™ mini glaucoma shunt	use Synthetic Substitute
Implantable Miniature Telescope™ (IMT)	use Synthetic Substitute, Intraocular Telescope for Replacement in Eye
Tissue bank graft	use Nonautologous Tissue Substitute

Device Aggregation Table Listings of Eye

See also Device Aggregation Table in Appendix E

Specific Device	For Operation	In Body System	General Device	
Epiretinal Visual Prosthesis	All applicable	Eye	J	Synthetic Substitute
Synthetic Substitute, Intraocular Telescope	Replacement	Eye	J	Synthetic Substitute

Coding Notes of Eye

Body System Specific PCS Reference Manual Exercises

PCS CODE	8 – EYE EXERCISES
085G3ZZ	Laser coagulation of right retinal vessel hemorrhage, percutaneous. (The "Retinal Vessel" body part values are in the "Eye" body system.)
087X7DZ	Trans-nasal dilation and stent placement in right lacrimal duct.
08C8XZZ	Removal of foreign body, right cornea.
08CX0ZZ	Incision and removal of right lacrimal duct stone.
08DJ3ZZ	Extraction of right intraocular lens without replacement, percutaneous.
08R83KZ	Penetrating keratoplasty of right cornea with donor matched cornea, percutaneous approach.
08RJ3JZ	Percutaneous phacoemulsification of right eye cataract with prosthetic lens insertion.
08U9X7Z	Onlay lamellar keratoplasty of left cornea using autograft, external approach.
08VX7DZ	Non-incisional, trans-nasal placement of restrictive stent in right lacrimal duct.

OTHER OBJECTIVES GROUP: Alteration, (Creation), (Fusion)
Root Operations that define other objectives.

- 1ST – **0** Medical and Surgical
- 2ND – **8** Eye
- 3RD – **0** ALTERATION

EXAMPLE: Cosmetic blepharoplasty   CMS Ex: Face lift

ALTERATION: Modifying the anatomic structure of a body part without affecting the function of the body part.

EXPLANATION: Principal purpose is to improve appearance

Body Part – 4TH	Approach – 5TH	Device – 6TH	Qualifier – 7TH
N Upper Eyelid, Right P Upper Eyelid, Left Q Lower Eyelid, Right R Lower Eyelid, Left	0 Open 3 Percutaneous X External	7 Autologous tissue substitute J Synthetic substitute K Nonautologous tissue substitute Z No device	Z No qualifier

TUBULAR GROUP: Bypass, Dilation, Occlusion, Restriction
Root Operations that alter the diameter/route of a tubular body part.

- 1ST – **0** Medical and Surgical
- 2ND – **8** Eye
- 3RD – **1** BYPASS

EXAMPLE: Dacryocystorhinostomy   CMS Ex: Coronary artery bypass

BYPASS: Altering the route of passage of the contents of a tubular body part.

EXPLANATION: Rerouting contents to a downstream part ...

Body Part – 4TH	Approach – 5TH	Device – 6TH	Qualifier – 7TH
2 Anterior Chamber, Right 3 Anterior Chamber, Left	3 Percutaneous	J Synthetic substitute K Nonautologous tissue substitute Z No device	4 Sclera
X Lacrimal Duct, Right Y Lacrimal Duct, Left	0 Open 3 Percutaneous	J Synthetic substitute K Nonautologous tissue substitute Z No device	3 Nasal Cavity

DEVICE GROUP: Change, Insertion, Removal, Replacement, Revision, Supplement
Root Operations that always involve a device.

- 1ST – **0** Medical and Surgical
- 2ND – **8** Eye
- 3RD – **2** CHANGE

EXAMPLE: Exchange drain tube   CMS Ex: Changing urinary catheter

CHANGE: Taking out or off a device from a body part and putting back an identical or similar device in or on the same body part without cutting or puncturing the skin or a mucous membrane.

EXPLANATION: ALL Changes use EXTERNAL approach only...

Body Part – 4TH	Approach – 5TH	Device – 6TH	Qualifier – 7TH
0 Eye, Right 1 Eye, Left	X External	0 Drainage device Y Other device	Z No qualifier

085

MEDICAL AND SURGICAL SECTION – 2016 ICD-10-PCS [2016.PCS]

EXCISION GROUP: Excision, Resection, Destruction, Extraction, (Detachment)
Root Operations that take out some or all of a body part.

- 1ST – **0** Medical and Surgical
- 2ND – **8** Eye
- 3RD – **5 DESTRUCTION**

EXAMPLE: Cryoablation eyelid lesion   CMS Ex: Fulguration polyp

DESTRUCTION: Physical eradication of all or a portion of a body part by the direct use of energy, force, or a destructive agent.

EXPLANATION: None of the body part is physically taken out

Body Part – 4TH	Approach – 5TH	Device – 6TH	Qualifier – 7TH
0 Eye, Right 1 Eye, Left 6 Sclera, Right 7 Sclera, Left 8 Cornea, Right 9 Cornea, Left S Conjunctiva, Right T Conjunctiva, Left	X External	Z No device	Z No qualifier
2 Anterior Chamber, Right 3 Anterior Chamber, Left 4 Vitreous, Right 5 Vitreous, Left C Iris, Right D Iris, Left E Retina, Right F Retina, Left G Retinal Vessel, Right H Retinal Vessel, Left J Lens, Right K Lens, Left	3 Percutaneous	Z No device	Z No qualifier
A Choroid, Right B Choroid, Left L Extraocular Muscle, Right M Extraocular Muscle, Left V Lacrimal Gland, Right W Lacrimal Gland, Left	0 Open 3 Percutaneous	Z No device	Z No qualifier
N Upper Eyelid, Right P Upper Eyelid, Left Q Lower Eyelid, Right R Lower Eyelid, Left	0 Open 3 Percutaneous X External	Z No device	Z No qualifier
X Lacrimal Duct, Right Y Lacrimal Duct, Left	0 Open 3 Percutaneous 7 Via natural or artificial opening 8 Via natural or artificial opening endoscopic	Z No device	Z No qualifier

TUBULAR GROUP: Bypass, Dilation, Occlusion, Restriction
Root Operations that alter the diameter/route of a tubular body part.

- 1ST – **0** Medical and Surgical
- 2ND – **8** Eye
- 3RD – **7 DILATION**

EXAMPLE: Dilation lacrimal duct   CMS Ex: Transluminal angioplasty

DILATION: Expanding an orifice or the lumen of a tubular body part.

EXPLANATION: By force (stretching) or cutting …

Body Part – 4TH	Approach – 5TH	Device – 6TH	Qualifier – 7TH
X Lacrimal Duct, Right Y Lacrimal Duct, Left	0 Open 3 Percutaneous 7 Via natural or artificial opening 8 Via natural or artificial opening endoscopic	D Intraluminal device Z No device	Z No qualifier

8 – EYE   089

DRAINAGE GROUP: Drainage, Extirpation, Fragmentation
Root Operations that take out solids/fluids/gases from a body part.

1ST – **0** Medical and Surgical
2ND – **8** Eye
3RD – **9** DRAINAGE

EXAMPLE: Drainage of lacrimal gland
CMS Ex: Thoracentesis

DRAINAGE: Taking or letting out fluids and/or gases from a body part.

EXPLANATION: Qualifier "X Diagnostic" indicates biopsy ...

Body Part – 4TH		Approach – 5TH	Device – 6TH	Qualifier – 7TH
0 Eye, Right 1 Eye, Left 6 Sclera, Right 7 Sclera, Left	8 Cornea, Right 9 Cornea, Left S Conjunctiva, Right T Conjunctiva, Left	X External	0 Drainage device	Z No qualifier
0 Eye, Right 1 Eye, Left 6 Sclera, Right 7 Sclera, Left	8 Cornea, Right 9 Cornea, Left S Conjunctiva, Right T Conjunctiva, Left	X External	Z No device	X Diagnostic Z No qualifier
2 Anterior Chamber, Right 3 Anterior Chamber, Left 4 Vitreous, Right 5 Vitreous, Left C Iris, Right D Iris, Left	E Retina, Right F Retina, Left G Retinal Vessel, Right H Retinal Vessel, Left J Lens, Right K Lens, Left	3 Percutaneous	0 Drainage device	Z No qualifier
2 Anterior Chamber, Right 3 Anterior Chamber, Left 4 Vitreous, Right 5 Vitreous, Left C Iris, Right D Iris, Left	E Retina, Right F Retina, Left G Retinal Vessel, Right H Retinal Vessel, Left J Lens, Right K Lens, Left	3 Percutaneous	Z No device	X Diagnostic Z No qualifier
A Choroid, Right B Choroid, Left L Extraocular Muscle, Right	M Extraocular Muscle, Left V Lacrimal Gland, Right W Lacrimal Gland, Left	0 Open 3 Percutaneous	0 Drainage device	Z No qualifier
A Choroid, Right B Choroid, Left L Extraocular Muscle, Right	M Extraocular Muscle, Left V Lacrimal Gland, Right W Lacrimal Gland, Left	0 Open 3 Percutaneous	Z No device	X Diagnostic Z No qualifier
N Upper Eyelid, Right P Upper Eyelid, Left Q Lower Eyelid, Right R Lower Eyelid, Left		0 Open 3 Percutaneous X External	0 Drainage device	Z No qualifier
N Upper Eyelid, Right P Upper Eyelid, Left Q Lower Eyelid, Right R Lower Eyelid, Left		0 Open 3 Percutaneous X External	Z No device	X Diagnostic Z No qualifier
X Lacrimal Duct, Right Y Lacrimal Duct, Left		0 Open 3 Percutaneous 7 Via natural or artificial opening 8 Via natural or artificial opening endoscopic	0 Drainage device	Z No qualifier
X Lacrimal Duct, Right Y Lacrimal Duct, Left		0 Open 3 Percutaneous 7 Via natural or artificial opening 8 Via natural or artificial opening endoscopic	Z No device	X Diagnostic Z No qualifier

0 8 B

MEDICAL AND SURGICAL SECTION – 2016 ICD-10-PCS

EXCISION GROUP: Excision, Resection, Destruction, Extraction, (Detachment)
Root Operations that take out some or all of a body part.

1ST - 0	Medical and Surgical
2ND - 8	Eye
3RD - B	EXCISION

EXAMPLE: Sclerectomy **CMS Ex:** Liver biopsy

EXCISION: Cutting out or off, without replacement, a portion of a body part.

EXPLANATION: Qualifier "X Diagnostic" indicates biopsy ...

Body Part – 4TH		Approach – 5TH	Device – 6TH	Qualifier – 7TH
0 Eye, Right 1 Eye, Left N Upper Eyelid, Right	P Upper Eyelid, Left Q Lower Eyelid, Right R Lower Eyelid, Left	0 Open 3 Percutaneous X External	Z No device	X Diagnostic Z No qualifier
4 Vitreous, Right 5 Vitreous, Left C Iris, Right D Iris, Left	E Retina, Right F Retina, Left J Lens, Right K Lens, Left	3 Percutaneous	Z No device	X Diagnostic Z No qualifier
6 Sclera, Right 7 Sclera, Left 8 Cornea, Right	9 Cornea, Left S Conjunctiva, Right T Conjunctiva, Left	X External	Z No device	X Diagnostic Z No qualifier
A Choroid, Right B Choroid, Left L Extraocular Muscle, Right	M Extraocular Muscle, Left V Lacrimal Gland, Right W Lacrimal Gland, Left	0 Open 3 Percutaneous	Z No device	X Diagnostic Z No qualifier
X Lacrimal Duct, Right Y Lacrimal Duct, Left		0 Open 3 Percutaneous 7 Via natural or artificial opening 8 Via natural or artificial opening endoscopic	Z No device	X Diagnostic Z No qualifier

252

08D

DRAINAGE GROUP: Drainage, Extirpation, Fragmentation
Root Operations that take out solids/fluids/gases from a body part.

- 1ST – **0** Medical and Surgical
- 2ND – **8** Eye
- 3RD – **C** EXTIRPATION

EXAMPLE: Magnetic extraction, metal splinter | CMS Ex: Choledocholithotomy

EXTIRPATION: Taking or cutting out solid matter from a body part.

EXPLANATION: Abnormal byproduct or foreign body ...

Body Part – 4TH		Approach – 5TH	Device – 6TH	Qualifier – 7TH
0 Eye, Right 1 Eye, Left 6 Sclera, Right 7 Sclera, Left	8 Cornea, Right 9 Cornea, Left S Conjunctiva, Right T Conjunctiva, Left	X External	Z No device	Z No qualifier
2 Anterior Chamber, Right 3 Anterior Chamber, Left 4 Vitreous, Right 5 Vitreous, Left C Iris, Right D Iris, Left	E Retina, Right F Retina, Left G Retinal Vessel, Right H Retinal Vessel, Left J Lens, Right K Lens, Left	3 Percutaneous X External	Z No device	Z No qualifier
A Choroid, Right B Choroid, Left L Extraocular Muscle, Right M Extraocular Muscle, Left N Upper Eyelid, Right	P Upper Eyelid, Left Q Lower Eyelid, Right R Lower Eyelid, Left V Lacrimal Gland, Right W Lacrimal Gland, Left	0 Open 3 Percutaneous X External	Z No device	Z No qualifier
X Lacrimal Duct, Right Y Lacrimal Duct, Left		0 Open 3 Percutaneous 7 Via natural or artificial opening 8 Via natural or artificial opening endoscopic	Z No device	Z No qualifier

EXCISION GROUP: Excision, Resection, Destruction, Extraction, (Detachment)
Root Operations that take out some or all of a body part.

- 1ST – **0** Medical and Surgical
- 2ND – **8** Eye
- 3RD – **D** EXTRACTION

EXAMPLE: Lens extraction without replacement | CMS Ex: D&C

EXTRACTION: Pulling or stripping out or off all or a portion of a body part by the use of force.

EXPLANATION: Qualifier "X Diagnostic" indicates biopsy ...

Body Part – 4TH	Approach – 5TH	Device – 6TH	Qualifier – 7TH
8 Cornea, Right 9 Cornea, Left	X External	Z No device	X Diagnostic Z No qualifier
J Lens, Right K Lens, Left	3 Percutaneous	Z No device	Z No qualifier

08F MEDICAL AND SURGICAL SECTION – 2016 ICD-10-PCS

DRAINAGE GROUP: Drainage, Extirpation, Fragmentation
Root Operations that take out solids/fluids/gases from a body part.

- 1ST – 0 Medical and Surgical
- 2ND – 8 Eye
- 3RD – F FRAGMENTATION

EXAMPLE: Lithotripsy, vitreous | CMS Ex: Extracorporeal shockwave lithotripsy

FRAGMENTATION: Breaking solid matter in a body part into pieces.

EXPLANATION: Pieces are not taken out during procedure ...

Body Part – 4TH	Approach – 5TH	Device – 6TH	Qualifier – 7TH
4 Vitreous, Right 5 Vitreous, Left	3 Percutaneous X External NC*	Z No device	Z No qualifier

NC* – Non-covered by Medicare. See current Medicare Code Editor for details.

DEVICE GROUP: Change, Insertion, Removal, Replacement, Revision, Supplement
Root Operations that always involve a device.

- 1ST – 0 Medical and Surgical
- 2ND – 8 Eye
- 3RD – H INSERTION

EXAMPLE: Implantation EpiRet | CMS Ex: Insertion central venous catheter

INSERTION: Putting in a nonbiological appliance that monitors, assists, performs, or prevents a physiological function but does not physically take the place of a body part.

EXPLANATION: None

Body Part – 4TH	Approach – 5TH	Device – 6TH	Qualifier – 7TH
0 Eye, Right 1 Eye, Left	0 Open	5 Epiretinal visual prosthesis	Z No qualifier
0 Eye, Right 1 Eye, Left	3 Percutaneous X External	1 Radioactive element 3 Infusion device	Z No qualifier

EXAMINATION GROUP: Inspection, (Map)
Root Operations involving examination only.

- 1ST – 0 Medical and Surgical
- 2ND – 8 Eye
- 3RD – J INSPECTION

EXAMPLE: Eye examination | CMS Ex: Colonoscopy

INSPECTION: Visually and/or manually exploring a body part.

EXPLANATION: Direct or instrumental visualization ...

Body Part – 4TH	Approach – 5TH	Device – 6TH	Qualifier – 7TH
0 Eye, Right 1 Eye, Left J Lens, Right K Lens, Left	X External	Z No device	Z No qualifier
L Extraocular Muscle, Right M Extraocular Muscle, Left	0 Open X External	Z No device	Z No qualifier

8 – EYE 08M

TUBULAR GROUP: Bypass, Dilation, Occlusion, Restriction
Root Operations that alter the diameter/route of a tubular body part.

- 1ST – **0** Medical and Surgical
- 2ND – **8** Eye
- 3RD – **L OCCLUSION**

EXAMPLE: Punctal occlusion **CMS Ex:** Fallopian tube ligation

OCCLUSION: Completely closing an orifice or lumen of a tubular body part.

EXPLANATION: Natural or artificially created orifice ...

Body Part – 4TH	Approach – 5TH	Device – 6TH	Qualifier – 7TH
X Lacrimal Duct, Right Y Lacrimal Duct, Left	0 Open 3 Percutaneous	C Extraluminal device D Intraluminal device Z No device	Z No qualifier
X Lacrimal Duct, Right Y Lacrimal Duct, Left	7 Via natural or artificial opening 8 Via natural or artificial opening endoscopic	D Intraluminal device Z No device	Z No qualifier

MOVE GROUP: Reattachment, Reposition, Transfer, (Transplantation)
Root Operations that put in/put back or move some/all of a body part.

- 1ST – **0** Medical and Surgical
- 2ND – **8** Eye
- 3RD – **M REATTACHMENT**

EXAMPLE: Reattachment avulsed eyelid **CMS Ex:** Reattachment hand

REATTACHMENT: Putting back in or on all or a portion of a separated body part to its normal location or other suitable location.

EXPLANATION: With/without reconnection of vessels/nerves...

Body Part – 4TH	Approach – 5TH	Device – 6TH	Qualifier – 7TH
N Upper Eyelid, Right P Upper Eyelid, Left Q Lower Eyelid, Right R Lower Eyelid, Left	X External	Z No device	Z No qualifier

08N MEDICAL AND SURGICAL SECTION – 2016 ICD-10-PCS

DIVISION GROUP: (Division), Release
Root Operations involving cutting or separation only.

- 1ST – **0** Medical and Surgical
- 2ND – **8** Eye
- 3RD – **N** RELEASE

EXAMPLE: Adhesiolysis lateral rectus **CMS Ex:** Carpal tunnel release

RELEASE: Freeing a body part from an abnormal physical constraint by cutting or by the use of force.

EXPLANATION: None of the body part is taken out ...

Body Part – 4TH		Approach – 5TH	Device – 6TH	Qualifier – 7TH
0 Eye, Right 1 Eye, Left 6 Sclera, Right 7 Sclera, Left	8 Cornea, Right 9 Cornea, Left S Conjunctiva, Right T Conjunctiva, Left	X External	Z No device	Z No qualifier
2 Anterior Chamber, Right 3 Anterior Chamber, Left 4 Vitreous, Right 5 Vitreous, Left C Iris, Right D Iris, Left	E Retina, Right F Retina, Left G Retinal Vessel, Right H Retinal Vessel, Left J Lens, Right K Lens, Left	3 Percutaneous	Z No device	Z No qualifier
A Choroid, Right B Choroid, Left L Extraocular Muscle, Right	M Extraocular Muscle, Left V Lacrimal Gland, Right W Lacrimal Gland, Left	0 Open 3 Percutaneous	Z No device	Z No qualifier
N Upper Eyelid, Right P Upper Eyelid, Left Q Lower Eyelid, Right R Lower Eyelid, Left		0 Open 3 Percutaneous X External	Z No device	Z No qualifier
X Lacrimal Duct, Right Y Lacrimal Duct, Left		0 Open 3 Percutaneous 7 Via natural or artificial opening 8 Via natural or artificial opening endoscopic	Z No device	Z No qualifier

08P

DEVICE GROUP: Change, Insertion, Removal, Replacement, Revision, Supplement
Root Operations that always involve a device.

1ST - **0** Medical and Surgical

2ND - **8** Eye

3RD - **P REMOVAL**

EXAMPLE: Removal eye drain tube

CMS Ex: Chest tube removal

REMOVAL: Taking out or off a device from a body part.

EXPLANATION: Removal without reinsertion ...

Body Part – 4TH	Approach – 5TH	Device – 6TH	Qualifier – 7TH
0 Eye, Right 1 Eye, Left	0 Open 3 Percutaneous 7 Via natural or artificial opening 8 Via natural or artificial opening endoscopic X External	0 Drainage device 1 Radioactive element 3 Infusion device 7 Autologous tissue substitute C Extraluminal device D Intraluminal device J Synthetic substitute K Nonautologous tissue substitute	Z No qualifier
J Lens, Right K Lens, Left	3 Percutaneous	J Synthetic substitute	Z No qualifier
L Extraocular Muscle, Right M Extraocular Muscle, Left	0 Open 3 Percutaneous	0 Drainage device 7 Autologous tissue substitute J Synthetic substitute K Nonautologous tissue substitute	Z No qualifier

08Q MEDICAL AND SURGICAL SECTION – 2016 ICD-10-PCS [2016.PCS]

OTHER REPAIRS GROUP: (Control), Repair
Root Operations that define other repairs.

1ST - **0** Medical and Surgical
2ND - **8** Eye
3RD - **Q REPAIR**

EXAMPLE: Iris mattress suture   CMS Ex: Suture laceration

REPAIR: Restoring, to the extent possible, a body part to its normal anatomic structure and function.

EXPLANATION: Only when no other root operation applies …

Body Part – 4TH		Approach – 5TH	Device – 6TH	Qualifier – 7TH
0 Eye, Right 1 Eye, Left 6 Sclera, Right 7 Sclera, Left	8 Cornea, Right NC* 9 Cornea, Left NC* S Conjunctiva, Right T Conjunctiva, Left	X External	Z No device	Z No qualifier
2 Anterior Chamber, Right 3 Anterior Chamber, Left 4 Vitreous, Right 5 Vitreous, Left C Iris, Right D Iris, Left	E Retina, Right F Retina, Left G Retinal Vessel, Right H Retinal Vessel, Left J Lens, Right K Lens, Left	3 Percutaneous	Z No device	Z No qualifier
A Choroid, Right B Choroid, Left L Extraocular Muscle, Right	M Extraocular Muscle, Left V Lacrimal Gland, Right W Lacrimal Gland, Left	0 Open 3 Percutaneous	Z No device	Z No qualifier
N Upper Eyelid, Right P Upper Eyelid, Left Q Lower Eyelid, Right R Lower Eyelid, Left		0 Open 3 Percutaneous X External	Z No device	Z No qualifier
X Lacrimal Duct, Right Y Lacrimal Duct, Left		0 Open 3 Percutaneous 7 Via natural or artificial opening 8 Via natural or artificial opening endoscopic	Z No device	Z No qualifier

NC* – Non-covered by Medicare. See current Medicare Code Editor for details.

08R

DEVICE GROUP: Change, Insertion, Removal, Replacement, Revision, Supplement
Root Operations that always involve a device.

1ST - 0 Medical and Surgical
2ND - 8 Eye
3RD - R REPLACEMENT

EXAMPLE: Extraction lens with prosthetic insertion **CMS Ex:** Total hip

REPLACEMENT: Putting in or on a biological or synthetic material that physically takes the place and/or function of all or a portion of a body part.

EXPLANATION: Includes taking out body part, or eradication...

Body Part – 4TH	Approach – 5TH	Device – 6TH	Qualifier – 7TH
0 Eye, Right 1 Eye, Left A Choroid, Right B Choroid, Left	0 Open 3 Percutaneous	7 Autologous tissue substitute J Synthetic substitute K Nonautologous tissue substitute	Z No qualifier
4 Vitreous, Right 5 Vitreous, Left C Iris, Right D Iris, Left G Retinal Vessel, Right H Retinal Vessel, Left	3 Percutaneous	7 Autologous tissue substitute J Synthetic substitute K Nonautologous tissue substitute	Z No qualifier
6 Sclera, Right 7 Sclera, Left S Conjunctiva, Right T Conjunctiva, Left	X External	7 Autologous tissue substitute J Synthetic substitute K Nonautologous tissue substitute	Z No qualifier
8 Cornea, Right 9 Cornea, Left	3 Percutaneous X External	7 Autologous tissue substitute J Synthetic substitute K Nonautologous tissue substitute	Z No qualifier
J Lens, Right K Lens, Left	3 Percutaneous	0 Synthetic substitute, intraocular telescope 7 Autologous tissue substitute J Synthetic substitute K Nonautologous tissue substitute	Z No qualifier
N Upper Eyelid, Right P Upper Eyelid, Left Q Lower Eyelid, Right R Lower Eyelid, Left	0 Open 3 Percutaneous X External	7 Autologous tissue substitute J Synthetic substitute K Nonautologous tissue substitute	Z No qualifier
X Lacrimal Duct, Right Y Lacrimal Duct, Left	0 Open 3 Percutaneous 7 Via natural or artificial opening 8 Via natural or artificial opening endoscopic	7 Autologous tissue substitute J Synthetic substitute K Nonautologous tissue substitute	Z No qualifier

08S

MEDICAL AND SURGICAL SECTION – 2016 ICD-10-PCS [2016.PCS]

MOVE GROUP: Reattachment, Reposition, Transfer, (Transplantation)
Root Operations that put in/put back or move some/all of a body part.

1ST – **0** Medical and Surgical
2ND – **8** Eye
3RD – **S** REPOSITION

EXAMPLE: Relocation eye muscle (strabismus) | **CMS Ex:** FX reduction

REPOSITION: Moving to its normal location, or other suitable location, all or a portion of a body part.

EXPLANATION: May or may not be cut to be moved ...

Body Part – 4TH	Approach – 5TH	Device – 6TH	Qualifier – 7TH
C Iris, Right D Iris, Left G Retinal Vessel, Right H Retinal Vessel, Left J Lens, Right K Lens, Left	3 Percutaneous	Z No device	Z No qualifier
L Extraocular Muscle, Right M Extraocular Muscle, Left V Lacrimal Gland, Right W Lacrimal Gland, Left	0 Open 3 Percutaneous	Z No device	Z No qualifier
N Upper Eyelid, Right P Upper Eyelid, Left Q Lower Eyelid, Right R Lower Eyelid, Left	0 Open 3 Percutaneous X External	Z No device	Z No qualifier
X Lacrimal Duct, Right Y Lacrimal Duct, Left	0 Open 3 Percutaneous 7 Via natural or artificial opening 8 Via natural or artificial opening endoscopic	Z No device	Z No qualifier

[2016.PCS] 8 – EYE 0 8 T

EXCISION GROUP: Excision, Resection, Destruction, Extraction, (Detachment)
Root Operations that take out some or all of a body part.

1ST - **0** Medical and Surgical
2ND - **8** Eye
3RD - **T** RESECTION

EXAMPLE: Enucleation eyeball   CMS Ex: Cholecystectomy

RESECTION: Cutting out or off, without replacement, all of a body part.

EXPLANATION: None

Body Part – 4TH		Approach – 5TH	Device – 6TH	Qualifier – 7TH
0 Eye, Right 1 Eye, Left	8 Cornea, Right 9 Cornea, Left	X External	Z No device	Z No qualifier
4 Vitreous, Right 5 Vitreous, Left C Iris, Right	D Iris, Left J Lens, Right K Lens, Left	3 Percutaneous	Z No device	Z No qualifier
L Extraocular Muscle, Right M Extraocular Muscle, Left V Lacrimal Gland, Right W Lacrimal Gland, Left		0 Open 3 Percutaneous	Z No device	Z No qualifier
N Upper Eyelid, Right P Upper Eyelid, Left Q Lower Eyelid, Right R Lower Eyelid, Left		0 Open X External	Z No device	Z No qualifier
X Lacrimal Duct, Right Y Lacrimal Duct, Left		0 Open 3 Percutaneous 7 Via natural or artificial opening 8 Via natural or artificial opening endoscopic	Z No device	Z No qualifier

0 8 U

DEVICE GROUP: Change, Insertion, Removal, Replacement, Revision, Supplement
Root Operations that always involve a device.

1ST – 0 Medical and Surgical
2ND – 8 Eye
3RD – U SUPPLEMENT

EXAMPLE: Scleral buckle with implant | CMS Ex: Hernia repair with mesh

SUPPLEMENT: Putting in or on biological or synthetic material that physically reinforces and/or augments the function of a portion of a body part.

EXPLANATION: Biological material from same individual ...

Body Part – 4TH	Approach – 5TH	Device – 6TH	Qualifier – 7TH
0 Eye, Right 1 Eye, Left C Iris, Right D Iris, Left E Retina, Right F Retina, Left G Retinal Vessel, Right H Retinal Vessel, Left L Extraocular Muscle, Right M Extraocular Muscle, Left	0 Open 3 Percutaneous	7 Autologous tissue substitute J Synthetic substitute K Nonautologous tissue substitute	Z No qualifier
8 Cornea, Right NC* 9 Cornea, Left NC* N Upper Eyelid, Right P Upper Eyelid, Left Q Lower Eyelid, Right R Lower Eyelid, Left	0 Open 3 Percutaneous X External	7 Autologous tissue substitute J Synthetic substitute K Nonautologous tissue substitute	Z No qualifier
X Lacrimal Duct, Right Y Lacrimal Duct, Left	0 Open 3 Percutaneous 7 Via natural or artificial opening 8 Via natural or artificial opening endoscopic	7 Autologous tissue substitute J Synthetic substitute K Nonautologous tissue substitute	Z No qualifier

NC* – Some procedures are considered non-covered by Medicare. See current Medicare Code Editor for details.

TUBULAR GROUP: Bypass, Dilation, Occlusion, Restriction
Root Operations that alter the diameter/route of a tubular body part.

1ST – 0 Medical and Surgical
2ND – 8 Eye
3RD – V RESTRICTION

EXAMPLE: Lacrimal duct restrictive stent | CMS Ex: Cervical cerclage

RESTRICTION: Partially closing an orifice or the lumen of a tubular body part.

EXPLANATION: Natural or artificially created orifice ...

Body Part – 4TH	Approach – 5TH	Device – 6TH	Qualifier – 7TH
X Lacrimal Duct, Right Y Lacrimal Duct, Left	0 Open 3 Percutaneous	C Extraluminal device D Intraluminal device Z No device	Z No qualifier
X Lacrimal Duct, Right Y Lacrimal Duct, Left	7 Via natural or artificial opening 8 Via natural or artificial opening endoscopic	D Intraluminal device Z No device	Z No qualifier

DEVICE GROUP: Change, Insertion, Removal, Replacement, Revision, Supplement
Root Operations that always involve a device.

1ST - 0 Medical and Surgical
2ND - 8 Eye
3RD - W REVISION

EXAMPLE: Reposition prosthetic lens | CMS Ex: Adjustment pacemaker lead

REVISION: Correcting, to the extent possible, a portion of a malfunctioning device or the position of a displaced device.

EXPLANATION: May replace components of a device ...

Body Part – 4TH	Approach – 5TH	Device – 6TH	Qualifier – 7TH
0 Eye, Right 1 Eye, Left	0 Open 3 Percutaneous 7 Via natural or artificial opening 8 Via natural or artificial opening endoscopic X External	0 Drainage device 3 Infusion device 7 Autologous tissue substitute C Extraluminal device D Intraluminal device J Synthetic substitute K Nonautologous tissue substitute	Z No qualifier
J Lens, Right K Lens, Left	3 Percutaneous X External	J Synthetic substitute	Z No qualifier
L Extraocular Muscle, Right M Extraocular Muscle, Left	0 Open 3 Percutaneous	0 Drainage device 7 Autologous tissue substitute J Synthetic substitute K Nonautologous tissue substitute	Z No qualifier

MOVE GROUP: Reattachment, Reposition, Transfer, (Transplantation)
Root Operations that put in/put back or move some/all of a body part.

1ST - 0 Medical and Surgical
2ND - 8 Eye
3RD - X TRANSFER

EXAMPLE: Transfer medial rectus muscle | CMS Ex: Tendon transfer

TRANSFER: Moving, without taking out, all or a portion of a body part to another location to take over the function of all or a portion of a body part.

EXPLANATION: The body part remains connected ...

Body Part – 4TH	Approach – 5TH	Device – 6TH	Qualifier – 7TH
L Extraocular Muscle, Right M Extraocular Muscle, Left	0 Open 3 Percutaneous	Z No device	Z No qualifier

NOTES

Educational Annotations | 9 – Ear, Nose, Sinus

Body System Specific Educational Annotations for the Ear, Nose, Sinus include:
- Anatomy and Physiology Review
- Anatomical Illustrations
- Definitions of Common Procedures
- AHA Coding Clinic® Reference Notations
- Body Part Key Listings
- Device Key Listings
- Device Aggregation Table Listings
- Coding Notes

Anatomy and Physiology Review of Ear, Nose, Sinus

BODY PART VALUES – 9 - EAR, NOSE, SINUS

Accessory Sinus – A paranasal sinus that is not identified as one of the four paired nasal sinuses (maxillary, frontal, ethmoid, and sphenoid).

Auditory Ossicle – ANATOMY – The three small bones of the middle ear (malleus, incus, and stapes). PHYSIOLOGY – These bones transfer the sound waves from the tympanic membrane to the oval window of the inner ear while modulating and amplifying the sound.

Ear – ANATOMY – The organ of hearing comprised of the external ear (auricle or pinna), middle ear (malleus, incus, and stapes bones), and inner ear (cochlea). PHYSIOLOGY – The external ear collects the sound, the middle ear transfers and amplifies the sound to the inner ear, and the inner ear converts it into neural impulses.

Ethmoid Sinus – The one of four paired, air-filled paranasal sinuses located within the ethmoid bone cavities that lies between the nose and the eyes.

Eustachian Tube – ANATOMY – The Eustachian (auditory) tube connects the middle ear with the nasopharynx. PHYSIOLOGY – The tube allows for proper equalization of atmospheric pressure between the atmosphere and the middle ear, and for mucous drainage from the middle ear.

External Auditory Canal – That cylindrical portion of the external ear that focuses the sound waves onto the tympanic membrane.

External Ear – ANATOMY – The visible outer portion of the ear (auricle or pinna) that includes the ear canal and outer tympanic membrane (ear drum). PHYSIOLOGY – The external ear collects the sound onto the tympanic membrane.

Frontal Sinus – The one of four paired, air-filled paranasal sinuses located above the eye in the frontal bone.

Inner Ear – ANATOMY – The fluid-filled (endolymph) inner ear is that portion behind the middle ear and comprised of the cochlea and the semicircular canals. PHYSIOLOGY – The sound waves travel through the endolymph of the cochlea stimulating millions of hairs that in turn send neural signals through the vestibulo-cochlear nerve to the brain where the brain interprets it as sound. The semicircular canals allow the individual to sense physical balance and motion.

Mastoid Sinus – The numerous, small air-filled cavities within the mastoid process of the temporal bone.

Maxillary Sinus – The largest of the one of four paired, air-filled paranasal sinuses located under the eye in the maxillary bone.

Middle Ear – ANATOMY – The middle ear is the air-filled space behind the tympanic membrane of the external ear that connects the inner ear, mastoid cells, and Eustachian tube. PHYSIOLOGY – The middle ear transfers, modulates, and amplifies the sound to the inner ear.

Nasal Septum – The bone and cartilage that divides the left and right nasal cavities and airways.

Nasal Turbinate – ANATOMY – The cartilage-like mucosal tissue grooves that divide the nasal airways into passages. PHYSIOLOGY – The turbinates assist in directing and smoothing the airflow through the nasal airways. They also sense heat and cold and help regulate the temperature and humidity of the inhaled air.

Nasopharynx – The upper portion of the pharynx from the base of skull and the nasal cavities to the top of the soft palate and the oral portion of the pharynx.

Nose – ANATOMY – The organ of sense of smell in the middle of the face and skull with the external portion extending out from the face. PHYSIOLOGY – The nose contains the organs and tissues (olfactory epithelium) that collect scent molecules and transmit impulses to the brain. The nose also warms, filters, and humidifies the air inhaled into the lungs.

Continued on next page

Educational Annotations
9 – Ear, Nose, Sinus

Anatomy and Physiology Review of Ear, Nose, Sinus

BODY PART VALUES – 9 - EAR, NOSE, SINUS
Continued from previous page

Sinus – ANATOMY – The group of four paired, air-filled mucous-membrane-lined skull bone cavities (maxillary, frontal, ethmoid, and sphenoid) that are linked to the nasal airways and the mastoid and accessory sinus bone cavities. PHYSIOLOGY – The sinuses function to warm and humidify the inhaled air, filter airborne pathogens, increase the resonance of the voice, lighten the weight of the skull, and provide a role in immunological response.

Sphenoid Sinus – The one of four paired, air-filled paranasal sinuses in the sphenoid bone and located behind the eye and nose.

Tympanic Membrane – ANATOMY – The membrane at the innermost portion of the ear canal that separates the external ear from the middle ear. PHYSIOLOGY – Transmits sound waves to the middle ear bones, and serves as a barrier to organisms and microorganisms.

Anatomical Illustrations of Ear, Nose, Sinus

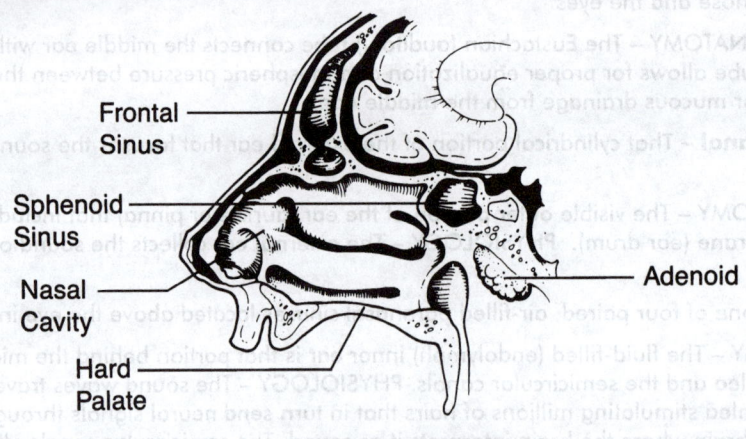

NASOPHARYNX

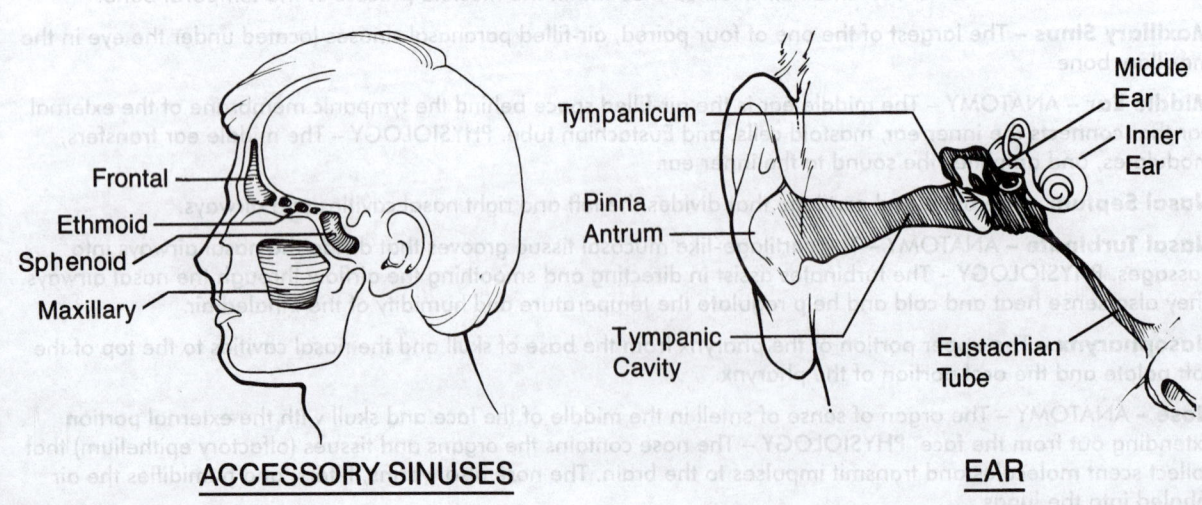

ACCESSORY SINUSES

EAR

Educational Annotations | 9 – Ear, Nose, Sinus

Definitions of Common Procedures of Ear, Nose, Sinus

Cochlear implant – The surgical implantation of a small, complex electronic hearing device (microphone, speech processor, transmitter, and electrical array) that can help to provide a sense of sound to individuals that are profoundly deaf. It is implanted behind the ear and connected to the auditory nerve.

Mastoidectomy – The surgical procedure to remove diseased mastoid air cells (chronic mastoiditis, cholesteatoma). A radical mastoidectomy also involves removing portions of the middle ear and tympanic membrane.

Rhinoplasty – The surgical repair of nasal defects or cosmetic reconstruction of the exterior shape of the nose.

Septoplasty – The surgical correction of a nasal septum defect (deviated nasal septum).

Sinusectomy – The surgical excision of paranasal sinus tissue to remove diseased or excessive tissue and/or to create a larger sinus cavity and promote more efficient drainage.

Sinusotomy (antrostomy) – The surgical incision/excision of paranasal sinus tissue to increase the drainage passage opening.

Stapedectomy/stapedotomy – The surgical correction of a dysfunctional stapes (middle ear) bone by implanting a small, movable prosthesis to allow the transfer of sound vibrations from the tympanic membrane to the middle ear and then on to the inner ear.

Turbinectomy – The surgical procedure to remove the turbinate bones of the nasal cavity that are causing nasal cavity obstruction.

AHA Coding Clinic® Reference Notations of Ear, Nose, Sinus

ROOT OPERATION - 9 - EAR, NOSE, SINUS
ALTERATION - 0
BYPASS - 1
CHANGE - 2
DESTRUCTION - 5
DILATION - 7
DIVISION - 8
DRAINAGE - 9
EXCISION - B
EXTIRPATION - C
EXTRACTION - D
INSERTION - H
INSPECTION - J
REATTACHMENT - M
RELEASE - N
REMOVAL - P
REPAIR - Q
    Endscopic balloon sinuplasty (dilation) ....AHA 13:4Q:p114
    Epistaxis control using sutures ....AHA 14:4Q:p20
    Fat graft to seal sphenoid sinus and sella ....AHA 14:3Q:p22
REPLACEMENT - R
REPOSITION - S
RESECTION - T
SUPPLEMENT - U
REVISION - W

Educational Annotations

9 – Ear, Nose, Sinus

Body Part Key Listings of Ear, Nose, Sinus

See also Body Part Key in Appendix C

Antihelix	*use* External Ear, Bilateral/Left/Right
Antitragus	*use* External Ear, Bilateral/Left/Right
Antrum of Highmore	*use* Maxillary Sinus, Left/Right
Auditory tube	*use* Eustachian Tube, Left/Right
Auricle	*use* External Ear, Bilateral/Left/Right
Bony labyrinth	*use* Inner Ear, Left/Right
Bony vestibule	*use* Inner Ear, Left/Right
Choana	*use* Nasopharynx
Cochlea	*use* Inner Ear, Left/Right
Columella	*use* Nose
Earlobe	*use* External Ear, Bilateral/Left/Right
Ethmoidal air cell	*use* Ethmoid Sinus, Left/Right
External auditory meatus	*use* External Auditory Canal, Left/Right
External naris	*use* Nose
Fossa of Rosenmuller	*use* Nasopharynx
Greater alar cartilage	*use* Nose
Helix	*use* External Ear, Bilateral/Left/Right
Incus	*use* Auditory Ossicle, Left/Right
Inferior turbinate	*use* Nasal Turbinate
Internal naris	*use* Nose
Lateral nasal cartilage	*use* Nose
Lesser alar cartilage	*use* Nose
Malleus	*use* Auditory Ossicle, Left/Right
Mastoid air cells	*use* Mastoid Sinus, Left/Right
Middle turbinate	*use* Nasal Turbinate
Nasal cavity	*use* Nose
Nasal concha	*use* Nasal Turbinate
Nostril	*use* Nose
Ossicular chain	*use* Auditory Ossicle, Left/Right
Oval window	*use* Middle Ear, Left/Right
Pars flaccida	*use* Tympanic Membrane, Left/Right
Pharyngeal recess	*use* Nasopharynx
Pharyngotympanic tube	*use* Eustachian Tube, Left/Right
Pinna	*use* External Ear, Bilateral/Left/Right
Quadrangular cartilage	*use* Nasal Septum
Rhinopharynx	*use* Nasopharynx
Round window	*use* Inner Ear, Left/Right
Semicircular canal	*use* Inner Ear, Left/Right
Septal cartilage	*use* Nasal Septum
Stapes	*use* Auditory Ossicle, Left/Right
Superior turbinate	*use* Nasal Turbinate
Tragus	*use* External Ear, Bilateral/Left/Right
Tympanic cavity	*use* Middle Ear, Left/Right
Vomer bone	*use* Nasal Septum

Educational Annotations | 9 – Ear, Nose, Sinus

Device Key Listings of Ear, Nose, Sinus

See also Device Key in Appendix D

Autograft	*use* Autologous Tissue Substitute
Bone anchored hearing device	*use* Hearing Device, Bone Conduction for Insertion in Ear, Nose, Sinus
Cochlear implant (CI), multiple channel (electrode)	*use* Hearing Device, Multiple Channel Cochlear Prosthesis for Insertion in Ear, Nose, Sinus
Cochlear implant (CI), single channel (electrode)	*use* Hearing Device, Single Channel Cochlear Prosthesis for Insertion in Ear, Nose, Sinus
Esteem® implantable hearing system	*use* Hearing Device in Ear, Nose, Sinus
Nasopharyngeal airway (NPA)	*use* Intraluminal Device, Airway in Ear, Nose, Sinus
Tissue bank graft	*use* Nonautologous Tissue Substitute

Device Aggregation Table Listings of Ear, Nose, Sinus

See also Device Aggregation Table in Appendix E

Specific Device	For Operation	In Body System		General Device
Hearing Device, Bone Conduction	Insertion	Ear, Nose, Sinus	S	Hearing Device
Hearing Device, Multiple Channel Cochlear Prosthesis	Insertion	Ear, Nose, Sinus	S	Hearing Device
Hearing Device, Single Channel Cochlear Prosthesis	Insertion	Ear, Nose, Sinus	S	Hearing Device
Intraluminal Device, Airway	All applicable	Ear, Nose, Sinus	D	Intraluminal Device

Coding Notes of Ear, Nose, Sinus

Body System Specific PCS Reference Manual Exercises

PCS CODE	9 – EAR, NOSE, SINUS EXERCISES
090K07Z	Cosmetic rhinoplasty with septal reduction and tip elevation using local tissue graft, open.
095KXZZ	Cautery of nosebleed.
099V4ZZ	Endoscopic drainage of left ethmoid sinus.
09CKXZZ	Forceps removal of foreign body in right nostril. (Nostril is coded to the "Nose" body part value.)
09D77ZZ	Removal of tattered right ear drum fragments with tweezers.
09HE06Z	Open insertion of multiple channel cochlear implant, left ear.
09M0XZZ	Reattachment of severed right ear.
09TQ4ZZ	Endoscopic bilateral total maxillary sinusectomy.
09TR4ZZ	

Educational Annotations

9 – Ear, Nose, Sinus

NOTES

9 – EAR NOSE SINUS

OTHER OBJECTIVES GROUP: Alteration, (Creation), (Fusion)
Root Operations that define other objectives.

- 1ST – **0** Medical and Surgical
- 2ND – **9** Ear, Nose, Sinus
- 3RD – **0** ALTERATION

EXAMPLE: Cosmetic rhinoplasty CMS Ex: Face lift

ALTERATION: Modifying the anatomic structure of a body part without affecting the function of the body part.

EXPLANATION: Principal purpose is to improve appearance

Body Part – 4TH	Approach – 5TH	Device – 6TH	Qualifier – 7TH
0 External Ear, Right 1 External Ear, Left 2 External Ear, Bilateral K Nose	0 Open 3 Percutaneous 4 Percutaneous endoscopic X External	7 Autologous tissue substitute J Synthetic substitute K Nonautologous tissue substitute Z No device	Z No qualifier

TUBULAR GROUP: Bypass, Dilation, (Occlusion), (Restriction)
Root Operations that alter the diameter/route of a tubular body part.

- 1ST – **0** Medical and Surgical
- 2ND – **9** Ear, Nose, Sinus
- 3RD – **1** BYPASS

EXAMPLE: Endolymphatic bypass CMS Ex: Coronary artery bypass

BYPASS: Altering the route of passage of the contents of a tubular body part.

EXPLANATION: Rerouting contents to a downstream part ...

Body Part – 4TH	Approach – 5TH	Device – 6TH	Qualifier – 7TH
D Inner Ear, Right E Inner Ear, Left	0 Open	7 Autologous tissue substitute J Synthetic substitute K Nonautologous tissue substitute Z No device	0 Endolymphatic

DEVICE GROUP: Change, Insertion, Removal, Replacement, Revision, Supplement
Root Operations that always involve a device.

- 1ST – **0** Medical and Surgical
- 2ND – **9** Ear, Nose, Sinus
- 3RD – **2** CHANGE

EXAMPLE: Exchange drain tube CMS Ex: Changing urinary catheter

CHANGE: Taking out or off a device from a body part and putting back an identical or similar device in or on the same body part without cutting or puncturing the skin or a mucous membrane.

EXPLANATION: ALL Changes use EXTERNAL approach only...

Body Part – 4TH	Approach – 5TH	Device – 6TH	Qualifier – 7TH
H Ear, Right J Ear, Left K Nose Y Sinus	X External	0 Drainage device Y Other device	Z No qualifier

MEDICAL AND SURGICAL SECTION – 2016 ICD-10-PCS

EXCISION GROUP: Excision, Resection, Destruction, Extraction, (Detachment)
Root Operations that take out some or all of a body part.

1ST - **0** Medical and Surgical	EXAMPLE: Cautery epistaxis		CMS Ex: Fulguration polyp
2ND - **9** Ear, Nose, Sinus	**DESTRUCTION:** Physical eradication of all or a portion of a body part by the direct use of energy, force, or a destructive agent.		
3RD - **5 DESTRUCTION**	EXPLANATION: None of the body part is physically taken out		

Body Part – 4TH		Approach – 5TH	Device – 6TH	Qualifier – 7TH
0 External Ear, Right 1 External Ear, Left K Nose		0 Open 3 Percutaneous 4 Percutaneous endoscopic X External	Z No device	Z No qualifier
3 External Auditory Canal, Right 4 External Auditory Canal, Left		0 Open 3 Percutaneous 4 Percutaneous endoscopic 7 Via natural or artificial opening 8 Via natural or artificial opening endoscopic X External	Z No device	Z No qualifier
5 Middle Ear, Right 6 Middle Ear, Left 9 Auditory Ossicle, Right	A Auditory Ossicle, Left D Inner Ear, Right E Inner Ear, Left	0 Open	Z No device	Z No qualifier
7 Tympanic Membrane, Right 8 Tympanic Membrane, Left F Eustachian Tube, Right G Eustachian Tube, Left L Nasal Turbinate N Nasopharynx		0 Open 3 Percutaneous 4 Percutaneous endoscopic 7 Via natural or artificial opening 8 Via natural or artificial opening endoscopic	Z No device	Z No qualifier
B Mastoid Sinus, Right C Mastoid Sinus, Left M Nasal Septum P Accessory Sinus Q Maxillary Sinus, Right R Maxillary Sinus, Left	S Frontal Sinus, Right T Frontal Sinus, Left U Ethmoid Sinus, Right V Ethmoid Sinus, Left W Sphenoid Sinus, Right X Sphenoid Sinus, Left	0 Open 3 Percutaneous 4 Percutaneous endoscopic	Z No device	Z No qualifier

9 – EAR NOSE SINUS

TUBULAR GROUP: Bypass, Dilation, (Occlusion), (Restriction)
Root Operations that alter the diameter/route of a tubular body part.

- 1ST – **0** Medical and Surgical
- 2ND – **9** Ear, Nose, Sinus
- 3RD – **7 DILATION**

EXAMPLE: Balloon dilation Eustachian   CMS Ex: Transluminal angioplasty

DILATION: Expanding an orifice or the lumen of a tubular body part.

EXPLANATION: By force (stretching) or cutting ...

Body Part – 4TH	Approach – 5TH	Device – 6TH	Qualifier – 7TH
F Eustachian Tube, Right G Eustachian Tube, Left	0 Open 7 Via natural or artificial opening 8 Via natural or artificial opening endoscopic	D Intraluminal device Z No device	Z No qualifier
F Eustachian Tube, Right G Eustachian Tube, Left	3 Percutaneous 4 Percutaneous endoscopic	Z No device	Z No qualifier

DIVISION GROUP: Division, Release
Root Operations involving cutting or separation only.

- 1ST – **0** Medical and Surgical
- 2ND – **9** Ear, Nose, Sinus
- 3RD – **8 DIVISION**

EXAMPLE: Division nasal turbinate   CMS Ex: Osteotomy

DIVISION: Cutting into a body part without draining fluids and/or gases from the body part in order to separate or transect a body part.

EXPLANATION: Separated into two or more portions ...

Body Part – 4TH	Approach – 5TH	Device – 6TH	Qualifier – 7TH
L Nasal Turbinate	0 Open 3 Percutaneous 4 Percutaneous endoscopic 7 Via natural or artificial opening 8 Via natural or artificial opening endoscopic	Z No device	Z No qualifier

273

099

MEDICAL AND SURGICAL SECTION – 2016 ICD-10-PCS

DRAINAGE GROUP: Drainage, Extirpation, (Fragmentation)
Root Operations that take out solids/fluids/gases from a body part.

1ST - **0** Medical and Surgical	EXAMPLE: Sinusotomy for drainage	CMS Ex: Thoracentesis
2ND - **9** Ear, Nose, Sinus	**DRAINAGE:** Taking or letting out fluids and/or gases from a body part.	
3RD - **9** DRAINAGE	EXPLANATION: Qualifier "X Diagnostic" indicates biopsy ...	

Body Part – 4TH	Approach – 5TH	Device – 6TH	Qualifier – 7TH
0 External Ear, Right 1 External Ear, Left K Nose	0 Open 3 Percutaneous 4 Percutaneous endoscopic X External	0 Drainage device	Z No qualifier
0 External Ear, Right 1 External Ear, Left K Nose	0 Open 3 Percutaneous 4 Percutaneous endoscopic X External	Z No device	X Diagnostic Z No qualifier
3 External Auditory Canal, Right 4 External Auditory Canal, Left	0 Open 3 Percutaneous 4 Percutaneous endoscopic 7 Via natural or artificial opening 8 Via natural or artificial opening endoscopic X External	0 Drainage device	Z No qualifier
3 External Auditory Canal, Right 4 External Auditory Canal, Left	0 Open 3 Percutaneous 4 Percutaneous endoscopic 7 Via natural or artificial opening 8 Via natural or artificial opening endoscopic X External	Z No device	X Diagnostic Z No qualifier
5 Middle Ear, Right A Auditory Ossicle, Left 6 Middle Ear, Left D Inner Ear, Right 9 Auditory Ossicle, Right E Inner Ear, Left	0 Open	0 Drainage device	Z No qualifier
5 Middle Ear, Right A Auditory Ossicle, Left 6 Middle Ear, Left D Inner Ear, Right 9 Auditory Ossicle, Right E Inner Ear, Left	0 Open	Z No device	X Diagnostic Z No qualifier

continued ⇨

0 9 9 DRAINAGE – continued

Body Part – 4ᵀᴴ		Approach – 5ᵀᴴ	Device – 6ᵀᴴ	Qualifier – 7ᵀᴴ
7 Tympanic Membrane, Right 8 Tympanic Membrane, Left F Eustachian Tube, Right G Eustachian Tube, Left L Nasal Turbinate N Nasopharynx		0 Open 3 Percutaneous 4 Percutaneous endoscopic 7 Via natural or artificial opening 8 Via natural or artificial opening endoscopic	0 Drainage device	Z No qualifier
7 Tympanic Membrane, Right 8 Tympanic Membrane, Left F Eustachian Tube, Right G Eustachian Tube, Left L Nasal Turbinate N Nasopharynx		0 Open 3 Percutaneous 4 Percutaneous endoscopic 7 Via natural or artificial opening 8 Via natural or artificial opening endoscopic	Z No device	X Diagnostic Z No qualifier
B Mastoid Sinus, Right C Mastoid Sinus, Left M Nasal Septum P Accessory Sinus Q Maxillary Sinus, Right R Maxillary Sinus, Left	S Frontal Sinus, Right T Frontal Sinus, Left U Ethmoid Sinus, Right V Ethmoid Sinus, Left W Sphenoid Sinus, Right X Sphenoid Sinus, Left	0 Open 3 Percutaneous 4 Percutaneous endoscopic	0 Drainage device	Z No qualifier
B Mastoid Sinus, Right C Mastoid Sinus, Left M Nasal Septum P Accessory Sinus Q Maxillary Sinus, Right R Maxillary Sinus, Left	S Frontal Sinus, Right T Frontal Sinus, Left U Ethmoid Sinus, Right V Ethmoid Sinus, Left W Sphenoid Sinus, Right X Sphenoid Sinus, Left	0 Open 3 Percutaneous 4 Percutaneous endoscopic	Z No device	X Diagnostic Z No qualifier

0 9 B

MEDICAL AND SURGICAL SECTION – 2016 ICD-10-PCS

EXCISION GROUP: Excision, Resection, Destruction, Extraction, (Detachment)
Root Operations that take out some or all of a body part.

- 1ST – **0** Medical and Surgical
- 2ND – **9** Ear, Nose, Sinus
- 3RD – **B** EXCISION

EXAMPLE: Excision lesion nose **CMS Ex:** Liver biopsy

EXCISION: Cutting out or off, without replacement, a portion of a body part.

EXPLANATION: Qualifier "X Diagnostic" indicates biopsy …

Body Part – 4TH	Approach – 5TH	Device – 6TH	Qualifier – 7TH
0 External Ear, Right 1 External Ear, Left K Nose	0 Open 3 Percutaneous 4 Percutaneous endoscopic X External	Z No device	X Diagnostic Z No qualifier
3 External Auditory Canal, Right 4 External Auditory Canal, Left	0 Open 3 Percutaneous 4 Percutaneous endoscopic 7 Via natural or artificial opening 8 Via natural or artificial opening endoscopic X External	Z No device	X Diagnostic Z No qualifier
5 Middle Ear, Right A Auditory Ossicle, Left 6 Middle Ear, Left D Inner Ear, Right 9 Auditory Ossicle, Right E Inner Ear, Left	0 Open	Z No device	X Diagnostic Z No qualifier
7 Tympanic Membrane, Right 8 Tympanic Membrane, Left F Eustachian Tube, Right G Eustachian Tube, Left L Nasal Turbinate N Nasopharynx	0 Open 3 Percutaneous 4 Percutaneous endoscopic 7 Via natural or artificial opening 8 Via natural or artificial opening endoscopic	Z No device	X Diagnostic Z No qualifier
B Mastoid Sinus, Right S Frontal Sinus, Right C Mastoid Sinus, Left T Frontal Sinus, Left M Nasal Septum U Ethmoid Sinus, Right P Accessory Sinus V Ethmoid Sinus, Left Q Maxillary Sinus, Right W Sphenoid Sinus, Right R Maxillary Sinus, Left X Sphenoid Sinus, Left	0 Open 3 Percutaneous 4 Percutaneous endoscopic	Z No device	X Diagnostic Z No qualifier

9 – EAR NOSE SINUS — 09C

DRAINAGE GROUP: Drainage, Extirpation, (Fragmentation)
Root Operations that take out solids/fluids/gases from a body part.

- 1ST – **0** Medical and Surgical
- 2ND – **9** Ear, Nose, Sinus
- 3RD – **C** EXTIRPATION

EXAMPLE: Removal foreign body nose CMS Ex: Choledocholithotomy

EXTIRPATION: Taking or cutting out solid matter from a body part.

EXPLANATION: Abnormal byproduct or foreign body ...

Body Part – 4TH	Approach – 5TH	Device – 6TH	Qualifier – 7TH
0 External Ear, Right 1 External Ear, Left K Nose	0 Open 3 Percutaneous 4 Percutaneous endoscopic X External	Z No device	Z No qualifier
3 External Auditory Canal, Right 4 External Auditory Canal, Left	0 Open 3 Percutaneous 4 Percutaneous endoscopic 7 Via natural or artificial opening 8 Via natural or artificial opening endoscopic X External	Z No device	Z No qualifier
5 Middle Ear, Right A Auditory Ossicle, Left 6 Middle Ear, Left D Inner Ear, Right 9 Auditory Ossicle, Right E Inner Ear, Left	0 Open	Z No device	Z No qualifier
7 Tympanic Membrane, Right 8 Tympanic Membrane, Left F Eustachian Tube, Right G Eustachian Tube, Left L Nasal Turbinate N Nasopharynx	0 Open 3 Percutaneous 4 Percutaneous endoscopic 7 Via natural or artificial opening 8 Via natural or artificial opening endoscopic	Z No device	Z No qualifier
B Mastoid Sinus, Right S Frontal Sinus, Right C Mastoid Sinus, Left T Frontal Sinus, Left M Nasal Septum U Ethmoid Sinus, Right P Accessory Sinus V Ethmoid Sinus, Left Q Maxillary Sinus, Right W Sphenoid Sinus, Right R Maxillary Sinus, Left X Sphenoid Sinus, Left	0 Open 3 Percutaneous 4 Percutaneous endoscopic	Z No device	Z No qualifier

09D MEDICAL AND SURGICAL SECTION – 2016 ICD-10-PCS

EXCISION GROUP: Excision, Resection, Destruction, Extraction, (Detachment)
Root Operations that take out some or all of a body part.

- 1ST - **0** Medical and Surgical
- 2ND - **9** Ear, Nose, Sinus
- 3RD - **D** EXTRACTION

EXAMPLE: Removal sinus lining membrane **CMS Ex: D&C**

EXTRACTION: Pulling or stripping out or off all or a portion of a body part by the use of force.

EXPLANATION: None for this Body System

Body Part – 4TH	Approach – 5TH	Device – 6TH	Qualifier – 7TH
7 Tympanic Membrane, Right 8 Tympanic Membrane, Left L Nasal Turbinate	0 Open 3 Percutaneous 4 Percutaneous endoscopic 7 Via natural or artificial opening 8 Via natural or artificial opening endoscopic	Z No device	Z No qualifier
9 Auditory Ossicle, Right A Auditory Ossicle, Left	0 Open	Z No device	Z No qualifier
B Mastoid Sinus, Right S Frontal Sinus, Right C Mastoid Sinus, Left T Frontal Sinus, Left M Nasal Septum U Ethmoid Sinus, Right P Accessory Sinus V Ethmoid Sinus, Left Q Maxillary Sinus, Right W Sphenoid Sinus, Right R Maxillary Sinus, Left X Sphenoid Sinus, Left	0 Open 3 Percutaneous 4 Percutaneous endoscopic	Z No device	Z No qualifier

9 – EAR NOSE SINUS 09H

DEVICE GROUP: Change, Insertion, Removal, Replacement, Revision, Supplement
Root Operations that always involve a device.

1ST - **0** Medical and Surgical
2ND - **9** Ear, Nose, Sinus
3RD - **H INSERTION**

EXAMPLE: Cochlear implant   CMS Ex: Insertion central venous catheter

INSERTION: Putting in a nonbiological appliance that monitors, assists, performs, or prevents a physiological function but does not physically take the place of a body part.

EXPLANATION: None

Body Part – 4TH	Approach – 5TH	Device – 6TH	Qualifier – 7TH
D Inner Ear, Right E Inner Ear, Left	0 Open 3 Percutaneous 4 Percutaneous endoscopic	4 Hearing device, bone conduction 5 Hearing device, single channel cochlear prosthesis 6 Hearing device, multiple channel cochlear prosthesis S Hearing device	Z No qualifier
N Nasopharynx	7 Via natural or artificial opening 8 Via natural or artificial opening endoscopic	B Intraluminal device, airway	Z No qualifier

09J

MEDICAL AND SURGICAL SECTION – 2016 ICD-10-PCS

EXAMINATION GROUP: Inspection, (Map)
Root Operations involving examination only.

1ST - 0	Medical and Surgical
2ND - 9	Ear, Nose, Sinus
3RD - J	INSPECTION

EXAMPLE: Sinus endoscopy CMS Ex: Colonoscopy

INSPECTION: Visually and/or manually exploring a body part.

EXPLANATION: Direct or instrumental visualization …

Body Part – 4TH	Approach – 5TH	Device – 6TH	Qualifier – 7TH
7 Tympanic Membrane, Right 8 Tympanic Membrane, Left H Ear, Right J Ear, Left	0 Open 3 Percutaneous 4 Percutaneous endoscopic 7 Via natural or artificial opening 8 Via natural or artificial opening endoscopic X External	Z No device	Z No qualifier
D Inner Ear, Right E Inner Ear, Left K Nose Y Sinus	0 Open 3 Percutaneous 4 Percutaneous endoscopic X External	Z No device	Z No qualifier

MOVE GROUP: Reattachment, Reposition, (Transfer), (Transplantation)
Root Operations that put in/put back or move some/all of a body part.

1ST - 0	Medical and Surgical
2ND - 9	Ear, Nose, Sinus
3RD - M	REATTACHMENT

EXAMPLE: Reattachment severed ear   CMS Ex: Reattachment hand

REATTACHMENT: Putting back in or on all or a portion of a separated body part to its normal location or other suitable location.

EXPLANATION: With/without reconnection of vessels/nerves…

Body Part – 4TH	Approach – 5TH	Device – 6TH	Qualifier – 7TH
0 External Ear, Right 1 External Ear, Left K Nose	X External	Z No device	Z No qualifier

9 – EAR NOSE SINUS

09N

DIVISION GROUP: Division, Release
Root Operations involving cutting or separation only.

1ST - 0	Medical and Surgical
2ND - 9	Ear, Nose, Sinus
3RD - N	RELEASE

EXAMPLE: Adhesiolysis middle ear   CMS Ex: Carpal tunnel release

RELEASE: Freeing a body part from an abnormal physical constraint by cutting or by the use of force.

EXPLANATION: None of the body part is taken out ...

Body Part – 4TH	Approach – 5TH	Device – 6TH	Qualifier – 7TH
0 External Ear, Right 1 External Ear, Left K Nose	0 Open 3 Percutaneous 4 Percutaneous endoscopic X External	Z No device	Z No qualifier
3 External Auditory Canal, Right 4 External Auditory Canal, Left	0 Open 3 Percutaneous 4 Percutaneous endoscopic 7 Via natural or artificial opening 8 Via natural or artificial opening endoscopic X External	Z No device	Z No qualifier
5 Middle Ear, Right A Auditory Ossicle, Left 6 Middle Ear, Left D Inner Ear, Right 9 Auditory Ossicle, Right E Inner Ear, Left	0 Open	Z No device	Z No qualifier
7 Tympanic Membrane, Right 8 Tympanic Membrane, Left F Eustachian Tube, Right G Eustachian Tube, Left L Nasal Turbinate N Nasopharynx	0 Open 3 Percutaneous 4 Percutaneous endoscopic 7 Via natural or artificial opening 8 Via natural or artificial opening endoscopic	Z No device	Z No qualifier
B Mastoid Sinus, Right S Frontal Sinus, Right C Mastoid Sinus, Left T Frontal Sinus, Left M Nasal Septum U Ethmoid Sinus, Right P Accessory Sinus V Ethmoid Sinus, Left Q Maxillary Sinus, Right W Sphenoid Sinus, Right R Maxillary Sinus, Left X Sphenoid Sinus, Left	0 Open 3 Percutaneous 4 Percutaneous endoscopic	Z No device	Z No qualifier

09P

MEDICAL AND SURGICAL SECTION – 2016 ICD-10-PCS

DEVICE GROUP: Change, Insertion, Removal, Replacement, Revision, Supplement
Root Operations that always involve a device.

1ST - **0** Medical and Surgical
2ND - **9** Ear, Nose, Sinus
3RD - **P REMOVAL**

EXAMPLE: Removal drain tube

CMS Ex: Chest tube removal

REMOVAL: Taking out or off a device from a body part.

EXPLANATION: Removal device without reinsertion ...

Body Part – 4TH	Approach – 5TH	Device – 6TH	Qualifier – 7TH
7 Tympanic Membrane, Right 8 Tympanic Membrane, Left	0 Open 7 Via natural or artificial opening 8 Via natural or artificial opening endoscopic X External	0 Drainage device	Z No qualifier
D Inner Ear, Right E Inner Ear, Left	0 Open 7 Via natural or artificial opening 8 Via natural or artificial opening endoscopic	S Hearing device	Z No qualifier
H Ear, Right J Ear, Left K Nose	0 Open 3 Percutaneous 4 Percutaneous endoscopic 7 Via natural or artificial opening 8 Via natural or artificial opening endoscopic X External	0 Drainage device 7 Autologous tissue substitute D Intraluminal device J Synthetic substitute K Nonautologous tissue substitute	Z No qualifier
Y Sinus	0 Open 3 Percutaneous 4 Percutaneous endoscopic X External	0 Drainage device	Z No qualifier

9 – EAR NOSE SINUS 09Q

OTHER REPAIRS GROUP: (Control), **Repair**
Root Operations that define other repairs.

1st - **0** Medical and Surgical
2nd - **9** Ear, Nose, Sinus
3rd - **Q REPAIR**

EXAMPLE: Epistaxis control using sutures CMS Ex: Suture laceration

REPAIR: Restoring, to the extent possible, a body part to its normal anatomic structure and function.

EXPLANATION: Only when no other root operation applies ...

Body Part – 4th	Approach – 5th	Device – 6th	Qualifier – 7th
0 External Ear, Right 1 External Ear, Left 2 External Ear, Bilateral K Nose	0 Open 3 Percutaneous 4 Percutaneous endoscopic X External	Z No device	Z No qualifier
3 External Auditory Canal, Right 4 External Auditory Canal, Left F Eustachian Tube, Right G Eustachian Tube, Left	0 Open 3 Percutaneous 4 Percutaneous endoscopic 7 Via natural or artificial opening 8 Via natural or artificial opening endoscopic X External	Z No device	Z No qualifier
5 Middle Ear, Right A Auditory Ossicle, Left 6 Middle Ear, Left D Inner Ear, Right 9 Auditory Ossicle, Right E Inner Ear, Left	0 Open	Z No device	Z No qualifier
7 Tympanic Membrane, Right 8 Tympanic Membrane, Left L Nasal Turbinate N Nasopharynx	0 Open 3 Percutaneous 4 Percutaneous endoscopic 7 Via natural or artificial opening 8 Via natural or artificial opening endoscopic	Z No device	Z No qualifier
B Mastoid Sinus, Right S Frontal Sinus, Right C Mastoid Sinus, Left T Frontal Sinus, Left M Nasal Septum U Ethmoid Sinus, Right P Accessory Sinus V Ethmoid Sinus, Left Q Maxillary Sinus, Right W Sphenoid Sinus, Right R Maxillary Sinus, Left X Sphenoid Sinus, Left	0 Open 3 Percutaneous 4 Percutaneous endoscopic	Z No device	Z No qualifier

0 9 R — MEDICAL AND SURGICAL SECTION – 2016 ICD-10-PCS

DEVICE GROUP: Change, Insertion, Removal, Replacement, Revision, Supplement
Root Operations that always involve a device.

- 1ST – **0** Medical and Surgical
- 2ND – **9** Ear, Nose, Sinus
- 3RD – **R** REPLACEMENT

EXAMPLE: External ear reconstruction   CMS Ex: Total hip

REPLACEMENT: Putting in or on a biological or synthetic material that physically takes the place and/or function of all or a portion of a body part.

EXPLANATION: Includes taking out body part, or eradication...

Body Part – 4TH	Approach – 5TH	Device – 6TH	Qualifier – 7TH
0 External Ear, Right 1 External Ear, Left 2 External Ear, Bilateral K Nose	0 Open X External	7 Autologous tissue substitute J Synthetic substitute K Nonautologous tissue substitute	Z No qualifier
5 Middle Ear, Right A Auditory Ossicle, Left 6 Middle Ear, Left D Inner Ear, Right 9 Auditory Ossicle, Right E Inner Ear, Left	0 Open	7 Autologous tissue substitute J Synthetic substitute K Nonautologous tissue substitute	Z No qualifier
7 Tympanic Membrane, Right 8 Tympanic Membrane, Left N Nasopharynx	0 Open 7 Via natural or artificial opening 8 Via natural or artificial opening endoscopic	7 Autologous tissue substitute J Synthetic substitute K Nonautologous tissue substitute	Z No qualifier
L Nasal Turbinate	0 Open 3 Percutaneous 4 Percutaneous endoscopic 7 Via natural or artificial opening 8 Via natural or artificial opening endoscopic	7 Autologous tissue substitute J Synthetic substitute K Nonautologous tissue substitute	Z No qualifier
M Nasal Septum	0 Open 3 Percutaneous 4 Percutaneous endoscopic	7 Autologous tissue substitute J Synthetic substitute K Nonautologous tissue substitute	Z No qualifier

MOVE GROUP: Reattachment, Reposition, (Transfer), (Transplantation)
Root Operations that put in/put back or move some/all of a body part.

1ST - 0 Medical and Surgical
2ND - 9 Ear, Nose, Sinus
3RD - S REPOSITION

EXAMPLE: Deviated septum septoplasty   CMS Ex: Fracture reduction

REPOSITION: Moving to its normal location, or other suitable location, all or a portion of a body part.

EXPLANATION: May or may not be cut to be moved ...

Body Part – 4TH	Approach – 5TH	Device – 6TH	Qualifier – 7TH
0 External Ear, Right 1 External Ear, Left 2 External Ear, Bilateral K Nose	0 Open 4 Percutaneous endoscopic X External	Z No device	Z No qualifier
7 Tympanic Membrane, Right 8 Tympanic Membrane, Left F Eustachian Tube, Right G Eustachian Tube, Left L Nasal Turbinate	0 Open 4 Percutaneous endoscopic 7 Via natural or artificial opening 8 Via natural or artificial opening endoscopic	Z No device	Z No qualifier
9 Auditory Ossicle, Right A Auditory Ossicle, Left M Nasal Septum	0 Open 4 Percutaneous endoscopic	Z No device	Z No qualifier

0 9 T

MEDICAL AND SURGICAL SECTION – 2016 ICD-10-PCS

[2016.PCS]

EXCISION GROUP: Excision, Resection, Destruction, Extraction, (Detachment)
Root Operations that take out some or all of a body part.

1ST - **0** Medical and Surgical
2ND - **9** Ear, Nose, Sinus
3RD - **T** RESECTION

EXAMPLE: Total maxillary sinusectomy   **CMS Ex:** Cholecystectomy

RESECTION: Cutting out or off, without replacement, all of a body part.

EXPLANATION: None

Body Part – 4TH		Approach – 5TH	Device – 6TH	Qualifier – 7TH
0 External Ear, Right 1 External Ear, Left K Nose		0 Open 4 Percutaneous endoscopic X External	Z No device	Z No qualifier
5 Middle Ear, Right 6 Middle Ear, Left 9 Auditory Ossicle, Right	A Auditory Ossicle, Left D Inner Ear, Right E Inner Ear, Left	0 Open	Z No device	Z No qualifier
7 Tympanic Membrane, Right 8 Tympanic Membrane, Left F Eustachian Tube, Right G Eustachian Tube, Left L Nasal Turbinate N Nasopharynx		0 Open 4 Percutaneous endoscopic 7 Via natural or artificial opening 8 Via natural or artificial opening endoscopic	Z No device	Z No qualifier
B Mastoid Sinus, Right C Mastoid Sinus, Left M Nasal Septum P Accessory Sinus Q Maxillary Sinus, Right R Maxillary Sinus, Left	S Frontal Sinus, Right T Frontal Sinus, Left U Ethmoid Sinus, Right V Ethmoid Sinus, Left W Sphenoid Sinus, Right X Sphenoid Sinus, Left	0 Open 4 Percutaneous endoscopic	Z No device	Z No qualifier

EAR NOSE SINUS 0 9 T

9 – EAR NOSE SINUS — 09U

DEVICE GROUP: Change, Insertion, Removal, Replacement, Revision, Supplement
Root Operations that always involve a device.

- 1ST – **0** Medical and Surgical
- 2ND – **9** Ear, Nose, Sinus
- 3RD – **U SUPPLEMENT**

EXAMPLE: Overlay graft myringoplasty | CMS Ex: Hernia repair with mesh

SUPPLEMENT: Putting in or on biological or synthetic material that physically reinforces and/or augments the function of a portion of a body part.

EXPLANATION: Biological material from same individual ...

Body Part – 4TH	Approach – 5TH	Device – 6TH	Qualifier – 7TH
0 External Ear, Right 1 External Ear, Left 2 External Ear, Bilateral K Nose	0 Open X External	7 Autologous tissue substitute J Synthetic substitute K Nonautologous tissue substitute	Z No qualifier
5 Middle Ear, Right A Auditory Ossicle, Left 6 Middle Ear, Left D Inner Ear, Right 9 Auditory Ossicle, Right E Inner Ear, Left	0 Open	7 Autologous tissue substitute J Synthetic substitute K Nonautologous tissue substitute	Z No qualifier
7 Tympanic Membrane, Right 8 Tympanic Membrane, Left N Nasopharynx	0 Open 7 Via natural or artificial opening 8 Via natural or artificial opening endoscopic	7 Autologous tissue substitute J Synthetic substitute K Nonautologous tissue substitute	Z No qualifier
L Nasal Turbinate	0 Open 3 Percutaneous 4 Percutaneous endoscopic 7 Via natural or artificial opening 8 Via natural or artificial opening endoscopic	7 Autologous tissue substitute J Synthetic substitute K Nonautologous tissue substitute	Z No qualifier
M Nasal Septum	0 Open 3 Percutaneous 4 Percutaneous endoscopic	7 Autologous tissue substitute J Synthetic substitute K Nonautologous tissue substitute	Z No qualifier

09W

MEDICAL AND SURGICAL SECTION – 2016 ICD-10-PCS [2016.PCS]

DEVICE GROUP: Change, Insertion, Removal, Replacement, Revision, Supplement
Root Operations that always involve a device.

1ST – 0	Medical and Surgical
2ND – 9	Ear, Nose, Sinus
3RD – W	REVISION

EXAMPLE: Reposition cochlear implant | CMS Ex: Adjustment pacemaker lead

REVISION: Correcting, to the extent possible, a portion of a malfunctioning device or the position of a displaced device.

EXPLANATION: May replace components of a device ...

Body Part – 4TH	Approach – 5TH	Device – 6TH	Qualifier – 7TH
7 Tympanic Membrane, Right 8 Tympanic Membrane, Left 9 Auditory Ossicle, Right A Auditory Ossicle, Left	0 Open 7 Via natural or artificial opening 8 Via natural or artificial opening endoscopic	7 Autologous tissue substitute J Synthetic substitute K Nonautologous tissue substitute	Z No qualifier
D Inner Ear, Right E Inner Ear, Left	0 Open 7 Via natural or artificial opening 8 Via natural or artificial opening endoscopic	S Hearing device	Z No qualifier
H Ear, Right J Ear, Left K Nose	0 Open 3 Percutaneous 4 Percutaneous endoscopic 7 Via natural or artificial opening 8 Via natural or artificial opening endoscopic X External	0 Drainage device 7 Autologous tissue substitute D Intraluminal device J Synthetic substitute K Nonautologous tissue substitute	Z No qualifier
Y Sinus	0 Open 3 Percutaneous 4 Percutaneous endoscopic X External	0 Drainage device	Z No qualifier

EAR NOSE SINUS 09W

B – Respiratory System

Educational Annotations

Body System Specific Educational Annotations for the Respiratory System include:
- Anatomy and Physiology Review
- Anatomical Illustrations
- Definitions of Common Procedures
- AHA Coding Clinic® Reference Notations
- Body Part Key Listings
- Device Key Listings
- Device Aggregation Table Listings
- Coding Notes

Anatomy and Physiology Review of Respiratory System

BODY PART VALUES – B - RESPIRATORY SYSTEM

Carina – ANATOMY – The carina is a ridge of cartilaginous tissue within the trachea at the tracheal bifurcation at the lower end of the trachea. PHYSIOLOGY – The sensitive mucous membrane of the carina is responsible for triggering a cough reflex.

Diaphragm – ANATOMY – The diaphragm is dome-shaped sheet of skeletal muscle between the thoracic and abdominal cavities. PHYSIOLOGY – The diaphragm is the primary muscle in respiration and when it contracts, air is drawn into the lungs.

Lingula Bronchus – The secondary bronchi serving a lung lingula.

Lower Lobe Bronchus – The secondary bronchi serving a lower lung lobe (left or right).

Lower Lobe Lung – The lower lung lobes are soft, spongy, cone-shaped organs of respiration (left or right).

Lung – ANATOMY – The lungs are soft, spongy, cone-shaped organs located in the thoracic cavity. The right and left lungs are separated medially by the heart and the mediastinum, and they are enclosed by the diaphragm and the thoracic cage. The right lung is divided into 3 lobes called the upper (superior), middle, and lower (inferior). The left lung is divided into 2 lobes, the upper and lower. The lobes are subdivided into lobules which are composed of bronchioles, alveolar sacs, alveoli, nerves, and associated blood and lymphatic vessels. The alveoli are thin-walled, microscopic air sacs that open only on the side communicating with the inhaled air. PHYSIOLOGY – The lungs are organs that perform pulmonary ventilation. The alveoli are the microscopic structures responsible for the exchange of oxygen into the blood and carbon dioxide out of the body. Inspiration (inhalation) and expiration (exhalation) are complex central nervous system functions. Two groups of nerve cell bodies in the medulla of the brain compose the inspiratory center and the expiratory center. These two centers act reciprocally; that is, when one is stimulated and discharging, the other is inhibited. Both centers discharge nerve impulses to the intercostal muscles. When the inspiration center discharges nerve impulses, the diaphragm moves down and the external intercostal muscles contract, causing inflation. Inflation of the lungs causes stimulation of stretch receptors, which send impulses to the medulla, which in turn stimulates the expiratory center. Two other respiratory centers are contained in the pons which modify and control the medullary centers' activities, and are called the apneustic center and the pneumotaxic center. In addition to the above centers, there is also a chemical reaction which helps to control pulmonary ventilation. The carbon dioxide level in the blood is directly measured by the medulla, and respiration is adjusted accordingly. A decrease in the oxygen level, sensed by nerve endings in the common carotid artery and the aortic arch, will also stimulate a respiratory adjustment, but it does not play a noticeable difference in pulmonary ventilation.

Lung Lingula – The downward projection of the upper lobe of the left lung.

Main Bronchus – ANATOMY – The bronchial tree consists of branched airways leading from the trachea to the microscopic air sacs. The two main branches, the right and left bronchi, subdivide into secondary or lobar bronchi, which in turn branch into finer tubes down to the bronchioles. PHYSIOLOGY – The trachea and bronchi allow for the rapid transport of air to and from the lung tissue.

Middle Lobe Bronchus – The secondary bronchi serving a middle lung lobe (right).

Middle Lobe Lung – The middle lung lobe is the soft, spongy, cone-shaped organ of respiration (right).

Pleura – ANATOMY – The pleura are closed, double-layered serous membranous sacs surrounding the lungs. The parietal pleura is the layer which lines the thoracic walls opposite to the visceral pleura. The visceral pleura is the layer which adheres to the lungs and together with the parietal, forms the pleural cavity. PHYSIOLOGY – The pleura functions to prevent friction of the lungs against the thoracic wall during respiration. There is a small amount of serous fluid in the pleural cavity which lubricates the facing membranes.

Continued on next page

B – Respiratory System

Educational Annotations

Anatomy and Physiology Review of Respiratory System

BODY PART VALUES – B - RESPIRATORY SYSTEM
Continued from previous page

Trachea – ANATOMY – The trachea is a cylindrical tube about 1 inch (2.5 cm) in diameter. It extends downward from the larynx in front of the esophagus and into the thoracic cavity, where it splits into the right and left main bronchi. PHYSIOLOGY – The trachea and bronchi allow for the rapid transport of air to and from the lung tissue.

Tracheobronchial Tree – The trachea, main bronchi, secondary (lobar) bronchi, and bronchioles.

Upper Lobe Bronchus – The secondary bronchi serving a lower lung lobe (left or right).

Upper Lobe Lung – The upper lung lobes are soft, spongy, cone-shaped organs of respiration (left or right).

Anatomical Illustrations of Respiratory System

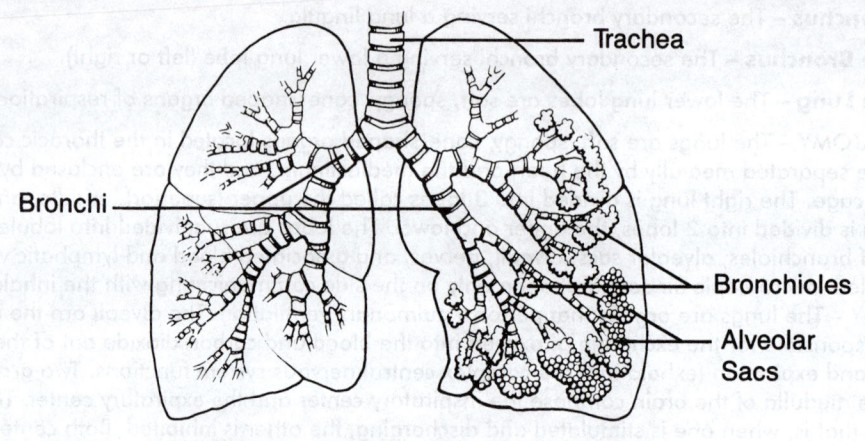

LUNGS — ANTERIOR (CUT-AWAY) VIEW

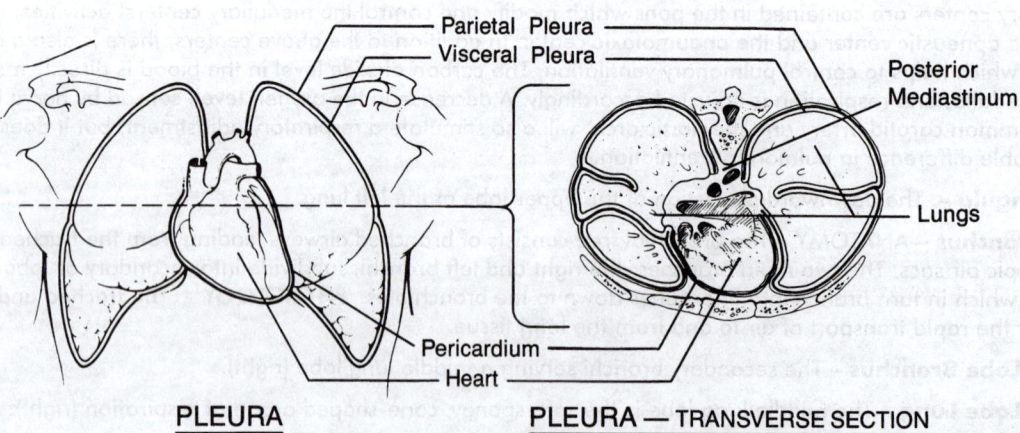

PLEURA   PLEURA — TRANSVERSE SECTION

Educational Annotations | B – Respiratory System

Definitions of Common Procedures of Respiratory System

Bronchoscopy – The use of a flexible bronchoscope to visualize and perform procedures on the bronchi and lungs.

Endobronchial valve insertion – The bronchoscopic placement of one-way bronchial airflow valves that prevent air from entering the designated lobe segments while allowing trapped air and secretions to flow out. The valves are used primarily to treat emphysema by not allowing that segment to inflate and thus allowing other healthier segments to inflate and exhale more easily and efficiently.

Endotracheal intubation – The placement of a flexible, plastic breathing tube into the trachea through the oral cavity and occasionally through the nose.

Lobectomy of lung – The surgical removal of an entire lobe of a lung.

Lung transplant – The surgical replacement of a diseased lung by implantation of a donor lung.

Pleurodesis – The medical procedure to eliminate the pleural cavity space by instilling a substance (chemical, talc, etc.) through a chest tube that adheres the visceral and parietal pleura together.

Tracheostomy – The creation of a surgical opening in the front of neck and into the trachea with the placement of a tube through the opening and into the trachea to maintain the patency of the new airway for breathing and secretion removal.

AHA Coding Clinic® Reference Notations of Respiratory System

ROOT OPERATION SPECIFIC - B - RESPIRATORY SYSTEM
BYPASS - 1
CHANGE - 2
DESTRUCTION - 5
DILATION - 7
DRAINAGE - 9
EXCISION - B
    Endoscopic transbronchial needle aspiration biopsy of right lung ....AHA 14:1Q:p20
    Cricotracheal resection ....AHA 15:1Q:p15
EXTIRPATION - C
EXTRACTION - D
FRAGMENTATION - F
INSERTION - H
    Endotracheal intubation...AHA 14:4Q:p3
INSPECTION - J
    Bronchoscopic placement of fiducial marker ....AHA 14:1Q:p20
    Endoscopic viewing of talc placement in pleural cavity ....AHA 15:2Q:p31
OCCLUSION - L
REATTACHMENT - M
RELEASE - N
REMOVAL - P
REPAIR - Q
    Repair of midline diaphragm (paraesophageal) hernia ....AHA 14:3Q:p28
REPOSITION - S
RESECTION - T
SUPPLEMENT - U
    Omental flap repair of bronchopleural fistula ....AHA 15:1Q:p28
RESTRICTION - V
REVISION - W
TRANSPLANTATION - Y

Educational Annotations | B – Respiratory System

Body Part Key Listings of Respiratory System

See also Body Part Key in Appendix C
Cricoid cartilage...*use* Trachea

Device Key Listings of Respiratory System

See also Device Key in Appendix D
Autograft ....*use* Autologous Tissue Substitute
Brachytherapy seeds ....*use* Radioactive Element
Endotracheal tube (cuffed) (double-lumen) ....*use* Intraluminal Device, Endotracheal Airway in Respiratory System
Phrenic nerve stimulator lead ....*use* Diaphragmatic Pacemaker Lead in Respiratory System
Spiration IBV™ Valve System ....*use* Intraluminal Device, Endobronchial Valve in Respiratory System
Tissue bank graft ....*use* Nonautologous Tissue Substitute
Tracheostomy tube..*use* Tracheostomy Device in Respiratory System

Device Aggregation Table Listings of Respiratory System

See also Device Aggregation Table in Appendix E

Specific Device	For Operation	In Body System	General Device
Intraluminal Device, Endobronchial Valve	All applicable	Respiratory System	D Intraluminal Device
Intraluminal Device, Endotracheal Airway	All applicable	Respiratory System	D Intraluminal Device

Coding Notes of Respiratory System

Body System Relevant Coding Guidelines

Branches of body parts
B4.2
Where a specific branch of a body part does not have its own body part value in PCS, the body part is coded to the closest proximal branch that has a specific body part value.
Example: A procedure performed on the mandibular branch of the trigeminal nerve is coded to the trigeminal nerve body part value.

Body System Specific PCS Reference Manual Exercises

PCS CODE	B – RESPIRATORY SYSTEM EXERCISES
0B113F4	Tracheostomy formation with tracheostomy tube placement, percutaneous.
0B21XFZ	Tracheostomy tube exchange.
0B5P4ZZ	Thoracoscopy with mechanical abrasion and application of talc for pleurodesis.
0B718ZZ	Tracheoscopy with intraluminal dilation of tracheal stenosis.
0BH081Z	Bronchoscopy with insertion of brachytherapy seeds, right main bronchus.
0BP1XDZ	Extubation, endotracheal tube.
0BYK0Z0	Right lung transplant, open, using organ donor match.

B – RESPIRATORY SYSTEM   0 B 2

TUBULAR GROUP: Bypass, Dilation, Occlusion, Restriction
Root Operations that alter the diameter/route of a tubular body part.

- 1ST – **0** Medical and Surgical
- 2ND – **B** Respiratory System
- 3RD – **1 BYPASS**

EXAMPLE: Tracheostomy tube placement **CMS Ex:** Coronary artery bypass

BYPASS: Altering the route of passage of the contents of a tubular body part.

EXPLANATION: Rerouting contents to a downstream part ...

Body Part – 4TH	Approach – 5TH	Device – 6TH	Qualifier – 7TH
1 Trachea	0 Open	D Intraluminal device	6 Esophagus
1 Trachea	0 Open	F Tracheostomy device Z No device	4 Cutaneous
1 Trachea	3 Percutaneous 4 Percutaneous endoscopic	F Tracheostomy device Z No device	4 Cutaneous

DEVICE GROUP: Change, Insertion, Removal, (Replacement), Revision, Supplement
Root Operations that always involve a device.

- 1ST – **0** Medical and Surgical
- 2ND – **B** Respiratory System
- 3RD – **2 CHANGE**

EXAMPLE: Exchange trachea tube **CMS Ex:** Changing urinary catheter

CHANGE: Taking out or off a device from a body part and putting back an identical or similar device in or on the same body part without cutting or puncturing the skin or a mucous membrane.

EXPLANATION: ALL Changes use EXTERNAL approach only...

Body Part – 4TH	Approach – 5TH	Device – 6TH	Qualifier – 7TH
0 Tracheobronchial Tree Q Pleura K Lung, Right T Diaphragm L Lung, Left	X External	0 Drainage device Y Other device	Z No qualifier
1 Trachea	X External	0 Drainage device E Intraluminial device, endotracheal airway F Tracheostomy device Y Other device	Z No qualifier

0B5 — MEDICAL AND SURGICAL SECTION – 2016 ICD-10-PCS

EXCISION GROUP: Excision, Resection, Destruction, Extraction, (Detachment)
Root Operations that take out some or all of a body part.

- 1ST – **0** Medical and Surgical
- 2ND – **B** Respiratory System
- 3RD – **5 DESTRUCTION**

EXAMPLE: Pleurodesis with talc   CMS Ex: Fulguration polyp

DESTRUCTION: Physical eradication of all or a portion of a body part by the direct use of energy, force, or a destructive agent.

EXPLANATION: None of the body part is physically taken out

Body Part – 4TH		Approach – 5TH	Device – 6TH	Qualifier – 7TH
1 Trachea	9 Lingula Bronchus	0 Open	Z No device	Z No qualifier
2 Carina	B Lower Lobe Bronchus, Left	3 Percutaneous		
3 Main Bronchus, Right	C Upper Lung Lobe, Right	4 Percutaneous endoscopic		
4 Upper Lobe Bronchus, Right	D Middle Lung Lobe, Right	7 Via natural or artificial opening		
5 Middle Lobe Bronchus, Right	F Lower Lung Lobe, Right	8 Via natural or artificial opening endoscopic		
6 Lower Lobe Bronchus, Right	G Upper Lung Lobe, Left			
7 Main Bronchus, Left	H Lung Lingula			
8 Upper Lobe Bronchus, Left	J Lower Lung Lobe, Left			
	K Lung, Right			
	L Lung, Left			
	M Lungs, Bilateral			
N Pleura, Right		0 Open	Z No device	Z No qualifier
P Pleura, Left		3 Percutaneous		
R Diaphragm, Right		4 Percutaneous endoscopic		
S Diaphragm, Left				

TUBULAR GROUP: Bypass, Dilation, Occlusion, Restriction
Root Operations that alter the diameter/route of a tubular body part.

- 1ST – **0** Medical and Surgical
- 2ND – **B** Respiratory System
- 3RD – **7 DILATION**

EXAMPLE: Dilation tracheal stenosis   CMS Ex: Transluminal angioplasty

DILATION: Expanding an orifice or the lumen of a tubular body part.

EXPLANATION: By force (stretching) or cutting ...

Body Part – 4TH	Approach – 5TH	Device – 6TH	Qualifier – 7TH
1 Trachea	0 Open	D Intraluminal device	Z No qualifier
2 Carina	3 Percutaneous	Z No device	
3 Main Bronchus, Right	4 Percutaneous endoscopic		
4 Upper Lobe Bronchus, Right	7 Via natural or artificial opening		
5 Middle Lobe Bronchus, Right	8 Via natural or artificial opening endoscopic		
6 Lower Lobe Bronchus, Right			
7 Main Bronchus, Left			
8 Upper Lobe Bronchus, Left			
9 Lingula Bronchus			
B Lower Lobe Bronchus, Left			

B – RESPIRATORY SYSTEM 0B9

DRAINAGE GROUP: Drainage, Extirpation, Fragmentation
Root Operations that take out solids/fluids/gases from a body part.

1ST - **0** Medical and Surgical
2ND - **B** Respiratory System
3RD - **9 DRAINAGE**

EXAMPLE: Needle aspiration lung abscess   CMS Ex: Thoracentesis

DRAINAGE: Taking or letting out fluids and/or gases from a body part.

EXPLANATION: Qualifier "X Diagnostic" indicates biopsy ...

Body Part – 4TH		Approach – 5TH	Device – 6TH	Qualifier – 7TH
1 Trachea 2 Carina 3 Main Bronchus, Right 4 Upper Lobe Bronchus, Right 5 Middle Lobe Bronchus, Right 6 Lower Lobe Bronchus, Right 7 Main Bronchus, Left 8 Upper Lobe Bronchus, Left	9 Lingula Bronchus B Lower Lobe Bronchus, Left C Upper Lung Lobe, Right D Middle Lung Lobe, Right F Lower Lung Lobe, Right G Upper Lung Lobe, Left H Lung Lingula J Lower Lung Lobe, Left K Lung, Right L Lung, Left M Lungs, Bilateral	0 Open 3 Percutaneous 4 Percutaneous endoscopic 7 Via natural or artificial opening 8 Via natural or artificial opening endoscopic	0 Drainage device	Z No qualifier
1 Trachea 2 Carina 3 Main Bronchus, Right 4 Upper Lobe Bronchus, Right 5 Middle Lobe Bronchus, Right 6 Lower Lobe Bronchus, Right 7 Main Bronchus, Left 8 Upper Lobe Bronchus, Left	9 Lingula Bronchus B Lower Lobe Bronchus, Left C Upper Lung Lobe, Right D Middle Lung Lobe, Right F Lower Lung Lobe, Right G Upper Lung Lobe, Left H Lung Lingula J Lower Lung Lobe, Left K Lung, Right L Lung, Left M Lungs, Bilateral	0 Open 3 Percutaneous 4 Percutaneous endoscopic 7 Via natural or artificial opening 8 Via natural or artificial opening endoscopic	Z No device	X Diagnostic Z No qualifier
N Pleura, Right P Pleura, Left R Diaphragm, Right S Diaphragm, Left		0 Open 3 Percutaneous 4 Percutaneous endoscopic	0 Drainage device	Z No qualifier
N Pleura, Right P Pleura, Left R Diaphragm, Right S Diaphragm, Left		0 Open 3 Percutaneous 4 Percutaneous endoscopic	Z No device	X Diagnostic Z No qualifier

0BB

MEDICAL AND SURGICAL SECTION – 2016 ICD-10-PCS

[2016.PCS]

EXCISION GROUP: Excision, Resection, Destruction, Extraction, (Detachment)
Root Operations that take out some or all of a body part.

- 1ST – **0** Medical and Surgical
- 2ND – **B** Respiratory System
- 3RD – **B EXCISION**

EXAMPLE: Endoscopic biopsy of lung   CMS Ex: Liver biopsy

EXCISION: Cutting out or off, without replacement, a portion of a body part.

EXPLANATION: Qualifier "X Diagnostic" indicates biopsy ...

Body Part – 4TH		Approach – 5TH	Device – 6TH	Qualifier – 7TH
1 Trachea	9 Lingula Bronchus	0 Open	Z No device	X Diagnostic
2 Carina	B Lower Lobe Bronchus, Left	3 Percutaneous		Z No qualifier
3 Main Bronchus, Right	C Upper Lung Lobe, Right	4 Percutaneous endoscopic		
4 Upper Lobe Bronchus, Right	D Middle Lung Lobe, Right			
5 Middle Lobe Bronchus, Right	F Lower Lung Lobe, Right	7 Via natural or artificial opening		
6 Lower Lobe Bronchus, Right	G Upper Lung Lobe, Left	8 Via natural or artificial opening endoscopic		
7 Main Bronchus, Left	H Lung Lingula			
8 Upper Lobe Bronchus, Left	J Lower Lung Lobe, Left			
	K Lung, Right			
	L Lung, Left			
	M Lungs, Bilateral			
N Pleura, Right		0 Open	Z No device	X Diagnostic
P Pleura, Left		3 Percutaneous		Z No qualifier
R Diaphragm, Right		4 Percutaneous endoscopic		
S Diaphragm, Left				

DRAINAGE GROUP: Drainage, Extirpation, Fragmentation
Root Operations that take out solids/fluids/gases from a body part.

- 1ST – **0** Medical and Surgical
- 2ND – **B** Respiratory System
- 3RD – **C EXTIRPATION**

EXAMPLE: Removal bronchial foreign body   CMS Ex: Choledocholithotomy

EXTIRPATION: Taking or cutting out solid matter from a body part.

EXPLANATION: Abnormal byproduct or foreign body ...

Body Part – 4TH		Approach – 5TH	Device – 6TH	Qualifier – 7TH
1 Trachea	9 Lingula Bronchus	0 Open	Z No device	Z No qualifier
2 Carina	B Lower Lobe Bronchus, Left	3 Percutaneous		
3 Main Bronchus, Right	C Upper Lung Lobe, Right	4 Percutaneous endoscopic		
4 Upper Lobe Bronchus, Right	D Middle Lung Lobe, Right			
5 Middle Lobe Bronchus, Right	F Lower Lung Lobe, Right	7 Via natural or artificial opening		
6 Lower Lobe Bronchus, Right	G Upper Lung Lobe, Left	8 Via natural or artificial opening endoscopic		
7 Main Bronchus, Left	H Lung Lingula			
8 Upper Lobe Bronchus, Left	J Lower Lung Lobe, Left			
	K Lung, Right			
	L Lung, Left			
	M Lungs, Bilateral			
N Pleura, Right		0 Open	Z No device	Z No qualifier
P Pleura, Left		3 Percutaneous		
R Diaphragm, Right		4 Percutaneous endoscopic		
S Diaphragm, Left				

B – RESPIRATORY SYSTEM   0BF

EXCISION GROUP: Excision, Resection, Destruction, Extraction, (Detachment)
Root Operations that take out some or all of a body part.

- 1ST – **0** Medical and Surgical
- 2ND – **B** Respiratory System
- 3RD – **D** EXTRACTION

EXAMPLE: Pleural extraction   CMS Ex: D&C

EXTRACTION: Pulling or stripping out or off all or a portion of a body part by the use of force.

EXPLANATION: Qualifier "X Diagnostic" indicates biopsy ...

Body Part – 4TH	Approach – 5TH	Device – 6TH	Qualifier – 7TH
N Pleura, Right P Pleura, Left	0 Open 3 Percutaneous 4 Percutaneous endoscopic	Z No device	X Diagnostic Z No qualifier

DRAINAGE GROUP: Drainage, Extirpation, Fragmentation
Root Operations that take out solids/fluids/gases from a body part.

- 1ST – **0** Medical and Surgical
- 2ND – **B** Respiratory System
- 3RD – **F** FRAGMENTATION

EXAMPLE: Lithotripsy broncholithiasis   CMS Ex: ESWL

FRAGMENTATION: Breaking solid matter in a body part into pieces.

EXPLANATION: Pieces are not taken out during procedure ...

Body Part – 4TH	Approach – 5TH	Device – 6TH	Qualifier – 7TH
1 Trachea 2 Carina 3 Main Bronchus, Right 4 Upper Lobe Bronchus, Right 5 Middle Lobe Bronchus, Right 6 Lower Lobe Bronchus, Right 7 Main Bronchus, Left 8 Upper Lobe Bronchus, Left 9 Lingula Bronchus B Lower Lobe Bronchus, Left	0 Open 3 Percutaneous 4 Percutaneous endoscopic 7 Via natural or artificial opening 8 Via natural or artificial opening endoscopic X External NC*	Z No device	Z No qualifier

NC* – Non-covered by Medicare. See current Medicare Code Editor for details.

0BH

MEDICAL AND SURGICAL SECTION – 2016 ICD-10-PCS [2016.PCS]

DEVICE GROUP: Change, Insertion, Removal, (Replacement), Revision, Supplement
Root Operations that always involve a device.

- 1ST – **0** Medical and Surgical
- 2ND – **B** Respiratory System
- 3RD – **H INSERTION**

EXAMPLE: Endotracheal intubation   CMS Ex: Central venous catheter

INSERTION: Putting in a nonbiological appliance that monitors, assists, performs, or prevents a physiological function but does not physically take the place of a body part.

EXPLANATION: None

Body Part – 4TH	Approach – 5TH	Device – 6TH	Qualifier – 7TH
0 Tracheobronchial Tree	0 Open 3 Percutaneous 4 Percutaneous endoscopic 7 Via natural or artificial opening 8 Via natural or artificial opening endoscopic	1 Radioactive element 2 Monitoring device 3 Infusion device D Intraluminal device	Z No qualifier
1 Trachea	0 Open	2 Monitoring device D Intraluminal device	Z No qualifier
1 Trachea	3 Percutaneous	D Intraluminal device E Intraluminal device, endotracheal airway	Z No qualifier
1 Trachea	4 Percutaneous endoscopic	D Intraluminal device	Z No qualifier
1 Trachea	7 Via natural or artificial opening 8 Via natural or artificial opening endoscopic	2 Monitoring device D Intraluminal device E Intraluminal device, endotracheal airway	Z No qualifier
3 Main Bronchus, Right 4 Upper Lobe Bronchus, Right 5 Middle Lobe Bronchus, Right 6 Lower Lobe Bronchus, Right 7 Main Bronchus, Left 8 Upper Lobe Bronchus, Left 9 Lingula Bronchus B Lower Lobe Bronchus, Left	0 Open 3 Percutaneous 4 Percutaneous endoscopic 7 Via natural or artificial opening 8 Via natural or artificial opening endoscopic	G Intraluminal device, endobronchial valve	Z No qualifier
K Lung, Right L Lung, Left	0 Open 3 Percutaneous 4 Percutaneous endoscopic 7 Via natural or artificial opening 8 Via natural or artificial opening endoscopic	1 Radioactive element 2 Monitoring device 3 Infusion device	Z No qualifier
R Diaphragm, Right S Diaphragm, Left	0 Open 3 Percutaneous 4 Percutaneous endoscopic	2 Monitoring device M Diaphragmatic pacemaker lead	Z No qualifier

B – RESPIRATORY SYSTEM   0 B L

EXAMINATION GROUP: Inspection, (Map)
Root Operations involving examination only.

1ST – **0** Medical and Surgical	EXAMPLE: Diagnostic bronchoscopy		CMS Ex: Colonoscopy
2ND – **B** Respiratory System	**INSPECTION:** Visually and/or manually exploring a body part.		
3RD – **J** INSPECTION	EXPLANATION: Direct or instrumental visualization ...		

Body Part – 4TH	Approach – 5TH	Device – 6TH	Qualifier – 7TH
0 Tracheobronchial Tree 1 Trachea K Lung, Right L Lung, Left Q Pleura T Diaphragm	0 Open 3 Percutaneous 4 Percutaneous endoscopic 7 Via natural or artificial opening 8 Via natural or artificial opening endoscopic X External	Z No device	Z No qualifier

TUBULAR GROUP: Bypass, Dilation, Occlusion, Restriction
Root Operations that alter the diameter/route of a tubular body part.

1ST – **0** Medical and Surgical	EXAMPLE: Suture closure bronchus		CMS Ex: Fallopian tube ligation
2ND – **B** Respiratory System	**OCCLUSION:** Completely closing an orifice or lumen of a tubular body part.		
3RD – **L** OCCLUSION	EXPLANATION: Natural or artificially created orifice ...		

Body Part – 4TH	Approach – 5TH	Device – 6TH	Qualifier – 7TH
1 Trachea 2 Carina 3 Main Bronchus, Right 4 Upper Lobe Bronchus, Right 5 Middle Lobe Bronchus, Right 6 Lower Lobe Bronchus, Right 7 Main Bronchus, Left 8 Upper Lobe Bronchus, Left 9 Lingula Bronchus B Lower Lobe Bronchus, Left	0 Open 3 Percutaneous 4 Percutaneous endoscopic	C Extraluminal device D Intraluminal device Z No device	Z No qualifier
1 Trachea 2 Carina 3 Main Bronchus, Right 4 Upper Lobe Bronchus, Right 5 Middle Lobe Bronchus, Right 6 Lower Lobe Bronchus, Right 7 Main Bronchus, Left 8 Upper Lobe Bronchus, Left 9 Lingula Bronchus B Lower Lobe Bronchus, Left	7 Via natural or artificial opening 8 Via natural or artificial opening endoscopic	D Intraluminal device Z No device	Z No qualifier

0BM

MEDICAL AND SURGICAL SECTION – 2016 ICD-10-PCS

MOVE GROUP: Reattachment, Reposition, (Transfer), Transplantation
Root Operations that put in/put back or move some/all of a body part.

- 1ST – **0** Medical and Surgical
- 2ND – **B** Respiratory System
- 3RD – **M REATTACHMENT**

EXAMPLE: Reattachment ruptured diaphragm CMS Ex: Reattach hand

REATTACHMENT: Putting back in or on all or a portion of a separated body part to its normal location or other suitable location.

EXPLANATION: With/without reconnection of vessels/nerves...

Body Part – 4TH		Approach – 5TH	Device – 6TH	Qualifier – 7TH
1 Trachea	B Lower Lobe Bronchus, Left	0 Open	Z No device	Z No qualifier
2 Carina	C Upper Lung Lobe, Right			
3 Main Bronchus, Right	D Middle Lung Lobe, Right			
4 Upper Lobe Bronchus, Right	F Lower Lung Lobe, Right			
5 Middle Lobe Bronchus, Right	G Upper Lung Lobe, Left			
6 Lower Lobe Bronchus, Right	H Lung Lingula			
7 Main Bronchus, Left	J Lower Lung Lobe, Left			
8 Upper Lobe Bronchus, Left	K Lung, Right			
9 Lingula Bronchus	L Lung, Left			
	R Diaphragm, Right			
	S Diaphragm, Left			

DIVISION GROUP: (Division), Release
Root Operations involving cutting or separation only.

- 1ST – **0** Medical and Surgical
- 2ND – **B** Respiratory System
- 3RD – **N RELEASE**

EXAMPLE: Lysis adhesions lung CMS Ex: Carpal tunnel release

RELEASE: Freeing a body part from an abnormal physical constraint by cutting or by the use of force.

EXPLANATION: None of the body part is taken out ...

Body Part – 4TH		Approach – 5TH	Device – 6TH	Qualifier – 7TH
1 Trachea	9 Lingula Bronchus	0 Open	Z No device	Z No qualifier
2 Carina	B Lower Lobe Bronchus, Left	3 Percutaneous		
3 Main Bronchus, Right	C Upper Lung Lobe, Right	4 Percutaneous endoscopic		
4 Upper Lobe Bronchus, Right	D Middle Lung Lobe, Right	7 Via natural or artificial opening		
5 Middle Lobe Bronchus, Right	F Lower Lung Lobe, Right	8 Via natural or artificial opening endoscopic		
6 Lower Lobe Bronchus, Right	G Upper Lung Lobe, Left			
7 Main Bronchus, Left	H Lung Lingula			
8 Upper Lobe Bronchus, Left	J Lower Lung Lobe, Left			
	K Lung, Right			
	L Lung, Left			
	M Lungs, Bilateral			
N Pleura, Right		0 Open	Z No device	Z No qualifier
P Pleura, Left		3 Percutaneous		
R Diaphragm, Right		4 Percutaneous endoscopic		
S Diaphragm, Left				

B – RESPIRATORY SYSTEM — 0BP

DEVICE GROUP: Change, Insertion, Removal, (Replacement), Revision, Supplement
Root Operations that always involve a device.

- 1ST – **0** Medical and Surgical
- 2ND – **B** Respiratory System
- 3RD – **P** REMOVAL

EXAMPLE: Removal tracheostomy tube
CMS Ex: Chest tube removal

REMOVAL: Taking out or off a device from a body part.

EXPLANATION: Removal device without reinsertion …

Body Part – 4TH	Approach – 5TH	Device – 6TH	Qualifier – 7TH
0 Tracheobronchial Tree	0 Open 3 Percutaneous 4 Percutaneous endoscopic 7 Via natural or artificial opening 8 Via natural or artificial opening endoscopic	0 Drainage device 1 Radioactive element 2 Monitoring device 3 Infusion device 7 Autologous tissue substitute C Extraluminal device D Intraluminal device J Synthetic substitute K Nonautologous tissue substitute	Z No qualifier
0 Tracheobronchial Tree	X External	0 Drainage device 1 Radioactive element 2 Monitoring device 3 Infusion device D Intraluminal device	Z No qualifier
1 Trachea	0 Open 3 Percutaneous 4 Percutaneous endoscopic 7 Via natural or artificial opening 8 Via natural or artificial opening endoscopic	0 Drainage device 2 Monitoring device 7 Autologous tissue substitute C Extraluminal device D Intraluminal device F Tracheostomy device J Synthetic substitute K Nonautologous tissue substitute	Z No qualifier
1 Trachea	X External	0 Drainage device 2 Monitoring device D Intraluminal device F Tracheostomy device	Z No qualifier

continued ➪

0BP REMOVAL – continued

Body Part – 4TH	Approach – 5TH	Device – 6TH	Qualifier – 7TH
K Lung, Right L Lung, Left	0 Open 3 Percutaneous 4 Percutaneous endoscopic 7 Via natural or artificial opening 8 Via natural or artificial opening endoscopic X External	0 Drainage device 1 Radioactive element 2 Monitoring device 3 Infusion device	Z No qualifier
Q Pleura	0 Open 3 Percutaneous 4 Percutaneous endoscopic 7 Via natural or artificial opening 8 Via natural or artificial opening endoscopic X External	0 Drainage device 1 Radioactive element 2 Monitoring device	Z No qualifier
T Diaphragm	0 Open 3 Percutaneous 4 Percutaneous endoscopic 7 Via natural or artificial opening 8 Via natural or artificial opening endoscopic	0 Drainage device 2 Monitoring device 7 Autologous tissue substitute J Synthetic substitute K Nonautologous tissue substitute M Diaphragmatic pacemaker lead	Z No qualifier
T Diaphragm	X External	0 Drainage device 2 Monitoring device M Diaphragmatic pacemaker lead	Z No qualifier

B – RESPIRATORY SYSTEM 0BS

OTHER REPAIRS GROUP: (Control), Repair
Root Operations that define other repairs.

- 1ST – **0** Medical and Surgical
- 2ND – **B** Respiratory System
- 3RD – **Q REPAIR**

EXAMPLE: Repair diaphragmatic hernia **CMS Ex:** Suture laceration

REPAIR: Restoring, to the extent possible, a body part to its normal anatomic structure and function.

EXPLANATION: Only when no other root operation applies ...

Body Part – 4TH		Approach – 5TH	Device – 6TH	Qualifier – 7TH
1 Trachea	9 Lingula Bronchus	0 Open	Z No device	Z No qualifier
2 Carina	B Lower Lobe Bronchus, Left	3 Percutaneous		
3 Main Bronchus, Right	C Upper Lung Lobe, Right	4 Percutaneous endoscopic		
4 Upper Lobe Bronchus, Right	D Middle Lung Lobe, Right	7 Via natural or artificial opening		
5 Middle Lobe Bronchus, Right	F Lower Lung Lobe, Right	8 Via natural or artificial opening endoscopic		
6 Lower Lobe Bronchus, Right	G Upper Lung Lobe, Left			
7 Main Bronchus, Left	H Lung Lingula			
8 Upper Lobe Bronchus, Left	J Lower Lung Lobe, Left			
	K Lung, Right			
	L Lung, Left			
	M Lungs, Bilateral			
N Pleura, Right		0 Open	Z No device	Z No qualifier
P Pleura, Left		3 Percutaneous		
R Diaphragm, Right		4 Percutaneous endoscopic		
S Diaphragm, Left				

MOVE GROUP: Reattachment, Reposition, (Transfer), Transplantation
Root Operations that put in/put back or move some/all of a body part.

- 1ST – **0** Medical and Surgical
- 2ND – **B** Respiratory System
- 3RD – **S REPOSITION**

EXAMPLE: Tracheal relocation **CMS Ex:** Fracture reduction

REPOSITION: Moving to its normal location, or other suitable location, all or a portion of a body part.

EXPLANATION: May or may not be cut to be moved ...

Body Part – 4TH		Approach – 5TH	Device – 6TH	Qualifier – 7TH
1 Trachea	B Lower Lobe Bronchus, Left	0 Open	Z No device	Z No qualifier
2 Carina	C Upper Lung Lobe, Right			
3 Main Bronchus, Right	D Middle Lung Lobe, Right			
4 Upper Lobe Bronchus, Right	F Lower Lung Lobe, Right			
5 Middle Lobe Bronchus, Right	G Upper Lung Lobe, Left			
6 Lower Lobe Bronchus, Right	H Lung Lingula			
7 Main Bronchus, Left	J Lower Lung Lobe, Left			
8 Upper Lobe Bronchus, Left	K Lung, Right			
9 Lingula Bronchus	L Lung, Left			
	R Diaphragm, Right			
	S Diaphragm, Left			

0BT

MEDICAL AND SURGICAL SECTION – 2016 ICD-10-PCS [2016.PCS]

EXCISION GROUP: Excision, Resection, Destruction, Extraction, (Detachment)
Root Operations that take out some or all of a body part.

- 1ST – **0** Medical and Surgical
- 2ND – **B** Respiratory System
- 3RD – **T** RESECTION

EXAMPLE: Lobectomy   CMS Ex: Cholecystectomy

RESECTION: Cutting out or off, without replacement, all of a body part.

EXPLANATION: None

Body Part – 4TH	Approach – 5TH	Device – 6TH	Qualifier – 7TH
1 Trachea	0 Open	Z No device	Z No qualifier
2 Carina	4 Percutaneous endoscopic		
3 Main Bronchus, Right			
4 Upper Lobe Bronchus, Right			
5 Middle Lobe Bronchus, Right			
6 Lower Lobe Bronchus, Right			
7 Main Bronchus, Left			
8 Upper Lobe Bronchus, Left			
9 Lingula Bronchus			
B Lower Lobe Bronchus, Left			
C Upper Lung Lobe, Right			
D Middle Lung Lobe, Right			
F Lower Lung Lobe, Right			
G Upper Lung Lobe, Left			
H Lung Lingula			
J Lower Lung Lobe, Left			
K Lung, Right			
L Lung, Left			
M Lungs, Bilateral			
R Diaphragm, Right			
S Diaphragm, Left			

DEVICE GROUP: Change, Insertion, Removal, (Replacement), Revision, Supplement
Root Operations that always involve a device.

- 1ST – **0** Medical and Surgical
- 2ND – **B** Respiratory System
- 3RD – **U** SUPPLEMENT

EXAMPLE: Graft repair diaphragm defect   CMS Ex: Hernia repair with mesh

SUPPLEMENT: Putting in or on biological or synthetic material that physically reinforces and/or augments the function of a portion of a body part.

EXPLANATION: Biological material from same individual …

Body Part – 4TH	Approach – 5TH	Device – 6TH	Qualifier – 7TH
1 Trachea	0 Open	7 Autologous tissue substitute	Z No qualifier
2 Carina	4 Percutaneous endoscopic	J Synthetic substitute	
3 Main Bronchus, Right		K Nonautologous tissue substitute	
4 Upper Lobe Bronchus, Right			
5 Middle Lobe Bronchus, Right			
6 Lower Lobe Bronchus, Right			
7 Main Bronchus, Left			
8 Upper Lobe Bronchus, Left			
9 Lingula Bronchus			
B Lower Lobe Bronchus, Left			
R Diaphragm, Right			
S Diaphragm, Left			

B – RESPIRATORY SYSTEM

0 B V

TUBULAR GROUP: Bypass, Dilation, Occlusion, Restriction
Root Operations that alter the diameter/route of a tubular body part.

1ST – **0** Medical and Surgical
2ND – **B** Respiratory System
3RD – **V RESTRICTION**

EXAMPLE: Bronchial restrictive stent | CMS Ex: Cervical cerclage

RESTRICTION: Partially closing an orifice or the lumen of a tubular body part.

EXPLANATION: Natural or artificially created orifice ...

Body Part – 4TH	Approach – 5TH	Device – 6TH	Qualifier – 7TH
1 Trachea 2 Carina 3 Main Bronchus, Right 4 Upper Lobe Bronchus, Right 5 Middle Lobe Bronchus, Right 6 Lower Lobe Bronchus, Right 7 Main Bronchus, Left 8 Upper Lobe Bronchus, Left 9 Lingula Bronchus B Lower Lobe Bronchus, Left	0 Open 3 Percutaneous 4 Percutaneous endoscopic	C Extraluminal device D Intraluminal device Z No device	Z No qualifier
1 Trachea 2 Carina 3 Main Bronchus, Right 4 Upper Lobe Bronchus, Right 5 Middle Lobe Bronchus, Right 6 Lower Lobe Bronchus, Right 7 Main Bronchus, Left 8 Upper Lobe Bronchus, Left 9 Lingula Bronchus B Lower Lobe Bronchus, Left	7 Via natural or artificial opening 8 Via natural or artificial opening endoscopic	D Intraluminal device Z No device	Z No qualifier

0BW

MEDICAL AND SURGICAL SECTION – 2016 ICD-10-PCS

[2016.PCS]

DEVICE GROUP: Change, Insertion, Removal, (Replacement), Revision, Supplement
Root Operations that always involve a device.

1ST - **0** Medical and Surgical
2ND - **B** Respiratory System
3RD - **W REVISION**

EXAMPLE: Reposition diaphragm lead **CMS Ex:** Adjustment pacemaker lead

REVISION: Correcting, to the extent possible, a portion of a malfunctioning device or the position of a displaced device.

EXPLANATION: May replace components of a device ...

Body Part – 4TH	Approach – 5TH	Device – 6TH	Qualifier – 7TH
0 Tracheobronchial Tree	0 Open 3 Percutaneous 4 Percutaneous endoscopic 7 Via natural or artificial opening 8 Via natural or artificial opening endoscopic X External	0 Drainage device 2 Monitoring device 3 Infusion device 7 Autologous tissue substitute C Extraluminal device D Intraluminal device J Synthetic substitute K Nonautologous tissue substitute	Z No qualifier
1 Trachea	0 Open 3 Percutaneous 4 Percutaneous endoscopic 7 Via natural or artificial opening 8 Via natural or artificial opening endoscopic X External	0 Drainage device 2 Monitoring device 7 Autologous tissue substitute C Extraluminal device D Intraluminal device F Tracheostomy device J Synthetic substitute K Nonautologous tissue substitute	Z No qualifier
K Lung, Right L Lung, Left	0 Open 3 Percutaneous 4 Percutaneous endoscopic 7 Via natural or artificial opening 8 Via natural or artificial opening endoscopic X External	0 Drainage device 2 Monitoring device 3 Infusion device	Z No qualifier
Q Pleura	0 Open 3 Percutaneous 4 Percutaneous endoscopic 7 Via natural or artificial opening 8 Via natural or artificial opening endoscopic X External	0 Drainage device 2 Monitoring device	Z No qualifier
T Diaphragm	0 Open 3 Percutaneous 4 Percutaneous endoscopic 7 Via natural or artificial opening 8 Via natural or artificial opening endoscopic X External	0 Drainage device 2 Monitoring device 7 Autologous tissue substitute J Synthetic substitute K Nonautologous tissue substitute M Diaphragmatic pacemaker lead	Z No qualifier

RESPIRATORY 0BW

B – RESPIRATORY SYSTEM — 0BY

MOVE GROUP: Reattachment, Reposition, (Transfer), Transplantation
Root Operations that put in/put back or move some/all of a body part.

1ST – **0** Medical and Surgical
2ND – **B** Respiratory System
3RD – **Y** TRANSPLANTATION

EXAMPLE: Lung transplant   **CMS Ex:** Kidney transplant

TRANSPLANTATION: Putting in or on all or a portion of a living body part taken from another individual or animal to physically take the place and/or function of all or a portion of a similar body part.

EXPLANATION: May take over all or part of its function …

Body Part – 4TH	Approach – 5TH	Device – 6TH	Qualifier – 7TH
C Upper Lung Lobe, Right LC*	0 Open	Z No device	0 Allogenic
D Middle Lung Lobe, Right LC*			1 Syngeneic
F Lower Lung Lobe, Right LC*			2 Zooplastic
G Upper Lung Lobe, Left LC*			
H Lung Lingula LC*			
J Lower Lung Lobe, Left LC*			
K Lung, Right LC*			
L Lung, Left LC*			
M Lungs, Bilateral LC*			

LC* – Some procedures are considered limited coverage by Medicare. See current Medicare Code Editor for details.

MEDICAL AND SURGICAL SECTION – 2016 ICD-10-PCS

NOTES

- 0 – Medical and Surgical
- B – Respiratory System
- Y – TRANSPLANTATION

TRANSPLANTATION: Putting in or on all or a portion of a living body part taken from another individual or animal to physically take the place and/or function of all or a portion of a similar body part

EXPLANATION: May take over all or part of its function

EXAMPLE: Lung transplant

CMS Ex.: Kidney transplant

Body Part – 4th	Approach – 5th	Device – 6th	Qualifier – 7th
C Upper Lung Lobe, Right ‡	0 Open	Z No device	0 Allogeneic
D Middle Lung Lobe, Right ‡			1 Syngeneic
F Lower Lung Lobe, Right ‡			2 Zooplastic
G Upper Lung Lobe, Left ‡			
H Lung Lingula ‡			
J Lower Lung Lobe, Left ‡			
K Lung, Right ‡			
L Lung, Left ‡			
M Lungs, Bilateral ‡			

‡ Some procedures are considered limited coverage by Medicare. See current Medicare Code Editor for details.

Educational Annotations | C – Mouth and Throat

Body System Specific Educational Annotations for the Mouth and Throat include:
- Anatomy and Physiology Review
- Anatomical Illustrations
- Definitions of Common Procedures
- AHA Coding Clinic® Reference Notations
- Body Part Key Listings
- Device Key Listings
- Device Aggregation Table Listings
- Coding Notes

Anatomy and Physiology Review of Mouth and Throat

BODY PART VALUES – C - MOUTH AND THROAT

Adenoids – ANATOMY – The adenoids (nasopharyngeal tonsils) are masses of lymphatic tissue located behind the nasal cavity and on roof of the nasopharynx. PHYSIOLOGY – The adenoids help in the prevention of bacteria entering the body.

Buccal Mucosa – The mucous membrane lining of the mouth and inside of cheeks.

Epiglottis – ANATOMY – The epiglottis is a mucous-membrane-covered flap of elastic cartilage tissue that is attached to the entrance of the larynx. PHYSIOLOGY – The epiglottis prevents food from going into the trachea and channels it into the esophagus.

Gingiva – ANATOMY – The gingiva (gums) are fibrous and mucous membrane tissue that surround the roots of erupted teeth and the crowns of unerupted teeth, and cover the alveolar process of the maxilla and mandible. PHYSIOLOGY – The gingiva (gums) function to help protect and support the roots of the teeth.

Hard Palate – The hard palate is the superior wall of the oral cavity formed by the palatine processes of the maxilla that separates the oral cavity from the nasal cavity.

Larynx – ANATOMY – The larynx is the musculocartilaginous structure, lined with mucous membrane located between the root of the tongue and the trachea. The glottis is the slit-like opening of the larynx formed by the true vocal cords. The supraglottis is that portion of the larynx situated above the glottis. There are nine laryngeal cartilages, three paired and three single. PHYSIOLOGY – The larynx functions to guard the entrance of the trachea from food and liquids, to control the expulsion of air, and to produce sound. The glottis produces sound, controls pitch, and when closed prevents food from entering the trachea. The supraglottis is an area of the larynx which helps to prevent food and liquid from entering the trachea. The laryngeal cartilages frame and support the larynx and its muscles.

Lip – ANATOMY – The soft tissue opening of the mouth comprised of skin, connective tissue, and muscle. PHYSIOLOGY – The lips contain sensitive nerve endings that provide sensory information about food. The lips secure the closure of the mouth during chewing and swallowing. They also are involved in sound production and facial expression.

Minor Salivary Gland – Any of the large number of small salivary glands in the oral mucosa of the mouth.

Parotid Duct – The tube (Stenson's ducts) beginning in the parotid gland and emptying into the oral cavity.

Parotid Gland – The two parotid glands lie above the mouth, and below and in front of the ears, with ducts (Stenson's ducts) that run down through the cheeks and empty into the roof of the mouth opposite of the second molar.

Pharynx – ANATOMY – The portion of the throat comprised of the oropharynx and the laryngopharynx. PHYSIOLOGY – The pharynx serves as a passageway for food and air.

Salivary Gland – ANATOMY – There are three pairs of major salivary glands; the parotids, the submandibular, and the sublingual glands. Both sympathetic and parasympathetic nerves stimulate the major salivary glands. PHYSIOLOGY – The major salivary glands function to secrete saliva which moistens food particles, help to bind them together, and begin digestion of carbohydrates. Saliva also dissolves various food chemicals so they can be tasted. There are two types of secretory cells. Serous cells produce a watery fluid which contain a digestive enzyme called amylase. Mucous cells produce a thick stringy liquid that bind food together and act as a lubricant during swallowing. Sympathetic nerves stimulate the glands to secrete a small quantity of saliva to keep the mouth moist. Parasympathetic nerves stimulate the glands reflexly when the person sees, smells, or even thinks about pleasant food.

Soft Palate – ANATOMY – The soft palate is the muscular extension of the hard palate in the superior-posterior oral cavity. PHYSIOLOGY – The soft palate contracts to allow swallowing and prevents food from entering the nasal cavity.

Continued on next page

Educational Annotations | C – Mouth and Throat

Anatomy and Physiology Review of Mouth and Throat

BODY PART VALUES – C - MOUTH AND THROAT
Continued from previous page

Sublingual Gland – The two sublingual glands lie beneath the tongue, with ducts opening near the frenulum of the tongue.

Submaxillary Gland – The two submaxillary (submandibular) glands lie in the floor of the mouth on the inside surface of the mandible, with ducts (Wharton's ducts) opening beneath the tongue, and with other ducts opening near the frenulum of the tongue.

Teeth – ANATOMY – The teeth consist of the bony substance dentine, which surround the soft inner pulp that contain blood vessels and nerves and are embedded in rows in the upper (maxilla) and lower (mandible) jaw bones. PHYSIOLOGY – The teeth function primarily to chew food into smaller parts in preparation for swallowing and digestion.

Tongue – ANATOMY – The tongue is the movable, muscular organ on the floor of the mouth. The lingual tonsils are a mass of lymphoid tissue at the root, and the frenulum is the mucous membrane fold which attaches the undersurface of the tongue to the floor of the mouth. PHYSIOLOGY – The tongue functions primarily as the organ of sense of taste, as well as aiding in the chewing and swallowing of food, and the articulation of sound. The lingual tonsils aid in the elimination of bacteria entering the oral cavity. The frenulum somewhat restricts the movement of the tongue.

Tonsils – ANATOMY – The tonsils (palatine tonsils) are masses of lymphatic tissue located on either side of the tongue in the posterior oral cavity. The tonsillar fossa is the depression in which the tonsils are located. The tonsillar pillars are the mucous membrane folds attached to the soft palate. PHYSIOLOGY – The tonsils function to help fight off bacteria by releasing bacteria-consuming phagocytes.

Uvula – The uvula is the cone-shaped projection of the soft palate.

Vocal Cord – ANATOMY – The vocal cords are folds of mucous membranes located within the larynx. PHYSIOLOGY – The vocal cords are primarily responsible for voice production. Sound is produced by the vibration of the folds as air is exhaled from the lungs.

Anatomical Illustrations of Mouth and Throat

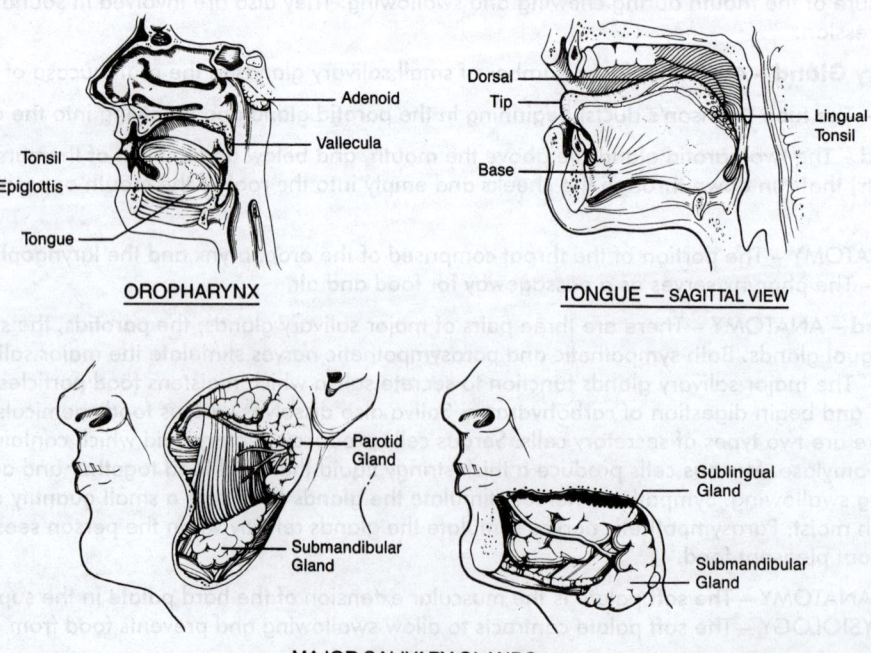

OROPHARYNX

TONGUE — SAGITTAL VIEW

MAJOR SALIVARY GLANDS

Continued on next page

Educational Annotations | C – Mouth and Throat

Anatomical Illustrations of Mouth and Throat

Continued from previous page

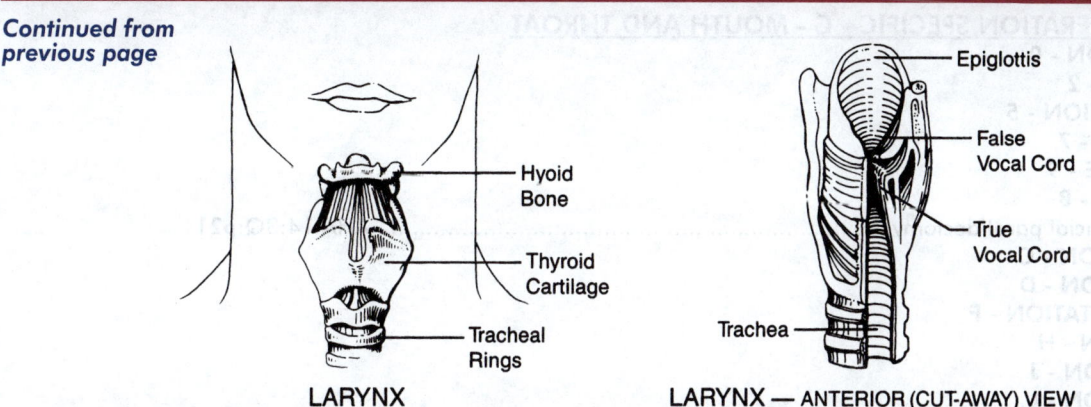

LARYNX

LARYNX — ANTERIOR (CUT-AWAY) VIEW

Definitions of Common Procedures of Mouth and Throat

Ablation of vocal cord lesion – The destruction of a vocal cord lesion using a tissue destroying technique (laser, radiofrequency heat, etc.).

Cleft palate repair – The reconstructing surgical repair of a cleft palate (defect in the roof of the mouth) by excising and moving tissue from the palate and other oral tissues and closing in layers while realigning the palatal muscles.

Glossectomy – The excision of all or a portion of the tongue.

Laser-assisted uvuloplasty – The use of repeated laser treatments to destroy and modify the uvula tissue in order to reduce or eliminate snoring.

Sialoadenectomy – The excision of a salivary gland.

Sialolithotomy – The incision of a salivary gland to remove a stone from the gland or its duct.

Tonsillectomy – The excision of the tonsils performed by a direct approach (external).

Total laryngectomy – The surgical removal of all of the larynx and usually with the insertion of an artificial voice box prosthesis.

Uvulopalatopharyngoplasty – The reconstructing surgical repair of the back of the oral cavity by removing the tonsils, and reshaping the uvula, pharynx, and soft palate to correct obstructive sleep apnea.

311

0C — C – Mouth and Throat

Educational Annotations

AHA Coding Clinic® Reference Notations of Mouth and Throat

ROOT OPERATION SPECIFIC - C - MOUTH AND THROAT

ALTERATION - 0
CHANGE - 2
DESTRUCTION - 5
DILATION - 7
DRAINAGE - 9
EXCISION - B
   Superficial parotidectomy..AHA 14:3Q:p21
EXTIRPATION - C
EXTRACTION - D
FRAGMENTATION - F
INSERTION - H
INSPECTION - J
OCCLUSION - L
REATTACHMENT - M
RELEASE - N
REMOVAL - P
REPAIR - Q
REPLACEMENT - R
   Intraoral graft using Oasis® acellular matrix ....AHA 14:2Q:p5,6
   Wide local excision of soft palate with placement of a maxillary
      surgical obturator ....AHA 14:3Q:p25
REPOSITION - S
RESECTION - T
   Extraction of impacted teeth ....AHA 14:3Q:p23
SUPPLEMENT - U
RESTRICTION - V
REVISION - W
TRANSFER - X

Body Part Key Listings of Mouth and Throat

See also Body Part Key in Appendix C

Anterior lingual gland	use Minor Salivary Gland
Aryepiglottic fold	use Larynx
Arytenoid cartilage	use Larynx
Buccal gland	use Buccal Mucosa
Corniculate cartilage	use Larynx
Cuneiform cartilage	use Larynx
False vocal cord	use Larynx
Frenulum labii inferioris	use Lower Lip
Frenulum labii superioris	use Upper Lip
Frenulum linguae	use Tongue
Glossoepiglottic fold	use Epiglottis
Glottis	use Larynx
Hypopharynx	use Pharynx
Labial gland	use Upper Lip, Lower Lip
Laryngopharynx	use Pharynx
Lingual tonsil	use Tongue
Molar gland	use Buccal Mucosa
Oropharynx	use Pharynx

Continued on next page

Educational Annotations | C – Mouth and Throat

Body Part Key Listings of Mouth and Throat

Continued from previous page

Palatine gland	*use* Buccal Mucosa
Palatine tonsil	*use* Tonsils
Palatine uvula	*use* Uvula
Pharyngeal tonsil	*use* Adenoids
Piriform recess (sinus)	*use* Pharynx
Rima glottidis	*use* Larynx
Stensen's duct	*use* Parotid Duct, Left/Right
Submandibular gland	*use* Submaxillary Gland, Left/Right
Thyroid cartilage	*use* Larynx
Ventricular fold	*use* Larynx
Vermilion border	*use* Upper Lip, Lower Lip
Vocal fold	*use* Vocal Cord, Left/Right

Device Key Listings of Mouth and Throat

See also Device Key in Appendix D

Autograft	*use* Autologous Tissue Substitute
Brachytherapy seeds	*use* Radioactive Element
Guedel airway	*use* Intraluminal Device, Airway in Mouth and Throat
Oropharyngeal airway (OPA)	*use* Intraluminal Device, Airway in Mouth and Throat
Tissue bank graft	*use* Nonautologous Tissue Substitute

Device Aggregation Table Listings of Mouth and Throat

See also Device Aggregation Table in Appendix E

Specific Device	For Operation	In Body System	General Device	
Intraluminal Device, Airway	All applicable	Mouth and Throat	D	Intraluminal Device

Educational Annotations | C – Mouth and Throat

Coding Notes of Mouth and Throat

Body System Specific PCS Reference Manual Exercises

PCS CODE	C – MOUTH AND THROAT EXERCISES
0C5T3ZZ	Percutaneous radiofrequency ablation of right vocal cord lesion.
0CB1XZZ	Excision of basal cell carcinoma of lower lip.
0CDWXZ2	Forceps total mouth extraction, upper and lower teeth.
0CDXXZ2	
0CJS8ZZ	Diagnostic laryngoscopy.
0CMXXZ1	Closed replantation of three avulsed teeth, lower jaw.
0CN7XZZ	Frenulotomy for treatment of tongue-tie syndrome. (The frenulum is coded to the body part value Tongue.)

C – MOUTH AND THROAT   0C2

OTHER OBJECTIVES GROUP: Alteration, (Creation), (Fusion)
Root Operations that define other objectives.

- 1ST – **0** Medical and Surgical
- 2ND – **C** Mouth and Throat
- 3RD – **0 ALTERATION**

EXAMPLE: Cosmetic lip augmentation   CMS Ex: Face lift

ALTERATION: Modifying the anatomic structure of a body part without affecting the function of the body part.

EXPLANATION: Principal purpose is to improve appearance

Body Part – 4TH	Approach – 5TH	Device – 6TH	Qualifier – 7TH
0 Upper Lip 1 Lower Lip	X External	7 Autologous tissue substitute J Synthetic substitute K Nonautologous tissue substitute Z No device	Z No qualifier

DEVICE GROUP: Change, Insertion, Removal, Replacement, Revision, Supplement
Root Operations that always involve a device.

- 1ST – **0** Medical and Surgical
- 2ND – **C** Mouth and Throat
- 3RD – **2 CHANGE**

EXAMPLE: Exchange drain tube   CMS Ex: Changing urinary catheter

CHANGE: Taking out or off a device from a body part and putting back an identical or similar device in or on the same body part without cutting or puncturing the skin or a mucous membrane.

EXPLANATION: ALL Changes use EXTERNAL approach only...

Body Part – 4TH	Approach – 5TH	Device – 6TH	Qualifier – 7TH
A Salivary Gland S Larynx Y Mouth and Throat	X External	0 Drainage device Y Other device	Z No qualifier

0C5 MEDICAL AND SURGICAL SECTION – 2016 ICD-10-PCS

EXCISION GROUP: Excision, Resection, Destruction, Extraction, (Detachment)
Root Operations that take out some or all of a body part.

- 1ST - **0** Medical and Surgical
- 2ND - **C** Mouth and Throat
- 3RD - **5 DESTRUCTION**

EXAMPLE: Ablation vocal cord lesion CMS Ex: Fulguration polyp

DESTRUCTION: Physical eradication of all or a portion of a body part by the direct use of energy, force, or a destructive agent.

EXPLANATION: None of the body part is physically taken out

Body Part – 4TH	Approach – 5TH	Device – 6TH	Qualifier – 7TH
0 Upper Lip 1 Lower Lip 2 Hard Palate 3 Soft Palate 4 Buccal Mucosa 5 Upper Gingiva 6 Lower Gingiva 7 Tongue N Uvula P Tonsils Q Adenoids	0 Open 3 Percutaneous X External	Z No device	Z No qualifier
8 Parotid Gland, Right 9 Parotid Gland, Left B Parotid Duct, Right C Parotid Duct, Left D Sublingual Gland, Right F Sublingual Gland, Left G Submaxillary Gland, Right H Submaxillary Gland, Left J Minor Salivary Gland	0 Open 3 Percutaneous	Z No device	Z No qualifier
M Pharynx R Epiglottis S Larynx T Vocal Cord, Right V Vocal Cord, Left	0 Open 3 Percutaneous 4 Percutaneous endoscopic 7 Via natural or artificial opening 8 Via natural or artificial opening endoscopic	Z No device	Z No qualifier
W Upper Tooth X Lower Tooth	0 Open X External	Z No device	0 Single 1 Multiple 2 All

C – MOUTH AND THROAT 0C7

TUBULAR GROUP: (Bypass), Dilation, Occlusion, Restriction
Root Operations that alter the diameter/route of a tubular body part.

1ST - 0 Medical and Surgical
2ND - C Mouth and Throat
3RD - 7 DILATION

EXAMPLE: Dilation laryngeal stenosis   CMS Ex: Transluminal angioplasty

DILATION: Expanding an orifice or the lumen of a tubular body part.

EXPLANATION: By force (stretching) or cutting ...

Body Part – 4TH	Approach – 5TH	Device – 6TH	Qualifier – 7TH
B Parotid Duct, Right C Parotid Duct, Left	0 Open 3 Percutaneous 7 Via natural or artificial opening	D Intraluminal device Z No device	Z No qualifier
M Pharynx	7 Via natural or artificial opening 8 Via natural or artificial opening endoscopic	D Intraluminal device Z No device	Z No qualifier
S Larynx	0 Open 3 Percutaneous 4 Percutaneous endoscopic 7 Via natural or artificial opening 8 Via natural or artificial opening endoscopic	D Intraluminal device Z No device	Z No qualifier

0C9 MEDICAL AND SURGICAL SECTION – 2016 ICD-10-PCS

DRAINAGE GROUP: Drainage, Extirpation, Fragmentation
Root Operations that take out solids/fluids/gases from a body part.

- 1ST – **0** Medical and Surgical
- 2ND – **C** Mouth and Throat
- 3RD – **9** DRAINAGE

EXAMPLE: I&D parotid gland abscess CMS Ex: Thoracentesis

DRAINAGE: Taking or letting out fluids and/or gases from a body part.

EXPLANATION: Qualifier "X Diagnostic" indicates biopsy ...

Body Part – 4TH	Approach – 5TH	Device – 6TH	Qualifier – 7TH
0 Upper Lip　　5 Upper Gingiva 1 Lower Lip　　6 Lower Gingiva 2 Hard Palate　7 Tongue 3 Soft Palate　　N Uvula 4 Buccal Mucosa　P Tonsils 　　　　　　　　Q Adenoids	0 Open 3 Percutaneous X External	0 Drainage device	Z No qualifier
0 Upper Lip　　5 Upper Gingiva 1 Lower Lip　　6 Lower Gingiva 2 Hard Palate　7 Tongue 3 Soft Palate　　N Uvula 4 Buccal Mucosa　P Tonsils 　　　　　　　　Q Adenoids	0 Open 3 Percutaneous X External	Z No device	X Diagnostic Z No qualifier
8 Parotid Gland, Right　D Sublingual Gland, Right 9 Parotid Gland, Left　F Sublingual Gland, Left B Parotid Duct, Right　G Submaxillary Gland, Right C Parotid Duct, Left　　H Submaxillary Gland, Left 　　　　　　　　　　J Minor Salivary Gland	0 Open 3 Percutaneous	0 Drainage device	Z No qualifier
8 Parotid Gland, Right　D Sublingual Gland, Right 9 Parotid Gland, Left　F Sublingual Gland, Left B Parotid Duct, Right　G Submaxillary Gland, Right C Parotid Duct, Left　　H Submaxillary Gland, Left 　　　　　　　　　　J Minor Salivary Gland	0 Open 3 Percutaneous	Z No device	X Diagnostic Z No qualifier
M Pharynx R Epiglottis S Larynx T Vocal Cord, Right V Vocal Cord, Left	0 Open 3 Percutaneous 4 Percutaneous endoscopic 7 Via natural or artificial opening 8 Via natural or artificial opening endoscopic	0 Drainage device	Z No qualifier
M Pharynx R Epiglottis S Larynx T Vocal Cord, Right V Vocal Cord, Left	0 Open 3 Percutaneous 4 Percutaneous endoscopic 7 Via natural or artificial opening 8 Via natural or artificial opening endoscopic	Z No device	X Diagnostic Z No qualifier
W Upper Tooth X Lower Tooth	0 Open X External	0 Drainage device Z No device	0 Single 1 Multiple 2 All

C – MOUTH AND THROAT   0CB

EXCISION GROUP: Excision, Resection, Destruction, Extraction, (Detachment)
Root Operations that take out some or all of a body part.

1ST - **0** Medical and Surgical
2ND - **C** Mouth and Throat
3RD - **B** EXCISION

EXAMPLE: Excision lesion lip   **CMS Ex:** Liver biopsy

EXCISION: Cutting out or off, without replacement, a portion of a body part.

EXPLANATION: Qualifier "X Diagnostic" indicates biopsy …

Body Part – 4TH		Approach – 5TH	Device – 6TH	Qualifier – 7TH
0 Upper Lip 1 Lower Lip 2 Hard Palate 3 Soft Palate 4 Buccal Mucosa	5 Upper Gingiva 6 Lower Gingiva 7 Tongue N Uvula P Tonsils Q Adenoids	0 Open 3 Percutaneous X External	Z No device	X Diagnostic Z No qualifier
8 Parotid Gland, Right 9 Parotid Gland, Left B Parotid Duct, Right C Parotid Duct, Left	D Sublingual Gland, Right F Sublingual Gland, Left G Submaxillary Gland, Right H Submaxillary Gland, Left J Minor Salivary Gland	0 Open 3 Percutaneous	Z No device	X Diagnostic Z No qualifier
M Pharynx R Epiglottis S Larynx T Vocal Cord, Right V Vocal Cord, Left		0 Open 3 Percutaneous 4 Percutaneous endoscopic 7 Via natural or artificial opening 8 Via natural or artificial opening endoscopic	Z No device	X Diagnostic Z No qualifier
W Upper Tooth X Lower Tooth		0 Open X External	Z No device	0 Single 1 Multiple 2 All

0CC

MEDICAL AND SURGICAL SECTION – 2016 ICD-10-PCS

[2016.PCS]

DRAINAGE GROUP: Drainage, Extirpation, Fragmentation
Root Operations that take out solids/fluids/gases from a body part.

1ST – **0** Medical and Surgical
2ND – **C** Mouth and Throat
3RD – **C EXTIRPATION**

EXAMPLE: Sialolithotomy   CMS Ex: Choledocholithotomy

EXTIRPATION: Taking or cutting out solid matter from a body part.

EXPLANATION: Abnormal byproduct or foreign body …

Body Part – 4TH	Approach – 5TH	Device – 6TH	Qualifier – 7TH
0 Upper Lip 1 Lower Lip 2 Hard Palate 3 Soft Palate 4 Buccal Mucosa 5 Upper Gingiva 6 Lower Gingiva 7 Tongue N Uvula P Tonsils Q Adenoids	0 Open 3 Percutaneous X External	Z No device	Z No qualifier
8 Parotid Gland, Right 9 Parotid Gland, Left B Parotid Duct, Right C Parotid Duct, Left D Sublingual Gland, Right F Sublingual Gland, Left G Submaxillary Gland, Right H Submaxillary Gland, Left J Minor Salivary Gland	0 Open 3 Percutaneous	Z No device	Z No qualifier
M Pharynx R Epiglottis S Larynx T Vocal Cord, Right V Vocal Cord, Left	0 Open 3 Percutaneous 4 Percutaneous endoscopic 7 Via natural or artificial opening 8 Via natural or artificial opening endoscopic	Z No device	Z No qualifier
W Upper Tooth X Lower Tooth	0 Open X External	Z No device	0 Single 1 Multiple 2 All

EXCISION GROUP: Excision, Resection, Destruction, Extraction, (Detachment)
Root Operations that take out some or all of a body part.

1ST – **0** Medical and Surgical
2ND – **C** Mouth and Throat
3RD – **D EXTRACTION**

EXAMPLE: Tooth extraction   CMS Ex: D&C

EXTRACTION: Pulling or stripping out or off all or a portion of a body part by the use of force.

EXPLANATION: None for this Body System

Body Part – 4TH	Approach – 5TH	Device – 6TH	Qualifier – 7TH
T Vocal Cord, Right V Vocal Cord, Left	0 Open 3 Percutaneous 4 Percutaneous endoscopic 7 Via natural or artificial opening 8 Via natural or artificial opening endoscopic	Z No device	Z No qualifier
W Upper Tooth X Lower Tooth	X External	Z No device	0 Single 1 Multiple 2 All

C – MOUTH AND THROAT   0 C H

DRAINAGE GROUP: Drainage, Extirpation, Fragmentation
Root Operations that take out solids/fluids/gases from a body part.

- 1ST – **0** Medical and Surgical
- 2ND – **C** Mouth and Throat
- 3RD – **F** FRAGMENTATION

EXAMPLE: Lithotripsy parotid stone   CMS Ex: Extracorporeal shockwave lithotripsy

FRAGMENTATION: Breaking solid matter in a body part into pieces.

EXPLANATION: Pieces are not taken out during procedure …

Body Part – 4TH	Approach – 5TH	Device – 6TH	Qualifier – 7TH
B Parotid Duct, Right C Parotid Duct, Left	0 Open 3 Percutaneous 7 Via natural or artificial opening X External NC*	Z No device	Z No qualifier

NC* – Non-covered by Medicare. See current Medicare Code Editor for details.

DEVICE GROUP: Change, Insertion, Removal, Replacement, Revision, Supplement
Root Operations that always involve a device.

- 1ST – **0** Medical and Surgical
- 2ND – **C** Mouth and Throat
- 3RD – **H** INSERTION

EXAMPLE: Insertion oral airway   CMS Ex: Central venous catheter

INSERTION: Putting in a nonbiological appliance that monitors, assists, performs, or prevents a physiological function but does not physically take the place of a body part.

EXPLANATION: None

Body Part – 4TH	Approach – 5TH	Device – 6TH	Qualifier – 7TH
7 Tongue	0 Open 3 Percutaneous X External	1 Radioactive element	Z No qualifier
Y Mouth and Throat	7 Via natural or artificial opening 8 Via natural or artificial opening endoscopic	B Intraluminal device, airway	Z No qualifier

0CJ

MEDICAL AND SURGICAL SECTION – 2016 ICD-10-PCS

EXAMINATION GROUP: Inspection, (Map)
Root Operations involving examination only.

- 1ST – **0** Medical and Surgical
- 2ND – **C** Mouth and Throat
- 3RD – **J** INSPECTION

EXAMPLE: Diagnostic laryngoscopy
CMS Ex: Colonoscopy

INSPECTION: Visually and/or manually exploring a body part.

EXPLANATION: Direct or instrumental visualization ...

Body Part – 4TH	Approach – 5TH	Device – 6TH	Qualifier – 7TH
A Salivary Gland	0 Open 3 Percutaneous X External	Z No device	Z No qualifier
S Larynx Y Mouth and Throat	0 Open 3 Percutaneous 4 Percutaneous endoscopic 7 Via natural or artificial opening 8 Via natural or artificial opening endoscopic X External	Z No device	Z No qualifier

TUBULAR GROUP: (Bypass), Dilation, Occlusion, Restriction
Root Operations that alter the diameter/route of a tubular body part.

- 1ST – **0** Medical and Surgical
- 2ND – **C** Mouth and Throat
- 3RD – **L** OCCLUSION

EXAMPLE: Ligation Stensen's duct
CMS Ex: Fallopian tube ligation

OCCLUSION: Completely closing an orifice or lumen of a tubular body part.

EXPLANATION: Natural or artificially created orifice ...

Body Part – 4TH	Approach – 5TH	Device – 6TH	Qualifier – 7TH
B Parotid Duct, Right C Parotid Duct, Left	0 Open 3 Percutaneous 4 Percutaneous endoscopic	C Extraluminal device D Intraluminal device Z No device	Z No qualifier
B Parotid Duct, Right C Parotid Duct, Left	7 Via natural or artificial opening 8 Via natural or artificial opening endoscopic	D Intraluminal device Z No device	Z No qualifier

C – MOUTH AND THROAT 0CN

MOVE GROUP: Reattachment, Reposition, Transfer, (Transplantation)
Root Operations that put in/put back or move some/all of a body part.

- 1ST – **0** Medical and Surgical
- 2ND – **C** Mouth and Throat
- 3RD – **M** REATTACHMENT

EXAMPLE: Replantation tooth   CMS Ex: Reattachment hand

REATTACHMENT: Putting back in or on all or a portion of a separated body part to its normal location or other suitable location.

EXPLANATION: With/without reconnection of vessels/nerves…

Body Part – 4TH	Approach – 5TH	Device – 6TH	Qualifier – 7TH
0 Upper Lip 1 Lower Lip 3 Soft Palate 7 Tongue N Uvula	0 Open	Z No device	Z No qualifier
W Upper Tooth X Lower Tooth	0 Open X External	Z No device	0 Single 1 Multiple 2 All

DIVISION GROUP: (Division), Release
Root Operations involving cutting or separation only.

- 1ST – **0** Medical and Surgical
- 2ND – **C** Mouth and Throat
- 3RD – **N** RELEASE

EXAMPLE: Lysis vocal cord adhesions   CMS Ex: Carpal tunnel release

RELEASE: Freeing a body part from an abnormal physical constraint by cutting or by the use of force.

EXPLANATION: None of the body part is taken out …

Body Part – 4TH	Approach – 5TH	Device – 6TH	Qualifier – 7TH
0 Upper Lip 1 Lower Lip 2 Hard Palate 3 Soft Palate 4 Buccal Mucosa 5 Upper Gingiva 6 Lower Gingiva 7 Tongue N Uvula P Tonsils Q Adenoids	0 Open 3 Percutaneous X External	Z No device	Z No qualifier
8 Parotid Gland, Right 9 Parotid Gland, Left B Parotid Duct, Right C Parotid Duct, Left D Sublingual Gland, Right F Sublingual Gland, Left G Submaxillary Gland, Right H Submaxillary Gland, Left J Minor Salivary Gland	0 Open 3 Percutaneous	Z No device	Z No qualifier
M Pharynx R Epiglottis S Larynx T Vocal Cord, Right V Vocal Cord, Left	0 Open 3 Percutaneous 4 Percutaneous endoscopic 7 Via natural or artificial opening 8 Via natural or artificial opening endoscopic	Z No device	Z No qualifier
W Upper Tooth X Lower Tooth	0 Open X External	Z No device	0 Single 1 Multiple 2 All

0CP

MEDICAL AND SURGICAL SECTION – 2016 ICD-10-PCS [2016.PCS]

DEVICE GROUP: Change, Insertion, Removal, Replacement, Revision, Supplement
Root Operations that always involve a device.

1ST – **0** Medical and Surgical
2ND – **C** Mouth and Throat
3RD – **P REMOVAL**

EXAMPLE: Removal drain tube   CMS Ex: Chest tube removal

REMOVAL: Taking out or off a device from a body part.

EXPLANATION: Removal device without reinsertion ...

Body Part – 4TH	Approach – 5TH	Device – 6TH	Qualifier – 7TH
A Salivary Gland	0 Open 3 Percutaneous	0 Drainage device C Extraluminal device	Z No qualifier
S Larynx	0 Open 3 Percutaneous 7 Via natural or artificial opening 8 Via natural or artificial opening endoscopic X External	0 Drainage device 7 Autologous tissue substitute D Intraluminal device J Synthetic substitute K Nonautologous tissue substitute	Z No qualifier
Y Mouth and Throat	0 Open 3 Percutaneous 7 Via natural or artificial opening 8 Via natural or artificial opening endoscopic X External	0 Drainage device 1 Radioactive element 7 Autologous tissue substitute D Intraluminal device J Synthetic substitute K Nonautologous tissue substitute	Z No qualifier

0CQ

C – MOUTH AND THROAT

OTHER REPAIRS GROUP: (Control), Repair
Root Operations that define other repairs.

1ST - 0	Medical and Surgical
2ND - C	Mouth and Throat
3RD - Q	REPAIR

EXAMPLE: Cleft palate repair **CMS Ex:** Suture laceration

REPAIR: Restoring, to the extent possible, a body part to its normal anatomic structure and function.

EXPLANATION: Only when no other root operation applies ...

Body Part – 4TH		Approach – 5TH	Device – 6TH	Qualifier – 7TH
0 Upper Lip	5 Upper Gingiva	0 Open	Z No device	Z No qualifier
1 Lower Lip	6 Lower Gingiva	3 Percutaneous		
2 Hard Palate	7 Tongue	X External		
3 Soft Palate	N Uvula			
4 Buccal Mucosa	P Tonsils			
	Q Adenoids			
8 Parotid Gland, Right	D Sublingual Gland, Right	0 Open	Z No device	Z No qualifier
9 Parotid Gland, Left	F Sublingual Gland, Left	3 Percutaneous		
B Parotid Duct, Right	G Submaxillary Gland, Right			
C Parotid Duct, Left	H Submaxillary Gland, Left			
	J Minor Salivary Gland			
M Pharynx		0 Open	Z No device	Z No qualifier
R Epiglottis		3 Percutaneous		
S Larynx		4 Percutaneous endoscopic		
T Vocal Cord, Right		7 Via natural or artificial opening		
V Vocal Cord, Left		8 Via natural or artificial opening endoscopic		
W Upper Tooth		0 Open	Z No device	0 Single
X Lower Tooth		X External		1 Multiple
				2 All

0CR

MEDICAL AND SURGICAL SECTION – 2016 ICD-10-PCS

DEVICE GROUP: Change, Insertion, Removal, Replacement, Revision, Supplement
Root Operations that always involve a device.

1ST – **0** Medical and Surgical
2ND – **C** Mouth and Throat
3RD – **R REPLACEMENT**

EXAMPLE: Parotid duct replacement   CMS Ex: Total hip

REPLACEMENT: Putting in or on a biological or synthetic material that physically takes the place and/or function of all or a portion of a body part.

EXPLANATION: Includes taking out body part, or eradication...

Body Part – 4TH	Approach – 5TH	Device – 6TH	Qualifier – 7TH
0 Upper Lip 1 Lower Lip 2 Hard Palate 3 Soft Palate 4 Buccal Mucosa 5 Upper Gingiva 6 Lower Gingiva 7 Tongue N Uvula	0 Open 3 Percutaneous X External	7 Autologous tissue substitute J Synthetic substitute K Nonautologous tissue substitute	Z No qualifier
B Parotid Duct, Right C Parotid Duct, Left	0 Open 3 Percutaneous	7 Autologous tissue substitute J Synthetic substitute K Nonautologous tissue substitute	Z No qualifier
M Pharynx R Epiglottis S Larynx T Vocal Cord, Right V Vocal Cord, Left	0 Open 7 Via natural or artificial opening 8 Via natural or artificial opening endoscopic	7 Autologous tissue substitute J Synthetic substitute K Nonautologous tissue substitute	Z No qualifier
W Upper Tooth X Lower Tooth	0 Open X External	7 Autologous tissue substitute J Synthetic substitute K Nonautologous tissue substitute	0 Single 1 Multiple 2 All

C – MOUTH AND THROAT 0CS

MOVE GROUP: Reattachment, Reposition, Transfer, (Transplantation)
Root Operations that put in/put back or move some/all of a body part.

1ST – **0** Medical and Surgical
2ND – **C** Mouth and Throat
3RD – **S** REPOSITION

EXAMPLE: Reposition tongue   **CMS Ex:** Fracture reduction

REPOSITION: Moving to its normal location, or other suitable location, all or a portion of a body part.

EXPLANATION: May or may not be cut to be moved ...

Body Part – 4TH	Approach – 5TH	Device – 6TH	Qualifier – 7TH
0 Upper Lip 1 Lower Lip 2 Hard Palate 3 Soft Palate 7 Tongue N Uvula	0 Open X External	Z No device	Z No qualifier
B Parotid Duct, Right C Parotid Duct, Left	0 Open 3 Percutaneous	Z No device	Z No qualifier
R Epiglottis T Vocal Cord, Right V Vocal Cord, Left	0 Open 7 Via natural or artificial opening 8 Via natural or artificial opening endoscopic	Z No device	Z No qualifier
W Upper Tooth X Lower Tooth	0 Open X External	5 External fixation device Z No device	0 Single 1 Multiple 2 All

0 C T

MEDICAL AND SURGICAL SECTION – 2016 ICD-10-PCS

EXCISION GROUP: Excision, Resection, Destruction, Extraction, (Detachment)
Root Operations that take out some or all of a body part.

EXAMPLE: Tonsillectomy	CMS Ex: Cholecystectomy

RESECTION: Cutting out or off, without replacement, all of a body part.

EXPLANATION: None

- 1ST – **0** Medical and Surgical
- 2ND – **C** Mouth and Throat
- 3RD – **T** RESECTION

Body Part – 4TH		Approach – 5TH	Device – 6TH	Qualifier – 7TH
0 Upper Lip 1 Lower Lip 2 Hard Palate 3 Soft Palate	7 Tongue N Uvula P Tonsils Q Adenoids	0 Open X External	Z No device	Z No qualifier
8 Parotid Gland, Right 9 Parotid Gland, Left B Parotid Duct, Right C Parotid Duct, Left	D Sublingual Gland, Right F Sublingual Gland, Left G Submaxillary Gland, Right H Submaxillary Gland, Left J Minor Salivary Gland	0 Open	Z No device	Z No qualifier
M Pharynx R Epiglottis S Larynx T Vocal Cord, Right V Vocal Cord, Left		0 Open 4 Percutaneous endoscopic 7 Via natural or artificial opening 8 Via natural or artificial opening endoscopic	Z No device	Z No qualifier
W Upper Tooth X Lower Tooth		0 Open	Z No device	0 Single 1 Multiple 2 All

---

DEVICE GROUP: Change, Insertion, Removal, Replacement, Revision, Supplement
Root Operations that always involve a device.

EXAMPLE: Palatoplasty with graft	CMS Ex: Hernia repair with mesh

SUPPLEMENT: Putting in or on biological or synthetic material that physically reinforces and/or augments the function of a portion of a body part.

EXPLANATION: Biological material from same individual …

- 1ST – **0** Medical and Surgical
- 2ND – **C** Mouth and Throat
- 3RD – **U** SUPPLEMENT

Body Part – 4TH		Approach – 5TH	Device – 6TH	Qualifier – 7TH
0 Upper Lip 1 Lower Lip 2 Hard Palate 3 Soft Palate 4 Buccal Mucosa	5 Upper Gingiva 6 Lower Gingiva 7 Tongue N Uvula	0 Open 3 Percutaneous X External	7 Autologous tissue substitute J Synthetic substitute K Nonautologous tissue substitute	Z No qualifier
M Pharynx R Epiglottis S Larynx T Vocal Cord, Right V Vocal Cord, Left		0 Open 7 Via natural or artificial opening 8 Via natural or artificial opening endoscopic	7 Autologous tissue substitute J Synthetic substitute K Nonautologous tissue substitute	Z No qualifier

TUBULAR GROUP: (Bypass), Dilation, Occlusion, Restriction
Root Operations that alter the diameter/route of a tubular body part.

1ST - **0** Medical and Surgical
2ND - **C** Mouth and Throat
3RD - **V** RESTRICTION

EXAMPLE: Parotid duct restrictive stent
CMS Ex: Cervical cerclage

RESTRICTION: Partially closing an orifice or the lumen of a tubular body part.

EXPLANATION: Natural or artificially created orifice ...

Body Part – 4TH	Approach – 5TH	Device – 6TH	Qualifier – 7TH
B Parotid Duct, Right C Parotid Duct, Left	0 Open 3 Percutaneous	C Extraluminal device D Intraluminal device Z No device	Z No qualifier
B Parotid Duct, Right C Parotid Duct, Left	7 Via natural or artificial opening 8 Via natural or artificial opening endoscopic	D Intraluminal device Z No device	Z No qualifier

DEVICE GROUP: Change, Insertion, Removal, Replacement, Revision, Supplement
Root Operations that always involve a device.

1ST - **0** Medical and Surgical
2ND - **C** Mouth and Throat
3RD - **W** REVISION

EXAMPLE: Trimming palatoplasty graft
CMS Ex: Adjustment pacemaker lead

REVISION: Correcting, to the extent possible, a portion of a malfunctioning device or the position of a displaced device.

EXPLANATION: May replace components of a device ...

Body Part – 4TH	Approach – 5TH	Device – 6TH	Qualifier – 7TH
A Salivary Gland	0 Open 3 Percutaneous X External	0 Drainage device C Extraluminal device	Z No qualifier
S Larynx	0 Open 3 Percutaneous 7 Via natural or artificial opening 8 Via natural or artificial opening endoscopic X External	0 Drainage device 7 Autologous tissue substitute D Intraluminal device J Synthetic substitute K Nonautologous tissue substitute	Z No qualifier
Y Mouth and Throat	0 Open 3 Percutaneous 7 Via natural or artificial opening 8 Via natural or artificial opening endoscopic X External	0 Drainage device 1 Radioactive element 7 Autologous tissue substitute D Intraluminal device J Synthetic substitute K Nonautologous tissue substitute	Z No qualifier

0CX

MEDICAL AND SURGICAL SECTION – 2016 ICD-10-PCS

MOVE GROUP: Reattachment, Reposition, Transfer, (Transplantation)
Root Operations that put in/put back or move some/all of a body part.

1ST - **0** Medical and Surgical	EXAMPLE: Gingival pedicle graft CMS Ex: Tendon transfer
2ND - **C** Mouth and Throat	**TRANSFER:** Moving, without taking out, all or a portion of a body part to another location to take over the function of all or a portion of a body part.
3RD - **X** TRANSFER	EXPLANATION: The body part remains connected ...

Body Part – 4TH		Approach – 5TH	Device – 6TH	Qualifier – 7TH
0 Upper Lip	5 Upper Gingiva	0 Open	Z No device	Z No qualifier
1 Lower Lip	6 Lower Gingiva	X External		
3 Soft Palate	7 Tongue			
4 Buccal Mucosa				

Educational Annotations | D – Gastrointestinal System

Body System Specific Educational Annotations for the Gastrointestinal System include:
- Anatomy and Physiology Review
- Anatomical Illustrations
- Definitions of Common Procedures
- AHA Coding Clinic® Reference Notations
- Body Part Key Listings
- Device Key Listings
- Device Aggregation Table Listings
- Coding Notes

Anatomy and Physiology Review of Gastrointestinal System

BODY PART VALUES – D - GASTROINTESTINAL SYSTEM

Anal Sphincter – ANATOMY – The anal sphincter is a group of muscles (internal and external) that surrounds the anus. PHYSIOLOGY – Maintains continence by controlling the release of stool from the rectum.

Anus – ANATOMY – The anus is the internal canal from the rectum which ends the alimentary tract at the anal opening. PHYSIOLOGY – The rectum and anus function to eliminate feces from the alimentary tract. A reflex signal is sent when the rectum fills and urgency to defecate is perceived. The external voluntary muscle is voluntarily relaxed to defecate.

Appendix – The appendix is a closed appendage of the colon and projects downward from the cecum.

Ascending Colon – The ascending colon arises from the cecum (the pouch-like structure) and continues upwards where it turns (hepatic flexure) and connects to the transverse colon.

Cecum – ANATOMY – The cecum is an enlarged pouch of the ascending intestine at the junction with the ileum. PHYSIOLOGY – Receives the contents from the small intestine.

Descending Colon – The descending colon extends downward to the rectum, and is called the sigmoid (flexure) colon where it makes an S-shaped curve over the pelvic brim.

Duodenum – The duodenum is the first portion about 10 inches (25 cm) long connected at its proximal end to the stomach.

Esophagogastric Junction – ANATOMY – The lower end of the esophagus at the transition to the stomach identified by the abrupt change from esophageal epithelium to the gastric folds.

Esophagus – ANATOMY – The esophagus, located between the pharynx and stomach, is a collapsible musculomembranous alimentary tract tube about 10 inches (25 cm) long. The esophagus is lined with mucous glands. PHYSIOLOGY – The esophagus is the passageway for food from the mouth to the stomach. The mucous glands moisten and lubricate the inner lining to facilitate the passage of food. Situated just above the stomach opening lie the contracted circular muscles which prevent regurgitation.

Esophagus, Lower – The distal lower one-third of the esophagus (also known as the abdominal esophagus).

Esophagus, Middle – The middle one-third of the esophagus (also known as the thoracic esophagus).

Esophagus, Upper – The proximal upper one-third of the esophagus (also known as the cervical esophagus).

Greater Omentum – The double layer of the peritoneum that extends from the greater curvature of the stomach to the transverse colon.

Ileocecal Valve – ANATOMY – The ileocecal valve is the sphincter muscle valve that separates the small intestine and the large intestine. PHYSIOLOGY – The ileocecal valve prevents contents from the large intestine from backflowing into the small intestine.

Ileum – The ileum is the distal portion of the small intestine which connects with the large intestine.

Jejunum – The jejunum is the middle portion of the small intestine, comprising approximately two-fifths of the intestine.

Large Intestine – ANATOMY – The large intestine (colon) is the tubular organ of the alimentary tract between the small intestine and the rectum, and is about 5 feet (1.5 m) long. The colon has four main segments: Ascending, transverse, descending, and sigmoid. The rectosigmoid junction is that portion of the alimentary tract between the distal end of the sigmoid colon and the proximal end of the rectum. PHYSIOLOGY – The large intestine (colon) functions to absorb water and electrolytes, and to move by peristalsis nonabsorbed substances to the rectum for defecation. Many bacteria normally inhabit the colon and serve to further break down substances for colonic absorption.

Large Intestine, Left – In general, the descending colon and part of the transverse colon.

Continued on next page

Educational Annotations | D – Gastrointestinal System

Anatomy and Physiology Review of Gastrointestinal System

BODY PART VALUES – D - GASTROINTESTINAL SYSTEM
Continued from previous page

Large Intestine, Right – In general, the ascending colon and part of the transverse colon.

Lesser Omentum – The double layer of the peritoneum that extends from the liver to lesser curvature of the stomach.

Lower Intestinal Tract – The gastrointestinal tract from the jejunum down to and including the rectum and anus (see Coding Guideline B4.8).

Mesentery – The mesentery is a fold of membranous tissue that arises from the posterior wall of the peritoneal cavity and attaches the intestine to the abdominal wall and holds it in place.

Omentum – The double layer of the peritoneum that encompasses most of the organs in the abdominal cavity.

Peritoneum – ANATOMY – The peritoneum is the serous membrane (visceral and parietal) which contains most of the abdominal contents, and where doubled upon itself forms supporting structures called ligaments. PHYSIOLOGY – The peritoneum encapsules and protects the abdominal visceral organs allowing them to move slightly without damaging function.

Rectum – ANATOMY – The rectum is the musculomembranous portion of the alimentary tract between the colon and anus, approximately 5 inches (13 cm) long. The rectosigmoid junction is that portion of the alimentary tract between the distal end of the sigmoid colon and the proximal end of the rectum. PHYSIOLOGY – The rectum and anus function to eliminate feces from the alimentary tract. A reflex signal is sent when the rectum fills and urgency to defecate is perceived. The external voluntary muscle is voluntarily relaxed to defecate.

Sigmoid Colon – The descending colon extends downward to the rectum, and is called the sigmoid (flexure) colon where it makes an S-shaped curve over the pelvic brim.

Small Intestine – ANATOMY – The small intestine is the tubular organ of the alimentary tract between the stomach and large intestine and is about 16 to 20 feet (5 to 6 m) long, and has 3 parts: Duodenum, jejunum, and ileum. Both the jejunum and ileum are suspended from the posterior abdominal wall by the mesentery. PHYSIOLOGY – The small intestine functions to absorb the nutrients produced through digestion. The food is passed through the small intestine by the contraction (peristalsis) of its circular smooth muscle layer. The duodenum releases several enzymes and mixes the pancreatic and bile juices with food from the stomach. The jejunum and ileum continue mixing and absorbing until the remaining substances pass into the large intestine.

Stomach – ANATOMY – The stomach, located in the upper abdomen, is a pouch-like organ of the alimentary tract connecting with the esophagus in the proximal (upper) portion and the duodenum in the distal (lower) portion and is about 10 to 12 inches (25 to 30 cm) long. The cardia lies at the opening of the esophagus at the fundus of the stomach. The fundus is the upper ballooned area of the stomach. The body is the main part of the stomach and is located between the fundus and the pyloric antrum and the duodenum. When empty, the mucous membrane on the interior surface forms longitudinal folds (rugae). There are three mucosal glands which secrete digestive juices and mucous. These are the gastric glands, which are located throughout the body of the stomach; the cardiac glands, which are found near the esophageal opening; and the pyloric glands, which are located in the pyloric (distal) region. The vagus nerve stimulates the gastric glands. There are three layers of smooth muscle and a serosal covering of the visceral peritoneum. The stomach has a rich arterial blood supply through the celiac artery. The venous blood is drained into the hepatic portal system. PHYSIOLOGY – The stomach functions to receive food from the esophagus, mixes it with the gastric juice, initiates the digestion of proteins with pepsin, carries on a limited amount of absorption, and moves food into the small intestine by peristaltic muscle action. The gastric glands produce mucous, digestive enzymes (pepsin), hydrochloric acid, and an intrinsic factor, forming the gastric juice. The mucous is thought to help prevent the pepsin and hydrochloric acid from digesting the stomach surface. The stomach may absorb small quantities of water, glucose, certain salts, and alcohol. The parasympathetic vagus nerve stimulates the gastric glands to secrete large amounts of gastric juice, which in turn releases gastrin, a hormone that causes the gastric glands to increase their secretory activity.

Stomach, Pylorus – The pylorus is the lower section of the stomach that connects to the duodenum and allows emptying of the contents into the small intestine.

Transverse Colon – The transverse colon extends horizontally and turns (splenic flexure) downward connecting to the descending colon.

Upper Intestinal Tract – The gastrointestinal tract from the esophagus down to and including the duodenum (see Coding Guideline B4.8).

D – Gastrointestinal System

Educational Annotations

Anatomical Illustrations of Gastrointestinal System

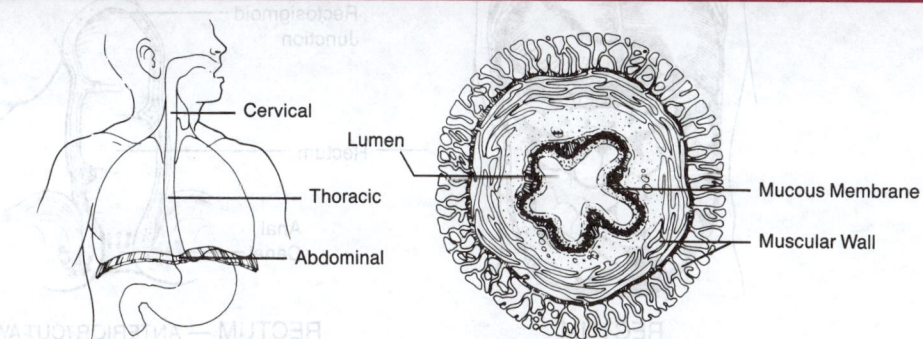

ESOPHAGUS — ANTERIOR VIEW   ESOPHAGUS — SECTION

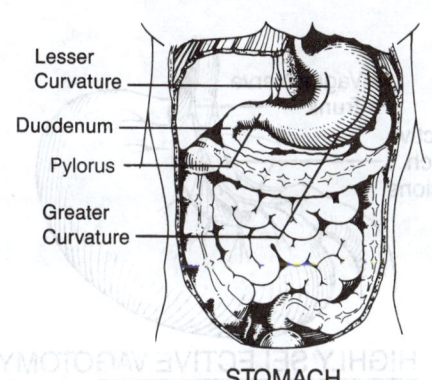

STOMACH

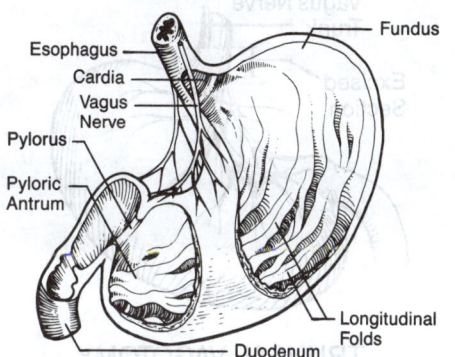

STOMACH — ANTERIOR (CUT-AWAY) VIEW

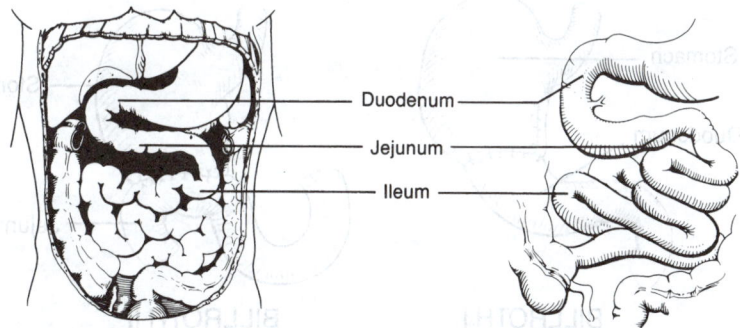

SMALL INTESTINE

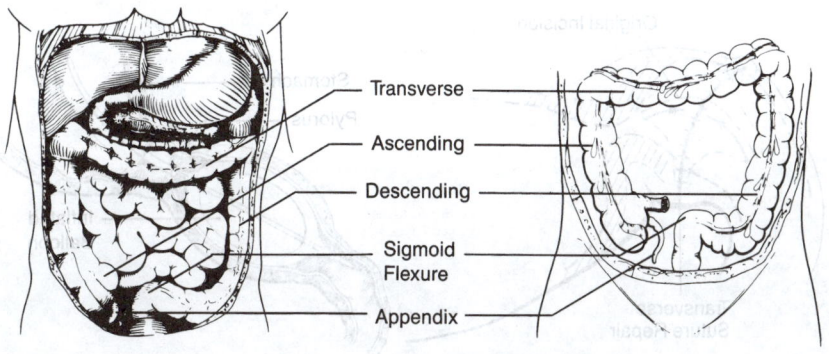

LARGE INTESTINE (COLON)

Continued on next page

Educational Annotations
D – Gastrointestinal System

Continued from previous page

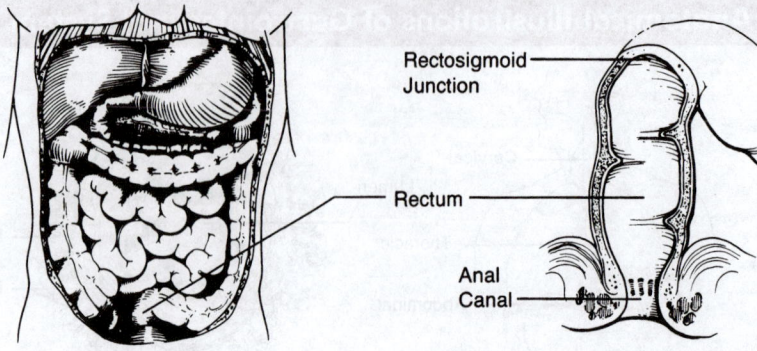

RECTUM

RECTUM — ANTERIOR (CUT-AWAY) VIEW

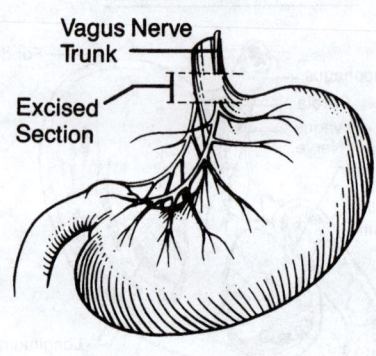

TRUNCAL VAGOTOMY

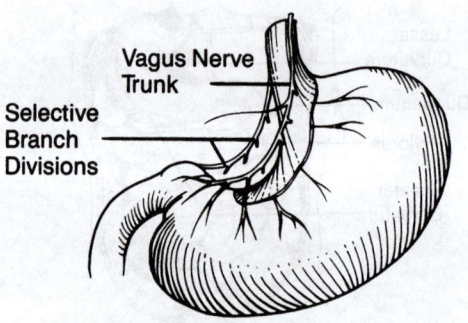

HIGHLY SELECTIVE VAGOTOMY

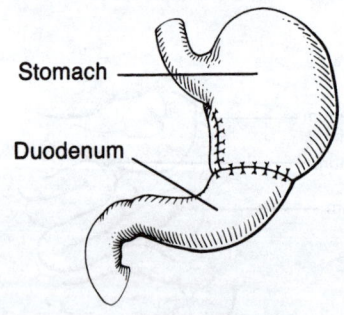

BILLROTH I

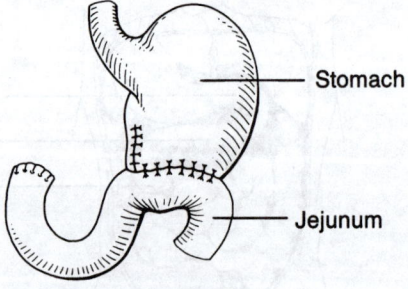

BILLROTH II

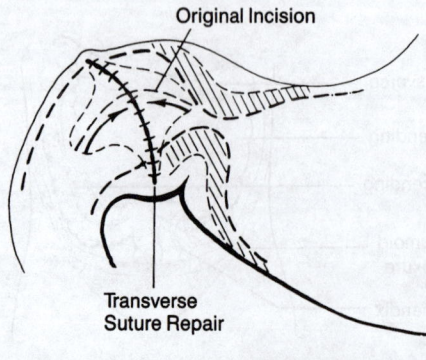

PYLOROPLASTY

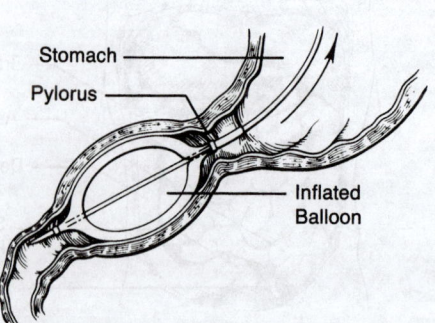

BALLOON DILATATION OF PYLORUS

Continued on next page

Educational Annotations | D – Gastrointestinal System

Continued from previous page

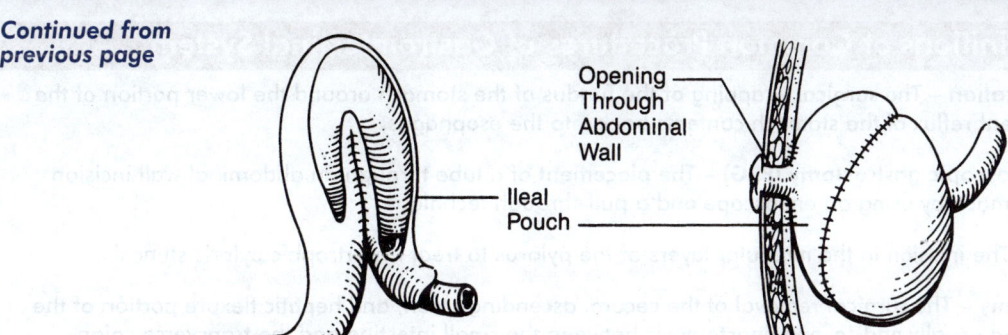

CONTINENT ILEOSTOMY

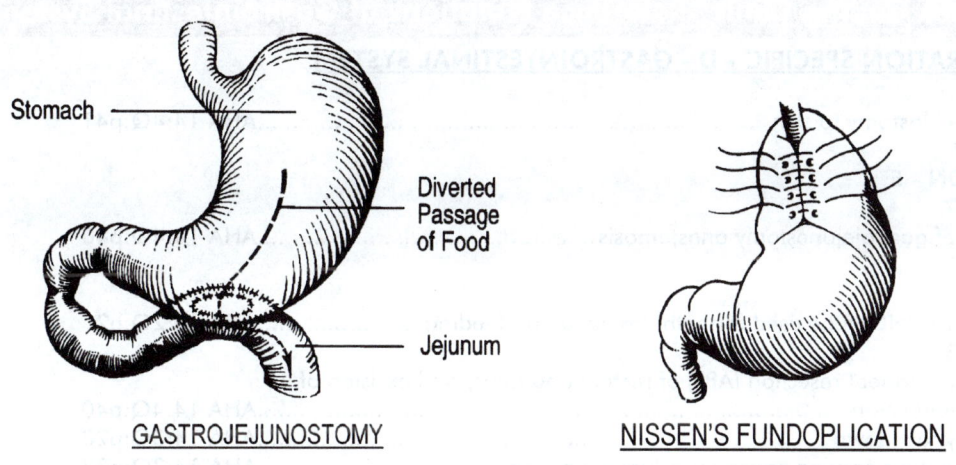

GASTROJEJUNOSTOMY   NISSEN'S FUNDOPLICATION

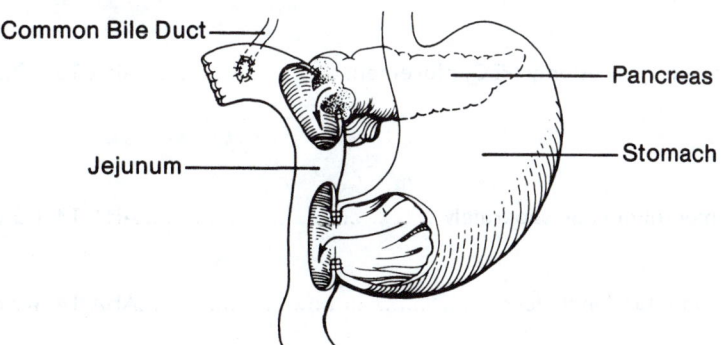

WHIPPLE PROCEDURE

Definitions of Common Procedures of Gastrointestinal System

Anal sphincterotomy – The incision of the anal sphincter muscle to prevent spasms and intentionally weaken the muscle during healing.

Colostomy – The creation of an artificial opening of the colon through the abdominal wall.

Gastrojejunostomy – The surgical creation of an anastomosis between the stomach and the jejunum (the second portion of the small intestine) to bypass and relieve gastric outlet obstruction.

Educational Annotations

D – Gastrointestinal System

Definitions of Common Procedures of Gastrointestinal System

Nissen's fundoplication – The surgical wrapping of the fundus of the stomach around the lower portion of the esophagus to prevent reflux of the stomach contents back into the esophagus.

Percutaneous endoscopic gastrostomy (PEG) – The placement of a tube through an abdominal wall incision from inside the stomach by using an endoscope and a pull-through technique.

Pyloromyotomy – The incision in the muscular layers of the pylorus to treat hypertrophic pyloric stenosis.

Right hemicolectomy – The surgical removal of the cecum, ascending colon, and hepatic flexure portion of the tranverse colon, and usually end-to-end anastomosis between the small intestine and the transverse colon.

Vertical sleeve gastrectomy – The surgical excision of a large portion of the stomach along a vertical line of the stomach to reduce the stomach volume and limit the amount of food that can be consumed at one time.

AHA Coding Clinic® Reference Notations of Gastrointestinal System

ROOT OPERATION SPECIFIC - D - GASTROINTESTINAL SYSTEM

BYPASS - 1
    Sigmoid colostomy to skin ....AHA 14:4Q:p41

CHANGE - 2

DESTRUCTION - 5

DILATION - 7
    Dilation of gastrojejunostomy anastomosis ....AHA 14:4Q:p40

DIVISION - 8

DRAINAGE - 9
    Nasogastric (NG) tube used for both drainage and feeding ....AHA 15:2Q:p2

EXCISION - B
    Abdominoperineal resection (APR) of rectum and anus, and excision of
        sigmoid colon ....AHA 14:4Q:p40
    Ileostomy takedown ....AHA 14:3Q:p28
    Whipple pyloric sparing pancreaticoduodenectomy............................AHA 14:3Q:p32

EXTIRPATION - C

FRAGMENTATION - F

INSERTION - H
    Percutaneous endoscopic gastrostomy (PEG) placement ....AHA 13:4Q:p117

INSPECTION - J

OCCLUSION - L

REATTACHMENT - M

RELEASE - N
    Lysis of adhesions, integral or code separately ....AHA 14:1Q:p3

REMOVAL - P

REPAIR - Q
    Clips to control bleeding duodenal ulcer ....AHA 14:4Q:p20

REPLACEMENT - R

REPOSITION - S

RESECTION - T
    Abdominoperineal resection (APR) of rectum and anus, and excision of
        sigmoid colon ....AHA 14:4Q:p40
    Colectomy, right...AHA 14:3Q:p6
    Colectomy with side-to-side anastomosis ....AHA 14:4Q:p42
    Ileocecectomy ....AHA 14:3Q:p6

SUPPLEMENT - U

RESTRICTION - V
    Nissen fundoplication ....AHA 14:3Q:p28

REVISION - W

TRANSFER - X

TRANSPLANTATION - Y

Educational Annotations | D – Gastrointestinal System

Body Part Key Listings of Gastrointestinal System

See also Body Part Key in Appendix C

Abdominal esophagus	*use* Esophagus, Lower
Anal orifice	*use* Anus
Anorectal junction	*use* Rectum
Cardia	*use* Esophagogastric Junction
Cardioesophageal junction	*use* Esophagogastric Junction
Cervical esophagus	*use* Esophagus, Upper
Duodenojejunal flexure	*use* Jejunum
Epiploic foramen	*use* Peritoneum
External anal sphincter	*use* Anal Sphincter
Gastrocolic ligament	*use* Greater Omentum
Gastrocolic omentum	*use* Greater Omentum
Gastroesophageal (GE) junction	*use* Esophagogastric Junction
Gastrohepatic omentum	*use* Lesser Omentum
Gastrophrenic ligament	*use* Greater Omentum
Gastrosplenic ligament	*use* Greater Omentum
Hepatic flexure	*use* Ascending Colon
Hepatogastric ligament	*use* Lesser Omentum
Internal anal sphincter	*use* Anal Sphincter
Mesoappendix	*use* Mesentery
Mesocolon	*use* Mesentery
Pyloric antrum	*use* Stomach, Pylorus
Pyloric canal	*use* Stomach, Pylorus
Pyloric sphincter	*use* Stomach, Pylorus
Rectosigmoid junction	*use* Sigmoid Colon
Sigmoid flexure	*use* Sigmoid Colon
Splenic flexure	*use* Transverse Colon
Thoracic esophagus	*use* Esophagus, Middle
Vermiform appendix	*use* Appendix

Device Key Listings of Gastrointestinal System

See also Device Key in Appendix D

Artificial anal sphincter (AAS)	*use* Artificial Sphincter in Gastrointestinal System
Artificial bowel sphincter (neosphincter)	*use* Artificial Sphincter in Gastrointestinal System
Autograft	*use* Autologous Tissue Substitute
Brachytherapy seeds	*use* Radioactive Element
Colonic Z-Stent®	*use* Intraluminal Device
Esophageal obturator airway (EOA)	*use* Intraluminal Device, Airway in Gastrointestinal System
Gastric electrical stimulation (GES) lead	*use* Stimulator Lead in Gastrointestinal System
Gastric pacemaker lead	*use* Stimulator Lead in Gastrointestinal System
LAP-BAND® adjustable gastric banding system	*use* Extraluminal Device
Percutaneous endoscopic gastrojejunostomy (PEG/J) tube	*use* Feeding Device in Gastrointestinal System
Percutaneous endoscopic gastrostomy (PEG) tube	*use* Feeding Device in Gastrointestinal System
REALIZE® Adjustable Gastric Band	*use* Extraluminal Device
Tissue bank graft	*use* Nonautologous Tissue Substitute
Ultraflex™ Precision Colonic Stent System	*use* Intraluminal Device

0D Educational Annotations | D – Gastrointestinal System

Device Aggregation Table Listings of Gastrointestinal System

See also Device Aggregation Table in Appendix E

Specific Device	For Operation	In Body System	General Device	
Intraluminal Device, Airway	All applicable	Gastrointestinal System	D	Intraluminal Device

Coding Notes of Gastrointestinal System

Body System Relevant Coding Guidelines

Upper and lower intestinal tract

B4.8
In the Gastrointestinal body system, the general body part values Upper Intestinal Tract and Lower Intestinal Tract are provided as an option for the root operations Change, Inspection, Removal and Revision. Upper Intestinal Tract includes the portion of the gastrointestinal tract from the esophagus down to and including the duodenum, and Lower Intestinal Tract includes the portion of the gastrointestinal tract from the jejunum down to and including the rectum and anus.
Example: In the root operation Change table, change of a device in the jejunum is coded using the body part Lower Intestinal Tract.

Body System Specific PCS Reference Manual Exercises

PCS CODE	D – GASTROINTESTINAL SYSTEM EXERCISES
0D160ZA	Open gastric bypass with Roux-en-Y limb to jejunum.
0D1L0Z4	Colostomy formation, open, transverse colon to abdominal wall.
0D717ZZ	Dilation of upper esophageal stricture, direct visualization, with Bougie sound.
0D848ZZ	EGD with esophagotomy of esophagogastric junction.
0D9QXZZ	Incision and drainage of external anal abscess.
0DB64Z3	Laparoscopic vertical sleeve gastrectomy.
0DB68ZX	EGD with gastric biopsy.
0DBN8ZZ	Sigmoidoscopy with sigmoid polypectomy.
0DC68ZZ	Esophagogastroscopy with removal of bezoar from stomach.
0DCV4ZZ	Laparoscopy with excision of old suture from mesentery.
0DJ08ZZ	EGD (esophagogastroduodenoscopy).
0DJD7ZZ	Digital rectal exam.
0DJD8ZZ	Colonoscopy, discontinued at sigmoid colon.
0DNW4ZZ	Laparoscopy with lysis of peritoneal adhesions.
0DP6X0Z	Removal of nasogastric drainage tube for decompression.
0DP6XUZ	Non-incisional PEG tube removal.
0DQ90ZZ	Laparotomy with suture repair of blunt force duodenal laceration.
0DS64ZZ	Laparoscopy with gastropexy for malrotation.
0DTH0ZZ	Open resection of cecum.
0DYE0Z0	Transplant of large intestine, organ donor match.

D – GASTROINTESTINAL SYSTEM 0D1

TUBULAR GROUP: Bypass, Dilation, Occlusion, Restriction
Root Operations that alter the diameter/route of a tubular body part.

1ST - **0** Medical and Surgical
2ND - **D** Gastrointestinal System
3RD - **1 BYPASS**

EXAMPLE: Colostomy formation CMS Ex: Coronary artery bypass

BYPASS: Altering the route of passage of the contents of a tubular body part.

EXPLANATION: Rerouting contents to a downstream part ...

Body Part – 4TH	Approach – 5TH	Device – 6TH	Qualifier – 7TH
1 Esophagus, Upper 2 Esophagus, Middle 3 Esophagus, Lower 5 Esophagus	0 Open 4 Percutaneous endoscopic 8 Via natural or artificial opening endoscopic	7 Autologous tissue substitute J Synthetic substitute K Nonautologous tissue substitute Z No device	4 Cutaneous 6 Stomach 9 Duodenum A Jejunum B Ileum
1 Esophagus, Upper 2 Esophagus, Middle 3 Esophagus, Lower 5 Esophagus	3 Percutaneous	J Synthetic substitute	4 Cutaneous
6 Stomach 9 Duodenum	0 Open 4 Percutaneous endoscopic 8 Via natural or artificial opening endoscopic	7 Autologous tissue substitute J Synthetic substitute K Nonautologous tissue substitute Z No device	4 Cutaneous 9 Duodenum A Jejunum B Ileum L Transverse Colon
6 Stomach 9 Duodenum	3 Percutaneous	J Synthetic substitute	4 Cutaneous
A Jejunum	0 Open 4 Percutaneous endoscopic 8 Via natural or artificial opening endoscopic	7 Autologous tissue substitute J Synthetic substitute K Nonautologous tissue substitute Z No device	4 Cutaneous A Jejunum B Ileum H Cecum K Ascending Colon L Transverse Colon M Descending Colon N Sigmoid Colon P Rectum Q Anus
A Jejunum	3 Percutaneous	J Synthetic substitute	4 Cutaneous

continued ⇒

0D1 BYPASS – continued

0 D 1

Body Part – 4TH	Approach – 5TH	Device – 6TH	Qualifier – 7TH
B Ileum	0 Open 4 Percutaneous endoscopic 8 Via natural or artificial opening endoscopic	7 Autologous tissue substitute J Synthetic substitute K Nonautologous tissue substitute Z No device	4 Cutaneous B Ileum H Cecum K Ascending Colon L Transverse Colon M Descending Colon N Sigmoid Colon P Rectum Q Anus
B Ileum	3 Percutaneous	J Synthetic substitute	4 Cutaneous
H Cecum	0 Open 4 Percutaneous endoscopic 8 Via natural or artificial opening endoscopic	7 Autologous tissue substitute J Synthetic substitute K Nonautologous tissue substitute Z No device	4 Cutaneous H Cecum K Ascending Colon L Transverse Colon M Descending Colon N Sigmoid Colon P Rectum
H Cecum	3 Percutaneous	J Synthetic substitute	4 Cutaneous
K Ascending Colon	0 Open 4 Percutaneous endoscopic 8 Via natural or artificial opening endoscopic	7 Autologous tissue substitute J Synthetic substitute K Nonautologous tissue substitute Z No device	4 Cutaneous K Ascending Colon L Transverse Colon M Descending Colon N Sigmoid Colon P Rectum
K Ascending Colon	3 Percutaneous	J Synthetic substitute	4 Cutaneous
L Transverse Colon	0 Open 4 Percutaneous endoscopic 8 Via natural or artificial opening endoscopic	7 Autologous tissue substitute J Synthetic substitute K Nonautologous tissue substitute Z No device	4 Cutaneous L Transverse Colon M Descending Colon N Sigmoid Colon P Rectum
L Transverse Colon	3 Percutaneous	J Synthetic substitute	4 Cutaneous

continued ➡

D – GASTROINTESTINAL SYSTEM

0D1 BYPASS – continued

Body Part – 4TH	Approach – 5TH	Device – 6TH	Qualifier – 7TH
M Descending Colon	0 Open 4 Percutaneous endoscopic 8 Via natural or artificial opening endoscopic	7 Autologous tissue substitute J Synthetic substitute K Nonautologous tissue substitute Z No device	4 Cutaneous M Descending Colon N Sigmoid Colon P Rectum
M Descending Colon	3 Percutaneous	J Synthetic substitute	4 Cutaneous
N Sigmoid Colon	0 Open 4 Percutaneous endoscopic 8 Via natural or artificial opening endoscopic	7 Autologous tissue substitute J Synthetic substitute K Nonautologous tissue substitute Z No device	4 Cutaneous N Sigmoid Colon P Rectum
N Sigmoid Colon	3 Percutaneous	J Synthetic substitute	4 Cutaneous

341

0D2

MEDICAL AND SURGICAL SECTION – 2016 ICD-10-PCS [2016.PCS]

DEVICE GROUP: Change, Insertion, Removal, Replacement, Revision, Supplement
Root Operations that always involve a device.

- 1ST – **0** Medical and Surgical
- 2ND – **D** Gastrointestinal System
- 3RD – **2 CHANGE**

EXAMPLE: Exchange feeding tube CMS Ex: Changing urinary catheter

CHANGE: Taking out or off a device from a body part and putting back an identical or similar device in or on the same body part without cutting or puncturing the skin or a mucous membrane.

EXPLANATION: ALL Changes use EXTERNAL approach only...

Body Part – 4TH	Approach – 5TH	Device – 6TH	Qualifier – 7TH
0 Upper Intestinal Tract D Lower Intestinal Tract	X External	0 Drainage device U Feeding device Y Other device	Z No qualifier
U Omentum V Mesentery W Peritoneum	X External	0 Drainage device Y Other device	Z No qualifier

EXCISION GROUP: Excision, Resection, Destruction, (Extraction), (Detachment)
Root Operations that take out some or all of a body part.

- 1ST – **0** Medical and Surgical
- 2ND – **D** Gastrointestinal System
- 3RD – **5 DESTRUCTION**

EXAMPLE: Ablation esophageal polyp CMS Ex: Fulguration polyp

DESTRUCTION: Physical eradication of all or a portion of a body part by the direct use of energy, force, or a destructive agent.

EXPLANATION: None of the body part is physically taken out

Body Part – 4TH	Approach – 5TH	Device – 6TH	Qualifier – 7TH
1 Esophagus, Upper 2 Esophagus, Middle 3 Esophagus, Lower 4 Esophagogastric Junction 5 Esophagus 6 Stomach 7 Stomach, Pylorus 8 Small Intestine 9 Duodenum A Jejunum B Ileum C Ileocecal Valve E Large Intestine F Large Intestine, Right G Large Intestine, Left H Cecum J Appendix K Ascending Colon L Transverse Colon M Descending Colon N Sigmoid Colon P Rectum	0 Open 3 Percutaneous 4 Percutaneous endoscopic 7 Via natural or artificial opening 8 Via natural or artificial opening endoscopic	Z No device	Z No qualifier
Q Anus	0 Open 3 Percutaneous 4 Percutaneous endoscopic 7 Via natural or artificial opening 8 Via natural or artificial opening endoscopic X External	Z No device	Z No qualifier
R Anal Sphincter S Greater Omentum T Lesser Omentum V Mesentery W Peritoneum	0 Open 3 Percutaneous 4 Percutaneous endoscopic	Z No device	Z No qualifier

D – GASTROINTESTINAL SYSTEM 0D8

TUBULAR GROUP: Bypass, Dilation, Occlusion, Restriction
Root Operations that alter the diameter/route of a tubular body part.

1ST - **0** Medical and Surgical
2ND - **D** Gastrointestinal System
3RD - **7 DILATION**

EXAMPLE: Dilation rectal stricture   CMS Ex: Transluminal angioplasty

DILATION: Expanding an orifice or the lumen of a tubular body part.

EXPLANATION: By force (stretching) or cutting ...

Body Part – 4TH	Approach – 5TH	Device – 6TH	Qualifier – 7TH
1 Esophagus, Upper 2 Esophagus, Middle 3 Esophagus, Lower 4 Esophagogastric Junction 5 Esophagus 6 Stomach 7 Stomach, Pylorus 8 Small Intestine 9 Duodenum A Jejunum B Ileum C Ileocecal Valve E Large Intestine F Large Intestine, Right G Large Intestine, Left H Cecum K Ascending Colon L Transverse Colon M Descending Colon N Sigmoid Colon P Rectum Q Anus	0 Open 3 Percutaneous 4 Percutaneous endoscopic 7 Via natural or artificial opening 8 Via natural or artificial opening endoscopic	D Intraluminal device Z No device	Z No qualifier

DIVISION GROUP: Division, Release
Root Operations involving cutting or separation only.

1ST - **0** Medical and Surgical
2ND - **D** Gastrointestinal System
3RD - **8 DIVISION**

EXAMPLE: Pyloromyotomy   CMS Ex: Osteotomy

DIVISION: Cutting into a body part without draining fluids and/or gases from the body part in order to separate or transect a body part.

EXPLANATION: Separated into two or more portions ...

Body Part – 4TH	Approach – 5TH	Device – 6TH	Qualifier – 7TH
4 Esophagogastric Junction 7 Stomach, Pylorus	0 Open 3 Percutaneous 4 Percutaneous endoscopic 7 Via natural or artificial opening 8 Via natural or artificial opening endoscopic	Z No device	Z No qualifier
R Anal Sphincter	0 Open 3 Percutaneous	Z No device	Z No qualifier

0D9 — MEDICAL AND SURGICAL SECTION – 2016 ICD-10-PCS

DRAINAGE GROUP: Drainage, Extirpation, Fragmentation
Root Operations that take out solids/fluids/gases from a body part.

- 1ST – **0** Medical and Surgical
- 2ND – **D** Gastrointestinal System
- 3RD – **9** DRAINAGE

EXAMPLE: I&D perianal abscess CMS Ex: Thoracentesis

DRAINAGE: Taking or letting out fluids and/or gases from a body part.

EXPLANATION: Qualifier "X Diagnostic" indicates biopsy ...

Body Part – 4TH		Approach – 5TH	Device – 6TH	Qualifier – 7TH
1 Esophagus, Upper 2 Esophagus, Middle 3 Esophagus, Lower 4 Esophagogastric Junction 5 Esophagus 6 Stomach 7 Stomach, Pylorus 8 Small Intestine 9 Duodenum A Jejunum B Ileum	C Ileocecal Valve E Large Intestine F Large Intestine, Right G Large Intestine, Left H Cecum J Appendix K Ascending Colon L Transverse Colon M Descending Colon N Sigmoid Colon P Rectum	0 Open 3 Percutaneous 4 Percutaneous endoscopic 7 Via natural or artificial opening 8 Via natural or artificial opening endoscopic	0 Drainage device	Z No qualifier
1 Esophagus, Upper 2 Esophagus, Middle 3 Esophagus, Lower 4 Esophagogastric Junction 5 Esophagus 6 Stomach 7 Stomach, Pylorus 8 Small Intestine 9 Duodenum A Jejunum B Ileum	C Ileocecal Valve E Large Intestine F Large Intestine, Right G Large Intestine, Left H Cecum J Appendix K Ascending Colon L Transverse Colon M Descending Colon N Sigmoid Colon P Rectum	0 Open 3 Percutaneous 4 Percutaneous endoscopic 7 Via natural or artificial opening 8 Via natural or artificial opening endoscopic	Z No device	X Diagnostic Z No qualifier
Q Anus		0 Open 3 Percutaneous 4 Percutaneous endoscopic 7 Via natural or artificial opening 8 Via natural or artificial opening endoscopic X External	0 Drainage device	Z No qualifier
Q Anus		0 Open 3 Percutaneous 4 Percutaneous endoscopic 7 Via natural or artificial opening 8 Via natural or artificial opening endoscopic X External	Z No device	X Diagnostic Z No qualifier

continued ⇨

0D9 DRAINAGE – continued

Body Part – 4ᵀᴴ	Approach – 5ᵀᴴ	Device – 6ᵀᴴ	Qualifier – 7ᵀᴴ
R Anal Sphincter S Greater Omentum T Lesser Omentum V Mesentery W Peritoneum	0 Open 3 Percutaneous 4 Percutaneous endoscopic	0 Drainage device	Z No qualifier
R Anal Sphincter S Greater Omentum T Lesser Omentum V Mesentery W Peritoneum	0 Open 3 Percutaneous 4 Percutaneous endoscopic	Z No device	X Diagnostic Z No qualifier

0DB

MEDICAL AND SURGICAL SECTION – 2016 ICD-10-PCS

EXCISION GROUP: Excision, Resection, Destruction, (Extraction), (Detachment)
Root Operations that take out some or all of a body part.

1ST - **0** Medical and Surgical	EXAMPLE: Vertical sleeve gastrectomy CMS Ex: Liver biopsy
2ND - **D** Gastrointestinal System	**EXCISION:** Cutting out or off, without replacement, a portion of a body part.
3RD - **B** EXCISION	EXPLANATION: Qualifier "X Diagnostic" indicates biopsy ...

Body Part – 4TH		Approach – 5TH	Device – 6TH	Qualifier – 7TH
1 Esophagus, Upper 2 Esophagus, Middle 3 Esophagus, Lower 4 Esophagogastric Junction 5 Esophagus 7 Stomach, Pylorus 8 Small Intestine 9 Duodenum A Jejunum B Ileum	C Ileocecal Valve E Large Intestine F Large Intestine, Right G Large Intestine, Left H Cecum J Appendix K Ascending Colon L Transverse Colon M Descending Colon N Sigmoid Colon P Rectum	0 Open 3 Percutaneous 4 Percutaneous endoscopic 7 Via natural or artificial opening 8 Via natural or artificial opening endoscopic	Z No device	X Diagnostic Z No qualifier
6 Stomach		0 Open 3 Percutaneous 4 Percutaneous endoscopic 7 Via natural or artificial opening 8 Via natural or artificial opening endoscopic	Z No device	3 Vertical X Diagnostic Z No qualifier
Q Anus		0 Open 3 Percutaneous 4 Percutaneous endoscopic 7 Via natural or artificial opening 8 Via natural or artificial opening endoscopic X External	Z No device	X Diagnostic Z No qualifier
R Anal Sphincter S Greater Omentum T Lesser Omentum V Mesentery W Peritoneum		0 Open 3 Percutaneous 4 Percutaneous endoscopic	Z No device	X Diagnostic Z No qualifier

GASTROINTESTINAL 0DB

[2016.PCS] **D – GASTROINTESTINAL SYSTEM** **0DF**

DRAINAGE GROUP: Drainage, Extirpation, Fragmentation
Root Operations that take out solids/fluids/gases from a body part.

1ST - 0 Medical and Surgical
2ND - D Gastrointestinal System
3RD - C EXTIRPATION

EXAMPLE: Removal gastric bezoar   CMS Ex: Choledocholithotomy

EXTIRPATION: Taking or cutting out solid matter from a body part.

EXPLANATION: Abnormal byproduct or foreign body …

Body Part – 4TH		Approach – 5TH	Device – 6TH	Qualifier – 7TH
1 Esophagus, Upper	C Ileocecal Valve	0 Open	Z No device	Z No qualifier
2 Esophagus, Middle	E Large Intestine	3 Percutaneous		
3 Esophagus, Lower	F Large Intestine, Right	4 Percutaneous endoscopic		
4 Esophagogastric Junction	G Large Intestine, Left	7 Via natural or artificial opening		
5 Esophagus	H Cecum	8 Via natural or artificial opening endoscopic		
6 Stomach	J Appendix			
7 Stomach, Pylorus	K Ascending Colon			
8 Small Intestine	L Transverse Colon			
9 Duodenum	M Descending Colon			
A Jejunum	N Sigmoid Colon			
B Ileum	P Rectum			
Q Anus		0 Open	Z No device	Z No qualifier
		3 Percutaneous		
		4 Percutaneous endoscopic		
		7 Via natural or artificial opening		
		8 Via natural or artificial opening endoscopic		
		X External		
R Anal Sphincter		0 Open	Z No device	Z No qualifier
S Greater Omentum		3 Percutaneous		
T Lesser Omentum		4 Percutaneous endoscopic		
V Mesentery				
W Peritoneum				

DRAINAGE GROUP: Drainage, Extirpation, Fragmentation
Root Operations that take out solids/fluids/gases from a body part.

1ST - 0 Medical and Surgical
2ND - D Gastrointestinal System
3RD - F FRAGMENTATION

EXAMPLE: Breaking apart gastric bezoar   CMS Ex: Shockwave lithotripsy

FRAGMENTATION: Breaking solid matter in a body part into pieces.

EXPLANATION: Pieces are not taken out during procedure …

Body Part – 4TH		Approach – 5TH	Device – 6TH	Qualifier – 7TH
5 Esophagus	H Cecum	0 Open	Z No device	Z No qualifier
6 Stomach	J Appendix	3 Percutaneous		
8 Small Intestine	K Ascending Colon	4 Percutaneous endoscopic		
9 Duodenum	L Transverse Colon	7 Via natural or artificial opening		
A Jejunum	M Descending Colon	8 Via natural or artificial opening endoscopic		
B Ileum	N Sigmoid Colon	X External NC*		
E Large Intestine	P Rectum			
F Large Intestine, Right	Q Anus			
G Large Intestine, Left				

NC* – Non-covered by Medicare. See current Medicare Code Editor for details.

0DH

MEDICAL AND SURGICAL SECTION – 2016 ICD-10-PCS [2016.PCS]

DEVICE GROUP: Change, Insertion, Removal, Replacement, Revision, Supplement
Root Operations that always involve a device.

1ST – **0** Medical and Surgical
2ND – **D** Gastrointestinal System
3RD – **H** INSERTION

EXAMPLE: Placement artificial anal sphincter   CMS Ex: CVP catheter

INSERTION: Putting in a nonbiological appliance that monitors, assists, performs, or prevents a physiological function but does not physically take the place of a body part.

EXPLANATION: None

Body Part – 4TH	Approach – 5TH	Device – 6TH	Qualifier – 7TH
5 Esophagus	0 Open 3 Percutaneous 4 Percutaneous endoscopic	1 Radioactive element 2 Monitoring device 3 Infusion device D Intraluminal device U Feeding device	Z No qualifier
5 Esophagus	7 Via natural or artificial opening 8 Via natural or artificial opening endoscopic	1 Radioactive element 2 Monitoring device 3 Infusion device B Intraluminal device, airway D Intraluminal device U Feeding device	Z No qualifier
6 Stomach	0 Open 3 Percutaneous 4 Percutaneous endoscopic	2 Monitoring device 3 Infusion device D Intraluminal device M Stimulator lead U Feeding device	Z No qualifier
6 Stomach	7 Via natural or artificial opening 8 Via natural or artificial opening endoscopic	2 Monitoring device 3 Infusion device D Intraluminal device U Feeding device	Z No qualifier
8 Small Intestine 9 Duodenum A Jejunum B Ileum	0 Open 3 Percutaneous 4 Percutaneous endoscopic 7 Via natural or artificial opening 8 Via natural or artificial opening endoscopic	2 Monitoring device 3 Infusion device D Intraluminal device U Feeding device	Z No qualifier

continued

0D H D – GASTROINTESTINAL SYSTEM

0 D H INSERTION – *continued*

Body Part – 4TH	Approach – 5TH	Device – 6TH	Qualifier – 7TH
E Large Intestine	0 Open 3 Percutaneous 4 Percutaneous endoscopic 7 Via natural or artificial opening 8 Via natural or artificial opening endoscopic	D Intraluminal device	Z No qualifier
P Rectum	0 Open 3 Percutaneous 4 Percutaneous endoscopic 7 Via natural or artificial opening 8 Via natural or artificial opening endoscopic	1 Radioactive element D Intraluminal device	Z No qualifier
Q Anus	0 Open 3 Percutaneous 4 Percutaneous endoscopic	D Intraluminal device L Artificial sphincter	Z No qualifier
Q Anus	7 Via natural or artificial opening 8 Via natural or artificial opening endoscopic	D Intraluminal device	Z No qualifier
R Anal Sphincter	0 Open 3 Percutaneous 4 Percutaneous endoscopic	M Stimulator lead	Z No qualifier

0DJ

MEDICAL AND SURGICAL SECTION – 2016 ICD-10-PCS

EXAMINATION GROUP: Inspection, (Map)
Root Operations involving examination only.

1ST - **0** Medical and Surgical
2ND - **D** Gastrointestinal System
3RD - **J** INSPECTION

EXAMPLE: Esophagogastroduodenoscopy
CMS Ex: Colonoscopy

INSPECTION: Visually and/or manually exploring a body part.

EXPLANATION: Direct or instrumental visualization …

Body Part – 4TH	Approach – 5TH	Device – 6TH	Qualifier – 7TH
0 Upper Intestinal Tract 6 Stomach D Lower Intestinal Tract	0 Open 3 Percutaneous 4 Percutaneous endoscopic 7 Via natural or artificial opening 8 Via natural or artificial opening endoscopic X External	Z No device	Z No qualifier
U Omentum V Mesentery W Peritoneum	0 Open 3 Percutaneous 4 Percutaneous endoscopic X External	Z No device	Z No qualifier

GASTROINTESTINAL 0DJ

D – GASTROINTESTINAL SYSTEM
0DL

TUBULAR GROUP: Bypass, Dilation, Occlusion, Restriction
Root Operations that alter the diameter/route of a tubular body part.

- 1ST – **0** Medical and Surgical
- 2ND – **D** Gastrointestinal System
- 3RD – **L** OCCLUSION

EXAMPLE: Closure of rectal stump
CMS Ex: Fallopian tube ligation

OCCLUSION: Completely closing an orifice or lumen of a tubular body part.

EXPLANATION: Natural or artificially created orifice ...

Body Part – 4TH	Approach – 5TH	Device – 6TH	Qualifier – 7TH
1 Esophagus, Upper 2 Esophagus, Middle 3 Esophagus, Lower 4 Esophagogastric Junction 5 Esophagus 6 Stomach 7 Stomach, Pylorus 8 Small Intestine 9 Duodenum A Jejunum B Ileum C Ileocecal Valve E Large Intestine F Large Intestine, Right G Large Intestine, Left H Cecum K Ascending Colon L Transverse Colon M Descending Colon N Sigmoid Colon P Rectum	0 Open 3 Percutaneous 4 Percutaneous endoscopic	C Extraluminal device D Intraluminal device Z No device	Z No qualifier
1 Esophagus, Upper 2 Esophagus, Middle 3 Esophagus, Lower 4 Esophagogastric Junction 5 Esophagus 6 Stomach 7 Stomach, Pylorus 8 Small Intestine 9 Duodenum A Jejunum B Ileum C Ileocecal Valve E Large Intestine F Large Intestine, Right G Large Intestine, Left H Cecum K Ascending Colon L Transverse Colon M Descending Colon N Sigmoid Colon P Rectum	7 Via natural or artificial opening 8 Via natural or artificial opening endoscopic	D Intraluminal device Z No device	Z No qualifier
Q Anus	0 Open 3 Percutaneous 4 Percutaneous endoscopic X External	C Extraluminal device D Intraluminal device Z No device	Z No qualifier
Q Anus	7 Via natural or artificial opening 8 Via natural or artificial opening endoscopic	D Intraluminal device Z No device	Z No qualifier

0DM

MEDICAL AND SURGICAL SECTION – 2016 ICD-10-PCS

MOVE GROUP: Reattachment, Reposition, Transfer, Transplantation
Root Operations that put in/put back or move some/all of a body part.

- 1ST – **0** Medical and Surgical
- 2ND – **D** Gastrointestinal System
- 3RD – **M REATTACHMENT**

EXAMPLE: Reattachment of avulsed esophagus | CMS Ex: Reattach hand

REATTACHMENT: Putting back in or on all or a portion of a separated body part to its normal location or other suitable location.

EXPLANATION: With/without reconnection of vessels/nerves...

Body Part – 4TH	Approach – 5TH	Device – 6TH	Qualifier – 7TH
5 Esophagus	0 Open	Z No device	Z No qualifier
6 Stomach	4 Percutaneous endoscopic		
8 Small Intestine			
9 Duodenum			
A Jejunum			
B Ileum			
E Large Intestine			
F Large Intestine, Right			
G Large Intestine, Left			
H Cecum			
K Ascending Colon			
L Transverse Colon			
M Descending Colon			
N Sigmoid Colon			
P Rectum			

D – GASTROINTESTINAL SYSTEM
0DN

DIVISION GROUP: Division, Release
Root Operations involving cutting or separation only.

1ST - **0** Medical and Surgical
2ND - **D** Gastrointestinal System
3RD - **N RELEASE**

EXAMPLE: Adhesiolysis colon CMS Ex: Carpal tunnel release

RELEASE: Freeing a body part from an abnormal physical constraint by cutting or by the use of force.

EXPLANATION: None of the body part is taken out ...

Body Part – 4TH	Approach – 5TH	Device – 6TH	Qualifier – 7TH
1 Esophagus, Upper 2 Esophagus, Middle 3 Esophagus, Lower 4 Esophagogastric Junction 5 Esophagus 6 Stomach 7 Stomach, Pylorus 8 Small Intestine 9 Duodenum A Jejunum B Ileum C Ileocecal Valve E Large Intestine F Large Intestine, Right G Large Intestine, Left H Cecum J Appendix K Ascending Colon L Transverse Colon M Descending Colon N Sigmoid Colon P Rectum	0 Open 3 Percutaneous 4 Percutaneous endoscopic 7 Via natural or artificial opening 8 Via natural or artificial opening endoscopic	Z No device	Z No qualifier
Q Anus	0 Open 3 Percutaneous 4 Percutaneous endoscopic 7 Via natural or artificial opening 8 Via natural or artificial opening endoscopic X External	Z No device	Z No qualifier
R Anal Sphincter S Greater Omentum T Lesser Omentum V Mesentery W Peritoneum	0 Open 3 Percutaneous 4 Percutaneous endoscopic	Z No device	Z No qualifier

0DP

MEDICAL AND SURGICAL SECTION – 2016 ICD-10-PCS

DEVICE GROUP: Change, Insertion, Removal, Replacement, Revision, Supplement
Root Operations that always involve a device.

1ST - **0** Medical and Surgical
2ND - **D** Gastrointestinal System
3RD - **P** REMOVAL

EXAMPLE: Removal artificial sphincter CMS Ex: Chest tube removal

REMOVAL: Taking out or off a device from a body part.

EXPLANATION: Removal device without reinsertion ...

Body Part – 4TH	Approach – 5TH	Device – 6TH	Qualifier – 7TH
0 Upper Intestinal Tract D Lower Intestinal Tract	0 Open 3 Percutaneous 4 Percutaneous endoscopic 7 Via natural or artificial opening 8 Via natural or artificial opening endoscopic	0 Drainage device 2 Monitoring device 3 Infusion device 7 Autologous tissue substitute C Extraluminal device D Intraluminal device J Synthetic substitute K Nonautologous tissue substitute U Feeding device	Z No qualifier
0 Upper Intestinal Tract D Lower Intestinal Tract	X External	0 Drainage device 2 Monitoring device 3 Infusion device D Intraluminal device U Feeding device	Z No qualifier
5 Esophagus	0 Open 3 Percutaneous 4 Percutaneous endoscopic	1 Radioactive element 2 Monitoring device 3 Infusion device U Feeding device	Z No qualifier
5 Esophagus	7 Via natural or artificial opening 8 Via natural or artificial opening endoscopic	1 Radioactive element D Intraluminal device	Z No qualifier
5 Esophagus	X External	1 Radioactive element 2 Monitoring device 3 Infusion device D Intraluminal device U Feeding device	Z No qualifier

continued ⇨

0 D P REMOVAL – continued

D – GASTROINTESTINAL SYSTEM — 0DP

Body Part – 4ᵀᴴ	Approach – 5ᵀᴴ	Device – 6ᵀᴴ	Qualifier – 7ᵀᴴ
6 Stomach	0 Open 3 Percutaneous 4 Percutaneous endoscopic	0 Drainage device 2 Monitoring device 3 Infusion device 7 Autologous tissue substitute C Extraluminal device D Intraluminal device J Synthetic substitute K Nonautologous tissue substitute M Stimulator lead U Feeding device	Z No qualifier
6 Stomach	7 Via natural or artificial opening 8 Via natural or artificial opening endoscopic	0 Drainage device 2 Monitoring device 3 Infusion device 7 Autologous tissue substitute C Extraluminal device D Intraluminal device J Synthetic substitute K Nonautologous tissue substitute U Feeding device	Z No qualifier
6 Stomach	X External	0 Drainage device 2 Monitoring device 3 Infusion device D Intraluminal device U Feeding device	Z No qualifier
P Rectum	0 Open 3 Percutaneous 4 Percutaneous endoscopic 7 Via natural or artificial opening 8 Via natural or artificial opening endoscopic X External	1 Radioactive element	Z No qualifier
Q Anus	0 Open 3 Percutaneous 4 Percutaneous endoscopic 7 Via natural or artificial opening 8 Via natural or artificial opening endoscopic	L Artificial sphincter	Z No qualifier
R Anal Sphincter	0 Open 3 Percutaneous 4 Percutaneous endoscopic	M Stimulator lead	Z No qualifier
U Omentum V Mesentery W Peritoneum	0 Open 3 Percutaneous 4 Percutaneous endoscopic	0 Drainage device 1 Radioactive element 7 Autologous tissue substitute J Synthetic substitute K Nonautologous tissue substitute	Z No qualifier

0DQ MEDICAL AND SURGICAL SECTION – 2016 ICD-10-PCS

OTHER REPAIRS GROUP: (Control), **Repair**
Root Operations that define other repairs.

1ST - **0** Medical and Surgical
2ND - **D** Gastrointestinal System
3RD - **Q REPAIR**

EXAMPLE: Suture duodenal laceration   CMS Ex: Suture laceration

REPAIR: Restoring, to the extent possible, a body part to its normal anatomic structure and function.

EXPLANATION: Only when no other root operation applies ...

Body Part – 4TH	Approach – 5TH	Device – 6TH	Qualifier – 7TH
1 Esophagus, Upper 2 Esophagus, Middle 3 Esophagus, Lower 4 Esophagogastric Junction 5 Esophagus 6 Stomach 7 Stomach, Pylorus 8 Small Intestine 9 Duodenum A Jejunum B Ileum C Ileocecal Valve E Large Intestine F Large Intestine, Right G Large Intestine, Left H Cecum J Appendix K Ascending Colon L Transverse Colon M Descending Colon N Sigmoid Colon P Rectum	0 Open 3 Percutaneous 4 Percutaneous endoscopic 7 Via natural or artificial opening 8 Via natural or artificial opening endoscopic	Z No device	Z No qualifier
Q Anus	0 Open 3 Percutaneous 4 Percutaneous endoscopic 7 Via natural or artificial opening 8 Via natural or artificial opening endoscopic X External	Z No device	Z No qualifier
R Anal Sphincter S Greater Omentum T Lesser Omentum V Mesentery W Peritoneum	0 Open 3 Percutaneous 4 Percutaneous endoscopic	Z No device	Z No qualifier

DEVICE GROUP: Change, Insertion, Removal, Replacement, Revision, Supplement
Root Operations that always involve a device.

1ST - 0 Medical and Surgical
2ND - D Gastrointestinal System
3RD - R REPLACEMENT

EXAMPLE: Esophageal segment replacement | CMS Ex: Total hip

REPLACEMENT: Putting in or on a biological or synthetic material that physically takes the place and/or function of all or a portion of a body part.

EXPLANATION: Includes taking out body part, or eradication...

Body Part – 4TH	Approach – 5TH	Device – 6TH	Qualifier – 7TH
5 Esophagus	0 Open 4 Percutaneous endoscopic 7 Via natural or artificial opening 8 Via natural or artificial opening endoscopic	7 Autologous tissue substitute J Synthetic substitute K Nonautologous tissue substitute	Z No qualifier
R Anal Sphincter S Greater Omentum T Lesser Omentum V Mesentery W Peritoneum	0 Open 4 Percutaneous endoscopic	7 Autologous tissue substitute J Synthetic substitute K Nonautologous tissue substitute	Z No qualifier

MOVE GROUP: Reattachment, Reposition, Transfer, Transplantation
Root Operations that put in/put back or move some/all of a body part.

1ST - 0 Medical and Surgical
2ND - D Gastrointestinal System
3RD - S REPOSITION

EXAMPLE: Gastropexy for malrotation | CMS Ex: Fracture reduction

REPOSITION: Moving to its normal location, or other suitable location, all or a portion of a body part.

EXPLANATION: May or may not be cut to be moved ...

Body Part – 4TH		Approach – 5TH	Device – 6TH	Qualifier – 7TH
5 Esophagus 6 Stomach 9 Duodenum A Jejunum B Ileum H Cecum	K Ascending Colon L Transverse Colon M Descending Colon N Sigmoid Colon P Rectum Q Anus	0 Open 4 Percutaneous endoscopic 7 Via natural or artificial opening 8 Via natural or artificial opening endoscopic X External	Z No device	Z No qualifier

0DT

MEDICAL AND SURGICAL SECTION – 2016 ICD-10-PCS

EXCISION GROUP: Excision, Resection, Destruction, (Extraction), (Detachment)
Root Operations that take out some or all of a body part.

- 1ST – **0** Medical and Surgical
- 2ND – **D** Gastrointestinal System
- 3RD – **T** RESECTION

EXAMPLE: Sigmoid colectomy

CMS Ex: Cholecystectomy

RESECTION: Cutting out or off, without replacement, all of a body part.

EXPLANATION: None

Body Part – 4TH		Approach – 5TH	Device – 6TH	Qualifier – 7TH
1 Esophagus, Upper 2 Esophagus, Middle 3 Esophagus, Lower 4 Esophagogastric Junction 5 Esophagus 6 Stomach 7 Stomach, Pylorus 8 Small Intestine 9 Duodenum A Jejunum B Ileum	C Ileocecal Valve E Large Intestine F Large Intestine, Right G Large Intestine, Left H Cecum J Appendix K Ascending Colon L Transverse Colon M Descending Colon N Sigmoid Colon P Rectum Q Anus	0 Open 4 Percutaneous endoscopic 7 Via natural or artificial opening 8 Via natural or artificial opening endoscopic	Z No device	Z No qualifier
R Anal Sphincter S Greater Omentum T Lesser Omentum		0 Open 4 Percutaneous endoscopic	Z No device	Z No qualifier

0DU

D – GASTROINTESTINAL SYSTEM

DEVICE GROUP: Change, Insertion, Removal, Replacement, Revision, Supplement
Root Operations that always involve a device.

- 1ST – **0** Medical and Surgical
- 2ND – **D** Gastrointestinal System
- 3RD – **U SUPPLEMENT**

EXAMPLE: Parastomal hernia repair with graft | **CMS Ex:** Hernia mesh

SUPPLEMENT: Putting in or on biological or synthetic material that physically reinforces and/or augments the function of a portion of a body part.

EXPLANATION: Biological material from same individual …

Body Part – 4TH	Approach – 5TH	Device – 6TH	Qualifier – 7TH
1 Esophagus, Upper 2 Esophagus, Middle 3 Esophagus, Lower 4 Esophagogastric Junction 5 Esophagus 6 Stomach 7 Stomach, Pylorus 8 Small Intestine 9 Duodenum A Jejunum B Ileum C Ileocecal Valve E Large Intestine F Large Intestine, Right G Large Intestine, Left H Cecum K Ascending Colon L Transverse Colon M Descending Colon N Sigmoid Colon P Rectum	0 Open 4 Percutaneous endoscopic 7 Via natural or artificial opening 8 Via natural or artificial opening endoscopic	7 Autologous tissue substitute J Synthetic substitute K Nonautologous tissue substitute	Z No qualifier
Q Anus	0 Open 4 Percutaneous endoscopic 7 Via natural or artificial opening 8 Via natural or artificial opening endoscopic X External	7 Autologous tissue substitute J Synthetic substitute K Nonautologous tissue substitute	Z No qualifier
R Anal Sphincter S Greater Omentum T Lesser Omentum V Mesentery W Peritoneum	0 Open 4 Percutaneous endoscopic	7 Autologous tissue substitute J Synthetic substitute K Nonautologous tissue substitute	Z No qualifier

0DV

MEDICAL AND SURGICAL SECTION – 2016 ICD-10-PCS

TUBULAR GROUP: Bypass, Dilation, Occlusion, Restriction
Root Operations that alter the diameter/route of a tubular body part.

1ST – **0** Medical and Surgical
2ND – **D** Gastrointestinal System
3RD – **V** RESTRICTION

EXAMPLE: Nissen fundoplication   CMS Ex: Cervical cerclage

RESTRICTION: Partially closing an orifice or the lumen of a tubular body part.

EXPLANATION: Natural or artificially created orifice ...

Body Part – 4TH		Approach – 5TH	Device – 6TH	Qualifier – 7TH
1 Esophagus, Upper 2 Esophagus, Middle 3 Esophagus, Lower 4 Esophagogastric Junction 5 Esophagus 6 Stomach 7 Stomach, Pylorus 8 Small Intestine 9 Duodenum A Jejunum B Ileum	C Ileocecal Valve E Large Intestine F Large Intestine, Right G Large Intestine, Left H Cecum K Ascending Colon L Transverse Colon M Descending Colon N Sigmoid Colon P Rectum	0 Open 3 Percutaneous 4 Percutaneous endoscopic	C Extraluminal device D Intraluminal device Z No device	Z No qualifier
1 Esophagus, Upper 2 Esophagus, Middle 3 Esophagus, Lower 4 Esophagogastric Junction 5 Esophagus 6 Stomach NC* 7 Stomach, Pylorus 8 Small Intestine 9 Duodenum A Jejunum B Ileum	C Ileocecal Valve E Large Intestine F Large Intestine, Right G Large Intestine, Left H Cecum K Ascending Colon L Transverse Colon M Descending Colon N Sigmoid Colon P Rectum	7 Via natural or artificial opening 8 Via natural or artificial opening endoscopic	D Intraluminal device Z No device	Z No qualifier
Q Anus		0 Open 3 Percutaneous 4 Percutaneous endoscopic X External	C Extraluminal device D Intraluminal device Z No device	Z No qualifier
Q Anus		7 Via natural or artificial opening 8 Via natural or artificial opening endoscopic	D Intraluminal device Z No device	Z No qualifier

NC* – Some procedures are considered non-covered by Medicare. See current Medicare Code Editor for details.

D – GASTROINTESTINAL SYSTEM — 0DW

DEVICE GROUP: Change, Insertion, Removal, Replacement, Revision, Supplement
Root Operations that always involve a device.

1ST - **0** Medical and Surgical
2ND - **D** Gastrointestinal System
3RD - **W** REVISION

EXAMPLE: Reposition artificial anal sphincter | CMS Ex: Adjustment lead

REVISION: Correcting, to the extent possible, a portion of a malfunctioning device or the position of a displaced device.

EXPLANATION: May replace components of a device ...

Body Part – 4TH	Approach – 5TH	Device – 6TH	Qualifier – 7TH
0 Upper Intestinal Tract D Lower Intestinal Tract	0 Open 3 Percutaneous 4 Percutaneous endoscopic 7 Via natural or artificial opening 8 Via natural or artificial opening endoscopic X External	0 Drainage device 2 Monitoring device 3 Infusion device 7 Autologous tissue substitute C Extraluminal device D Intraluminal device J Synthetic substitute K Nonautologous tissue substitute U Feeding device	Z No qualifier
5 Esophagus	7 Via natural or artificial opening 8 Via natural or artificial opening endoscopic X External	D Intraluminal device	Z No qualifier
6 Stomach	0 Open 3 Percutaneous 4 Percutaneous endoscopic	0 Drainage device 2 Monitoring device 3 Infusion device 7 Autologous tissue substitute C Extraluminal device D Intraluminal device J Synthetic substitute K Nonautologous tissue substitute M Stimulator lead U Feeding device	Z No qualifier
6 Stomach	7 Via natural or artificial opening 8 Via natural or artificial opening endoscopic X External	0 Drainage device 2 Monitoring device 3 Infusion device 7 Autologous tissue substitute C Extraluminal device D Intraluminal device J Synthetic substitute K Nonautologous tissue substitute U Feeding device	Z No qualifier
8 Small Intestine E Large Intestine	0 Open 4 Percutaneous endoscopic 7 Via natural or artificial opening 8 Via natural or artificial opening endoscopic	7 Autologous tissue substitute J Synthetic substitute K Nonautologous tissue substitute	Z No qualifier
Q Anus	0 Open 3 Percutaneous 4 Percutaneous endoscopic 7 Via natural or artificial opening 8 Via natural or artificial opening endoscopic	L Artificial sphincter	Z No qualifier

continued ➡

0DW

REVISION – continued

Body Part – 4TH	Approach – 5TH	Device – 6TH	Qualifier – 7TH
R Anal Sphincter	0 Open 3 Percutaneous 4 Percutaneous endoscopic	M Stimulator lead	Z No qualifier
U Omentum V Mesentery W Peritoneum	0 Open 3 Percutaneous 4 Percutaneous endoscopic	0 Drainage device 7 Autologous tissue substitute J Synthetic substitute K Nonautologous tissue substitute	Z No qualifier

MOVE GROUP: Reattachment, Reposition, Transfer, Transplantation
Root Operations that put in/put back or move some/all of a body part.

- 1ST – **0** Medical and Surgical
- 2ND – **D** Gastrointestinal System
- 3RD – **X** TRANSFER

EXAMPLE: Colon-interposition esophagus **CMS Ex:** Tendon transfer

TRANSFER: Moving, without taking out, all or a portion of a body part to another location to take over the function of all or a portion of a body part.

EXPLANATION: The body part remains connected …

Body Part – 4TH	Approach – 5TH	Device – 6TH	Qualifier – 7TH
6 Stomach 8 Small Intestine E Large Intestine	0 Open 4 Percutaneous endoscopic	Z No device	5 Esophagus

MOVE GROUP: Reattachment, Reposition, Transfer, Transplantation
Root Operations that put in/put back or move some/all of a body part.

- 1ST – **0** Medical and Surgical
- 2ND – **D** Gastrointestinal System
- 3RD – **Y** TRANSPLANTATION

EXAMPLE: Esophagus transplant **CMS Ex:** Kidney transplant

TRANSPLANTATION: Putting in or on all or a portion of a living body part taken from another individual or animal to physically take the place and/or function of all or a portion of a similar body part.

EXPLANATION: May take over all or part of its function …

Body Part – 4TH	Approach – 5TH	Device – 6TH	Qualifier – 7TH
5 Esophagus 6 Stomach 8 Small Intestine LC* E Large Intestine LC*	0 Open	Z No device	0 Allogenic 1 Syngeneic 2 Zooplastic

LC* – Some procedures are considered limited coverage by Medicare. See current Medicare Code Editor for details.

Educational Annotations | F – Hepatobiliary System and Pancreas

Body System Specific Educational Annotations for the Hepatobiliary System and Pancreas include:

- Anatomy and Physiology Review
- Anatomical Illustrations
- Definitions of Common Procedures
- AHA Coding Clinic® Reference Notations
- Body Part Key Listings
- Device Key Listings
- Device Aggregation Table Listings
- Coding Notes

Anatomy and Physiology Review of Hepatobiliary System and Pancreas

BODY PART VALUES – F - HEPATOBILIARY SYSTEM AND PANCREAS

Ampulla of Vater – The common bile duct merges with the pancreatic duct in the dilated area known as the ampulla of Vater.

Common Bile Duct – ANATOMY – The common bile duct is formed by the merger of the cystic duct from the gallbladder and the common hepatic duct. PHYSIOLOGY – The cystic duct, hepatic duct, and common bile duct convey the bile into the duodenum.

Cystic Duct – ANATOMY – The cystic duct is the tubular drain of the gallbladder which merges with the hepatic duct to form the common bile duct. PHYSIOLOGY – The cystic duct, hepatic duct, and common bile duct convey the bile into the duodenum.

Gallbladder – ANATOMY – The gallbladder is the musculomembranous, pear-shaped bile reservoir located on the undersurface of the liver. PHYSIOLOGY – The gallbladder functions to store and concentrate the bile and release the bile on demand to the small intestine for the digestion of fats.

Hepatic Duct – ANATOMY – The common hepatic duct is formed by the merger of the right and left hepatic ducts that drain the smaller intrahepatic ducts. PHYSIOLOGY – The cystic duct, hepatic duct, and common bile duct convey the bile into the duodenum.

Hepatobiliary Duct – The ducts of the hepatobiliary system including the cystic duct, hepatic ducts, and common bile duct.

Liver – ANATOMY – The liver is the largest organ in the body, weighing about 3 pounds (1 kg) in the adult. Located in the upper right quadrant of the abdominal cavity, its superior surface lies under the dome of the diaphragm. There are 4 lobes of the liver; the left, right (the right lobe has two smaller lobes, the caudate and quadrate). The common bile duct is formed by the joining of the hepatic duct, which carries bile from the liver, and the cystic duct, which carries bile from the gallbladder. The common duct then carries the bile into the duodenum through an opening on the duodenal papilla. The hepatic artery furnishes arterial blood for the nourishment of the liver cells. The portal vein carries blood containing products of digestion from the intestinal tract into the liver. Internally, the liver lobules are the functional units of liver substance. Bile is secreted by the liver cells into tiny canals, or canaliculi, and then emptied into a bile duct. PHYSIOLOGY – One of the regulatory functions of the liver is controlling the blood sugar level. The liver is able to both absorb excess sugar and dispense it into the blood. The liver also stores and secretes other essential nutrients. It chemically processes these materials and detoxifies many substances that could be harmful if allowed to accumulate in the body. Its bile salts are necessary for the absorption of vitamin K from the gastrointestinal tract, which in turn are needed for the production of prothrombin. Another important liver function is producing bile. A brownish-yellow fluid, it is secreted continuously by the liver in amounts averaging about 20 fluid ounces (600 ml) per day. Bile contains the bile salts which are very important in the digestion of fat.

Liver, Left Lobe – One of the two common lobes of the liver.

Liver, Right Lobe – One of the two common lobes of the liver.

Continued on next page

0F — Hepatobiliary System and Pancreas

Educational Annotations | **F – Hepatobiliary System and Pancreas**

MEDICAL AND SURGICAL SECTION – 2016 ICD-10-PCS

Anatomy and Physiology Review of Hepatobiliary System and Pancreas

BODY PART VALUES – F - HEPATOBILIARY SYSTEM AND PANCREAS
Continued from previous page

Pancreas – ANATOMY – The pancreas is a slender organ about 6 to 9 inches (15 to 23 cm) long lying horizontally and located in the abdomen behind and under the stomach. The pancreas is divided into 3 areas: The head, lying in the curve formed by the duodenum; the body, the main portion lying between the head and tail; and the tail, the most lateral portion blunting up against the spleen. The cells that produce pancreatic juice are called pancreatic acinar cells, and they make up the bulk of the pancreas. These cells are clustered around tiny tubes which drain into the pancreatic duct (duct of Wirsung). This duct connects with the duodenum at the same place where the bile ducts join the duodenum. The second type of pancreatic cells are arranged in groups closely associated with blood vessels and are called islets of Langerhans. The pancreas arterial blood is supplied via the common hepatic artery, the gastroduodenal artery, the pancreatico-duodenal arches, the splenic artery, and also from the superior mesenteric artery. PHYSIOLOGY – The pancreas functions as both an exocrine gland, producing pancreatic juice, and as an endocrine gland, producing the hormones insulin and glucagon. The pancreatic juice contains enzymes capable of digesting carbohydrates, fats, proteins, and nucleic acids, and is produced by the pancreatic acinar cells. This juice is drained into the duodenum. The pancreatic hormones which are produced by the islets of Langerhans cells regulate blood glucose level.

Pancreatic Duct – The pancreatic duct connects with the duodenum at the dilated area known as the ampulla of Vater.

Pancreatic Duct, Accessory – The presence of an additional pancreatic duct that connects directly with the duodenum.

Anatomical Illustrations of Hepatobiliary System and Pancreas

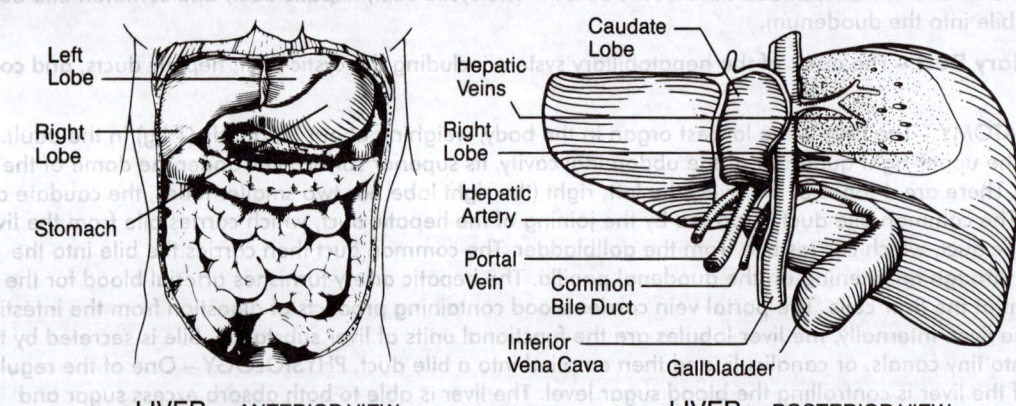

LIVER — ANTERIOR VIEW

LIVER — POSTERIOR VIEW

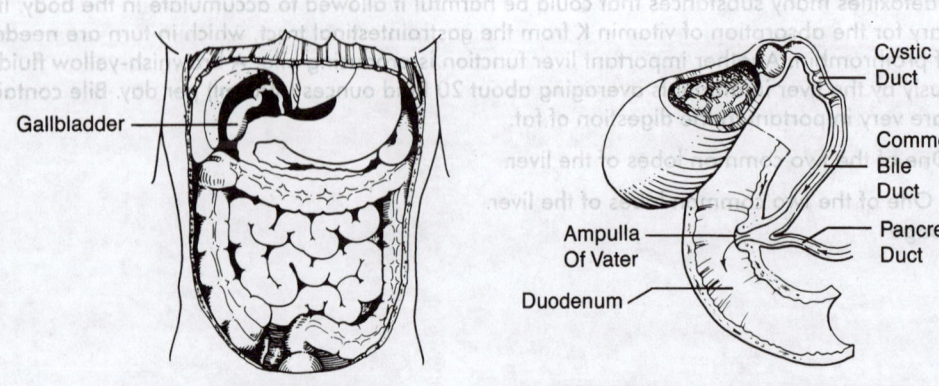

GALLBLADDER

GALLBLADDER — ANTERIOR (CUT-AWAY) VIEW

Continued on next page

Educational Annotations | F – Hepatobiliary System and Pancreas

Anatomical Illustrations of Hepatobiliary System and Pancreas

Continued from previous page

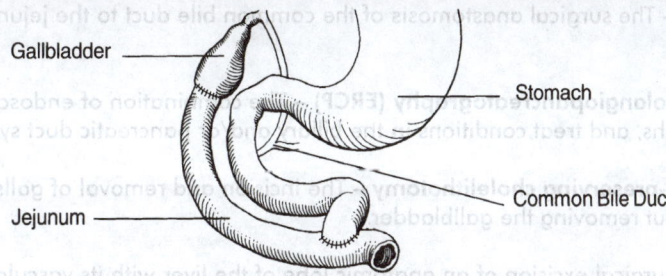

ANASTOMOSIS OF GALLBLADDER TO INTESTINE

AHA Coding Clinic® Reference Notations of Hepatobiliary System and Pancreas

ROOT OPERATION SPECIFIC – F – HEPATOBILIARY SYSTEM AND PANCREAS

BYPASS – 1
CHANGE – 2
DESTRUCTION – 5
DILATION – 7
  Dilation of common bile duct ....AHA 14:3Q:p15
DIVISION – 8
DRAINAGE – 9
  ERCP with pseudocyst drainage ....AHA 14:3Q:p15
  Placement of external-internal biliary drainage catheter ....AHA 15:1Q:p32
EXCISION – B
  Whipple pyloric sparing pancreaticoduodenectomy...................................AHA 14:3Q:p32
EXTIRPATION – C
FRAGMENTATION – F
INSERTION – H
INSPECTION – J
OCCLUSION – L
REATTACHMENT – M
RELEASE – N
REMOVAL – P
REPAIR – Q
REPLACEMENT – R
REPOSITION – S
RESECTION – T
  Resection of liver to capture "domino liver transplant" ....AHA 12:4Q:p99
SUPPLEMENT – U
RESTRICTION – V
REVISION – W
TRANSPLANTATION – Y
  "Domino liver transplant"..AHA 12:4Q:p99
  Orthotopic liver allotransplant ....AHA 14:3Q:p13

Educational Annotations | F – Hepatobiliary System and Pancreas

Definitions of Common Procedures of Hepatobiliary System and Pancreas

Choledochojejunostomy – The surgical anastomosis of the common bile duct to the jejunum to relieve biliary obstruction symptoms.

Endoscopic retrograde cholangiopancreatography (ERCP) – The combination of endoscopic and fluoroscopy to visualize, obtain radiographs, and treat conditions in the biliary and/or pancreatic duct systems.

Laparoscopic gallbladder-preserving cholelithotomy – The incision and removal of gallstones that is performed laparoscopically and without removing the gallbladder.

Lobectomy of liver – The surgical excision of an anatomic lobe of the liver with its vascular connections.

Wedge resection of liver – The surgical excision of less than a whole anatomic liver segment or parts of two anatomic segments.

Whipple procedure (pancreatoduodenectomy) – The surgical excision of the head of the pancreas that usually includes a duodenectomy, cholecystectomy, and a portion of the stomach including the pylorus, with anastomosis of the common bile duct, pancreas, and stomach to the jejunum. A pyloric-sparing version keeps the stomach and pylorus intact.

Body Part Key Listings of Hepatobiliary System and Pancreas

See also Body Part Key in Appendix C

Duct of Santorini	*use* Pancreatic Duct, Accessory
Duct of Wirsung	*use* Pancreatic Duct
Duodenal ampulla	*use* Ampulla of Vater
Hepatopancreatic ampulla	*use* Ampulla of Vater
Quadrate lobe	*use* Liver

Device Key Listings of Hepatobiliary System and Pancreas

See also Device Key in Appendix D

Autograft	*use* Autologous Tissue Substitute
Brachytherapy seeds	*use* Radioactive Element
Stent, intraluminal (cardiovascular) (gastrointestinal) (hepatobiliary) (urinary)	*use* Intraluminal Device
Tissue bank graft	*use* Nonautologous Tissue Substitute

Device Aggregation Table Listings of Hepatobiliary System and Pancreas

See also Device Aggregation Table in Appendix E

Specific Device	For Operation	In Body System	General Device
None Listed in Device Aggregation Table for this Body System			

Educational Annotations | F – Hepatobiliary System and Pancreas

Coding Notes of Hepatobiliary System and Pancreas

Body System Specific PCS Reference Manual Exercises

PCS CODE	F – HEPATOBILIARY SYSTEM AND PANCREAS EXERCISES
0F798ZZ	ERCP with balloon dilation of common bile duct.
0F9100Z	Laparotomy with drain placement for liver abscess, right lobe.
0FB20ZZ	Laparotomy with wedge resection of left lateral segment of liver.
0FBG0ZZ	Open excision of tail of pancreas.
0FF98ZZ	Endoscopic Retrograde Cholangiopancreatography (ERCP) with lithotripsy of common bile duct stone. (ERCP is performed through the mouth to the biliary system via the duodenum, so the approach value is Via Natural or Artificial Opening Endoscopic.)
0FJ00ZZ	Laparotomy with palpation of liver.
0FPG00Z	Laparotomy with removal of pancreatic drain.
0FT44ZZ	Laparoscopic cholecystectomy.
0FY00Z0	Liver transplant with donor matched liver.
0FYG0Z0	Left kidney/pancreas organ bank transplant.
0TY10Z0	

Educational Annotations

F – Hepatobiliary System and Pancreas

NOTES

F – HEPATOBILIARY SYSTEM AND PANCREAS — 0F2

TUBULAR GROUP: Bypass, Dilation, Occlusion, Restriction
Root Operations that alter the diameter/route of a tubular body part.

1ST – **0** Medical and Surgical
2ND – **F** Hepatobiliary System and Pancreas
3RD – **1 BYPASS**

EXAMPLE: Choledochojejunostomy   CMS Ex: Coronary artery bypass

BYPASS: Altering the route of passage of the contents of a tubular body part.

EXPLANATION: Rerouting contents to a downstream part …

Body Part – 4TH	Approach – 5TH	Device – 6TH	Qualifier – 7TH
4 Gallbladder 5 Hepatic Duct, Right 6 Hepatic Duct, Left 8 Cystic Duct 9 Common Bile Duct	0 Open 4 Percutaneous endoscopic	D Intraluminal device Z No device	3 Duodenum 4 Stomach 5 Hepatic Duct, Right 6 Hepatic Duct, Left 7 Hepatic Duct, Caudate 8 Cystic Duct 9 Common Bile Duct B Small Intestine
D Pancreatic Duct F Pancreatic Duct, Accessory G Pancreas	0 Open 4 Percutaneous endoscopic	D Intraluminal device Z No device	3 Duodenum B Small Intestine C Large Intestine

DEVICE GROUP: Change, Insertion, Removal, Replacement, Revision, Supplement
Root Operations that always involve a device.

1ST – **0** Medical and Surgical
2ND – **F** Hepatobiliary System and Pancreas
3RD – **2 CHANGE**

EXAMPLE: Exchange drain tube   CMS Ex: Changing urinary catheter

CHANGE: Taking out or off a device from a body part and putting back an identical or similar device in or on the same body part without cutting or puncturing the skin or a mucous membrane.

EXPLANATION: ALL Changes use EXTERNAL approach only…

Body Part – 4TH	Approach – 5TH	Device – 6TH	Qualifier – 7TH
0 Liver 4 Gallbladder B Hepatobiliary Duct D Pancreatic Duct G Pancreas	X External	0 Drainage device Y Other device	Z No qualifier

0F5

MEDICAL AND SURGICAL SECTION – 2016 ICD-10-PCS

EXCISION GROUP: Excision, Resection, Destruction, (Extraction), (Detachment)
Root Operations that take out some or all of a body part.

1ST – 0	Medical and Surgical
2ND – F	Hepatobiliary System and Pancreas
3RD – 5	**DESTRUCTION**

EXAMPLE: RF ablation liver lesion   CMS Ex: Fulguration polyp

DESTRUCTION: Physical eradication of all or a portion of a body part by the direct use of energy, force, or a destructive agent.

EXPLANATION: None of the body part is physically taken out

Body Part – 4TH	Approach – 5TH	Device – 6TH	Qualifier – 7TH
0 Liver 1 Liver, Right Lobe 2 Liver, Left Lobe 4 Gallbladder G Pancreas	0 Open 3 Percutaneous 4 Percutaneous endoscopic	Z No device	Z No qualifier
5 Hepatic Duct, Right 6 Hepatic Duct, Left 8 Cystic Duct 9 Common Bile Duct C Ampulla of Vater D Pancreatic Duct F Pancreatic Duct, Accessory	0 Open 3 Percutaneous 4 Percutaneous endoscopic 7 Via natural or artificial opening 8 Via natural or artificial opening endoscopic	Z No device	Z No qualifier

---

TUBULAR GROUP: Bypass, Dilation, Occlusion, Restriction
Root Operations that alter the diameter/route of a tubular body part.

1ST – 0	Medical and Surgical
2ND – F	Hepatobiliary System and Pancreas
3RD – 7	**DILATION**

EXAMPLE: ERCP dilation pancreatic duct   CMS Ex: Transluminal angioplasty

DILATION: Expanding an orifice or the lumen of a tubular body part.

EXPLANATION: By force (stretching) or cutting ...

Body Part – 4TH	Approach – 5TH	Device – 6TH	Qualifier – 7TH
5 Hepatic Duct, Right 6 Hepatic Duct, Left 8 Cystic Duct 9 Common Bile Duct C Ampulla of Vater D Pancreatic Duct F Pancreatic Duct, Accessory	0 Open 3 Percutaneous 4 Percutaneous endoscopic 7 Via natural or artificial opening 8 Via natural or artificial opening endoscopic	D Intraluminal device Z No device	Z No qualifier

F – HEPATOBILIARY SYSTEM AND PANCREAS — 0F9

DIVISION GROUP: Division, Release
Root Operations involving cutting or separation only.

- 1ST – **0** Medical and Surgical
- 2ND – **F** Hepatobiliary System and Pancreas
- 3RD – **8 DIVISION**

EXAMPLE: Pancreatotomy CMS Ex: Osteotomy

DIVISION: Cutting into a body part without draining fluids and/or gases from the body part in order to separate or transect a body part.

EXPLANATION: Separated into two or more portions ...

Body Part – 4TH	Approach – 5TH	Device – 6TH	Qualifier – 7TH
G Pancreas	0 Open 3 Percutaneous 4 Percutaneous endoscopic	Z No device	Z No qualifier

DRAINAGE GROUP: Drainage, Extirpation, Fragmentation
Root Operations that take out solids/fluids/gases from a body part.

- 1ST – **0** Medical and Surgical
- 2ND – **F** Hepatobiliary System and Pancreas
- 3RD – **9 DRAINAGE**

EXAMPLE: ERCP pseudocyst drainage CMS Ex: Thoracentesis

DRAINAGE: Taking or letting out fluids and/or gases from a body part.

EXPLANATION: Qualifier "X Diagnostic" indicates biopsy ...

Body Part – 4TH	Approach – 5TH	Device – 6TH	Qualifier – 7TH
0 Liver 1 Liver, Right Lobe 2 Liver, Left Lobe 4 Gallbladder G Pancreas	0 Open 3 Percutaneous 4 Percutaneous endoscopic	0 Drainage device	Z No qualifier
0 Liver 1 Liver, Right Lobe 2 Liver, Left Lobe 4 Gallbladder G Pancreas	0 Open 3 Percutaneous 4 Percutaneous endoscopic	Z No device	X Diagnostic Z No qualifier
5 Hepatic Duct, Right 6 Hepatic Duct, Left 8 Cystic Duct 9 Common Bile Duct C Ampulla of Vater D Pancreatic Duct F Pancreatic Duct, Accessory	0 Open 3 Percutaneous 4 Percutaneous endoscopic 7 Via natural or artificial opening 8 Via natural or artificial opening endoscopic	0 Drainage device	Z No qualifier
5 Hepatic Duct, Right 6 Hepatic Duct, Left 8 Cystic Duct 9 Common Bile Duct C Ampulla of Vater D Pancreatic Duct F Pancreatic Duct, Accessory	0 Open 3 Percutaneous 4 Percutaneous endoscopic 7 Via natural or artificial opening 8 Via natural or artificial opening endoscopic	Z No device	X Diagnostic Z No qualifier

0FB

MEDICAL AND SURGICAL SECTION – 2016 ICD-10-PCS

[2016.PCS]

Hepatobiliary 0FB

EXCISION GROUP: Excision, Resection, Destruction, (Extraction), (Detachment)
Root Operations that take out some or all of a body part.

- 1ST – **0** Medical and Surgical
- 2ND – **F** Hepatobiliary System and Pancreas
- 3RD – **B EXCISION**

EXAMPLE: Wedge resection liver
CMS Ex: Liver biopsy

EXCISION: Cutting out or off, without replacement, a portion of a body part.

EXPLANATION: Qualifier "X Diagnostic" indicates biopsy ...

Body Part – 4TH	Approach – 5TH	Device – 6TH	Qualifier – 7TH
0 Liver 1 Liver, Right Lobe 2 Liver, Left Lobe 4 Gallbladder G Pancreas	0 Open 3 Percutaneous 4 Percutaneous endoscopic	Z No device	X Diagnostic Z No qualifier
5 Hepatic Duct, Right 6 Hepatic Duct, Left 8 Cystic Duct 9 Common Bile Duct C Ampulla of Vater D Pancreatic Duct F Pancreatic Duct, Accessory	0 Open 3 Percutaneous 4 Percutaneous endoscopic 7 Via natural or artificial opening 8 Via natural or artificial opening endoscopic	Z No device	X Diagnostic Z No qualifier

DRAINAGE GROUP: Drainage, Extirpation, Fragmentation
Root Operations that take out solids/fluids/gases from a body part.

- 1ST – **0** Medical and Surgical
- 2ND – **F** Hepatobiliary System and Pancreas
- 3RD – **C EXTIRPATION**

EXAMPLE: Cholelithotomy
CMS Ex: Choledocholithotomy

EXTIRPATION: Taking or cutting out solid matter from a body part.

EXPLANATION: Abnormal byproduct or foreign body ...

Body Part – 4TH	Approach – 5TH	Device – 6TH	Qualifier – 7TH
0 Liver 1 Liver, Right Lobe 2 Liver, Left Lobe 4 Gallbladder G Pancreas	0 Open 3 Percutaneous 4 Percutaneous endoscopic	Z No device	Z No qualifier
5 Hepatic Duct, Right 6 Hepatic Duct, Left 8 Cystic Duct 9 Common Bile Duct C Ampulla of Vater D Pancreatic Duct F Pancreatic Duct, Accessory	0 Open 3 Percutaneous 4 Percutaneous endoscopic 7 Via natural or artificial opening 8 Via natural or artificial opening endoscopic	Z No device	Z No qualifier

F – HEPATOBILIARY SYSTEM AND PANCREAS 0 F H

DRAINAGE GROUP: Drainage, Extirpation, Fragmentation
Root Operations that take out solids/fluids/gases from a body part.

1ST - 0 Medical and Surgical
2ND - F Hepatobiliary System and Pancreas
3RD - F FRAGMENTATION

EXAMPLE: Lithotripsy gallstones   CMS Ex: Extracorporeal shockwave lithotripsy

FRAGMENTATION: Breaking solid matter in a body part into pieces.

EXPLANATION: Pieces are not taken out during procedure …

Body Part – 4TH	Approach – 5TH	Device – 6TH	Qualifier – 7TH
4 Gallbladder	0 Open	Z No device	Z No qualifier
5 Hepatic Duct, Right	3 Percutaneous		
6 Hepatic Duct, Left	4 Percutaneous endoscopic		
8 Cystic Duct	7 Via natural or artificial opening		
9 Common Bile Duct	8 Via natural or artificial opening endoscopic		
C Ampulla of Vater	X External NC*		
D Pancreatic Duct			
F Pancreatic Duct, Accessory			

NC* – Non-covered by Medicare. See current Medicare Code Editor for details.

DEVICE GROUP: Change, Insertion, Removal, Replacement, Revision, Supplement
Root Operations that always involve a device.

1ST - 0 Medical and Surgical
2ND - F Hepatobiliary System and Pancreas
3RD - H INSERTION

EXAMPLE: Insertion infusion pump pancreas   CMS Ex: CVP catheter

INSERTION: Putting in a nonbiological appliance that monitors, assists, performs, or prevents a physiological function but does not physically take the place of a body part.

EXPLANATION: None

Body Part – 4TH	Approach – 5TH	Device – 6TH	Qualifier – 7TH
0 Liver	0 Open	2 Monitoring device	Z No qualifier
1 Liver, Right Lobe	3 Percutaneous	3 Infusion device	
2 Liver, Left Lobe	4 Percutaneous endoscopic		
4 Gallbladder			
G Pancreas			
B Hepatobiliary Duct	0 Open	1 Radioactive element	Z No qualifier
D Pancreatic Duct	3 Percutaneous	2 Monitoring device	
	4 Percutaneous endoscopic	3 Infusion device	
	7 Via natural or artificial opening	D Intraluminal device	
	8 Via natural or artificial opening endoscopic		

0FJ MEDICAL AND SURGICAL SECTION – 2016 ICD-10-PCS

EXAMINATION GROUP: Inspection, (Map)
Root Operations involving examination only.

- 1ST – **0** Medical and Surgical
- 2ND – **F** Hepatobiliary System and Pancreas
- 3RD – **J** INSPECTION

EXAMPLE: Exploration of common bile duct CMS Ex: Colonoscopy

INSPECTION: Visually and/or manually exploring a body part.

EXPLANATION: Direct or instrumental visualization ...

Body Part – 4TH	Approach – 5TH	Device – 6TH	Qualifier – 7TH
0 Liver 4 Gallbladder G Pancreas	0 Open 3 Percutaneous 4 Percutaneous endoscopic X External	Z No device	Z No qualifier
B Hepatobiliary Duct D Pancreatic Duct	0 Open 3 Percutaneous 4 Percutaneous endoscopic 7 Via natural or artificial opening 8 Via natural or artificial opening endoscopic	Z No device	Z No qualifier

TUBULAR GROUP: Bypass, Dilation, Occlusion, Restriction
Root Operations that alter the diameter/route of a tubular body part.

- 1ST – **0** Medical and Surgical
- 2ND – **F** Hepatobiliary System and Pancreas
- 3RD – **L** OCCLUSION

EXAMPLE: Clipping accessory pancreatic duct CMS Ex: Tubal ligation

OCCLUSION: Completely closing an orifice or lumen of a tubular body part.

EXPLANATION: Natural or artificially created orifice ...

Body Part – 4TH	Approach – 5TH	Device – 6TH	Qualifier – 7TH
5 Hepatic Duct, Right 6 Hepatic Duct, Left 8 Cystic Duct 9 Common Bile Duct C Ampulla of Vater D Pancreatic Duct F Pancreatic Duct, Accessory	0 Open 3 Percutaneous 4 Percutaneous endoscopic	C Extraluminal device D Intraluminal device Z No device	Z No qualifier
5 Hepatic Duct, Right 6 Hepatic Duct, Left 8 Cystic Duct 9 Common Bile Duct C Ampulla of Vater D Pancreatic Duct F Pancreatic Duct, Accessory	7 Via natural or artificial opening 8 Via natural or artificial opening endoscopic	D Intraluminal device Z No device	Z No qualifier

F – HEPATOBILIARY SYSTEM AND PANCREAS 0 F N

MOVE GROUP: Reattachment, Reposition, (Transfer), Transplantation
Root Operations that put in/put back or move some/all of a body part.

- 1ST – **0** Medical and Surgical
- 2ND – **F** Hepatobiliary System and Pancreas
- 3RD – **M REATTACHMENT**

EXAMPLE: Reattachment avulsed pancreas | CMS Ex: Reattachment hand

REATTACHMENT: Putting back in or on all or a portion of a separated body part to its normal location or other suitable location.

EXPLANATION: With/without reconnection of vessels/nerves...

Body Part – 4TH	Approach – 5TH	Device – 6TH	Qualifier – 7TH
0 Liver 1 Liver, Right Lobe 2 Liver, Left Lobe 4 Gallbladder 5 Hepatic Duct, Right 6 Hepatic Duct, Left 8 Cystic Duct 9 Common Bile Duct C Ampulla of Vater D Pancreatic Duct F Pancreatic Duct, Accessory G Pancreas	0 Open 4 Percutaneous endoscopic	Z No device	Z No qualifier

---

DIVISION GROUP: Division, Release
Root Operations involving cutting or separation only.

- 1ST – **0** Medical and Surgical
- 2ND – **F** Hepatobiliary System and Pancreas
- 3RD – **N RELEASE**

EXAMPLE: Lysis adhesions gallbladder | CMS Ex: Carpal tunnel release

RELEASE: Freeing a body part from an abnormal physical constraint by cutting or by the use of force.

EXPLANATION: None of the body part is taken out ...

Body Part – 4TH	Approach – 5TH	Device – 6TH	Qualifier – 7TH
0 Liver 1 Liver, Right Lobe 2 Liver, Left Lobe 4 Gallbladder G Pancreas	0 Open 3 Percutaneous 4 Percutaneous endoscopic	Z No device	Z No qualifier
5 Hepatic Duct, Right 6 Hepatic Duct, Left 8 Cystic Duct 9 Common Bile Duct C Ampulla of Vater D Pancreatic Duct F Pancreatic Duct, Accessory	0 Open 3 Percutaneous 4 Percutaneous endoscopic 7 Via natural or artificial opening 8 Via natural or artificial opening endoscopic	Z No device	Z No qualifier

0 F P   MEDICAL AND SURGICAL SECTION – 2016 ICD-10-PCS

DEVICE GROUP: Change, Insertion, Removal, Replacement, Revision, Supplement
Root Operations that always involve a device.

- 1ST – **0** Medical and Surgical
- 2ND – **F** Hepatobiliary System and Pancreas
- 3RD – **P** REMOVAL

EXAMPLE: Removal drain tube   CMS Ex: Chest tube removal

REMOVAL: Taking out or off a device from a body part.

EXPLANATION: Removal device without reinsertion ...

Body Part – 4TH	Approach – 5TH	Device – 6TH	Qualifier – 7TH
0 Liver	0 Open 3 Percutaneous 4 Percutaneous endoscopic X External	0 Drainage device 2 Monitoring device 3 Infusion device	Z No qualifier
4 Gallbladder G Pancreas	0 Open 3 Percutaneous 4 Percutaneous endoscopic X External	0 Drainage device 2 Monitoring device 3 Infusion device D Intraluminal device	Z No qualifier
B Hepatobiliary Duct D Pancreatic Duct	0 Open 3 Percutaneous 4 Percutaneous endoscopic 7 Via natural or artificial opening 8 Via natural or artificial opening endoscopic	0 Drainage device 1 Radioactive element 2 Monitoring device 3 Infusion device 7 Autologous tissue substitute C Extraluminal device D Intraluminal device J Synthetic substitute K Nonautologous tissue substitute	Z No qualifier
B Hepatobiliary Duct D Pancreatic Duct	X External	0 Drainage device 1 Radioactive element 2 Monitoring device 3 Infusion device D Intraluminal device	Z No qualifier

376

F – HEPATOBILIARY SYSTEM AND PANCREAS — 0FR

OTHER REPAIRS GROUP: (Control), Repair
Root Operations that define other repairs.

- 1ST – **0** Medical and Surgical
- 2ND – **F** Hepatobiliary System and Pancreas
- 3RD – **Q** REPAIR

EXAMPLE: Repair liver laceration
CMS Ex: Suture laceration

REPAIR: Restoring, to the extent possible, a body part to its normal anatomic structure and function.

EXPLANATION: Only when no other root operation applies …

Body Part – 4TH	Approach – 5TH	Device – 6TH	Qualifier – 7TH
0 Liver 1 Liver, Right Lobe 2 Liver, Left Lobe 4 Gallbladder G Pancreas	0 Open 3 Percutaneous 4 Percutaneous endoscopic	Z No device	Z No qualifier
5 Hepatic Duct, Right 6 Hepatic Duct, Left 8 Cystic Duct 9 Common Bile Duct C Ampulla of Vater D Pancreatic Duct F Pancreatic Duct, Accessory	0 Open 3 Percutaneous 4 Percutaneous endoscopic 7 Via natural or artificial opening 8 Via natural or artificial opening endoscopic	Z No device	Z No qualifier

DEVICE GROUP: Change, Insertion, Removal, Replacement, Revision, Supplement
Root Operations that always involve a device.

- 1ST – **0** Medical and Surgical
- 2ND – **F** Hepatobiliary System and Pancreas
- 3RD – **R** REPLACEMENT

EXAMPLE: Hepatic duct replacement
CMS Ex: Total hip

REPLACEMENT: Putting in or on a biological or synthetic material that physically takes the place and/or function of all or a portion of a body part.

EXPLANATION: Includes taking out body part, or eradication…

Body Part – 4TH	Approach – 5TH	Device – 6TH	Qualifier – 7TH
5 Hepatic Duct, Right 6 Hepatic Duct, Left 8 Cystic Duct 9 Common Bile Duct C Ampulla of Vater D Pancreatic Duct F Pancreatic Duct, Accessory	0 Open 4 Percutaneous endoscopic	7 Autologous tissue substitute J Synthetic substitute K Nonautologous tissue substitute	Z No qualifier

0FS

MEDICAL AND SURGICAL SECTION – 2016 ICD-10-PCS

[2016.PCS]

MOVE GROUP: Reattachment, Reposition, (Transfer), Transplantation
Root Operations that put in/put back or move some/all of a body part.

1ST - **0** Medical and Surgical	EXAMPLE: Relocation cystic duct	CMS Ex: Fracture reduction
2ND - **F** Hepatobiliary System and Pancreas	**REPOSITION:** Moving to its normal location, or other suitable location, all or a portion of a body part.	
3RD - **S** REPOSITION	EXPLANATION: May or may not be cut to be moved ...	

Body Part – 4TH	Approach – 5TH	Device – 6TH	Qualifier – 7TH
0 Liver 4 Gallbladder 5 Hepatic Duct, Right 6 Hepatic Duct, Left 8 Cystic Duct 9 Common Bile Duct C Ampulla of Vater D Pancreatic Duct F Pancreatic Duct, Accessory G Pancreas	0 Open 4 Percutaneous endoscopic	Z No device	Z No qualifier

EXCISION GROUP: Excision, Resection, Destruction, (Extraction), (Detachment)
Root Operations that take out some or all of a body part.

1ST - **0** Medical and Surgical	EXAMPLE: Liver lobectomy	CMS Ex: Cholecystectomy
2ND - **F** Hepatobiliary System and Pancreas	**RESECTION:** Cutting out or off, without replacement, all of a body part.	
3RD - **T** RESECTION	EXPLANATION: None	

Body Part – 4TH	Approach – 5TH	Device – 6TH	Qualifier – 7TH
0 Liver 1 Liver, Right Lobe 2 Liver, Left Lobe 4 Gallbladder G Pancreas	0 Open 4 Percutaneous endoscopic	Z No device	Z No qualifier
5 Hepatic Duct, Right 6 Hepatic Duct, Left 8 Cystic Duct 9 Common Bile Duct C Ampulla of Vater D Pancreatic Duct F Pancreatic Duct, Accessory	0 Open 4 Percutaneous endoscopic 7 Via natural or artificial opening 8 Via natural or artificial opening endoscopic	Z No device	Z No qualifier

Hepatobiliary 0FS

F – HEPATOBILIARY SYSTEM AND PANCREAS — 0FV

DEVICE GROUP: Change, Insertion, Removal, Replacement, Revision, Supplement
Root Operations that always involve a device.

- 1ST – **0** Medical and Surgical
- 2ND – **F** Hepatobiliary System and Pancreas
- 3RD – **U SUPPLEMENT**

EXAMPLE: Tissue graft ductal repair | CMS Ex: Hernia repair with mesh

SUPPLEMENT: Putting in or on biological or synthetic material that physically reinforces and/or augments the function of a portion of a body part.

EXPLANATION: Biological material from same individual ...

Body Part – 4TH	Approach – 5TH	Device – 6TH	Qualifier – 7TH
5 Hepatic Duct, Right 6 Hepatic Duct, Left 8 Cystic Duct 9 Common Bile Duct C Ampulla of Vater D Pancreatic Duct F Pancreatic Duct, Accessory	0 Open 3 Percutaneous 4 Percutaneous endoscopic	7 Autologous tissue substitute J Synthetic substitute K Nonautologous tissue substitute	Z No qualifier

TUBULAR GROUP: Bypass, Dilation, Occlusion, Restriction
Root Operations that alter the diameter/route of a tubular body part.

- 1ST – **0** Medical and Surgical
- 2ND – **F** Hepatobiliary System and Pancreas
- 3RD – **V RESTRICTION**

EXAMPLE: Restrictive ductal stent | CMS Ex: Cervical cerclage

RESTRICTION: Partially closing an orifice or the lumen of a tubular body part.

EXPLANATION: Natural or artificially created orifice ...

Body Part – 4TH	Approach – 5TH	Device – 6TH	Qualifier – 7TH
5 Hepatic Duct, Right 6 Hepatic Duct, Left 8 Cystic Duct 9 Common Bile Duct C Ampulla of Vater D Pancreatic Duct F Pancreatic Duct, Accessory	0 Open 3 Percutaneous 4 Percutaneous endoscopic	C Extraluminal device D Intraluminal device Z No device	Z No qualifier
5 Hepatic Duct, Right 6 Hepatic Duct, Left 8 Cystic Duct 9 Common Bile Duct C Ampulla of Vater D Pancreatic Duct F Pancreatic Duct, Accessory	7 Via natural or artificial opening 8 Via natural or artificial opening endoscopic	D Intraluminal device Z No device	Z No qualifier

0 F W — MEDICAL AND SURGICAL SECTION – 2016 ICD-10-PCS

DEVICE GROUP: Change, Insertion, Removal, Replacement, Revision, Supplement
Root Operations that always involve a device.

- 1ST – **0** Medical and Surgical
- 2ND – **F** Hepatobiliary System and Pancreas
- 3RD – **W** REVISION

EXAMPLE: Reposition drainage tube | CMS Ex: Adjustment pacemaker lead

REVISION: Correcting, to the extent possible, a portion of a malfunctioning device or the position of a displaced device.

EXPLANATION: May replace components of a device ...

Body Part – 4TH	Approach – 5TH	Device – 6TH	Qualifier – 7TH
0 Liver	0 Open 3 Percutaneous 4 Percutaneous endoscopic X External	0 Drainage device 2 Monitoring device 3 Infusion device	Z No qualifier
4 Gallbladder G Pancreas	0 Open 3 Percutaneous 4 Percutaneous endoscopic X External	0 Drainage device 2 Monitoring device 3 Infusion device D Intraluminal device	Z No qualifier
B Hepatobiliary Duct D Pancreatic Duct	0 Open 3 Percutaneous 4 Percutaneous endoscopic 7 Via natural or artificial opening 8 Via natural or artificial opening endoscopic X External	0 Drainage device 2 Monitoring device 3 Infusion device 7 Autologous tissue substitute C Extraluminal device D Intraluminal device J Synthetic substitute K Nonautologous tissue substitute	Z No qualifier

MOVE GROUP: Reattachment, Reposition, (Transfer), Transplantation
Root Operations that put in/put back or move some/all of a body part.

- 1ST – **0** Medical and Surgical
- 2ND – **F** Hepatobiliary System and Pancreas
- 3RD – **Y** TRANSPLANTATION

EXAMPLE: Liver transplant | CMS Ex: Kidney transplant

TRANSPLANTATION: Putting in or on all or a portion of a living body part taken from another individual or animal to physically take the place and/or function of all or a portion of a similar body part.

EXPLANATION: May take over all or part of its function ...

Body Part – 4TH	Approach – 5TH	Device – 6TH	Qualifier – 7TH
0 Liver G Pancreas NC*	0 Open	Z No device	0 Allogenic 1 Syngeneic 2 Zooplastic NC*

NC* – Some procedures are considered non-covered by Medicare. See current Medicare Code Editor for details.

Educational Annotations | G – Endocrine System

Body System Specific Educational Annotations for the Endocrine System include:
- Anatomy and Physiology Review
- Anatomical Illustrations
- Definitions of Common Procedures
- AHA Coding Clinic® Reference Notations
- Body Part Key Listings
- Device Key Listings
- Device Aggregation Table Listings
- Coding Notes

Anatomy and Physiology Review of Endocrine System

BODY PART VALUES – G - ENDOCRINE SYSTEM

Adrenal Gland – ANATOMY – The adrenal gland is the highly vascular, pyramid-shaped endocrine gland that sits upon the top of each kidney. PHYSIOLOGY – The adrenal gland produces several important hormones, among them: Adrenalin, noradrenalin, aldosterone, cortisol, and some sex hormones.

Aortic Body – ANATOMY – The aortic body is the small neurovascular structure located at the aortic arch. PHYSIOLOGY – The aortic body monitors and regulates the reflex respiration and blood pressure.

Carotid Body – ANATOMY – The carotid bodies are small neurovascular structures at the carotid bifurcation. PHYSIOLOGY – The carotid bodies function as a blood oxygen, carbon dioxide, and Ph sensor.

Coccygeal Glomus – The coccygeal glomus is a very small (2.5mm), oval mass exocrine gland tissue located beneath the coccyx tip.

Endocrine Gland – A gland that secretes hormones.

Glomus Jugulare – A mass of neuroendocrine cells in the jugular foramen area of the temporal bone near the middle and inner ear.

Para-aortic Body – ANATOMY – The para-aortic body is the small mass of chromaffin tissue located alongside the abdominal aorta. PHYSIOLOGY – The para-aortic body produces catecholamines.

Paraganglion Extremity – Groups of extra-adrenal neuroendocrine cells usually found in the peripheral nervous system that produce adrenaline.

Parathyroid Gland – ANATOMY – The parathyroid glands are 4 small glands, 2 on the posterior surface of the thyroid lobes. PHYSIOLOGY – The parathyroid gland secretes one hormone, the parathyroid hormone which causes an increase in the blood calcium level and a decrease in the blood phosphate level.

Pineal Gland – ANATOMY – The pineal gland is the small endocrine gland located below the posterior base of the corpus callosum, and attached to the upper portion of the thalamus. PHYSIOLOGY – The pineal gland produces the hormone melatonin.

Pituitary Gland – ANATOMY – The pituitary gland is the small endocrine gland with two lobes located in the sella turcica of the sphenoid bone at the base of the cerebrum, and is about 0.4 inches (1 cm) in diameter. PHYSIOLOGY – The pituitary gland functions as the central endocrine gland by producing hormones which stimulate many of the other endocrine glands, and has two lobes. The anterior lobe (adenohypophysis) produces the growth hormone (prolactin), thyroid-stimulating hormone, follicle-stimulating and luteinizing hormones, and adrenocorticotropic hormone. The posterior lobe (neurohypophysis) secretes the antidiuretic hormone and oxytocin.

Thyroid Gland – ANATOMY – The thyroid gland is the bi-lobed endocrine gland of the front of the neck and is connected by a narrow isthmus. PHYSIOLOGY – The thyroid gland produces the hormones thyroxine and triiodothyronine that help to regulate the metabolic rate of the body.

Thyroid Gland Isthmus – The narrow, middle portion connecting the two thyroid lobes.

Educational Annotations | G – Endocrine System

Anatomical Illustrations of Endocrine System

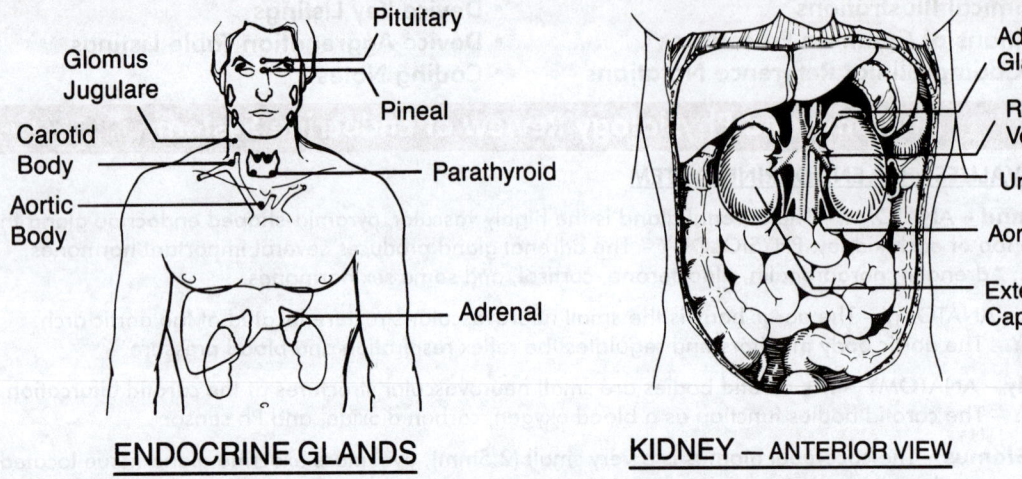

ENDOCRINE GLANDS

KIDNEY — ANTERIOR VIEW

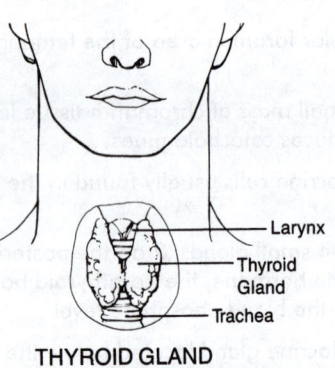

THYROID GLAND

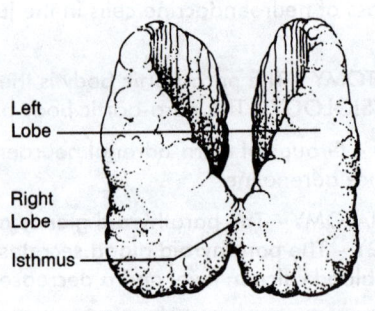

THYROID GLAND — ANTERIOR (DETAIL) VIEW

Definitions of Common Procedures of Endocrine System

Adrenalectomy – The surgical removal of one or both of the adrenal glands.

Hypophysectomy – The surgical removal of the pituitary gland (hypophysis).

Thyroid lobectomy – The surgical removal of one of the two lobes of the thyroid.

Total thyroidectomy – The surgical removal of both lobes and the isthmus of the thyroid.

Educational Annotations | G – Endocrine System

AHA Coding Clinic® Reference Notations of Endocrine System

ROOT OPERATION SPECIFIC - G - ENDOCRINE SYSTEM
CHANGE - 2
DESTRUCTION - 5
DIVISION - 8
DRAINAGE - 9
EXCISION - B
    Removal of pituitary tumor ....AHA 14:3Q:p22
EXTIRPATION - C
INSERTION - H
INSPECTION - J
REATTACHMENT - M
RELEASE - N
REMOVAL - P
REPAIR - Q
REPOSITION - S
RESECTION - T
REVISION - W

Body Part Key Listings of Endocrine System

See also Body Part Key in Appendix C

Adenohypophysis	*use* Pituitary Gland
Carotid glomus	*use* Carotid Body, Bilateral/Left/Right
Coccygeal body	*use* Coccygeal Glomus
Hypophysis	*use* Pituitary Gland
Jugular body	*use* Glomus Jugulare
Neurohypophysis	*use* Pituitary Gland
Suprarenal gland	*use* Adrenal Gland, Bilateral/Left/Right

Device Key Listings of Endocrine System

See also Device Key in Appendix D

Autograft	*use* Autologous Tissue Substitute
Tissue bank graft	*use* Nonautologous Tissue Substitute

Device Aggregation Table Listings of Endocrine System

See also Device Aggregation Table in Appendix E

Specific Device	For Operation	In Body System	General Device
None Listed in Device Aggregation Table for this Body System			

G – Endocrine System

Educational Annotations

Coding Notes of Endocrine System

Body System Specific PCS Reference Manual Exercises

PCS CODE	G – ENDOCRINE SYSTEM EXERCISES
0GT00ZZ	Total excision of pituitary gland, open.

Removal of pituitary tumor...AHA 14:3Q;22

G – ENDOCRINE SYSTEM   0G5

DEVICE GROUP: Change, Insertion, Removal, (Replacement), Revision, (Supplement)
Root Operations that always involve a device.

1ST - 0 Medical and Surgical
2ND - G Endocrine System
3RD - 2 CHANGE

EXAMPLE: Exchange drain tube   CMS Ex: Changing urinary catheter

CHANGE: Taking out or off a device from a body part and putting back an identical or similar device in or on the same body part without cutting or puncturing the skin or a mucous membrane.

EXPLANATION: ALL Changes use EXTERNAL approach only...

Body Part – 4TH	Approach – 5TH	Device – 6TH	Qualifier – 7TH
0 Pituitary Gland	X External	0 Drainage device	Z No qualifier
1 Pineal Body		Y Other device	
5 Adrenal Gland			
K Thyroid Gland			
R Parathyroid Gland			
S Endocrine Gland			

EXCISION GROUP: Excision, Resection, Destruction, (Extraction), (Detachment)
Root Operations that take out some or all of a body part.

1ST - 0 Medical and Surgical
2ND - G Endocrine System
3RD - 5 DESTRUCTION

EXAMPLE: Radiofrequency ablation   CMS Ex: Fulguration polyp

DESTRUCTION: Physical eradication of all or a portion of a body part by the direct use of energy, force, or a destructive agent.

EXPLANATION: None of the body part is physically taken out

Body Part – 4TH		Approach – 5TH	Device – 6TH	Qualifier – 7TH
0 Pituitary Gland	G Thyroid Gland Lobe, Left	0 Open	Z No device	Z No qualifier
1 Pineal Body	H Thyroid Gland Lobe, Right	3 Percutaneous		
2 Adrenal Gland, Left	K Thyroid Gland	4 Percutaneous endoscopic		
3 Adrenal Gland, Right	L Superior Parathyroid Gland, Right			
4 Adrenal Glands, Bilateral	M Superior Parathyroid Gland, Left			
6 Carotid Body, Left	N Inferior Parathyroid Gland, Right			
7 Carotid Body, Right	P Inferior Parathyroid Gland, Left			
8 Carotid Bodies, Bilateral	Q Parathyroid Glands, Multiple			
9 Para-aortic Body	R Parathyroid Gland			
B Coccygeal Glomus				
C Glomus Jugulare				
D Aortic Body				
F Paraganglion Extremity				

0 G 8

MEDICAL AND SURGICAL SECTION – 2016 ICD-10-PCS

[2016.PCS]

DIVISION GROUP: Division, Release
Root Operations involving cutting or separation only.

1ST - **0** Medical and Surgical
2ND - **G** Endocrine System
3RD - **8 DIVISION**

EXAMPLE: Transection thyroid isthmus **CMS Ex:** Osteotomy

DIVISION: Cutting into a body part without draining fluids and/or gases from the body part in order to separate or transect a body part.

EXPLANATION: Separated into two or more portions ...

Body Part – 4TH	Approach – 5TH	Device – 6TH	Qualifier – 7TH
0 Pituitary Gland J Thyroid Gland Isthmus	0 Open 3 Percutaneous 4 Percutaneous endoscopic	Z No device	Z No qualifier

DRAINAGE GROUP: Drainage, Extirpation, (Fragmentation)
Root Operations that take out solids/fluids/gases from a body part.

1ST - **0** Medical and Surgical
2ND - **G** Endocrine System
3RD - **9 DRAINAGE**

EXAMPLE: Needle aspiration adrenal abscess **CMS Ex:** Thoracentesis

DRAINAGE: Taking or letting out fluids and/or gases from a body part.

EXPLANATION: Qualifier "X Diagnostic" indicates biopsy ...

Body Part – 4TH		Approach – 5TH	Device – 6TH	Qualifier – 7TH
0 Pituitary Gland 1 Pineal Body 2 Adrenal Gland, Left 3 Adrenal Gland, Right 4 Adrenal Glands, Bilateral 6 Carotid Body, Left 7 Carotid Body, Right 8 Carotid Bodies, Bilateral 9 Para-aortic Body B Coccygeal Glomus C Glomus Jugulare D Aortic Body F Paraganglion Extremity	G Thyroid Gland Lobe, Left H Thyroid Gland Lobe, Right K Thyroid Gland L Superior Parathyroid Gland, Right M Superior Parathyroid Gland, Left N Inferior Parathyroid Gland, Right P Inferior Parathyroid Gland, Left Q Parathyroid Glands, Multiple R Parathyroid Gland	0 Open 3 Percutaneous 4 Percutaneous endoscopic	0 Drainage device	Z No qualifier
0 Pituitary Gland 1 Pineal Body 2 Adrenal Gland, Left 3 Adrenal Gland, Right 4 Adrenal Glands, Bilateral 6 Carotid Body, Left 7 Carotid Body, Right 8 Carotid Bodies, Bilateral 9 Para-aortic Body B Coccygeal Glomus C Glomus Jugulare D Aortic Body F Paraganglion Extremity	G Thyroid Gland Lobe, Left H Thyroid Gland Lobe, Right K Thyroid Gland L Superior Parathyroid Gland, Right M Superior Parathyroid Gland, Left N Inferior Parathyroid Gland, Right P Inferior Parathyroid Gland, Left Q Parathyroid Glands, Multiple R Parathyroid Gland	0 Open 3 Percutaneous 4 Percutaneous endoscopic	Z No device	X Diagnostic Z No qualifier

G – ENDOCRINE SYSTEM 0GC

EXCISION GROUP: Excision, Resection, Destruction, (Extraction), (Detachment)
Root Operations that take out some or all of a body part.

- 1ST – **0** Medical and Surgical
- 2ND – **G** Endocrine System
- 3RD – **B EXCISION**

EXAMPLE: Needle biopsy parathyroid gland   **CMS Ex:** Liver biopsy

EXCISION: Cutting out or off, without replacement, a portion of a body part.

EXPLANATION: Qualifier "X Diagnostic" indicates biopsy …

Body Part – 4TH	Approach – 5TH	Device – 6TH	Qualifier – 7TH
0 Pituitary Gland	0 Open	Z No device	X Diagnostic
1 Pineal Body	3 Percutaneous		Z No qualifier
2 Adrenal Gland, Left	4 Percutaneous endoscopic		
3 Adrenal Gland, Right			
4 Adrenal Glands, Bilateral			
6 Carotid Body, Left			
7 Carotid Body, Right			
8 Carotid Bodies, Bilateral			
9 Para-aortic Body			
B Coccygeal Glomus			
C Glomus Jugulare			
D Aortic Body			
F Paraganglion Extremity			
G Thyroid Gland Lobe, Left			
H Thyroid Gland Lobe, Right			
L Superior Parathyroid Gland, Right			
M Superior Parathyroid Gland, Left			
N Inferior Parathyroid Gland, Right			
P Inferior Parathyroid Gland, Left			
Q Parathyroid Glands, Multiple			
R Parathyroid Gland			

DRAINAGE GROUP: Drainage, Extirpation, (Fragmentation)
Root Operations that take out solids/fluids/gases from a body part.

- 1ST – **0** Medical and Surgical
- 2ND – **G** Endocrine System
- 3RD – **C EXTIRPATION**

EXAMPLE: Removal foreign body   **CMS Ex:** Choledocholithotomy

EXTIRPATION: Taking or cutting out solid matter from a body part.

EXPLANATION: Abnormal byproduct or foreign body …

Body Part – 4TH	Approach – 5TH	Device – 6TH	Qualifier – 7TH
0 Pituitary Gland	0 Open	Z No device	Z No qualifier
1 Pineal Body	3 Percutaneous		
2 Adrenal Gland, Left	4 Percutaneous endoscopic		
3 Adrenal Gland, Right			
4 Adrenal Glands, Bilateral			
6 Carotid Body, Left			
7 Carotid Body, Right			
8 Carotid Bodies, Bilateral			
9 Para-aortic Body			
B Coccygeal Glomus			
C Glomus Jugulare			
D Aortic Body			
F Paraganglion Extremity			
G Thyroid Gland Lobe, Left			
H Thyroid Gland Lobe, Right			
K Thyroid Gland			
L Superior Parathyroid Gland, Right			
M Superior Parathyroid Gland, Left			
N Inferior Parathyroid Gland, Right			
P Inferior Parathyroid Gland, Left			
Q Parathyroid Glands, Multiple			
R Parathyroid Gland			

0 G H — MEDICAL AND SURGICAL SECTION – 2016 ICD-10-PCS

DEVICE GROUP: Change, Insertion, Removal, (Replacement), Revision, (Supplement)
Root Operations that always involve a device.

- **1ST - 0** Medical and Surgical
- **2ND - G** Endocrine System
- **3RD - H** INSERTION

EXAMPLE: Insertion infusion device   CMS Ex: Insertion CV catheter

INSERTION: Putting in a nonbiological appliance that monitors, assists, performs, or prevents a physiological function but does not physically take the place of a body part.

EXPLANATION: None

Body Part – 4TH	Approach – 5TH	Device – 6TH	Qualifier – 7TH
S Endocrine Gland	0 Open 3 Percutaneous 4 Percutaneous endoscopic	2 Monitoring device 3 Infusion device	Z No qualifier

EXAMINATION GROUP: Inspection, (Map)
Root Operations involving examination only.

- **1ST - 0** Medical and Surgical
- **2ND - G** Endocrine System
- **3RD - J** INSPECTION

EXAMPLE: Examination adrenal gland   CMS Ex: Colonoscopy

INSPECTION: Visually and/or manually exploring a body part.

EXPLANATION: Direct or instrumental visualization ...

Body Part – 4TH		Approach – 5TH	Device – 6TH	Qualifier – 7TH
0 Pituitary Gland 1 Pineal Body 5 Adrenal Gland	K Thyroid Gland R Parathyroid Gland S Endocrine Gland	0 Open 3 Percutaneous 4 Percutaneous endoscopic	Z No device	Z No qualifier

MOVE GROUP: Reattachment, Reposition, (Transfer), (Transplantation)
Root Operations that put in/put back or move some/all of a body part.

- **1ST - 0** Medical and Surgical
- **2ND - G** Endocrine System
- **3RD - M** REATTACHMENT

EXAMPLE: Reattachment thyroid   CMS Ex: Reattachment hand

REATTACHMENT: Putting back in or on all or a portion of a separated body part to its normal location or other suitable location.

EXPLANATION: With/without reconnection of vessels/nerves...

Body Part – 4TH	Approach – 5TH	Device – 6TH	Qualifier – 7TH
2 Adrenal Gland, Left 3 Adrenal Gland, Right G Thyroid Gland Lobe, Left H Thyroid Gland Lobe, Right L Superior Parathyroid Gland, Right M Superior Parathyroid Gland, Left N Inferior Parathyroid Gland, Right P Inferior Parathyroid Gland, Left Q Parathyroid Glands, Multiple R Parathyroid Gland	0 Open 4 Percutaneous endoscopic	Z No device	Z No qualifier

G – ENDOCRINE SYSTEM

0GP

DIVISION GROUP: Division, Release
Root Operations involving cutting or separation only.

- 1ST – **0** Medical and Surgical
- 2ND – **G** Endocrine System
- 3RD – **N** RELEASE

EXAMPLE: Adhesiolysis adrenal gland   CMS Ex: Carpal tunnel release

RELEASE: Freeing a body part from an abnormal physical constraint by cutting or by the use of force.

EXPLANATION: None of the body part is taken out ...

Body Part – 4TH		Approach – 5TH	Device – 6TH	Qualifier – 7TH
0 Pituitary Gland	G Thyroid Gland Lobe, Left	0 Open	Z No device	Z No qualifier
1 Pineal Body	H Thyroid Gland Lobe, Right	3 Percutaneous		
2 Adrenal Gland, Left	K Thyroid Gland	4 Percutaneous endoscopic		
3 Adrenal Gland, Right	L Superior Parathyroid Gland, Right			
4 Adrenal Glands, Bilateral	M Superior Parathyroid Gland, Left			
6 Carotid Body, Left	N Inferior Parathyroid Gland, Right			
7 Carotid Body, Right	P Inferior Parathyroid Gland, Left			
8 Carotid Bodies, Bilateral	Q Parathyroid Glands, Multiple			
9 Para-aortic Body	R Parathyroid Gland			
B Coccygeal Glomus				
C Glomus Jugulare				
D Aortic Body				
F Paraganglion Extremity				

DEVICE GROUP: Change, Insertion, Removal, (Replacement), Revision, (Supplement)
Root Operations that always involve a device.

- 1ST – **0** Medical and Surgical
- 2ND – **G** Endocrine System
- 3RD – **P** REMOVAL

EXAMPLE: Removal drain tube   CMS Ex: Chest tube removal

REMOVAL: Taking out or off a device from a body part.

EXPLANATION: Removal device without reinsertion ...

Body Part – 4TH	Approach – 5TH	Device – 6TH	Qualifier – 7TH
0 Pituitary Gland	0 Open	0 Drainage device	Z No qualifier
1 Pineal Body	3 Percutaneous		
5 Adrenal Gland	4 Percutaneous endoscopic		
K Thyroid Gland	X External		
R Parathyroid Gland			
S Endocrine Gland	0 Open	0 Drainage device	Z No qualifier
	3 Percutaneous	2 Monitoring device	
	4 Percutaneous endoscopic	3 Infusion device	
	X External		

0GQ MEDICAL AND SURGICAL SECTION – 2016 ICD-10-PCS

OTHER REPAIRS GROUP: (Control), Repair
Root Operations that define other repairs.

- 1ST – **0** Medical and Surgical
- 2ND – **G** Endocrine System
- 3RD – **Q REPAIR**

EXAMPLE: Suture thyroid laceration   CMS Ex: Suture laceration

REPAIR: Restoring, to the extent possible, a body part to its normal anatomic structure and function.

EXPLANATION: Only when no other root operation applies …

Body Part – 4TH		Approach – 5TH	Device – 6TH	Qualifier – 7TH
0 Pituitary Gland	J Thyroid Gland Isthmus	0 Open	Z No device	Z No qualifier
1 Pineal Body	K Thyroid Gland	3 Percutaneous		
2 Adrenal Gland, Left	L Superior Parathyroid Gland, Right	4 Percutaneous endoscopic		
3 Adrenal Gland, Right				
4 Adrenal Glands, Bilateral	M Superior Parathyroid Gland, Left			
6 Carotid Body, Left				
7 Carotid Body, Right	N Inferior Parathyroid Gland, Right			
8 Carotid Bodies, Bilateral				
9 Para-aortic Body	P Inferior Parathyroid Gland, Left			
B Coccygeal Glomus				
C Glomus Jugulare	Q Parathyroid Glands, Multiple			
D Aortic Body				
F Paraganglion Extremity	R Parathyroid Gland			
G Thyroid Gland Lobe, Left				
H Thyroid Gland Lobe, Right				

MOVE GROUP: Reattachment, Reposition, (Transfer), (Transplantation)
Root Operations that put in/put back or move some/all of a body part.

- 1ST – **0** Medical and Surgical
- 2ND – **G** Endocrine System
- 3RD – **S REPOSITION**

EXAMPLE: Relocation parathyroid glands   CMS Ex: Fracture reduction

REPOSITION: Moving to its normal location, or other suitable location, all or a portion of a body part.

EXPLANATION: May or may not be cut to be moved …

Body Part – 4TH		Approach – 5TH	Device – 6TH	Qualifier – 7TH
2 Adrenal Gland, Left	Q Parathyroid Glands, Multiple	0 Open	Z No device	Z No qualifier
3 Adrenal Gland, Right		4 Percutaneous endoscopic		
G Thyroid Gland Lobe, Left	R Parathyroid Gland			
H Thyroid Gland Lobe, Right				
L Superior Parathyroid Gland, Right				
M Superior Parathyroid Gland, Left				
N Inferior Parathyroid Gland, Right				
P Inferior Parathyroid Gland, Left				

G – ENDOCRINE SYSTEM — 0GW

EXCISION GROUP: Excision, Resection, Destruction, (Extraction), (Detachment)
Root Operations that take out some or all of a body part.

- 1ST – **0** Medical and Surgical
- 2ND – **G** Endocrine System
- 3RD – **T** RESECTION

EXAMPLE: Thyroid lobectomy
CMS Ex: Cholecystectomy

RESECTION: Cutting out or off, without replacement, all of a body part.

EXPLANATION: None

Body Part – 4TH		Approach – 5TH	Device – 6TH	Qualifier – 7TH
0 Pituitary Gland	G Thyroid Gland Lobe, Left	0 Open	Z No device	Z No qualifier
1 Pineal Body	H Thyroid Gland Lobe, Right	4 Percutaneous endoscopic		
2 Adrenal Gland, Left	K Thyroid Gland			
3 Adrenal Gland, Right	L Superior Parathyroid Gland, Right			
4 Adrenal Glands, Bilateral				
6 Carotid Body, Left	M Superior Parathyroid Gland, Left			
7 Carotid Body, Right				
8 Carotid Bodies, Bilateral	N Inferior Parathyroid Gland, Right			
9 Para-aortic Body				
B Coccygeal Glomus	P Inferior Parathyroid Gland, Left			
C Glomus Jugulare				
D Aortic Body	Q Parathyroid Glands, Multiple			
F Paraganglion Extremity				
	R Parathyroid Gland			

DEVICE GROUP: Change, Insertion, Removal, (Replacement), Revision, (Supplement)
Root Operations that always involve a device.

- 1ST – **0** Medical and Surgical
- 2ND – **G** Endocrine System
- 3RD – **W** REVISION

EXAMPLE: Reposition drainage tube
CMS Ex: Adjustment pacemaker lead

REVISION: Correcting, to the extent possible, a portion of a malfunctioning device or the position of a displaced device.

EXPLANATION: May replace components of a device ...

Body Part – 4TH	Approach – 5TH	Device – 6TH	Qualifier – 7TH
0 Pituitary Gland 1 Pineal Body 5 Adrenal Gland K Thyroid Gland R Parathyroid Gland	0 Open 3 Percutaneous 4 Percutaneous endoscopic X External	0 Drainage device	Z No qualifier
S Endocrine Gland	0 Open 3 Percutaneous 4 Percutaneous endoscopic X External	0 Drainage device 2 Monitoring device 3 Infusion device	Z No qualifier

0GW

MEDICAL AND SURGICAL SECTION – 2016 ICD-10-PCS

NOTES

1st 0 Medical and Surgical
2nd G Endocrine System
3rd T RESECTION

EXCISION GROUP: Excision, Resection, Destruction, Extirpation, Extraction
Root Operations that take out some or all of a body part

RESECTION: Cutting out or off, without replacement, all of a body part

EXPLANATION: None

EXAMPLE: Thyroid lobectomy

Body Part – 4th	Approach – 5th	Device – 6th	Qualifier – 7th
0 Pituitary Gland	0 Open	Z No device	Z No qualifier
1 Pineal Body	4 Percutaneous endoscopic		
2 Adrenal Gland, Left			
3 Adrenal Gland, Right			
4 Adrenal Glands, Bilateral			
6 Carotid Body, Left			
7 Carotid Body, Right			
8 Carotid Bodies, Bilateral			
9 Para-aortic Body			
B Coccygeal Glomus			
C Glomus Jugulare			
D Aortic Body			
F Paraganglion Extremity			
G Thyroid Gland Lobe, Left			
H Thyroid Gland Lobe, Right			
K Thyroid Gland			
L Superior Parathyroid Gland, Right			
M Superior Parathyroid Gland, Left			
N Inferior Parathyroid Gland, Right			
P Inferior Parathyroid Gland, Left			
Q Parathyroid Glands, Multiple			
R Parathyroid Gland			

1st 0 Medical and Surgical
2nd G Endocrine System
3rd W REVISION

DEVICE GROUP: Change, Insertion, Removal, Replacement, Revision, Supplement
Root Operations that always involve a device

REVISION: Correcting, to the extent possible, a portion of a malfunctioning device or the position of a displaced device

EXPLANATION: May replace components of a device

EXAMPLE: Reposition drainage tube, Adjustment pacemaker lead

Body Part – 4th	Approach – 5th	Device – 6th	Qualifier – 7th
0 Pituitary Gland	0 Open	0 Drainage device	Z No qualifier
1 Pineal Body	3 Percutaneous		
5 Adrenal Gland	4 Percutaneous endoscopic		
K Thyroid Gland	X External		
R Parathyroid Gland			
S Endocrine Gland	0 Open	0 Drainage device	Z No qualifier
	3 Percutaneous	2 Monitoring device	
	4 Percutaneous endoscopic	3 Infusion device	
	X External		

ENDOCRINE 0G

Educational Annotations | H – Skin and Breast

Body System Specific Educational Annotations for the Skin and Breast include:
- Anatomy and Physiology Review
- Anatomical Illustrations
- Definitions of Common Procedures
- AHA Coding Clinic® Reference Notations
- Body Part Key Listings
- Device Key Listings
- Device Aggregation Table Listings
- Coding Notes

Anatomy and Physiology Review of Skin and Breast

BODY PART VALUES – H - SKIN AND BREAST

Breast, Female – ANATOMY – The female breast is the modified cutaneous glandular cone-shaped prominence overlying the pectoral muscles on the anterior chest, and contains the milk-producing mammary glands. PHYSIOLOGY – The female breast functions to secrete nourishing milk for the newborn. During pregnancy, hormones increase the size of the mammary glands, and following delivery, the pituitary gland secretes prolactin, which stimulates the mammary glands to produce milk. The mammary ducts convey the milk to the nipple.

Breast, Male – ANATOMY – The male breast is the modified cutaneous glandular structure overlying the pectoral muscles of the anterior chest. PHYSIOLOGY – The male breast fails to develop due to the lack of ovarian hormones.

Finger Nail – ANATOMY – The tough keratin covering of the top and end of the fingers. PHYSIOLOGY – The nail functions to protect the end of the finger.

Hair – ANATOMY – Hair is a threadlike structure that grows from follicles found in the dermis and is made of protein. PHYSIOLOGY – Hair serves multiple functions depending on location, including: Sensory transmission, heat retention, skin protection, and protection from particles and organisms.

Nipple – ANATOMY – The nipple is the pigmented projection of the breast and contains the ends of the mammary ducts. The areola is the circular pigmented area around the nipple.

Skin – ANATOMY – The skin is the outer covering of the body, consisting of the epidermis and dermis, that rests upon the subcutaneous tissue. The epidermis is the outermost layer of the skin which develops keratin, a tough, fibrous waterproof protein, and lacks blood vessels. The dermis is the tough, elastic vascular connective tissue layer of the skin which contains the sebaceous and sweat glands. PHYSIOLOGY – The skin functions to protect the body from invading microorganisms, limits the loss of water from deep tissues, assists homeostasis, aids in the regulation of body temperature, acts as the sense organ for the cutaneous senses, and is a source of vitamin D when it is exposed to light.

Supernumerary Breast – The presence of an additional breast (accessory breast) that may or may not have an associated areola and nipple.

Toe Nail – ANATOMY – The tough keratin covering of the top and end of the toes. PHYSIOLOGY – The nail functions to protect the end of the toe.

Anatomical Illustrations of Skin and Breast

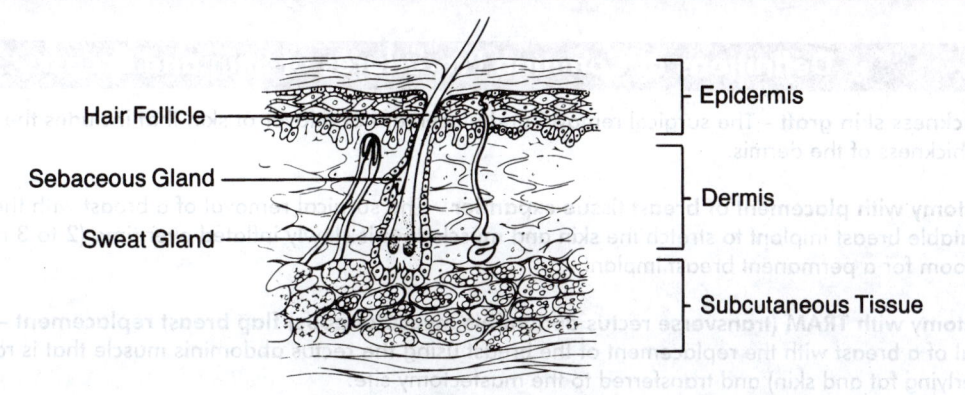

SKIN

Continued on next page

0H — Skin and Breast

Educational Annotations

Anatomical Illustrations of Skin and Breast

Continued from previous page

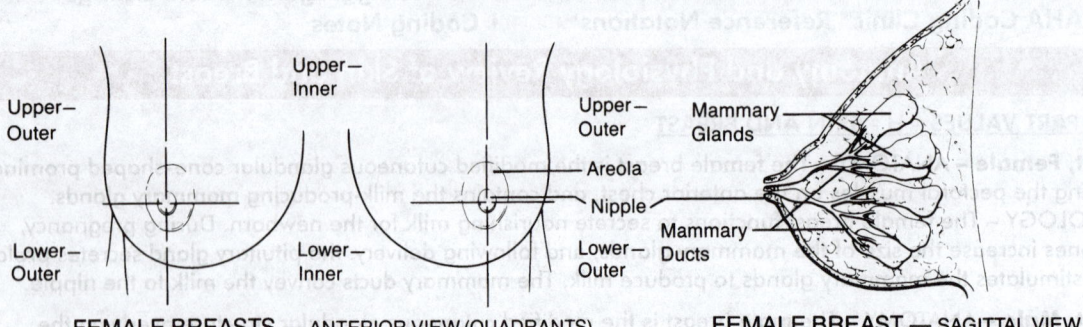

FEMALE BREASTS — ANTERIOR VIEW (QUADRANTS): Upper-Outer, Upper-Inner, Lower-Outer, Lower-Inner, Areola, Nipple

FEMALE BREAST — SAGITTAL VIEW: Mammary Glands, Mammary Ducts

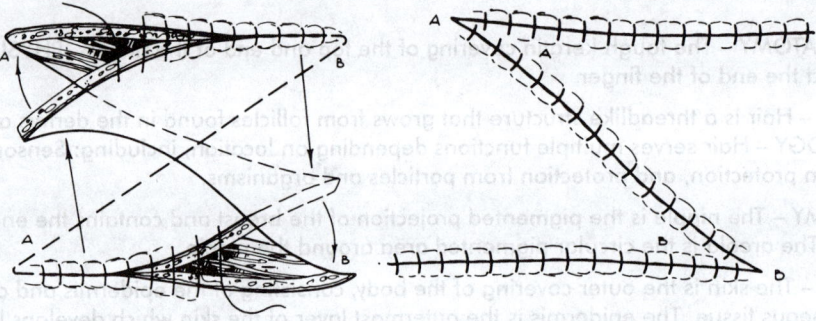

Z-PLASTY — Stage I • Z-PLASTY — Stage II

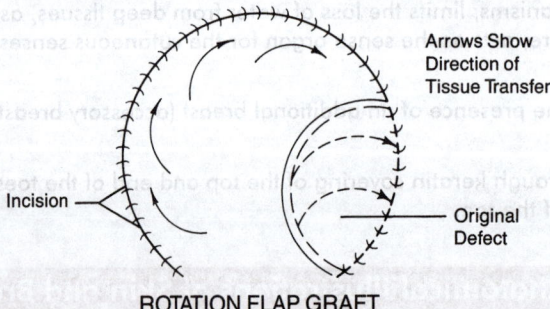

ROTATION FLAP GRAFT — Incision, Original Defect, Arrows Show Direction of Tissue Transfer

Definitions of Common Procedures of Skin and Breast

Full-thickness skin graft – The surgical removal and placement of a layer of skin that includes the epidermis and entire thickness of the dermis.

Mastectomy with placement of breast tissue expander – The surgical removal of a breast with the placement of an inflatable breast implant to stretch the skin and muscle that is slowly inflated over time (2 to 3 months) to make room for a permanent breast implant.

Mastectomy with TRAM (transverse rectus abdominis myocutaneous) flap breast replacement – The surgical removal of a breast with the replacement of the breast using the rectus abdominis muscle that is raised (including the overlying fat and skin) and transferred to the mastectomy site.

Split-thickness skin graft – The surgical removal and placement of a layer of skin that includes the epidermis and part of the dermis.

Educational Annotations | H – Skin and Breast

AHA Coding Clinic® Reference Notations of Skin and Breast

ROOT OPERATION SPECIFIC - H - SKIN AND BREAST
ALTERATION - 0
CHANGE - 2
DESTRUCTION - 5
DIVISION - 8
DRAINAGE - 9
EXCISION - B
EXTIRPATION - C
EXTRACTION - D
INSERTION - H
    Bilateral breast tissue expanders .... AHA 14:2Q:p12
    Breast tissue expander using acellular dermal matrix .... AHA 13:4Q:p107
INSPECTION - J
REATTACHMENT - M
RELEASE - N
REMOVAL - P
REPAIR - Q
    Delayed closure of wound using skin clips .... AHA 14:4Q:p31
REPLACEMENT - R
    Application of TheraSkin® .... AHA 14:3Q:p14
    Biologically derived skin substitutes .... AHA 14:2Q:p5
REPOSITION - S
RESECTION - T
    Skin-sparing mastectomy .... AHA 14:4Q:p34
SUPPLEMENT - U
REVISION - W
TRANSFER - X

Body Part Key Listings of Skin and Breast

See also Body Part Key in Appendix C
Areola .... *use* Nipple, Left/Right
Dermis .... *use* Skin
Epidermis .... *use* Skin
Mammary duct .... *use* Breast, Bilateral/Left/Right
Mammary gland .... *use* Breast, Bilateral/Left/Right
Nail bed, Nail plate .... *use* Finger Nail, Toe Nail
Sebaceous gland .... *use* Skin
Sweat gland .... *use* Skin

0H

MEDICAL AND SURGICAL SECTION – 2016 ICD-10-PCS

Educational Annotations | H – Skin and Breast

Device Key Listings of Skin and Breast

See also Device Key in Appendix D

Acellular Hydrated Dermis	*use* Nonautologous Tissue Substitute
Autograft	*use* Autologous Tissue Substitute
Blood glucose monitoring system	*use* Monitoring Device
Brachytherapy seeds	*use* Radioactive Element
Continuous Glucose Monitoring (CGM) device	*use* Monitoring Device
Cultured epidermal cell autograft	*use* Autologous Tissue Substitute
Epicel® cultured epidermal autograft	*use* Autologous Tissue Substitute
Implantable glucose monitoring device	*use* Monitoring Device
Tissue bank graft	*use* Nonautologous Tissue Substitute
Tissue expander (inflatable) (injectable)	*use* Tissue Expander in Skin and Breast

Device Aggregation Table Listings of Skin and Breast

See also Device Aggregation Table in Appendix E

Specific Device	For Operation	In Body System	General Device
None Listed in Device Aggregation Table for this Body System			

Coding Notes of Skin and Breast

Body System Relevant Coding Guidelines

Skin, subcutaneous tissue and fascia overlying a joint

B4.6

If a procedure is performed on the skin, subcutaneous tissue or fascia overlying a joint, the procedure is coded to the following body part:
- Shoulder is coded to Upper Arm
- Elbow is coded to Lower Arm
- Wrist is coded to Lower Arm
- Hip is coded to Upper Leg
- Knee is coded to Lower Leg
- Ankle is coded to Foot

Body System Specific PCS Reference Manual Exercises

PCS CODE	H – SKIN AND BREAST EXERCISES
0H0V0JZ	Bilateral breast augmentation with silicone implants, open.
0H5GXZZ	Cryotherapy of wart on left hand.
0HB2XZZ	Excision of malignant melanoma from skin of right ear.
0HCGXZZ	Foreign body removal, skin of left thumb. (There is no specific value for thumb skin, so the procedure is coded to the hand.)
0HDMXZZ	Non-excisional debridement of skin ulcer, right foot.
0HDQXZZ	Removal of left thumbnail. (No separate body part value is given for thumbnail, so this is coded to Fingernail.)
0HM0XZZ	Replantation of avulsed scalp.
0HNDXZZ	Incision of scar contracture, right elbow. (The skin of the elbow region is coded to the lower arm.)
0HRDX73	Full-thickness skin graft to right lower arm, autograft (graft harvest not coded for this exercise example).
0HRV076	Bilateral mastectomy with free TRAM flap reconstruction.
0HRV0JZ	Bilateral mastectomy with concomitant saline breast implants, open.

Continued on next page

H – Skin and Breast

Educational Annotations

Continued from previous page

0HTT0ZZ Right total mastectomy, open.
0HX0XZZ Right scalp advancement flap to right temple.
0HX6XZZ Skin transfer flap closure of complex open wound, left lower back.

H – Skin and Breast

Educational Annotations

NOTES

H – SKIN AND BREAST 0H2

OTHER OBJECTIVES GROUP: Alteration, (Creation), (Fusion)
Root Operations that define other objectives.

- 1ST - **0** Medical and Surgical
- 2ND - **H** Skin and Breast
- 3RD - **0 ALTERATION**

EXAMPLE: Breast augmentation with implants CMS Ex: Face lift

ALTERATION: Modifying the anatomic structure of a body part without affecting the function of the body part.

EXPLANATION: Principal purpose is to improve appearance

Body Part – 4TH	Approach – 5TH	Device – 6TH	Qualifier – 7TH
T Breast, Right U Breast, Left V Breast, Bilateral	0 Open 3 Percutaneous X External	7 Autologous tissue substitute J Synthetic substitute K Nonautologous tissue substitute Z No device	Z No qualifier

DEVICE GROUP: Change, Insertion, Removal, Replacement, Revision, Supplement
Root Operations that always involve a device.

- 1ST - **0** Medical and Surgical
- 2ND - **H** Skin and Breast
- 3RD - **2 CHANGE**

EXAMPLE: Exchange drain tube CMS Ex: Changing urinary catheter

CHANGE: Taking out or off a device from a body part and putting back an identical or similar device in or on the same body part without cutting or puncturing the skin or a mucous membrane.

EXPLANATION: ALL Changes use EXTERNAL approach only …

Body Part – 4TH	Approach – 5TH	Device – 6TH	Qualifier – 7TH
P Skin T Breast, Right U Breast, Left	X External	0 Drainage device Y Other device	Z No qualifier

0H5

MEDICAL AND SURGICAL SECTION – 2016 ICD-10-PCS

EXCISION GROUP: Excision, Resection, Destruction, Extraction, (Detachment)
Root Operations that take out some or all of a body part.

- 1ST – **0** Medical and Surgical
- 2ND – **H** Skin and Breast
- 3RD – **5 DESTRUCTION**

EXAMPLE: Cryoablation skin lesion CMS Ex: Fulguration polyp

DESTRUCTION: Physical eradication of all or a portion of a body part by the direct use of energy, force, or a destructive agent.

EXPLANATION: None of the body part is physically taken out

Body Part – 4TH		Approach – 5TH	Device – 6TH	Qualifier – 7TH
0 Skin, Scalp	B Skin, Right Upper Arm	X External	Z No device	D Multiple
1 Skin, Face	C Skin, Left Upper Arm			Z No qualifier
2 Skin, Right Ear	D Skin, Right Lower Arm			
3 Skin, Left Ear	E Skin, Left Lower Arm			
4 Skin, Neck	F Skin, Right Hand			
5 Skin, Chest	G Skin, Left Hand			
6 Skin, Back	H Skin, Right Upper Leg			
7 Skin, Abdomen	J Skin, Left Upper Leg			
8 Skin, Buttock	K Skin, Right Lower Leg			
9 Skin, Perineum	L Skin, Left Lower Leg			
A Skin, Genitalia	M Skin, Right Foot			
	N Skin, Left Foot			
Q Finger Nail		X External	Z No device	Z No qualifier
R Toe Nail				
T Breast, Right		0 Open	Z No device	Z No qualifier
U Breast, Left		3 Percutaneous		
V Breast, Bilateral		7 Via natural or artificial opening		
W Nipple, Right		8 Via natural or artificial opening endoscopic		
X Nipple, Left		X External		

DIVISION GROUP: Division, Release
Root Operations involving cutting or separation only.

- 1ST – **0** Medical and Surgical
- 2ND – **H** Skin and Breast
- 3RD – **8 DIVISION**

EXAMPLE: Division skin CMS Ex: Osteotomy

DIVISION: Cutting into a body part without draining fluids and/or gases from the body part in order to separate or transect a body part.

EXPLANATION: Separated into two or more portions …

Body Part – 4TH		Approach – 5TH	Device – 6TH	Qualifier – 7TH
0 Skin, Scalp	B Skin, Right Upper Arm	X External	Z No device	Z No qualifier
1 Skin, Face	C Skin, Left Upper Arm			
2 Skin, Right Ear	D Skin, Right Lower Arm			
3 Skin, Left Ear	E Skin, Left Lower Arm			
4 Skin, Neck	F Skin, Right Hand			
5 Skin, Chest	G Skin, Left Hand			
6 Skin, Back	H Skin, Right Upper Leg			
7 Skin, Abdomen	J Skin, Left Upper Leg			
8 Skin, Buttock	K Skin, Right Lower Leg			
9 Skin, Perineum	L Skin, Left Lower Leg			
A Skin, Genitalia	M Skin, Right Foot			
	N Skin, Left Foot			

0 H 9

H – SKIN AND BREAST

DRAINAGE GROUP: Drainage, Extirpation, (Fragmentation)
Root Operations that take out solids/fluids/gases from a body part.

1ST - **0** Medical and Surgical
2ND - **H** Skin and Breast
3RD - **9 DRAINAGE**

EXAMPLE: Incision and drainage boil **CMS Ex:** Thoracentesis

DRAINAGE: Taking or letting out fluids and/or gases from a body part.

EXPLANATION: Qualifier "X Diagnostic" indicates biopsy …

Body Part – 4TH		Approach – 5TH	Device – 6TH	Qualifier – 7TH
0 Skin, Scalp 1 Skin, Face 2 Skin, Right Ear 3 Skin, Left Ear 4 Skin, Neck 5 Skin, Chest 6 Skin, Back 7 Skin, Abdomen 8 Skin, Buttock 9 Skin, Perineum A Skin, Genitalia B Skin, Right Upper Arm C Skin, Left Upper Arm	D Skin, Right Lower Arm E Skin, Left Lower Arm F Skin, Right Hand G Skin, Left Hand H Skin, Right Upper Leg J Skin, Left Upper Leg K Skin, Right Lower Leg L Skin, Left Lower Leg M Skin, Right Foot N Skin, Left Foot Q Finger Nail R Toe Nail	X External	0 Drainage device	Z No qualifier
0 Skin, Scalp 1 Skin, Face 2 Skin, Right Ear 3 Skin, Left Ear 4 Skin, Neck 5 Skin, Chest 6 Skin, Back 7 Skin, Abdomen 8 Skin, Buttock 9 Skin, Perineum A Skin, Genitalia B Skin, Right Upper Arm C Skin, Left Upper Arm	D Skin, Right Lower Arm E Skin, Left Lower Arm F Skin, Right Hand G Skin, Left Hand H Skin, Right Upper Leg J Skin, Left Upper Leg K Skin, Right Lower Leg L Skin, Left Lower Leg M Skin, Right Foot N Skin, Left Foot Q Finger Nail R Toe Nail	X External	Z No device	X Diagnostic Z No qualifier
T Breast, Right U Breast, Left V Breast, Bilateral W Nipple, Right X Nipple, Left		0 Open 3 Percutaneous 7 Via natural or artificial opening 8 Via natural or artificial opening endoscopic X External	0 Drainage device	Z No qualifier
T Breast, Right U Breast, Left V Breast, Bilateral W Nipple, Right X Nipple, Left		0 Open 3 Percutaneous 7 Via natural or artificial opening 8 Via natural or artificial opening endoscopic X External	Z No device	X Diagnostic Z No qualifier

0HB — MEDICAL AND SURGICAL SECTION – 2016 ICD-10-PCS

EXCISION GROUP: Excision, Resection, Destruction, Extraction, (Detachment)
Root Operations that take out some or all of a body part.

1ST - 0 Medical and Surgical
2ND - H Skin and Breast
3RD - B EXCISION

EXAMPLE: Partial mastectomy **CMS Ex:** Liver biopsy

EXCISION: Cutting out or off, without replacement, a portion of a body part.

EXPLANATION: Qualifier "X Diagnostic" indicates biopsy ...

Body Part – 4TH		Approach – 5TH	Device – 6TH	Qualifier – 7TH
0 Skin, Scalp	D Skin, Right Lower Arm	X External	Z No device	X Diagnostic
1 Skin, Face	E Skin, Left Lower Arm			Z No qualifier
2 Skin, Right Ear	F Skin, Right Hand			
3 Skin, Left Ear	G Skin, Left Hand			
4 Skin, Neck	H Skin, Right Upper Leg			
5 Skin, Chest	J Skin, Left Upper Leg			
6 Skin, Back	K Skin, Right Lower Leg			
7 Skin, Abdomen	L Skin, Left Lower Leg			
8 Skin, Buttock	M Skin, Right Foot			
9 Skin, Perineum	N Skin, Left Foot			
A Skin, Genitalia	Q Finger Nail			
B Skin, Right Upper Arm	R Toe Nail			
C Skin, Left Upper Arm				
T Breast, Right		0 Open	Z No device	X Diagnostic
U Breast, Left		3 Percutaneous		Z No qualifier
V Breast, Bilateral		7 Via natural or artificial opening		
W Nipple, Right		8 Via natural or artificial opening endoscopic		
X Nipple, Left		X External		
Y Supernumerary Breast				

H – SKIN AND BREAST 0HD

DRAINAGE GROUP: Drainage, Extirpation, (Fragmentation)
Root Operations that take out solids/fluids/gases from a body part.

1ST - 0 Medical and Surgical	EXAMPLE: Removal splinter skin	CMS Ex: Choledocholithotomy
2ND - H Skin and Breast	**EXTIRPATION:** Taking or cutting out solid matter from a body part.	
3RD - C EXTIRPATION	EXPLANATION: Abnormal byproduct or foreign body ...	

Body Part – 4TH		Approach – 5TH	Device – 6TH	Qualifier – 7TH
0 Skin, Scalp	D Skin, Right Lower Arm	X External	Z No device	Z No qualifier
1 Skin, Face	E Skin, Left Lower Arm			
2 Skin, Right Ear	F Skin, Right Hand			
3 Skin, Left Ear	G Skin, Left Hand			
4 Skin, Neck	H Skin, Right Upper Leg			
5 Skin, Chest	J Skin, Left Upper Leg			
6 Skin, Back	K Skin, Right Lower Leg			
7 Skin, Abdomen	L Skin, Left Lower Leg			
8 Skin, Buttock	M Skin, Right Foot			
9 Skin, Perineum	N Skin, Left Foot			
A Skin, Genitalia	Q Finger Nail			
B Skin, Right Upper Arm	R Toe Nail			
C Skin, Left Upper Arm				

T Breast, Right		0 Open	Z No device	Z No qualifier
U Breast, Left		3 Percutaneous		
V Breast, Bilateral		7 Via natural or artificial opening		
W Nipple, Right		8 Via natural or artificial opening endoscopic		
X Nipple, Left		X External		

EXCISION GROUP: Excision, Resection, Destruction, Extraction, (Detachment)
Root Operations that take out some or all of a body part.

1ST - 0 Medical and Surgical	EXAMPLE: Non-excisional debridement skin	CMS Ex: D&C
2ND - H Skin and Breast	**EXTRACTION:** Pulling or stripping out or off all or a portion of a body part by the use of force.	
3RD - D EXTRACTION	EXPLANATION: None for this Body System	

Body Part – 4TH		Approach – 5TH	Device – 6TH	Qualifier – 7TH
0 Skin, Scalp	D Skin, Right Lower Arm	X External	Z No device	Z No qualifier
1 Skin, Face	E Skin, Left Lower Arm			
2 Skin, Right Ear	F Skin, Right Hand			
3 Skin, Left Ear	G Skin, Left Hand			
4 Skin, Neck	H Skin, Right Upper Leg			
5 Skin, Chest	J Skin, Left Upper Leg			
6 Skin, Back	K Skin, Right Lower Leg			
7 Skin, Abdomen	L Skin, Left Lower Leg			
8 Skin, Buttock	M Skin, Right Foot			
9 Skin, Perineum	N Skin, Left Foot			
A Skin, Genitalia	Q Finger Nail			
B Skin, Right Upper Arm	R Toe Nail			
C Skin, Left Upper Arm	S Hair			

0 H H   MEDICAL AND SURGICAL SECTION – 2016 ICD-10-PCS   [2016.PCS]

DEVICE GROUP: Change, Insertion, Removal, Replacement, Revision, Supplement
Root Operations that always involve a device.

1ST – 0 Medical and Surgical
2ND – H Skin and Breast
3RD – H INSERTION

EXAMPLE: Insertion breast tissue expander   CMS Ex: Venous catheter

INSERTION: Putting in a nonbiological appliance that monitors, assists, performs, or prevents a physiological function but does not physically take the place of a body part.

EXPLANATION: None

Body Part – 4TH	Approach – 5TH	Device – 6TH	Qualifier – 7TH
T Breast, Right U Breast, Left V Breast, Bilateral W Nipple, Right X Nipple, Left	0 Open 3 Percutaneous 7 Via natural or artificial opening 8 Via natural or artificial opening endoscopic	1 Radioactive element N Tissue expander	Z No qualifier
T Breast, Right U Breast, Left V Breast, Bilateral W Nipple, Right X Nipple, Left	X External	1 Radioactive element	Z No qualifier

EXAMINATION GROUP: Inspection, (Map)
Root Operations involving examination only.

1ST – 0 Medical and Surgical
2ND – H Skin and Breast
3RD – J INSPECTION

EXAMPLE: Breast exam   CMS Ex: Colonoscopy

INSPECTION: Visually and/or manually exploring a body part.

EXPLANATION: Direct or instrumental visualization ...

Body Part – 4TH	Approach – 5TH	Device – 6TH	Qualifier – 7TH
P Skin Q Finger Nail R Toe Nail	X External	Z No device	Z No qualifier
T Breast, Right U Breast, Left	0 Open 3 Percutaneous 7 Via natural or artificial opening 8 Via natural or artificial opening endoscopic X External	Z No device	Z No qualifier

H – SKIN AND BREAST

MOVE GROUP: Reattachment, Reposition, Transfer, (Transplantation)
Root Operations that put in/put back or move some/all of a body part.

1ST - 0 Medical and Surgical
2ND - H Skin and Breast
3RD - M REATTACHMENT

EXAMPLE: Replantation avulsed scalp CMS Ex: Reattachment hand

REATTACHMENT: Putting back in or on all or a portion of a separated body part to its normal location or other suitable location.

EXPLANATION: With/without reconnection of vessels/nerves...

Body Part – 4TH		Approach – 5TH	Device – 6TH	Qualifier – 7TH
0 Skin, Scalp	F Skin, Right Hand	X External	Z No device	Z No qualifier
1 Skin, Face	G Skin, Left Hand			
2 Skin, Right Ear	H Skin, Right Upper Leg			
3 Skin, Left Ear	J Skin, Left Upper Leg			
4 Skin, Neck	K Skin, Right Lower Leg			
5 Skin, Chest	L Skin, Left Lower Leg			
6 Skin, Back	M Skin, Right Foot			
7 Skin, Abdomen	N Skin, Left Foot			
8 Skin, Buttock	T Breast, Right			
9 Skin, Perineum	U Breast, Left			
A Skin, Genitalia	V Breast, Bilateral			
B Skin, Right Upper Arm	W Nipple, Right			
C Skin, Left Upper Arm	X Nipple, Left			
D Skin, Right Lower Arm				
E Skin, Left Lower Arm				

DIVISION GROUP: Division, Release
Root Operations involving cutting or separation only.

1ST - 0 Medical and Surgical
2ND - H Skin and Breast
3RD - N RELEASE

EXAMPLE: Incision scar contracture CMS Ex: Carpal tunnel release

RELEASE: Freeing a body part from an abnormal physical constraint by cutting or by the use of force.

EXPLANATION: None of the body part is taken out ...

Body Part – 4TH		Approach – 5TH	Device – 6TH	Qualifier – 7TH
0 Skin, Scalp	D Skin, Right Lower Arm	X External	Z No device	Z No qualifier
1 Skin, Face	E Skin, Left Lower Arm			
2 Skin, Right Ear	F Skin, Right Hand			
3 Skin, Left Ear	G Skin, Left Hand			
4 Skin, Neck	H Skin, Right Upper Leg			
5 Skin, Chest	J Skin, Left Upper Leg			
6 Skin, Back	K Skin, Right Lower Leg			
7 Skin, Abdomen	L Skin, Left Lower Leg			
8 Skin, Buttock	M Skin, Right Foot			
9 Skin, Perineum	N Skin, Left Foot			
A Skin, Genitalia	Q Finger Nail			
B Skin, Right Upper Arm	R Toe Nail			
C Skin, Left Upper Arm				
T Breast, Right		0 Open	Z No device	Z No qualifier
U Breast, Left		3 Percutaneous		
V Breast, Bilateral		7 Via natural or artificial opening		
W Nipple, Right		8 Via natural or artificial opening endoscopic		
X Nipple, Left		X External		

0HP MEDICAL AND SURGICAL SECTION – 2016 ICD-10-PCS

DEVICE GROUP: Change, Insertion, Removal, Replacement, Revision, Supplement
Root Operations that always involve a device.

- 1ST – **0** Medical and Surgical
- 2ND – **H** Skin and Breast
- 3RD – **P** REMOVAL

EXAMPLE: Removal tissue expander **CMS Ex:** Chest tube removal

REMOVAL: Taking out or off a device from a body part.

EXPLANATION: Removal device without reinsertion …

Body Part – 4TH	Approach – 5TH	Device – 6TH	Qualifier – 7TH
P Skin Q Finger Nail R Toe Nail	X External	0 Drainage device 7 Autologous tissue substitute J Synthetic substitute K Nonautologous tissue substitute	Z No qualifier
S Hair	X External	7 Autologous tissue substitute J Synthetic substitute K Nonautologous tissue substitute	Z No qualifier
T Breast, Right U Breast, Left	0 Open 3 Percutaneous 7 Via natural or artificial opening 8 Via natural or artificial opening endoscopic	0 Drainage device 1 Radioactive element 7 Autologous tissue substitute J Synthetic substitute K Nonautologous tissue substitute N Tissue expander	Z No qualifier
T Breast, Right U Breast, Left	X External	0 Drainage device 1 Radioactive element 7 Autologous tissue substitute J Synthetic substitute K Nonautologous tissue substitute	Z No qualifier

H – SKIN AND BREAST 0HQ

OTHER REPAIRS GROUP: (Control), **Repair**
Root Operations that define other repairs.

1ST - **0** Medical and Surgical
2ND - **H** Skin and Breast
3RD - **Q REPAIR**

EXAMPLE: Repair first degree perineum laceration | **CMS Ex:** Suture

REPAIR: Restoring, to the extent possible, a body part to its normal anatomic structure and function.

EXPLANATION: Only when no other root operation applies …

Body Part – 4TH		Approach – 5TH	Device – 6TH	Qualifier – 7TH
0 Skin, Scalp	D Skin, Right Lower Arm	X External	Z No device	Z No qualifier
1 Skin, Face	E Skin, Left Lower Arm			
2 Skin, Right Ear	F Skin, Right Hand			
3 Skin, Left Ear	G Skin, Left Hand			
4 Skin, Neck	H Skin, Right Upper Leg			
5 Skin, Chest	J Skin, Left Upper Leg			
6 Skin, Back	K Skin, Right Lower Leg			
7 Skin, Abdomen	L Skin, Left Lower Leg			
8 Skin, Buttock	M Skin, Right Foot			
9 Skin, Perineum	N Skin, Left Foot			
A Skin, Genitalia	Q Finger Nail			
B Skin, Right Upper Arm	R Toe Nail			
C Skin, Left Upper Arm				
T Breast, Right		0 Open	Z No device	Z No qualifier
U Breast, Left		3 Percutaneous		
V Breast, Bilateral		7 Via natural or artificial opening		
W Nipple, Right		8 Via natural or artificial opening endoscopic		
X Nipple, Left		X External		
Y Supernumerary Breast				

0HR — Medical and Surgical Section – 2016 ICD-10-PCS

DEVICE GROUP: Change, Insertion, Removal, Replacement, Revision, Supplement
Root Operations that always involve a device.

- 1ST – **0** Medical and Surgical
- 2ND – **H** Skin and Breast
- 3RD – **R** REPLACEMENT

EXAMPLE: Mastectomy with implant   CMS Ex: Total hip

REPLACEMENT: Putting in or on a biological or synthetic material that physically takes the place and/or function of all or a portion of a body part.

EXPLANATION: Includes taking out body part, or eradication...

Body Part – 4TH		Approach – 5TH	Device – 6TH	Qualifier – 7TH
0 Skin, Scalp 1 Skin, Face 2 Skin, Right Ear 3 Skin, Left Ear 4 Skin, Neck 5 Skin, Chest 6 Skin, Back 7 Skin, Abdomen 8 Skin, Buttock 9 Skin, Perineum A Skin, Genitalia	B Skin, Right Upper Arm C Skin, Left Upper Arm D Skin, Right Lower Arm E Skin, Left Lower Arm F Skin, Right Hand G Skin, Left Hand H Skin, Right Upper Leg J Skin, Left Upper Leg K Skin, Right Lower Leg L Skin, Left Lower Leg M Skin, Right Foot N Skin, Left Foot	X External	7 Autologous tissue substitute K Nonautologous tissue substitute	3 Full thickness 4 Partial thickness
0 Skin, Scalp 1 Skin, Face 2 Skin, Right Ear 3 Skin, Left Ear 4 Skin, Neck 5 Skin, Chest 6 Skin, Back 7 Skin, Abdomen 8 Skin, Buttock 9 Skin, Perineum A Skin, Genitalia	B Skin, Right Upper Arm C Skin, Left Upper Arm D Skin, Right Lower Arm E Skin, Left Lower Arm F Skin, Right Hand G Skin, Left Hand H Skin, Right Upper Leg J Skin, Left Upper Leg K Skin, Right Lower Leg L Skin, Left Lower Leg M Skin, Right Foot N Skin, Left Foot	X External	J Synthetic substitute	3 Full thickness 4 Partial thickness Z No qualifier
Q Finger Nail R Toe Nail S Hair		X External	7 Autologous tissue substitute J Synthetic substitute K Nonautologous tissue substitute	Z No qualifier

continued ➡

0 H R REPLACEMENT — continued

Body Part – 4TH	Approach – 5TH	Device – 6TH	Qualifier – 7TH
T Breast, Right U Breast, Left V Breast, Bilateral	0 Open	7 Autologous tissue substitute	5 Latissimus Dorsi Myocutaneous Flap 6 Transverse Rectus Abdominis Myocutaneous Flap 7 Deep Inferior Epigastric Artery Perforator Flap 8 Superficial Inferior Epigastric Artery Flap 9 Gluteal Artery Perforator Flap Z No qualifier
T Breast, Right U Breast, Left V Breast, Bilateral	0 Open	J Synthetic substitute K Nonautologous tissue substitute	Z No qualifier
T Breast, Right U Breast, Left V Breast, Bilateral	3 Percutaneous X External	7 Autologous tissue substitute J Synthetic substitute K Nonautologous tissue substitute	Z No qualifier
W Nipple, Right X Nipple, Left	0 Open 3 Percutaneous X External	7 Autologous tissue substitute J Synthetic substitute K Nonautologous tissue substitute	Z No qualifier

MOVE GROUP: Reattachment, Reposition, Transfer, (Transplantation)
Root Operations that put in/put back or move some/all of a body part.

- 1ST – **0** Medical and Surgical
- 2ND – **H** Skin and Breast
- 3RD – **S** REPOSITION

EXAMPLE: Reposition nipple location   CMS Ex: Fracture reduction

REPOSITION: Moving to its normal location, or other suitable location, all or a portion of a body part.

EXPLANATION: May or may not be cut to be moved ...

Body Part – 4TH	Approach – 5TH	Device – 6TH	Qualifier – 7TH
S Hair W Nipple, Right X Nipple, Left	X External	Z No device	Z No qualifier
T Breast, Right U Breast, Left V Breast, Bilateral	0 Open	Z No device	Z No qualifier

0HT

MEDICAL AND SURGICAL SECTION – 2016 ICD-10-PCS [2016.PCS]

EXCISION GROUP: Excision, Resection, Destruction, Extraction, (Detachment)
Root Operations that take out some or all of a body part.

1ST - **0** Medical and Surgical
2ND - **H** Skin and Breast
3RD - **T RESECTION**

EXAMPLE: Skin-sparing total mastectomy CMS Ex: Cholecystectomy

RESECTION: Cutting out or off, without replacement, all of a body part.

EXPLANATION: None

Body Part – 4TH	Approach – 5TH	Device – 6TH	Qualifier – 7TH
Q Finger Nail R Toe Nail W Nipple, Right X Nipple, Left	X External	Z No device	Z No qualifier
T Breast, Right U Breast, Left V Breast, Bilateral Y Supernumerary Breast	0 Open	Z No device	Z No qualifier

DEVICE GROUP: Change, Insertion, Removal, Replacement, Revision, Supplement
Root Operations that always involve a device.

1ST - **0** Medical and Surgical
2ND - **H** Skin and Breast
3RD - **U SUPPLEMENT**

EXAMPLE: Repair inverted nipple with graft CMS Ex: Hernia mesh

SUPPLEMENT: Putting in or on biological or synthetic material that physically reinforces and/or augments the function of a portion of a body part.

EXPLANATION: Biological material from same individual ...

Body Part – 4TH	Approach – 5TH	Device – 6TH	Qualifier – 7TH
T Breast, Right U Breast, Left V Breast, Bilateral W Nipple, Right X Nipple, Left	0 Open 3 Percutaneous 7 Via natural or artificial opening 8 Via natural or artificial opening endoscopic X External	7 Autologous tissue substitute J Synthetic substitute K Nonautologous tissue substitute	Z No qualifier

H – SKIN AND BREAST

0 H W

DEVICE GROUP: Change, Insertion, Removal, Replacement, Revision, Supplement
Root Operations that always involve a device.

- 1ST – **0** Medical and Surgical
- 2ND – **H** Skin and Breast
- 3RD – **W** REVISION

EXAMPLE: Reposition tissue expander | CMS Ex: Adjustment pacemaker lead

REVISION: Correcting, to the extent possible, a portion of a malfunctioning device or the position of a displaced device.

EXPLANATION: May replace components of a device ...

Body Part – 4TH	Approach – 5TH	Device – 6TH	Qualifier – 7TH
P Skin Q Finger Nail R Toe Nail	X External	0 Drainage device 7 Autologous tissue substitute J Synthetic substitute K Nonautologous tissue substitute	Z No qualifier
S Hair	X External	7 Autologous tissue substitute J Synthetic substitute K Nonautologous tissue substitute	Z No qualifier
T Breast, Right U Breast, Left	0 Open 3 Percutaneous 7 Via natural or artificial opening 8 Via natural or artificial opening endoscopic	0 Drainage device 7 Autologous tissue substitute J Synthetic substitute K Nonautologous tissue substitute N Tissue expander	Z No qualifier
T Breast, Right U Breast, Left	X External	0 Drainage device 7 Autologous tissue substitute J Synthetic substitute K Nonautologous tissue substitute	Z No qualifier

0HX

MEDICAL AND SURGICAL SECTION – 2016 ICD-10-PCS

MOVE GROUP: Reattachment, Reposition, Transfer, (Transplantation)
Root Operations that put in/put back or move some/all of a body part.

- 1ST – **0** Medical and Surgical
- 2ND – **H** Skin and Breast
- 3RD – **X** TRANSFER

EXAMPLE: Scalp advancement flap **CMS Ex:** Tendon transfer

TRANSFER: Moving, without taking out, all or a portion of a body part to another location to take over the function of all or a portion of a body part.

EXPLANATION: The body part remains connected ...

Body Part – 4TH		Approach – 5TH	Device – 6TH	Qualifier – 7TH
0 Skin, Scalp	B Skin, Right Upper Arm	X External	Z No device	Z No qualifier
1 Skin, Face	C Skin, Left Upper Arm			
2 Skin, Right Ear	D Skin, Right Lower Arm			
3 Skin, Left Ear	E Skin, Left Lower Arm			
4 Skin, Neck	F Skin, Right Hand			
5 Skin, Chest	G Skin, Left Hand			
6 Skin, Back	H Skin, Right Upper Leg			
7 Skin, Abdomen	J Skin, Left Upper Leg			
8 Skin, Buttock	K Skin, Right Lower Leg			
9 Skin, Perineum	L Skin, Left Lower Leg			
A Skin, Genitalia	M Skin, Right Foot			
	N Skin, Left Foot			

Educational Annotations | J – Subcutaneous Tissue and Fascia

Body System Specific Educational Annotations for the Subcutaneous Tissue and Fascia include:
- Anatomy and Physiology Review
- Anatomical Illustrations
- Definitions of Common Procedures
- AHA Coding Clinic® Reference Notations
- Body Part Key Listings
- Device Key Listings
- Device Aggregation Table Listings
- Coding Notes

Anatomy and Physiology Review of Subcutaneous Tissue and Fascia

BODY PART VALUES – J - SUBCUTANEOUS TISSUE AND FASCIA

Fascia – ANATOMY – The sheets or bands of dense connective tissue located beneath the skin between muscles, organs, and other structures. PHYSIOLOGY – The fascia is strong but flexible and functions to separate, protect, and reduce friction of muscle movement on the organs, blood vessels, nerves, muscles, and other structures within the body.

Subcutaneous Tissue – ANATOMY – The innermost layer of the three layers of the skin (also known as the hypodermis) and comprised of fibous tissue, adipose tissue, elastic fibers, connective tissue, and hair follicle roots. PHYSIOLOGY – The subcutaneous tissue is responsible for regulating body temperature, plays a role in pigmentation, and protects the inner organs and bones.

Anatomical Illustrations of Subcutaneous Tissue and Fascia

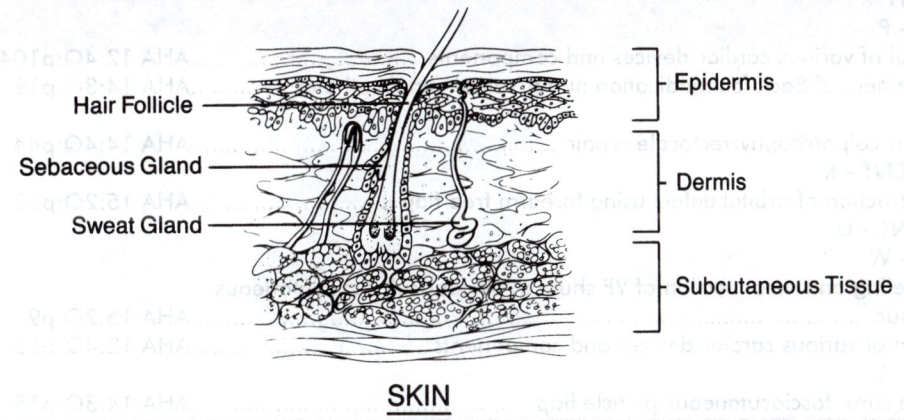

SKIN

Definitions of Common Procedures of Subcutaneous Tissue and Fascia

Free fascia graft – The implantation of fascia to fill a defect using an allograft or donor tissue.

Insertion of pacemaker generator – The surgical placement of a pacemaker generator just under the skin in the subcutaneous tissue.

Liposuction – The surgical removal of excess fat deposits using a hollow cannula that is connected to a strong suction pump.

Pedicle fascia graft – The transfer of fascia to fill a defect without dissecting the graft tissue free from its vascular and nervous supply.

Educational Annotations | J – Subcutaneous Tissue and Fascia

AHA Coding Clinic® Reference Notations of Subcutaneous Tissue and Fascia

ROOT OPERATION SPECIFIC - J - SUBCUTANEOUS TISSUE AND FASCIA

ALTERATION - 0
CHANGE - 2
DESTRUCTION - 5
DIVISION - 8
DRAINAGE - 9
EXCISION - B
- Excision of abdominal subcutaneous fat during hernia repair ....AHA 14:4Q:p38
- Excision of inclusion cyst of perineum ....AHA 13:4Q:p119
- Excisional repair of perineal fistula ....AHA 15:1Q:p29
- Graft excision, forearm free flap ....AHA 15:2Q:p13
- Harvesting of fat graft from abdomen ....AHA 14:3Q:p22

EXTIRPATION - C
EXTRACTION - D
- Non-excisional debridement using Pulsavac ....AHA 15:1Q:p23

INSERTION - H
- Insertion of various cardiac devices and components ....AHA 12:4Q:p104
- Insertion of venous access port ....AHA 13:4Q:p116
    - Official Clarification of 13:4Q:p116 ....AHA 15:2Q:p34
- Replacement of Baclofen medication pump/spinal canal catheter ....AHA 14:3Q:p19

INSPECTION - J
RELEASE - N
REMOVAL - P
- Removal of various cardiac devices and components ....AHA 12:4Q:p104
- Replacement of Baclofen medication pump/spinal canal catheter ....AHA 14:3Q:p19

REPAIR - Q
- Posterior colporrhaphy/rectocele repair ....AHA 14:4Q:p44

REPLACEMENT - R
- Reconstruction of orbital defect using forearm free flap ....AHA 15:2Q:p13

SUPPLEMENT - U
REVISION - W
- Retunneling and reconnection of VP shunt in periauricular subcutaneous tissue ....AHA 15:2Q:p9
- Revision of various cardiac devices and components ....AHA 12:4Q:p104

TRANSFER - X
- Reverse sural fasciocutaneous pedicle flap ....AHA 14:3Q:p18

Body Part Key Listings of Subcutaneous Tissue and Fascia

See also Body Part Key in Appendix C

Antebrachial fascia	*use* Subcutaneous Tissue and Fascia, Lower Arm, Left/Right
Axillary fascia	*use* Subcutaneous Tissue and Fascia, Upper Arm, Left/Right
Bicipital aponeurosis	*use* Subcutaneous Tissue and Fascia, Lower Arm, Left/Right
Crural fascia	*use* Subcutaneous Tissue and Fascia, Upper Leg, Left/Right
Deep cervical fascia	*use* Subcutaneous Tissue and Fascia, Anterior Neck
Deltoid fascia	*use* Subcutaneous Tissue and Fascia, Upper Arm, Left/Right
External oblique aponeurosis	*use* Subcutaneous Tissue and Fascia, Trunk
Fascia lata	*use* Subcutaneous Tissue and Fascia, Upper Leg, Left/Right
Galea aponeurotica	*use* Subcutaneous Tissue and Fascia, Scalp
Iliac fascia	*use* Subcutaneous Tissue and Fascia, Upper Leg, Left/Right
Iliotibial tract (band)	*use* Subcutaneous Tissue and Fascia, Upper Leg, Left/Right
Infraspinatus fascia	*use* Subcutaneous Tissue and Fascia, Upper Arm, Left/Right
Masseteric fascia	*use* Subcutaneous Tissue and Fascia, Face
Orbital fascia	*use* Subcutaneous Tissue and Fascia, Face
Palmar fascia (aponeurosis)	*use* Subcutaneous Tissue and Fascia, Hand, Left/Right

Continued on next page

Educational Annotations | J – Subcutaneous Tissue and Fascia

Body Part Key Listings of Subcutaneous Tissue and Fascia

Continued from previous page

Pectoral fascia	*use* Subcutaneous Tissue and Fascia, Chest
Plantar fascia (aponeurosis)	*use* Subcutaneous Tissue and Fascia, Foot, Left/Right
Pretracheal fascia	*use* Subcutaneous Tissue and Fascia, Anterior Neck
Prevertebral fascia	*use* Subcutaneous Tissue and Fascia, Posterior Neck
Subscapular aponeurosis	*use* Subcutaneous Tissue and Fascia, Upper Arm, Left/Right
Supraspinatus fascia	*use* Subcutaneous Tissue and Fascia, Upper Arm, Left/Right
Transversalis fascia	*use* Subcutaneous Tissue and Fascia, Trunk

Device Key Listings of Subcutaneous Tissue and Fascia

See also Device Key in Appendix D

Activa PC neurostimulator	*use* Stimulator Generator, Multiple Array for Insertion in Subcutaneous Tissue and Fascia
Activa RC neurostimulator	*use* Stimulator Generator, Multiple Array Rechargeable for Insertion in Subcutaneous Tissue and Fascia
Activa SC neurostimulator	*use* Stimulator Generator, Single Array for Insertion in Subcutaneous Tissue and Fascia
Advisa (MRI)	*use* Pacemaker, Dual Chamber for Insertion in Subcutaneous Tissue and Fascia
Autograft	*use* Autologous Tissue Substitute
Baroreflex Activation Therapy® (BAT®)	*use* Stimulator Generator in Subcutaneous Tissue and Fascia
Brachytherapy seeds	*use* Radioactive Element
COGNIS® CRT-D	*use* Cardiac Resynchronization Defibrillator Pulse Generator for Insertion in Subcutaneous Tissue and Fascia
Concerto II CRT-D	*use* Cardiac Resynchronization Defibrillator Pulse Generator for Insertion in Subcutaneous Tissue and Fascia
Consulta CRT-D	*use* Cardiac Resynchronization Defibrillator Pulse Generator for Insertion in Subcutaneous Tissue and Fascia
Consulta CRT-P	*use* Cardiac Resynchronization Pacemaker Pulse Generator for Insertion in Subcutaneous Tissue and Fascia
CONTAK RENEWAL® 3 RF (HE) CRT-D	*use* Cardiac Resynchronization Defibrillator Pulse Generator for Insertion in Subcutaneous Tissue and Fascia
Diaphragmatic pacemaker generator	*use* Stimulator Generator in Subcutaneous Tissue and Fascia
EnRhythm	*use* Pacemaker, Dual Chamber for Insertion in Subcutaneous Tissue and Fascia
Enterra gastric neurostimulator	*use* Stimulator Generator, Multiple Array for Insertion in Subcutaneous Tissue and Fascia
Evera (XT) (S) (DR/VR)	*use* Defibrillator Generator for Insertion in Subcutaneous Tissue and Fascia
Implantable cardioverter-defibrillator (ICD)	*use* Defibrillator Generator for Insertion in Subcutaneous Tissue and Fascia
Implantable drug infusion pump (anti-spasmodic) (chemotherapy) (pain)	*use* Infusion Device, Pump in Subcutaneous Tissue and Fascia
Implantable hemodynamic monitor (IHM)	*use* Monitoring Device, Hemodynamic for Insertion in Subcutaneous Tissue and Fascia
Implantable hemodynamic monitoring system (IHMS)	*use* Monitoring Device, Hemodynamic for Insertion in Subcutaneous Tissue and Fascia
Implanted (venous) (access) port	*use* Vascular Access Device, Reservoir in Subcutaneous Tissue and Fascia

Continued on next page

J – Subcutaneous Tissue and Fascia

Educational Annotations

Device Key Listings of Subcutaneous Tissue and Fascia

Continued from previous page

Injection reservoir, port	*use* Vascular Access Device, Reservoir in Subcutaneous Tissue and Fascia
Injection reservoir, pump	*use* Infusion Device, Pump in Subcutaneous Tissue and Fascia
InterStim® Therapy neurostimulator	*use* Stimulator Generator, Single Array for Insertion in Subcutaneous Tissue and Fascia
Itrel (3) (4) neurostimulator	*use* Stimulator Generator, Single Array for Insertion in Subcutaneous Tissue and Fascia
Kappa	*use* Pacemaker, Dual Chamber for Insertion in Subcutaneous Tissue and Fascia
LIVIAN™ CRT-D	*use* Cardiac Resynchronization Defibrillator Pulse Generator for Insertion in Subcutaneous Tissue and Fascia
Loop recorder, implantable	*use* Monitoring Device
Mark IV Breathing Pacemaker System	*use* Stimulator Generator in Subcutaneous Tissue and Fascia
Maximo II DR (VR)	*use* Defibrillator Generator for Insertion in Subcutaneous Tissue and Fascia
Maximo II DR CRT-D	*use* Cardiac Resynchronization Defibrillator Pulse Generator for Insertion in Subcutaneous Tissue and Fascia
Neurostimulator generator, multiple channel	*use* Stimulator Generator, Multiple Array for Insertion in Subcutaneous Tissue and Fascia
Neurostimulator generator, multiple channel rechargeable	*use* Stimulator Generator, Multiple Array Rechargeable for Insertion in Subcutaneous Tissue and Fascia
Neurostimulator generator, single channel	*use* Stimulator Generator, Single Array for Insertion in Subcutaneous Tissue and Fascia
Neurostimulator generator, single channel rechargeable	*use* Stimulator Generator, Single Array Rechargeable for Insertion in Subcutaneous Tissue and Fascia
Optimizer™ III implantable pulse generator	*use* Contractility Modulation Device for Insertion in Subcutaneous Tissue and Fascia
Ovatio™ CRT-D	*use* Cardiac Resynchronization Defibrillator Pulse Generator for Insertion in Subcutaneous Tissue and Fascia
Phrenic nerve stimulator generator	*use* Stimulator Generator in Subcutaneous Tissue and Fascia
PrimeAdvanced neurostimulator (SureScan) (MRI Safe)	*use* Stimulator Generator, Multiple Array for Insertion in Subcutaneous Tissue and Fascia
Protecta XT CRT-D	*use* Cardiac Resynchronization Defibrillator Pulse Generator for Insertion in Subcutaneous Tissue and Fascia
Protecta XT DR (XT VR)	*use* Defibrillator Generator for Insertion in Subcutaneous Tissue and Fascia
Pump reservoir	*use* Infusion Device, Pump in Subcutaneous Tissue and Fascia
RestoreAdvanced neurostimulator (SureScan) (MRI Safe)	*use* Stimulator Generator, Multiple Array Rechargeable for Insertion in Subcutaneous Tissue and Fascia
RestoreSensor neurostimulator (SureScan) (MRI Safe)	*use* Stimulator Generator, Multiple Array Rechargeable for Insertion in Subcutaneous Tissue and Fascia
RestoreUltra neurostimulator (SureScan) (MRI Safe)	*use* Stimulator Generator, Multiple Array Rechargeable for Insertion in Subcutaneous Tissue and Fascia

Continued on next page

Educational Annotations | J – Subcutaneous Tissue and Fascia

Device Key Listings of Subcutaneous Tissue and Fascia

Continued from previous page

Reveal (DX) (XT)	use Monitoring Device
Revo MRI™ SureScan® pacemaker	use Pacemaker, Dual Chamber for Insertion in Subcutaneous Tissue and Fascia
Rheos® System device	use Stimulator Generator in Subcutaneous Tissue and Fascia
Secura (DR) (VR)	use Defibrillator Generator for Insertion in Subcutaneous Tissue and Fascia
Single lead pacemaker (atrium) (ventricle)	use Pacemaker, Single Chamber for Insertion in Subcutaneous Tissue and Fascia
Single lead rate responsive pacemaker (atrium) (ventricle)	use Pacemaker, Single Chamber Rate Responsive for Insertion in Subcutaneous Tissue and Fascia
Stratos LV	use Cardiac Resynchronization Pacemaker Pulse Generator for Insertion in Subcutaneous Tissue and Fascia
Subcutaneous injection reservoir, port	use Vascular Access Device, Reservoir in Subcutaneous Tissue and Fascia
Subcutaneous injection reservoir, pump	use Infusion Device, Pump in Subcutaneous Tissue and Fascia
Subdermal progesterone implant	use Contraceptive Device in Subcutaneous Tissue and Fascia
Synchra CRT-P	use Cardiac Resynchronization Pacemaker Pulse Generator for Insertion in Subcutaneous Tissue and Fascia
SynchroMed pump	use Infusion Device, Pump in Subcutaneous Tissue and Fascia
Tissue bank graft	use Nonautologous Tissue Substitute
Tissue expander (inflatable) (injectable)	use Tissue Expander in Subcutaneous Tissue and Fascia
Tunneled central venous catheter	use Vascular Access Device in Subcutaneous Tissue and Fascia
Two lead pacemaker	use Pacemaker, Dual Chamber for Insertion in Subcutaneous Tissue and Fascia
Vectra® Vascular Access Graft	use Vascular Access Device in Subcutaneous Tissue and Fascia
Versa	use Pacemaker, Dual Chamber for Insertion in Subcutaneous Tissue and Fascia
Virtuoso (II) (DR) (VR)	use Defibrillator Generator for Insertion in Subcutaneous Tissue and Fascia
Viva (XT) (S)	use Cardiac Resynchronization Defibrillator Pulse Generator for Insertion in Subcutaneous Tissue and Fascia

Device Aggregation Table Listings of Subcutaneous Tissue and Fascia

See also Device Aggregation Table in Appendix E

Specific Device	For Operation	In Body System		General Device
Cardiac Resynchronization Defibrillator Pulse Generator	Insertion	Subcutaneous Tissue and Fascia	P	Cardiac Rhythm Related Device
Cardiac Resynchronization Pacemaker Pulse Generator	Insertion	Subcutaneous Tissue and Fascia	P	Cardiac Rhythm Related Device
Contractility Modulation Device	Insertion	Subcutaneous Tissue and Fascia	P	Cardiac Rhythm Related Device
Defibrillator Generator	Insertion	Subcutaneous Tissue and Fascia	P	Cardiac Rhythm Related Device
Monitoring Device, Hemodynamic	Insertion	Subcutaneous Tissue and Fascia	2	Monitoring Device
Pacemaker, Dual Chamber	Insertion	Subcutaneous Tissue and Fascia	P	Cardiac Rhythm Related Device
Pacemaker, Single Chamber	Insertion	Subcutaneous Tissue and Fascia	P	Cardiac Rhythm Related Device
Pacemaker, Single Chamber Rate Responsive	Insertion	Subcutaneous Tissue and Fascia	P	Cardiac Rhythm Related Device
Stimulator Generator, Multiple Array	Insertion	Subcutaneous Tissue and Fascia	M	Stimulator Generator
Stimulator Generator, Multiple Array Rechargeable	Insertion	Subcutaneous Tissue and Fascia	M	Stimulator Generator
Stimulator Generator, Single Array	Insertion	Subcutaneous Tissue and Fascia	M	Stimulator Generator
Stimulator Generator, Single Array Rechargeable	Insertion	Subcutaneous Tissue and Fascia	M	Stimulator Generator

Educational Annotations | J – Subcutaneous Tissue and Fascia

Coding Notes of Subcutaneous Tissue and Fascia

Body System Relevant Coding Guidelines

Tendons, ligaments, bursae and fascia near a joint
B4.5
Procedures performed on tendons, ligaments, bursae and fascia supporting a joint are coded to the body part in the respective body system that is the focus of the procedure. Procedures performed on joint structures themselves are coded to the body part in the joint body systems.
Example: Repair of the anterior cruciate ligament of the knee is coded to the knee bursae and ligament body part in the bursae and ligaments body system. Knee arthroscopy with shaving of articular cartilage is coded to the knee joint body part in the Lower Joints body system.

Skin, subcutaneous tissue and fascia overlying a joint
B4.6
If a procedure is performed on the skin, subcutaneous tissue or fascia overlying a joint, the procedure is coded to the following body part:
- Shoulder is coded to Upper Arm
- Elbow is coded to Lower Arm
- Wrist is coded to Lower Arm
- Hip is coded to Upper Leg
- Knee is coded to Lower Leg
- Ankle is coded to Foot

Body System Specific PCS Reference Manual Exercises

PCS CODE	J – SUBCUTANEOUS TISSUE AND FASCIA EXERCISES
0JOL3ZZ	Liposuction of bilateral thighs.
0JOM3ZZ	
0JD80ZZ	Open stripping of abdominal fascia, right side.
0JDF3ZZ	Liposuction for medical purposes, left upper arm. (The Percutaneous approach is inherent in the liposuction technique.)
0JH606Z	Open placement of dual chamber pacemaker generator in chest wall.
0JH80DZ	End-of-life replacement of spinal neurostimulator generator, multiple array, in lower abdomen. (Taking out the old generator is coded separately to the root operation Removal.)
0JUC0JZ	Anterior colporrhaphy with polypropylene mesh reinforcement, open approach.
0JWT0XZ	Revision of totally implantable VAD port placement in chest wall, causing patient discomfort, open.
0JX43ZZ	Percutaneous fascia transfer to fill defect, anterior neck.
0JXM0ZC	Fasciocutaneous flap closure of left thigh, open. (The qualifier identifies the body layers in addition to fascia included in the procedure.)

J – SUBCUTANEOUS TISSUE AND FASCIA — 0J2

OTHER OBJECTIVES GROUP: Alteration, (Creation), (Fusion)
Root Operations that define other objectives.

1ST - 0 Medical and Surgical
2ND - J Subcutaneous Tissue and Fascia
3RD - 0 ALTERATION

EXAMPLE: Liposuction thighs CMS Ex: Face lift

ALTERATION: Modifying the anatomic structure of a body part without affecting the function of the body part.

EXPLANATION: Principal purpose is to improve appearance

Body Part – 4TH	Approach – 5TH	Device – 6TH	Qualifier – 7TH
1 Subcutaneous Tissue and Fascia, Face	0 Open	Z No device	Z No qualifier
4 Subcutaneous Tissue and Fascia, Anterior Neck	3 Percutaneous		
5 Subcutaneous Tissue and Fascia, Posterior Neck			
6 Subcutaneous Tissue and Fascia, Chest			
7 Subcutaneous Tissue and Fascia, Back			
8 Subcutaneous Tissue and Fascia, Abdomen			
9 Subcutaneous Tissue and Fascia, Buttock			
D Subcutaneous Tissue and Fascia, Right Upper Arm			
F Subcutaneous Tissue and Fascia, Left Upper Arm			
G Subcutaneous Tissue and Fascia, Right Lower Arm			
H Subcutaneous Tissue and Fascia, Left Lower Arm			
L Subcutaneous Tissue and Fascia, Right Upper Leg			
M Subcutaneous Tissue and Fascia, Left Upper Leg			
N Subcutaneous Tissue and Fascia, Right Lower Leg			
P Subcutaneous Tissue and Fascia, Left Lower Leg			

DEVICE GROUP: Change, Insertion, Removal, Replacement, Revision, Supplement
Root Operations that always involve a device.

1ST - 0 Medical and Surgical
2ND - J Subcutaneous Tissue and Fascia
3RD - 2 CHANGE

EXAMPLE: Exchange drain tube CMS Ex: Changing urinary catheter

CHANGE: Taking out or off a device from a body part and putting back an identical or similar device in or on the same body part without cutting or puncturing the skin or a mucous membrane.

EXPLANATION: ALL Changes use EXTERNAL approach only …

Body Part – 4TH	Approach – 5TH	Device – 6TH	Qualifier – 7TH
S Subcutaneous Tissue and Fascia, Head and Neck	X External	0 Drainage device	Z No qualifier
T Subcutaneous Tissue and Fascia, Trunk		Y Other device	
V Subcutaneous Tissue and Fascia, Upper Extremity			
W Subcutaneous Tissue and Fascia, Lower Extremity			

0J5

EXCISION GROUP: Excision, (Resection), Destruction, Extraction (Detachment)
Root Operations that take out some or all of a body part.

1ST - 0	Medical and Surgical
2ND - J	Subcutaneous Tissue and Fascia
3RD - 5	DESTRUCTION

EXAMPLE: Radiofrequency ablation   **CMS Ex:** Fulguration polyp

DESTRUCTION: Physical eradication of all or a portion of a body part by the direct use of energy, force, or a destructive agent.

EXPLANATION: None of the body part is physically taken out

Body Part – 4TH	Approach – 5TH	Device – 6TH	Qualifier – 7TH
0 Subcutaneous Tissue and Fascia, Scalp	0 Open	Z No device	Z No qualifier
1 Subcutaneous Tissue and Fascia, Face	3 Percutaneous		
4 Subcutaneous Tissue and Fascia, Anterior Neck			
5 Subcutaneous Tissue and Fascia, Posterior Neck			
6 Subcutaneous Tissue and Fascia, Chest			
7 Subcutaneous Tissue and Fascia, Back			
8 Subcutaneous Tissue and Fascia, Abdomen			
9 Subcutaneous Tissue and Fascia, Buttock			
B Subcutaneous Tissue and Fascia, Perineum			
C Subcutaneous Tissue and Fascia, Pelvic Region			
D Subcutaneous Tissue and Fascia, Right Upper Arm			
F Subcutaneous Tissue and Fascia, Left Upper Arm			
G Subcutaneous Tissue and Fascia, Right Lower Arm			
H Subcutaneous Tissue and Fascia, Left Lower Arm			
J Subcutaneous Tissue and Fascia, Right Hand			
K Subcutaneous Tissue and Fascia, Left Hand			
L Subcutaneous Tissue and Fascia, Right Upper Leg			
M Subcutaneous Tissue and Fascia, Left Upper Leg			
N Subcutaneous Tissue and Fascia, Right Lower Leg			
P Subcutaneous Tissue and Fascia, Left Lower Leg			
Q Subcutaneous Tissue and Fascia, Right Foot			
R Subcutaneous Tissue and Fascia, Left Foot			

J – SUBCUTANEOUS TISSUE AND FASCIA 0J8

DIVISION GROUP: Division, Release
Root Operations involving cutting or separation only.

- 1ST – **0** Medical and Surgical
- 2ND – **J** Subcutaneous Tissue and Fascia
- 3RD – **8 DIVISION**

EXAMPLE: Division plantar fascia **CMS Ex:** Osteotomy

DIVISION: Cutting into a body part without draining fluids and/or gases from the body part in order to separate or transect a body part.

EXPLANATION: Separated into two or more portions ...

Body Part – 4TH	Approach – 5TH	Device – 6TH	Qualifier – 7TH
0 Subcutaneous Tissue and Fascia, Scalp	0 Open	Z No device	Z No qualifier
1 Subcutaneous Tissue and Fascia, Face	3 Percutaneous		
4 Subcutaneous Tissue and Fascia, Anterior Neck			
5 Subcutaneous Tissue and Fascia, Posterior Neck			
6 Subcutaneous Tissue and Fascia, Chest			
7 Subcutaneous Tissue and Fascia, Back			
8 Subcutaneous Tissue and Fascia, Abdomen			
9 Subcutaneous Tissue and Fascia, Buttock			
B Subcutaneous Tissue and Fascia, Perineum			
C Subcutaneous Tissue and Fascia, Pelvic Region			
D Subcutaneous Tissue and Fascia, Right Upper Arm			
F Subcutaneous Tissue and Fascia, Left Upper Arm			
G Subcutaneous Tissue and Fascia, Right Lower Arm			
H Subcutaneous Tissue and Fascia, Left Lower Arm			
J Subcutaneous Tissue and Fascia, Right Hand			
K Subcutaneous Tissue and Fascia, Left Hand			
L Subcutaneous Tissue and Fascia, Right Upper Leg			
M Subcutaneous Tissue and Fascia, Left Upper Leg			
N Subcutaneous Tissue and Fascia, Right Lower Leg			
P Subcutaneous Tissue and Fascia, Left Lower Leg			
Q Subcutaneous Tissue and Fascia, Right Foot			
R Subcutaneous Tissue and Fascia, Left Foot			
S Subcutaneous Tissue and Fascia, Head and Neck			
T Subcutaneous Tissue and Fascia, Trunk			
V Subcutaneous Tissue and Fascia, Upper Extremity			
W Subcutaneous Tissue and Fascia, Lower Extremity			

0J9 MEDICAL AND SURGICAL SECTION – 2016 ICD-10-PCS [2016.PCS]

DRAINAGE GROUP: Drainage, Extirpation, (Fragmentation)
Root Operations that take out solids/fluids/gases from a body part.

1ST - **0** Medical and Surgical
2ND - **J** Subcutaneous Tissue and Fascia
3RD - **9** DRAINAGE

EXAMPLE: I&D fascial abscess   CMS Ex: Thoracentesis

DRAINAGE: Taking or letting out fluids and/or gases from a body part.

EXPLANATION: Qualifier "X Diagnostic" indicates biopsy …

Body Part – 4TH	Approach – 5TH	Device – 6TH	Qualifier – 7TH
0 Subcutaneous Tissue and Fascia, Scalp	0 Open	0 Drainage device	Z No qualifier
1 Subcutaneous Tissue and Fascia, Face	3 Percutaneous		
4 Subcutaneous Tissue and Fascia, Anterior Neck			
5 Subcutaneous Tissue and Fascia, Posterior Neck			
6 Subcutaneous Tissue and Fascia, Chest			
7 Subcutaneous Tissue and Fascia, Back			
8 Subcutaneous Tissue and Fascia, Abdomen			
9 Subcutaneous Tissue and Fascia, Buttock			
B Subcutaneous Tissue and Fascia, Perineum			
C Subcutaneous Tissue and Fascia, Pelvic Region			
D Subcutaneous Tissue and Fascia, Right Upper Arm			
F Subcutaneous Tissue and Fascia, Left Upper Arm			
G Subcutaneous Tissue and Fascia, Right Lower Arm			
H Subcutaneous Tissue and Fascia, Left Lower Arm			
J Subcutaneous Tissue and Fascia, Right Hand			
K Subcutaneous Tissue and Fascia, Left Hand			
L Subcutaneous Tissue and Fascia, Right Upper Leg			
M Subcutaneous Tissue and Fascia, Left Upper Leg			
N Subcutaneous Tissue and Fascia, Right Lower Leg			
P Subcutaneous Tissue and Fascia, Left Lower Leg			
Q Subcutaneous Tissue and Fascia, Right Foot			
R Subcutaneous Tissue and Fascia, Left Foot			
0 Subcutaneous Tissue and Fascia, Scalp	0 Open	Z No device	X Diagnostic
1 Subcutaneous Tissue and Fascia, Face	3 Percutaneous		Z No qualifier
4 Subcutaneous Tissue and Fascia, Anterior Neck			
5 Subcutaneous Tissue and Fascia, Posterior Neck			
6 Subcutaneous Tissue and Fascia, Chest			
7 Subcutaneous Tissue and Fascia, Back			
8 Subcutaneous Tissue and Fascia, Abdomen			
9 Subcutaneous Tissue and Fascia, Buttock			
B Subcutaneous Tissue and Fascia, Perineum			
C Subcutaneous Tissue and Fascia, Pelvic Region			
D Subcutaneous Tissue and Fascia, Right Upper Arm			
F Subcutaneous Tissue and Fascia, Left Upper Arm			
G Subcutaneous Tissue and Fascia, Right Lower Arm			
H Subcutaneous Tissue and Fascia, Left Lower Arm			
J Subcutaneous Tissue and Fascia, Right Hand			
K Subcutaneous Tissue and Fascia, Left Hand			
L Subcutaneous Tissue and Fascia, Right Upper Leg			
M Subcutaneous Tissue and Fascia, Left Upper Leg			
N Subcutaneous Tissue and Fascia, Right Lower Leg			
P Subcutaneous Tissue and Fascia, Left Lower Leg			
Q Subcutaneous Tissue and Fascia, Right Foot			
R Subcutaneous Tissue and Fascia, Left Foot			

J – SUBCUTANEOUS TISSUE AND FASCIA — 0JB

EXCISION GROUP: Excision, (Resection), Destruction, Extraction (Detachment)
Root Operations that take out some or all of a body part.

- 1ST – **0** Medical and Surgical
- 2ND – **J** Subcutaneous Tissue and Fascia
- 3RD – **B** EXCISION

EXAMPLE: Harvesting fat for graft
CMS Ex: Liver biopsy

EXCISION: Cutting out or off, without replacement, a portion of a body part.

EXPLANATION: Qualifier "X Diagnostic" indicates biopsy …

Body Part – 4TH	Approach – 5TH	Device – 6TH	Qualifier – 7TH
0 Subcutaneous Tissue and Fascia, Scalp	0 Open	Z No device	X Diagnostic
1 Subcutaneous Tissue and Fascia, Face	3 Percutaneous		Z No qualifier
4 Subcutaneous Tissue and Fascia, Anterior Neck			
5 Subcutaneous Tissue and Fascia, Posterior Neck			
6 Subcutaneous Tissue and Fascia, Chest			
7 Subcutaneous Tissue and Fascia, Back			
8 Subcutaneous Tissue and Fascia, Abdomen			
9 Subcutaneous Tissue and Fascia, Buttock			
B Subcutaneous Tissue and Fascia, Perineum			
C Subcutaneous Tissue and Fascia, Pelvic Region			
D Subcutaneous Tissue and Fascia, Right Upper Arm			
F Subcutaneous Tissue and Fascia, Left Upper Arm			
G Subcutaneous Tissue and Fascia, Right Lower Arm			
H Subcutaneous Tissue and Fascia, Left Lower Arm			
J Subcutaneous Tissue and Fascia, Right Hand			
K Subcutaneous Tissue and Fascia, Left Hand			
L Subcutaneous Tissue and Fascia, Right Upper Leg			
M Subcutaneous Tissue and Fascia, Left Upper Leg			
N Subcutaneous Tissue and Fascia, Right Lower Leg			
P Subcutaneous Tissue and Fascia, Left Lower Leg			
Q Subcutaneous Tissue and Fascia, Right Foot			
R Subcutaneous Tissue and Fascia, Left Foot			

0JC

MEDICAL AND SURGICAL SECTION – 2016 ICD-10-PCS [2016.PCS]

DRAINAGE GROUP: Drainage, Extirpation, (Fragmentation)
Root Operations that take out solids/fluids/gases from a body part.

- 1ST – **0** Medical and Surgical
- 2ND – **J** Subcutaneous Tissue and Fascia
- 3RD – **C** EXTIRPATION

EXAMPLE: Removal foreign body CMS Ex: Choledocholithotomy

EXTIRPATION: Taking or cutting out solid matter from a body part.

EXPLANATION: Abnormal byproduct or foreign body …

Body Part – 4TH	Approach – 5TH	Device – 6TH	Qualifier – 7TH
0 Subcutaneous Tissue and Fascia, Scalp	0 Open	Z No device	Z No qualifier
1 Subcutaneous Tissue and Fascia, Face	3 Percutaneous		
4 Subcutaneous Tissue and Fascia, Anterior Neck			
5 Subcutaneous Tissue and Fascia, Posterior Neck			
6 Subcutaneous Tissue and Fascia, Chest			
7 Subcutaneous Tissue and Fascia, Back			
8 Subcutaneous Tissue and Fascia, Abdomen			
9 Subcutaneous Tissue and Fascia, Buttock			
B Subcutaneous Tissue and Fascia, Perineum			
C Subcutaneous Tissue and Fascia, Pelvic Region			
D Subcutaneous Tissue and Fascia, Right Upper Arm			
F Subcutaneous Tissue and Fascia, Left Upper Arm			
G Subcutaneous Tissue and Fascia, Right Lower Arm			
H Subcutaneous Tissue and Fascia, Left Lower Arm			
J Subcutaneous Tissue and Fascia, Right Hand			
K Subcutaneous Tissue and Fascia, Left Hand			
L Subcutaneous Tissue and Fascia, Right Upper Leg			
M Subcutaneous Tissue and Fascia, Left Upper Leg			
N Subcutaneous Tissue and Fascia, Right Lower Leg			
P Subcutaneous Tissue and Fascia, Left Lower Leg			
Q Subcutaneous Tissue and Fascia, Right Foot			
R Subcutaneous Tissue and Fascia, Left Foot			

SUBCUTANEOUS 0JC

0JD

J – SUBCUTANEOUS TISSUE AND FASCIA

EXCISION GROUP: Excision, (Resection), Destruction, Extraction (Detachment)
Root Operations that take out some or all of a body part.

1ST - 0	Medical and Surgical
2ND - J	Subcutaneous Tissue and Fascia
3RD - D	EXTRACTION

EXAMPLE: Non-excisional debridement **CMS Ex:** D&C

EXTRACTION: Pulling or stripping out or off all or a portion of a body part by the use of force.

EXPLANATION: None for this Body System

Body Part – 4TH	Approach – 5TH	Device – 6TH	Qualifier – 7TH
0 Subcutaneous Tissue and Fascia, Scalp	0 Open	Z No device	Z No qualifier
1 Subcutaneous Tissue and Fascia, Face	3 Percutaneous		
4 Subcutaneous Tissue and Fascia, Anterior Neck			
5 Subcutaneous Tissue and Fascia, Posterior Neck			
6 Subcutaneous Tissue and Fascia, Chest			
7 Subcutaneous Tissue and Fascia, Back			
8 Subcutaneous Tissue and Fascia, Abdomen			
9 Subcutaneous Tissue and Fascia, Buttock			
B Subcutaneous Tissue and Fascia, Perineum			
C Subcutaneous Tissue and Fascia, Pelvic Region			
D Subcutaneous Tissue and Fascia, Right Upper Arm			
F Subcutaneous Tissue and Fascia, Left Upper Arm			
G Subcutaneous Tissue and Fascia, Right Lower Arm			
H Subcutaneous Tissue and Fascia, Left Lower Arm			
J Subcutaneous Tissue and Fascia, Right Hand			
K Subcutaneous Tissue and Fascia, Left Hand			
L Subcutaneous Tissue and Fascia, Right Upper Leg			
M Subcutaneous Tissue and Fascia, Left Upper Leg			
N Subcutaneous Tissue and Fascia, Right Lower Leg			
P Subcutaneous Tissue and Fascia, Left Lower Leg			
Q Subcutaneous Tissue and Fascia, Right Foot			
R Subcutaneous Tissue and Fascia, Left Foot			

0JH MEDICAL AND SURGICAL SECTION – 2016 ICD-10-PCS

DEVICE GROUP: Change, Insertion, Removal, Replacement, Revision, Supplement
Root Operations that always involve a device.

1ST - **0** Medical and Surgical
2ND - **J** Subcutaneous Tissue and Fascia
3RD - **H INSERTION**

EXAMPLE: Placement pacemaker generator   CMS Ex: CVP catheter

INSERTION: Putting in a nonbiological appliance that monitors, assists, performs, or prevents a physiological function but does not physically take the place of a body part.

EXPLANATION: None

Body Part – 4TH	Approach – 5TH	Device – 6TH	Qualifier – 7TH
0 Subcutaneous Tissue and Fascia, Scalp 1 Subcutaneous Tissue and Fascia, Face 4 Subcutaneous Tissue and Fascia, Anterior Neck 5 Subcutaneous Tissue and Fascia, Posterior Neck 9 Subcutaneous Tissue and Fascia, Buttock B Subcutaneous Tissue and Fascia, Perineum C Subcutaneous Tissue and Fascia, Pelvic Region J Subcutaneous Tissue and Fascia, Right Hand K Subcutaneous Tissue and Fascia, Left Hand Q Subcutaneous Tissue and Fascia, Right Foot R Subcutaneous Tissue and Fascia, Left Foot	0 Open 3 Percutaneous	N Tissue Expander	Z No qualifier
6 Subcutaneous Tissue and Fascia, Chest 8 Subcutaneous Tissue and Fascia, Abdomen	0 Open 3 Percutaneous	0 Monitoring device, hemodynamic 2 Monitoring device 4 Pacemaker, single chamber 5 Pacemaker, single chamber rate responsive 6 Pacemaker, dual chamber 7 Cardiac resynchronization pacemaker pulse generator 8 Defibrillator generator 9 Cardiac resynchronization defibrillator pulse generator A Contractility modulation device B Stimulator generator, single array C Stimulator generator, single array rechargeable D Stimulator generator, multiple array E Stimulator generator, multiple array rechargeable H Contraceptive device M Stimulator generator NC* N Tissue expander P Cardiac rhythm related device V Infusion device, pump W Vascular access device, reservoir X Vascular access device	Z No qualifier

continued

J – SUBCUTANEOUS TISSUE AND FASCIA   0JJ

0 J H INSERTION – *continued*

Body Part – 4ᵀᴴ	Approach – 5ᵀᴴ	Device – 6ᵀᴴ	Qualifier – 7ᵀᴴ
7 Subcutaneous Tissue and Fascia, Back	0 Open 3 Percutaneous	B Stimulator generator, single array C Stimulator generator, single array rechargeable D Stimulator generator, multiple array E Stimulator generator, multiple array rechargeable M Stimulator generator ᴺᶜ* N Tissue expander V Infusion device, pump	Z No qualifier
D Subcutaneous Tissue and Fascia, Right Upper Arm F Subcutaneous Tissue and Fascia, Left Upper Arm G Subcutaneous Tissue and Fascia, Right Lower Arm H Subcutaneous Tissue and Fascia, Left Lower Arm L Subcutaneous Tissue and Fascia, Right Upper Leg M Subcutaneous Tissue and Fascia, Left Upper Leg N Subcutaneous Tissue and Fascia, Right Lower Leg P Subcutaneous Tissue and Fascia, Left Lower Leg	0 Open 3 Percutaneous	H Contraceptive device N Tissue expander V Infusion device, pump W Vascular access device, reservoir X Vascular access device	Z No qualifier
S Subcutaneous Tissue and Fascia, Head and Neck V Subcutaneous Tissue and Fascia, Upper Extremity W Subcutaneous Tissue and Fascia, Lower Extremity	0 Open 3 Percutaneous	1 Radioactive element 3 Infusion device	Z No qualifier
T Subcutaneous Tissue and Fascia, Trunk	0 Open 3 Percutaneous	1 Radioactive element 3 Infusion device V Infusion device, pump	Z No qualifier

NC* – Some procedures are considered non-covered by Medicare. See current Medicare Code Editor for details.

EXAMINATION GROUP: Inspection, (Map)
Root Operations involving examination only.

1ˢᵀ – **0** Medical and Surgical
2ᴺᴰ – **J** Subcutaneous Tissue and Fascia
3ᴿᴰ – **J** INSPECTION

EXAMPLE: Exploration abdominal fascia   CMS Ex: Colonoscopy

INSPECTION: Visually and/or manually exploring a body part.

EXPLANATION: Direct or instrumental visualization ...

Body Part – 4ᵀᴴ	Approach – 5ᵀᴴ	Device – 6ᵀᴴ	Qualifier – 7ᵀᴴ
S Subcutaneous Tissue and Fascia, Head and Neck T Subcutaneous Tissue and Fascia, Trunk V Subcutaneous Tissue and Fascia, Upper Extremity W Subcutaneous Tissue and Fascia, Lower Extremity	0 Open 3 Percutaneous X External	Z No device	Z No qualifier

0JN

MEDICAL AND SURGICAL SECTION – 2016 ICD-10-PCS

DIVISION GROUP: Division, Release
Root Operations involving cutting or separation only.

- 1ST – **0** Medical and Surgical
- 2ND – **J** Subcutaneous Tissue and Fascia
- 3RD – **N** RELEASE

EXAMPLE: Lysis fascial adhesions CMS Ex: Carpal tunnel release

RELEASE: Freeing a body part from an abnormal physical constraint by cutting or by the use of force.

EXPLANATION: None of the body part is taken out ...

Body Part – 4TH	Approach – 5TH	Device – 6TH	Qualifier – 7TH
0 Subcutaneous Tissue and Fascia, Scalp	0 Open	Z No device	Z No qualifier
1 Subcutaneous Tissue and Fascia, Face	3 Percutaneous		
4 Subcutaneous Tissue and Fascia, Anterior Neck	X External		
5 Subcutaneous Tissue and Fascia, Posterior Neck			
6 Subcutaneous Tissue and Fascia, Chest			
7 Subcutaneous Tissue and Fascia, Back			
8 Subcutaneous Tissue and Fascia, Abdomen			
9 Subcutaneous Tissue and Fascia, Buttock			
B Subcutaneous Tissue and Fascia, Perineum			
C Subcutaneous Tissue and Fascia, Pelvic Region			
D Subcutaneous Tissue and Fascia, Right Upper Arm			
F Subcutaneous Tissue and Fascia, Left Upper Arm			
G Subcutaneous Tissue and Fascia, Right Lower Arm			
H Subcutaneous Tissue and Fascia, Left Lower Arm			
J Subcutaneous Tissue and Fascia, Right Hand			
K Subcutaneous Tissue and Fascia, Left Hand			
L Subcutaneous Tissue and Fascia, Right Upper Leg			
M Subcutaneous Tissue and Fascia, Left Upper Leg			
N Subcutaneous Tissue and Fascia, Right Lower Leg			
P Subcutaneous Tissue and Fascia, Left Lower Leg			
Q Subcutaneous Tissue and Fascia, Right Foot			
R Subcutaneous Tissue and Fascia, Left Foot			

J – SUBCUTANEOUS TISSUE AND FASCIA

0 J P

DEVICE GROUP: Change, Insertion, Removal, Replacement, Revision, Supplement
Root Operations that always involve a device.

- 1ST - **0** Medical and Surgical
- 2ND - **J** Subcutaneous Tissue and Fascia
- 3RD - **P REMOVAL**

EXAMPLE: Removal VAD reservoir
CMS Ex: Chest tube removal

REMOVAL: Taking out or off a device from a body part.

EXPLANATION: Removal device without reinsertion ...

Body Part – 4TH	Approach – 5TH	Device – 6TH	Qualifier – 7TH
S Subcutaneous Tissue and Fascia, Head and Neck	0 Open 3 Percutaneous	0 Drainage device 1 Radioactive element 3 Infusion device 7 Autologous tissue substitute J Synthetic substitute K Nonautologous tissue substitute N Tissue expander	Z No qualifier
S Subcutaneous Tissue and Fascia, Head and Neck	X External	0 Drainage device 1 Radioactive element 3 Infusion device	Z No qualifier
T Subcutaneous Tissue and Fascia, Trunk	0 Open 3 Percutaneous	0 Drainage device 1 Radioactive element 2 Monitoring device 3 Infusion device 7 Autologous tissue substitute H Contraceptive device J Synthetic substitute K Nonautologous tissue substitute M Stimulator generator N Tissue expander P Cardiac rhythm related device V Infusion device, pump W Vascular access device, reservoir X Vascular access device	Z No qualifier
T Subcutaneous Tissue and Fascia, Trunk	X External	0 Drainage device 1 Radioactive element 2 Monitoring device 3 Infusion device H Contraceptive device V Infusion device, pump X Vascular access device	Z No qualifier

continued ⇨

0JP MEDICAL AND SURGICAL SECTION – 2016 ICD-10-PCS [2016.PCS]

0 J P REMOVAL – *continued*

Body Part – 4ᵀᴴ	Approach – 5ᵀᴴ	Device – 6ᵀᴴ	Qualifier – 7ᵀᴴ
V Subcutaneous Tissue and Fascia, Upper Extremity W Subcutaneous Tissue and Fascia, Lower Extremity	0 Open 3 Percutaneous	0 Drainage device 1 Radioactive element 2 Monitoring device 3 Infusion device 7 Autologous tissue substitute H Contraceptive device J Synthetic substitute K Nonautologous tissue substitute N Tissue expander V Infusion device, pump W Vascular access device, reservoir X Vascular access device	Z No qualifier
V Subcutaneous Tissue and Fascia, Upper Extremity W Subcutaneous Tissue and Fascia, Lower Extremity	X External	0 Drainage device 1 Radioactive element 3 Infusion device H Contraceptive device V Infusion device, pump X Vascular access device	Z No qualifier

---

OTHER REPAIRS GROUP: (Control), **Repair**
Root Operations that define other repairs.

1ˢᵀ - 0 Medical and Surgical
2ᴺᴰ - J Subcutaneous Tissue and Fascia
3ᴿᴰ - Q REPAIR

EXAMPLE: Rectocele repair with sutures   **CMS Ex:** Suture laceration

REPAIR: Restoring, to the extent possible, a body part to its normal anatomic structure and function.

EXPLANATION: Only when no other root operation applies ...

Body Part – 4ᵀᴴ	Approach – 5ᵀᴴ	Device – 6ᵀᴴ	Qualifier – 7ᵀᴴ
0 Subcutaneous Tissue and Fascia, Scalp 1 Subcutaneous Tissue and Fascia, Face 4 Subcutaneous Tissue and Fascia, Anterior Neck 5 Subcutaneous Tissue and Fascia, Posterior Neck 6 Subcutaneous Tissue and Fascia, Chest 7 Subcutaneous Tissue and Fascia, Back 8 Subcutaneous Tissue and Fascia, Abdomen 9 Subcutaneous Tissue and Fascia, Buttock B Subcutaneous Tissue and Fascia, Perineum C Subcutaneous Tissue and Fascia, Pelvic Region D Subcutaneous Tissue and Fascia, Right Upper Arm F Subcutaneous Tissue and Fascia, Left Upper Arm G Subcutaneous Tissue and Fascia, Right Lower Arm H Subcutaneous Tissue and Fascia, Left Lower Arm J Subcutaneous Tissue and Fascia, Right Hand K Subcutaneous Tissue and Fascia, Left Hand L Subcutaneous Tissue and Fascia, Right Upper Leg M Subcutaneous Tissue and Fascia, Left Upper Leg N Subcutaneous Tissue and Fascia, Right Lower Leg P Subcutaneous Tissue and Fascia, Left Lower Leg Q Subcutaneous Tissue and Fascia, Right Foot R Subcutaneous Tissue and Fascia, Left Foot	0 Open 3 Percutaneous	Z No device	Z No qualifier

J – SUBCUTANEOUS TISSUE AND FASCIA

0JR

DEVICE GROUP: Change, Insertion, Removal, Replacement, Revision, Supplement
Root Operations that always involve a device.

1ST – **0** Medical and Surgical
2ND – **J** Subcutaneous Tissue and Fascia
3RD – **R** REPLACEMENT

EXAMPLE: Free fascia lata graft   CMS Ex: Total hip

REPLACEMENT: Putting in or on a biological or synthetic material that physically takes the place and/or function of all or a portion of a body part.

EXPLANATION: Includes taking out body part, or eradication...

Body Part – 4TH	Approach – 5TH	Device – 6TH	Qualifier – 7TH
0 Subcutaneous Tissue and Fascia, Scalp	0 Open	7 Autologous tissue substitute	Z No qualifier
1 Subcutaneous Tissue and Fascia, Face	3 Percutaneous	J Synthetic substitute	
4 Subcutaneous Tissue and Fascia, Anterior Neck		K Nonautologous tissue substitute	
5 Subcutaneous Tissue and Fascia, Posterior Neck			
6 Subcutaneous Tissue and Fascia, Chest			
7 Subcutaneous Tissue and Fascia, Back			
8 Subcutaneous Tissue and Fascia, Abdomen			
9 Subcutaneous Tissue and Fascia, Buttock			
B Subcutaneous Tissue and Fascia, Perineum			
C Subcutaneous Tissue and Fascia, Pelvic Region			
D Subcutaneous Tissue and Fascia, Right Upper Arm			
F Subcutaneous Tissue and Fascia, Left Upper Arm			
G Subcutaneous Tissue and Fascia, Right Lower Arm			
H Subcutaneous Tissue and Fascia, Left Lower Arm			
J Subcutaneous Tissue and Fascia, Right Hand			
K Subcutaneous Tissue and Fascia, Left Hand			
L Subcutaneous Tissue and Fascia, Right Upper Leg			
M Subcutaneous Tissue and Fascia, Left Upper Leg			
N Subcutaneous Tissue and Fascia, Right Lower Leg			
P Subcutaneous Tissue and Fascia, Left Lower Leg			
Q Subcutaneous Tissue and Fascia, Right Foot			
R Subcutaneous Tissue and Fascia, Left Foot			

0JU

MEDICAL AND SURGICAL SECTION – 2016 ICD-10-PCS

DEVICE GROUP: Change, Insertion, Removal, Replacement, Revision, Supplement
Root Operations that always involve a device.

- 1ST – **0** Medical and Surgical
- 2ND – **J** Subcutaneous Tissue and Fascia
- 3RD – **U SUPPLEMENT**

EXAMPLE: Rectocele repair with mesh | **CMS Ex:** Hernia repair with mesh

SUPPLEMENT: Putting in or on biological or synthetic material that physically reinforces and/or augments the function of a portion of a body part.

EXPLANATION: Biological material from same individual ...

Body Part – 4TH	Approach – 5TH	Device – 6TH	Qualifier – 7TH
0 Subcutaneous Tissue and Fascia, Scalp	0 Open	7 Autologous tissue substitute	Z No qualifier
1 Subcutaneous Tissue and Fascia, Face	3 Percutaneous	J Synthetic substitute	
4 Subcutaneous Tissue and Fascia, Anterior Neck		K Nonautologous tissue substitute	
5 Subcutaneous Tissue and Fascia, Posterior Neck			
6 Subcutaneous Tissue and Fascia, Chest			
7 Subcutaneous Tissue and Fascia, Back			
8 Subcutaneous Tissue and Fascia, Abdomen			
9 Subcutaneous Tissue and Fascia, Buttock			
B Subcutaneous Tissue and Fascia, Perineum			
C Subcutaneous Tissue and Fascia, Pelvic Region			
D Subcutaneous Tissue and Fascia, Right Upper Arm			
F Subcutaneous Tissue and Fascia, Left Upper Arm			
G Subcutaneous Tissue and Fascia, Right Lower Arm			
H Subcutaneous Tissue and Fascia, Left Lower Arm			
J Subcutaneous Tissue and Fascia, Right Hand			
K Subcutaneous Tissue and Fascia, Left Hand			
L Subcutaneous Tissue and Fascia, Right Upper Leg			
M Subcutaneous Tissue and Fascia, Left Upper Leg			
N Subcutaneous Tissue and Fascia, Right Lower Leg			
P Subcutaneous Tissue and Fascia, Left Lower Leg			
Q Subcutaneous Tissue and Fascia, Right Foot			
R Subcutaneous Tissue and Fascia, Left Foot			

J – SUBCUTANEOUS TISSUE AND FASCIA — 0JW

DEVICE GROUP: Change, Insertion, Removal, Replacement, Revision, Supplement
Root Operations that always involve a device.

- 1ST – **0** Medical and Surgical
- 2ND – **J** Subcutaneous Tissue and Fascia
- 3RD – **W** REVISION

EXAMPLE: Reposition stimulator generator CMS Ex: Adjustment lead

REVISION: Correcting, to the extent possible, a portion of a malfunctioning device or the position of a displaced device.

EXPLANATION: May replace components of a device ...

Body Part – 4TH	Approach – 5TH	Device – 6TH	Qualifier – 7TH
S Subcutaneous Tissue and Fascia, Head and Neck	0 Open 3 Percutaneous X External	0 Drainage device 3 Infusion device 7 Autologous tissue substitute J Synthetic substitute K Nonautologous tissue substitute N Tissue expander	Z No qualifier
T Subcutaneous Tissue and Fascia, Trunk	0 Open 3 Percutaneous X External	0 Drainage device 2 Monitoring device 3 Infusion device 7 Autologous tissue substitute H Contraceptive device J Synthetic substitute K Nonautologous tissue substitute M Stimulator generator N Tissue expander P Cardiac rhythm related device V Infusion device, pump W Vascular access device, reservoir X Vascular access device	Z No qualifier
V Subcutaneous Tissue and Fascia, Upper Extremity W Subcutaneous Tissue and Fascia, Lower Extremity	0 Open 3 Percutaneous X External	0 Drainage device 3 Infusion device 7 Autologous tissue substitute H Contraceptive device J Synthetic substitute K Nonautologous tissue substitute N Tissue expander V Infusion device, pump W Vascular access device, reservoir X Vascular access device	Z No qualifier

0JX

MEDICAL AND SURGICAL SECTION – 2016 ICD-10-PCS

MOVE GROUP: (Reattachment), (Reposition), **Transfer,** (Transplantation)
Root Operations that put in/put back or move some/all of a body part.

- 1ST – **0** Medical and Surgical
- 2ND – **J** Subcutaneous Tissue and Fascia
- 3RD – **X TRANSFER**

EXAMPLE: Fasciocutaneous pedicle flap **CMS Ex:** Tendon transfer

TRANSFER: Moving, without taking out, all or a portion of a body part to another location to take over the function of all or a portion of a body part.

EXPLANATION: The body part remains connected ...

Body Part – 4TH	Approach – 5TH	Device – 6TH	Qualifier – 7TH
0 Subcutaneous Tissue and Fascia, Scalp 1 Subcutaneous Tissue and Fascia, Face 4 Subcutaneous Tissue and Fascia, Anterior Neck 5 Subcutaneous Tissue and Fascia, Posterior Neck 6 Subcutaneous Tissue and Fascia, Chest 7 Subcutaneous Tissue and Fascia, Back 8 Subcutaneous Tissue and Fascia, Abdomen 9 Subcutaneous Tissue and Fascia, Buttock B Subcutaneous Tissue and Fascia, Perineum C Subcutaneous Tissue and Fascia, Pelvic Region D Subcutaneous Tissue and Fascia, Right Upper Arm F Subcutaneous Tissue and Fascia, Left Upper Arm G Subcutaneous Tissue and Fascia, Right Lower Arm H Subcutaneous Tissue and Fascia, Left Lower Arm J Subcutaneous Tissue and Fascia, Right Hand K Subcutaneous Tissue and Fascia, Left Hand L Subcutaneous Tissue and Fascia, Right Upper Leg M Subcutaneous Tissue and Fascia, Left Upper Leg N Subcutaneous Tissue and Fascia, Right Lower Leg P Subcutaneous Tissue and Fascia, Left Lower Leg Q Subcutaneous Tissue and Fascia, Right Foot R Subcutaneous Tissue and Fascia, Left Foot	0 Open 3 Percutaneous	Z No device	B Skin and Subcutaneous Tissue C Skin, Subcutaneous Tissue and Fascia Z No qualifier

Educational Annotations | K – Muscles

Body System Specific Educational Annotations for the Muscles include:
- Anatomy and Physiology Review
- Anatomical Illustrations
- Definitions of Common Procedures
- AHA Coding Clinic® Reference Notations
- Body Part Key Listings
- Device Key Listings
- Device Aggregation Table Listings
- Coding Notes

Anatomy and Physiology Review of Muscles

BODY PART VALUES – K - MUSCLES

Lower Muscle – The muscles located below the diaphragm (see Coding Guideline B2.1b).

Muscle – ANATOMY – Muscles are groups of skeletal muscle tissue, blood vessels, and nerves that are attached to the skeletal bones. Cardiac and smooth muscle tissue is also found in the heart and other organs. PHYSIOLOGY – The muscles contract to allow the movement of the human body.

Upper Muscle – The muscles located above the diaphragm (see Coding Guideline B2.1b).

Anatomical Illustrations of Muscles

None for the Muscles Body System

Definitions of Common Procedures of Muscles

Muscle transfer – The surgical detachment of the distal end of a muscle and subsequent connection to another nearby site while maintaining its vascular and nervous supply.

Muscle transplant – The surgical removal of a muscle with transplantation to a different site and, through microsurgery, connected to blood vessels and a nerve.

TRAM (transverse rectus abdominis myocutaneous) flap breast reconstruction – The post-mastectomy reconstruction of the breast using the transverse rectus abdominis muscle that is raised (including the overlying fat and skin) and transferred to the mastectomy site.

AHA Coding Clinic® Reference Notations of Muscles

ROOT OPERATION SPECIFIC - K - MUSCLES
CHANGE - 2
DESTRUCTION - 5
DIVISION - 8
DRAINAGE - 9
EXCISION - B
EXTIRPATION - C
INSERTION - H
INSPECTION - J
REATTACHMENT - M
RELEASE - N
    Biceps tenotomy...AHA 15:2Q:p22
    Repair of incisional hernia with component release and mesh..................AHA 14:4Q:p39
REMOVAL - P
REPAIR - Q
    Repair of second degree perineal laceration...AHA 14:4Q:p43
    Repair of second degree perineal laceration including muscle...................AHA 13:4Q:p120
REPOSITION - S
RESECTION - T
    Resection of perineum muscle ....AHA 15:1Q:p38
SUPPLEMENT - U
REVISION - W
TRANSFER - X
    Ipsilateral pedicle transverse abdominomyocutaneous (TRAM) flap
        breast reconstruction...AHA 14:2Q:p10
    Pedicle latissimus myocutaneous flap breast reconstruction.....................AHA 14:2Q:p12
    Perineal myocutaneous flap closure of abdominoperineal resection..........AHA 14:4Q:p41
    Posterior pharyngeal flap to the soft palate..AHA 15:2Q:p26

0K

MEDICAL AND SURGICAL SECTION – 2016 ICD-10-PCS

Educational Annotations | K – Muscles

Body Part Key Listings of Muscles

See also Body Part Key in Appendix C

Abductor hallucis muscle	*use* Foot Muscle, Left/Right
Adductor brevis muscle	*use* Upper Leg Muscle, Left/Right
Adductor hallucis muscle	*use* Foot Muscle, Left/Right
Adductor longus muscle	*use* Upper Leg Muscle, Left/Right
Adductor magnus muscle	*use* Upper Leg Muscle, Left/Right
Anatomical snuffbox	*use* Lower Arm and Wrist Muscle, Left/Right
Anterior vertebral muscle	*use* Neck Muscle, Left/Right
Arytenoid muscle	*use* Neck Muscle, Left/Right
Auricularis muscle	*use* Head Muscle
Biceps brachii muscle	*use* Upper Arm Muscle, Left/Right
Biceps femoris muscle	*use* Upper Leg Muscle, Left/Right
Brachialis muscle	*use* Upper Arm Muscle, Left/Right
Brachioradialis muscle	*use* Lower Arm and Wrist Muscle, Left/Right
Buccinator muscle	*use* Facial Muscle
Bulbospongiosus muscle	*use* Perineum Muscle
Chondroglossus muscle	*use* Tongue, Palate, Pharynx Muscle
Coccygeus muscle	*use* Trunk Muscle, Left/Right
Coracobrachialis muscle	*use* Upper Arm Muscle, Left/Right
Corrugator supercilii muscle	*use* Facial Muscle
Cremaster muscle	*use* Perineum Muscle
Cricothyroid muscle	*use* Neck Muscle, Left/Right
Deep transverse perineal muscle	*use* Perineum Muscle
Deltoid muscle	*use* Shoulder Muscle, Left/Right
Depressor anguli oris muscle	*use* Facial Muscle
Depressor labii inferioris muscle	*use* Facial Muscle
Depressor septi nasi muscle	*use* Facial Muscle
Depressor supercilii muscle	*use* Facial Muscle
Erector spinae muscle	*use* Trunk Muscle, Left/Right
Extensor carpi radialis muscle	*use* Lower Arm and Wrist Muscle, Left/Right
Extensor carpi ulnaris muscle	*use* Lower Arm and Wrist Muscle, Left/Right
Extensor digitorum brevis muscle	*use* Foot Muscle, Left/Right
Extensor digitorum longus muscle	*use* Lower Leg Muscle, Left/Right
Extensor hallucis brevis muscle	*use* Foot Muscle, Left/Right
Extensor hallucis longus muscle	*use* Lower Leg Muscle, Left/Right
External oblique muscle	*use* Abdomen Muscle, Left/Right
Fibularis brevis muscle	*use* Lower Leg Muscle, Left/Right
Fibularis longus muscle	*use* Lower Leg Muscle, Left/Right
Flexor carpi radialis muscle	*use* Lower Arm and Wrist Muscle, Left/Right
Flexor carpi ulnaris muscle	*use* Lower Arm and Wrist Muscle, Left/Right
Flexor digitorum brevis muscle	*use* Foot Muscle, Left/Right
Flexor digitorum longus muscle	*use* Lower Leg Muscle, Left/Right
Flexor hallucis brevis muscle	*use* Foot Muscle, Left/Right
Flexor hallucis longus muscle	*use* Lower Leg Muscle, Left/Right
Flexor pollicis longus muscle	*use* Lower Arm and Wrist Muscle, Left/Right
Gastrocnemius muscle	*use* Lower Leg Muscle, Left/Right
Gemellus muscle	*use* Hip Muscle, Left/Right
Genioglossus muscle	*use* Tongue, Palate, Pharynx Muscle
Gluteus maximus muscle	*use* Hip Muscle, Left/Right

Continued on next page

Educational Annotations

K – Muscles

Body Part Key Listings of Muscles

Continued from previous page

Gluteus medius muscle	*use* Hip Muscle, Left/Right
Gluteus minimus muscle	*use* Hip Muscle, Left/Right
Gracilis muscle	*use* Upper Leg Muscle, Left/Right
Hyoglossus muscle	*use* Tongue, Palate, Pharynx Muscle
Hypothenar muscle	*use* Hand Muscle, Left/Right
Iliacus muscle	*use* Hip Muscle, Left/Right
Inferior longitudinal muscle	*use* Tongue, Palate, Pharynx Muscle
Infrahyoid muscle	*use* Neck Muscle, Left/Right
Infraspinatus muscle	*use* Shoulder Muscle, Left/Right
Intercostal muscle	*use* Thorax Muscle, Left/Right
Internal oblique muscle	*use* Abdomen Muscle, Left/Right
Interspinalis muscle	*use* Trunk Muscle, Left/Right
Intertransversarius muscle	*use* Trunk Muscle, Left/Right
Ischiocavernosus muscle	*use* Perineum Muscle
Latissimus dorsi muscle	*use* Trunk Muscle, Left/Right
Levator anguli oris muscle	*use* Facial Muscle
Levator ani muscle	*use* Trunk Muscle, Left/Right
Levator labii superioris alaeque nasi muscle	*use* Facial Muscle
Levator labii superioris muscle	*use* Facial Muscle
Levator scapulae muscle	*use* Neck Muscle, Left/Right
Levator veli palatini muscle	*use* Tongue, Palate, Pharynx Muscle
Levatores costarum muscle	*use* Thorax Muscle, Left/Right
Masseter muscle	*use* Head Muscle
Mentalis muscle	*use* Facial Muscle
Nasalis muscle	*use* Facial Muscle
Obturator muscle	*use* Hip Muscle, Left/Right
Occipitofrontalis muscle	*use* Facial Muscle
Orbicularis oris muscle	*use* Facial Muscle
Palatoglossal muscle	*use* Tongue, Palate, Pharynx Muscle
Palatopharyngeal muscle	*use* Tongue, Palate, Pharynx Muscle
Palmar interosseous muscle	*use* Hand Muscle, Left/Right
Palmaris longus muscle	*use* Lower Arm and Wrist Muscle, Left/Right
Pectineus muscle	*use* Upper Leg Muscle, Left/Right
Pectoralis major muscle	*use* Thorax Muscle, Left/Right
Pectoralis minor muscle	*use* Thorax Muscle, Left/Right
Peroneus brevis muscle	*use* Lower Leg Muscle, Left/Right
Peroneus longus muscle	*use* Lower Leg Muscle, Left/Right
Pharyngeal constrictor muscle	*use* Tongue, Palate, Pharynx Muscle
Piriformis muscle	*use* Hip Muscle, Left/Right
Platysma muscle	*use* Neck Muscle, Left/Right
Popliteus muscle	*use* Lower Leg Muscle, Left/Right
Procerus muscle	*use* Facial Muscle
Pronator quadratus muscle	*use* Lower Arm and Wrist Muscle, Left/Right
Pronator teres muscle	*use* Lower Arm and Wrist Muscle, Left/Right
Psoas muscle	*use* Hip Muscle, Left/Right
Pterygoid muscle	*use* Head Muscle
Pyramidalis muscle	*use* Abdomen Muscle, Left/Right
Quadratus femoris muscle	*use* Hip Muscle, Left/Right
Quadratus lumborum muscle	*use* Trunk Muscle, Left/Right

Continued on next page

Educational Annotations

K – Muscles

Body Part Key Listings of Muscles

Continued from previous page

Quadratus plantae muscle	*use* Foot Muscle, Left/Right
Quadriceps (femoris)	*use* Upper Leg Muscle, Left/Right
Rectus abdominis muscle	*use* Abdomen Muscle, Left/Right
Rectus femoris muscle	*use* Upper Leg Muscle, Left/Right
Rhomboid major muscle	*use* Trunk Muscle, Left/Right
Rhomboid minor muscle	*use* Trunk Muscle, Left/Right
Risorius muscle	*use* Facial Muscle
Salpingopharyngeus muscle	*use* Tongue, Palate, Pharynx Muscle
Sartorius muscle	*use* Upper Leg Muscle, Left/Right
Scalene muscle	*use* Neck Muscle, Left/Right
Semimembranosus muscle	*use* Upper Leg Muscle, Left/Right
Semitendinosus muscle	*use* Upper Leg Muscle, Left/Right
Serratus anterior muscle	*use* Thorax Muscle, Left/Right
Serratus posterior muscle	*use* Trunk Muscle, Left/Right
Soleus muscle	*use* Lower Leg Muscle, Left/Right
Splenius capitis muscle	*use* Head Muscle
Splenius cervicis muscle	*use* Neck Muscle, Left/Right
Sternocleidomastoid muscle	*use* Neck Muscle, Left/Right
Styloglossus muscle	*use* Tongue, Palate, Pharynx Muscle
Stylopharyngeus muscle	*use* Tongue, Palate, Pharynx Muscle
Subclavius muscle	*use* Thorax Muscle, Left/Right
Subcostal muscle	*use* Thorax Muscle, Left/Right
Subscapularis muscle	*use* Shoulder Muscle, Left/Right
Superficial transverse perineal muscle	*use* Perineum Muscle
Superior longitudinal muscle	*use* Tongue, Palate, Pharynx Muscle
Suprahyoid muscle	*use* Neck Muscle, Left/Right
Supraspinatus muscle	*use* Shoulder Muscle, Left/Right
Temporalis muscle	*use* Head Muscle
Temporoparietalis muscle	*use* Head Muscle
Tensor fasciae latae muscle	*use* Hip Muscle, Left/Right
Tensor veli palatini muscle	*use* Tongue, Palate, Pharynx Muscle
Teres major muscle	*use* Shoulder Muscle, Left/Right
Teres minor muscle	*use* Shoulder Muscle, Left/Right
Thenar muscle	*use* Hand Muscle, Left/Right
Thyroarytenoid muscle	*use* Neck Muscle, Left/Right
Tibialis anterior muscle	*use* Lower Leg Muscle, Left/Right
Tibialis posterior muscle	*use* Lower Leg Muscle, Left/Right
Transverse thoracis muscle	*use* Thorax Muscle, Left/Right
Transversospinalis muscle	*use* Trunk Muscle, Left/Right
Transversus abdominis muscle	*use* Abdomen Muscle, Left/Right
Trapezius muscle	*use* Trunk Muscle, Left/Right
Triceps brachii muscle	*use* Upper Arm Muscle, Left/Right
Vastus intermedius muscle	*use* Upper Leg Muscle, Left/Right
Vastus lateralis muscle	*use* Upper Leg Muscle, Left/Right
Vastus medialis muscle	*use* Upper Leg Muscle, Left/Right
Zygomaticus muscle	*use* Facial Muscle

Educational Annotations

K – Muscles

Device Key Listings of Muscles

See also Device Key in Appendix D

Autograft ....*use* Autologous Tissue Substitute
Electrical muscle stimulation (EMS) lead ....*use* Stimulator Lead in Muscles
Electronic muscle stimulator lead ....*use* Stimulator Lead in Muscles
Neuromuscular electrical stimulation (NEMS) lead *use* Stimulator Lead in Muscles
Tissue bank graft ....*use* Nonautologous Tissue Substitute

Device Aggregation Table Listings of Muscles

See also Device Aggregation Table in Appendix E

Specific Device	For Operation	In Body System	General Device
None Listed in Device Aggregation Table for this Body System			

Coding Notes of Muscles

Body System Relevant Coding Guidelines

General Guidelines

B2.1b
  Where the general body part values "upper" and "lower" are provided as an option in the Upper Arteries, Lower Arteries, Upper Veins, Lower Veins, Muscles and Tendons body systems, "upper" and "lower" specifies body parts located above or below the diaphragm respectively.
  Example: Vein body parts above the diaphragm are found in the Upper Veins body system; vein body parts below the diaphragm are found in the Lower Veins body system.

Body System Specific PCS Reference Manual Exercises

PCS CODE	K – MUSCLES EXERCISES
0KBS3ZX	Percutaneous biopsy of right gastrocnemius muscle.
0KMT0ZZ	Reattachment of traumatic left gastrocnemius avulsion, open.
0KXK0Z6	Bilateral TRAM pedicle flap reconstruction status post mastectomy, muscle only, open. (The
0KXL0Z6	transverse rectus abdominus muscle (TRAM) flap is coded for each flap developed.)

Educational Annotations

K – Muscles

NOTES

Devices - Character 6

See also Device Key in Appendix D
Autograft .... use Autologous Tissue Substitute
Electrical muscle stimulation (EMS) lead .... use Stimulator Lead in Muscles
Electronic muscle stimulator lead .... use Stimulator Lead in Muscles
Neuromuscular electrical stimulation (NEMS) lead use Stimulator Lead in Muscles
Tissue bank graft .... use Nonautologous Tissue Substitute

Device Aggregation Table - Character 6

See also Device Aggregation Table in Appendix E

Specific Device	For Operation	In Body System	General Device

None Listed in Device Aggregation Table for this Body System

Coding Notes - Muscles

Body System Relevant Coding Guidelines

General Guidelines

B2.1b

Where the general body part values "upper" and "lower" are provided as an option in the Upper Arteries, Lower Arteries, Upper Veins, Lower Veins, Muscles and Tendons body systems, "upper" and "lower" specifies body parts located above or below the diaphragm respectively.

Example: Vein body parts above the diaphragm are found in the Upper Veins body system; vein body parts below the diaphragm are found in the Lower Veins body system.

Body System Specific PCS Reference Manual Exercises

PCS CODE	K – MUSCLES EXERCISES
0KB32ZX	Percutaneous biopsy of right gastrocnemius muscle.
0KMT0ZZ	Reattachment of traumatic left gastrocnemius avulsion, open.
0KXK0Z6	Bilateral TRAM pedicle flap reconstruction status post mastectomy, muscle only, open. (The transverse rectus abdominis muscle (TRAM) flap is coded for each flap developed.)
0KXL0Z6	

K – MUSCLES 0K5

DEVICE GROUP: Change, Insertion, Removal, (Replacement), Revision, Supplement
Root Operations that always involve a device.

1ST - **0** Medical and Surgical
2ND - **K** Muscles
3RD - **2 CHANGE**

EXAMPLE: Exchange drain tube
CMS Ex: Changing urinary catheter

CHANGE: Taking out or off a device from a body part and putting back an identical or similar device in or on the same body part without cutting or puncturing the skin or a mucous membrane.

EXPLANATION: ALL Changes use EXTERNAL approach only ...

Body Part – 4TH	Approach – 5TH	Device – 6TH	Qualifier – 7TH
X Upper Muscle Y Lower Muscle	X External	0 Drainage device Y Other device	Z No qualifier

EXCISION GROUP: Excision, Resection, Destruction, (Extraction), (Detachment)
Root Operations that take out some or all of a body part.

1ST - **0** Medical and Surgical
2ND - **K** Muscles
3RD - **5 DESTRUCTION**

EXAMPLE: Radiofrequency ablation
CMS Ex: Fulguration polyp

DESTRUCTION: Physical eradication of all or a portion of a body part by the direct use of energy, force, or a destructive agent.

EXPLANATION: None of the body part is physically taken out

Body Part – 4TH		Approach – 5TH	Device – 6TH	Qualifier – 7TH
0 Head Muscle 1 Facial Muscle 2 Neck Muscle, Right 3 Neck Muscle, Left 4 Tongue, Palate, Pharynx Muscle 5 Shoulder Muscle, Right 6 Shoulder Muscle, Left 7 Upper Arm Muscle, Right 8 Upper Arm Muscle, Left 9 Lower Arm and Wrist Muscle, Right B Lower Arm and Wrist Muscle, Left	C Hand Muscle, Right D Hand Muscle, Left F Trunk Muscle, Right G Trunk Muscle, Left H Thorax Muscle, Right J Thorax Muscle, Left K Abdomen Muscle, Right L Abdomen Muscle, Left M Perineum Muscle N Hip Muscle, Right P Hip Muscle, Left Q Upper Leg Muscle, Right R Upper Leg Muscle, Left S Lower Leg Muscle, Right T Lower Leg Muscle, Left V Foot Muscle, Right W Foot Muscle, Left	0 Open 3 Percutaneous 4 Percutaneous endoscopic	Z No device	Z No qualifier

0K8

MEDICAL AND SURGICAL SECTION – 2016 ICD-10-PCS

DIVISION GROUP: Division, Release
Root Operations involving cutting or separation only.

- 1ST – **0** Medical and Surgical
- 2ND – **K** Muscles
- 3RD – **8 DIVISION**

EXAMPLE: Myotomy hand muscle   CMS Ex: Osteotomy

DIVISION: Cutting into a body part without draining fluids and/or gases from the body part in order to separate or transect a body part.

EXPLANATION: Separated into two or more portions ...

Body Part – 4TH		Approach – 5TH	Device – 6TH	Qualifier – 7TH
0 Head Muscle	C Hand Muscle, Right	0 Open	Z No device	Z No qualifier
1 Facial Muscle	D Hand Muscle, Left	3 Percutaneous		
2 Neck Muscle, Right	F Trunk Muscle, Right	4 Percutaneous endoscopic		
3 Neck Muscle, Left	G Trunk Muscle, Left			
4 Tongue, Palate, Pharynx Muscle	H Thorax Muscle, Right			
	J Thorax Muscle, Left			
5 Shoulder Muscle, Right	K Abdomen Muscle, Right			
6 Shoulder Muscle, Left	L Abdomen Muscle, Left			
7 Upper Arm Muscle, Right	M Perineum Muscle			
8 Upper Arm Muscle, Left	N Hip Muscle, Right			
9 Lower Arm and Wrist Muscle, Right	P Hip Muscle, Left			
	Q Upper Leg Muscle, Right			
B Lower Arm and Wrist Muscle, Left	R Upper Leg Muscle, Left			
	S Lower Leg Muscle, Right			
	T Lower Leg Muscle, Left			
	V Foot Muscle, Right			
	W Foot Muscle, Left			

K – MUSCLES 0K9

DRAINAGE GROUP: Drainage, Extirpation, (Fragmentation)
Root Operations that take out solids/fluids/gases from a body part.

1ST - **0** Medical and Surgical
2ND - **K** Muscles
3RD - **9** DRAINAGE

EXAMPLE: Aspiration psoas muscle abscess   CMS Ex: Thoracentesis

DRAINAGE: Taking or letting out fluids and/or gases from a body part.

EXPLANATION: Qualifier "X Diagnostic" indicates biopsy ...

Body Part – 4TH		Approach – 5TH	Device – 6TH	Qualifier – 7TH
0 Head Muscle	C Hand Muscle, Right	0 Open	0 Drainage device	Z No qualifier
1 Facial Muscle	D Hand Muscle, Left	3 Percutaneous		
2 Neck Muscle, Right	F Trunk Muscle, Right	4 Percutaneous endoscopic		
3 Neck Muscle, Left	G Trunk Muscle, Left			
4 Tongue, Palate, Pharynx Muscle	H Thorax Muscle, Right			
	J Thorax Muscle, Left			
5 Shoulder Muscle, Right	K Abdomen Muscle, Right			
6 Shoulder Muscle, Left	L Abdomen Muscle, Left			
7 Upper Arm Muscle, Right	M Perineum Muscle			
8 Upper Arm Muscle, Left	N Hip Muscle, Right			
9 Lower Arm and Wrist Muscle, Right	P Hip Muscle, Left			
	Q Upper Leg Muscle, Right			
B Lower Arm and Wrist Muscle, Left	R Upper Leg Muscle, Left			
	S Lower Leg Muscle, Right			
	T Lower Leg Muscle, Left			
	V Foot Muscle, Right			
	W Foot Muscle, Left			
0 Head Muscle	C Hand Muscle, Right	0 Open	Z No device	X Diagnostic
1 Facial Muscle	D Hand Muscle, Left	3 Percutaneous		Z No qualifier
2 Neck Muscle, Right	F Trunk Muscle, Right	4 Percutaneous endoscopic		
3 Neck Muscle, Left	G Trunk Muscle, Left			
4 Tongue, Palate, Pharynx Muscle	H Thorax Muscle, Right			
	J Thorax Muscle, Left			
5 Shoulder Muscle, Right	K Abdomen Muscle, Right			
6 Shoulder Muscle, Left	L Abdomen Muscle, Left			
7 Upper Arm Muscle, Right	M Perineum Muscle			
8 Upper Arm Muscle, Left	N Hip Muscle, Right			
9 Lower Arm and Wrist Muscle, Right	P Hip Muscle, Left			
	Q Upper Leg Muscle, Right			
B Lower Arm and Wrist Muscle, Left	R Upper Leg Muscle, Left			
	S Lower Leg Muscle, Right			
	T Lower Leg Muscle, Left			
	V Foot Muscle, Right			
	W Foot Muscle, Left			

0KB — MEDICAL AND SURGICAL SECTION – 2016 ICD-10-PCS

EXCISION GROUP: Excision, Resection, Destruction, (Extraction), (Detachment)
Root Operations that take out some or all of a body part.

- 1ST – **0** Medical and Surgical
- 2ND – **K** Muscles
- 3RD – **B** EXCISION

EXAMPLE: Muscle biopsy CMS Ex: Liver biopsy

EXCISION: Cutting out or off, without replacement, a portion of a body part.

EXPLANATION: Qualifier "X Diagnostic" indicates biopsy …

Body Part – 4TH	Approach – 5TH	Device – 6TH	Qualifier – 7TH
0 Head Muscle 1 Facial Muscle 2 Neck Muscle, Right 3 Neck Muscle, Left 4 Tongue, Palate, Pharynx Muscle 5 Shoulder Muscle, Right 6 Shoulder Muscle, Left 7 Upper Arm Muscle, Right 8 Upper Arm Muscle, Left 9 Lower Arm and Wrist Muscle, Right B Lower Arm and Wrist Muscle, Left C Hand Muscle, Right D Hand Muscle, Left F Trunk Muscle, Right G Trunk Muscle, Left H Thorax Muscle, Right J Thorax Muscle, Left K Abdomen Muscle, Right L Abdomen Muscle, Left M Perineum Muscle N Hip Muscle, Right P Hip Muscle, Left Q Upper Leg Muscle, Right R Upper Leg Muscle, Left S Lower Leg Muscle, Right T Lower Leg Muscle, Left V Foot Muscle, Right W Foot Muscle, Left	0 Open 3 Percutaneous 4 Percutaneous endoscopic	Z No device	X Diagnostic Z No qualifier

DRAINAGE GROUP: Drainage, Extirpation, (Fragmentation)
Root Operations that take out solids/fluids/gases from a body part.

- 1ST – **0** Medical and Surgical
- 2ND – **K** Muscles
- 3RD – **C** EXTIRPATION

EXAMPLE: Removal foreign body CMS Ex: Choledocholithotomy

EXTIRPATION: Taking or cutting out solid matter from a body part.

EXPLANATION: Abnormal byproduct or foreign body …

Body Part – 4TH	Approach – 5TH	Device – 6TH	Qualifier – 7TH
0 Head Muscle 1 Facial Muscle 2 Neck Muscle, Right 3 Neck Muscle, Left 4 Tongue, Palate, Pharynx Muscle 5 Shoulder Muscle, Right 6 Shoulder Muscle, Left 7 Upper Arm Muscle, Right 8 Upper Arm Muscle, Left 9 Lower Arm and Wrist Muscle, Right B Lower Arm and Wrist Muscle, Left C Hand Muscle, Right D Hand Muscle, Left F Trunk Muscle, Right G Trunk Muscle, Left H Thorax Muscle, Right J Thorax Muscle, Left K Abdomen Muscle, Right L Abdomen Muscle, Left M Perineum Muscle N Hip Muscle, Right P Hip Muscle, Left Q Upper Leg Muscle, Right R Upper Leg Muscle, Left S Lower Leg Muscle, Right T Lower Leg Muscle, Left V Foot Muscle, Right W Foot Muscle, Left	0 Open 3 Percutaneous 4 Percutaneous endoscopic	Z No device	Z No qualifier

0 K J

K – MUSCLES

DEVICE GROUP: Change, Insertion, Removal, (Replacement), Revision, Supplement
Root Operations that always involve a device.

- 1ST – **0** Medical and Surgical
- 2ND – **K** Muscles
- 3RD – **H** INSERTION

EXAMPLE: Insertion stimulator lead	CMS Ex: Central venous catheter

INSERTION: Putting in a nonbiological appliance that monitors, assists, performs, or prevents a physiological function but does not physically take the place of a body part.

EXPLANATION: None

Body Part – 4TH	Approach – 5TH	Device – 6TH	Qualifier – 7TH
X Upper Muscle Y Lower Muscle	0 Open 3 Percutaneous 4 Percutaneous endoscopic	M Stimulator lead	Z No qualifier

EXAMINATION GROUP: Inspection, (Map)
Root Operations involving examination only.

- 1ST – **0** Medical and Surgical
- 2ND – **K** Muscles
- 3RD – **J** INSPECTION

EXAMPLE: Examination pelvic floor muscle	CMS Ex: Colonoscopy

INSPECTION: Visually and/or manually exploring a body part.

EXPLANATION: Direct or instrumental visualization …

Body Part – 4TH	Approach – 5TH	Device – 6TH	Qualifier – 7TH
X Upper Muscle Y Lower Muscle	0 Open 3 Percutaneous 4 Percutaneous endoscopic X External	Z No device	Z No qualifier

445

0KM MEDICAL AND SURGICAL SECTION – 2016 ICD-10-PCS [2016.PCS]

MOVE GROUP: Reattachment, Reposition, Transfer, (Transplantation)
Root Operations that put in/put back or move some/all of a body part.

1ST - **0** Medical and Surgical	EXAMPLE: Reattachment arm muscle	CMS Ex: Reattachment hand
2ND - **K** Muscles	**REATTACHMENT:** Putting back in or on all or a portion of a separated body part to its normal location or other suitable location.	
3RD - **M REATTACHMENT**	EXPLANATION: With/without reconnection of vessels/nerves...	

Body Part – 4TH		Approach – 5TH	Device – 6TH	Qualifier – 7TH
0 Head Muscle	C Hand Muscle, Right	0 Open	Z No device	Z No qualifier
1 Facial Muscle	D Hand Muscle, Left	4 Percutaneous endoscopic		
2 Neck Muscle, Right	F Trunk Muscle, Right			
3 Neck Muscle, Left	G Trunk Muscle, Left			
4 Tongue, Palate, Pharynx Muscle	H Thorax Muscle, Right			
	J Thorax Muscle, Left			
5 Shoulder Muscle, Right	K Abdomen Muscle, Right			
6 Shoulder Muscle, Left	L Abdomen Muscle, Left			
7 Upper Arm Muscle, Right	M Perineum Muscle			
8 Upper Arm Muscle, Left	N Hip Muscle, Right			
9 Lower Arm and Wrist Muscle, Right	P Hip Muscle, Left			
	Q Upper Leg Muscle, Right			
B Lower Arm and Wrist Muscle, Left	R Upper Leg Muscle, Left			
	S Lower Leg Muscle, Right			
	T Lower Leg Muscle, Left			
	V Foot Muscle, Right			
	W Foot Muscle, Left			

MUSCLES

0KN

DIVISION GROUP: Division, Release
Root Operations involving cutting or separation only.

1ST - **0** Medical and Surgical	EXAMPLE: Component muscle separation	CMS Ex: Carpal tunnel release
2ND - **K** Muscles	**RELEASE:** Freeing a body part from an abnormal physical constraint by cutting or by the use of force.	
3RD - **N RELEASE**	EXPLANATION: None of the body part is taken out ...	

Body Part – 4TH		Approach – 5TH	Device – 6TH	Qualifier – 7TH
0 Head Muscle	C Hand Muscle, Right	0 Open	Z No device	Z No qualifier
1 Facial Muscle	D Hand Muscle, Left	3 Percutaneous		
2 Neck Muscle, Right	F Trunk Muscle, Right	4 Percutaneous endoscopic		
3 Neck Muscle, Left	G Trunk Muscle, Left	X External		
4 Tongue, Palate, Pharynx Muscle	H Thorax Muscle, Right			
	J Thorax Muscle, Left			
5 Shoulder Muscle, Right	K Abdomen Muscle, Right			
6 Shoulder Muscle, Left	L Abdomen Muscle, Left			
7 Upper Arm Muscle, Right	M Perineum Muscle			
8 Upper Arm Muscle, Left	N Hip Muscle, Right			
9 Lower Arm and Wrist Muscle, Right	P Hip Muscle, Left			
	Q Upper Leg Muscle, Right			
B Lower Arm and Wrist Muscle, Left	R Upper Leg Muscle, Left			
	S Lower Leg Muscle, Right			
	T Lower Leg Muscle, Left			
	V Foot Muscle, Right			
	W Foot Muscle, Left			

K – MUSCLES 0KQ

DEVICE GROUP: Change, Insertion, Removal, (Replacement), Revision, Supplement
Root Operations that always involve a device.

1ST - 0 Medical and Surgical
2ND - K Muscles
3RD - P REMOVAL

EXAMPLE: Removal stimulator lead | CMS Ex: Chest tube removal

REMOVAL: Taking out or off a device from a body part.

EXPLANATION: Removal device without reinsertion ...

Body Part – 4TH	Approach – 5TH	Device – 6TH	Qualifier – 7TH
X Upper Muscle Y Lower Muscle	0 Open 3 Percutaneous 4 Percutaneous endoscopic	0 Drainage device 7 Autologous tissue substitute J Synthetic substitute K Nonautologous tissue substitute M Stimulator lead	Z No qualifier
X Upper Muscle Y Lower Muscle	X External	0 Drainage device M Stimulator lead	Z No qualifier

OTHER REPAIRS GROUP: (Control), Repair
Root Operations that define other repairs.

1ST - 0 Medical and Surgical
2ND - K Muscles
3RD - Q REPAIR

EXAMPLE: Repair second degree perineum muscle | CMS Ex: Suture

REPAIR: Restoring, to the extent possible, a body part to its normal anatomic structure and function.

EXPLANATION: Only when no other root operation applies ...

Body Part – 4TH	Approach – 5TH	Device – 6TH	Qualifier – 7TH
0 Head Muscle 1 Facial Muscle 2 Neck Muscle, Right 3 Neck Muscle, Left 4 Tongue, Palate, Pharynx Muscle 5 Shoulder Muscle, Right 6 Shoulder Muscle, Left 7 Upper Arm Muscle, Right 8 Upper Arm Muscle, Left 9 Lower Arm and Wrist Muscle, Right B Lower Arm and Wrist Muscle, Left C Hand Muscle, Right D Hand Muscle, Left F Trunk Muscle, Right G Trunk Muscle, Left H Thorax Muscle, Right J Thorax Muscle, Left K Abdomen Muscle, Right L Abdomen Muscle, Left M Perineum Muscle N Hip Muscle, Right P Hip Muscle, Left Q Upper Leg Muscle, Right R Upper Leg Muscle, Left S Lower Leg Muscle, Right T Lower Leg Muscle, Left V Foot Muscle, Right W Foot Muscle, Left	0 Open 3 Percutaneous 4 Percutaneous endoscopic	Z No device	Z No qualifier

0KS — MEDICAL AND SURGICAL SECTION – 2016 ICD-10-PCS

MOVE GROUP: Reattachment, Reposition, Transfer, (Transplantation)
Root Operations that put in/put back or move some/all of a body part.

- 1ST - **0** Medical and Surgical
- 2ND - **K** Muscles
- 3RD - **S** REPOSITION

EXAMPLE: Relocation shoulder muscle
CMS Ex: Fracture reduction

REPOSITION: Moving to its normal location, or other suitable location, all or a portion of a body part.

EXPLANATION: May or may not be cut to be moved …

Body Part – 4TH	Approach – 5TH	Device – 6TH	Qualifier – 7TH
0 Head Muscle 1 Facial Muscle 2 Neck Muscle, Right 3 Neck Muscle, Left 4 Tongue, Palate, Pharynx Muscle 5 Shoulder Muscle, Right 6 Shoulder Muscle, Left 7 Upper Arm Muscle, Right 8 Upper Arm Muscle, Left 9 Lower Arm and Wrist Muscle, Right B Lower Arm and Wrist Muscle, Left C Hand Muscle, Right D Hand Muscle, Left F Trunk Muscle, Right G Trunk Muscle, Left H Thorax Muscle, Right J Thorax Muscle, Left K Abdomen Muscle, Right L Abdomen Muscle, Left M Perineum Muscle N Hip Muscle, Right P Hip Muscle, Left Q Upper Leg Muscle, Right R Upper Leg Muscle, Left S Lower Leg Muscle, Right T Lower Leg Muscle, Left V Foot Muscle, Right W Foot Muscle, Left	0 Open 4 Percutaneous endoscopic	Z No device	Z No qualifier

EXCISION GROUP: Excision, Resection, Destruction, (Extraction), (Detachment)
Root Operations that take out some or all of a body part.

- 1ST - **0** Medical and Surgical
- 2ND - **K** Muscles
- 3RD - **T** RESECTION

EXAMPLE: Resection perineum muscle
CMS Ex: Cholecystectomy

RESECTION: Cutting out or off, without replacement, all of a body part.

EXPLANATION: None

Body Part – 4TH	Approach – 5TH	Device – 6TH	Qualifier – 7TH
0 Head Muscle 1 Facial Muscle 2 Neck Muscle, Right 3 Neck Muscle, Left 4 Tongue, Palate, Pharynx Muscle 5 Shoulder Muscle, Right 6 Shoulder Muscle, Left 7 Upper Arm Muscle, Right 8 Upper Arm Muscle, Left 9 Lower Arm and Wrist Muscle, Right B Lower Arm and Wrist Muscle, Left C Hand Muscle, Right D Hand Muscle, Left F Trunk Muscle, Right G Trunk Muscle, Left H Thorax Muscle, Right J Thorax Muscle, Left K Abdomen Muscle, Right L Abdomen Muscle, Left M Perineum Muscle N Hip Muscle, Right P Hip Muscle, Left Q Upper Leg Muscle, Right R Upper Leg Muscle, Left S Lower Leg Muscle, Right T Lower Leg Muscle, Left V Foot Muscle, Right W Foot Muscle, Left	0 Open 4 Percutaneous endoscopic	Z No device	Z No qualifier

0KW K – MUSCLES

DEVICE GROUP: Change, Insertion, Removal, (Replacement), Revision, Supplement
Root Operations that always involve a device.

1ST - 0 Medical and Surgical
2ND - K Muscles
3RD - U SUPPLEMENT

EXAMPLE: Gracilis muscle graft to face | CMS Ex: Hernia repair with mesh

SUPPLEMENT: Putting in or on biological or synthetic material that physically reinforces and/or augments the function of a portion of a body part.

EXPLANATION: Biological material from same individual ...

Body Part – 4TH	Approach – 5TH	Device – 6TH	Qualifier – 7TH
0 Head Muscle	0 Open	7 Autologous tissue substitute	Z No qualifier
1 Facial Muscle	4 Percutaneous endoscopic	J Synthetic substitute	
2 Neck Muscle, Right		K Nonautologous tissue substitute	
3 Neck Muscle, Left			
4 Tongue, Palate, Pharynx Muscle			
5 Shoulder Muscle, Right			
6 Shoulder Muscle, Left			
7 Upper Arm Muscle, Right			
8 Upper Arm Muscle, Left			
9 Lower Arm and Wrist Muscle, Right			
B Lower Arm and Wrist Muscle, Left			
C Hand Muscle, Right			
D Hand Muscle, Left			
F Trunk Muscle, Right			
G Trunk Muscle, Left			
H Thorax Muscle, Right			
J Thorax Muscle, Left			
K Abdomen Muscle, Right			
L Abdomen Muscle, Left			
M Perineum Muscle			
N Hip Muscle, Right			
P Hip Muscle, Left			
Q Upper Leg Muscle, Right			
R Upper Leg Muscle, Left			
S Lower Leg Muscle, Right			
T Lower Leg Muscle, Left			
V Foot Muscle, Right			
W Foot Muscle, Left			

DEVICE GROUP: Change, Insertion, Removal, (Replacement), Revision, Supplement
Root Operations that always involve a device.

1ST - 0 Medical and Surgical
2ND - K Muscles
3RD - W REVISION

EXAMPLE: Reposition stimulator lead | CMS Ex: Adjustment pacemaker lead

REVISION: Correcting, to the extent possible, a portion of a malfunctioning device or the position of a displaced device.

EXPLANATION: May replace components of a device ...

Body Part – 4TH	Approach – 5TH	Device – 6TH	Qualifier – 7TH
X Upper Muscle	0 Open	0 Drainage device	Z No qualifier
Y Lower Muscle	3 Percutaneous	7 Autologous tissue substitute	
	4 Percutaneous endoscopic	J Synthetic substitute	
	X External	K Nonautologous tissue substitute	
		M Stimulator lead	

0KX

MEDICAL AND SURGICAL SECTION – 2016 ICD-10-PCS

MOVE GROUP: Reattachment, Reposition, Transfer, (Transplantation)
Root Operations that put in/put back or move some/all of a body part.

1ST - **0** Medical and Surgical
2ND - **K** Muscles
3RD - **X** TRANSFER

EXAMPLE: TRAM flap breast reconstruction | **CMS Ex:** Tendon transfer

TRANSFER: Moving, without taking out, all or a portion of a body part to another location to take over the function of all or a portion of a body part.

EXPLANATION: The body part remains connected ...

Body Part – 4TH		Approach – 5TH	Device – 6TH	Qualifier – 7TH
0 Head Muscle 1 Facial Muscle 2 Neck Muscle, Right 3 Neck Muscle, Left 4 Tongue, Palate, Pharynx Muscle 5 Shoulder Muscle, Right 6 Shoulder Muscle, Left 7 Upper Arm Muscle, Right 8 Upper Arm Muscle, Left 9 Lower Arm and Wrist Muscle, Right B Lower Arm and Wrist Muscle, Left	C Hand Muscle, Right D Hand Muscle, Left F Trunk Muscle, Right G Trunk Muscle, Left H Thorax Muscle, Right J Thorax Muscle, Left M Perineum Muscle N Hip Muscle, Right P Hip Muscle, Left Q Upper Leg Muscle, Right R Upper Leg Muscle, Left S Lower Leg Muscle, Right T Lower Leg Muscle, Left V Foot Muscle, Right W Foot Muscle, Left	0 Open 4 Percutaneous endoscopic	Z No device	0 Skin 1 Subcutaneous Tissue 2 Skin and Subcutaneous Tissue Z No qualifier
K Abdomen Muscle, Right L Abdomen Muscle, Left		0 Open 4 Percutaneous endoscopic	Z No device	0 Skin 1 Subcutaneous Tissue 2 Skin and Subcutaneous Tissue 6 Transverse Rectus Abdominis Myocutaneous Flap Z No qualifier

Educational Annotations

L – Tendons

Body System Specific Educational Annotations for the Tendons include:
- Anatomy and Physiology Review
- Anatomical Illustrations
- Definitions of Common Procedures
- AHA Coding Clinic® Reference Notations
- Body Part Key Listings
- Device Key Listings
- Device Aggregation Table Listings
- Coding Notes

Anatomy and Physiology Review of Tendons

BODY PART VALUES – L - TENDONS

Lower Tendon – The tendons located below the diaphragm (see Coding Guideline B2.1b).

Tendon – ANATOMY – A tendon is a strong, yet somewhat flexible cord or band of fibrous connective tissue that most often connects muscle to bone. PHYSIOLOGY – Tendons and muscles work together to move the bones.

Upper Tendon – The tendons located above the diaphragm (see Coding Guideline B2.1b).

Anatomical Illustrations of Tendons

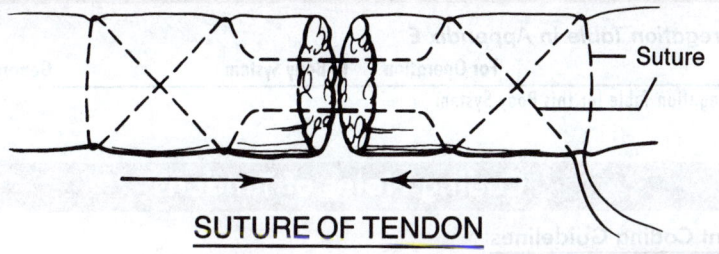

SUTURE OF TENDON

Definitions of Common Procedures of Tendons

Bridle procedure tendon transfer – The surgical transfer of the distal ends of the posterior tibial, peroneus longus, and the anterior tibialis tendons in a "bridle" configuration to correct the condition of foot drop.

Free tendon graft – The surgical placement of a section of tendon (from another part of the body or donor) to repair a damaged tendon.

AHA Coding Clinic® Reference Notations of Tendons

ROOT OPERATION SPECIFIC - L - TENDONS
CHANGE - 2
DESTRUCTION - 5
DIVISION - 8
DRAINAGE - 9
EXCISION - B
    Excisional debridement of nonhealing wound that included tendon............AHA 14:3Q:p18
    Excisional debridement of ulceration that included tendon ....AHA 14:3Q:p14
EXTIRPATION - C
INSPECTION - H
REATTACHMENT - M
RELEASE - N
REMOVAL - P
REPAIR - Q
    Arthroscopic rotator cuff suture repair ....AHA 13:3Q:p20
REPLACEMENT - R
REPOSITION - S
RESECTION - T
SUPPLEMENT - U
    Patellar tendon augmentation with allograft...AHA 15:2Q:p11
REVISION - W
TRANSFER - X

Educational Annotations | L – Tendons

Body Part Key Listings of Tendons

See also Body Part Key in Appendix C
Achilles tendon .... *use* Lower Leg Tendon, Left/Right
Patellar tendon .... *use* Knee Tendon, Left/Right

Device Key Listings of Tendons

See also Device Key in Appendix D
Autograft .... *use* Autologous Tissue Substitute
Tissue bank graft .... *use* Nonautologous Tissue Substitute

Device Aggregation Table Listings of Tendons

See also Device Aggregation Table in Appendix E

Specific Device	For Operation	In Body System	General Device
None Listed in Device Aggregation Table for this Body System			

Coding Notes of Tendons

Body System Relevant Coding Guidelines

General Guidelines
  B2.1b
    Where the general body part values "upper" and "lower" are provided as an option in the Upper Arteries, Lower Arteries, Upper Veins, Lower Veins, Muscles and Tendons body systems, "upper" and "lower" specifies body parts located above or below the diaphragm respectively.
    Example: Vein body parts above the diaphragm are found in the Upper Veins body system; vein body parts below the diaphragm are found in the Lower Veins body system.

Tendons, ligaments, bursae and fascia near a joint
  B4.5
    Procedures performed on tendons, ligaments, bursae and fascia supporting a joint are coded to the body part in the respective body system that is the focus of the procedure. Procedures performed on joint structures themselves are coded to the body part in the joint body systems.
    Example: Repair of the anterior cruciate ligament of the knee is coded to the knee bursae and ligament body part in the bursae and ligaments body system. Knee arthroscopy with shaving of articular cartilage is coded to the knee joint body part in the Lower Joints body system.

Body System Specific PCS Reference Manual Exercises

PCS CODE	L – TENDONS EXERCISES
0L8V3ZZ	Division of right foot tendon, percutaneous.
0LBN0ZZ	Open excision of lesion from right Achilles tendon.
0LNP3ZZ	Percutaneous left Achilles tendon release.
0LQ30ZZ	Suture repair of right biceps tendon laceration, open.
0LRS0KZ	Tenonectomy with graft to right ankle using cadaver graft, open.
0LU207Z	Tendon graft to strengthen injured left shoulder using autograft, open (do not code graft harvest for this exercise).
0LX70ZZ	Right hand open palmaris longus tendon transfer.
0LXP4ZZ	Endoscopic left leg flexor hallucis longus tendon transfer.

L – TENDONS

DEVICE GROUP: Change, (Insertion), Removal, Replacement, Revision, Supplement
Root Operations that always involve a device.

1ST - 0 Medical and Surgical
2ND - L Tendons
3RD - 2 CHANGE

EXAMPLE: Exchange drain tube
CMS Ex: Changing urinary catheter

CHANGE: Taking out or off a device from a body part and putting back an identical or similar device in or on the same body part without cutting or puncturing the skin or a mucous membrane.

EXPLANATION: ALL Changes use EXTERNAL approach only …

Body Part – 4TH	Approach – 5TH	Device – 6TH	Qualifier – 7TH
X Upper Tendon	X External	0 Drainage device	Z No qualifier
Y Lower Tendon		Y Other device	

EXCISION GROUP: Excision, Resection, Destruction, (Extraction), (Detachment)
Root Operations that take out some or all of a body part.

1ST - 0 Medical and Surgical
2ND - L Tendons
3RD - 5 DESTRUCTION

EXAMPLE: Radiofrequency ablation
CMS Ex: Fulguration polyp

DESTRUCTION: Physical eradication of all or a portion of a body part by the direct use of energy, force, or a destructive agent.

EXPLANATION: None of the body part is physically taken out

Body Part – 4TH		Approach – 5TH	Device – 6TH	Qualifier – 7TH
0 Head and Neck Tendon	F Abdomen Tendon, Right	0 Open	Z No device	Z No qualifier
1 Shoulder Tendon, Right	G Abdomen Tendon, Left	3 Percutaneous		
2 Shoulder Tendon, Left	H Perineum Tendon	4 Percutaneous endoscopic		
3 Upper Arm Tendon, Right	J Hip Tendon, Right			
4 Upper Arm Tendon, Left	K Hip Tendon, Left			
5 Lower Arm and Wrist Tendon, Right	L Upper Leg Tendon, Right			
	M Upper Leg Tendon, Left			
6 Lower Arm and Wrist Tendon, Left	N Lower Leg Tendon, Right			
	P Lower Leg Tendon, Left			
7 Hand Tendon, Right	Q Knee Tendon, Right			
8 Hand Tendon, Left	R Knee Tendon, Left			
9 Trunk Tendon, Right	S Ankle Tendon, Right			
B Trunk Tendon, Left	T Ankle Tendon, Left			
C Thorax Tendon, Right	V Foot Tendon, Right			
D Thorax Tendon, Left	W Foot Tendon, Left			

0L8

MEDICAL AND SURGICAL SECTION – 2016 ICD-10-PCS

DIVISION GROUP: Division, Release
Root Operations involving cutting or separation only.

1ST - **0** Medical and Surgical
2ND - **L** Tendons
3RD - **8** DIVISION

EXAMPLE: Division Achilles tendon   CMS Ex: Osteotomy

DIVISION: Cutting into a body part without draining fluids and/or gases from the body part in order to separate or transect a body part.

EXPLANATION: Separated into two or more portions ...

Body Part – 4TH		Approach – 5TH	Device – 6TH	Qualifier – 7TH
0 Head and Neck Tendon	F Abdomen Tendon, Right	0 Open	Z No device	Z No qualifier
1 Shoulder Tendon, Right	G Abdomen Tendon, Left	3 Percutaneous		
2 Shoulder Tendon, Left	H Perineum Tendon	4 Percutaneous endoscopic		
3 Upper Arm Tendon, Right	J Hip Tendon, Right			
4 Upper Arm Tendon, Left	K Hip Tendon, Left			
5 Lower Arm and Wrist Tendon, Right	L Upper Leg Tendon, Right			
	M Upper Leg Tendon, Left			
6 Lower Arm and Wrist Tendon, Left	N Lower Leg Tendon, Right			
	P Lower Leg Tendon, Left			
7 Hand Tendon, Right	Q Knee Tendon, Right			
8 Hand Tendon, Left	R Knee Tendon, Left			
9 Trunk Tendon, Right	S Ankle Tendon, Right			
B Trunk Tendon, Left	T Ankle Tendon, Left			
C Thorax Tendon, Right	V Foot Tendon, Right			
D Thorax Tendon, Left	W Foot Tendon, Left			

L – TENDONS 0L9

DRAINAGE GROUP: Drainage, Extirpation, (Fragmentation)
Root Operations that take out solids/fluids/gases from a body part.

1ST - **0** Medical and Surgical
2ND - **L** Tendons
3RD - **9 DRAINAGE**

EXAMPLE: I&D tendon sheath abscess
CMS Ex: Thoracentesis

DRAINAGE: Taking or letting out fluids and/or gases from a body part.

EXPLANATION: Qualifier "X Diagnostic" indicates biopsy …

Body Part – 4TH		Approach – 5TH	Device – 6TH	Qualifier – 7TH
0 Head and Neck Tendon	F Abdomen Tendon, Right	0 Open	0 Drainage device	Z No qualifier
1 Shoulder Tendon, Right	G Abdomen Tendon, Left	3 Percutaneous		
2 Shoulder Tendon, Left	H Perineum Tendon	4 Percutaneous endoscopic		
3 Upper Arm Tendon, Right	J Hip Tendon, Right			
4 Upper Arm Tendon, Left	K Hip Tendon, Left			
5 Lower Arm and Wrist Tendon, Right	L Upper Leg Tendon, Right			
	M Upper Leg Tendon, Left			
6 Lower Arm and Wrist Tendon, Left	N Lower Leg Tendon, Right			
	P Lower Leg Tendon, Left			
7 Hand Tendon, Right	Q Knee Tendon, Right			
8 Hand Tendon, Left	R Knee Tendon, Left			
9 Trunk Tendon, Right	S Ankle Tendon, Right			
B Trunk Tendon, Left	T Ankle Tendon, Left			
C Thorax Tendon, Right	V Foot Tendon, Right			
D Thorax Tendon, Left	W Foot Tendon, Left			
0 Head and Neck Tendon	F Abdomen Tendon, Right	0 Open	Z No device	X Diagnostic
1 Shoulder Tendon, Right	G Abdomen Tendon, Left	3 Percutaneous		Z No qualifier
2 Shoulder Tendon, Left	H Perineum Tendon	4 Percutaneous endoscopic		
3 Upper Arm Tendon, Right	J Hip Tendon, Right			
4 Upper Arm Tendon, Left	K Hip Tendon, Left			
5 Lower Arm and Wrist Tendon, Right	L Upper Leg Tendon, Right			
	M Upper Leg Tendon, Left			
6 Lower Arm and Wrist Tendon, Left	N Lower Leg Tendon, Right			
	P Lower Leg Tendon, Left			
7 Hand Tendon, Right	Q Knee Tendon, Right			
8 Hand Tendon, Left	R Knee Tendon, Left			
9 Trunk Tendon, Right	S Ankle Tendon, Right			
B Trunk Tendon, Left	T Ankle Tendon, Left			
C Thorax Tendon, Right	V Foot Tendon, Right			
D Thorax Tendon, Left	W Foot Tendon, Left			

0LB

MEDICAL AND SURGICAL SECTION – 2016 ICD-10-PCS

EXCISION GROUP: Excision, Resection, Destruction, (Extraction), (Detachment)
Root Operations that take out some or all of a body part.

- 1ST – **0** Medical and Surgical
- 2ND – **L** Tendons
- 3RD – **B EXCISION**

EXAMPLE: Ganglionectomy tendon sheath **CMS Ex:** Liver biopsy

EXCISION: Cutting out or off, without replacement, a portion of a body part.

EXPLANATION: Qualifier "X Diagnostic" indicates biopsy …

Body Part – 4TH		Approach – 5TH	Device – 6TH	Qualifier – 7TH
0 Head and Neck Tendon	F Abdomen Tendon, Right	0 Open	Z No device	X Diagnostic
1 Shoulder Tendon, Right	G Abdomen Tendon, Left	3 Percutaneous		Z No qualifier
2 Shoulder Tendon, Left	H Perineum Tendon	4 Percutaneous endoscopic		
3 Upper Arm Tendon, Right	J Hip Tendon, Right			
4 Upper Arm Tendon, Left	K Hip Tendon, Left			
5 Lower Arm and Wrist Tendon, Right	L Upper Leg Tendon, Right			
	M Upper Leg Tendon, Left			
6 Lower Arm and Wrist Tendon, Left	N Lower Leg Tendon, Right			
	P Lower Leg Tendon, Left			
7 Hand Tendon, Right	Q Knee Tendon, Right			
8 Hand Tendon, Left	R Knee Tendon, Left			
9 Trunk Tendon, Right	S Ankle Tendon, Right			
B Trunk Tendon, Left	T Ankle Tendon, Left			
C Thorax Tendon, Right	V Foot Tendon, Right			
D Thorax Tendon, Left	W Foot Tendon, Left			

DRAINAGE GROUP: Drainage, Extirpation, (Fragmentation)
Root Operations that take out solids/fluids/gases from a body part.

- 1ST – **0** Medical and Surgical
- 2ND – **L** Tendons
- 3RD – **C EXTIRPATION**

EXAMPLE: Removal calcium tendon deposits **CMS Ex:** Choledocholithotomy

EXTIRPATION: Taking or cutting out solid matter from a body part.

EXPLANATION: Abnormal byproduct or foreign body …

Body Part – 4TH		Approach – 5TH	Device – 6TH	Qualifier – 7TH
0 Head and Neck Tendon	F Abdomen Tendon, Right	0 Open	Z No device	Z No qualifier
1 Shoulder Tendon, Right	G Abdomen Tendon, Left	3 Percutaneous		
2 Shoulder Tendon, Left	H Perineum Tendon	4 Percutaneous endoscopic		
3 Upper Arm Tendon, Right	J Hip Tendon, Right			
4 Upper Arm Tendon, Left	K Hip Tendon, Left			
5 Lower Arm and Wrist Tendon, Right	L Upper Leg Tendon, Right			
	M Upper Leg Tendon, Left			
6 Lower Arm and Wrist Tendon, Left	N Lower Leg Tendon, Right			
	P Lower Leg Tendon, Left			
7 Hand Tendon, Right	Q Knee Tendon, Right			
8 Hand Tendon, Left	R Knee Tendon, Left			
9 Trunk Tendon, Right	S Ankle Tendon, Right			
B Trunk Tendon, Left	T Ankle Tendon, Left			
C Thorax Tendon, Right	V Foot Tendon, Right			
D Thorax Tendon, Left	W Foot Tendon, Left			

0LM

L – TENDONS

EXAMINATION GROUP: Inspection, (Map)
Root Operations involving examination only.

- 1ST – **0** Medical and Surgical
- 2ND – **L** Tendons
- 3RD – **J** INSPECTION

EXAMPLE: Exploration tendon attachments
CMS Ex: Colonoscopy

INSPECTION: Visually and/or manually exploring a body part.

EXPLANATION: Direct or instrumental visualization ...

Body Part – 4TH	Approach – 5TH	Device – 6TH	Qualifier – 7TH
X Upper Tendon Y Lower Tendon	0 Open 3 Percutaneous 4 Percutaneous endoscopic X External	Z No device	Z No qualifier

MOVE GROUP: Reattachment, Reposition, Transfer, (Transplantation)
Root Operations that put in/put back or move some/all of a body part.

- 1ST – **0** Medical and Surgical
- 2ND – **L** Tendons
- 3RD – **M** REATTACHMENT

EXAMPLE: Re-anchor torn tendon
CMS Ex: Reattachment hand

REATTACHMENT: Putting back in or on all or a portion of a separated body part to its normal location or other suitable location.

EXPLANATION: With/without reconnection of vessels/nerves...

Body Part – 4TH		Approach – 5TH	Device – 6TH	Qualifier – 7TH
0 Head and Neck Tendon 1 Shoulder Tendon, Right 2 Shoulder Tendon, Left 3 Upper Arm Tendon, Right 4 Upper Arm Tendon, Left 5 Lower Arm and Wrist Tendon, Right 6 Lower Arm and Wrist Tendon, Left 7 Hand Tendon, Right 8 Hand Tendon, Left 9 Trunk Tendon, Right B Trunk Tendon, Left C Thorax Tendon, Right D Thorax Tendon, Left	F Abdomen Tendon, Right G Abdomen Tendon, Left H Perineum Tendon J Hip Tendon, Right K Hip Tendon, Left L Upper Leg Tendon, Right M Upper Leg Tendon, Left N Lower Leg Tendon, Right P Lower Leg Tendon, Left Q Knee Tendon, Right R Knee Tendon, Left S Ankle Tendon, Right T Ankle Tendon, Left V Foot Tendon, Right W Foot Tendon, Left	0 Open 4 Percutaneous endoscopic	Z No device	Z No qualifier

0LN

MEDICAL AND SURGICAL SECTION – 2016 ICD-10-PCS

DIVISION GROUP: Division, Release
Root Operations involving cutting or separation only.

- 1ST – **0** Medical and Surgical
- 2ND – **L** Tendons
- 3RD – **N** RELEASE

EXAMPLE: Extensor tenolysis CMS Ex: Carpal tunnel release

RELEASE: Freeing a body part from an abnormal physical constraint by cutting or by the use of force.

EXPLANATION: None of the body part is taken out ...

Body Part – 4TH		Approach – 5TH	Device – 6TH	Qualifier – 7TH
0 Head and Neck Tendon	F Abdomen Tendon, Right	0 Open	Z No device	Z No qualifier
1 Shoulder Tendon, Right	G Abdomen Tendon, Left	3 Percutaneous		
2 Shoulder Tendon, Left	H Perineum Tendon	4 Percutaneous endoscopic		
3 Upper Arm Tendon, Right	J Hip Tendon, Right	X External		
4 Upper Arm Tendon, Left	K Hip Tendon, Left			
5 Lower Arm and Wrist Tendon, Right	L Upper Leg Tendon, Right			
	M Upper Leg Tendon, Left			
6 Lower Arm and Wrist Tendon, Left	N Lower Leg Tendon, Right			
	P Lower Leg Tendon, Left			
7 Hand Tendon, Right	Q Knee Tendon, Right			
8 Hand Tendon, Left	R Knee Tendon, Left			
9 Trunk Tendon, Right	S Ankle Tendon, Right			
B Trunk Tendon, Left	T Ankle Tendon, Left			
C Thorax Tendon, Right	V Foot Tendon, Right			
D Thorax Tendon, Left	W Foot Tendon, Left			

DEVICE GROUP: Change, (Insertion), Removal, Replacement, Revision, Supplement
Root Operations that always involve a device.

- 1ST – **0** Medical and Surgical
- 2ND – **L** Tendons
- 3RD – **P** REMOVAL

EXAMPLE: Removal drain tube CMS Ex: Chest tube removal

REMOVAL: Taking out or off a device from a body part.

EXPLANATION: Removal device without reinsertion ...

Body Part – 4TH	Approach – 5TH	Device – 6TH	Qualifier – 7TH
X Upper Tendon	0 Open	0 Drainage device	Z No qualifier
Y Lower Tendon	3 Percutaneous	7 Autologous tissue substitute	
	4 Percutaneous endoscopic	J Synthetic substitute	
		K Nonautologous tissue substitute	
X Upper Tendon	X External	0 Drainage device	Z No qualifier
Y Lower Tendon			

0LR

L – TENDONS

OTHER REPAIRS GROUP: (Control), Repair
Root Operations that define other repairs.

- 1ST – **0** Medical and Surgical
- 2ND – **L** Tendons
- 3RD – **Q REPAIR**

EXAMPLE: Tenorrhaphy **CMS Ex:** Suture laceration

REPAIR: Restoring, to the extent possible, a body part to its normal anatomic structure and function.

EXPLANATION: Only when no other root operation applies ...

Body Part – 4TH		Approach – 5TH	Device – 6TH	Qualifier – 7TH
0 Head and Neck Tendon	F Abdomen Tendon, Right	0 Open	Z No device	Z No qualifier
1 Shoulder Tendon, Right	G Abdomen Tendon, Left	3 Percutaneous		
2 Shoulder Tendon, Left	H Perineum Tendon	4 Percutaneous endoscopic		
3 Upper Arm Tendon, Right	J Hip Tendon, Right			
4 Upper Arm Tendon, Left	K Hip Tendon, Left			
5 Lower Arm and Wrist Tendon, Right	L Upper Leg Tendon, Right			
	M Upper Leg Tendon, Left			
6 Lower Arm and Wrist Tendon, Left	N Lower Leg Tendon, Right			
	P Lower Leg Tendon, Left			
7 Hand Tendon, Right	Q Knee Tendon, Right			
8 Hand Tendon, Left	R Knee Tendon, Left			
9 Trunk Tendon, Right	S Ankle Tendon, Right			
B Trunk Tendon, Left	T Ankle Tendon, Left			
C Thorax Tendon, Right	V Foot Tendon, Right			
D Thorax Tendon, Left	W Foot Tendon, Left			

DEVICE GROUP: Change, (Insertion), Removal, Replacement, Revision, Supplement
Root Operations that always involve a device.

- 1ST – **0** Medical and Surgical
- 2ND – **L** Tendons
- 3RD – **R REPLACEMENT**

EXAMPLE: Tendon replacement with cadaver graft **CMS Ex:** Total hip

REPLACEMENT: Putting in or on a biological or synthetic material that physically takes the place and/or function of all or a portion of a body part.

EXPLANATION: Includes taking out body part, or eradication...

Body Part – 4TH		Approach – 5TH	Device – 6TH	Qualifier – 7TH
0 Head and Neck Tendon	F Abdomen Tendon, Right	0 Open	7 Autologous tissue substitute	Z No qualifier
1 Shoulder Tendon, Right	G Abdomen Tendon, Left	4 Percutaneous endoscopic	J Synthetic substitute	
2 Shoulder Tendon, Left	H Perineum Tendon		K Nonautologous tissue substitute	
3 Upper Arm Tendon, Right	J Hip Tendon, Right			
4 Upper Arm Tendon, Left	K Hip Tendon, Left			
5 Lower Arm and Wrist Tendon, Right	L Upper Leg Tendon, Right			
	M Upper Leg Tendon, Left			
6 Lower Arm and Wrist Tendon, Left	N Lower Leg Tendon, Right			
	P Lower Leg Tendon, Left			
7 Hand Tendon, Right	Q Knee Tendon, Right			
8 Hand Tendon, Left	R Knee Tendon, Left			
9 Trunk Tendon, Right	S Ankle Tendon, Right			
B Trunk Tendon, Left	T Ankle Tendon, Left			
C Thorax Tendon, Right	V Foot Tendon, Right			
D Thorax Tendon, Left	W Foot Tendon, Left			

0LS — MEDICAL AND SURGICAL SECTION – 2016 ICD-10-PCS

MOVE GROUP: Reattachment, Reposition, Transfer, (Transplantation)
Root Operations that put in/put back or move some/all of a body part.

1ST – 0 Medical and Surgical
2ND – L Tendons
3RD – S REPOSITION

EXAMPLE: Relocation extensor tendon hand   CMS Ex: Fracture reduction

REPOSITION: Moving to its normal location, or other suitable location, all or a portion of a body part.

EXPLANATION: May or may not be cut to be moved ...

Body Part – 4TH		Approach – 5TH	Device – 6TH	Qualifier – 7TH
0 Head and Neck Tendon	F Abdomen Tendon, Right	0 Open	Z No device	Z No qualifier
1 Shoulder Tendon, Right	G Abdomen Tendon, Left	4 Percutaneous endoscopic		
2 Shoulder Tendon, Left	H Perineum Tendon			
3 Upper Arm Tendon, Right	J Hip Tendon, Right			
4 Upper Arm Tendon, Left	K Hip Tendon, Left			
5 Lower Arm and Wrist Tendon, Right	L Upper Leg Tendon, Right			
6 Lower Arm and Wrist Tendon, Left	M Upper Leg Tendon, Left			
	N Lower Leg Tendon, Right			
	P Lower Leg Tendon, Left			
7 Hand Tendon, Right	Q Knee Tendon, Right			
8 Hand Tendon, Left	R Knee Tendon, Left			
9 Trunk Tendon, Right	S Ankle Tendon, Right			
B Trunk Tendon, Left	T Ankle Tendon, Left			
C Thorax Tendon, Right	V Foot Tendon, Right			
D Thorax Tendon, Left	W Foot Tendon, Left			

EXCISION GROUP: Excision, Resection, Destruction, (Extraction), (Detachment)
Root Operations that take out some or all of a body part.

1ST – 0 Medical and Surgical
2ND – L Tendons
3RD – T RESECTION

EXAMPLE: Resection flexor tendon hand   CMS Ex: Cholecystectomy

RESECTION: Cutting out or off, without replacement, all of a body part.

EXPLANATION: None

Body Part – 4TH		Approach – 5TH	Device – 6TH	Qualifier – 7TH
0 Head and Neck Tendon	F Abdomen Tendon, Right	0 Open	Z No device	Z No qualifier
1 Shoulder Tendon, Right	G Abdomen Tendon, Left	4 Percutaneous endoscopic		
2 Shoulder Tendon, Left	H Perineum Tendon			
3 Upper Arm Tendon, Right	J Hip Tendon, Right			
4 Upper Arm Tendon, Left	K Hip Tendon, Left			
5 Lower Arm and Wrist Tendon, Right	L Upper Leg Tendon, Right			
6 Lower Arm and Wrist Tendon, Left	M Upper Leg Tendon, Left			
	N Lower Leg Tendon, Right			
	P Lower Leg Tendon, Left			
7 Hand Tendon, Right	Q Knee Tendon, Right			
8 Hand Tendon, Left	R Knee Tendon, Left			
9 Trunk Tendon, Right	S Ankle Tendon, Right			
B Trunk Tendon, Left	T Ankle Tendon, Left			
C Thorax Tendon, Right	V Foot Tendon, Right			
D Thorax Tendon, Left	W Foot Tendon, Left			

L – TENDONS

0LW

DEVICE GROUP: Change, (Insertion), Removal, Replacement, Revision, Supplement
Root Operations that always involve a device.

1ST - 0 Medical and Surgical
2ND - L Tendons
3RD - U SUPPLEMENT

EXAMPLE: Tenoplasty augmentation graft | CMS Ex: Hernia repair mesh

SUPPLEMENT: Putting in or on biological or synthetic material that physically reinforces and/or augments the function of a portion of a body part.

EXPLANATION: Biological material from same individual ...

Body Part – 4TH		Approach – 5TH	Device – 6TH	Qualifier – 7TH
0 Head and Neck Tendon	F Abdomen Tendon, Right	0 Open	7 Autologous tissue substitute	Z No qualifier
1 Shoulder Tendon, Right	G Abdomen Tendon, Left	4 Percutaneous endoscopic	J Synthetic substitute	
2 Shoulder Tendon, Left	H Perineum Tendon		K Nonautologous tissue substitute	
3 Upper Arm Tendon, Right	J Hip Tendon, Right			
4 Upper Arm Tendon, Left	K Hip Tendon, Left			
5 Lower Arm and Wrist Tendon, Right	L Upper Leg Tendon, Right			
6 Lower Arm and Wrist Tendon, Left	M Upper Leg Tendon, Left			
7 Hand Tendon, Right	N Lower Leg Tendon, Right			
8 Hand Tendon, Left	P Lower Leg Tendon, Left			
9 Trunk Tendon, Right	Q Knee Tendon, Right			
B Trunk Tendon, Left	R Knee Tendon, Left			
C Thorax Tendon, Right	S Ankle Tendon, Right			
D Thorax Tendon, Left	T Ankle Tendon, Left			
	V Foot Tendon, Right			
	W Foot Tendon, Left			

DEVICE GROUP: Change, (Insertion), Removal, Replacement, Revision, Supplement
Root Operations that always involve a device.

1ST - 0 Medical and Surgical
2ND - L Tendons
3RD - W REVISION

EXAMPLE: Reposition drainage tube | CMS Ex: Adjustment pacemaker lead

REVISION: Correcting, to the extent possible, a portion of a malfunctioning device or the position of a displaced device.

EXPLANATION: May replace components of a device ...

Body Part – 4TH	Approach – 5TH	Device – 6TH	Qualifier – 7TH
X Upper Tendon	0 Open	0 Drainage device	Z No qualifier
Y Lower Tendon	3 Percutaneous	7 Autologous tissue substitute	
	4 Percutaneous endoscopic	J Synthetic substitute	
	X External	K Nonautologous tissue substitute	

0LX — MEDICAL AND SURGICAL SECTION – 2016 ICD-10-PCS

MOVE GROUP: Reattachment, Reposition, Transfer, (Transplantation)
Root Operations that put in/put back or move some/all of a body part.

- 1ST - **0** Medical and Surgical
- 2ND - **L** Tendons
- 3RD - **X** TRANSFER

EXAMPLE: Pedicled tendon graft   **CMS Ex:** Tendon transfer

TRANSFER: Moving, without taking out, all or a portion of a body part to another location to take over the function of all or a portion of a body part.

EXPLANATION: The body part remains connected ...

Body Part – 4TH		Approach – 5TH	Device – 6TH	Qualifier – 7TH
0 Head and Neck Tendon	F Abdomen Tendon, Right	0 Open	Z No device	Z No qualifier
1 Shoulder Tendon, Right	G Abdomen Tendon, Left	4 Percutaneous endoscopic		
2 Shoulder Tendon, Left	H Perineum Tendon			
3 Upper Arm Tendon, Right	J Hip Tendon, Right			
4 Upper Arm Tendon, Left	K Hip Tendon, Left			
5 Lower Arm and Wrist Tendon, Right	L Upper Leg Tendon, Right			
	M Upper Leg Tendon, Left			
6 Lower Arm and Wrist Tendon, Left	N Lower Leg Tendon, Right			
	P Lower Leg Tendon, Left			
7 Hand Tendon, Right	Q Knee Tendon, Right			
8 Hand Tendon, Left	R Knee Tendon, Left			
9 Trunk Tendon, Right	S Ankle Tendon, Right			
B Trunk Tendon, Left	T Ankle Tendon, Left			
C Thorax Tendon, Right	V Foot Tendon, Right			
D Thorax Tendon, Left	W Foot Tendon, Left			

Educational Annotations | M – Bursae and Ligaments

Body System Specific Educational Annotations for the Bursae and Ligaments include:
- Anatomy and Physiology Review
- Anatomical Illustrations
- Definitions of Common Procedures
- AHA Coding Clinic® Reference Notations
- Body Part Key Listings
- Device Key Listings
- Device Aggregation Table Listings
- Coding Notes

Anatomy and Physiology Review of Bursae and Ligaments

BODY PART VALUES – M - BURSAE AND LIGAMENTS

Bursa – ANATOMY – Bursa are small, synovial fluid-filled sacs that lie between bones, tendons, and muscles around joints. PHYSIOLOGY – Bursa function to allow less friction between the bones, tendons, and muscles around joints during movement.

Ligament – ANATOMY – A ligament is a strong band or sheath of connective tissue that connects bones to bones. PHYSIOLOGY – Ligaments hold bones and joints in proper alignment and allow some flexibility.

Lower Bursa and Ligament – The bursa and ligaments located below the diaphragm (see Coding Guideline B2.1b)

Upper Bursa and Ligament – The bursa and ligaments located above the diaphragm (see Coding Guideline B2.1b).

Anatomical Illustrations of Bursae and Ligaments

None for the Bursae and Ligaments Body System

Definitions of Common Procedures of Bursae and Ligaments

Prepatellar bursectomy – The surgical removal of a prepatellar (knee) bursal sac.

Reattach severed ankle ligament – The repair of a torn ankle ligament using sutures to a small hole drilled in the fibula.

Tommy John surgery – The surgical reconstruction of a torn ulnar collateral ligament by using a tendon graft sewn through small drill holes in the medial epicondyle of the humerus and sublime tubercle of the ulna in a figure 8 pattern with any remnants of the original ligament attached to the tendon.

AHA Coding Clinic® Reference Notations of Bursae and Ligaments

ROOT OPERATION SPECIFIC - M - BURSAE AND LIGAMENTS
CHANGE - 2
DESTRUCTION - 5
DIVISION - 7
DRAINAGE - 9
EXCISION - B
EXTIRPATION - C
EXTRACTION - D
INSPECTION - J
REATTACHMENT - M
    Arthroscopic type 2 SLAP repair ....AHA 13:3Q:p20
RELEASE - N
REMOVAL - P
REPAIR - Q
    Cervical interspinous ligamentoplasty...AHA 14:3Q:p9
REPOSITION - S
RESECTION - T
SUPPLEMENT - U
REVISION - W
TRANSFER - X

M – Bursae and Ligaments

Educational Annotations

Body Part Key Listings of Bursae and Ligaments

See also Body Part Key in Appendix C

Acromioclavicular ligament	*use* Shoulder Bursa and Ligament, Left/Right
Alar ligament of axis	*use* Head and Neck Bursa and Ligament
Annular ligament	*use* Elbow Bursa and Ligament, Left/Right
Anterior cruciate ligament (ACL)	*use* Knee Bursa and Ligament, Left/Right
Calcaneocuboid ligament	*use* Foot Bursa and Ligament, Left/Right
Calcaneofibular ligament	*use* Ankle Bursa and Ligament, Left/Right
Carpometacarpal ligament	*use* Hand Bursa and Ligament, Left/Right
Cervical interspinous ligament	*use* Head and Neck Bursa and Ligament
Cervical intertransverse ligament	*use* Head and Neck Bursa and Ligament
Cervical ligamentum flavum	*use* Head and Neck Bursa and Ligament
Coracoacromial ligament	*use* Shoulder Bursa and Ligament, Left/Right
Coracoclavicular ligament	*use* Shoulder Bursa and Ligament, Left/Right
Coracohumeral ligament	*use* Shoulder Bursa and Ligament, Left/Right
Costoclavicular ligament	*use* Shoulder Bursa and Ligament, Left/Right
Costotransverse ligament	*use* Thorax Bursa and Ligament, Left/Right
Costoxiphoid ligament	*use* Thorax Bursa and Ligament, Left/Right
Cuneonavicular ligament	*use* Foot Bursa and Ligament, Left/Right
Deltoid ligament	*use* Ankle Bursa and Ligament, Left/Right
Glenohumeral ligament	*use* Shoulder Bursa and Ligament, Left/Right
Iliofemoral ligament	*use* Hip Bursa and Ligament, Left/Right
Iliolumbar ligament	*use* Trunk Bursa and Ligament, Left/Right
Intercarpal ligament	*use* Hand Bursa and Ligament, Left/Right
Interclavicular ligament	*use* Shoulder Bursa and Ligament, Left/Right
Intercuneiform ligament	*use* Foot Bursa and Ligament, Left/Right
Interphalangeal ligament	*use* Hand Bursa and Ligament, Left/Right
	use Foot Bursa and Ligament, Left/Right
Interspinous ligament	*use* Head and Neck Bursa and Ligament
	use Trunk Bursa and Ligament, Left/Right
Intertransverse ligament	*use* Trunk Bursa and Ligament, Left/Right
Ischiofemoral ligament	*use* Hip Bursa and Ligament, Left/Right
Lateral collateral ligament (LCL)	*use* Knee Bursa and Ligament, Left/Right
Lateral temporomandibular ligament	*use* Head and Neck Bursa and Ligament
Ligament of head of fibula	*use* Knee Bursa and Ligament, Left/Right
Ligament of the lateral malleolus	*use* Ankle Bursa and Ligament, Left/Right
Ligamentum flavum	*use* Trunk Bursa and Ligament, Left/Right
Lunotriquetral ligament	*use* Hand Bursa and Ligament, Left/Right
Medial collateral ligament (MCL)	*use* Knee Bursa and Ligament, Left/Right
Metacarpal ligament	*use* Hand Bursa and Ligament, Left/Right
Metacarpophalangeal ligament	*use* Hand Bursa and Ligament, Left/Right
Metatarsal ligament	*use* Foot Bursa and Ligament, Left/Right
Metatarsophalangeal ligament	*use* Foot Bursa and Ligament, Left/Right
Olecranon bursa	*use* Elbow Bursa and Ligament, Left/Right
Palmar ulnocarpal ligament	*use* Wrist Bursa and Ligament, Left/Right
Patellar ligament	*use* Knee Bursa and Ligament, Left/Right
Pisohamate ligament	*use* Hand Bursa and Ligament, Left/Right
Pisometacarpal ligament	*use* Hand Bursa and Ligament, Left/Right
Popliteal ligament	*use* Knee Bursa and Ligament, Left/Right
Posterior cruciate ligament (PCL)	*use* Knee Bursa and Ligament, Left/Right

Continued on next page

Educational Annotations

M – Bursae and Ligaments

Body Part Key Listings of Bursae and Ligaments

Continued from previous page

Prepatellar bursa	*use* Knee Bursa and Ligament, Left/Right
Pubic ligament	*use* Trunk Bursa and Ligament, Left/Right
Pubofemoral ligament	*use* Hip Bursa and Ligament, Left/Right
Radial collateral carpal ligament	*use* Wrist Bursa and Ligament, Left/Right
Radial collateral ligament	*use* Elbow Bursa and Ligament, Left/Right
Radiocarpal ligament	*use* Wrist Bursa and Ligament, Left/Right
Radioulnar ligament	*use* Wrist Bursa and Ligament, Left/Right
Sacrococcygeal ligament	*use* Trunk Bursa and Ligament, Left/Right
Sacroiliac ligament	*use* Trunk Bursa and Ligament, Left/Right
Sacrospinous ligament	*use* Trunk Bursa and Ligament, Left/Right
Sacrotuberous ligament	*use* Trunk Bursa and Ligament, Left/Right
Scapholunate ligament	*use* Hand Bursa and Ligament, Left/Right
Scaphotrapezium ligament	*use* Hand Bursa and Ligament, Left/Right
Sphenomandibular ligament	*use* Head and Neck Bursa and Ligament
Sternoclavicular ligament	*use* Shoulder Bursa and Ligament, Left/Right
Sternocostal ligament	*use* Thorax Bursa and Ligament, Left/Right
Stylomandibular ligament	*use* Head and Neck Bursa and Ligament
Subacromial bursa	*use* Shoulder Bursa and Ligament, Left/Right
Subtalar ligament	*use* Foot Bursa and Ligament, Left/Right
Supraspinous ligament	*use* Trunk Bursa and Ligament, Left/Right
Talocalcaneal ligament	*use* Foot Bursa and Ligament, Left/Right
Talocalcaneonavicular ligament	*use* Foot Bursa and Ligament, Left/Right
Talofibular ligament	*use* Ankle Bursa and Ligament, Left/Right
Tarsometatarsal ligament	*use* Foot Bursa and Ligament, Left/Right
Transverse acetabular ligament	*use* Hip Bursa and Ligament, Left/Right
Transverse humeral ligament	*use* Shoulder Bursa and Ligament, Left/Right
Transverse ligament of atlas	*use* Head and Neck Bursa and Ligament
Transverse scapular ligament	*use* Shoulder Bursa and Ligament, Left/Right
Trochanteric bursa	*use* Hip Bursa and Ligament, Left/Right
Ulnar collateral carpal ligament	*use* Wrist Bursa and Ligament, Left/Right
Ulnar collateral ligament	*use* Elbow Bursa and Ligament, Left/Right

Device Key Listings of Bursae and Ligaments

See also Device Key in Appendix D

Autograft	*use* Autologous Tissue Substitute
Tissue bank graft	*use* Nonautologous Tissue Substitute

Device Aggregation Table Listings of Bursae and Ligaments

See also Device Aggregation Table in Appendix E

Specific Device	For Operation	In Body System	General Device
None Listed in Device Aggregation Table for this Body System			

Educational Annotations | M – Bursae and Ligaments

Coding Notes of Bursae and Ligaments

Body System Relevant Coding Guidelines

General Guidelines

B2.1b

Where the general body part values "upper" and "lower" are provided as an option in the Upper Arteries, Lower Arteries, Upper Veins, Lower Veins, Muscles and Tendons body systems, "upper" and "lower" specifies body parts located above or below the diaphragm respectively.

Example: Vein body parts above the diaphragm are found in the Upper Veins body system; vein body parts below the diaphragm are found in the Lower Veins body system.

Tendons, ligaments, bursae and fascia near a joint

B4.5

Procedures performed on tendons, ligaments, bursae and fascia supporting a joint are coded to the body part in the respective body system that is the focus of the procedure. Procedures performed on joint structures themselves are coded to the body part in the joint body systems.

Example: Repair of the anterior cruciate ligament of the knee is coded to the knee bursa and ligament body part in the bursa and ligaments body system. Knee arthroscopy with shaving of articular cartilage is coded to the knee joint body part in the Lower Joints body system.

Body System Specific PCS Reference Manual Exercises

PCS CODE	M – BURSAE AND LIGAMENTS EXERCISES
0MN14ZZ	Right shoulder arthroscopy with coracoacromial ligament release.
0MSP4ZZ	Left knee arthroscopy with reposition of anterior cruciate ligament.

M – BURSAE AND LIGAMENTS

0M5

DEVICE GROUP: Change, (Insertion), Removal, (Replacement), Revision, Supplement
Root Operations that always involve a device.

- 1ST – **0** Medical and Surgical
- 2ND – **M** Bursae and Ligaments
- 3RD – **2 CHANGE**

EXAMPLE: Exchange drain tube | CMS Ex: Changing urinary catheter

CHANGE: Taking out or off a device from a body part and putting back an identical or similar device in or on the same body part without cutting or puncturing the skin or a mucous membrane.

EXPLANATION: ALL Changes use EXTERNAL approach only ...

Body Part – 4TH	Approach – 5TH	Device – 6TH	Qualifier – 7TH
X Upper Bursa and Ligament Y Lower Bursa and Ligament	X External	0 Drainage device Y Other device	Z No qualifier

EXCISION GROUP: Excision, Resection, Destruction, Extraction, (Detachment)
Root Operations that take out some or all of a body part.

- 1ST – **0** Medical and Surgical
- 2ND – **M** Bursae and Ligaments
- 3RD – **5 DESTRUCTION**

EXAMPLE: Radiofrequency ablation | CMS Ex: Fulguration polyp

DESTRUCTION: Physical eradication of all or a portion of a body part by the direct use of energy, force, or a destructive agent.

EXPLANATION: None of the body part is physically taken out

Body Part – 4TH	Approach – 5TH	Device – 6TH	Qualifier – 7TH
0 Head and Neck Bursa and Ligament 1 Shoulder Bursa and Ligament, Right 2 Shoulder Bursa and Ligament, Left 3 Elbow Bursa and Ligament, Right 4 Elbow Bursa and Ligament, Left 5 Wrist Bursa and Ligament, Right 6 Wrist Bursa and Ligament, Left 7 Hand Bursa and Ligament, Right 8 Hand Bursa and Ligament, Left 9 Upper Extremity Bursa and Ligament, Right B Upper Extremity Bursa and Ligament, Left C Trunk Bursa and Ligament, Right D Trunk Bursa and Ligament, Left F Thorax Bursa and Ligament, Right G Thorax Bursa and Ligament, Left H Abdomen Bursa and Ligament, Right J Abdomen Bursa and Ligament, Left K Perineum Bursa and Ligament L Hip Bursa and Ligament, Right M Hip Bursa and Ligament, Left N Knee Bursa and Ligament, Right P Knee Bursa and Ligament, Left Q Ankle Bursa and Ligament, Right R Ankle Bursa and Ligament, Left S Foot Bursa and Ligament, Right T Foot Bursa and Ligament, Left V Lower Extremity Bursa and Ligament, Right W Lower Extremity Bursa and Ligament, Left	0 Open 3 Percutaneous 4 Percutaneous endoscopic	Z No device	Z No qualifier

0 M 8

MEDICAL AND SURGICAL SECTION – 2016 ICD-10-PCS

DIVISION GROUP: Division, Release
Root Operations involving cutting or separation only.

- 1ST – **0** Medical and Surgical
- 2ND – **M** Bursae and Ligaments
- 3RD – **8** DIVISION

EXAMPLE: Ligament transection   CMS Ex: Osteotomy

DIVISION: Cutting into a body part without draining fluids and/or gases from the body part in order to separate or transect a body part.

EXPLANATION: Separated into two or more portions ...

Body Part – 4TH	Approach – 5TH	Device – 6TH	Qualifier – 7TH
0 Head and Neck Bursa and Ligament	0 Open	Z No device	Z No qualifier
1 Shoulder Bursa and Ligament, Right	3 Percutaneous		
2 Shoulder Bursa and Ligament, Left	4 Percutaneous endoscopic		
3 Elbow Bursa and Ligament, Right			
4 Elbow Bursa and Ligament, Left			
5 Wrist Bursa and Ligament, Right			
6 Wrist Bursa and Ligament, Left			
7 Hand Bursa and Ligament, Right			
8 Hand Bursa and Ligament, Left			
9 Upper Extremity Bursa and Ligament, Right			
B Upper Extremity Bursa and Ligament, Left			
C Trunk Bursa and Ligament, Right			
D Trunk Bursa and Ligament, Left			
F Thorax Bursa and Ligament, Right			
G Thorax Bursa and Ligament, Left			
H Abdomen Bursa and Ligament, Right			
J Abdomen Bursa and Ligament, Left			
K Perineum Bursa and Ligament			
L Hip Bursa and Ligament, Right			
M Hip Bursa and Ligament, Left			
N Knee Bursa and Ligament, Right			
P Knee Bursa and Ligament, Left			
Q Ankle Bursa and Ligament, Right			
R Ankle Bursa and Ligament, Left			
S Foot Bursa and Ligament, Right			
T Foot Bursa and Ligament, Left			
V Lower Extremity Bursa and Ligament, Right			
W Lower Extremity Bursa and Ligament, Left			

M – BURSAE AND LIGAMENTS 0 M 9

DRAINAGE GROUP: Drainage, Extirpation, (Fragmentation)
Root Operations that take out solids/fluids/gases from a body part.

1ST - **0** Medical and Surgical
2ND - **M** Bursae and Ligaments
3RD - **9 DRAINAGE**

EXAMPLE: Aspiration prepatellar bursa   **CMS Ex:** Thoracentesis

DRAINAGE: Taking or letting out fluids and/or gases from a body part.

EXPLANATION: Qualifier "X Diagnostic" indicates biopsy ...

Body Part – 4TH	Approach – 5TH	Device – 6TH	Qualifier – 7TH
0 Head and Neck Bursa and Ligament	0 Open	0 Drainage device	Z No qualifier
1 Shoulder Bursa and Ligament, Right	3 Percutaneous		
2 Shoulder Bursa and Ligament, Left	4 Percutaneous endoscopic		
3 Elbow Bursa and Ligament, Right			
4 Elbow Bursa and Ligament, Left			
5 Wrist Bursa and Ligament, Right			
6 Wrist Bursa and Ligament, Left			
7 Hand Bursa and Ligament, Right			
8 Hand Bursa and Ligament, Left			
9 Upper Extremity Bursa and Ligament, Right			
B Upper Extremity Bursa and Ligament, Left			
C Trunk Bursa and Ligament, Right			
D Trunk Bursa and Ligament, Left			
F Thorax Bursa and Ligament, Right			
G Thorax Bursa and Ligament, Left			
H Abdomen Bursa and Ligament, Right			
J Abdomen Bursa and Ligament, Left			
K Perineum Bursa and Ligament			
L Hip Bursa and Ligament, Right			
M Hip Bursa and Ligament, Left			
N Knee Bursa and Ligament, Right			
P Knee Bursa and Ligament, Left			
Q Ankle Bursa and Ligament, Right			
R Ankle Bursa and Ligament, Left			
S Foot Bursa and Ligament, Right			
T Foot Bursa and Ligament, Left			
V Lower Extremity Bursa and Ligament, Right			
W Lower Extremity Bursa and Ligament, Left			

continued ⇨

0 M 9 DRAINAGE – continued

Body Part – 4ᵀᴴ	Approach – 5ᵀᴴ	Device – 6ᵀᴴ	Qualifier – 7ᵀᴴ
0 Head and Neck Bursa and Ligament 1 Shoulder Bursa and Ligament, Right 2 Shoulder Bursa and Ligament, Left 3 Elbow Bursa and Ligament, Right 4 Elbow Bursa and Ligament, Left 5 Wrist Bursa and Ligament, Right 6 Wrist Bursa and Ligament, Left 7 Hand Bursa and Ligament, Right 8 Hand Bursa and Ligament, Left 9 Upper Extremity Bursa and Ligament, Right B Upper Extremity Bursa and Ligament, Left C Trunk Bursa and Ligament, Right D Trunk Bursa and Ligament, Left F Thorax Bursa and Ligament, Right G Thorax Bursa and Ligament, Left H Abdomen Bursa and Ligament, Right J Abdomen Bursa and Ligament, Left K Perineum Bursa and Ligament L Hip Bursa and Ligament, Right M Hip Bursa and Ligament, Left N Knee Bursa and Ligament, Right P Knee Bursa and Ligament, Left Q Ankle Bursa and Ligament, Right R Ankle Bursa and Ligament, Left S Foot Bursa and Ligament, Right T Foot Bursa and Ligament, Left V Lower Extremity Bursa and Ligament, Right W Lower Extremity Bursa and Ligament, Left	0 Open 3 Percutaneous 4 Percutaneous endoscopic	Z No device	X Diagnostic Z No qualifier

M – BURSAE AND LIGAMENTS

0MB

EXCISION GROUP: Excision, Resection, Destruction, Extraction, (Detachment)
Root Operations that take out some or all of a body part.

- 1ST – **0** Medical and Surgical
- 2ND – **M** Bursae and Ligaments
- 3RD – **B** EXCISION

EXAMPLE: Partial bursectomy elbow   **CMS Ex:** Liver biopsy

EXCISION: Cutting out or off, without replacement, a portion of a body part.

EXPLANATION: Qualifier "X Diagnostic" indicates biopsy …

Body Part – 4TH	Approach – 5TH	Device – 6TH	Qualifier – 7TH
0 Head and Neck Bursa and Ligament	0 Open	Z No device	X Diagnostic
1 Shoulder Bursa and Ligament, Right	3 Percutaneous		Z No qualifier
2 Shoulder Bursa and Ligament, Left	4 Percutaneous endoscopic		
3 Elbow Bursa and Ligament, Right			
4 Elbow Bursa and Ligament, Left			
5 Wrist Bursa and Ligament, Right			
6 Wrist Bursa and Ligament, Left			
7 Hand Bursa and Ligament, Right			
8 Hand Bursa and Ligament, Left			
9 Upper Extremity Bursa and Ligament, Right			
B Upper Extremity Bursa and Ligament, Left			
C Trunk Bursa and Ligament, Right			
D Trunk Bursa and Ligament, Left			
F Thorax Bursa and Ligament, Right			
G Thorax Bursa and Ligament, Left			
H Abdomen Bursa and Ligament, Right			
J Abdomen Bursa and Ligament, Left			
K Perineum Bursa and Ligament			
L Hip Bursa and Ligament, Right			
M Hip Bursa and Ligament, Left			
N Knee Bursa and Ligament, Right			
P Knee Bursa and Ligament, Left			
Q Ankle Bursa and Ligament, Right			
R Ankle Bursa and Ligament, Left			
S Foot Bursa and Ligament, Right			
T Foot Bursa and Ligament, Left			
V Lower Extremity Bursa and Ligament, Right			
W Lower Extremity Bursa and Ligament, Left			

0MC

MEDICAL AND SURGICAL SECTION – 2016 ICD-10-PCS

DRAINAGE GROUP: Drainage, Extirpation, (Fragmentation)
Root Operations that take out solids/fluids/gases from a body part.

- 1ST – **0** Medical and Surgical
- 2ND – **M** Bursae and Ligaments
- 3RD – **C** EXTIRPATION

EXAMPLE: Removal calcification   CMS Ex: Choledocholithotomy

EXTIRPATION: Taking or cutting out solid matter from a body part.

EXPLANATION: Abnormal byproduct or foreign body …

Body Part – 4TH	Approach – 5TH	Device – 6TH	Qualifier – 7TH
0 Head and Neck Bursa and Ligament	0 Open	Z No device	Z No qualifier
1 Shoulder Bursa and Ligament, Right	3 Percutaneous		
2 Shoulder Bursa and Ligament, Left	4 Percutaneous endoscopic		
3 Elbow Bursa and Ligament, Right			
4 Elbow Bursa and Ligament, Left			
5 Wrist Bursa and Ligament, Right			
6 Wrist Bursa and Ligament, Left			
7 Hand Bursa and Ligament, Right			
8 Hand Bursa and Ligament, Left			
9 Upper Extremity Bursa and Ligament, Right			
B Upper Extremity Bursa and Ligament, Left			
C Trunk Bursa and Ligament, Right			
D Trunk Bursa and Ligament, Left			
F Thorax Bursa and Ligament, Right			
G Thorax Bursa and Ligament, Left			
H Abdomen Bursa and Ligament, Right			
J Abdomen Bursa and Ligament, Left			
K Perineum Bursa and Ligament			
L Hip Bursa and Ligament, Right			
M Hip Bursa and Ligament, Left			
N Knee Bursa and Ligament, Right			
P Knee Bursa and Ligament, Left			
Q Ankle Bursa and Ligament, Right			
R Ankle Bursa and Ligament, Left			
S Foot Bursa and Ligament, Right			
T Foot Bursa and Ligament, Left			
V Lower Extremity Bursa and Ligament, Right			
W Lower Extremity Bursa and Ligament, Left			

M – BURSAE AND LIGAMENTS 0MJ

EXCISION GROUP: Excision, Resection, Destruction, Extraction, (Detachment)
Root Operations that take out some or all of a body part.

1ST – **0** Medical and Surgical
2ND – **M** Bursae and Ligaments
3RD – **D** EXTRACTION

EXAMPLE: Extraction bursal sac CMS Ex: D&C

EXTRACTION: Pulling or stripping out or off all or a portion of a body part by the use of force.

EXPLANATION: None for this Body System

Body Part – 4TH	Approach – 5TH	Device – 6TH	Qualifier – 7TH
0 Head and Neck Bursa and Ligament	0 Open	Z No device	Z No qualifier
1 Shoulder Bursa and Ligament, Right	3 Percutaneous		
2 Shoulder Bursa and Ligament, Left	4 Percutaneous endoscopic		
3 Elbow Bursa and Ligament, Right			
4 Elbow Bursa and Ligament, Left			
5 Wrist Bursa and Ligament, Right			
6 Wrist Bursa and Ligament, Left			
7 Hand Bursa and Ligament, Right			
8 Hand Bursa and Ligament, Left			
9 Upper Extremity Bursa and Ligament, Right			
B Upper Extremity Bursa and Ligament, Left			
C Trunk Bursa and Ligament, Right			
D Trunk Bursa and Ligament, Left			
F Thorax Bursa and Ligament, Right			
G Thorax Bursa and Ligament, Left			
H Abdomen Bursa and Ligament, Right			
J Abdomen Bursa and Ligament, Left			
K Perineum Bursa and Ligament			
L Hip Bursa and Ligament, Right			
M Hip Bursa and Ligament, Left			
N Knee Bursa and Ligament, Right			
P Knee Bursa and Ligament, Left			
Q Ankle Bursa and Ligament, Right			
R Ankle Bursa and Ligament, Left			
S Foot Bursa and Ligament, Right			
T Foot Bursa and Ligament, Left			
V Lower Extremity Bursa and Ligament, Right			
W Lower Extremity Bursa and Ligament, Left			

EXAMINATION GROUP: Inspection, (Map)
Root Operations involving examination only.

1ST – **0** Medical and Surgical
2ND – **M** Bursae and Ligaments
3RD – **J** INSPECTION

EXAMPLE: Examination ligament attachments CMS Ex: Colonoscopy

INSPECTION: Visually and/or manually exploring a body part.

EXPLANATION: Direct or instrumental visualization ...

Body Part – 4TH	Approach – 5TH	Device – 6TH	Qualifier – 7TH
X Upper Bursa and Ligament	0 Open	Z No device	Z No qualifier
Y Lower Bursa and Ligament	3 Percutaneous		
	4 Percutaneous endoscopic		
	X External		

0MM

MEDICAL AND SURGICAL SECTION – 2016 ICD-10-PCS

MOVE GROUP: Reattachment, Reposition, Transfer, (Transplantation)
Root Operations that put in/put back or move some/all of a body part.

- 1ST – **0** Medical and Surgical
- 2ND – **M** Bursae and Ligaments
- 3RD – **M REATTACHMENT**

EXAMPLE: Reattach torn ligament **CMS Ex:** Reattachment hand

REATTACHMENT: Putting back in or on all or a portion of a separated body part to its normal location or other suitable location.

EXPLANATION: With/without reconnection of vessels/nerves...

Body Part – 4TH	Approach – 5TH	Device – 6TH	Qualifier – 7TH
0 Head and Neck Bursa and Ligament	0 Open	Z No device	Z No qualifier
1 Shoulder Bursa and Ligament, Right	4 Percutaneous endoscopic		
2 Shoulder Bursa and Ligament, Left			
3 Elbow Bursa and Ligament, Right			
4 Elbow Bursa and Ligament, Left			
5 Wrist Bursa and Ligament, Right			
6 Wrist Bursa and Ligament, Left			
7 Hand Bursa and Ligament, Right			
8 Hand Bursa and Ligament, Left			
9 Upper Extremity Bursa and Ligament, Right			
B Upper Extremity Bursa and Ligament, Left			
C Trunk Bursa and Ligament, Right			
D Trunk Bursa and Ligament, Left			
F Thorax Bursa and Ligament, Right			
G Thorax Bursa and Ligament, Left			
H Abdomen Bursa and Ligament, Right			
J Abdomen Bursa and Ligament, Left			
K Perineum Bursa and Ligament			
L Hip Bursa and Ligament, Right			
M Hip Bursa and Ligament, Left			
N Knee Bursa and Ligament, Right			
P Knee Bursa and Ligament, Left			
Q Ankle Bursa and Ligament, Right			
R Ankle Bursa and Ligament, Left			
S Foot Bursa and Ligament, Right			
T Foot Bursa and Ligament, Left			
V Lower Extremity Bursa and Ligament, Right			
W Lower Extremity Bursa and Ligament, Left			

M – BURSAE AND LIGAMENTS 0MP

DIVISION GROUP: Division, Release
Root Operations involving cutting or separation only.

1ST – 0	Medical and Surgical
2ND – M	Bursae and Ligaments
3RD – N	RELEASE

EXAMPLE: Coracoacromial ligament release **CMS Ex:** Carpal tunnel

RELEASE: Freeing a body part from an abnormal physical constraint by cutting or by the use of force.

EXPLANATION: None of the body part is taken out ...

Body Part – 4TH	Approach – 5TH	Device – 6TH	Qualifier – 7TH
0 Head and Neck Bursa and Ligament	0 Open	Z No device	Z No qualifier
1 Shoulder Bursa and Ligament, Right	3 Percutaneous		
2 Shoulder Bursa and Ligament, Left	4 Percutaneous endoscopic		
3 Elbow Bursa and Ligament, Right	X External		
4 Elbow Bursa and Ligament, Left			
5 Wrist Bursa and Ligament, Right			
6 Wrist Bursa and Ligament, Left			
7 Hand Bursa and Ligament, Right			
8 Hand Bursa and Ligament, Left			
9 Upper Extremity Bursa and Ligament, Right			
B Upper Extremity Bursa and Ligament, Left			
C Trunk Bursa and Ligament, Right			
D Trunk Bursa and Ligament, Left			
F Thorax Bursa and Ligament, Right			
G Thorax Bursa and Ligament, Left			
H Abdomen Bursa and Ligament, Right			
J Abdomen Bursa and Ligament, Left			
K Perineum Bursa and Ligament			
L Hip Bursa and Ligament, Right			
M Hip Bursa and Ligament, Left			
N Knee Bursa and Ligament, Right			
P Knee Bursa and Ligament, Left			
Q Ankle Bursa and Ligament, Right			
R Ankle Bursa and Ligament, Left			
S Foot Bursa and Ligament, Right			
T Foot Bursa and Ligament, Left			
V Lower Extremity Bursa and Ligament, Right			
W Lower Extremity Bursa and Ligament, Left			

DEVICE GROUP: Change, (Insertion), Removal, (Replacement), Revision, Supplement
Root Operations that always involve a device.

1ST – 0	Medical and Surgical
2ND – M	Bursae and Ligaments
3RD – P	REMOVAL

EXAMPLE: Removal drain tube **CMS Ex:** Chest tube removal

REMOVAL: Taking out or off a device from a body part.

EXPLANATION: Removal device without reinsertion ...

Body Part – 4TH	Approach – 5TH	Device – 6TH	Qualifier – 7TH
X Upper Bursa and Ligament	0 Open	0 Drainage device	Z No qualifier
Y Lower Bursa and Ligament	3 Percutaneous	7 Autologous tissue substitute	
	4 Percutaneous endoscopic	J Synthetic substitute	
		K Nonautologous tissue substitute	
X Upper Bursa and Ligament	X External	0 Drainage device	Z No qualifier
Y Lower Bursa and Ligament			

0MQ MEDICAL AND SURGICAL SECTION – 2016 ICD-10-PCS [2016.PCS]

OTHER REPAIRS GROUP: (Control), **Repair**
Root Operations that define other repairs.

1ST – **0** Medical and Surgical
2ND – **M** Bursae and Ligaments
3RD – **Q REPAIR**

EXAMPLE: Suture torn ligament **CMS Ex:** Suture laceration

REPAIR: Restoring, to the extent possible, a body part to its normal anatomic structure and function.

EXPLANATION: Only when no other root operation applies ...

Body Part – 4TH	Approach – 5TH	Device – 6TH	Qualifier – 7TH
0 Head and Neck Bursa and Ligament	0 Open	Z No device	Z No qualifier
1 Shoulder Bursa and Ligament, Right	3 Percutaneous		
2 Shoulder Bursa and Ligament, Left	4 Percutaneous endoscopic		
3 Elbow Bursa and Ligament, Right			
4 Elbow Bursa and Ligament, Left			
5 Wrist Bursa and Ligament, Right			
6 Wrist Bursa and Ligament, Left			
7 Hand Bursa and Ligament, Right			
8 Hand Bursa and Ligament, Left			
9 Upper Extremity Bursa and Ligament, Right			
B Upper Extremity Bursa and Ligament, Left			
C Trunk Bursa and Ligament, Right			
D Trunk Bursa and Ligament, Left			
F Thorax Bursa and Ligament, Right			
G Thorax Bursa and Ligament, Left			
H Abdomen Bursa and Ligament, Right			
J Abdomen Bursa and Ligament, Left			
K Perineum Bursa and Ligament			
L Hip Bursa and Ligament, Right			
M Hip Bursa and Ligament, Left			
N Knee Bursa and Ligament, Right			
P Knee Bursa and Ligament, Left			
Q Ankle Bursa and Ligament, Right			
R Ankle Bursa and Ligament, Left			
S Foot Bursa and Ligament, Right			
T Foot Bursa and Ligament, Left			
V Lower Extremity Bursa and Ligament, Right			
W Lower Extremity Bursa and Ligament, Left			

476

0MS

M – BURSAE AND LIGAMENTS

MOVE GROUP: Reattachment, Reposition, Transfer, (Transplantation)
Root Operations that put in/put back or move some/all of a body part.

- 1ST - **0** Medical and Surgical
- 2ND - **M** Bursae and Ligaments
- 3RD - **S** REPOSITION

EXAMPLE: Reposition ACL ligament **CMS Ex:** Fracture reduction

REPOSITION: Moving to its normal location, or other suitable location, all or a portion of a body part.

EXPLANATION: May or may not be cut to be moved ...

Body Part – 4TH	Approach – 5TH	Device – 6TH	Qualifier – 7TH
0 Head and Neck Bursa and Ligament	0 Open	Z No device	Z No qualifier
1 Shoulder Bursa and Ligament, Right	4 Percutaneous endoscopic		
2 Shoulder Bursa and Ligament, Left			
3 Elbow Bursa and Ligament, Right			
4 Elbow Bursa and Ligament, Left			
5 Wrist Bursa and Ligament, Right			
6 Wrist Bursa and Ligament, Left			
7 Hand Bursa and Ligament, Right			
8 Hand Bursa and Ligament, Left			
9 Upper Extremity Bursa and Ligament, Right			
B Upper Extremity Bursa and Ligament, Left			
C Trunk Bursa and Ligament, Right			
D Trunk Bursa and Ligament, Left			
F Thorax Bursa and Ligament, Right			
G Thorax Bursa and Ligament, Left			
H Abdomen Bursa and Ligament, Right			
J Abdomen Bursa and Ligament, Left			
K Perineum Bursa and Ligament			
L Hip Bursa and Ligament, Right			
M Hip Bursa and Ligament, Left			
N Knee Bursa and Ligament, Right			
P Knee Bursa and Ligament, Left			
Q Ankle Bursa and Ligament, Right			
R Ankle Bursa and Ligament, Left			
S Foot Bursa and Ligament, Right			
T Foot Bursa and Ligament, Left			
V Lower Extremity Bursa and Ligament, Right			
W Lower Extremity Bursa and Ligament, Left			

OMT — MEDICAL AND SURGICAL SECTION – 2016 ICD-10-PCS

[2016.PCS]

EXCISION GROUP: Excision, Resection, Destruction, Extraction, (Detachment)
Root Operations that take out some or all of a body part.

- 1ST – **0** Medical and Surgical
- 2ND – **M** Bursae and Ligaments
- 3RD – **T RESECTION**

EXAMPLE: Collateral ligament resection
CMS Ex: Cholecystectomy

RESECTION: Cutting out or off, without replacement, all of a body part.

EXPLANATION: None

Body Part – 4TH	Approach – 5TH	Device – 6TH	Qualifier – 7TH
0 Head and Neck Bursa and Ligament	0 Open	Z No device	Z No qualifier
1 Shoulder Bursa and Ligament, Right	4 Percutaneous endoscopic		
2 Shoulder Bursa and Ligament, Left			
3 Elbow Bursa and Ligament, Right			
4 Elbow Bursa and Ligament, Left			
5 Wrist Bursa and Ligament, Right			
6 Wrist Bursa and Ligament, Left			
7 Hand Bursa and Ligament, Right			
8 Hand Bursa and Ligament, Left			
9 Upper Extremity Bursa and Ligament, Right			
B Upper Extremity Bursa and Ligament, Left			
C Trunk Bursa and Ligament, Right			
D Trunk Bursa and Ligament, Left			
F Thorax Bursa and Ligament, Right			
G Thorax Bursa and Ligament, Left			
H Abdomen Bursa and Ligament, Right			
J Abdomen Bursa and Ligament, Left			
K Perineum Bursa and Ligament			
L Hip Bursa and Ligament, Right			
M Hip Bursa and Ligament, Left			
N Knee Bursa and Ligament, Right			
P Knee Bursa and Ligament, Left			
Q Ankle Bursa and Ligament, Right			
R Ankle Bursa and Ligament, Left			
S Foot Bursa and Ligament, Right			
T Foot Bursa and Ligament, Left			
V Lower Extremity Bursa and Ligament, Right			
W Lower Extremity Bursa and Ligament, Left			

M – BURSAE AND LIGAMENTS 0MW

DEVICE GROUP: Change, (Insertion), Removal, (Replacement), Revision, Supplement
Root Operations that always involve a device.

1ST – **0** Medical and Surgical
2ND – **M** Bursae and Ligaments
3RD – **U SUPPLEMENT**

EXAMPLE: Augmentation ligamentoplasty | CMS Ex: Hernia repair mesh

SUPPLEMENT: Putting in or on biological or synthetic material that physically reinforces and/or augments the function of a portion of a body part.

EXPLANATION: Biological material from same individual ...

Body Part – 4TH	Approach – 5TH	Device – 6TH	Qualifier – 7TH
0 Head and Neck Bursa and Ligament	0 Open	7 Autologous tissue substitute	Z No qualifier
1 Shoulder Bursa and Ligament, Right	4 Percutaneous endoscopic	J Synthetic substitute	
2 Shoulder Bursa and Ligament, Left		K Nonautologous tissue substitute	
3 Elbow Bursa and Ligament, Right			
4 Elbow Bursa and Ligament, Left			
5 Wrist Bursa and Ligament, Right			
6 Wrist Bursa and Ligament, Left			
7 Hand Bursa and Ligament, Right			
8 Hand Bursa and Ligament, Left			
9 Upper Extremity Bursa and Ligament, Right			
B Upper Extremity Bursa and Ligament, Left			
C Trunk Bursa and Ligament, Right			
D Trunk Bursa and Ligament, Left			
F Thorax Bursa and Ligament, Right			
G Thorax Bursa and Ligament, Left			
H Abdomen Bursa and Ligament, Right			
J Abdomen Bursa and Ligament, Left			
K Perineum Bursa and Ligament			
L Hip Bursa and Ligament, Right			
M Hip Bursa and Ligament, Left			
N Knee Bursa and Ligament, Right			
P Knee Bursa and Ligament, Left			
Q Ankle Bursa and Ligament, Right			
R Ankle Bursa and Ligament, Left			
S Foot Bursa and Ligament, Right			
T Foot Bursa and Ligament, Left			
V Lower Extremity Bursa and Ligament, Right			
W Lower Extremity Bursa and Ligament, Left			

DEVICE GROUP: Change, (Insertion), Removal, (Replacement), Revision, Supplement
Root Operations that always involve a device.

1ST – **0** Medical and Surgical
2ND – **M** Bursae and Ligaments
3RD – **W REVISION**

EXAMPLE: Resuture ligament graft | CMS Ex: Adjustment pacemaker lead

REVISION: Correcting, to the extent possible, a portion of a malfunctioning device or the position of a displaced device.

EXPLANATION: May replace components of a device ...

Body Part – 4TH	Approach – 5TH	Device – 6TH	Qualifier – 7TH
X Upper Bursa and Ligament	0 Open	0 Drainage device	Z No qualifier
Y Lower Bursa and Ligament	3 Percutaneous	7 Autologous tissue substitute	
	4 Percutaneous endoscopic	J Synthetic substitute	
	X External	K Nonautologous tissue substitute	

0MX

MEDICAL AND SURGICAL SECTION – 2016 ICD-10-PCS [2016.PCS]

MOVE GROUP: Reattachment, Reposition, Transfer, (Transplantation)
Root Operations that put in/put back or move some/all of a body part.

1ST - 0 Medical and Surgical
2ND - M Bursae and Ligaments
3RD - X TRANSFER

EXAMPLE: Carpal ligament transfer CMS Ex: Tendon transfer

TRANSFER: Moving, without taking out, all or a portion of a body part to another location to take over the function of all or a portion of a body part.

EXPLANATION: The body part remains connected ...

Body Part – 4TH	Approach – 5TH	Device – 6TH	Qualifier – 7TH
0 Head and Neck Bursa and Ligament	0 Open	Z No device	Z No qualifier
1 Shoulder Bursa and Ligament, Right	4 Percutaneous endoscopic		
2 Shoulder Bursa and Ligament, Left			
3 Elbow Bursa and Ligament, Right			
4 Elbow Bursa and Ligament, Left			
5 Wrist Bursa and Ligament, Right			
6 Wrist Bursa and Ligament, Left			
7 Hand Bursa and Ligament, Right			
8 Hand Bursa and Ligament, Left			
9 Upper Extremity Bursa and Ligament, Right			
B Upper Extremity Bursa and Ligament, Left			
C Trunk Bursa and Ligament, Right			
D Trunk Bursa and Ligament, Left			
F Thorax Bursa and Ligament, Right			
G Thorax Bursa and Ligament, Left			
H Abdomen Bursa and Ligament, Right			
J Abdomen Bursa and Ligament, Left			
K Perineum Bursa and Ligament			
L Hip Bursa and Ligament, Right			
M Hip Bursa and Ligament, Left			
N Knee Bursa and Ligament, Right			
P Knee Bursa and Ligament, Left			
Q Ankle Bursa and Ligament, Right			
R Ankle Bursa and Ligament, Left			
S Foot Bursa and Ligament, Right			
T Foot Bursa and Ligament, Left			
V Lower Extremity Bursa and Ligament, Right			
W Lower Extremity Bursa and Ligament, Left			

Educational Annotations | N – Head and Facial Bones

Body System Specific Educational Annotations for the Head and Facial Bones include:
- Anatomy and Physiology Review
- Anatomical Illustrations
- Definitions of Common Procedures
- AHA Coding Clinic® Reference Notations
- Body Part Key Listings
- Device Key Listings
- Device Aggregation Table Listings
- Coding Notes

Anatomy and Physiology Review of Head and Facial Bones

BODY PART VALUES – N - HEAD AND FACIAL BONES

Conchae Bone – The 2 small paired bones of the nasal cavity that are attached to the maxilla.

Ethmoid Bone – The single bone located between the orbits that forms the roof of the nasal cavity, part of the floor of the cranial cavity, and part of the orbit.

Facial Bone – Any one of the 14 bones of the facial area below the cranium (2 nasal bones, vomer, 2 conchae, 2 maxilla, mandible, 2 palatine bones, 2 zygomatic bones, 2 lacrimal bones).

Frontal Bone – The single bone in the front of the skull that also forms part of the roof of the nasal cavity and part of the orbit.

Hyoid Bone – The single horseshoe-shaped bone that lies in the front of the neck and just under the chin and aids in tongue movement and swallowing. It is not directly articulated with any other bone and not considered part of the skull.

Lacrimal Bone – The 2 small paired bones that form the medial side of the orbit and the nasolacrimal canal.

Mandible – The single horseshoe-shaped bone forming the lower jaw.

Maxilla – The 2 fused irregularly-shaped bones that form the upper jaw, the roof of the mouth, and a part of the orbit.

Nasal Bone – The 2 small paired bones that form the bridge of the nose.

Occipital Bone – The single bone of the base and back of the skull.

Orbit – The bones (7) which form the orbit (eye socket): Zygomatic, sphenoid, ethmoid, maxilla, lacrimal, palatine, and frontal.

Palatine Bone – The 2 small paired bones at the back of the nasal cavity that form the floor and lateral wall of the nasal cavity, part of the roof of the mouth, and part of the floor of the orbit.

Parietal Bone – The 2 paired bones that form the top and sides of the skull.

Skull – The skull consists of all (22) of the cranial and facial bones. Eight of these bones form the cranium (occipital bone, frontal bone, 2 temporal bones, 2 parietal bones, sphenoid bone, ethmoid bone), and 14 of these bones form the skull below the cranium (2 nasal bones, vomer, 2 conchae, 2 maxilla, mandible, 2 palatine bones, 2 zygomatic bones, 2 lacrimal bones).

Sphenoid Bone – The single winged-shaped bone of the skull floor that forms part of the base of the cranial cavity, sides of the skull, and part of the orbital floor and side.

Temporal Bone – The 2 paired bones that form the lower sides and base of the skull and contain the internal organs and structures of hearing.

Vomer Bone – The single bone of the inferior nasal septum.

Zygomatic Bone – The 2 paired quadrangular bones of the cheeks (also known as the malar bones) that form the cheek prominence and lower-outer part of the orbit.

N – Head and Facial Bones

Educational Annotations

Anatomical Illustrations of Head and Facial Bones

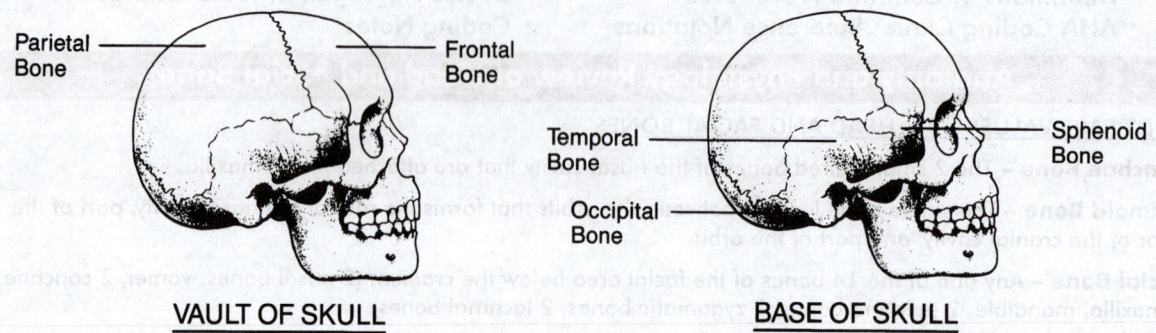

VAULT OF SKULL

BASE OF SKULL

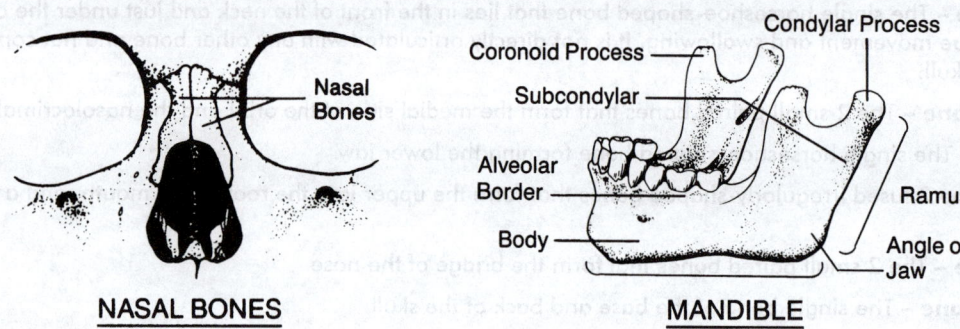

NASAL BONES

MANDIBLE

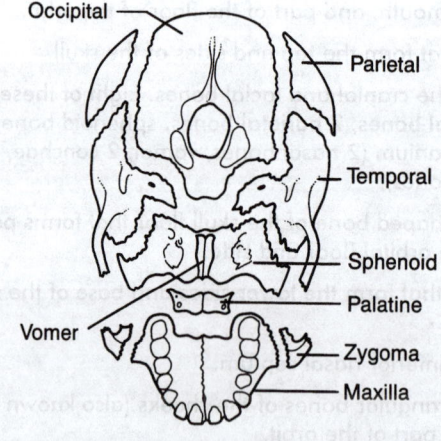

ORBITAL FLOOR AND MALAR BONES

Continued on next page

Educational Annotations

N – Head and Facial Bones

Continued from previous page

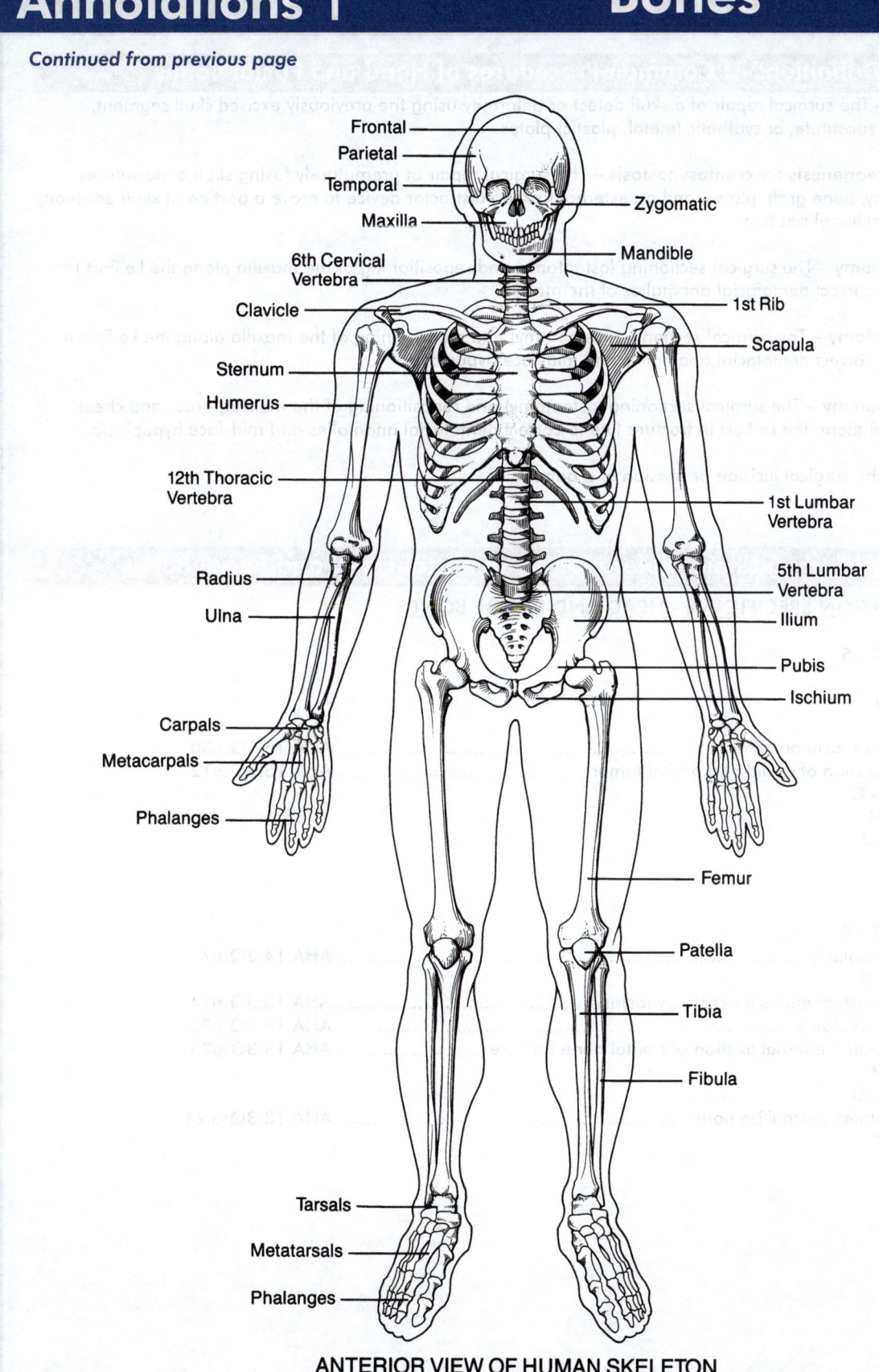

ANTERIOR VIEW OF HUMAN SKELETON

Educational Annotations | N – Head and Facial Bones

Definitions of Common Procedures of Head and Facial Bones

Cranioplasty – The surgical repair of a skull defect or deformity using the previously excised skull segment, synthetic bone substitute, or synthetic (metal, plastic) plates.

Distraction osteogenesis for craniosynostosis – The surgical repair of prematurely fusing skull bone sutures using osteotomy, bone graft, plates, and an external fixation distractor device to move a portion of skull gradually into a more functional position.

Le Fort I osteotomy – The surgical sectioning (osteotomy) and repositioning of the maxilla along the Le Fort I fracture line to correct dentofacial anomalies of the maxilla.

Le Fort II osteotomy – The surgical sectioning (osteotomy) and repositioning of the maxilla along the Le Fort II fracture line to correct dentofacial anomalies and mid-face hypoplasia.

Le Fort III osteotomy – The surgical sectioning (osteotomy) and repositioning of the maxilla, nose, and cheek bones (zygoma) along the Le Fort III fracture line to correct dentofacial anomalies and mid-face hypoplasia.

Osteotomy – The surgical incision or division of a bone.

AHA Coding Clinic® Reference Notations of Head and Facial Bones

ROOT OPERATION SPECIFIC - N - HEAD AND FACIAL BONES
CHANGE - 2
DESTRUCTION - 5
DIVISION - 8
DRAINAGE - 9
EXCISION - B
    Harvesting of local bone for graft ....AHA 15:1Q:p30
    Radical resection of eyelid and orbital tumor ....AHA 15:2Q:p12
EXTIRPATION - C
INSERTION - H
INSPECTION - J
RELEASE - N
REMOVAL - P
REPAIR - Q
REPLACEMENT - R
    Hemi-cranioplasty ....AHA 14:3Q:p7
REPOSITION - S
    Distraction osteogenesis for craniosynostosis ....AHA 13:3Q:p24
    Le Fort 1 osteotomy ....AHA 14:3Q:p23
    Open reduction internal fixation of frontal bone fracture ....AHA 13:3Q:p25
RESECTION - T
SUPPLEMENT - U
    Titanium plates to stabilize bone ....AHA 13:3Q:p 24
REVISION - W

Educational Annotations | N – Head and Facial Bones

Body Part Key Listings of Head and Facial Bones

See also Body Part Key in Appendix C

Alveolar process of mandible	*use* Mandible, Left/Right
Alveolar process of maxilla	*use* Maxilla, Left/Right
Bony orbit	*use* Orbit, Left/Right
Condyloid process	*use* Mandible, Left/Right
Cribriform plate	*use* Ethmoid Bone, Left/Right
Foramen magnum	*use* Occipital Bone, Left/Right
Greater wing	*use* Sphenoid Bone, Left/Right
Lesser wing	*use* Sphenoid Bone, Left/Right
Mandibular notch	*use* Mandible, Left/Right
Mastoid process	*use* Temporal Bone, Left/Right
Mental foramen	*use* Mandible, Left/Right
Optic foramen	*use* Sphenoid Bone, Left/Right
Orbital portion of ethmoid bone	*use* Orbit, Left/Right
Orbital portion of frontal bone	*use* Orbit, Left/Right
Orbital portion of lacrimal bone	*use* Orbit, Left/Right
Orbital portion of maxilla	*use* Orbit, Left/Right
Orbital portion of palatine bone	*use* Orbit, Left/Right
Orbital portion of sphenoid bone	*use* Orbit, Left/Right
Orbital portion of zygomatic bone	*use* Orbit, Left/Right
Petrous part of temporal bone	*use* Temporal Bone, Left/Right
Pterygoid process	*use* Sphenoid Bone, Left/Right
Sella turcica	*use* Sphenoid Bone, Left/Right
Tympanic part of temporal bone	*use* Temporal Bone, Left/Right
Vomer of nasal septum	*use* Nasal Bone
Zygomatic process of frontal bone	*use* Frontal Bone, Left/Right
Zygomatic process of temporal bone	*use* Temporal Bone, Left/Right

Device Key Listings of Head and Facial Bones

See also Device Key in Appendix D

Autograft	*use* Autologous Tissue Substitute
Bone anchored hearing device	*use* Hearing Device in Head and Facial Bones
Bone bank bone graft	*use* Nonautologous Tissue Substitute
Bone screw (interlocking) (lag) (pedicle) (recessed)	*use* Internal Fixation Device in Head and Facial Bones, Upper Bones, Lower Bones
Electrical bone growth stimulator (EBGS)	*use* Bone Growth Stimulator in Head and Facial Bones, Upper Bones, Lower Bones
External fixator	*use* External Fixation Device in Head and Facial Bones, Upper Bones, Lower Bones, Upper Joints, Lower Joints
Kirschner wire (K-wire)	*use* Internal Fixation Device in Head and Facial Bones, Upper Bones, Lower Bones, Upper Joints, Lower Joints
Neutralization plate	*use* Internal Fixation Device in Head and Facial Bones, Upper Bones, Lower Bones
Polymethylmethacrylate (PMMA)	*use* Synthetic Substitute
RNS system neurostimulator generator	*use* Neurostimulator Generator in Head and Facial Bones
Tissue bank graft	*use* Nonautologous Tissue Substitute
Ultrasonic osteogenic stimulator	*use* Bone Growth Stimulator in Head and Facial Bones, Upper Bones, Lower Bones
Ultrasound bone healing system	*use* Bone Growth Stimulator in Head and Facial Bones, Upper Bones, Lower Bones

Educational Annotations

N – Head and Facial Bones

Device Aggregation Table Listings of Head and Facial Bones

See also Device Aggregation Table in Appendix E

Specific Device	For Operation	In Body System	General Device
None Listed in Device Aggregation Table for this Body System			

Coding Notes of Head and Facial Bones

Body System Relevant Coding Guidelines

Reposition for fracture treatment
  B3.15
  Reduction of a displaced fracture is coded to the root operation Reposition and the application of a cast or splint in conjunction with the Reposition procedure is not coded separately. Treatment of a nondisplaced fracture is coded to the procedure performed.
  Examples: Putting a pin in a nondisplaced fracture is coded to the root operation Insertion.
  Casting of a nondisplaced fracture is coded to the root operation Immobilization in the Placement section.

Body System Specific PCS Reference Manual Exercises

PCS CODE   N – HEAD AND FACIAL BONES EXERCISES

None for this Body System

N – HEAD AND FACIAL BONES 0N5

DEVICE GROUP: Change, Insertion, Removal, Replacement, Revision, Supplement
Root Operations that always involve a device.

1ST - 0 Medical and Surgical
2ND - N Head and Facial Bones
3RD - 2 CHANGE

EXAMPLE: Exchange drain tube | CMS Ex: Changing urinary catheter

CHANGE: Taking out or off a device from a body part and putting back an identical or similar device in or on the same body part without cutting or puncturing the skin or a mucous membrane.

EXPLANATION: ALL Changes use EXTERNAL approach only …

Body Part – 4TH	Approach – 5TH	Device – 6TH	Qualifier – 7TH
0 Skull	X External	0 Drainage device	Z No qualifier
B Nasal Bone		Y Other device	
W Facial Bone			

EXCISION GROUP: Excision, Resection, Destruction, (Extraction), (Detachment)
Root Operations that take out some or all of a body part.

1ST - 0 Medical and Surgical
2ND - N Head and Facial Bones
3RD - 5 DESTRUCTION

EXAMPLE: Cryoablation bone cyst | CMS Ex: Fulguration polyp

DESTRUCTION: Physical eradication of all or a portion of a body part by the direct use of energy, force, or a destructive agent.

EXPLANATION: None of the body part is physically taken out

Body Part – 4TH		Approach – 5TH	Device – 6TH	Qualifier – 7TH
0 Skull	H Lacrimal Bone, Right	0 Open	Z No device	Z No qualifier
1 Frontal Bone, Right	J Lacrimal Bone, Left	3 Percutaneous		
2 Frontal Bone, Left	K Palatine Bone, Right	4 Percutaneous endoscopic		
3 Parietal Bone, Right	L Palatine Bone, Left			
4 Parietal Bone, Left	M Zygomatic Bone, Right			
5 Temporal Bone, Right	N Zygomatic Bone, Left			
6 Temporal Bone, Left	P Orbit, Right			
7 Occipital Bone, Right	Q Orbit, Left			
8 Occipital Bone, Left	R Maxilla, Right			
B Nasal Bone	S Maxilla, Left			
C Sphenoid Bone, Right	T Mandible, Right			
D Sphenoid Bone, Left	V Mandible, Left			
F Ethmoid Bone, Right	X Hyoid Bone			
G Ethmoid Bone, Left				

0N8

DIVISION GROUP: Division, Release
Root Operations involving cutting or separation only.

- 1ST - **0** Medical and Surgical
- 2ND - **N** Head and Facial Bones
- 3RD - **8 DIVISION**

EXAMPLE: Mandibular osteotomy **CMS Ex:** Osteotomy

DIVISION: Cutting into a body part without draining fluids and/or gases from the body part in order to separate or transect a body part.

EXPLANATION: Separated into two or more portions ...

Body Part – 4TH		Approach – 5TH	Device – 6TH	Qualifier – 7TH
0 Skull	H Lacrimal Bone, Right	0 Open	Z No device	Z No qualifier
1 Frontal Bone, Right	J Lacrimal Bone, Left	3 Percutaneous		
2 Frontal Bone, Left	K Palatine Bone, Right	4 Percutaneous endoscopic		
3 Parietal Bone, Right	L Palatine Bone, Left			
4 Parietal Bone, Left	M Zygomatic Bone, Right			
5 Temporal Bone, Right	N Zygomatic Bone, Left			
6 Temporal Bone, Left	P Orbit, Right			
7 Occipital Bone, Right	Q Orbit, Left			
8 Occipital Bone, Left	R Maxilla, Right			
B Nasal Bone	S Maxilla, Left			
C Sphenoid Bone, Right	T Mandible, Right			
D Sphenoid Bone, Left	V Mandible, Left			
F Ethmoid Bone, Right	X Hyoid Bone			
G Ethmoid Bone, Left				

N – HEAD AND FACIAL BONES

0N9

DRAINAGE GROUP: Drainage, Extirpation, (Fragmentation)
Root Operations that take out solids/fluids/gases from a body part.

- 1ST – **0** Medical and Surgical
- 2ND – **N** Head and Facial Bones
- 3RD – **9** DRAINAGE

EXAMPLE: Aspiration bone cyst   **CMS Ex:** Thoracentesis

DRAINAGE: Taking or letting out fluids and/or gases from a body part.

EXPLANATION: Qualifier "X Diagnostic" indicates biopsy …

Body Part – 4TH		Approach – 5TH	Device – 6TH	Qualifier – 7TH
0 Skull	H Lacrimal Bone, Right	0 Open	0 Drainage device	Z No qualifier
1 Frontal Bone, Right	J Lacrimal Bone, Left	3 Percutaneous		
2 Frontal Bone, Left	K Palatine Bone, Right	4 Percutaneous endoscopic		
3 Parietal Bone, Right	L Palatine Bone, Left			
4 Parietal Bone, Left	M Zygomatic Bone, Right			
5 Temporal Bone, Right	N Zygomatic Bone, Left			
6 Temporal Bone, Left	P Orbit, Right			
7 Occipital Bone, Right	Q Orbit, Left			
8 Occipital Bone, Left	R Maxilla, Right			
B Nasal Bone	S Maxilla, Left			
C Sphenoid Bone, Right	T Mandible, Right			
D Sphenoid Bone, Left	V Mandible, Left			
F Ethmoid Bone, Right	X Hyoid Bone			
G Ethmoid Bone, Left				

Body Part – 4TH		Approach – 5TH	Device – 6TH	Qualifier – 7TH
0 Skull	H Lacrimal Bone, Right	0 Open	Z No device	X Diagnostic
1 Frontal Bone, Right	J Lacrimal Bone, Left	3 Percutaneous		Z No qualifier
2 Frontal Bone, Left	K Palatine Bone, Right	4 Percutaneous endoscopic		
3 Parietal Bone, Right	L Palatine Bone, Left			
4 Parietal Bone, Left	M Zygomatic Bone, Right			
5 Temporal Bone, Right	N Zygomatic Bone, Left			
6 Temporal Bone, Left	P Orbit, Right			
7 Occipital Bone, Right	Q Orbit, Left			
8 Occipital Bone, Left	R Maxilla, Right			
B Nasal Bone	S Maxilla, Left			
C Sphenoid Bone, Right	T Mandible, Right			
D Sphenoid Bone, Left	V Mandible, Left			
F Ethmoid Bone, Right	X Hyoid Bone			
G Ethmoid Bone, Left				

0NB MEDICAL AND SURGICAL SECTION – 2016 ICD-10-PCS

EXCISION GROUP: Excision, Resection, Destruction, (Extraction), (Detachment)
Root Operations that take out some or all of a body part.

1ST - 0 Medical and Surgical
2ND - N Head and Facial Bones
3RD - B EXCISION

EXAMPLE: Mandibular sequestrectomy CMS Ex: Liver biopsy

EXCISION: Cutting out or off, without replacement, a portion of a body part.

EXPLANATION: Qualifier "X Diagnostic" indicates biopsy …

Body Part – 4TH		Approach – 5TH	Device – 6TH	Qualifier – 7TH
0 Skull	H Lacrimal Bone, Right	0 Open	Z No device	X Diagnostic
1 Frontal Bone, Right	J Lacrimal Bone, Left	3 Percutaneous		Z No qualifier
2 Frontal Bone, Left	K Palatine Bone, Right	4 Percutaneous endoscopic		
3 Parietal Bone, Right	L Palatine Bone, Left			
4 Parietal Bone, Left	M Zygomatic Bone, Right			
5 Temporal Bone, Right	N Zygomatic Bone, Left			
6 Temporal Bone, Left	P Orbit, Right			
7 Occipital Bone, Right	Q Orbit, Left			
8 Occipital Bone, Left	R Maxilla, Right			
B Nasal Bone	S Maxilla, Left			
C Sphenoid Bone, Right	T Mandible, Right			
D Sphenoid Bone, Left	V Mandible, Left			
F Ethmoid Bone, Right	X Hyoid Bone			
G Ethmoid Bone, Left				

DRAINAGE GROUP: Drainage, Extirpation, (Fragmentation)
Root Operations that take out solids/fluids/gases from a body part.

1ST - 0 Medical and Surgical
2ND - N Head and Facial Bones
3RD - C EXTIRPATION

EXAMPLE: Removal foreign body CMS Ex: Choledocholithotomy

EXTIRPATION: Taking or cutting out solid matter from a body part.

EXPLANATION: Abnormal byproduct or foreign body …

Body Part – 4TH		Approach – 5TH	Device – 6TH	Qualifier – 7TH
1 Frontal Bone, Right	H Lacrimal Bone, Right	0 Open	Z No device	Z No qualifier
2 Frontal Bone, Left	J Lacrimal Bone, Left	3 Percutaneous		
3 Parietal Bone, Right	K Palatine Bone, Right	4 Percutaneous endoscopic		
4 Parietal Bone, Left	L Palatine Bone, Left			
5 Temporal Bone, Right	M Zygomatic Bone, Right			
6 Temporal Bone, Left	N Zygomatic Bone, Left			
7 Occipital Bone, Right	P Orbit, Right			
8 Occipital Bone, Left	Q Orbit, Left			
B Nasal Bone	R Maxilla, Right			
C Sphenoid Bone, Right	S Maxilla, Left			
D Sphenoid Bone, Left	T Mandible, Right			
F Ethmoid Bone, Right	V Mandible, Left			
G Ethmoid Bone, Left	X Hyoid Bone			

N – HEAD AND FACIAL BONES

0NH

DEVICE GROUP: Change, Insertion, Removal, Replacement, Revision, Supplement
Root Operations that always involve a device.

- 1ST – **0** Medical and Surgical
- 2ND – **N** Head and Facial Bones
- 3RD – **H** INSERTION

EXAMPLE: Bone growth stimulator **CMS Ex:** Central venous catheter

INSERTION: Putting in a nonbiological appliance that monitors, assists, performs, or prevents a physiological function but does not physically take the place of a body part.

EXPLANATION: None

Body Part – 4TH	Approach – 5TH	Device – 6TH	Qualifier – 7TH
0 Skull	0 Open	4 Internal fixation device 5 External fixation device M Bone growth stimulator N Neurostimulator generator	Z No qualifier
0 Skull	3 Percutaneous 4 Percutaneous endoscopic	4 Internal fixation device 5 External fixation device M Bone growth stimulator	Z No qualifier
1 Frontal Bone, Right 2 Frontal Bone, Left 3 Parietal Bone, Right 4 Parietal Bone, Left 7 Occipital Bone, Right 8 Occipital Bone, Left C Sphenoid Bone, Right D Sphenoid Bone, Left F Ethmoid Bone, Right G Ethmoid Bone, Left H Lacrimal Bone, Right J Lacrimal Bone, Left K Palatine Bone, Right L Palatine Bone, Left M Zygomatic Bone, Right N Zygomatic Bone, Left P Orbit, Right Q Orbit, Left X Hyoid Bone	0 Open 3 Percutaneous 4 Percutaneous endoscopic	4 Internal fixation device	Z No qualifier
5 Temporal Bone, Right 6 Temporal Bone, Left	0 Open 3 Percutaneous 4 Percutaneous endoscopic	4 Internal fixation device S Hearing device	Z No qualifier
B Nasal Bone	0 Open 3 Percutaneous 4 Percutaneous endoscopic	4 Internal fixation device M Bone growth stimulator	Z No qualifier
R Maxilla, Right S Maxilla, Left T Mandible, Right V Mandible, Left	0 Open 3 Percutaneous 4 Percutaneous endoscopic	4 Internal fixation device 5 External fixation device	Z No qualifier
W Facial Bone	0 Open 3 Percutaneous 4 Percutaneous endoscopic	M Bone growth stimulator	Z No qualifier

0 N J MEDICAL AND SURGICAL SECTION – 2016 ICD-10-PCS [2016.PCS]

EXAMINATION GROUP: Inspection, (Map)
Root Operations involving examination only.

- 1ST – **0** Medical and Surgical
- 2ND – **N** Head and Facial Bones
- 3RD – **J** INSPECTION

EXAMPLE: Examination bone   CMS Ex: Colonoscopy

INSPECTION: Visually and/or manually exploring a body part.

EXPLANATION: Direct or instrumental visualization ...

Body Part – 4TH	Approach – 5TH	Device – 6TH	Qualifier – 7TH
0 Skull	0 Open	Z No device	Z No qualifier
B Nasal Bone	3 Percutaneous		
W Facial Bone	4 Percutaneous endoscopic		
	X External		

DIVISION GROUP: Division, Release
Root Operations involving cutting or separation only.

- 1ST – **0** Medical and Surgical
- 2ND – **N** Head and Facial Bones
- 3RD – **N** RELEASE

EXAMPLE: Extra-articular bone adhesiolysis   CMS Ex: Carpal tunnel release

RELEASE: Freeing a body part from an abnormal physical constraint by cutting or by the use of force.

EXPLANATION: None of the body part is taken out ...

Body Part – 4TH		Approach – 5TH	Device – 6TH	Qualifier – 7TH
1 Frontal Bone, Right	H Lacrimal Bone, Right	0 Open	Z No device	Z No qualifier
2 Frontal Bone, Left	J Lacrimal Bone, Left	3 Percutaneous		
3 Parietal Bone, Right	K Palatine Bone, Right	4 Percutaneous endoscopic		
4 Parietal Bone, Left	L Palatine Bone, Left			
5 Temporal Bone, Right	M Zygomatic Bone, Right			
6 Temporal Bone, Left	N Zygomatic Bone, Left			
7 Occipital Bone, Right	P Orbit, Right			
8 Occipital Bone, Left	Q Orbit, Left			
B Nasal Bone	R Maxilla, Right			
C Sphenoid Bone, Right	S Maxilla, Left			
D Sphenoid Bone, Left	T Mandible, Right			
F Ethmoid Bone, Right	V Mandible, Left			
G Ethmoid Bone, Left	X Hyoid Bone			

N – HEAD AND FACIAL BONES   0NP

DEVICE GROUP: Change, Insertion, Removal, Replacement, Revision, Supplement
Root Operations that always involve a device.

1ST - **0** Medical and Surgical
2ND - **N** Head and Facial Bones
3RD - **P REMOVAL**

EXAMPLE: Removal bone growth stimulator CMS Ex: Chest tube removal

REMOVAL: Taking out or off a device from a body part.

EXPLANATION: Removal device without reinsertion ...

Body Part – 4TH	Approach – 5TH	Device – 6TH	Qualifier – 7TH
0 Skull	0 Open	0 Drainage device 4 Internal fixation device 5 External fixation device 7 Autologous tissue substitute J Synthetic substitute K Nonautologous tissue substitute M Bone growth stimulator N Neurostimulator generator S Hearing device	Z No qualifier
0 Skull	3 Percutaneous 4 Percutaneous endoscopic	0 Drainage device 4 Internal fixation device 5 External fixation device 7 Autologous tissue substitute J Synthetic substitute K Nonautologous tissue substitute M Bone growth stimulator S Hearing device	Z No qualifier
0 Skull	X External	0 Drainage device 4 Internal fixation device 5 External fixation device M Bone growth stimulator S Hearing device	Z No qualifier
B Nasal Bone W Facial Bone	0 Open 3 Percutaneous 4 Percutaneous endoscopic	0 Drainage device 4 Internal fixation device 7 Autologous tissue substitute J Synthetic substitute K Nonautologous tissue substitute M Bone growth stimulator	Z No qualifier
B Nasal Bone W Facial Bone	X External	0 Drainage device 4 Internal fixation device M Bone growth stimulator	Z No qualifier

0NQ MEDICAL AND SURGICAL SECTION – 2016 ICD-10-PCS

OTHER REPAIRS GROUP: (Control), Repair
Root Operations that define other repairs.

1ST - 0 Medical and Surgical
2ND - N Head and Facial Bones
3RD - Q REPAIR

EXAMPLE: Orbital osteoplasty CMS Ex: Suture laceration

REPAIR: Restoring, to the extent possible, a body part to its normal anatomic structure and function.

EXPLANATION: Only when no other root operation applies …

Body Part – 4TH		Approach – 5TH	Device – 6TH	Qualifier – 7TH
0 Skull	H Lacrimal Bone, Right	0 Open	Z No device	Z No qualifier
1 Frontal Bone, Right	J Lacrimal Bone, Left	3 Percutaneous		
2 Frontal Bone, Left	K Palatine Bone, Right	4 Percutaneous endoscopic		
3 Parietal Bone, Right	L Palatine Bone, Left	X External		
4 Parietal Bone, Left	M Zygomatic Bone, Right			
5 Temporal Bone, Right	N Zygomatic Bone, Left			
6 Temporal Bone, Left	P Orbit, Right			
7 Occipital Bone, Right	Q Orbit, Left			
8 Occipital Bone, Left	R Maxilla, Right			
B Nasal Bone	S Maxilla, Left			
C Sphenoid Bone, Right	T Mandible, Right			
D Sphenoid Bone, Left	V Mandible, Left			
F Ethmoid Bone, Right	X Hyoid Bone			
G Ethmoid Bone, Left				

DEVICE GROUP: Change, Insertion, Removal, Replacement, Revision, Supplement
Root Operations that always involve a device.

1ST - 0 Medical and Surgical
2ND - N Head and Facial Bones
3RD - R REPLACEMENT

EXAMPLE: Hemi-cranioplasty defect repair CMS Ex: Total hip

REPLACEMENT: Putting in or on a biological or synthetic material that physically takes the place and/or function of all or a portion of a body part.

EXPLANATION: Includes taking out body part, or eradication…

Body Part – 4TH		Approach – 5TH	Device – 6TH	Qualifier – 7TH
0 Skull	H Lacrimal Bone, Right	0 Open	7 Autologous tissue substitute	Z No qualifier
1 Frontal Bone, Right	J Lacrimal Bone, Left	3 Percutaneous	J Synthetic substitute	
2 Frontal Bone, Left	K Palatine Bone, Right	4 Percutaneous endoscopic	K Nonautologous tissue substitute	
3 Parietal Bone, Right	L Palatine Bone, Left			
4 Parietal Bone, Left	M Zygomatic Bone, Right			
5 Temporal Bone, Right	N Zygomatic Bone, Left			
6 Temporal Bone, Left	P Orbit, Right			
7 Occipital Bone, Right	Q Orbit, Left			
8 Occipital Bone, Left	R Maxilla, Right			
B Nasal Bone	S Maxilla, Left			
C Sphenoid Bone, Right	T Mandible, Right			
D Sphenoid Bone, Left	V Mandible, Left			
F Ethmoid Bone, Right	X Hyoid Bone			
G Ethmoid Bone, Left				

N – HEAD AND FACIAL BONES   0 N S

MOVE GROUP: (Reattachment), **Reposition**, (Transfer), (Transplantation)
Root Operations that put in/put back or move some/all of a body part.

1ST - 0 Medical and Surgical
2ND - N Head and Facial Bones
3RD - S REPOSITION

EXAMPLE: Le Fort 1 maxillary osteotomy | **CMS Ex:** Fracture reduction

REPOSITION: Moving to its normal location, or other suitable location, all or a portion of a body part.

EXPLANATION: May or may not be cut to be moved ...

Body Part – 4TH		Approach – 5TH	Device – 6TH	Qualifier – 7TH
0 Skull R Maxilla, Right S Maxilla, Left T Mandible, Right V Mandible, Left		0 Open 3 Percutaneous 4 Percutaneous endoscopic	4 Internal fixation device 5 External fixation device Z No device	Z No qualifier
0 Skull R Maxilla, Right S Maxilla, Left T Mandible, Right V Mandible, Left		X External	Z No device	Z No qualifier
1 Frontal Bone, Right 2 Frontal Bone, Left 3 Parietal Bone, Right 4 Parietal Bone, Left 5 Temporal Bone, Right 6 Temporal Bone, Left 7 Occipital Bone, Right 8 Occipital Bone, Left B Nasal Bone C Sphenoid Bone, Right D Sphenoid Bone, Left	F Ethmoid Bone, Right G Ethmoid Bone, Left H Lacrimal Bone, Right J Lacrimal Bone, Left K Palatine Bone, Right L Palatine Bone, Left M Zygomatic Bone, Right N Zygomatic Bone, Left P Orbit, Right Q Orbit, Left X Hyoid Bone	0 Open 3 Percutaneous 4 Percutaneous endoscopic	4 Internal fixation device Z No device	Z No qualifier
1 Frontal Bone, Right 2 Frontal Bone, Left 3 Parietal Bone, Right 4 Parietal Bone, Left 5 Temporal Bone, Right 6 Temporal Bone, Left 7 Occipital Bone, Right 8 Occipital Bone, Left B Nasal Bone C Sphenoid Bone, Right D Sphenoid Bone, Left	F Ethmoid Bone, Right G Ethmoid Bone, Left H Lacrimal Bone, Right J Lacrimal Bone, Left K Palatine Bone, Right L Palatine Bone, Left M Zygomatic Bone, Right N Zygomatic Bone, Left P Orbit, Right Q Orbit, Left X Hyoid Bone	X External	Z No device	Z No qualifier

0NT

MEDICAL AND SURGICAL SECTION – 2016 ICD-10-PCS [2016.PCS]

EXCISION GROUP: Excision, Resection, Destruction, (Extraction), (Detachment)
Root Operations that take out some or all of a body part.

- 1ST – **0** Medical and Surgical
- 2ND – **N** Head and Facial Bones
- 3RD – **T RESECTION**

EXAMPLE: Total removal hyoid bone CMS Ex: Cholecystectomy

RESECTION: Cutting out or off, without replacement, all of a body part.

EXPLANATION: None

Body Part – 4TH		Approach – 5TH	Device – 6TH	Qualifier – 7TH
1 Frontal Bone, Right	H Lacrimal Bone, Right	0 Open	Z No device	Z No qualifier
2 Frontal Bone, Left	J Lacrimal Bone, Left			
3 Parietal Bone, Right	K Palatine Bone, Right			
4 Parietal Bone, Left	L Palatine Bone, Left			
5 Temporal Bone, Right	M Zygomatic Bone, Right			
6 Temporal Bone, Left	N Zygomatic Bone, Left			
7 Occipital Bone, Right	P Orbit, Right			
8 Occipital Bone, Left	Q Orbit, Left			
B Nasal Bone	R Maxilla, Right			
C Sphenoid Bone, Right	S Maxilla, Left			
D Sphenoid Bone, Left	T Mandible, Right			
F Ethmoid Bone, Right	V Mandible, Left			
G Ethmoid Bone, Left	X Hyoid Bone			

DEVICE GROUP: Change, Insertion, Removal, Replacement, Revision, Supplement
Root Operations that always involve a device.

- 1ST – **0** Medical and Surgical
- 2ND – **N** Head and Facial Bones
- 3RD – **U SUPPLEMENT**

EXAMPLE: Stabilizing plate for defect CMS Ex: Hernia repair with mesh

SUPPLEMENT: Putting in or on biological or synthetic material that physically reinforces and/or augments the function of a portion of a body part.

EXPLANATION: Biological material from same individual ...

Body Part – 4TH		Approach – 5TH	Device – 6TH	Qualifier – 7TH
0 Skull	H Lacrimal Bone, Right	0 Open	7 Autologous tissue substitute	Z No qualifier
1 Frontal Bone, Right	J Lacrimal Bone, Left	3 Percutaneous	J Synthetic substitute	
2 Frontal Bone, Left	K Palatine Bone, Right	4 Percutaneous endoscopic	K Nonautologous tissue substitute	
3 Parietal Bone, Right	L Palatine Bone, Left			
4 Parietal Bone, Left	M Zygomatic Bone, Right			
5 Temporal Bone, Right	N Zygomatic Bone, Left			
6 Temporal Bone, Left	P Orbit, Right			
7 Occipital Bone, Right	Q Orbit, Left			
8 Occipital Bone, Left	R Maxilla, Right			
B Nasal Bone	S Maxilla, Left			
C Sphenoid Bone, Right	T Mandible, Right			
D Sphenoid Bone, Left	V Mandible, Left			
F Ethmoid Bone, Right	X Hyoid Bone			
G Ethmoid Bone, Left				

Head & Facial Bones 0NU

N – HEAD AND FACIAL BONES   0 N W

DEVICE GROUP: Change, Insertion, Removal, Replacement, Revision, Supplement
Root Operations that always involve a device.

1ST - **0** Medical and Surgical
2ND - **N** Head and Facial Bones
3RD - **W REVISION**

EXAMPLE: Reposition bone stimulator | CMS Ex: Adjustment pacemaker lead

REVISION: Correcting, to the extent possible, a portion of a malfunctioning device or the position of a displaced device.

EXPLANATION: May replace components of a device ...

Body Part – 4TH	Approach – 5TH	Device – 6TH	Qualifier – 7TH
0 Skull	0 Open	0 Drainage device 4 Internal fixation device 5 External fixation device 7 Autologous tissue substitute J Synthetic substitute K Nonautologous tissue substitute M Bone growth stimulator N Neurostimulator generator S Hearing device	Z No qualifier
0 Skull	3 Percutaneous 4 Percutaneous endoscopic X External	0 Drainage device 4 Internal fixation device 5 External fixation device 7 Autologous tissue substitute J Synthetic substitute K Nonautologous tissue substitute M Bone growth stimulator S Hearing device	Z No qualifier
B Nasal Bone W Facial Bone	0 Open 3 Percutaneous 4 Percutaneous endoscopic X External	0 Drainage device 4 Internal fixation device 7 Autologous tissue substitute J Synthetic substitute K Nonautologous tissue substitute M Bone growth stimulator	Z No qualifier

0N MEDICAL AND SURGICAL SECTION – 2016 ICD-10-PCS

NOTES

Educational Annotations | P – Upper Bones

Body System Specific Educational Annotations for the Upper Bones include:
- Anatomy and Physiology Review
- Anatomical Illustrations
- Definitions of Common Procedures
- AHA Coding Clinic® Reference Notations
- Body Part Key Listings
- Device Key Listings
- Device Aggregation Table Listings
- Coding Notes

Anatomy and Physiology Review of Upper Bones

BODY PART VALUES – P - UPPER BONES

Carpal – The 8 compact bones of the wrist, forming 2 rows of 4 bones each. The proximal row contains the scaphoid, lunate, pisiform, and triquetrum. The distal row contains the trapezium, trapezoid, capitate, and hamate.

Cervical Vertebra – The cervical section of the spinal vertebral column comprised of 7 vertebra, C1-C7.

Clavicle – The paired, straightened S-shaped bones (also known as the collarbones) that connect the sternum with the scapula.

Finger Phalanx – The digital bones of the fingers. Each finger contains three bones: Proximal phalanx, intermediate (middle) phalanx, and distal phalanx.

Glenoid Cavity – The shallow, round depression of the scapula that articulates with the humeral head.

Humeral Head – The upper end of the humerus that is part of the shoulder joint.

Humeral Shaft – The middle, long portion of the humerus.

Humerus – The paired, long bones of the upper arm that articulate at the shoulder and the elbow. The capitulum of the humerus articulates with the head of the radius, and the trochlea of the humerus articulates with the trochlear notch of the ulna.

Metacarpal – One of the 5 cylindrical bones of the palm of the hand connecting the carpals to the phalanges of the hand.

Radius – The paired long bones of the forearms that are further away from the body than the ulnas.

Rib – The 12 paired arched bones of the rib cage that partially enclose and protect the chest cavity.

Scapula – The paired flat, triangular bones located in the upper back behind the shoulder (also called the shoulder blade).

Sternum – The long flat bone (also known as the breast bone) of the chest that connects to the clavicles and most of the ribs.

Thoracic Vertebra – The thoracic section of the spinal vertebral column comprised of 12 vertebra, T1-T12.

Thumb Phalanx – The digital bones of the thumb. The thumb contains two bones: Proximal phalanx and distal phalanx.

Ulna – The paired long bones of the forearms that are closer to the side of the body than the radii.

Upper Bone – Any of the bones designated in the Upper Bones PCS Body System.

Educational Annotations | P – Upper Bones

Anatomical Illustrations of Upper Bones

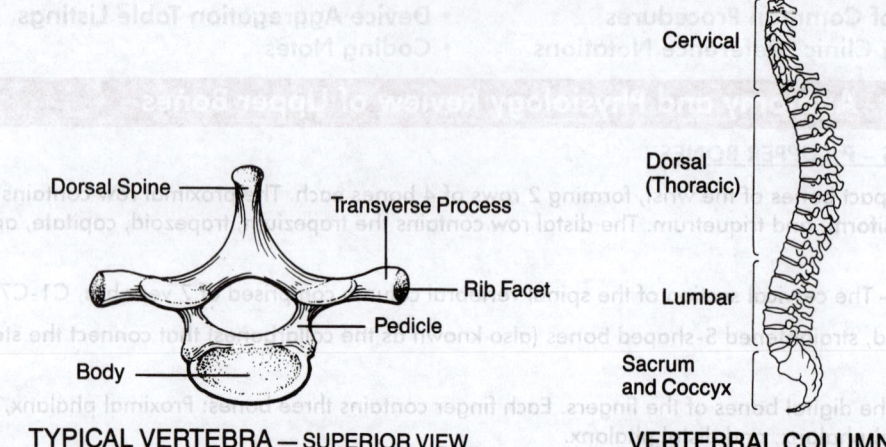

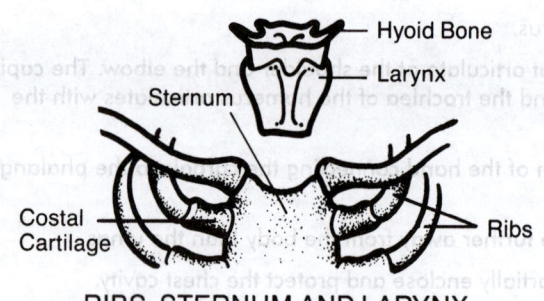

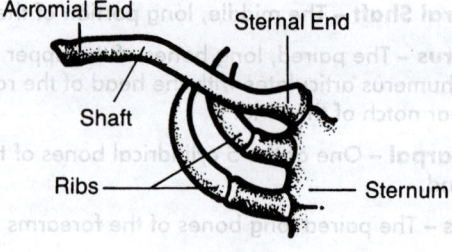

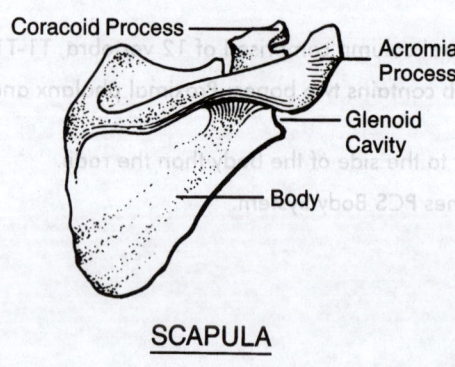

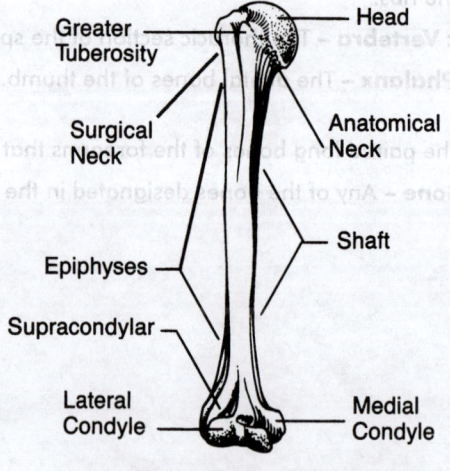

Continued on next page

Educational Annotations | P – Upper Bones

Anatomical Illustrations of Upper Bones

Continued from previous page

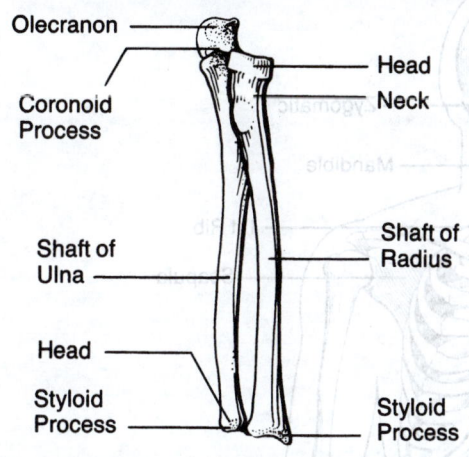
RADIUS AND ULNA — ANTERIOR VIEW

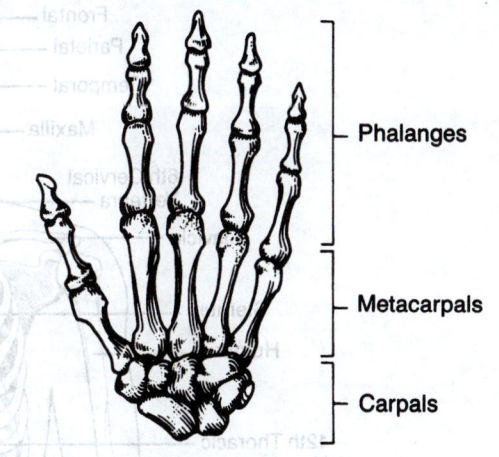
RIGHT HAND — DORSAL VIEW

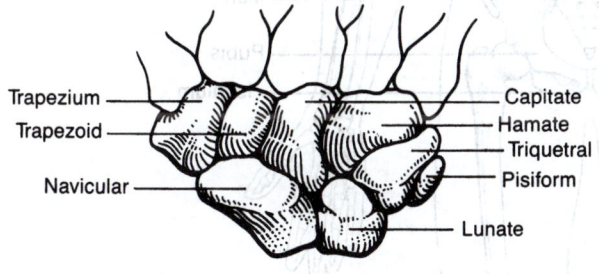
CARPAL BONES — DORSAL VIEW

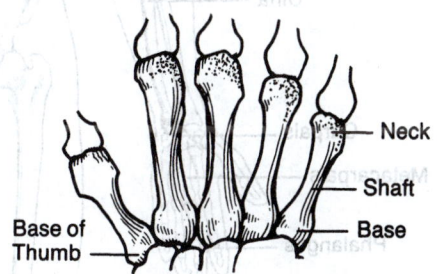
METACARPAL BONES

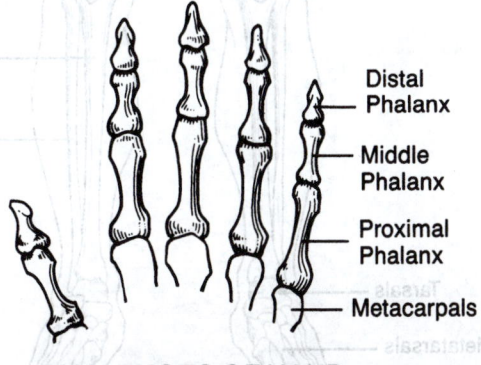
PHALANGES OF HAND

Continued on next page

Educational Annotations

P – Upper Bones

Anatomical Illustrations of Upper Bones

Continued from previous page

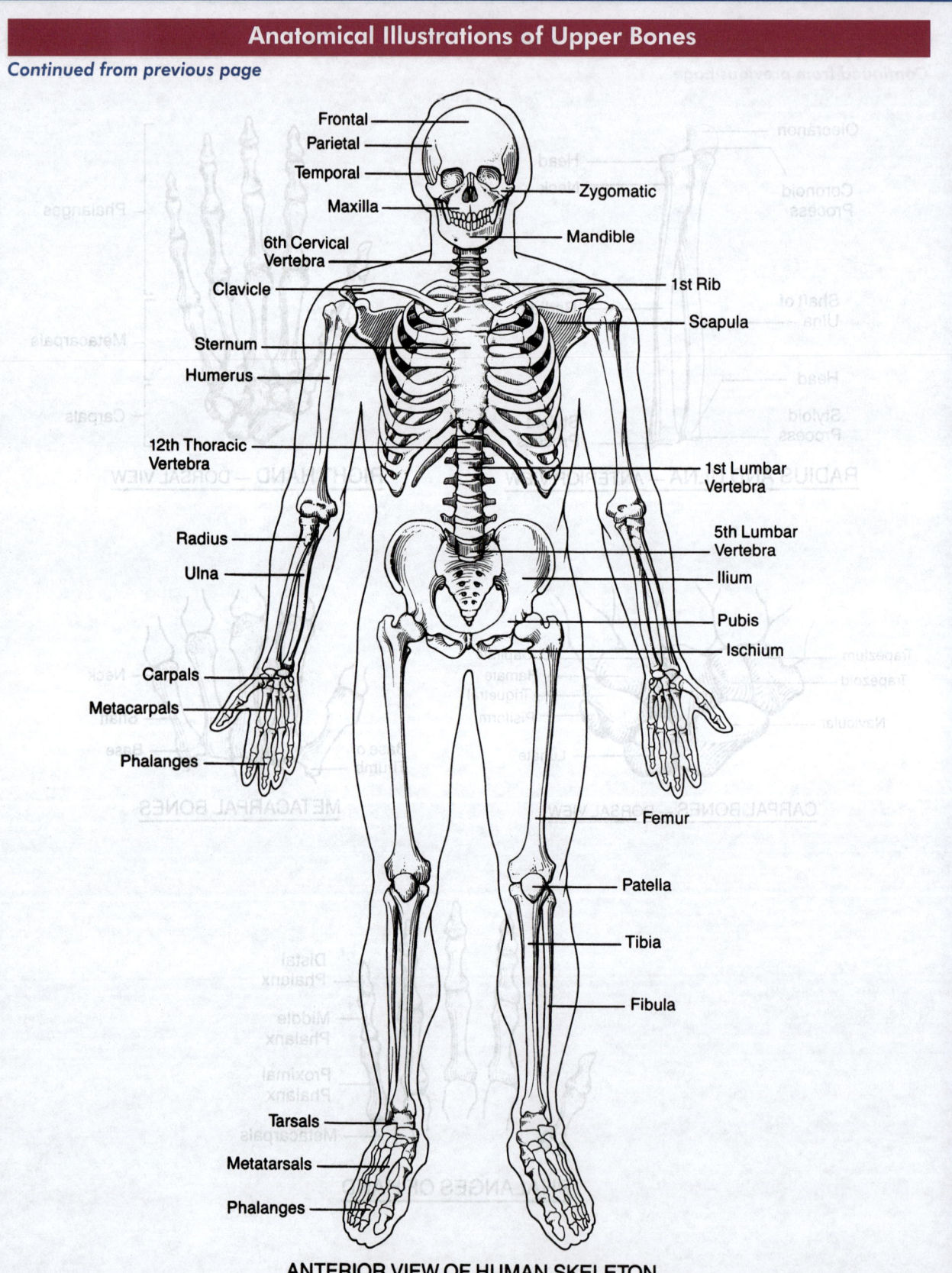

ANTERIOR VIEW OF HUMAN SKELETON

Continued on next page

Educational Annotations | P – Upper Bones

Anatomical Illustrations of Upper Bones

Continued from previous page

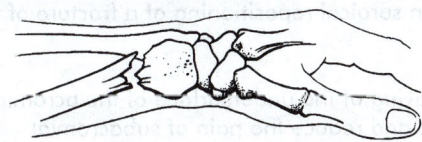
COLLES'

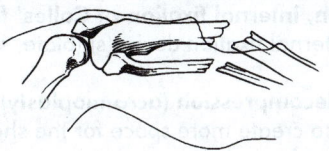
COMPOUND

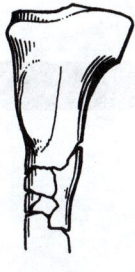
COMMINUTED

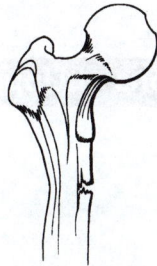
GREENSTICK

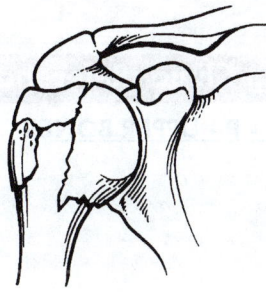
IMPACTED

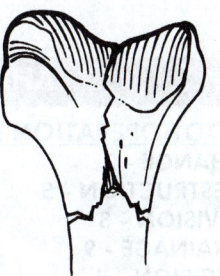
INTERCONDYLAR

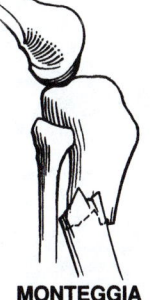
MONTEGGIA

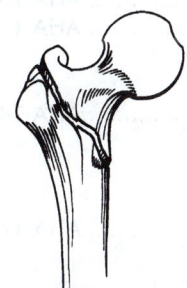
PERTROCHANTERIC

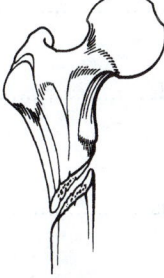
SPIRAL

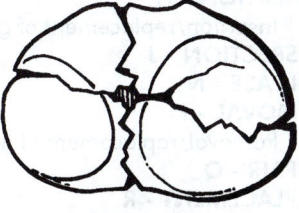
STELLATE

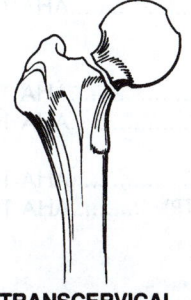
TRANSCERVICAL

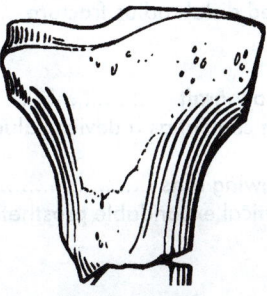
TRANSVERSE

FRACTURE TYPES

Educational Annotations | P – Upper Bones

Definitions of Common Procedures of Upper Bones

Laminectomy – The surgical excision of the lamina of a vertebra, usually to relieve spinal cord compression.

Open reduction, internal fixation of Colles' fracture – The open surgical repositioning of a fracture of the distal radius using internal fixation device(s) (plate, screws, pins).

Subacromial decompression (acromioplasty) – The surgical shaving of the undersurface of the acromial process of the scapula to create more space for the shoulder's soft tissue and reduce the pain of subacromial impingement syndrome.

Total claviculectomy – The surgical removal of the entire clavicle bone.

Vertebroplasty – The surgical injection of bone cement into a fractured vertebra.

AHA Coding Clinic® Reference Notations of Upper Bones

ROOT OPERATION SPECIFIC - P - UPPER BONES
CHANGE - 2
DESTRUCTION - 5
DIVISION - 8
DRAINAGE - 9
EXCISION - B
    Harvesting of local bone for graft ....AHA 15:1Q:p30
    Resection of rib segment ....AHA 12:4Q:p101
    Spinal decompression meaning laminectomy ....AHA 13:4Q:p116
        Official Clarification of 13:4Q:p116 ....AHA 15:2Q:p34
    Subacromial decompression..AHA 13:3Q:p20
EXTIRPATION - C
INSERTION - H
    Insertion/replacement of growing rods ....AHA 14:4Q:p28
INSPECTION - J
RELEASE - N
REMOVAL - P
    Removal/replacement of growing rods ....AHA 14:4Q:p28
REPAIR - Q
REPLACEMENT - R
REPOSITION - S
    Open reduction internal fixation (ORIF) of forearm bones ....AHA 14:4Q:p32
    Placement of vertical expandable prosthetic titanium rib (VEPTR).............AHA 14:4Q:p26
    Reposition of cervical vertebra fracture ....AHA 15:2Q:p34
    Reposition of healed distal radius fracture ....AHA 14:3Q:p33
RESECTION - T
SUPPLEMENT - U
    Laminoplasty with allograft ....AHA 15:2Q:p20
    Vertebroplasty with cement as a device value ....AHA 14:2Q:p12
REVISION - W
    Lengthening of growing rods ....AHA 14:4Q:p27
    Lengthening of vertical expandable prosthetic titanium rib (VEPTR) ....AHA 14:4Q:p26

Educational Annotations

P – Upper Bones

Body Part Key Listings of Upper Bones

See also Body Part Key in Appendix C

Acromion (process)	*use* Scapula, Left/Right
Capitate bone	*use* Carpal, Left/Right
Coracoid process	*use* Scapula, Left/Right
Distal humerus	*use* Humeral Shaft, Left/Right
Glenoid fossa (of scapula)	*use* Glenoid Cavity, Left/Right
Greater tuberosity	*use* Humeral Head, Left/Right
Hamate bone	*use* Carpal, Left/Right
Humerus, distal	*use* Humeral Shaft, Left/Right
Lateral epicondyle of humerus	*use* Humeral Shaft, Left/Right
Lesser tuberosity	*use* Humeral Head, Left/Right
Lunate bone	*use* Carpal, Left/Right
Manubrium	*use* Sternum
Medial epicondyle of humerus	*use* Humeral Shaft, Left/Right
Neck of humerus (anatomical) (surgical)	*use* Humeral Head, Left/Right
Olecranon process	*use* Ulna, Left/Right
Pisiform bone	*use* Carpal, Left/Right
Radial notch	*use* Ulna, Left/Right
Scaphoid bone	*use* Carpal, Left/Right
Spinous process	*use* Cervical, Thoracic, Lumbar Vertebra
Suprasternal notch	*use* Sternum
Trapezium bone	*use* Carpal, Left/Right
Trapezoid bone	*use* Carpal, Left/Right
Triquetral bone	*use* Carpal, Left/Right
Ulnar notch	*use* Radius, Left/Right
Vertebral arch	*use* Cervical, Thoracic, Lumbar Vertebra
Vertebral foramen	*use* Cervical, Thoracic, Lumbar Vertebra
Vertebral lamina	*use* Cervical, Thoracic, Lumbar Vertebra
Vertebral pedicle	*use* Cervical, Thoracic, Lumbar Vertebra
Xiphoid process	*use* Sternum

Device Key Listings of Upper Bones

See also Device Key in Appendix D

Autograft	*use* Autologous Tissue Substitute
Bone bank bone graft	*use* Nonautologous Tissue Substitute
Bone screw (interlocking) (lag) (pedicle) (recessed)	*use* Internal Fixation Device in Head and Facial Bones, Upper Bones, Lower Bones
Clamp and rod internal fixation system (CRIF)	*use* Internal Fixation Device in Upper Bones, Lower Bones
Delta frame external fixator	*use* External Fixation Device, Hybrid for Insertion in Upper Bones, Lower Bones
	use External Fixation Device, Hybrid for Reposition in Upper Bones, Lower Bones
Electrical bone growth stimulator (EBGS)	*use* Bone Growth Stimulator in Head and Facial Bones, Upper Bones, Lower Bones
External fixator	*use* External Fixation Device in Head and Facial Bones, Upper Bones, Lower Bones, Upper Joints, Lower Joints

Continued on next page

Educational Annotations

P – Upper Bones

Device Key Listings of Upper Bones

Continued from previous page

Ilizarov external fixator	*use* External Fixation Device, Ring for Insertion in Upper Bones, Lower Bones
	use External Fixation Device, Ring for Reposition in Upper Bones, Lower Bones
Ilizarov-Vecklich device	*use* External Fixation Device, Limb Lengthening for Insertion in Upper Bones, Lower Bones
Intramedullary (IM) rod (nail)	*use* Internal Fixation Device, Intramedullary in Upper Bones, Lower Bones
Intramedullary skeletal kinetic distractor (ISKD)	*use* Internal Fixation Device, Intramedullary in Upper Bones, Lower Bones
Kirschner wire (K-wire)	*use* Internal Fixation Device in Head and Facial Bones, Upper Bones, Lower Bones, Upper Joints, Lower Joints
Kuntscher nail	*use* Internal Fixation Device, Intramedullary in Upper Bones, Lower Bones
Neutralization plate	*use* Internal Fixation Device in Head and Facial Bones, Upper Bones, Lower Bones
Polymethylmethacrylate (PMMA)	*use* Synthetic Substitute
Sheffield hybrid external fixator	*use* External Fixation Device, Hybrid for Insertion in Upper Bones, Lower Bones
	use External Fixation Device, Hybrid for Reposition in Upper Bones, Lower Bones
Sheffield ring external fixator	*use* External Fixation Device, Ring for Insertion in Upper Bones, Lower Bones
	use External Fixation Device, Ring for Reposition in Upper Bones, Lower Bones
Tissue bank graft	*use* Nonautologous Tissue Substitute
Titanium Sternal Fixation System (TSFS)	*use* Internal Fixation Device, Rigid Plate for Insertion in Upper Bones
	use Internal Fixation Device, Rigid Plate for Reposition in Upper Bones
Ultrasonic osteogenic stimulator	*use* Bone Growth Stimulator in Head and Facial Bones, Upper Bones, Lower Bones
Ultrasound bone healing system	*use* Bone Growth Stimulator in Head and Facial Bones, Upper Bones, Lower Bones
Uniplanar external fixator	*use* External Fixation Device, Monoplanar for Insertion in Upper Bones, Lower Bones
	use External Fixation Device, Monoplanar for Reposition in Upper Bones, Lower Bones

Educational Annotations | P – Upper Bones

Device Aggregation Table Listings of Upper Bones

See also Device Aggregation Table in Appendix E

Specific Device	For Operation	In Body System		General Device
External Fixation Device, Hybrid	Insertion	Upper Bones	5	External Fixation Device
External Fixation Device, Hybrid	Reposition	Upper Bones	5	External Fixation Device
External Fixation Device, Limb Lengthening	Insertion	Upper Bones	5	External Fixation Device
External Fixation Device, Monoplanar	Insertion	Upper Bones	5	External Fixation Device
External Fixation Device, Monoplanar	Reposition	Upper Bones	5	External Fixation Device
External Fixation Device, Ring	Insertion	Upper Bones	5	External Fixation Device
External Fixation Device, Ring	Reposition	Upper Bones	5	External Fixation Device
Internal Fixation Device, Intramedullary	All applicable	Upper Bones	4	Internal Fixation Device
Internal Fixation Device, Rigid Plate	Insertion	Upper Bones	4	Internal Fixation Device
Internal Fixation Device, Rigid Plate	Reposition	Upper Bones	4	Internal Fixation Device

Coding Notes of Upper Bones

Body System Relevant Coding Guidelines

Reposition for fracture treatment
B3.15
   Reduction of a displaced fracture is coded to the root operation Reposition and the application of a cast or splint in conjunction with the Reposition procedure is not coded separately. Treatment of a nondisplaced fracture is coded to the procedure performed.
   Examples: Putting a pin in a nondisplaced fracture is coded to the root operation Insertion.
   Casting of a nondisplaced fracture is coded to the root operation Immobilization in the Placement section.

Body System Specific PCS Reference Manual Exercises

PCS CODE	P – UPPER BONES EXERCISES
0P8N0ZZ	Open osteotomy of capitate, left hand. (The capitate is one of the carpal bones of the hand.)
0PPJX5Z	Removal of external fixator, left radial fracture.

Educational Annotations

P – Upper Bones

NOTES

P – UPPER BONES 0P5

DEVICE GROUP: Change, Insertion, Removal, Replacement, Revision, Supplement
Root Operations that always involve a device.

- 1ST – **0** Medical and Surgical
- 2ND – **P** Upper Bones
- 3RD – **2 CHANGE**

EXAMPLE: Exchange drain tube
CMS Ex: Changing urinary catheter

CHANGE: Taking out or off a device from a body part and putting back an identical or similar device in or on the same body part without cutting or puncturing the skin or a mucous membrane.

EXPLANATION: ALL Changes use EXTERNAL approach only ...

Body Part – 4TH	Approach – 5TH	Device – 6TH	Qualifier – 7TH
Y Upper Bone	X External	0 Drainage device Y Other device	Z No qualifier

EXCISION GROUP: Excision, Resection, Destruction, (Extraction), (Detachment)
Root Operations that take out some or all of a body part.

- 1ST – **0** Medical and Surgical
- 2ND – **P** Upper Bones
- 3RD – **5 DESTRUCTION**

EXAMPLE: Cryoablation bone cyst
CMS Ex: Fulguration polyp

DESTRUCTION: Physical eradication of all or a portion of a body part by the direct use of energy, force, or a destructive agent.

EXPLANATION: None of the body part is physically taken out

Body Part – 4TH		Approach – 5TH	Device – 6TH	Qualifier – 7TH
0 Sternum	H Radius, Right	0 Open	Z No device	Z No qualifier
1 Rib, Right	J Radius, Left	3 Percutaneous		
2 Rib, Left	K Ulna, Right	4 Percutaneous endoscopic		
3 Cervical Vertebra	L Ulna, Left			
4 Thoracic Vertebra	M Carpal, Right			
5 Scapula, Right	N Carpal, Left			
6 Scapula, Left	P Metacarpal, Right			
7 Glenoid Cavity, Right	Q Metacarpal, Left			
8 Glenoid Cavity, Left	R Thumb Phalanx, Right			
9 Clavicle, Right	S Thumb Phalanx, Left			
B Clavicle, Left	T Finger Phalanx, Right			
C Humeral Head, Right	V Finger Phalanx, Left			
D Humeral Head, Left				
F Humeral Shaft, Right				
G Humeral Shaft, Left				

0P8 — MEDICAL AND SURGICAL SECTION – 2016 ICD-10-PCS

DIVISION GROUP: Division, Release
Root Operations involving cutting or separation only.

- 1ST – **0** Medical and Surgical
- 2ND – **P** Upper Bones
- 3RD – **8** DIVISION

EXAMPLE: Carpal osteotomy CMS Ex: Osteotomy

DIVISION: Cutting into a body part without draining fluids and/or gases from the body part in order to separate or transect a body part.

EXPLANATION: Separated into two or more portions ...

Body Part – 4TH	Approach – 5TH	Device – 6TH	Qualifier – 7TH
0 Sternum	0 Open	Z No device	Z No qualifier
1 Rib, Right	3 Percutaneous		
2 Rib, Left	4 Percutaneous endoscopic		
3 Cervical Vertebra			
4 Thoracic Vertebra			
5 Scapula, Right			
6 Scapula, Left			
7 Glenoid Cavity, Right			
8 Glenoid Cavity, Left			
9 Clavicle, Right			
B Clavicle, Left			
C Humeral Head, Right			
D Humeral Head, Left			
F Humeral Shaft, Right			
G Humeral Shaft, Left			
H Radius, Right			
J Radius, Left			
K Ulna, Right			
L Ulna, Left			
M Carpal, Right			
N Carpal, Left			
P Metacarpal, Right			
Q Metacarpal, Left			
R Thumb Phalanx, Right			
S Thumb Phalanx, Left			
T Finger Phalanx, Right			
V Finger Phalanx, Left			

P – UPPER BONES

0P9

DRAINAGE GROUP: Drainage, Extirpation, (Fragmentation)
Root Operations that take out solids/fluids/gases from a body part.

- 1ST – **0** Medical and Surgical
- 2ND – **P** Upper Bones
- 3RD – **9 DRAINAGE**

EXAMPLE: Aspiration bone cyst

CMS Ex: Thoracentesis

DRAINAGE: Taking or letting out fluids and/or gases from a body part.

EXPLANATION: Qualifier "X Diagnostic" indicates biopsy ...

Body Part – 4TH		Approach – 5TH	Device – 6TH	Qualifier – 7TH
0 Sternum 1 Rib, Right 2 Rib, Left 3 Cervical Vertebra 4 Thoracic Vertebra 5 Scapula, Right 6 Scapula, Left 7 Glenoid Cavity, Right 8 Glenoid Cavity, Left 9 Clavicle, Right B Clavicle, Left C Humeral Head, Right D Humeral Head, Left F Humeral Shaft, Right G Humeral Shaft, Left	H Radius, Right J Radius, Left K Ulna, Right L Ulna, Left M Carpal, Right N Carpal, Left P Metacarpal, Right Q Metacarpal, Left R Thumb Phalanx, Right S Thumb Phalanx, Left T Finger Phalanx, Right V Finger Phalanx, Left	0 Open 3 Percutaneous 4 Percutaneous endoscopic	0 Drainage device	Z No qualifier
0 Sternum 1 Rib, Right 2 Rib, Left 3 Cervical Vertebra 4 Thoracic Vertebra 5 Scapula, Right 6 Scapula, Left 7 Glenoid Cavity, Right 8 Glenoid Cavity, Left 9 Clavicle, Right B Clavicle, Left C Humeral Head, Right D Humeral Head, Left F Humeral Shaft, Right G Humeral Shaft, Left	H Radius, Right J Radius, Left K Ulna, Right L Ulna, Left M Carpal, Right N Carpal, Left P Metacarpal, Right Q Metacarpal, Left R Thumb Phalanx, Right S Thumb Phalanx, Left T Finger Phalanx, Right V Finger Phalanx, Left	0 Open 3 Percutaneous 4 Percutaneous endoscopic	Z No device	X Diagnostic Z No qualifier

0PB

MEDICAL AND SURGICAL SECTION – 2016 ICD-10-PCS

EXCISION GROUP: Excision, Resection, Destruction, (Extraction), (Detachment)
Root Operations that take out some or all of a body part.

- 1ST – **0** Medical and Surgical
- 2ND – **P** Upper Bones
- 3RD – **B** EXCISION

EXAMPLE: Vertebral laminectomy   CMS Ex: Liver biopsy

EXCISION: Cutting out or off, without replacement, a portion of a body part.

EXPLANATION: Qualifier "X Diagnostic" indicates biopsy …

Body Part – 4TH		Approach – 5TH	Device – 6TH	Qualifier – 7TH
0 Sternum	H Radius, Right	0 Open	Z No device	X Diagnostic
1 Rib, Right	J Radius, Left	3 Percutaneous		Z No qualifier
2 Rib, Left	K Ulna, Right	4 Percutaneous endoscopic		
3 Cervical Vertebra	L Ulna, Left			
4 Thoracic Vertebra	M Carpal, Right			
5 Scapula, Right	N Carpal, Left			
6 Scapula, Left	P Metacarpal, Right			
7 Glenoid Cavity, Right	Q Metacarpal, Left			
8 Glenoid Cavity, Left	R Thumb Phalanx, Right			
9 Clavicle, Right	S Thumb Phalanx, Left			
B Clavicle, Left	T Finger Phalanx, Right			
C Humeral Head, Right	V Finger Phalanx, Left			
D Humeral Head, Left				
F Humeral Shaft, Right				
G Humeral Shaft, Left				

DRAINAGE GROUP: Drainage, Extirpation, (Fragmentation)
Root Operations that take out solids/fluids/gases from a body part.

- 1ST – **0** Medical and Surgical
- 2ND – **P** Upper Bones
- 3RD – **C** EXTIRPATION

EXAMPLE: Removal foreign body   CMS Ex: Choledocholithotomy

EXTIRPATION: Taking or cutting out solid matter from a body part.

EXPLANATION: Abnormal byproduct or foreign body …

Body Part – 4TH		Approach – 5TH	Device – 6TH	Qualifier – 7TH
0 Sternum	H Radius, Right	0 Open	Z No device	Z No qualifier
1 Rib, Right	J Radius, Left	3 Percutaneous		
2 Rib, Left	K Ulna, Right	4 Percutaneous endoscopic		
3 Cervical Vertebra	L Ulna, Left			
4 Thoracic Vertebra	M Carpal, Right			
5 Scapula, Right	N Carpal, Left			
6 Scapula, Left	P Metacarpal, Right			
7 Glenoid Cavity, Right	Q Metacarpal, Left			
8 Glenoid Cavity, Left	R Thumb Phalanx, Right			
9 Clavicle, Right	S Thumb Phalanx, Left			
B Clavicle, Left	T Finger Phalanx, Right			
C Humeral Head, Right	V Finger Phalanx, Left			
D Humeral Head, Left				
F Humeral Shaft, Right				
G Humeral Shaft, Left				

0PH

P – UPPER BONES

DEVICE GROUP: Change, Insertion, Removal, Replacement, Revision, Supplement
Root Operations that always involve a device.

- 1ST – **0** Medical and Surgical
- 2ND – **P** Upper Bones
- 3RD – **H** INSERTION

EXAMPLE: Insertion external fixation pin | **CMS Ex:** Central venous catheter

INSERTION: Putting in a nonbiological appliance that monitors, assists, performs, or prevents a physiological function but does not physically take the place of a body part.
EXPLANATION: None

Body Part – 4TH		Approach – 5TH	Device – 6TH	Qualifier – 7TH
0 Sternum		0 Open 3 Percutaneous 4 Percutaneous endoscopic	0 Internal fixation device, rigid plate 4 Internal fixation device	Z No qualifier
1 Rib, Right 2 Rib, Left 3 Cervical Vertebra 4 Thoracic Vertebra 5 Scapula, Right 6 Scapula, Left	7 Glenoid Cavity, Right 8 Glenoid Cavity, Left 9 Clavicle, Right B Clavicle, Left	0 Open 3 Percutaneous 4 Percutaneous endoscopic	4 Internal fixation device	Z No qualifier
C Humeral Head, Right D Humeral Head, Left F Humeral Shaft, Right G Humeral Shaft, Left	H Radius, Right J Radius, Left K Ulna, Right L Ulna, Left	0 Open 3 Percutaneous 4 Percutaneous endoscopic	4 Internal fixation device 5 External fixation device 6 Internal fixation device, intramedullary 8 External fixation device, limb lengthening B External fixation device, monoplanar C External fixation device, ring D External fixation device, hybrid	Z No qualifier
M Carpal, Right N Carpal, Left P Metacarpal, Right Q Metacarpal, Left	R Thumb Phalanx, Right S Thumb Phalanx, Left T Finger Phalanx, Right V Finger Phalanx, Left	0 Open 3 Percutaneous 4 Percutaneous endoscopic	4 Internal fixation device 5 External fixation device	Z No qualifier
Y Upper Bone		0 Open 3 Percutaneous 4 Percutaneous endoscopic	M Bone growth stimulator	Z No qualifier

0PJ — MEDICAL AND SURGICAL SECTION – 2016 ICD-10-PCS

EXAMINATION GROUP: Inspection, (Map)
Root Operations involving examination only.

- 1ST – **0** Medical and Surgical
- 2ND – **P** Upper Bones
- 3RD – **J** INSPECTION

EXAMPLE: Examination bone
CMS Ex: Colonoscopy

INSPECTION: Visually and/or manually exploring a body part.

EXPLANATION: Direct or instrumental visualization …

Body Part – 4TH	Approach – 5TH	Device – 6TH	Qualifier – 7TH
Y Upper Bone	0 Open 3 Percutaneous 4 Percutaneous endoscopic X External	Z No device	Z No qualifier

DIVISION GROUP: Division, Release
Root Operations involving cutting or separation only.

- 1ST – **0** Medical and Surgical
- 2ND – **P** Upper Bones
- 3RD – **N** RELEASE

EXAMPLE: Extra-articular bone adhesiolysis
CMS Ex: Carpal tunnel release

RELEASE: Freeing a body part from an abnormal physical constraint by cutting or by the use of force.

EXPLANATION: None of the body part is taken out …

Body Part – 4TH		Approach – 5TH	Device – 6TH	Qualifier – 7TH
0 Sternum	H Radius, Right	0 Open	Z No device	Z No qualifier
1 Rib, Right	J Radius, Left	3 Percutaneous		
2 Rib, Left	K Ulna, Right	4 Percutaneous endoscopic		
3 Cervical Vertebra	L Ulna, Left			
4 Thoracic Vertebra	M Carpal, Right			
5 Scapula, Right	N Carpal, Left			
6 Scapula, Left	P Metacarpal, Right			
7 Glenoid Cavity, Right	Q Metacarpal, Left			
8 Glenoid Cavity, Left	R Thumb Phalanx, Right			
9 Clavicle, Right	S Thumb Phalanx, Left			
B Clavicle, Left	T Finger Phalanx, Right			
C Humeral Head, Right	V Finger Phalanx, Left			
D Humeral Head, Left				
F Humeral Shaft, Right				
G Humeral Shaft, Left				

P – UPPER BONES

0PP

DEVICE GROUP: Change, Insertion, Removal, Replacement, Revision, Supplement
Root Operations that always involve a device.

- 1ST – **0** Medical and Surgical
- 2ND – **P** Upper Bones
- 3RD – **P** REMOVAL

EXAMPLE: Removal external fixation pin CMS Ex: Chest tube removal

REMOVAL: Taking out or off a device from a body part.

EXPLANATION: Removal device without reinsertion ...

Body Part – 4TH		Approach – 5TH	Device – 6TH	Qualifier – 7TH
0 Sternum 1 Rib, Right 2 Rib, Left 3 Cervical Vertebra 4 Thoracic Vertebra 5 Scapula, Right 6 Scapula, Left	7 Glenoid Cavity, Right 8 Glenoid Cavity, Left 9 Clavicle, Right B Clavicle, Left	0 Open 3 Percutaneous 4 Percutaneous endoscopic	4 Internal fixation device 7 Autologous tissue substitute J Synthetic substitute K Nonautologous tissue substitute	Z No qualifier
0 Sternum 1 Rib, Right 2 Rib, Left 3 Cervical Vertebra 4 Thoracic Vertebra 5 Scapula, Right 6 Scapula, Left	7 Glenoid Cavity, Right 8 Glenoid Cavity, Left 9 Clavicle, Right B Clavicle, Left	X External	4 Internal fixation device	Z No qualifier
C Humeral Head, Right D Humeral Head, Left F Humeral Shaft, Right G Humeral Shaft, Left H Radius, Right J Radius, Left K Ulna, Right L Ulna, Left	M Carpal, Right N Carpal, Left P Metacarpal, Right Q Metacarpal, Left R Thumb Phalanx, Right S Thumb Phalanx, Left T Finger Phalanx, Right V Finger Phalanx, Left	0 Open 3 Percutaneous 4 Percutaneous endoscopic	4 Internal fixation device 5 External fixation device 7 Autologous tissue substitute J Synthetic substitute K Nonautologous tissue substitute	Z No qualifier
C Humeral Head, Right D Humeral Head, Left F Humeral Shaft, Right G Humeral Shaft, Left H Radius, Right J Radius, Left K Ulna, Right L Ulna, Left	M Carpal, Right N Carpal, Left P Metacarpal, Right Q Metacarpal, Left R Thumb Phalanx, Right S Thumb Phalanx, Left T Finger Phalanx, Right V Finger Phalanx, Left	X External	4 Internal fixation device 5 External fixation device	Z No qualifier
Y Upper Bone		0 Open 3 Percutaneous 4 Percutaneous endoscopic X External	0 Drainage device M Bone growth stimulator	Z No qualifier

0PQ MEDICAL AND SURGICAL SECTION – 2016 ICD-10-PCS

OTHER REPAIRS GROUP: (Control), Repair
Root Operations that define other repairs.

- 1ST – **0** Medical and Surgical
- 2ND – **P** Upper Bones
- 3RD – **Q REPAIR**

EXAMPLE: Vertebral laminoplasty CMS Ex: Suture laceration

REPAIR: Restoring, to the extent possible, a body part to its normal anatomic structure and function.

EXPLANATION: Only when no other root operation applies …

Body Part – 4TH		Approach – 5TH	Device – 6TH	Qualifier – 7TH
0 Sternum	H Radius, Right	0 Open	Z No device	Z No qualifier
1 Rib, Right	J Radius, Left	3 Percutaneous		
2 Rib, Left	K Ulna, Right	4 Percutaneous endoscopic		
3 Cervical Vertebra	L Ulna, Left	X External		
4 Thoracic Vertebra	M Carpal, Right			
5 Scapula, Right	N Carpal, Left			
6 Scapula, Left	P Metacarpal, Right			
7 Glenoid Cavity, Right	Q Metacarpal, Left			
8 Glenoid Cavity, Left	R Thumb Phalanx, Right			
9 Clavicle, Right	S Thumb Phalanx, Left			
B Clavicle, Left	T Finger Phalanx, Right			
C Humeral Head, Right	V Finger Phalanx, Left			
D Humeral Head, Left				
F Humeral Shaft, Right				
G Humeral Shaft, Left				

DEVICE GROUP: Change, Insertion, Removal, Replacement, Revision, Supplement
Root Operations that always involve a device.

- 1ST – **0** Medical and Surgical
- 2ND – **P** Upper Bones
- 3RD – **R REPLACEMENT**

EXAMPLE: Humeral head replacement CMS Ex: Total hip

REPLACEMENT: Putting in or on a biological or synthetic material that physically takes the place and/or function of all or a portion of a body part.

EXPLANATION: Includes taking out body part, or eradication…

Body Part – 4TH		Approach – 5TH	Device – 6TH	Qualifier – 7TH
0 Sternum	H Radius, Right	0 Open	7 Autologous tissue substitute	Z No qualifier
1 Rib, Right	J Radius, Left	3 Percutaneous	J Synthetic substitute	
2 Rib, Left	K Ulna, Right	4 Percutaneous endoscopic	K Nonautologous tissue substitute	
3 Cervical Vertebra	L Ulna, Left			
4 Thoracic Vertebra	M Carpal, Right			
5 Scapula, Right	N Carpal, Left			
6 Scapula, Left	P Metacarpal, Right			
7 Glenoid Cavity, Right	Q Metacarpal, Left			
8 Glenoid Cavity, Left	R Thumb Phalanx, Right			
9 Clavicle, Right	S Thumb Phalanx, Left			
B Clavicle, Left	T Finger Phalanx, Right			
C Humeral Head, Right	V Finger Phalanx, Left			
D Humeral Head, Left				
F Humeral Shaft, Right				
G Humeral Shaft, Left				

0 P S

P – UPPER BONES

MOVE GROUP: (Reattachment), **Reposition**, (Transfer), (Transplantation)
Root Operations that put in/put back or move some/all of a body part.

- 1ST – **0** Medical and Surgical
- 2ND – **P** Upper Bones
- 3RD – **S** REPOSITION

EXAMPLE: ORIF Colles' fracture **CMS Ex:** Fracture reduction

REPOSITION: Moving to its normal location, or other suitable location, all or a portion of a body part.

EXPLANATION: May or may not be cut to be moved ...

Body Part – 4TH		Approach – 5TH	Device – 6TH	Qualifier – 7TH
0 Sternum		0 Open 3 Percutaneous 4 Percutaneous endoscopic	4 Internal fixation device, rigid plate 4 Internal fixation device Z No device	Z No qualifier
0 Sternum		X External	Z No device	Z No qualifier
1 Rib, Right 2 Rib, Left 3 Cervical Vertebra 4 Thoracic Vertebra 5 Scapula, Right	6 Scapula, Left 7 Glenoid Cavity, Right 8 Glenoid Cavity, Left 9 Clavicle, Right B Clavicle, Left	0 Open 3 Percutaneous 4 Percutaneous endoscopic	4 Internal fixation device Z No device	Z No qualifier
1 Rib, Right 2 Rib, Left 3 Cervical Vertebra 4 Thoracic Vertebra 5 Scapula, Right	6 Scapula, Left 7 Glenoid Cavity, Right 8 Glenoid Cavity, Left 9 Clavicle, Right B Clavicle, Left	X External	Z No device	Z No qualifier
C Humeral Head, Right D Humeral Head, Left F Humeral Shaft, Right G Humeral Shaft, Left	H Radius, Right J Radius, Left K Ulna, Right L Ulna, Left	0 Open 3 Percutaneous 4 Percutaneous endoscopic	4 Internal fixation device 5 External fixation device 6 Internal fixation device, intramedullary B External fixation device, monoplanar C External fixation device, ring D External fixation device, hybrid Z No device	Z No qualifier
C Humeral Head, Right D Humeral Head, Left F Humeral Shaft, Right G Humeral Shaft, Left	H Radius, Right J Radius, Left K Ulna, Right L Ulna, Left	X External	Z No device	Z No qualifier
M Carpal, Right N Carpal, Left P Metacarpal, Right Q Metacarpal, Left	R Thumb Phalanx, Right S Thumb Phalanx, Left T Finger Phalanx, Right V Finger Phalanx, Left	0 Open 3 Percutaneous 4 Percutaneous endoscopic	4 Internal fixation device 5 External fixation device Z No device	Z No qualifier
M Carpal, Right N Carpal, Left P Metacarpal, Right Q Metacarpal, Left	R Thumb Phalanx, Right S Thumb Phalanx, Left T Finger Phalanx, Right V Finger Phalanx, Left	X External	Z No device	Z No qualifier

0 P T — MEDICAL AND SURGICAL SECTION – 2016 ICD-10-PCS

EXCISION GROUP: Excision, Resection, Destruction, (Extraction), (Detachment)
Root Operations that take out some or all of a body part.

- 1ST – **0** Medical and Surgical
- 2ND – **P** Upper Bones
- 3RD – **T** RESECTION

EXAMPLE: Total claviculectomy   CMS Ex: Cholecystectomy

RESECTION: Cutting out or off, without replacement, all of a body part.

EXPLANATION: None

Body Part – 4TH		Approach – 5TH	Device – 6TH	Qualifier – 7TH
0 Sternum	H Radius, Right	0 Open	Z No device	Z No qualifier
1 Rib, Right	J Radius, Left			
2 Rib, Left	K Ulna, Right			
5 Scapula, Right	L Ulna, Left			
6 Scapula, Left	M Carpal, Right			
7 Glenoid Cavity, Right	N Carpal, Left			
8 Glenoid Cavity, Left	P Metacarpal, Right			
9 Clavicle, Right	Q Metacarpal, Left			
B Clavicle, Left	R Thumb Phalanx, Right			
C Humeral Head, Right	S Thumb Phalanx, Left			
D Humeral Head, Left	T Finger Phalanx, Right			
F Humeral Shaft, Right	V Finger Phalanx, Left			
G Humeral Shaft, Left				

DEVICE GROUP: Change, Insertion, Removal, Replacement, Revision, Supplement
Root Operations that always involve a device.

- 1ST – **0** Medical and Surgical
- 2ND – **P** Upper Bones
- 3RD – **U** SUPPLEMENT

EXAMPLE: Application bone void filler   CMS Ex: Hernia repair with mesh

SUPPLEMENT: Putting in or on biological or synthetic material that physically reinforces and/or augments the function of a portion of a body part.

EXPLANATION: Biological material from same individual …

Body Part – 4TH		Approach – 5TH	Device – 6TH	Qualifier – 7TH
0 Sternum	H Radius, Right	0 Open	7 Autologous tissue substitute	Z No qualifier
1 Rib, Right	J Radius, Left	3 Percutaneous	J Synthetic substitute	
2 Rib, Left	K Ulna, Right	4 Percutaneous endoscopic	K Nonautologous tissue substitute	
3 Cervical Vertebra	L Ulna, Left			
4 Thoracic Vertebra	M Carpal, Right			
5 Scapula, Right	N Carpal, Left			
6 Scapula, Left	P Metacarpal, Right			
7 Glenoid Cavity, Right	Q Metacarpal, Left			
8 Glenoid Cavity, Left	R Thumb Phalanx, Right			
9 Clavicle, Right	S Thumb Phalanx, Left			
B Clavicle, Left	T Finger Phalanx, Right			
C Humeral Head, Right	V Finger Phalanx, Left			
D Humeral Head, Left				
F Humeral Shaft, Right				
G Humeral Shaft, Left				

P – UPPER BONES

0PW

DEVICE GROUP: Change, Insertion, Removal, Replacement, Revision, Supplement
Root Operations that always involve a device.

1ST – **0** Medical and Surgical
2ND – **P** Upper Bones
3RD – **W REVISION**

EXAMPLE: Lengthening growing rods | **CMS Ex:** Adjustment pacemaker lead

REVISION: Correcting, to the extent possible, a portion of a malfunctioning device or the position of a displaced device.

EXPLANATION: May replace components of a device …

Body Part – 4TH		Approach – 5TH	Device – 6TH	Qualifier – 7TH
0 Sternum 1 Rib, Right 2 Rib, Left 3 Cervical Vertebra 4 Thoracic Vertebra 5 Scapula, Right 6 Scapula, Left	7 Glenoid Cavity, Right 8 Glenoid Cavity, Left 9 Clavicle, Right B Clavicle, Left	0 Open 3 Percutaneous 4 Percutaneous endoscopic X External	4 Internal fixation device 7 Autologous tissue substitute J Synthetic substitute K Nonautologous tissue substitute	Z No qualifier
C Humeral Head, Right D Humeral Head, Left F Humeral Shaft, Right G Humeral Shaft, Left H Radius, Right J Radius, Left K Ulna, Right L Ulna, Left	M Carpal, Right N Carpal, Left P Metacarpal, Right Q Metacarpal, Left R Thumb Phalanx, Right S Thumb Phalanx, Left T Finger Phalanx, Right V Finger Phalanx, Left	0 Open 3 Percutaneous 4 Percutaneous endoscopic X External	4 Internal fixation device 5 External fixation device 7 Autologous tissue substitute J Synthetic substitute K Nonautologous tissue substitute	Z No qualifier
Y Upper Bone		0 Open 3 Percutaneous 4 Percutaneous endoscopic X External	0 Drainage device M Bone growth stimulator	Z No qualifier

0P0 Medical and Surgical

0 Medical and Surgical
P Upper Bones
W Revision

DEVICE GROUP: Change, Insertion, Removal, Replacement, Revision, Supplement
Root Operations that always involve a device.

EXAMPLE: Lengthening growing rods, CNS Ex: Adjustment pacemaker lead

REVISION: Correcting, to the extent possible, a portion of a malfunctioning device or the position of a displaced device

EXPLANATION: May replace components of a device

Body Part – 4ᵗʰ	Approach – 5ᵗʰ	Device – 6ᵗʰ	Qualifier – 7ᵗʰ
0 Sternum 1 Rib, Right 2 Rib, Left 3 Cervical Vertebra 4 Thoracic Vertebra 5 Scapula, Right 6 Scapula, Left 7 Glenoid Cavity, Right 8 Glenoid Cavity, Left 9 Clavicle, Right B Clavicle, Left	0 Open 3 Percutaneous 4 Percutaneous endoscopic X External	4 Internal fixation device 7 Autologous tissue substitute J Synthetic substitute K Nonautologous tissue substitute	Z No qualifier
C Humeral Head, Right D Humeral Head, Left F Humeral Shaft, Right G Humeral Shaft, Left H Radius, Right J Radius, Left K Ulna, Right L Ulna, Left M Carpal, Right N Carpal, Left P Metacarpal, Right Q Metacarpal, Left R Thumb Phalanx, Right S Thumb Phalanx, Left T Finger Phalanx, Right V Finger Phalanx, Left	0 Open 3 Percutaneous 4 Percutaneous endoscopic X External	4 Internal fixation device 5 External fixation device 7 Autologous tissue substitute J Synthetic substitute K Nonautologous tissue substitute	Z No qualifier
Y Upper Bone	0 Open 3 Percutaneous 4 Percutaneous endoscopic X External	0 Drainage device M Bone growth stimulator	Z No qualifier

Q – Lower Bones

Educational Annotations

Body System Specific Educational Annotations for the Lower Bones include:
- Anatomy and Physiology Review
- Anatomical Illustrations
- Definitions of Common Procedures
- AHA Coding Clinic® Reference Notations
- Body Part Key Listings
- Device Key Listings
- Device Aggregation Table Listings
- Coding Notes

Anatomy and Physiology Review of Lower Bones

BODY PART VALUES – Q - LOWER BONES

Acetabulum – The round, concave depression in the pelvic bone that articulates with the femoral head forming the hip joint.

Coccyx – The small wedge-shaped bone (also known as the tailbone) at the end of the spinal column.

Femoral Shaft – The middle long portion of the femur.

Femur – The paired long bones (also known as the thigh bone) that articulate at the hip and the knee. It is the longest bone in the body.

Fibula – The paired long slender bones of the lower leg located toward the outside of the lower leg that articulate at the knee and the ankle.

Lower Bone – Any of the bones designated in the Lower Bones PCS Body System.

Lower Femur – The distal end of the femur that articulates with the knee joint.

Lumbar Vertebra – The lumbar section of the spinal vertebral column comprised of 5 vertebra, S1-S5.

Metatarsal – One of the 5 cylindrical bones connecting the tarsals and the phalanges of the foot.

Patella – The paired triangular-shaped bones situated at the front of the knee.

Pelvic Bone – Any of the three bones (ilium, ischium, pubis) that connect with the sacrum to form the pelvic girdle.

Sacrum – The large wedge-shaped vertebra at the lower end of the spine that connects with S5.

Tarsal – The seven bones of the foot (calcaneus, talus, cuboid, navicular, and the medial, intermediate, and lateral cuneiform bones) distal to the tibia and fibula and proximal to the metatarsal bones.

Tibia – The paired long bones of the lower leg (also known as the shin bone) that is the innermost bone of the lower leg supporting and articulating with the knee and with the ankle.

Toe Phalanx – The digital bones of the toes. Each toe contains three bones: Proximal phalanx, intermediate (middle) phalanx, and distal phalanx, except the great toe which only has proximal and distal phalanx bones.

Upper Femur – The proximal end of the femur (head) that articulates with the acetabulum to form the hip joint.

Educational Annotations

Q – Lower Bones

Anatomical Illustrations of Lower Bones

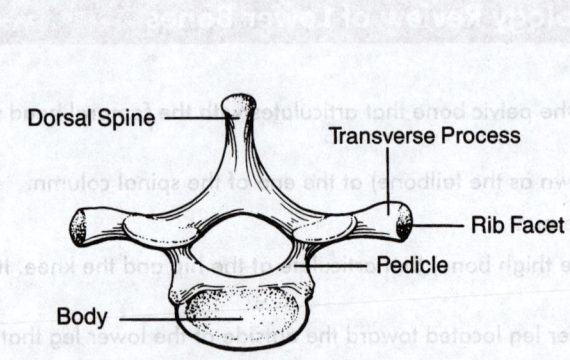
TYPICAL VERTEBRA — SUPERIOR VIEW

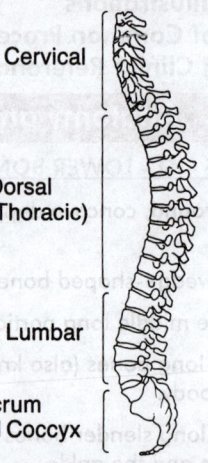
VERTEBRAL COLUMN

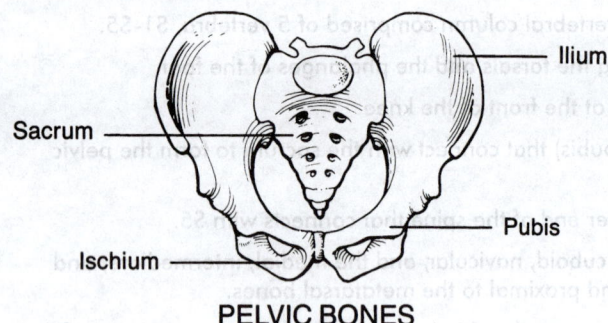
PELVIC BONES

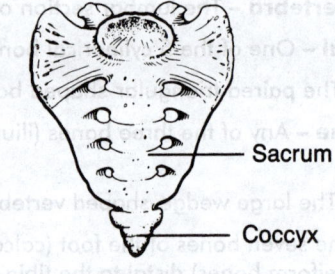
SACRUM AND COCCYX

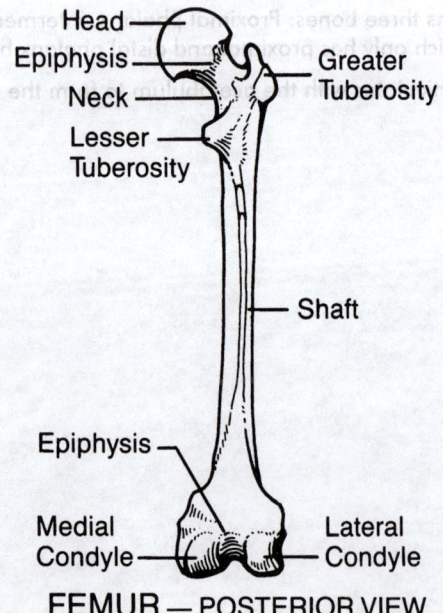
FEMUR — POSTERIOR VIEW

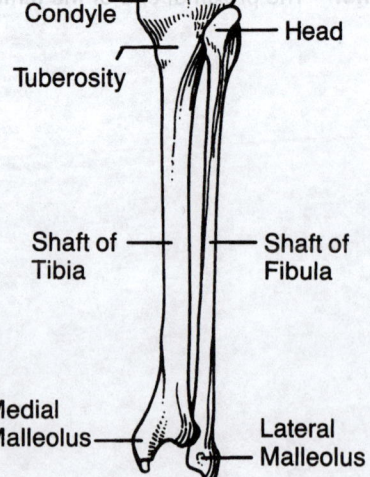
TIBIA AND FIBULA — POSTERIOR VIEW

Continued on next page

Educational Annotations | Q – Lower Bones

Anatomical Illustrations of Lower Bones

Continued from previous page

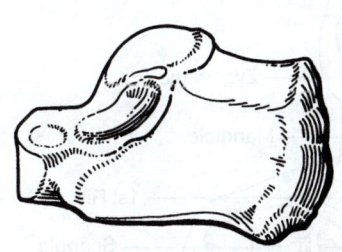

CALCANEUS — MEDIAL VIEW

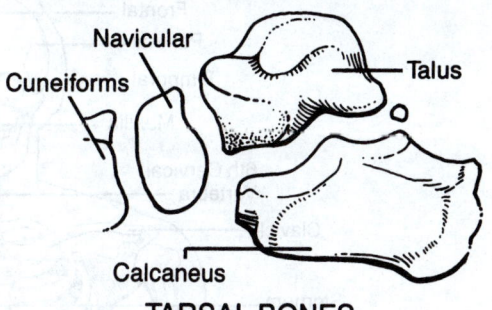

TARSAL BONES

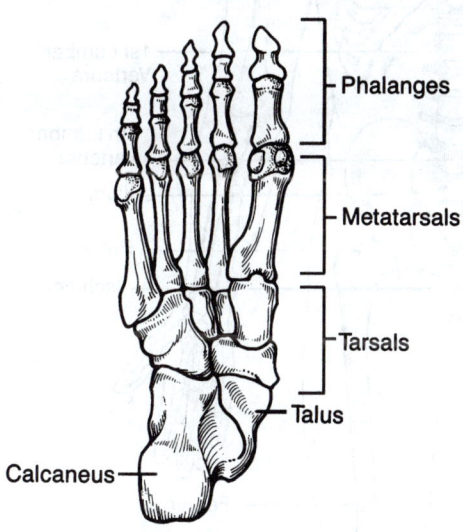

RIGHT FOOT — PLANTAR VIEW

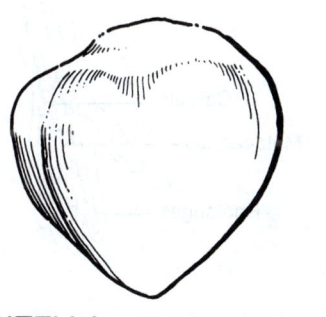

PATELLA — ANTERIOR VIEW

Continued on next page

Q – Lower Bones

Anatomical Illustrations of Lower Bones

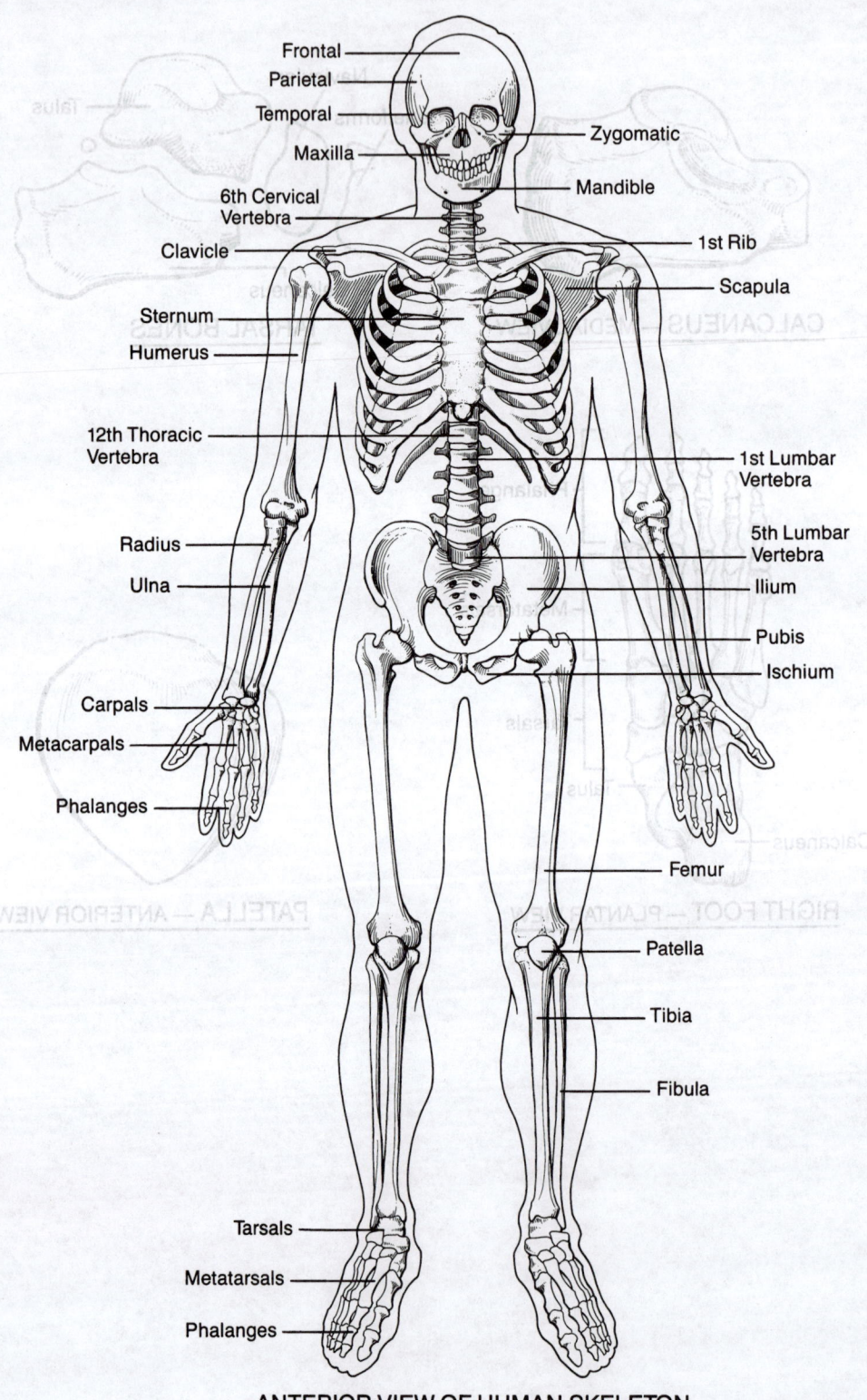

ANTERIOR VIEW OF HUMAN SKELETON

Educational Annotations

Q – Lower Bones

Anatomical Illustrations of Lower Bones

Continued from previous page

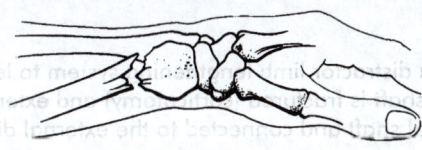
COLLES'

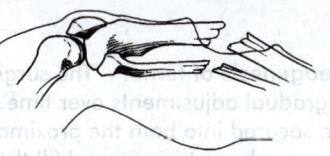
COMPOUND

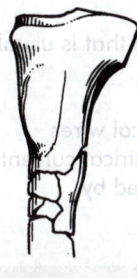
COMMINUTED

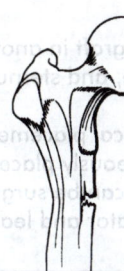
GREENSTICK

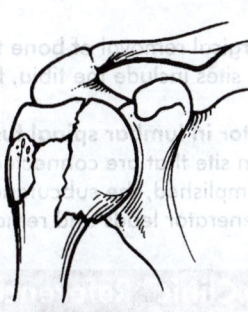
IMPACTED

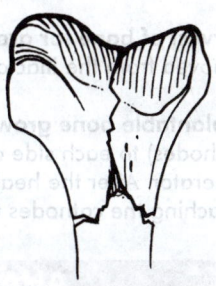
INTERCONDYLAR

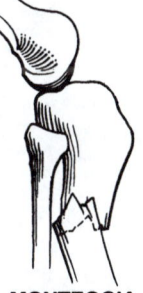
MONTEGGIA

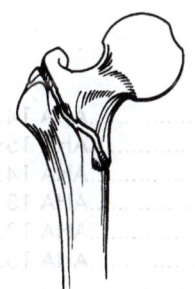
PERTROCHANTERIC

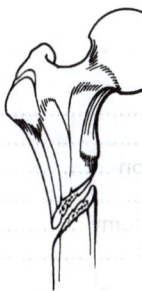
SPIRAL

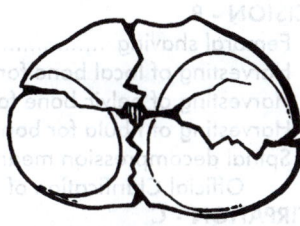
STELLATE

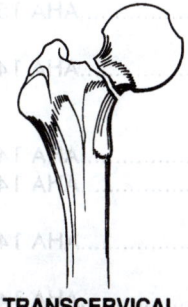
TRANSCERVICAL

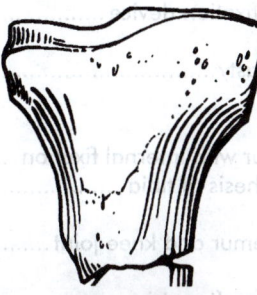
TRANSVERSE

FRACTURE TYPES

Educational Annotations | Q – Lower Bones

Definitions of Common Procedures of Lower Bones

Bone void filler to iliac crest defect – The surgical placement of a bone void filler (usually synthetic bone material) to fill in a defect in the natural shape of the iliac crest and to enhance the stability and strength of the bone.

Distraction osteogenesis of femur – The surgical placement of a distractor limb lengthening system to lengthen the femur with gradual adjustments over time. The mid-femoral shaft is fractured (corticotomy) and external fixation pins are secured into both the proximal and distal femoral shaft and connected to the external distraction system, allowing new bone to grow and fill the gap.

Femoral head shaving – The surgical grinding down of the femoral head bone that is causing the pain and impaired range of motion (femoroacetabular impingement syndrome). Procedures on the joint tissues often accompany this procedure.

Harvest of bone for graft – The surgical removal of bone to be used as a graft in another location that is usually removed from the iliac crest. Other sites include the tibia, fibula, mandible, and sternum.

Implantable bone growth stimulator in lumbar spinal fusion – The surgical placement of electrical wires (cathodes) to each side of the fusion site that are connected to a subcutaneously placed direct electrical current generator. After the healing is accomplished, the subcutaneous generator can be surgically removed by detaching the cathodes from the generator leads and removing the generator and leads.

AHA Coding Clinic® Reference Notations of Lower Bones

ROOT OPERATION SPECIFIC - Q - LOWER BONES
CHANGE - 2
DESTRUCTION - 5
DIVISION - 8
DRAINAGE - 9
EXCISION - B
- Femoral shaving ....AHA 14:4Q:p25
- Harvesting of local bone for graft..AHA 15:1Q:p30
- Harvesting of pelvic bone for spinal fusion ....AHA 14:2Q:p6
- Harvesting of fibula for bone graft ....AHA 13:2Q:p39
- Spinal decompression meaning laminectomy ....AHA 13:4Q:p116
  - Official Clarification of 13:4Q:p116 ....AHA 15:2Q:p34

EXTIRPATION - C
INSERTION - H
INSPECTION - J
RELEASE - N
REMOVAL - P
- Removal of internal fixation device ....AHA 15:2Q:p6

REPAIR - Q
- Sacrum S1 laminoplasty...AHA 14:3Q:p24

REPLACEMENT - R
REPOSITION - S
- Realignment of femur with internal fixation ....AHA 14:4Q:p31
- Rotational osteosynthesis of tibia ....AHA 14:4Q:p29

RESECTION - T
- Resection of lower femur and knee joint..AHA 14:4Q:p29

SUPPLEMENT - U
- Application of bone graft matrix ....AHA 14:4Q:p31
- Bone void filler..AHA 13:2Q:p35
- Vertebroplasty with cement as a device value ....AHA 14:2Q:p12

REVISION - W

Q – Lower Bones

Educational Annotations

Body Part Key Listings of Lower Bones

See also Body Part Key in Appendix C

Body of femur	*use* Femoral Shaft, Left/Right
Body of fibula	*use* Fibula, Left/Right
Calcaneus	*use* Tarsal, Left/Right
Cuboid bone	*use* Tarsal, Left/Right
Femoral head	*use* Upper Femur, Left/Right
Greater trochanter	*use* Upper Femur, Left/Right
Head of fibula	*use* Fibula, Left/Right
Iliac crest	*use* Pelvic Bone, Left/Right
Ilium	*use* Pelvic Bone, Left/Right
Intermediate cuneiform bone	*use* Tarsal, Left/Right
Ischium	*use* Pelvic Bone, Left/Right
Lateral condyle of femur	*use* Lower Femur, Left/Right
Lateral condyle of tibia	*use* Tibia, Left/Right
Lateral cuneiform bone	*use* Tarsal, Left/Right
Lateral epicondyle of femur	*use* Lower Femur, Left/Right
Lateral malleolus	*use* Fibula, Left/Right
Lesser trochanter	*use* Upper Femur, Left/Right
Medial condyle of femur	*use* Lower Femur, Left/Right
Medial condyle of tibia	*use* Tibia, Left/Right
Medial cuneiform bone	*use* Tarsal, Left/Right
Medial epicondyle of femur	*use* Lower Femur, Left/Right
Medial malleolus	*use* Tibia, Left/Right
Navicular bone	*use* Tarsal, Left/Right
Neck of femur	*use* Upper Femur, Left/Right
Pubis	*use* Pelvic Bone, Left/Right
Spinous process	*use* Cervical, Thoracic, Lumbar Vertebra
Talus bone	*use* Tarsal, Left/Right
Vertebral arch	*use* Cervical, Thoracic, Lumbar Vertebra
Vertebral foramen	*use* Cervical, Thoracic, Lumbar Vertebra
Vertebral lamina	*use* Cervical, Thoracic, Lumbar Vertebra
Vertebral pedicle	*use* Cervical, Thoracic, Lumbar Vertebra

Device Key Listings of Lower Bones

See also Device Key in Appendix D

Autograft	*use* Autologous Tissue Substitute
Bone bank bone graft	*use* Nonautologous Tissue Substitute
Bone screw (interlocking) (lag) (pedicle) (recessed)	*use* Internal Fixation Device in Head and Facial Bones, Upper Bones, Lower Bones
Clamp and rod internal fixation system (CRIF)	*use* Internal Fixation Device in Upper Bones, Lower Bones
Delta frame external fixator	*use* External Fixation Device, Hybrid for Insertion in Upper Bones, Lower Bones
	use External Fixation Device, Hybrid for Reposition in Upper Bones, Lower Bones
Electrical bone growth stimulator (EBGS)	*use* Bone Growth Stimulator in Head and Facial Bones, Upper Bones, Lower Bones
External fixator	*use* External Fixation Device in Head and Facial Bones, Upper Bones, Lower Bones, Upper Joints, Lower Joints

Continued on next page

Educational Annotations

Q – Lower Bones

Device Key Listings of Lower Bones

Continued from previous page

Ilizarov external fixator	*use* External Fixation Device, Ring for Insertion in Upper Bones, Lower Bones
	use External Fixation Device, Ring for Reposition in Upper Bones, Lower Bones
Ilizarov-Vecklich device	*use* External Fixation Device, Limb Lengthening for Insertion in Upper Bones, Lower Bones
Intramedullary (IM) rod (nail)	*use* Internal Fixation Device, Intramedullary in Upper Bones, Lower Bones
Intramedullary skeletal kinetic distractor (ISKD)	*use* Internal Fixation Device, Intramedullary in Upper Bones, Lower Bones
Kirschner wire (K-wire)	*use* Internal Fixation Device in Head and Facial Bones, Upper Bones, Lower Bones, Upper Joints, Lower Joints
Kuntscher nail	*use* Internal Fixation Device, Intramedullary in Upper Bones, Lower Bones
Neutralization plate	*use* Internal Fixation Device in Head and Facial Bones, Upper Bones, Lower Bones
Polymethylmethacrylate (PMMA)	*use* Synthetic Substitute
Sheffield hybrid external fixator	*use* External Fixation Device, Hybrid for Insertion in Upper Bones, Lower Bones
	use External Fixation Device, Hybrid for Reposition in Upper Bones, Lower Bones
Sheffield ring external fixator	*use* External Fixation Device, Ring for Insertion in Upper Bones, Lower Bones
	use External Fixation Device, Ring for Reposition in Upper Bones, Lower Bones
Tissue bank graft	*use* Nonautologous Tissue Substitute
Ultrasonic osteogenic stimulator	*use* Bone Growth Stimulator in Head and Facial Bones, Upper Bones, Lower Bones
Ultrasound bone healing system	*use* Bone Growth Stimulator in Head and Facial Bones, Upper Bones, Lower Bones
Uniplanar external fixator	*use* External Fixation Device, Monoplanar for Insertion in Upper Bones, Lower Bones
	use External Fixation Device, Monoplanar for Reposition in Upper Bones, Lower Bones

Device Aggregation Table Listings of Lower Bones

See also Device Aggregation Table in Appendix E

Specific Device	For Operation	In Body System		General Device
External Fixation Device, Hybrid	Insertion	Lower Bones	5	External Fixation Device
External Fixation Device, Hybrid	Reposition	Lower Bones	5	External Fixation Device
External Fixation Device, Limb Lengthening	Insertion	Lower Bones	5	External Fixation Device
External Fixation Device, Monoplanar	Insertion	Lower Bones	5	External Fixation Device
External Fixation Device, Monoplanar	Reposition	Lower Bones	5	External Fixation Device
External Fixation Device, Ring	Insertion	Lower Bones	5	External Fixation Device
External Fixation Device, Ring	Reposition	Lower Bones	5	External Fixation Device
Internal Fixation Device, Intramedullary	All applicable	Lower Bones	4	Internal Fixation Device

Educational Annotations

Q – Lower Bones

Coding Notes of Lower Bones

Body System Relevant Coding Guidelines

Reposition for fracture treatment
B3.15
Reduction of a displaced fracture is coded to the root operation Reposition and the application of a cast or splint in conjunction with the Reposition procedure is not coded separately. Treatment of a nondisplaced fracture is coded to the procedure performed.
Examples: Putting a pin in a nondisplaced fracture is coded to the root operation Insertion.
Casting of a nondisplaced fracture is coded to the root operation Immobilization in the Placement section.

Body System Specific PCS Reference Manual Exercises

PCS CODE	Q – LOWER BONES EXERCISES
0QHY0MZ	Open placement of bone growth stimulator, left femoral shaft.
0QPN04Z	Incision with removal of K-wire fixation, right first metatarsal.
0QR70KZ	Excision of necrosed left femoral head with bone bank bone graft to fill the defect, open.
0QS634Z	Closed reduction with percutaneous internal fixation of right femoral neck fracture.
0QSG0ZZ	Open fracture reduction, right tibia.
0QWH04Z	Taking out loose screw and putting larger screw in fracture repair plate, left tibia.

Q – Lower Bones

NOTES

Q – LOWER BONES

0Q5

DEVICE GROUP: Change, Insertion, Removal, Replacement, Revision, Supplement
Root Operations that always involve a device.

- 1ST – **0** Medical and Surgical
- 2ND – **Q** Lower Bones
- 3RD – **2 CHANGE**

EXAMPLE: Exchange drain tube | CMS Ex: Changing urinary catheter

CHANGE: Taking out or off a device from a body part and putting back an identical or similar device in or on the same body part without cutting or puncturing the skin or a mucous membrane.

EXPLANATION: ALL Changes use EXTERNAL approach only …

Body Part – 4TH	Approach – 5TH	Device – 6TH	Qualifier – 7TH
Y Lower Bone	X External	0 Drainage device Y Other device	Z No qualifier

---

EXCISION GROUP: Excision, Resection, Destruction, (Extraction), (Detachment)
Root Operations that take out some or all of a body part.

- 1ST – **0** Medical and Surgical
- 2ND – **Q** Lower Bones
- 3RD – **5 DESTRUCTION**

EXAMPLE: Cryoablation bone cyst | CMS Ex: Fulguration polyp

DESTRUCTION: Physical eradication of all or a portion of a body part by the direct use of energy, force, or a destructive agent.

EXPLANATION: None of the body part is physically taken out

Body Part – 4TH		Approach – 5TH	Device – 6TH	Qualifier – 7TH
0 Lumbar Vertebra	D Patella, Right	0 Open	Z No device	Z No qualifier
1 Sacrum	F Patella, Left	3 Percutaneous		
2 Pelvic Bone, Right	G Tibia, Right	4 Percutaneous endoscopic		
3 Pelvic Bone, Left	H Tibia, Left			
4 Acetabulum, Right	J Fibula, Right			
5 Acetabulum, Left	K Fibula, Left			
6 Upper Femur, Right	L Tarsal, Right			
7 Upper Femur, Left	M Tarsal, Left			
8 Femoral Shaft, Right	N Metatarsal, Right			
9 Femoral Shaft, Left	P Metatarsal, Left			
B Lower Femur, Right	Q Toe Phalanx, Right			
C Lower Femur, Left	R Toe Phalanx, Left			
	S Coccyx			

0Q8 MEDICAL AND SURGICAL SECTION – 2016 ICD-10-PCS

DIVISION GROUP: Division, Release
Root Operations involving cutting or separation only.

1ST - **0** Medical and Surgical
2ND - **Q** Lower Bones
3RD - **8 DIVISION**

EXAMPLE: Tarsal osteotomy
CMS Ex: Osteotomy

DIVISION: Cutting into a body part without draining fluids and/or gases from the body part in order to separate or transect a body part.

EXPLANATION: Separated into two or more portions ...

Body Part – 4TH		Approach – 5TH	Device – 6TH	Qualifier – 7TH
0 Lumbar Vertebra	D Patella, Right	0 Open	Z No device	Z No qualifier
1 Sacrum	F Patella, Left	3 Percutaneous		
2 Pelvic Bone, Right	G Tibia, Right	4 Percutaneous endoscopic		
3 Pelvic Bone, Left	H Tibia, Left			
4 Acetabulum, Right	J Fibula, Right			
5 Acetabulum, Left	K Fibula, Left			
6 Upper Femur, Right	L Tarsal, Right			
7 Upper Femur, Left	M Tarsal, Left			
8 Femoral Shaft, Right	N Metatarsal, Right			
9 Femoral Shaft, Left	P Metatarsal, Left			
B Lower Femur, Right	Q Toe Phalanx, Right			
C Lower Femur, Left	R Toe Phalanx, Left			
	S Coccyx			

Q – LOWER BONES 0Q9

DRAINAGE GROUP: Drainage, Extirpation, (Fragmentation)
Root Operations that take out solids/fluids/gases from a body part.

1ST - **0** Medical and Surgical	EXAMPLE: Aspiration bone cyst	CMS Ex: Thoracentesis
2ND - **Q** Lower Bones	**DRAINAGE:** Taking or letting out fluids and/or gases from a body part.	
3RD - **9 DRAINAGE**	EXPLANATION: Qualifier "X Diagnostic" indicates biopsy ...	

Body Part – 4TH		Approach – 5TH	Device – 6TH	Qualifier – 7TH
0 Lumbar Vertebra	D Patella, Right	0 Open	0 Drainage device	Z No qualifier
1 Sacrum	F Patella, Left	3 Percutaneous		
2 Pelvic Bone, Right	G Tibia, Right	4 Percutaneous endoscopic		
3 Pelvic Bone, Left	H Tibia, Left			
4 Acetabulum, Right	J Fibula, Right			
5 Acetabulum, Left	K Fibula, Left			
6 Upper Femur, Right	L Tarsal, Right			
7 Upper Femur, Left	M Tarsal, Left			
8 Femoral Shaft, Right	N Metatarsal, Right			
9 Femoral Shaft, Left	P Metatarsal, Left			
B Lower Femur, Right	Q Toe Phalanx, Right			
C Lower Femur, Left	R Toe Phalanx, Left			
	S Coccyx			
0 Lumbar Vertebra	D Patella, Right	0 Open	Z No device	X Diagnostic
1 Sacrum	F Patella, Left	3 Percutaneous		Z No qualifier
2 Pelvic Bone, Right	G Tibia, Right	4 Percutaneous endoscopic		
3 Pelvic Bone, Left	H Tibia, Left			
4 Acetabulum, Right	J Fibula, Right			
5 Acetabulum, Left	K Fibula, Left			
6 Upper Femur, Right	L Tarsal, Right			
7 Upper Femur, Left	M Tarsal, Left			
8 Femoral Shaft, Right	N Metatarsal, Right			
9 Femoral Shaft, Left	P Metatarsal, Left			
B Lower Femur, Right	Q Toe Phalanx, Right			
C Lower Femur, Left	R Toe Phalanx, Left			
	S Coccyx			

0QB MEDICAL AND SURGICAL SECTION – 2016 ICD-10-PCS [2016.PCS]

EXCISION GROUP: Excision, Resection, Destruction, (Extraction), (Detachment)
Root Operations that take out some or all of a body part.

1ST - 0 Medical and Surgical
2ND - Q Lower Bones
3RD - B EXCISION

EXAMPLE: Harvest bone for graft CMS Ex: Liver biopsy

EXCISION: Cutting out or off, without replacement, a portion of a body part.

EXPLANATION: Qualifier "X Diagnostic" indicates biopsy …

Body Part – 4TH		Approach – 5TH	Device – 6TH	Qualifier – 7TH
0 Lumbar Vertebra	D Patella, Right	0 Open	Z No device	X Diagnostic
1 Sacrum	F Patella, Left	3 Percutaneous		Z No qualifier
2 Pelvic Bone, Right	G Tibia, Right	4 Percutaneous endoscopic		
3 Pelvic Bone, Left	H Tibia, Left			
4 Acetabulum, Right	J Fibula, Right			
5 Acetabulum, Left	K Fibula, Left			
6 Upper Femur, Right	L Tarsal, Right			
7 Upper Femur, Left	M Tarsal, Left			
8 Femoral Shaft, Right	N Metatarsal, Right			
9 Femoral Shaft, Left	P Metatarsal, Left			
B Lower Femur, Right	Q Toe Phalanx, Right			
C Lower Femur, Left	R Toe Phalanx, Left			
	S Coccyx			

DRAINAGE GROUP: Drainage, Extirpation, (Fragmentation)
Root Operations that take out solids/fluids/gases from a body part.

1ST - 0 Medical and Surgical
2ND - Q Lower Bones
3RD - C EXTIRPATION

EXAMPLE: Removal foreign body CMS Ex: Choledocholithotomy

EXTIRPATION: Taking or cutting out solid matter from a body part.

EXPLANATION: Abnormal byproduct or foreign body …

Body Part – 4TH		Approach – 5TH	Device – 6TH	Qualifier – 7TH
0 Lumbar Vertebra	D Patella, Right	0 Open	Z No device	Z No qualifier
1 Sacrum	F Patella, Left	3 Percutaneous		
2 Pelvic Bone, Right	G Tibia, Right	4 Percutaneous endoscopic		
3 Pelvic Bone, Left	H Tibia, Left			
4 Acetabulum, Right	J Fibula, Right			
5 Acetabulum, Left	K Fibula, Left			
6 Upper Femur, Right	L Tarsal, Right			
7 Upper Femur, Left	M Tarsal, Left			
8 Femoral Shaft, Right	N Metatarsal, Right			
9 Femoral Shaft, Left	P Metatarsal, Left			
B Lower Femur, Right	Q Toe Phalanx, Right			
C Lower Femur, Left	R Toe Phalanx, Left			
	S Coccyx			

Q – LOWER BONES   0QH

DEVICE GROUP: Change, Insertion, Removal, Replacement, Revision, Supplement
Root Operations that always involve a device.

1ST - **0** Medical and Surgical
2ND - **Q** Lower Bones
3RD - **H INSERTION**

EXAMPLE: Insertion growing rods   CMS Ex: Central venous catheter

INSERTION: Putting in a nonbiological appliance that monitors, assists, performs, or prevents a physiological function but does not physically take the place of a body part.

EXPLANATION: None

Body Part – 4TH	Approach – 5TH	Device – 6TH	Qualifier – 7TH
0 Lumbar Vertebra 1 Sacrum 2 Pelvic Bone, Right 3 Pelvic Bone, Left 4 Acetabulum, Right 5 Acetabulum, Left D Patella, Right F Patella, Left L Tarsal, Right M Tarsal, Left N Metatarsal, Right P Metatarsal, Left Q Toe Phalanx, Right R Toe Phalanx, Left S Coccyx	0 Open 3 Percutaneous 4 Percutaneous endoscopic	4 Internal fixation device 5 External fixation device	Z No qualifier
6 Upper Femur, Right 7 Upper Femur, Left 8 Femoral Shaft, Right 9 Femoral Shaft, Left B Lower Femur, Right C Lower Femur, Left G Tibia, Right H Tibia, Left J Fibula, Right K Fibula, Left	0 Open 3 Percutaneous 4 Percutaneous endoscopic	4 Internal fixation device 5 External fixation device 6 Internal fixation device, intramedullary 8 External fixation device, limb lengthening B External fixation device, monoplanar C External fixation device, ring D External fixation device, hybrid	Z No qualifier
Y Lower Bone	0 Open 3 Percutaneous 4 Percutaneous endoscopic	M Bone growth stimulator	Z No qualifier

0QJ MEDICAL AND SURGICAL SECTION – 2016 ICD-10-PCS

EXAMINATION GROUP: Inspection, (Map)
Root Operations involving examination only.

- 1ST – **0** Medical and Surgical
- 2ND – **Q** Lower Bones
- 3RD – **J** INSPECTION

EXAMPLE: Examination bone | CMS Ex: Colonoscopy

INSPECTION: Visually and/or manually exploring a body part.

EXPLANATION: Direct or instrumental visualization ...

Body Part – 4TH	Approach – 5TH	Device – 6TH	Qualifier – 7TH
Y Lower Bone	0 Open 3 Percutaneous 4 Percutaneous endoscopic X External	Z No device	Z No qualifier

DIVISION GROUP: Division, Release
Root Operations involving cutting or separation only.

- 1ST – **0** Medical and Surgical
- 2ND – **Q** Lower Bones
- 3RD – **N** RELEASE

EXAMPLE: Extra-articular bone adhesiolysis | CMS Ex: Carpal tunnel release

RELEASE: Freeing a body part from an abnormal physical constraint by cutting or by the use of force.

EXPLANATION: None of the body part is taken out ...

Body Part – 4TH		Approach – 5TH	Device – 6TH	Qualifier – 7TH
0 Lumbar Vertebra	D Patella, Right	0 Open	Z No device	Z No qualifier
1 Sacrum	F Patella, Left	3 Percutaneous		
2 Pelvic Bone, Right	G Tibia, Right	4 Percutaneous endoscopic		
3 Pelvic Bone, Left	H Tibia, Left			
4 Acetabulum, Right	J Fibula, Right			
5 Acetabulum, Left	K Fibula, Left			
6 Upper Femur, Right	L Tarsal, Right			
7 Upper Femur, Left	M Tarsal, Left			
8 Femoral Shaft, Right	N Metatarsal, Right			
9 Femoral Shaft, Left	P Metatarsal, Left			
B Lower Femur, Right	Q Toe Phalanx, Right			
C Lower Femur, Left	R Toe Phalanx, Left			
	S Coccyx			

Q – LOWER BONES 0QP

DEVICE GROUP: Change, Insertion, Removal, Replacement, Revision, Supplement
Root Operations that always involve a device.

1ST – **0** Medical and Surgical
2ND – **Q** Lower Bones
3RD – **P REMOVAL**

EXAMPLE: Removal growing rods   CMS Ex: Chest tube removal

REMOVAL: Taking out or off a device from a body part.

EXPLANATION: Removal device without reinsertion ...

Body Part – 4TH	Approach – 5TH	Device – 6TH	Qualifier – 7TH
0 Lumbar Vertebra 1 Sacrum 4 Acetabulum, Right 5 Acetabulum, Left S Coccyx	0 Open 3 Percutaneous 4 Percutaneous endoscopic	4 Internal fixation device 7 Autologous tissue substitute J Synthetic substitute K Nonautologous tissue substitute	Z No qualifier
0 Lumbar Vertebra 1 Sacrum 4 Acetabulum, Right 5 Acetabulum, Left S Coccyx	X External	4 Internal fixation device	Z No qualifier
2 Pelvic Bone, Right 3 Pelvic Bone, Left 6 Upper Femur, Right 7 Upper Femur, Left 8 Femoral Shaft, Right 9 Femoral Shaft, Left B Lower Femur, Right C Lower Femur, Left D Patella, Right F Patella, Left G Tibia, Right H Tibia, Left J Fibula, Right K Fibula, Left L Tarsal, Right M Tarsal, Left N Metatarsal, Right P Metatarsal, Left Q Toe Phalanx, Right R Toe Phalanx, Left	0 Open 3 Percutaneous 4 Percutaneous endoscopic	4 Internal fixation device 5 External fixation device 7 Autologous tissue substitute J Synthetic substitute K Nonautologous tissue substitute	Z No qualifier
2 Pelvic Bone, Right 3 Pelvic Bone, Left 6 Upper Femur, Right 7 Upper Femur, Left 8 Femoral Shaft, Right 9 Femoral Shaft, Left B Lower Femur, Right C Lower Femur, Left D Patella, Right F Patella, Left G Tibia, Right H Tibia, Left J Fibula, Right K Fibula, Left L Tarsal, Right M Tarsal, Left N Metatarsal, Right P Metatarsal, Left Q Toe Phalanx, Right R Toe Phalanx, Left	X External	4 Internal fixation device 5 External fixation device	Z No qualifier
Y Lower Bone	0 Open 3 Percutaneous 4 Percutaneous endoscopic X External	0 Drainage device M Bone growth stimulator	Z No qualifier

0QQ MEDICAL AND SURGICAL SECTION – 2016 ICD-10-PCS

OTHER REPAIRS GROUP: (Control), Repair
Root Operations that define other repairs.

- 1ST – **0** Medical and Surgical
- 2ND – **Q** Lower Bones
- 3RD – **Q REPAIR**

EXAMPLE: Vertebral laminoplasty CMS Ex: Suture laceration

REPAIR: Restoring, to the extent possible, a body part to its normal anatomic structure and function.

EXPLANATION: Only when no other root operation applies ...

Body Part – 4TH		Approach – 5TH	Device – 6TH	Qualifier – 7TH
0 Lumbar Vertebra	D Patella, Right	0 Open	Z No device	Z No qualifier
1 Sacrum	F Patella, Left	3 Percutaneous		
2 Pelvic Bone, Right	G Tibia, Right	4 Percutaneous endoscopic		
3 Pelvic Bone, Left	H Tibia, Left	X External		
4 Acetabulum, Right	J Fibula, Right			
5 Acetabulum, Left	K Fibula, Left			
6 Upper Femur, Right	L Tarsal, Right			
7 Upper Femur, Left	M Tarsal, Left			
8 Femoral Shaft, Right	N Metatarsal, Right			
9 Femoral Shaft, Left	P Metatarsal, Left			
B Lower Femur, Right	Q Toe Phalanx, Right			
C Lower Femur, Left	R Toe Phalanx, Left			
	S Coccyx			

DEVICE GROUP: Change, Insertion, Removal, Replacement, Revision, Supplement
Root Operations that always involve a device.

- 1ST – **0** Medical and Surgical
- 2ND – **Q** Lower Bones
- 3RD – **R REPLACEMENT**

EXAMPLE: Patella replacement CMS Ex: Total hip

REPLACEMENT: Putting in or on a biological or synthetic material that physically takes the place and/or function of all or a portion of a body part.

EXPLANATION: Includes taking out body part, or eradication...

Body Part – 4TH		Approach – 5TH	Device – 6TH	Qualifier – 7TH
0 Lumbar Vertebra	D Patella, Right	0 Open	7 Autologous tissue substitute	Z No qualifier
1 Sacrum	F Patella, Left	3 Percutaneous	J Synthetic substitute	
2 Pelvic Bone, Right	G Tibia, Right	4 Percutaneous endoscopic	K Nonautologous tissue substitute	
3 Pelvic Bone, Left	H Tibia, Left			
4 Acetabulum, Right	J Fibula, Right			
5 Acetabulum, Left	K Fibula, Left			
6 Upper Femur, Right	L Tarsal, Right			
7 Upper Femur, Left	M Tarsal, Left			
8 Femoral Shaft, Right	N Metatarsal, Right			
9 Femoral Shaft, Left	P Metatarsal, Left			
B Lower Femur, Right	Q Toe Phalanx, Right			
C Lower Femur, Left	R Toe Phalanx, Left			
	S Coccyx			

Q – LOWER BONES
0QS

MOVE GROUP: (Reattachment), **Reposition**, (Transfer), (Transplantation)
Root Operations that put in/put back or move some/all of a body part.

1ST – **0** Medical and Surgical
2ND – **Q** Lower Bones
3RD – **S REPOSITION**

EXAMPLE: Reduction with hybrid device **CMS Ex:** Fracture reduction

REPOSITION: Moving to its normal location, or other suitable location, all or a portion of a body part.

EXPLANATION: May or may not be cut to be moved ...

Body Part – 4TH		Approach – 5TH	Device – 6TH	Qualifier – 7TH
0 Lumbar Vertebra 1 Sacrum	4 Acetabulum, Right 5 Acetabulum, Left S Coccyx	0 Open 3 Percutaneous 4 Percutaneous endoscopic	4 Internal fixation device Z No device	Z No qualifier
0 Lumbar Vertebra 1 Sacrum	4 Acetabulum, Right 5 Acetabulum, Left S Coccyx	X External	Z No device	Z No qualifier
2 Pelvic Bone, Right 3 Pelvic Bone, Left D Patella, Right F Patella, Left L Tarsal, Right M Tarsal, Left	N Metatarsal, Right P Metatarsal, Left Q Toe Phalanx, Right R Toe Phalanx, Left	0 Open 3 Percutaneous 4 Percutaneous endoscopic	4 Internal fixation device 5 External fixation device Z No device	Z No qualifier
2 Pelvic Bone, Right 3 Pelvic Bone, Left D Patella, Right F Patella, Left L Tarsal, Right M Tarsal, Left	N Metatarsal, Right P Metatarsal, Left Q Toe Phalanx, Right R Toe Phalanx, Left	X External	Z No device	Z No qualifier
6 Upper Femur, Right 7 Upper Femur, Left 8 Femoral Shaft, Right 9 Femoral Shaft, Left B Lower Femur, Right C Lower Femur, Left	G Tibia, Right H Tibia, Left J Fibula, Right K Fibula, Left	0 Open 3 Percutaneous 4 Percutaneous endoscopic	4 Internal fixation device 5 External fixation device 6 Internal fixation device, intramedullary B External fixation device, monoplanar C External fixation device, ring D External fixation device, hybrid Z No device	Z No qualifier
6 Upper Femur, Right 7 Upper Femur, Left 8 Femoral Shaft, Right 9 Femoral Shaft, Left B Lower Femur, Right C Lower Femur, Left	G Tibia, Right H Tibia, Left J Fibula, Right K Fibula, Left	X External	Z No device	Z No qualifier

0QT

MEDICAL AND SURGICAL SECTION – 2016 ICD-10-PCS

EXCISION GROUP: Excision, Resection, Destruction, (Extraction), (Detachment)
Root Operations that take out some or all of a body part.

- 1ST – **0** Medical and Surgical
- 2ND – **Q** Lower Bones
- 3RD – **T** RESECTION

EXAMPLE: Total patellectomy   CMS Ex: Cholecystectomy

RESECTION: Cutting out or off, without replacement, all of a body part.

EXPLANATION: None

Body Part – 4TH		Approach – 5TH	Device – 6TH	Qualifier – 7TH
2 Pelvic Bone, Right	G Tibia, Right	0 Open	Z No device	Z No qualifier
3 Pelvic Bone, Left	H Tibia, Left			
4 Acetabulum, Right	J Fibula, Right			
5 Acetabulum, Left	K Fibula, Left			
6 Upper Femur, Right	L Tarsal, Right			
7 Upper Femur, Left	M Tarsal, Left			
8 Femoral Shaft, Right	N Metatarsal, Right			
9 Femoral Shaft, Left	P Metatarsal, Left			
B Lower Femur, Right	Q Toe Phalanx, Right			
C Lower Femur, Left	R Toe Phalanx, Left			
D Patella, Right	S Coccyx			
F Patella, Left				

DEVICE GROUP: Change, Insertion, Removal, Replacement, Revision, Supplement
Root Operations that always involve a device.

- 1ST – **0** Medical and Surgical
- 2ND – **Q** Lower Bones
- 3RD – **U** SUPPLEMENT

EXAMPLE: Application bone void filler   CMS Ex: Hernia repair with mesh

UPPLEMENT: Putting in or on biological or synthetic material that physically reinforces and/or augments the function of a portion of a body part.

EXPLANATION: Biological material from same individual ...

Body Part – 4TH		Approach – 5TH	Device – 6TH	Qualifier – 7TH
0 Lumbar Vertebra	D Patella, Right	0 Open	7 Autologous tissue substitute	Z No qualifier
1 Sacrum	F Patella, Left	3 Percutaneous	J Synthetic substitute	
2 Pelvic Bone, Right	G Tibia, Right	4 Percutaneous endoscopic	K Nonautologous tissue substitute	
3 Pelvic Bone, Left	H Tibia, Left			
4 Acetabulum, Right	J Fibula, Right			
5 Acetabulum, Left	K Fibula, Left			
6 Upper Femur, Right	L Tarsal, Right			
7 Upper Femur, Left	M Tarsal, Left			
8 Femoral Shaft, Right	N Metatarsal, Right			
9 Femoral Shaft, Left	P Metatarsal, Left			
B Lower Femur, Right	Q Toe Phalanx, Right			
C Lower Femur, Left	R Toe Phalanx, Left			
	S Coccyx			

LOWER BONES 0QT

0QW

Q – LOWER BONES

DEVICE GROUP: Change, Insertion, Removal, Replacement, Revision, Supplement
Root Operations that always involve a device.

- 1ST – **0** Medical and Surgical
- 2ND – **Q** Lower Bones
- 3RD – **W REVISION**

EXAMPLE: Lengthening growing rods | CMS Ex: Adjustment pacemaker lead

REVISION: Correcting, to the extent possible, a portion of a malfunctioning device or the position of a displaced device.

EXPLANATION: May replace components of a device …

Body Part – 4TH		Approach – 5TH	Device – 6TH	Qualifier – 7TH
0 Lumbar Vertebra 1 Sacrum	4 Acetabulum, Right 5 Acetabulum, Left S Coccyx	0 Open 3 Percutaneous 4 Percutaneous endoscopic X External	4 Internal fixation device 7 Autologous tissue substitute J Synthetic substitute K Nonautologous tissue substitute	Z No qualifier
2 Pelvic Bone, Right 3 Pelvic Bone, Left 6 Upper Femur, Right 7 Upper Femur, Left 8 Femoral Shaft, Right 9 Femoral Shaft, Left B Lower Femur, Right C Lower Femur, Left D Patella, Right F Patella, Left	G Tibia, Right H Tibia, Left J Fibula, Right K Fibula, Left L Tarsal, Right M Tarsal, Left N Metatarsal, Right P Metatarsal, Left Q Toe Phalanx, Right R Toe Phalanx, Left	0 Open 3 Percutaneous 4 Percutaneous endoscopic X External	4 Internal fixation device 5 External fixation device 7 Autologous tissue substitute J Synthetic substitute K Nonautologous tissue substitute	Z No qualifier
Y Lower Bone		0 Open 3 Percutaneous 4 Percutaneous endoscopic X External	0 Drainage device M Bone growth stimulator	Z No qualifier

0Q Lower Bones

MEDICAL AND SURGICAL SECTION – 2016 ICD-10-PCS

0 Medical and Surgical
Q Lower Bones
W Revision

DEVICE GROUP: Change, Insertion, Removal, Replacement, Revision, Supplement
Root Operations that always involve a device

EXAMPLE: Lengthening growing rods (CMS-Br. Adjustment pacemaker lead)

REVISION: Correcting, to the extent possible, a portion of a malfunctioning device or the position of a displaced device

EXPLANATION: May replace components of a device

Body Part – 4ᵗʰ	Approach – 5ᵗʰ	Device – 6ᵗʰ	Qualifier – 7ᵗʰ
0 Lumbar Vertebra 1 Sacrum 4 Acetabulum, Right 5 Acetabulum, Left S Coccyx	0 Open 3 Percutaneous 4 Percutaneous endoscopic X External	4 Internal fixation device 7 Autologous tissue substitute J Synthetic substitute K Nonautologous tissue substitute	Z No qualifier
2 Pelvic Bone, Right 3 Pelvic Bone, Left 6 Upper Femur, Right 7 Upper Femur, Left 8 Femoral Shaft, Right 9 Femoral Shaft, Left B Lower Femur, Right C Lower Femur, Left D Patella, Right F Patella, Left G Tibia, Right H Tibia, Left J Fibula, Right K Fibula, Left L Tarsal, Right M Tarsal, Left N Metatarsal, Right P Metatarsal, Left Q Toe Phalanx, Right R Toe Phalanx, Left	0 Open 3 Percutaneous 4 Percutaneous endoscopic X External	4 Internal fixation device 5 External fixation device 7 Autologous tissue substitute J Synthetic substitute K Nonautologous tissue substitute	Z No qualifier
Y Lower Bone	0 Open 3 Percutaneous 4 Percutaneous endoscopic X External	0 Drainage device M Bone growth stimulator	Z No qualifier

542

Educational Annotations | R – Upper Joints

Body System Specific Educational Annotations for the Upper Joints include:
- Anatomy and Physiology Review
- Anatomical Illustrations
- Definitions of Common Procedures
- AHA Coding Clinic® Reference Notations
- Body Part Key Listings
- Device Key Listings
- Device Aggregation Table Listings
- Coding Notes

Anatomy and Physiology Review of Upper Joints

BODY PART VALUES – R - UPPER JOINTS

Acromioclavicular Joint – The joint formed between the acromion portion of the scapula and the distal end of the clavicle.

Carpal Joint – A complex collection of joints formed by the interconnection of the 8 carpal bones in the hand.

Cervical Vertebral Disc – The disc-shaped fibrocartilage pad between the cervical spine vertebral bodies comprised of a tough outer portion (annulus fibrosus) and a gel-like inner portion (nucleus pulposus).

Cervical Vertebral Joint – The synovial and cartilaginous joints connecting the vertebra of the cervical spine.

Cervicothoracic Vertebral Disc – The disc-shaped fibrocartilage pad between the C7 vertebral body of the cervical spine and the T1 vertebral body of the thoracic spine comprised of a tough outer portion (annulus fibrosus) and a gel-like inner portion (nucleus pulposus).

Cervicothoracic Vertebral Joint – The synovial and cartilaginous joints connecting the C7 vertebra of the cervical spine and the T1 vertebra of the thoracic spine.

Elbow Joint – A hinge joint between the humerus in the upper arm and the radius and ulna in the forearm.

Finger Phalangeal Joint – Any of 9 hinge joints in the fingers between the proximal and intermediate phalanges (PIP), and the intermediate and distal phalanges (DIP). The thumb has only two phalanges and therefore only one phalangeal joint.

Metacarpocarpal Joint – Any of the 5 joints in the hand that articulate the distal row of carpal bones and the proximal bases of the five metacarpal bones.

Metacarpophalangeal Joint – Any of 5 condyloid joints (except the hinge joint of the thumb) in the hand that articulate the distal heads of the five metacarpal bones and the proximal phalanx of each finger.

Occipital-cervical Joint – The joint formed between the C1 vertebra and the base of the skull (occipital bone).

Shoulder Joint – A multiaxial ball-and-socket joint (also known as the glenohumeral joint) between the head of the humerus and the rounded depression (glenoid fossa) of the scapula.

Sternoclavicular Joint – The joint formed between the upper portion of the sternum and the medial end of the clavicle.

Temporomandibular Joint – The joint formed between the mandible and temporal bone.

Thoracic Vertebral Disc – The disc-shaped fibrocartilage pad between the thoracic spine vertebral bodies comprised of a tough outer portion (annulus fibrosus) and a gel-like inner portion (nucleus pulposus).

Thoracic Vertebral Joint – The synovial and cartilaginous joints connecting the vertebra of the thoracic spine.

Thoracolumbar Vertebral Disc – The disc-shaped fibrocartilage pad between the T12 vertebral body of the thoracic spine and the L1 vertebral body of the lumbar spine comprised of a tough outer portion (annulus fibrosus) and a gel-like inner portion (nucleus pulposus).

Thoracolumbar Vertebral Joint – The synovial and cartilaginous joints connecting the T12 vertebra of the thoracic spine and the L1 vertebra of the lumbar spine.

Upper Joint – Any of the joints designated in the Upper Joints PCS Body System.

Wrist Joint – A pivot joint between the distal radius and the carpus.

Educational Annotations | R – Upper Joints

MEDICAL AND SURGICAL SECTION – 2016 ICD-10-PCS

Anatomical Illustrations of Upper Joints

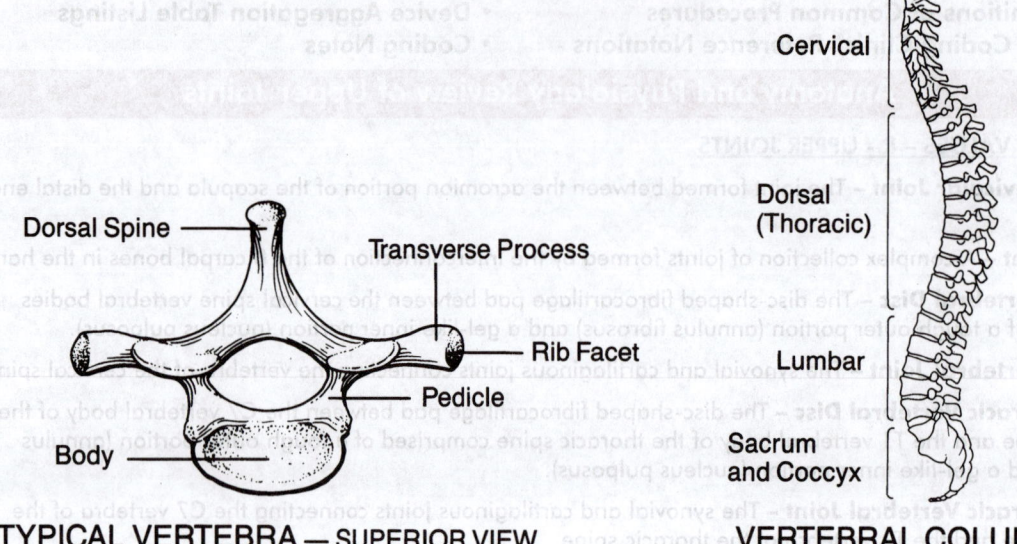

TYPICAL VERTEBRA — SUPERIOR VIEW (labels: Dorsal Spine, Transverse Process, Rib Facet, Pedicle, Body)

VERTEBRAL COLUMN (labels: Cervical, Dorsal (Thoracic), Lumbar, Sacrum and Coccyx)

Definitions of Common Procedures of Upper Joints

Arthroscopy – The surgical visualization and examination of a joint using an endoscope and often the approach used for joint procedures.

Cervical interbody spinal fusion – The permanent surgical joining of two or more cervical vertebrae together using bone graft placed between the intervertebral space after the disc(s) have been removed and using metal or plastic cage to support the spine while the bone graft hardens.

Cervical spinal fusion – The permanent surgical joining of two or more cervical vertebrae together using a bone graft and immobilization by using plates, rods, screws, and/or wires.

Discectomy – The surgical removal of all (total) or a portion of an intervertebral disc.

Reverse total shoulder arthroplasty – The surgical replacement of the shoulder joint by reversing the cup and head replacement. The cup is placed onto the humerus and the ball is placed in the socket. This procedure is done for patients with severe rotator cuff damage.

Total shoulder arthroplasty – The surgical replacement of the shoulder joint socket (glenoid) cup and humeral head in the normal anatomical configuration.

Type 2 SLAP (superior labral tear from anterior to posterior) repair – The surgical repair of the glenoid labrum of the shoulder joint.

Educational Annotations | R – Upper Joints

AHA Coding Clinic® Reference Notations of Upper Joints

ROOT OPERATION SPECIFIC - R - UPPER JOINTS
CHANGE - 2
DESTRUCTION - 5
DRAINAGE - 9
EXCISION - B
    Spinal fusion with discectomy .... AHA 14:2Q:p6
EXTIRPATION - C
FUSION - G
    Components in fusion procedures included in Fusion root operation .... AHA 14:3Q:p30
    Fusion of cervicothoracic vertebral joint with interbody fusion device .... AHA 13:1Q:p29
    .... AHA 14:2Q:p7
    Fusion of multiple vertebral joints .... AHA 13:1Q:p21
INSERTION - H
INSPECTION - J
RELEASE - N
    Release of shoulder joint .... AHA 15:2Q:p23
    Subacromial and rotator cuff decompression .... AHA 15:2Q:p22
REMOVAL - P
REPAIR - Q
REPLACEMENT - R
    Reverse total shoulder arthroplasty .... AHA 15:1Q:p27
REPOSITION - S
    Manipulation of radioulnar joint dislocation .... AHA 14:4Q:p32
    Reposition of carpal joint .... AHA 14:3Q:p33
    Tongs used to stabilize cervical fracture .... AHA 13:2Q:p39
        Official Correction of 13:2Q:p39 .... AHA 15:2Q:p34
RESECTION - T
    Spinal fusion with total discectomy .... AHA 14:2Q:p7
SUPPLEMENT - U
REVISION - W

Body Part Key Listings of Upper Joints

See also Body Part Key in Appendix C

Atlantoaxial joint	*use* Cervical Vertebral Joint
Carpometacarpal (CMC) joint	*use* Metacarpocarpal Joint, Left/Right
Cervical facet joint	*use* Cervical Vertebral Joint(s)
Cervicothoracic facet joint	*use* Cervicothoracic Vertebral Joint
Costotransverse joint	*use* Thoracic Vertebral Joint
Costovertebral joint	*use* Thoracic Vertebral Joint
Distal humerus, involving joint	*use* Elbow Joint, Left/Right
Distal radioulnar joint	*use* Wrist Joint, Left/Right
Glenohumeral joint	*use* Shoulder Joint, Left/Right
Glenoid ligament (labrum)	*use* Shoulder Joint, Left/Right
Humeroradial joint	*use* Elbow Joint, Left/Right
Humeroulnar joint	*use* Elbow Joint, Left/Right
Intercarpal joint	*use* Carpal Joint, Left/Right
Interphalangeal (IP) joint	*use* Finger Phalangeal Joint, Left/Right
Midcarpal joint	*use* Carpal Joint, Left/Right
Proximal radioulnar joint	*use* Elbow Joint, Left/Right
Radiocarpal joint	*use* Wrist Joint, Left/Right
Thoracic facet joint	*use* Thoracic Vertebral Joint
Thoracolumbar facet joint	*use* Thoracolumbar Vertebral Joint

Educational Annotations | R – Upper Joints

Device Key Listings of Upper Joints

See also Device Key in Appendix D

Autograft	*use* Autologous Tissue Substitute
BAK/C® Interbody Cervical Fusion System	*use* Interbody Fusion Device in Upper Joints
BRYAN® Cervical Disc System	*use* Synthetic Substitute
Delta III Reverse shoulder prosthesis	*use* Synthetic Substitute, Reverse Ball and Socket for Replacement in Upper Joints
Dynesys® Dynamic Stabilization System	*use* Spinal Stabilization Device, Pedicle-Based for Insertion in Upper Joints, Lower Joints
External fixator	*use* External Fixation Device in Head and Facial Bones, Upper Bones, Lower Bones, Upper Joints, Lower Joints
Facet replacement spinal stabilization device	*use* Spinal Stabilization Device, Facet Replacement for Insertion in Upper Joints, Lower Joints
Fusion screw (compression) (lag) (locking)	*use* Internal Fixation Device in Upper Joints, Lower Joints
Interbody fusion (spine) cage	*use* Interbody Fusion Device in Upper Joints, Lower Joints
Interspinous process spinal stabilization device	*use* Spinal Stabilization Device, Interspinous Process for Insertion in Upper Joints, Lower Joints
Joint fixation plate	*use* Internal Fixation Device in Upper Joints, Lower Joints
Joint spacer (antibiotic)	*use* Spacer in Upper Joints, Lower Joints
Kirschner wire (K-wire)	*use* Internal Fixation Device in Head and Facial Bones, Upper Bones, Lower Bones, Upper Joints, Lower Joints
Pedicle-based dynamic stabilization device	*use* Spinal Stabilization Device, Pedicle-Based for Insertion in Upper Joints, Lower Joints
Polymethylmethacrylate (PMMA)	*use* Synthetic Substitute
PRESTIGE® Cervical Disc	*use* Synthetic Substitute
Prodisc-C	*use* Synthetic Substitute
Reverse® Shoulder Prosthesis	*use* Synthetic Substitute, Reverse Ball and Socket for Replacement in Upper Joints
Tissue bank graft	*use* Nonautologous Tissue Substitute
X-STOP® Spacer	*use* Spinal Stabilization Device, Interspinous Process for Insertion in Upper Joints, Lower Joints

Device Aggregation Table Listings of Upper Joints

See also Device Aggregation Table in Appendix E

Specific Device	For Operation	In Body System	General Device	
Spinal Stabilization Device, Facet Replacement	Insertion	Upper Joints	4	Internal Fixation Device
Spinal Stabilization Device, Interspinous Process	Insertion	Upper Joints	4	Internal Fixation Device
Spinal Stabilization Device, Pedicle-Based	Insertion	Upper Joints	4	Internal Fixation Device

Educational Annotations | R – Upper Joints

Coding Notes of Upper Joints

Body System Relevant Coding Guidelines

Fusion procedures of the spine

B3.10a
The body part coded for a spinal vertebral joint(s) rendered immobile by a spinal fusion procedure is classified by the level of the spine (e.g. thoracic). There are distinct body part values for a single vertebral joint and for multiple vertebral joints at each spinal level.
Example: Body part values specify Lumbar Vertebral Joint, Lumbar Vertebral Joints, 2 or More and Lumbosacral Vertebral Joint.

B3.10b
If multiple vertebral joints are fused, a separate procedure is coded for each vertebral joint that uses a different device and/or qualifier.
Example: Fusion of lumbar vertebral joint, posterior approach, anterior column and fusion of lumbar vertebral joint, posterior approach, posterior column are coded separately.

B3.10c
Combinations of devices and materials are often used on a vertebral joint to render the joint immobile. When combinations of devices are used on the same vertebral joint, the device value coded for the procedure is as follows:
- If an interbody fusion device is used to render the joint immobile (alone or containing other material like bone graft), the procedure is coded with the device value Interbody Fusion Device
- If bone graft is the only device used to render the joint immobile, the procedure is coded with the device value Nonautologous Tissue Substitute or Autologous Tissue Substitute
- If a mixture of autologous and nonautologous bone graft (with or without biological or synthetic extenders or binders) is used to render the joint immobile, code the procedure with the device value Autologous Tissue Substitute

Examples: Fusion of a vertebral joint using a cage style interbody fusion device containing morsellized bone graft is coded to the device Interbody Fusion Device.
Fusion of a vertebral joint using a bone dowel interbody fusion device made of cadaver bone and packed with a mixture of local morsellized bone and demineralized bone matrix is coded to the device Interbody Fusion Device.
Fusion of a vertebral joint using both autologous bone graft and bone bank bone graft is coded to the device Autologous Tissue Substitute.

Tendons, ligaments, bursae and fascia near a joint

B4.5
Procedures performed on tendons, ligaments, bursae and fascia supporting a joint are coded to the body part in the respective body system that is the focus of the procedure. Procedures performed on joint structures themselves are coded to the body part in the joint body systems.
Example: Repair of the anterior cruciate ligament of the knee is coded to the knee bursae and ligament body part in the bursae and ligaments body system. Knee arthroscopy with shaving of articular cartilage is coded to the knee joint body part in the Lower Joints body system.

Body System Specific PCS Reference Manual Exercises

PCS CODE	R – UPPER JOINTS EXERCISES
0RGP04Z	Radiocarpal fusion of left hand with internal fixation, open.
0RGQ0KZ	Intercarpal fusion of right hand with bone bank bone graft, open.
0RJJ4ZZ	Diagnostic arthroscopy of right shoulder.
0RNJXZZ	Manual rupture of right shoulder joint adhesions under general anesthesia.

Educational Annotations

R – Upper Joints

NOTES

R – UPPER JOINTS

0R2 CHANGE

DEVICE GROUP: Change, Insertion, Removal, Replacement, Revision, Supplement
Root Operations that always involve a device.

- 1ST – **0** Medical and Surgical
- 2ND – **R** Upper Joints
- 3RD – **2 CHANGE**

EXAMPLE: Exchange drain tube | CMS Ex: Changing urinary catheter

CHANGE: Taking out or off a device from a body part and putting back an identical or similar device in or on the same body part without cutting or puncturing the skin or a mucous membrane.

EXPLANATION: ALL Changes use EXTERNAL approach only …

Body Part – 4TH	Approach – 5TH	Device – 6TH	Qualifier – 7TH
Y Upper Joint	X External	0 Drainage device Y Other device	Z No qualifier

0R5 DESTRUCTION

EXCISION GROUP: Excision, Resection, Destruction, (Extraction), (Detachment)
Root Operations that take out some or all of a body part.

- 1ST – **0** Medical and Surgical
- 2ND – **R** Upper Joints
- 3RD – **5 DESTRUCTION**

EXAMPLE: Radiofrequency ablation | CMS Ex: Fulguration polyp

DESTRUCTION: Physical eradication of all or a portion of a body part by the direct use of energy, force, or a destructive agent.

EXPLANATION: None of the body part is physically taken out

Body Part – 4TH	Approach – 5TH	Device – 6TH	Qualifier – 7TH
0 Occipital-cervical Joint 1 Cervical Vertebral Joint 3 Cervical Vertebral Disc 4 Cervicothoracic Vertebral Joint 5 Cervicothoracic Vertebral Disc 6 Thoracic Vertebral Joint 9 Thoracic Vertebral Disc A Thoracolumbar Vertebral Joint B Thoracolumbar Vertebral Disc C Temporomandibular Joint, Right D Temporomandibular Joint, Left E Sternoclavicular Joint, Right F Sternoclavicular Joint, Left G Acromioclavicular Joint, Right H Acromioclavicular Joint, Left J Shoulder Joint, Right K Shoulder Joint, Left L Elbow Joint, Right M Elbow Joint, Left N Wrist Joint, Right P Wrist Joint, Left Q Carpal Joint, Right R Carpal Joint, Left S Metacarpocarpal Joint, Right T Metacarpocarpal Joint, Left U Metacarpophalangeal Joint, Right V Metacarpophalangeal Joint, Left W Finger Phalangeal Joint, Right X Finger Phalangeal Joint, Left	0 Open 3 Percutaneous 4 Percutaneous endoscopic	Z No device	Z No qualifier

0R9

MEDICAL AND SURGICAL SECTION – 2016 ICD-10-PCS

DRAINAGE GROUP: Drainage, Extirpation, (Fragmentation)
Root Operations that take out solids/fluids/gases from a body part.

- 1ST – **0** Medical and Surgical
- 2ND – **R** Upper Joints
- 3RD – **9 DRAINAGE**

EXAMPLE: Aspiration elbow joint   CMS Ex: Thoracentesis

DRAINAGE: Taking or letting out fluids and/or gases from a body part.

EXPLANATION: Qualifier "X Diagnostic" indicates biopsy …

Body Part – 4TH	Approach – 5TH	Device – 6TH	Qualifier – 7TH
0 Occipital-cervical Joint	0 Open	0 Drainage device	Z No qualifier
1 Cervical Vertebral Joint	3 Percutaneous		
3 Cervical Vertebral Disc	4 Percutaneous endoscopic		
4 Cervicothoracic Vertebral Joint			
5 Cervicothoracic Vertebral Disc			
6 Thoracic Vertebral Joint			
9 Thoracic Vertebral Disc			
A Thoracolumbar Vertebral Joint			
B Thoracolumbar Vertebral Disc			
C Temporomandibular Joint, Right			
D Temporomandibular Joint, Left			
E Sternoclavicular Joint, Right			
F Sternoclavicular Joint, Left			
G Acromioclavicular Joint, Right			
H Acromioclavicular Joint, Left			
J Shoulder Joint, Right			
K Shoulder Joint, Left			
L Elbow Joint, Right			
M Elbow Joint, Left			
N Wrist Joint, Right			
P Wrist Joint, Left			
Q Carpal Joint, Right			
R Carpal Joint, Left			
S Metacarpocarpal Joint, Right			
T Metacarpocarpal Joint, Left			
U Metacarpophalangeal Joint, Right			
V Metacarpophalangeal Joint, Left			
W Finger Phalangeal Joint, Right			
X Finger Phalangeal Joint, Left			

continued ⇨

0 R 9 DRAINAGE – continued

Body Part – 4ᵀᴴ	Approach – 5ᵀᴴ	Device – 6ᵀᴴ	Qualifier – 7ᵀᴴ
0 Occipital-cervical Joint 1 Cervical Vertebral Joint 3 Cervical Vertebral Disc 4 Cervicothoracic Vertebral Joint 5 Cervicothoracic Vertebral Disc 6 Thoracic Vertebral Joint 9 Thoracic Vertebral Disc A Thoracolumbar Vertebral Joint B Thoracolumbar Vertebral Disc C Temporomandibular Joint, Right D Temporomandibular Joint, Left E Sternoclavicular Joint, Right F Sternoclavicular Joint, Left G Acromioclavicular Joint, Right H Acromioclavicular Joint, Left J Shoulder Joint, Right K Shoulder Joint, Left L Elbow Joint, Right M Elbow Joint, Left N Wrist Joint, Right P Wrist Joint, Left Q Carpal Joint, Right R Carpal Joint, Left S Metacarpocarpal Joint, Right T Metacarpocarpal Joint, Left U Metacarpophalangeal Joint, Right V Metacarpophalangeal Joint, Left W Finger Phalangeal Joint, Right X Finger Phalangeal Joint, Left	0 Open 3 Percutaneous 4 Percutaneous endoscopic	Z No device	X Diagnostic Z No qualifier

0RB — MEDICAL AND SURGICAL SECTION – 2016 ICD-10-PCS

EXCISION GROUP: Excision, Resection, Destruction, (Extraction), (Detachment)
Root Operations that take out some or all of a body part.

EXAMPLE: Partial cervical discectomy **CMS Ex:** Liver biopsy

- 1ST – **0** Medical and Surgical
- 2ND – **R** Upper Joints
- 3RD – **B** EXCISION

EXCISION: Cutting out or off, without replacement, a portion of a body part.

EXPLANATION: Qualifier "X Diagnostic" indicates biopsy ...

Body Part – 4TH	Approach – 5TH	Device – 6TH	Qualifier – 7TH
0 Occipital-cervical Joint	0 Open	Z No device	X Diagnostic
1 Cervical Vertebral Joint	3 Percutaneous		Z No qualifier
3 Cervical Vertebral Disc	4 Percutaneous endoscopic		
4 Cervicothoracic Vertebral Joint			
5 Cervicothoracic Vertebral Disc			
6 Thoracic Vertebral Joint			
9 Thoracic Vertebral Disc			
A Thoracolumbar Vertebral Joint			
B Thoracolumbar Vertebral Disc			
C Temporomandibular Joint, Right			
D Temporomandibular Joint, Left			
E Sternoclavicular Joint, Right			
F Sternoclavicular Joint, Left			
G Acromioclavicular Joint, Right			
H Acromioclavicular Joint, Left			
J Shoulder Joint, Right			
K Shoulder Joint, Left			
L Elbow Joint, Right			
M Elbow Joint, Left			
N Wrist Joint, Right			
P Wrist Joint, Left			
Q Carpal Joint, Right			
R Carpal Joint, Left			
S Metacarpocarpal Joint, Right			
T Metacarpocarpal Joint, Left			
U Metacarpophalangeal Joint, Right			
V Metacarpophalangeal Joint, Left			
W Finger Phalangeal Joint, Right			
X Finger Phalangeal Joint, Left			

R – UPPER JOINTS 0RC

DRAINAGE GROUP: Drainage, Extirpation, (Fragmentation)
Root Operations that take out solids/fluids/gases from a body part.

1ST - **0** Medical and Surgical	EXAMPLE: Removal loose bodies elbow CMS Ex: Choledocholithotomy
2ND - **R** Upper Joints	**EXTIRPATION:** Taking or cutting out solid matter from a body part.
3RD - **C EXTIRPATION**	EXPLANATION: Abnormal byproduct or foreign body ...

Body Part – 4TH	Approach – 5TH	Device – 6TH	Qualifier – 7TH
0 Occipital-cervical Joint	0 Open	Z No device	Z No qualifier
1 Cervical Vertebral Joint	3 Percutaneous		
3 Cervical Vertebral Disc	4 Percutaneous endoscopic		
4 Cervicothoracic Vertebral Joint			
5 Cervicothoracic Vertebral Disc			
6 Thoracic Vertebral Joint			
9 Thoracic Vertebral Disc			
A Thoracolumbar Vertebral Joint			
B Thoracolumbar Vertebral Disc			
C Temporomandibular Joint, Right			
D Temporomandibular Joint, Left			
E Sternoclavicular Joint, Right			
F Sternoclavicular Joint, Left			
G Acromioclavicular Joint, Right			
H Acromioclavicular Joint, Left			
J Shoulder Joint, Right			
K Shoulder Joint, Left			
L Elbow Joint, Right			
M Elbow Joint, Left			
N Wrist Joint, Right			
P Wrist Joint, Left			
Q Carpal Joint, Right			
R Carpal Joint, Left			
S Metacarpocarpal Joint, Right			
T Metacarpocarpal Joint, Left			
U Metacarpophalangeal Joint, Right			
V Metacarpophalangeal Joint, Left			
W Finger Phalangeal Joint, Right			
X Finger Phalangeal Joint, Left			

0RG MEDICAL AND SURGICAL SECTION – 2016 ICD-10-PCS

OTHER OBJECTIVES GROUP: (Alteration), (Creation), **Fusion**
Root Operations that define other objectives.

- 1ST – **0** Medical and Surgical
- 2ND – **R** Upper Joints
- 3RD – **G FUSION**

EXAMPLE: C3-C5 spinal fusion   CMS Ex: Spinal fusion

FUSION: Joining together portions of an articular body part, rendering the articular body part immobile.

EXPLANATION: Use of fixation device, graft, or other means ...

Body Part – 4TH	Approach – 5TH	Device – 6TH	Qualifier – 7TH
0 Occipital-cervical Joint 1 Cervical Vertebral Joint 2 Cervical Vertebral Joints, 2 or more 4 Cervicothoracic Vertebral Joint 6 Thoracic Vertebral Joint 7 Thoracic Vertebral Joints, 2 to 7 8 Thoracic Vertebral Joints, 8 or more A Thoracolumbar Vertebral Joint	0 Open 3 Percutaneous 4 Percutaneous endoscopic	7 Autologous tissue substitute A Interbody fusion device J Synthetic substitute K Nonautologous tissue substitute Z No device	0 Anterior approach, anterior column 1 Posterior approach, posterior column J Posterior approach, anterior column
C Temporomandibular Joint, Right D Temporomandibular Joint, Left E Sternoclavicular Joint, Right F Sternoclavicular Joint, Left G Acromioclavicular Joint, Right H Acromioclavicular Joint, Left J Shoulder Joint, Right K Shoulder Joint, Left	0 Open 3 Percutaneous 4 Percutaneous endoscopic	4 Internal fixation device 7 Autologous tissue substitute J Synthetic substitute K Nonautologous tissue substitute Z No device	Z No qualifier
L Elbow Joint, Right M Elbow Joint, Left N Wrist Joint, Right P Wrist Joint, Left Q Carpal Joint, Right R Carpal Joint, Left S Metacarpocarpal Joint, Right T Metacarpocarpal Joint, Left U Metacarpophalangeal Joint, Right V Metacarpophalangeal Joint, Left W Finger Phalangeal Joint, Right X Finger Phalangeal Joint, Left	0 Open 3 Percutaneous 4 Percutaneous endoscopic	4 Internal fixation device 5 External fixation device 7 Autologous tissue substitute J Synthetic substitute K Nonautologous tissue substitute Z No device	Z No qualifier

R – UPPER JOINTS — 0RH

DEVICE GROUP: Change, Insertion, Removal, Replacement, Revision, Supplement
Root Operations that always involve a device.

1ST - 0 Medical and Surgical
2ND - R Upper Joints
3RD - H INSERTION

EXAMPLE: Implantation joint spacer **CMS Ex:** Central venous catheter

INSERTION: Putting in a nonbiological appliance that monitors, assists, performs, or prevents a physiological function but does not physically take the place of a body part.

EXPLANATION: None

Body Part – 4TH	Approach – 5TH	Device – 6TH	Qualifier – 7TH
0 Occipital-cervical Joint 1 Cervical Vertebral Joint 4 Cervicothoracic Vertebral Joint 6 Thoracic Vertebral Joint A Thoracolumbar Vertebral Joint	0 Open 3 Percutaneous 4 Percutaneous endoscopic	3 Infusion device 4 Internal fixation device 8 Spacer B Spinal stabilization device, interspinous process C Spinal stabilization device, pedicle-based D Spinal stabilization device, facet replacement	Z No qualifier
3 Cervical Vertebral Disc 5 Cervicothoracic Vertebral Disc 9 Thoracic Vertebral Disc B Thoracolumbar Vertebral Disc	0 Open 3 Percutaneous 4 Percutaneous endoscopic	3 Infusion device	Z No qualifier
C Temporomandibular Joint, Right D Temporomandibular Joint, Left E Sternoclavicular Joint, Right F Sternoclavicular Joint, Left G Acromioclavicular Joint, Right H Acromioclavicular Joint, Left J Shoulder Joint, Right K Shoulder Joint, Left	0 Open 3 Percutaneous 4 Percutaneous endoscopic	3 Infusion device 4 Internal fixation device 8 Spacer	Z No qualifier
L Elbow Joint, Right M Elbow Joint, Left N Wrist Joint, Right P Wrist Joint, Left Q Carpal Joint, Right R Carpal Joint, Left S Metacarpocarpal Joint, Right T Metacarpocarpal Joint, Left U Metacarpophalangeal Joint, Right V Metacarpophalangeal Joint, Left W Finger Phalangeal Joint, Right X Finger Phalangeal Joint, Left	0 Open 3 Percutaneous 4 Percutaneous endoscopic	3 Infusion device 4 Internal fixation device 5 External fixation device 8 Spacer	Z No qualifier

0RJ

MEDICAL AND SURGICAL SECTION – 2016 ICD-10-PCS

EXAMINATION GROUP: Inspection, (Map)
Root Operations involving examination only.

- 1ST – **0** Medical and Surgical
- 2ND – **R** Upper Joints
- 3RD – **J** INSPECTION

EXAMPLE: Diagnostic arthroscopy shoulder
CMS Ex: Colonoscopy

INSPECTION: Visually and/or manually exploring a body part.

EXPLANATION: Direct or instrumental visualization ...

Body Part – 4TH	Approach – 5TH	Device – 6TH	Qualifier – 7TH
0 Occipital-cervical Joint	0 Open	Z No device	Z No qualifier
1 Cervical Vertebral Joint	3 Percutaneous		
3 Cervical Vertebral Disc	4 Percutaneous endoscopic		
4 Cervicothoracic Vertebral Joint	X External		
5 Cervicothoracic Vertebral Disc			
6 Thoracic Vertebral Joint			
9 Thoracic Vertebral Disc			
A Thoracolumbar Vertebral Joint			
B Thoracolumbar Vertebral Disc			
C Temporomandibular Joint, Right			
D Temporomandibular Joint, Left			
E Sternoclavicular Joint, Right			
F Sternoclavicular Joint, Left			
G Acromioclavicular Joint, Right			
H Acromioclavicular Joint, Left			
J Shoulder Joint, Right			
K Shoulder Joint, Left			
L Elbow Joint, Right			
M Elbow Joint, Left			
N Wrist Joint, Right			
P Wrist Joint, Left			
Q Carpal Joint, Right			
R Carpal Joint, Left			
S Metacarpocarpal Joint, Right			
T Metacarpocarpal Joint, Left			
U Metacarpophalangeal Joint, Right			
V Metacarpophalangeal Joint, Left			
W Finger Phalangeal Joint, Right			
X Finger Phalangeal Joint, Left			

UPPER JOINTS 0RJ

0RN

R – UPPER JOINTS

DIVISION GROUP: (Division), Release
Root Operations involving cutting or separation only.

1ST - 0	Medical and Surgical
2ND - R	Upper Joints
3RD - N	**RELEASE**

EXAMPLE: Manual rupture joint adhesions | **CMS Ex:** Carpal tunnel release

RELEASE: Freeing a body part from an abnormal physical constraint by cutting or by the use of force.

EXPLANATION: None of the body part is taken out ...

Body Part – 4TH	Approach – 5TH	Device – 6TH	Qualifier – 7TH
0 Occipital-cervical Joint	0 Open	Z No device	Z No qualifier
1 Cervical Vertebral Joint	3 Percutaneous		
3 Cervical Vertebral Disc	4 Percutaneous endoscopic		
4 Cervicothoracic Vertebral Joint	X External		
5 Cervicothoracic Vertebral Disc			
6 Thoracic Vertebral Joint			
9 Thoracic Vertebral Disc			
A Thoracolumbar Vertebral Joint			
B Thoracolumbar Vertebral Disc			
C Temporomandibular Joint, Right			
D Temporomandibular Joint, Left			
E Sternoclavicular Joint, Right			
F Sternoclavicular Joint, Left			
G Acromioclavicular Joint, Right			
H Acromioclavicular Joint, Left			
J Shoulder Joint, Right			
K Shoulder Joint, Left			
L Elbow Joint, Right			
M Elbow Joint, Left			
N Wrist Joint, Right			
P Wrist Joint, Left			
Q Carpal Joint, Right			
R Carpal Joint, Left			
S Metacarpocarpal Joint, Right			
T Metacarpocarpal Joint, Left			
U Metacarpophalangeal Joint, Right			
V Metacarpophalangeal Joint, Left			
W Finger Phalangeal Joint, Right			
X Finger Phalangeal Joint, Left			

UPPER JOINTS 0RN

0RP

MEDICAL AND SURGICAL SECTION – 2016 ICD-10-PCS

DEVICE GROUP: Change, Insertion, Removal, Replacement, Revision, Supplement
Root Operations that always involve a device.

1ST – 0	Medical and Surgical
2ND – R	Upper Joints
3RD – P	REMOVAL

EXAMPLE: Removal fixation device   CMS Ex: Chest tube removal

REMOVAL: Taking out or off a device from a body part.

EXPLANATION: Removal device without reinsertion ...

Body Part – 4TH	Approach – 5TH	Device – 6TH	Qualifier – 7TH
0 Occipital-cervical Joint 1 Cervical Vertebral Joint 4 Cervicothoracic Vertebral Joint 6 Thoracic Vertebral Joint A Thoracolumbar Vertebral Joint	0 Open 3 Percutaneous 4 Percutaneous endoscopic	0 Drainage device 3 Infusion device 4 Internal fixation device 7 Autologous tissue substitute 8 Spacer A Interbody fusion device J Synthetic substitute K Nonautologous tissue substitute	Z No qualifier
0 Occipital-cervical Joint 1 Cervical Vertebral Joint 4 Cervicothoracic Vertebral Joint 6 Thoracic Vertebral Joint A Thoracolumbar Vertebral Joint	X External	0 Drainage device 3 Infusion device 4 Internal fixation device	Z No qualifier
3 Cervical Vertebral Disc 5 Cervicothoracic Vertebral Disc 9 Thoracic Vertebral Disc B Thoracolumbar Vertebral Disc	0 Open 3 Percutaneous 4 Percutaneous endoscopic	0 Drainage device 3 Infusion device 7 Autologous tissue substitute J Synthetic substitute K Nonautologous tissue substitute	Z No qualifier
3 Cervical Vertebral Disc 5 Cervicothoracic Vertebral Disc 9 Thoracic Vertebral Disc B Thoracolumbar Vertebral Disc	X External	0 Drainage device 3 Infusion device	Z No qualifier

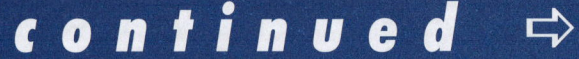

continued ⇨

0RP REMOVAL – continued

Body Part – 4TH	Approach – 5TH	Device – 6TH	Qualifier – 7TH
C Temporomandibular Joint, Right D Temporomandibular Joint, Left E Sternoclavicular Joint, Right F Sternoclavicular Joint, Left G Acromioclavicular Joint, Right H Acromioclavicular Joint, Left J Shoulder Joint, Right K Shoulder Joint, Left	0 Open 3 Percutaneous 4 Percutaneous endoscopic	0 Drainage device 3 Infusion device 4 Internal fixation device 7 Autologous tissue substitute 8 Spacer J Synthetic substitute K Nonautologous tissue substitute	Z No qualifier
C Temporomandibular Joint, Right D Temporomandibular Joint, Left E Sternoclavicular Joint, Right F Sternoclavicular Joint, Left G Acromioclavicular Joint, Right H Acromioclavicular Joint, Left J Shoulder Joint, Right K Shoulder Joint, Left	X External	0 Drainage device 3 Infusion device 4 Internal fixation device	Z No qualifier
L Elbow Joint, Right M Elbow Joint, Left N Wrist Joint, Right P Wrist Joint, Left Q Carpal Joint, Right R Carpal Joint, Left S Metacarpocarpal Joint, Right T Metacarpocarpal Joint, Left U Metacarpophalangeal Joint, Right V Metacarpophalangeal Joint, Left W Finger Phalangeal Joint, Right X Finger Phalangeal Joint, Left	0 Open 3 Percutaneous 4 Percutaneous endoscopic	0 Drainage device 3 Infusion device 4 Internal fixation device 5 External fixation device 7 Autologous tissue substitute 8 Spacer J Synthetic dubstitute K Nonautologous tissue substitute	Z No qualifier
L Elbow Joint, Right M Elbow Joint, Left N Wrist Joint, Right P Wrist Joint, Left Q Carpal Joint, Right R Carpal Joint, Left S Metacarpocarpal Joint, Right T Metacarpocarpal Joint, Left U Metacarpophalangeal Joint, Right V Metacarpophalangeal Joint, Left W Finger Phalangeal Joint, Right X Finger Phalangeal Joint, Left	X External	0 Drainage device 3 Infusion device 4 Internal fixation device 5 External fixation device	Z No qualifier

0RQ

OTHER REPAIRS GROUP: (Control), Repair
Root Operations that define other repairs.

1ST - 0 Medical and Surgical
2ND - R Upper Joints
3RD - Q REPAIR

EXAMPLE: Suture arthroplasty wrist   CMS Ex: Suture laceration

REPAIR: Restoring, to the extent possible, a body part to its normal anatomic structure and function.

EXPLANATION: Only when no other root operation applies ...

Body Part – 4TH	Approach – 5TH	Device – 6TH	Qualifier – 7TH
0 Occipital-cervical Joint	0 Open	Z No device	Z No qualifier
1 Cervical Vertebral Joint	3 Percutaneous		
3 Cervical Vertebral Disc	4 Percutaneous endoscopic		
4 Cervicothoracic Vertebral Joint	X External		
5 Cervicothoracic Vertebral Disc			
6 Thoracic Vertebral Joint			
9 Thoracic Vertebral Disc			
A Thoracolumbar Vertebral Joint			
B Thoracolumbar Vertebral Disc			
C Temporomandibular Joint, Right			
D Temporomandibular Joint, Left			
E Sternoclavicular Joint, Right			
F Sternoclavicular Joint, Left			
G Acromioclavicular Joint, Right			
H Acromioclavicular Joint, Left			
J Shoulder Joint, Right			
K Shoulder Joint, Left			
L Elbow Joint, Right			
M Elbow Joint, Left			
N Wrist Joint, Right			
P Wrist Joint, Left			
Q Carpal Joint, Right			
R Carpal Joint, Left			
S Metacarpocarpal Joint, Right			
T Metacarpocarpal Joint, Left			
U Metacarpophalangeal Joint, Right			
V Metacarpophalangeal Joint, Left			
W Finger Phalangeal Joint, Right			
X Finger Phalangeal Joint, Left			

R – UPPER JOINTS

0RR

DEVICE GROUP: Change, Insertion, Removal, Replacement, Revision, Supplement
Root Operations that always involve a device.

1ST - **0** Medical and Surgical
2ND - **R** Upper Joints
3RD - **R** REPLACEMENT

EXAMPLE: Reverse total shoulder arthroplasty | **CMS Ex:** Total hip

REPLACEMENT: Putting in or on a biological or synthetic material that physically takes the place and/or function of all or a portion of a body part.

EXPLANATION: Includes taking out body part, or eradication...

Body Part – 4TH	Approach – 5TH	Device – 6TH	Qualifier – 7TH
0 Occipital-cervical Joint 1 Cervical Vertebral Joint 3 Cervical Vertebral Disc 4 Cervicothoracic Vertebral Joint 5 Cervicothoracic Vertebral Disc 6 Thoracic Vertebral Joint 9 Thoracic Vertebral Disc A Thoracolumbar Vertebral Joint B Thoracolumbar Vertebral Disc C Temporomandibular Joint, Right D Temporomandibular Joint, Left E Sternoclavicular Joint, Right F Sternoclavicular Joint, Left G Acromioclavicular Joint, Right H Acromioclavicular Joint, Left L Elbow Joint, Right M Elbow Joint, Left N Wrist Joint, Right P Wrist Joint, Left Q Carpal Joint, Right R Carpal Joint, Left S Metacarpocarpal Joint, Right T Metacarpocarpal Joint, Left U Metacarpophalangeal Joint, Right V Metacarpophalangeal Joint, Left W Finger Phalangeal Joint, Right X Finger Phalangeal Joint, Left	0 Open	7 Autologous tissue substitute J Synthetic substitute K Nonautologous tissue substitute	Z No qualifier
J Shoulder Joint, Right K Shoulder Joint, Left	0 Open	0 Synthetic substitute, reverse ball and socket 7 Autologous tissue substitute K Nonautologous tissue substitute	Z No qualifier
J Shoulder Joint, Right K Shoulder Joint, Left	0 Open	J Synthetic substitute	6 Humeral Surface 7 Glenoid Surface Z No qualifier

0RS

MEDICAL AND SURGICAL SECTION – 2016 ICD-10-PCS

[2016.PCS]

MOVE GROUP: (Reattachment), **Reposition**, (Transfer), (Transplantation)
Root Operations that put in/put back or move some/all of a body part.

1ST – **0** Medical and Surgical	**EXAMPLE:** Closed reduction elbow joint	**CMS Ex:** Fracture reduction
2ND – **R** Upper Joints	**REPOSITION:** Moving to its normal location, or other suitable location, all or a portion of a body part.	
3RD – **S** REPOSITION	**EXPLANATION:** May or may not be cut to be moved ...	

Body Part – 4TH	Approach – 5TH	Device – 6TH	Qualifier – 7TH
0 Occipital-cervical Joint 1 Cervical Vertebral Joint 4 Cervicothoracic Vertebral Joint 6 Thoracic Vertebral Joint A Thoracolumbar Vertebral Joint C Temporomandibular Joint, Right D Temporomandibular Joint, Left E Sternoclavicular Joint, Right F Sternoclavicular Joint, Left G Acromioclavicular Joint, Right H Acromioclavicular Joint, Left J Shoulder Joint, Right K Shoulder Joint, Left	0 Open 3 Percutaneous 4 Percutaneous endoscopic X External	4 Internal fixation device Z No device	Z No qualifier
L Elbow Joint, Right M Elbow Joint, Left N Wrist Joint, Right P Wrist Joint, Left Q Carpal Joint, Right R Carpal Joint, Left S Metacarpocarpal Joint, Right T Metacarpocarpal Joint, Left U Metacarpophalangeal Joint, Right V Metacarpophalangeal Joint, Left W Finger Phalangeal Joint, Right X Finger Phalangeal Joint, Left	0 Open 3 Percutaneous 4 Percutaneous endoscopic X External	4 Internal fixation device 5 External fixation device Z No device	Z No qualifier

0RT

R – UPPER JOINTS

EXCISION GROUP: Excision, Resection, Destruction, (Extraction), (Detachment)
Root Operations that take out some or all of a body part.

1ST - **0** Medical and Surgical	**EXAMPLE:** Total cervical discectomy **CMS Ex:** Cholecystectomy
2ND - **R** Upper Joints	**RESECTION:** Cutting out or off, without replacement, all of a body part.
3RD - **T** RESECTION	**EXPLANATION:** None

Body Part – 4TH	Approach – 5TH	Device – 6TH	Qualifier – 7TH
3 Cervical Vertebral Disc	0 Open	Z No device	Z No qualifier
4 Cervicothoracic Vertebral Joint			
5 Cervicothoracic Vertebral Disc			
9 Thoracic Vertebral Disc			
B Thoracolumbar Vertebral Disc			
C Temporomandibular Joint, Right			
D Temporomandibular Joint, Left			
E Sternoclavicular Joint, Right			
F Sternoclavicular Joint, Left			
G Acromioclavicular Joint, Right			
H Acromioclavicular Joint, Left			
J Shoulder Joint, Right			
K Shoulder Joint, Left			
L Elbow Joint, Right			
M Elbow Joint, Left			
N Wrist Joint, Right			
P Wrist Joint, Left			
Q Carpal Joint, Right			
R Carpal Joint, Left			
S Metacarpocarpal Joint, Right			
T Metacarpocarpal Joint, Left			
U Metacarpophalangeal Joint, Right			
V Metacarpophalangeal Joint, Left			
W Finger Phalangeal Joint, Right			
X Finger Phalangeal Joint, Left			

UPPER JOINTS 0RT

0RU

MEDICAL AND SURGICAL SECTION – 2016 ICD-10-PCS

DEVICE GROUP: Change, Insertion, Removal, Replacement, Revision, Supplement
Root Operations that always involve a device.

1ST - 0	Medical and Surgical
2ND - R	Upper Joints
3RD - U	SUPPLEMENT

EXAMPLE: Shoulder joint resurfacing **CMS Ex:** Hernia repair with mesh

SUPPLEMENT: Putting in or on biological or synthetic material that physically reinforces and/or augments the function of a portion of a body part.

EXPLANATION: Biological material from same individual …

Body Part – 4TH	Approach – 5TH	Device – 6TH	Qualifier – 7TH
0 Occipital-cervical Joint	0 Open	7 Autologous tissue substitute	Z No qualifier
1 Cervical Vertebral Joint	3 Percutaneous	J Synthetic substitute	
3 Cervical Vertebral Disc	4 Percutaneous endoscopic	K Nonautologous tissue substitute	
4 Cervicothoracic Vertebral Joint			
5 Cervicothoracic Vertebral Disc			
6 Thoracic Vertebral Joint			
9 Thoracic Vertebral Disc			
A Thoracolumbar Vertebral Joint			
B Thoracolumbar Vertebral Disc			
C Temporomandibular Joint, Right			
D Temporomandibular Joint, Left			
E Sternoclavicular Joint, Right			
F Sternoclavicular Joint, Left			
G Acromioclavicular Joint, Right			
H Acromioclavicular Joint, Left			
J Shoulder Joint, Right			
K Shoulder Joint, Left			
L Elbow Joint, Right			
M Elbow Joint, Left			
N Wrist Joint, Right			
P Wrist Joint, Left			
Q Carpal Joint, Right			
R Carpal Joint, Left			
S Metacarpocarpal Joint, Right			
T Metacarpocarpal Joint, Left			
U Metacarpophalangeal Joint, Right			
V Metacarpophalangeal Joint, Left			
W Finger Phalangeal Joint, Right			
X Finger Phalangeal Joint, Left			

0RW — R – UPPER JOINTS

DEVICE GROUP: Change, Insertion, Removal, Replacement, Revision, Supplement
Root Operations that always involve a device.

1ST - 0	Medical and Surgical
2ND - R	Upper Joints
3RD - W	REVISION

EXAMPLE: Reposition joint spacer   CMS Ex: Adjustment pacemaker lead

REVISION: Correcting, to the extent possible, a portion of a malfunctioning device or the position of a displaced device.

EXPLANATION: May replace components of a device ...

Body Part – 4TH	Approach – 5TH	Device – 6TH	Qualifier – 7TH
0 Occipital-cervical Joint 1 Cervical Vertebral Joint 4 Cervicothoracic Vertebral Joint 6 Thoracic Vertebral Joint A Thoracolumbar Vertebral Joint	0 Open 3 Percutaneous 4 Percutaneous endoscopic X External	0 Drainage device 3 Infusion device 4 Internal fixation device 7 Autologous tissue substitute 8 Spacer A Interbody fusion device J Synthetic substitute K Nonautologous tissue substitute	Z No qualifier
3 Cervical Vertebral Disc 5 Cervicothoracic Vertebral Disc 9 Thoracic Vertebral Disc B Thoracolumbar Vertebral Disc	0 Open 3 Percutaneous 4 Percutaneous endoscopic X External	0 Drainage device 3 Infusion device 7 Autologous tissue substitute J Synthetic substitute K Nonautologous tissue substitute	Z No qualifier
C Temporomandibular Joint, Right D Temporomandibular Joint, Left E Sternoclavicular Joint, Right F Sternoclavicular Joint, Left G Acromioclavicular Joint, Right H Acromioclavicular Joint, Left J Shoulder Joint, Right K Shoulder Joint, Left	0 Open 3 Percutaneous 4 Percutaneous endoscopic X External	0 Drainage device 3 Infusion device 4 Internal fixation device 7 Autologous tissue substitute 8 Spacer J Synthetic substitute K Nonautologous tissue substitute	Z No qualifier
L Elbow Joint, Right M Elbow Joint, Left N Wrist Joint, Right P Wrist Joint, Left Q Carpal Joint, Right R Carpal Joint, Left S Metacarpocarpal Joint, Right T Metacarpocarpal Joint, Left U Metacarpophalangeal Joint, Right V Metacarpophalangeal Joint, Left W Finger Phalangeal Joint, Right X Finger Phalangeal Joint, Left	0 Open 3 Percutaneous 4 Percutaneous endoscopic X External	0 Drainage device 3 Infusion device 4 Internal fixation device 5 External fixation device 7 Autologous tissue substitute 8 Spacer J Synthetic substitute K Nonautologous tissue substitute	Z No qualifier

0R — MEDICAL AND SURGICAL SECTION – 2016 ICD-10-PCS

UPPER JOINTS

0 Medical and Surgical
R Upper Joints
W Revision: Correcting, to the extent possible, a portion of a malfunctioning device or the position of a displaced device

EXPLANATION: May include correction by taking out and/or putting back a portion of the device

EXAMPLE: Reposition of joint spacer

Body Part – 4	Approach – 5	Device – 6	Qualifier – 7
0 Occipital-cervical Joint 1 Cervical Vertebral Joint 2 Cervicothoracic Vertebral Joint 6 Thoracic Vertebral Joint A Thoracolumbar Vertebral Joint	0 Open 3 Percutaneous 4 Percutaneous Endoscopic X External	0 Drainage Device 3 Infusion Device 4 Internal Fixation Device 7 Autologous Tissue Substitute 8 Spacer A Interbody Fusion Device J Synthetic Substitute K Nonautologous Tissue Substitute	Z No Qualifier
3 Cervical Vertebral Disc 5 Cervicothoracic Vertebral Disc 9 Thoracic Vertebral Disc B Thoracolumbar Vertebral Disc	0 Open 3 Percutaneous 4 Percutaneous Endoscopic X External	0 Drainage Device 3 Infusion Device 7 Autologous Tissue Substitute J Synthetic Substitute K Nonautologous Tissue Substitute	Z No Qualifier
C Temporomandibular Joint, Right D Temporomandibular Joint, Left E Sternoclavicular Joint, Right F Sternoclavicular Joint, Left G Acromioclavicular Joint, Right H Acromioclavicular Joint, Left J Shoulder Joint, Right K Shoulder Joint, Left	0 Open 3 Percutaneous 4 Percutaneous Endoscopic X External	0 Drainage Device 3 Infusion Device 5 Internal Fixation Device 7 Autologous Tissue Substitute 8 Spacer J Synthetic Substitute K Nonautologous Tissue Substitute	Z No Qualifier
L Elbow Joint, Right M Elbow Joint, Left N Wrist Joint, Right P Wrist Joint, Left Q Carpal Joint, Right R Carpal Joint, Left S Metacarpocarpal Joint, Right T Metacarpocarpal Joint, Left U Metacarpophalangeal Joint, Right V Metacarpophalangeal Joint, Left W Finger Phalangeal Joint, Right X Finger Phalangeal Joint, Left	0 Open 3 Percutaneous 4 Percutaneous Endoscopic X External	0 Drainage Device 3 Infusion Device 4 Internal Fixation Device 7 Autologous Tissue Substitute 8 Spacer J Synthetic Substitute K Nonautologous Tissue Substitute	Z No Qualifier

Educational Annotations | S – Lower Joints

Body System Specific Educational Annotations for the Lower Joints include:
- Anatomy and Physiology Review
- Anatomical Illustrations
- Definitions of Common Procedures
- AHA Coding Clinic® Reference Notations
- Body Part Key Listings
- Device Key Listings
- Device Aggregation Table Listings
- Coding Notes

Anatomy and Physiology Review of Lower Joints

BODY PART VALUES – S - LOWER JOINTS

Ankle Joint – The hinge joint formed between the distal tibia and fibula and the talus.

Coccygeal Joint – The joints formed between the several (3-5) very small bones that make up the coccyx.

Hip Joint – A ball-and-socket joint between the head of the femur and the acetabulum of the pelvis.

Hip Joint, Acetabular Surface – The surface of the acetabulum of the pelvis.

Hip Joint, Femoral Surface – The surface of the femoral head.

Knee Joint – The large hinge joint between the femur and the tibia.

Knee Joint, Femoral Surface – The surface of the femoral condyles.

Knee Joint, Tibial Surface – The surface of the tibial head.

Lower Joint – Any of the joints designated in the Lower Joints PCS Body System.

Lumbar Vertebral Disc – The disc-shaped fibrocartilage pad between the lumbar spine vertebral bodies comprised of a tough outer portion (annulus fibrosus) and a gel-like inner portion (nucleus pulposus).

Lumbar Vertebral Joint – The synovial and cartilaginous joints connecting the vertebra of the lumbar spine.

Lumbosacral Disc – The disc-shaped fibrocartilage pad between the S5 vertebral body of the lumbar spine and the sacrum comprised of a tough outer portion (annulus fibrosus) and a gel-like inner portion (nucleus pulposus).

Lumbosacral Joint – The synovial and cartilaginous joints connecting the S5 vertebra of the thoracic spine and the sacrum.

Metatarsal-Phalangeal Joint – Any of 5 condyloid joints in the foot that articulate the distal heads of the five metatarsal bones and the proximal phalanx of each toe.

Metatarsal-Tarsal Joint – Any of the 5 joints in the foot that articulate the tarsal bones and the proximal bases of the five metatarsal bones.

Sacrococcygeal Joint – The joint formed between the sacrum and coccyx.

Sacroiliac Joint – The strong joint joining the sacrum to the ilium bones that form the rigid pelvis.

Tarsal Joint – A complex collection of joints formed by the interconnection of the 7 tarsal bones in the foot.

Toe Phalangeal Joint – Any of 9 hinge joints in the toes between the proximal and intermediate phalanges (PIP), and the intermediate and distal phalanges (DIP). The great toe has only two phalanges and therefore only one phalangeal joint.

Educational Annotations | S – Lower Joints

Anatomical Illustrations of Lower Joints

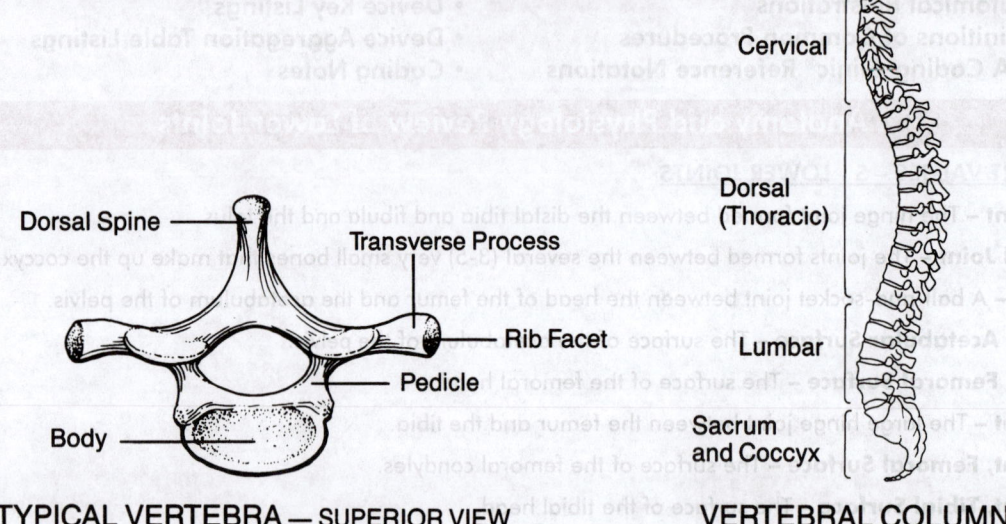

TYPICAL VERTEBRA — SUPERIOR VIEW

VERTEBRAL COLUMN

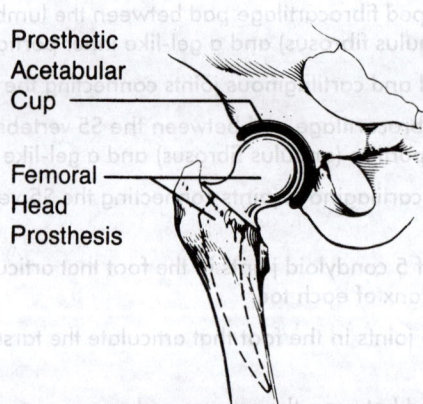

TOTAL HIP REPLACEMENT

Definitions of Common Procedures of Lower Joints

Arthroscopy – The surgical visualization and examination of a joint using an endoscope and often the approach used for joint procedures.

Discectomy – The surgical removal of all (total) or a portion of an intervertebral disc.

Interspinous process spacer – The surgical placement of a device between the spinous processes of vertebrae to relieve pressure on the spinal nerve roots.

Lumbar interbody spinal fusion – The permanent surgical joining of two or more lumbar vertebrae together using bone graft placed between the intervertebral space after the discs have been removed using metal or plastic cage to support the spine while the bone graft hardens.

Lumbar spinal fusion – The permanent surgical joining of two or more lumbar vertebrae together using a bone graft and immobilization by using plates, rods, screws, and/or wires.

Educational Annotations

S – Lower Joints

AHA Coding Clinic® Reference Notations of Lower Joints

ROOT OPERATION SPECIFIC - S - LOWER JOINTS
CHANGE - 2
DESTRUCTION - 5
DRAINAGE - 9
EXCISION - B
    Menisectomy and abrasion chondroplasty with synovectomy......................AHA 15:1Q:p34
    Spinal fusion with discectomy ....AHA 14:2Q:p6
EXTIRPATION - C
FUSION - G
    360-degree spinal fusion ....AHA 13:3Q:p25
    Ankle fusion with bone graft and internal fixation ....AHA 13:2Q:p39
    Components in fusion procedures included in Fusion root operation ....AHA 14:3Q:p30
    Fusion of multiple vertebral joints ....AHA 13:1Q:p21
    Lumbar spinal fusion at two levels with pelvic bone graft ....AHA 14:2Q:p6
        (see also AHA Correction Notice at 14:3Q:p36)
INSERTION - H
INSPECTION - J
RELEASE - N
REMOVAL - P
    Removal of previous total knee replacement components ....AHA 15:2Q:p18
    Removal of retained ankle screws..AHA 13:2Q:p39
    Removal of synthetic joint components ....AHA 15:2Q:p19
REPAIR - Q
    Osteoplasty and labral refixation of hip joint ....AHA 14:4Q:p25
REPLACEMENT - R
    Replacement of femoral surface component ....AHA 15:2Q:p19
    Replacement of previous total knee replacement ....AHA 15:2Q:p18
REPOSITION - S
RESECTION - T
    Resection of lower femur and knee joint..AHA 14:4Q:p29
    Spinal fusion with total discectomy ....AHA 14:2Q:p7
SUPPLEMENT - U
    Placement of new liner..AHA 15:2Q:p19
REVISION - W

Body Part Key Listings of Lower Joints

See also Body Part Key in Appendix C
Acetabulofemoral joint ....*use* Hip Joint, Left/Right
Calcaneocuboid joint ....*use* Tarsal Joint, Left/Right
Cuboideonavicular joint..*use* Tarsal Joint, Left/Right
Cuneonavicular joint ....*use* Tarsal Joint, Left/Right
Femoropatellar joint ....*use* Knee Joint, Left/Right
    ....*use* Knee Joint, Femoral Surface, Left/Right
Femorotibial joint..*use* Knee Joint, Left/Right
    ....*use* Knee Joint, Tibial Surface, Left/Right

Continued on next page

Educational Annotations

S – Lower Joints

Body Part Key Listings of Lower Joints

Continued from previous page

Inferior tibiofibular joint	*use* Ankle Joint, Left/Right
Intercuneiform joint	*use* Tarsal Joint, Left/Right
Interphalangeal (IP) joint	*use* Toe Phalangeal Joint, Left/Right
Lateral meniscus	*use* Knee Joint, Left/Right
Lumbar facet joint	*use* Lumbar Vertebral Joint
Lumbosacral facet joint	*use* Lumbosacral Joint
Medial meniscus	*use* Knee Joint, Left/Right
Metatarsophalangeal (MTP) joint	*use* Metatarsal-Phalangeal Joint, Left/Right
Patellofemoral joint	*use* Knee Joint, Left/Right
	use Knee Joint, Femoral Surface, Left/Right
Sacrococcygeal symphysis	*use* Sacrococcygeal Joint
Subtalar (talocalcaneal) joint	*use* Tarsal Joint, Left/Right
Talocalcaneal (subtalar) joint	*use* Tarsal Joint, Left/Right
Talocalcaneonavicular joint	*use* Tarsal Joint, Left/Right
Talocrural joint	*use* Ankle Joint, Left/Right
Tarsometatarsal joint	*use* Metatarsal-Tarsal Joint, Left/Right
Tibiofemoral joint	*use* Knee Joint, Left/Right
	use Knee Joint, Tibial Surface, Left/Right

Device Key Listings of Lower Joints

See also Device Key in Appendix D

Acetabular cup	*use* Liner in Lower Joints
Autograft	*use* Autologous Tissue Substitute
Axial Lumbar Interbody Fusion System	*use* Interbody Fusion Device in Lower Joints
AxiaLIF® System	*use* Interbody Fusion Device in Lower Joints
Cobalt/chromium head and polyethylene socket	*use* Synthetic Substitute, Metal on Polyethylene for Replacement in Lower Joints
Cobalt/chromium head and socket	*use* Synthetic Substitute, Metal for Replacement in Lower Joints
CONSERVE® PLUS Total Resurfacing Hip System	*use* Resurfacing Device in Lower Joints
Cormet Hip Resurfacing System	*use* Resurfacing Device in Lower Joints
CoRoent® XL	*use* Interbody Fusion Device in Lower Joints
Direct Lateral Interbody Fusion (DLIF) device	*use* Interbody Fusion Device in Lower Joints
Dynesys® Dynamic Stabilization System	*use* Spinal Stabilization Device, Pedicle-Based for Insertion in Upper Joints, Lower Joints
External fixator	*use* External Fixation Device in Head and Facial Bones, Upper Bones, Lower Bones, Upper Joints, Lower Joints
EXtreme Lateral Interbody Fusion (XLIF) device	*use* Interbody Fusion Device in Lower Joints
Facet replacement spinal stabilization device	*use* Spinal Stabilization Device, Facet Replacement for Insertion in Upper Joints, Lower Joints
Fusion screw (compression) (lag) (locking)	*use* Internal Fixation Device in Upper Joints, Lower Joints
Hip (joint) liner	*use* Liner in Lower Joints
Interbody fusion (spine) cage	*use* Interbody Fusion Device in Upper Joints, Lower Joints
Interspinous process spinal stabilization device	*use* Spinal Stabilization Device, Interspinous Process for Insertion in Upper Joints, Lower Joints
Joint fixation plate	*use* Internal Fixation Device in Upper Joints, Lower Joints
Joint liner (insert)	*use* Liner in Lower Joints
Joint spacer (antibiotic)	*use* Spacer in Upper Joints, Lower Joints

Continued on next page

Educational Annotations | S – Lower Joints

Device Key Listings of Lower Joints

Continued from previous page

Kirschner wire (K-wire)	*use* Internal Fixation Device in Head and Facial Bones, Upper Bones, Lower Bones, Upper Joints, Lower Joints
Knee (implant) insert	*use* Liner in Lower Joints
Novation® Ceramic AHS® (Articulation Hip System)	*use* Synthetic Substitute, Ceramic for Replacement in Lower Joints
Oxidized zirconium ceramic hip bearing surface	*use* Synthetic Substitute, Ceramic on Polyethylene for Replacement in Lower Joints
Pedicle-based dynamic stabilization device	*use* Spinal Stabilization Device, Pedicle-Based for Insertion in Upper Joints, Lower Joints
Polyethylene socket	*use* Synthetic Substitute, Polyethylene for Replacement in Lower Joints
Polymethylmethacrylate (PMMA)	*use* Synthetic Substitute
Prodisc-L	*use* Synthetic Substitute
Tibial insert	*use* Liner in Lower Joints
Tissue bank graft	*use* Nonautologous Tissue Substitute
X-STOP® Spacer	*use* Spinal Stabilization Device, Interspinous Process for Insertion in Upper Joints, Lower Joints
XLIF® System	*use* Interbody Fusion Device in Lower Joints
Zimmer® NexGen® LPS Mobile Bearing Knee	*use* Synthetic Substitute
Zimmer® NexGen® LPS-Flex Mobile Knee	*use* Synthetic Substitute

Device Aggregation Table Listings of Lower Joints

See also Device Aggregation Table in Appendix E

Specific Device	For Operation	In Body System	General Device	
Spinal Stabilization Device, Facet Replacement	Insertion	Lower Joints	4	Internal Fixation Device
Spinal Stabilization Device, Interspinous Process	Insertion	Lower Joints	4	Internal Fixation Device
Spinal Stabilization Device, Pedicle-Based	Insertion	Lower Joints	4	Internal Fixation Device
Synthetic Substitute, Ceramic	Replacement	Lower Joints	J	Synthetic Substitute
Synthetic Substitute, Ceramic on Polyethylene	Replacement	Lower Joints	J	Synthetic Substitute
Synthetic Substitute, Metal	Replacement	Lower Joints	J	Synthetic Substitute
Synthetic Substitute, Metal on Polyethylene	Replacement	Lower Joints	J	Synthetic Substitute
Synthetic Substitute, Polyethylene	Replacement	Lower Joints	J	Synthetic Substitute

Coding Notes of Lower Joints

Body System Relevant Coding Guidelines

Fusion procedures of the spine

B3.10a

The body part coded for a spinal vertebral joint(s) rendered immobile by a spinal fusion procedure is classified by the level of the spine (e.g. thoracic). There are distinct body part values for a single vertebral joint and for multiple vertebral joints at each spinal level.

Example: Body part values specify Lumbar Vertebral Joint, Lumbar Vertebral Joints, 2 or More and Lumbosacral Vertebral Joint.

B3.10b

If multiple vertebral joints are fused, a separate procedure is coded for each vertebral joint that uses a different device and/or qualifier.

Example: Fusion of lumbar vertebral joint, posterior approach, anterior column and fusion of lumbar vertebral joint, posterior approach, posterior column are coded separately.

Continued on next page

Educational Annotations
S – Lower Joints

Coding Notes of Lower Joints

Body System Relevant Coding Guidelines

Continued from previous page

B3.10c
Combinations of devices and materials are often used on a vertebral joint to render the joint immobile. When combinations of devices are used on the same vertebral joint, the device value coded for the procedure is as follows:
- If an interbody fusion device is used to render the joint immobile (alone or containing other material like bone graft), the procedure is coded with the device value Interbody Fusion Device
- If bone graft is the only device used to render the joint immobile, the procedure is coded with the device value Nonautologous Tissue Substitute or Autologous Tissue Substitute
- If a mixture of autologous and nonautologous bone graft (with or without biological or synthetic extenders or binders) is used to render the joint immobile, code the procedure with the device value Autologous Tissue Substitute

Examples: Fusion of a vertebral joint using a cage style interbody fusion device containing morsellized bone graft is coded to the device Interbody Fusion Device.

Fusion of a vertebral joint using a bone dowel interbody fusion device made of cadaver bone and packed with a mixture of local morsellized bone and demineralized bone matrix is coded to the device Interbody Fusion Device.

Fusion of a vertebral joint using both autologous bone graft and bone bank bone graft is coded to the device Autologous Tissue Substitute.

Tendons, ligaments, bursae and fascia near a joint

B4.5
Procedures performed on tendons, ligaments, bursae and fascia supporting a joint are coded to the body part in the respective body system that is the focus of the procedure. Procedures performed on joint structures themselves are coded to the body part in the joint body systems.

Example: Repair of the anterior cruciate ligament of the knee is coded to the knee bursae and ligament body part in the bursae and ligaments body system. Knee arthroscopy with shaving of articular cartilage is coded to the knee joint body part in the Lower Joints body system.

Body System Specific PCS Reference Manual Exercises

PCS CODE	S – LOWER JOINTS EXERCISES
0S2YX0Z	Exchange of drainage tube from right hip joint.
0S9C00Z	Right knee arthrotomy with drain placement.
0SG10AJ	Posterior spinal fusion at L1-L3 level with BAK cage interbody fusion device, open.
0SG507Z	Sacrococcygeal fusion with bone graft from same operative site, open.
0SGQ34Z	Interphalangeal fusion of left great toe, percutaneous pin fixation.
0SJD0ZZ	Exploratory arthrotomy of left knee.
0SRB03A	Total left hip replacement using ceramic on ceramic prosthesis, without bone cement.
0SRC0JZ	Total right knee arthroplasty with insertion of total knee prosthesis.
0SUR0BZ	Resurfacing procedure on right femoral head, open approach.
0SUS09Z	Exchange of liner in femoral component of previous left hip replacement, open approach. (Taking out the old liner is coded separately to the root operation Removal.)
0SW90JZ	Open revision of right hip replacement, with recementing of the prosthesis.

S – LOWER JOINTS 0S5

DEVICE GROUP: Change, Insertion, Removal, Replacement, Revision, Supplement
Root Operations that always involve a device.

1ST - 0 Medical and Surgical
2ND - S Lower Joints
3RD - 2 CHANGE

EXAMPLE: Exchange drain tube | CMS Ex: Changing urinary catheter

CHANGE: Taking out or off a device from a body part and putting back an identical or similar device in or on the same body part without cutting or puncturing the skin or a mucous membrane.

EXPLANATION: ALL Changes use EXTERNAL approach only ...

Body Part – 4TH	Approach – 5TH	Device – 6TH	Qualifier – 7TH
Y Lower Joint	X External	0 Drainage device Y Other device	Z No qualifier

---

EXCISION GROUP: Excision, Resection, Destruction, (Extraction), (Detachment)
Root Operations that take out some or all of a body part.

1ST - 0 Medical and Surgical
2ND - S Lower Joints
3RD - 5 DESTRUCTION

EXAMPLE: Radiofrequency ablation | CMS Ex: Fulguration polyp

DESTRUCTION: Physical eradication of all or a portion of a body part by the direct use of energy, force, or a destructive agent.

EXPLANATION: None of the body part is physically taken out

Body Part – 4TH		Approach – 5TH	Device – 6TH	Qualifier – 7TH
0 Lumbar Vertebral Joint	H Tarsal Joint, Right	0 Open	Z No device	Z No qualifier
2 Lumbar Vertebral Disc	J Tarsal Joint, Left	3 Percutaneous		
3 Lumbosacral Joint	K Metatarsal-Tarsal Joint, Right	4 Percutaneous endoscopic		
4 Lumbosacral Disc	L Metatarsal-Tarsal Joint, Left			
5 Sacrococcygeal Joint	M Metatarsal-Phalangeal Joint, Right			
6 Coccygeal Joint	N Metatarsal-Phalangeal Joint, Left			
7 Sacroiliac Joint, Right	P Toe Phalangeal Joint, Right			
8 Sacroiliac Joint, Left	Q Toe Phalangeal Joint, Left			
9 Hip Joint, Right				
B Hip Joint, Left				
C Knee Joint, Right				
D Knee Joint, Left				
F Ankle Joint, Right				
G Ankle Joint, Left				

0S9

MEDICAL AND SURGICAL SECTION – 2016 ICD-10-PCS

DRAINAGE GROUP: Drainage, Extirpation, (Fragmentation)
Root Operations that take out solids/fluids/gases from a body part.

- 1ST – **0** Medical and Surgical
- 2ND – **S** Lower Joints
- 3RD – **9** DRAINAGE

EXAMPLE: Aspiration knee joint   CMS Ex: Thoracentesis

DRAINAGE: Taking or letting out fluids and/or gases from a body part.

EXPLANATION: Qualifier "X Diagnostic" indicates biopsy …

Body Part – 4TH		Approach – 5TH	Device – 6TH	Qualifier – 7TH
0 Lumbar Vertebral Joint 2 Lumbar Vertebral Disc 3 Lumbosacral Joint 4 Lumbosacral Disc 5 Sacrococcygeal Joint 6 Coccygeal Joint 7 Sacroiliac Joint, Right 8 Sacroiliac Joint, Left 9 Hip Joint, Right B Hip Joint, Left C Knee Joint, Right D Knee Joint, Left F Ankle Joint, Right G Ankle Joint, Left	H Tarsal Joint, Right J Tarsal Joint, Left K Metatarsal-Tarsal Joint, Right L Metatarsal-Tarsal Joint, Left M Metatarsal-Phalangeal Joint, Right N Metatarsal-Phalangeal Joint, Left P Toe Phalangeal Joint, Right Q Toe Phalangeal Joint, Left	0 Open 3 Percutaneous 4 Percutaneous endoscopic	0 Drainage device	Z No qualifier
0 Lumbar Vertebral Joint 2 Lumbar Vertebral Disc 3 Lumbosacral Joint 4 Lumbosacral Disc 5 Sacrococcygeal Joint 6 Coccygeal Joint 7 Sacroiliac Joint, Right 8 Sacroiliac Joint, Left 9 Hip Joint, Right B Hip Joint, Left C Knee Joint, Right D Knee Joint, Left F Ankle Joint, Right G Ankle Joint, Left	H Tarsal Joint, Right J Tarsal Joint, Left K Metatarsal-Tarsal Joint, Right L Metatarsal-Tarsal Joint, Left M Metatarsal-Phalangeal Joint, Right N Metatarsal-Phalangeal Joint, Left P Toe Phalangeal Joint, Right Q Toe Phalangeal Joint, Left	0 Open 3 Percutaneous 4 Percutaneous endoscopic	Z No device	X Diagnostic Z No qualifier

LOWER JOINTS 0S9

S – LOWER JOINTS 0SC

EXCISION GROUP: Excision, Resection, Destruction, (Extraction), (Detachment)
Root Operations that take out some or all of a body part.

- 1ST – **0** Medical and Surgical
- 2ND – **S** Lower Joints
- 3RD – **B** EXCISION

EXAMPLE: Partial medial meniscectomy   CMS Ex: Liver biopsy

EXCISION: Cutting out or off, without replacement, a portion of a body part.

EXPLANATION: Qualifier "X Diagnostic" indicates biopsy ...

Body Part – 4TH	Approach – 5TH	Device – 6TH	Qualifier – 7TH
0 Lumbar Vertebral Joint	0 Open	Z No device	X Diagnostic
2 Lumbar Vertebral Disc	3 Percutaneous		Z No qualifier
3 Lumbosacral Joint	4 Percutaneous endoscopic		
4 Lumbosacral Disc			
5 Sacrococcygeal Joint			
6 Coccygeal Joint			
7 Sacroiliac Joint, Right			
8 Sacroiliac Joint, Left			
9 Hip Joint, Right			
B Hip Joint, Left			
C Knee Joint, Right			
D Knee Joint, Left			
F Ankle Joint, Right			
G Ankle Joint, Left			
H Tarsal Joint, Right			
J Tarsal Joint, Left			
K Metatarsal-Tarsal Joint, Right			
L Metatarsal-Tarsal Joint, Left			
M Metatarsal-Phalangeal Joint, Right			
N Metatarsal-Phalangeal Joint, Left			
P Toe Phalangeal Joint, Right			
Q Toe Phalangeal Joint, Left			

DRAINAGE GROUP: Drainage, Extirpation, (Fragmentation)
Root Operations that take out solids/fluids/gases from a body part.

- 1ST – **0** Medical and Surgical
- 2ND – **S** Lower Joints
- 3RD – **C** EXTIRPATION

EXAMPLE: Removal loose bodies knee   CMS Ex: Choledocholithotomy

EXTIRPATION: Taking or cutting out solid matter from a body part.

EXPLANATION: Abnormal byproduct or foreign body ...

Body Part – 4TH	Approach – 5TH	Device – 6TH	Qualifier – 7TH
0 Lumbar Vertebral Joint	0 Open	Z No device	Z No qualifier
2 Lumbar Vertebral Disc	3 Percutaneous		
3 Lumbosacral Joint	4 Percutaneous endoscopic		
4 Lumbosacral Disc			
5 Sacrococcygeal Joint			
6 Coccygeal Joint			
7 Sacroiliac Joint, Right			
8 Sacroiliac Joint, Left			
9 Hip Joint, Right			
B Hip Joint, Left			
C Knee Joint, Right			
D Knee Joint, Left			
F Ankle Joint, Right			
G Ankle Joint, Left			
H Tarsal Joint, Right			
J Tarsal Joint, Left			
K Metatarsal-Tarsal Joint, Right			
L Metatarsal-Tarsal Joint, Left			
M Metatarsal-Phalangeal Joint, Right			
N Metatarsal-Phalangeal Joint, Left			
P Toe Phalangeal Joint, Right			
Q Toe Phalangeal Joint, Left			

0SG — MEDICAL AND SURGICAL SECTION – 2016 ICD-10-PCS

OTHER OBJECTIVES GROUP: (Alteration), (Creation), **Fusion**
Root Operations that define other objectives.

- 1ST – **0** Medical and Surgical
- 2ND – **S** Lower Joints
- 3RD – **G FUSION**

EXAMPLE: Lumbosacral spinal fusion   **CMS Ex:** Spinal fusion

FUSION: Joining together portions of an articular body part, rendering the articular body part immobile.

EXPLANATION: Use of fixation device, graft, or other means …

Body Part – 4TH	Approach – 5TH	Device – 6TH	Qualifier – 7TH
0 Lumbar Vertebral Joint 1 Lumbar Vertebral Joints, 2 or more 3 Lumbosacral Joint	0 Open 3 Percutaneous 4 Percutaneous endoscopic	7 Autologous tissue substitute A Interbody fusion device J Synthetic substitute K Nonautologous tissue substitute Z No Device	0 Anterior approach, anterior column 1 Posterior approach, posterior column J Posterior approach, anterior column
5 Sacrococcygeal Joint 6 Coccygeal Joint 7 Sacroiliac Joint, Right 8 Sacroiliac Joint, Left	0 Open 3 Percutaneous 4 Percutaneous endoscopic	4 Internal fixation device 7 Autologous tissue substitute J Synthetic substitute K Nonautologous tissue substitute Z No device	Z No qualifier
9 Hip Joint, Right B Hip Joint, Left C Knee Joint, Right D Knee Joint, Left F Ankle Joint, Right G Ankle Joint, Left H Tarsal Joint, Right J Tarsal Joint, Left K Metatarsal-Tarsal Joint, Right L Metatarsal-Tarsal Joint, Left M Metatarsal-Phalangeal Joint, Right N Metatarsal-Phalangeal Joint, Left P Toe Phalangeal Joint, Right Q Toe Phalangeal Joint, Left	0 Open 3 Percutaneous 4 Percutaneous endoscopic	4 Internal fixation device 5 External fixation device 7 Autologous tissue substitute J Synthetic substitute K Nonautologous tissue substitute Z No device	Z No qualifier

S – LOWER JOINTS 0SH

DEVICE GROUP: Change, Insertion, Removal, Replacement, Revision, Supplement
Root Operations that always involve a device.

1ST - 0 Medical and Surgical
2ND - S Lower Joints
3RD - H INSERTION

EXAMPLE: Implantation joint spacer   CMS Ex: Central venous catheter

INSERTION: Putting in a nonbiological appliance that monitors, assists, performs, or prevents a physiological function but does not physically take the place of a body part.
EXPLANATION: None

Body Part – 4TH	Approach – 5TH	Device – 6TH	Qualifier – 7TH
0 Lumbar Vertebral Joint 3 Lumbosacral Joint	0 Open 3 Percutaneous 4 Percutaneous endoscopic	3 Infusion device 4 Internal fixation device 8 Spacer B Spinal stabilization device, interspinous process C Spinal stabilization device, pedicle-based D Spinal stabilization device, facet replacement	Z No qualifier
2 Lumbar Vertebral Disc 4 Lumbosacral Disc	0 Open 3 Percutaneous 4 Percutaneous endoscopic	3 Infusion device 8 Spacer	Z No qualifier
5 Sacrococcygeal Joint 6 Coccygeal Joint 7 Sacroiliac Joint, Right 8 Sacroiliac Joint, Left	0 Open 3 Percutaneous 4 Percutaneous endoscopic	3 Infusion device 4 Internal fixation device 8 Spacer	Z No qualifier
9 Hip Joint, Right B Hip Joint, Left C Knee Joint, Right D Knee Joint, Left F Ankle Joint, Right G Ankle Joint, Left H Tarsal Joint, Right J Tarsal Joint, Left K Metatarsal-Tarsal Joint, Right L Metatarsal-Tarsal Joint, Left M Metatarsal-Phalangeal Joint, Right N Metatarsal-Phalangeal Joint, Left P Toe Phalangeal Joint, Right Q Toe Phalangeal Joint, Left	0 Open 3 Percutaneous 4 Percutaneous endoscopic	3 Infusion device 4 Internal fixation device 5 External fixation device 8 Spacer	Z No qualifier

0SJ   MEDICAL AND SURGICAL SECTION – 2016 ICD-10-PCS   [2016.PCS]

EXAMINATION GROUP: Inspection, (Map)
Root Operations involving examination only.

- 1ST - **0** Medical and Surgical
- 2ND - **S** Lower Joints
- 3RD - **J** INSPECTION

EXAMPLE: Diagnostic arthroscopy knee   CMS Ex: Colonoscopy

INSPECTION: Visually and/or manually exploring a body part.

EXPLANATION: Direct or instrumental visualization …

Body Part – 4TH	Approach – 5TH	Device – 6TH	Qualifier – 7TH
0 Lumbar Vertebral Joint	0 Open	Z No device	Z No qualifier
2 Lumbar Vertebral Disc	3 Percutaneous		
3 Lumbosacral Joint	4 Percutaneous endoscopic		
4 Lumbosacral Disc	X External		
5 Sacrococcygeal Joint			
6 Coccygeal Joint			
7 Sacroiliac Joint, Right			
8 Sacroiliac Joint, Left			
9 Hip Joint, Right			
B Hip Joint, Left			
C Knee Joint, Right			
D Knee Joint, Left			
F Ankle Joint, Right			
G Ankle Joint, Left			
H Tarsal Joint, Right			
J Tarsal Joint, Left			
K Metatarsal-Tarsal Joint, Right			
L Metatarsal-Tarsal Joint, Left			
M Metatarsal-Phalangeal Joint, Right			
N Metatarsal-Phalangeal Joint, Left			
P Toe Phalangeal Joint, Right			
Q Toe Phalangeal Joint, Left			

DIVISION GROUP: (Division), Release
Root Operations involving cutting or separation only.

- 1ST - **0** Medical and Surgical
- 2ND - **S** Lower Joints
- 3RD - **N** RELEASE

EXAMPLE: Manual rupture joint adhesions   CMS Ex: Carpal tunnel release

RELEASE: Freeing a body part from an abnormal physical constraint by cutting or by the use of force.

EXPLANATION: None of the body part is taken out …

Body Part – 4TH	Approach – 5TH	Device – 6TH	Qualifier – 7TH
0 Lumbar Vertebral Joint	0 Open	Z No device	Z No qualifier
2 Lumbar Vertebral Disc	3 Percutaneous		
3 Lumbosacral Joint	4 Percutaneous endoscopic		
4 Lumbosacral Disc	X External		
5 Sacrococcygeal Joint			
6 Coccygeal Joint			
7 Sacroiliac Joint, Right			
8 Sacroiliac Joint, Left			
9 Hip Joint, Right			
B Hip Joint, Left			
C Knee Joint, Right			
D Knee Joint, Left			
F Ankle Joint, Right			
G Ankle Joint, Left			
H Tarsal Joint, Right			
J Tarsal Joint, Left			
K Metatarsal-Tarsal Joint, Right			
L Metatarsal-Tarsal Joint, Left			
M Metatarsal-Phalangeal Joint, Right			
N Metatarsal-Phalangeal Joint, Left			
P Toe Phalangeal Joint, Right			
Q Toe Phalangeal Joint, Left			

S – LOWER JOINTS 0 S P

DEVICE GROUP: Change, Insertion, Removal, Replacement, Revision, Supplement
Root Operations that always involve a device.

1ST - 0 Medical and Surgical
2ND - S Lower Joints
3RD - P REMOVAL

EXAMPLE: Removal fixation device   CMS Ex: Chest tube removal

REMOVAL: Taking out or off a device from a body part.

EXPLANATION: Removal device without reinsertion ...

Body Part – 4TH	Approach – 5TH	Device – 6TH	Qualifier – 7TH
0 Lumbar Vertebral Joint 3 Lumbosacral Joint	0 Open 3 Percutaneous 4 Percutaneous endoscopic	0 Drainage device 3 Infusion device 4 Internal fixation device 7 Autologous tissue substitute 8 Spacer A Interbody fusion device J Synthetic substitute K Nonautologous tissue substitute	Z No qualifier
0 Lumbar Vertebral Joint 3 Lumbosacral Joint	X External	0 Drainage device 3 Infusion device 4 Internal fixation device	Z No qualifier
2 Lumbar Vertebral Disc 4 Lumbosacral Disc	0 Open 3 Percutaneous 4 Percutaneous endoscopic	0 Drainage device 3 Infusion device 7 Autologous tissue substitute J Synthetic substitute K Nonautologous tissue substitute	Z No qualifier
2 Lumbar Vertebral Disc 4 Lumbosacral Disc	X External	0 Drainage device 3 Infusion device	Z No qualifier
5 Sacrococcygeal Joint 6 Coccygeal Joint 7 Sacroiliac Joint, Right 8 Sacroiliac Joint, Left	0 Open 3 Percutaneous 4 Percutaneous endoscopic	0 Drainage device 3 Infusion device 4 Internal fixation device 7 Autologous tissue substitute 8 Spacer J Synthetic substitute K Nonautologous tissue substitute	Z No qualifier
5 Sacrococcygeal Joint 6 Coccygeal Joint 7 Sacroiliac Joint, Right 8 Sacroiliac Joint, Left	X External	0 Drainage device 3 Infusion device 4 Internal fixation device	Z No qualifier

continued ⇨

0SP

MEDICAL AND SURGICAL SECTION – 2016 ICD-10-PCS

0 S P REMOVAL – continued

Lower Joints

Body Part – 4TH	Approach – 5TH	Device – 6TH	Qualifier – 7TH
9 Hip Joint, Right B Hip Joint, Left	0 Open	0 Drainage device 3 Infusion device 4 Internal fixation device 5 External fixation device 7 Autologous tissue substitute 8 Spacer 9 Liner B Resurfacing device J Synthetic substitute K Nonautologous tissue substitute	Z No qualifier
9 Hip Joint, Right B Hip Joint, Left	3 Percutaneous 4 Percutaneous endoscopic	0 Drainage device 3 Infusion device 4 Internal fixation device 5 External fixation device 7 Autologous tissue substitute 8 Spacer J Synthetic substitute K Nonautologous tissue substitute	Z No qualifier
9 Hip Joint, Right B Hip Joint, Left	X External	0 Drainage device 3 Infusion device 4 Internal fixation device 5 External fixation device	Z No qualifier
C Knee Joint, Right D Knee Joint, Left	0 Open	0 Drainage device 3 Infusion device 4 Internal fixation device 5 External fixation device 7 Autologous tissue substitute 8 Spacer 9 Liner J Synthetic substitute K Nonautologous tissue substitute	Z No qualifier

continued

0 S P REMOVAL – continued

Body Part – 4TH	Approach – 5TH	Device – 6TH	Qualifier – 7TH
C Knee Joint, Right D Knee Joint, Left	3 Percutaneous 4 Percutaneous endoscopic	0 Drainage device 3 Infusion device 4 Internal fixation device 5 External fixation device 7 Autologous tissue substitute 8 Spacer J Synthetic Substitute K Nonautologous tissue substitute	Z No qualifier
C Knee Joint, Right D Knee Joint, Left	X External	0 Drainage device 3 Infusion device 4 Internal fixation device 5 External fixation device	Z No qualifier
F Ankle Joint, Right G Ankle Joint, Left H Tarsal Joint, Right J Tarsal Joint, Left K Metatarsal-Tarsal Joint, Right L Metatarsal-Tarsal Joint, Left M Metatarsal-Phalangeal Joint, Right N Metatarsal-Phalangeal Joint, Left P Toe Phalangeal Joint, Right Q Toe Phalangeal Joint, Left	0 Open 3 Percutaneous 4 Percutaneous endoscopic	0 Drainage device 3 Infusion device 4 Internal fixation device 5 External fixation device 7 Autologous tissue substitute 8 Spacer J Synthetic substitute K Nonautologous tissue substitute	Z No qualifier
F Ankle Joint, Right G Ankle Joint, Left H Tarsal Joint, Right J Tarsal Joint, Left K Metatarsal-Tarsal Joint, Right L Metatarsal-Tarsal Joint, Left M Metatarsal-Phalangeal Joint, Right N Metatarsal-Phalangeal Joint, Left P Toe Phalangeal Joint, Right Q Toe Phalangeal Joint, Left	X External	0 Drainage device 3 Infusion device 4 Internal fixation device 5 External fixation device	Z No qualifier

0SQ

MEDICAL AND SURGICAL SECTION – 2016 ICD-10-PCS

OTHER REPAIRS GROUP: (Control), **Repair**
Root Operations that define other repairs.

1ST - **0** Medical and Surgical
2ND - **S** Lower Joints
3RD - **Q REPAIR**

EXAMPLE: Suture arthroplasty ankle   **CMS Ex:** Suture laceration

REPAIR: Restoring, to the extent possible, a body part to its normal anatomic structure and function.

EXPLANATION: Only when no other root operation applies ...

Body Part – 4TH		Approach – 5TH	Device – 6TH	Qualifier – 7TH
0 Lumbar Vertebral Joint	H Tarsal Joint, Right	0 Open	Z No device	Z No qualifier
2 Lumbar Vertebral Disc	J Tarsal Joint, Left	3 Percutaneous		
3 Lumbosacral Joint	K Metatarsal-Tarsal Joint, Right	4 Percutaneous endoscopic		
4 Lumbosacral Disc	L Metatarsal-Tarsal Joint, Left	X External		
5 Sacrococcygeal Joint				
6 Coccygeal Joint	M Metatarsal-Phalangeal Joint, Right			
7 Sacroiliac Joint, Right	N Metatarsal-Phalangeal Joint, Left			
8 Sacroiliac Joint, Left				
9 Hip Joint, Right	P Toe Phalangeal Joint, Right			
B Hip Joint, Left	Q Toe Phalangeal Joint, Left			
C Knee Joint, Right				
D Knee Joint, Left				
F Ankle Joint, Right				
G Ankle Joint, Left				

0SR

S – LOWER JOINTS

DEVICE GROUP: Change, Insertion, Removal, Replacement, Revision, Supplement
Root Operations that always involve a device.

1ST - **0** Medical and Surgical
2ND - **S** Lower Joints
3RD - **R** REPLACEMENT

EXAMPLE: Total knee replacement   **CMS Ex:** Total hip

REPLACEMENT: Putting in or on a biological or synthetic material that physically takes the place and/or function of all or a portion of a body part.

EXPLANATION: Includes taking out body part, or eradication...

Body Part – 4TH	Approach – 5TH	Device – 6TH	Qualifier – 7TH
0 Lumbar Vertebral Joint 2 Lumbar Vertebral Disc NC* 3 Lumbosacral Joint 4 Lumbosacral Disc NC* 5 Sacrococcygeal Joint 6 Coccygeal Joint 7 Sacroiliac Joint, Right 8 Sacroiliac Joint, Left H Tarsal Joint, Right J Tarsal Joint, Left K Metatarsal-Tarsal Joint, Right L Metatarsal-Tarsal Joint, Left M Metatarsal-Phalangeal Joint, Right N Metatarsal-Phalangeal Joint, Left P Toe Phalangeal Joint, Right Q Toe Phalangeal Joint, Left	0 Open	7 Autologous tissue substitute J Synthetic substitute K Nonautologous tissue substitute	Z No qualifier
9 Hip Joint, Right B Hip Joint, Left	0 Open	1 Synthetic substitute, metal 2 Synthetic substitute, metal on polyethylene 3 Synthetic substitute, ceramic 4 Synthetic substitute, ceramic on polyethylene J Synthetic substitute	9 Cemented A Uncemented Z No qualifier
9 Hip Joint, Right B Hip Joint, Left	0 Open	7 Autologous tissue substitute K Nonautologous tissue substitute	Z No qualifier

NC* – Some procedures are considered non-covered by Medicare. See current Medicare Code Editor (patient over 60 years with Synthetic substitute) for details.

continued ⇨

0SR REPLACEMENT – continued

Lower Joints 0SR

Body Part – 4ᵀᴴ	Approach – 5ᵀᴴ	Device – 6ᵀᴴ	Qualifier – 7ᵀᴴ
A Hip Joint, Acetabular Surface, Right E Hip Joint, Acetabular Surface, Left	0 Open	0 Synthetic substitute, polyethylene 1 Synthetic substitute, metal 3 Synthetic substitute, ceramic J Synthetic substitute	9 Cemented A Uncemented Z No qualifier
A Hip Joint, Acetabular Surface, Right E Hip Joint, Acetabular Surface, Left	0 Open	7 Autologous tissue substitute K Nonautologous tissue substitute	Z No qualifier
C Knee Joint, Right D Knee Joint, Left F Ankle Joint, Right G Ankle Joint, Left T Knee Joint, Femoral Surface, Right U Knee Joint, Femoral Surface, Left V Knee Joint, Tibial Surface, Right W Knee Joint, Tibial Surface, Left	0 Open	7 Autologous tissue substitute K Nonautologous tissue substitute	Z No qualifier
C Knee Joint, Right D Knee Joint, Left F Ankle Joint, Right G Ankle Joint, Left T Knee Joint, Femoral Surface, Right U Knee Joint, Femoral Surface, Left V Knee Joint, Tibial Surface, Right W Knee Joint, Tibial Surface, Left	0 Open	J Synthetic substitute	9 Cemented A Uncemented Z No qualifier
R Hip Joint, Femoral Surface, Right S Hip Joint, Femoral Surface, Left	0 Open	1 Synthetic substitute, metal 3 Synthetic substitute, ceramic J Synthetic substitute	9 Cemented A Uncemented Z No qualifier
R Hip Joint, Femoral Surface, Right S Hip Joint, Femoral Surface, Left	0 Open	7 Autologous tissue substitute K Nonautologous tissue substitute	Z No qualifier

0ST

S – LOWER JOINTS

MOVE GROUP: (Reattachment), **Reposition**, (Transfer), (Transplantation)
Root Operations that put in/put back or move some/all of a body part.

- 1ST – **0** Medical and Surgical
- 2ND – **S** Lower Joints
- 3RD – **S** REPOSITION

EXAMPLE: Closed reduction hip joint **CMS Ex:** Fracture reduction

REPOSITION: Moving to its normal location, or other suitable location, all or a portion of a body part.

EXPLANATION: May or may not be cut to be moved ...

Body Part – 4TH	Approach – 5TH	Device – 6TH	Qualifier – 7TH
0 Lumbar Vertebral Joint 3 Lumbosacral Joint 5 Sacrococcygeal Joint 6 Coccygeal Joint 7 Sacroiliac Joint, Right 8 Sacroiliac Joint, Left	0 Open 3 Percutaneous 4 Percutaneous endoscopic X External	4 Internal fixation device Z No device	Z No qualifier
9 Hip Joint, Right B Hip Joint, Left C Knee Joint, Right D Knee Joint, Left F Ankle Joint, Right G Ankle Joint, Left H Tarsal Joint, Right J Tarsal Joint, Left K Metatarsal-Tarsal Joint, Right L Metatarsal-Tarsal Joint, Left M Metatarsal-Phalangeal Joint, Right N Metatarsal-Phalangeal Joint, Left P Toe Phalangeal Joint, Right Q Toe Phalangeal Joint, Left	0 Open 3 Percutaneous 4 Percutaneous endoscopic X External	4 Internal fixation device 5 External fixation device Z No device	Z No qualifier

---

EXCISION GROUP: **Excision**, **Resection**, **Destruction**, (Extraction), (Detachment)
Root Operations that take out some or all of a body part.

- 1ST – **0** Medical and Surgical
- 2ND – **S** Lower Joints
- 3RD – **T** RESECTION

EXAMPLE: Total lumbar discectomy **CMS Ex:** Cholecystectomy

RESECTION: Cutting out or off, without replacement, all of a body part.

EXPLANATION: None

Body Part – 4TH		Approach – 5TH	Device – 6TH	Qualifier – 7TH
2 Lumbar Vertebral Disc 4 Lumbosacral Disc 5 Sacrococcygeal Joint 6 Coccygeal Joint 7 Sacroiliac Joint, Right 8 Sacroiliac Joint, Left 9 Hip Joint, Right B Hip Joint, Left C Knee Joint, Right D Knee Joint, Left F Ankle Joint, Right G Ankle Joint, Left	H Tarsal Joint, Right J Tarsal Joint, Left K Metatarsal-Tarsal Joint, Right L Metatarsal-Tarsal Joint, Left M Metatarsal-Phalangeal Joint, Right N Metatarsal-Phalangeal Joint, Left P Toe Phalangeal Joint, Right Q Toe Phalangeal Joint, Left	0 Open	Z No device	Z No qualifier

0SU

MEDICAL AND SURGICAL SECTION – 2016 ICD-10-PCS [2016.PCS]

DEVICE GROUP: Change, Insertion, Removal, Replacement, Revision, Supplement
Root Operations that always involve a device.

EXAMPLE: Femoral resurfacing hip joint | **CMS Ex:** Hernia repair with mesh

1ST – **0** Medical and Surgical
2ND – **S** Lower Joints
3RD – **U SUPPLEMENT**

SUPPLEMENT: Putting in or on biological or synthetic material that physically reinforces and/or augments the function of a portion of a body part.

EXPLANATION: Biological material from same individual ...

Body Part – 4TH	Approach – 5TH	Device – 6TH	Qualifier – 7TH
0 Lumbar Vertebral Joint 2 Lumbar Vertebral Disc 3 Lumbosacral Joint 4 Lumbosacral Disc 5 Sacrococcygeal Joint 6 Coccygeal Joint 7 Sacroiliac Joint, Right 8 Sacroiliac Joint, Left F Ankle Joint, Right G Ankle Joint, Left H Tarsal Joint, Right J Tarsal Joint, Left K Metatarsal-Tarsal Joint, Right L Metatarsal-Tarsal Joint, Left M Metatarsal-Phalangeal Joint, Right N Metatarsal-Phalangeal Joint, Left P Toe Phalangeal Joint, Right Q Toe Phalangeal Joint, Left	0 Open 3 Percutaneous 4 Percutaneous endoscopic	7 Autologous tissue substitute J Synthetic substitute K Nonautologous tissue substitute	Z No qualifier
9 Hip Joint, Right B Hip Joint, Left	0 Open	7 Autologous tissue substitute 9 Liner B Resurfacing device J Synthetic substitute K Nonautologous tissue substitute	Z No qualifier
9 Hip Joint, Right B Hip Joint, Left	3 Percutaneous 4 Percutaneous endoscopic	7 Autologous tissue substitute J Synthetic substitute K Nonautologous tissue substitute	Z No qualifier
A Hip Joint, Acetabular Surface, Right E Hip Joint, Acetabular Surface, Left R Hip Joint, Femoral Surface, Right S Hip Joint, Femoral Surface, Left	0 Open	9 Liner B Resurfacing device	Z No qualifier
C Knee Joint, Right D Knee Joint, Left	0 Open	7 Autologous tissue substitute J Synthetic substitute K Nonautologous tissue substitute	Z No qualifier
C Knee Joint, Right D Knee Joint, Left	0 Open	9 Liner	C Patellar Surface Z No qualifier
C Knee Joint, Right D Knee Joint, Left	3 Percutaneous 4 Percutaneous endoscopic	7 Autologous tissue substitute J Synthetic substitute K Nonautologous tissue substitute	Z No qualifier
T Knee Joint, Femoral Surface, Right U Knee Joint, Femoral Surface, Left V Knee Joint, Tibial Surface, Right W Knee Joint, Tibial Surface, Left	0 Open	9 Liner	Z No qualifier

0SW S – LOWER JOINTS

DEVICE GROUP: Change, Insertion, Removal, Replacement, Revision, Supplement
Root Operations that always involve a device.

- 1ST – **0** Medical and Surgical
- 2ND – **S** Lower Joints
- 3RD – **W REVISION**

EXAMPLE: Reposition joint spacer **CMS Ex:** Adjustment pacemaker lead

REVISION: Correcting, to the extent possible, a portion of a malfunctioning device or the position of a displaced device.

EXPLANATION: May replace components of a device ...

Body Part – 4TH	Approach – 5TH	Device – 6TH	Qualifier – 7TH
0 Lumbar Vertebral Joint 3 Lumbosacral Joint	0 Open 3 Percutaneous 4 Percutaneous endoscopic X External	0 Drainage device 3 Infusion device 4 Internal fixation device 7 Autologous tissue substitute 8 Spacer A Interbody infusion device J Synthetic substitute K Nonautologous tissue substitute	Z No qualifier
2 Lumbar Vertebral Disc 4 Lumbosacral Disc	0 Open 3 Percutaneous 4 Percutaneous endoscopic X External	0 Drainage device 3 Infusion device 7 Autologous tissue substitute J Synthetic substitute K Nonautologous tissue substitute	Z No qualifier
5 Sacrococcygeal Joint 6 Coccygeal Joint 7 Sacroiliac Joint, Right 8 Sacroiliac Joint, Left	0 Open 3 Percutaneous 4 Percutaneous endoscopic X External	0 Drainage device 3 Infusion device 4 Internal fixation device 7 Autologous tissue substitute 8 Spacer J Synthetic substitute K Nonautologous tissue substitute	Z No qualifier
9 Hip Joint, Right B Hip Joint, Left	0 Open	0 Drainage device 3 Infusion device 4 Internal fixation device 5 External fixation device 7 Autologous tissue substitute 8 Spacer 9 Liner B Resufacing device J Synthetic substitute K Nonautologous tissue substitute	Z No qualifier

continued ➡

0SW REVISION – continued

LOWER JOINTS 0SW

Body Part – 4ᵀᴴ	Approach – 5ᵀᴴ	Device – 6ᵀᴴ	Qualifier – 7ᵀᴴ
9 Hip Joint, Right B Hip Joint, Left	3 Percutaneous 4 Percutaneous endoscopic X External	0 Drainage device 3 Infusion device 4 Internal fixation device 5 External fixation device 7 Autologous tissue substitute 8 Spacer J Synthetic substitute K Nonautologous tissue substitute	Z No qualifier
C Knee Joint, Right D Knee Joint, Left	0 Open	0 Drainage device 3 Infusion device 4 Internal fixation device 5 External fixation device 7 Autologous tissue substitute 8 Spacer 9 Liner J Synthetic substitute K Nonautologous tissue substitute	Z No qualifier
C Knee Joint, Right D Knee Joint, Left	3 Percutaneous 4 Percutaneous endoscopic X External	0 Drainage device 3 Infusion device 4 Internal fixation device 5 External fixation device 7 Autologous tissue substitute 8 Spacer J Synthetic substitute K Nonautologous tissue substitute	Z No qualifier
F Ankle Joint, Right G Ankle Joint, Left H Tarsal Joint, Right J Tarsal Joint, Left K Metatarsal-Tarsal Joint, Right L Metatarsal-Tarsal Joint, Left M Metatarsal-Phalangeal Joint, Right N Metatarsal-Phalangeal Joint, Left P Toe Phalangeal Joint, Right Q Toe Phalangeal Joint, Left	0 Open 3 Percutaneous 4 Percutaneous endoscopic X External	0 Drainage device 3 Infusion device 4 Internal fixation device 5 External fixation device 7 Autologous tissue substitute 8 Spacer J Synthetic substitute K Nonautologous tissue substitute	Z No qualifier

Educational Annotations | T – Urinary System

Body System Specific Educational Annotations for the Urinary System include:
- Anatomy and Physiology Review
- Anatomical Illustrations
- Definitions of Common Procedures
- AHA Coding Clinic® Reference Notations
- Body Part Key Listings
- Device Key Listings
- Device Aggregation Table Listings
- Coding Notes

Anatomy and Physiology Review of Urinary System

BODY PART VALUES – T - URINARY SYSTEM

Bladder – ANATOMY – The urinary bladder is a hollow, collapsible musculomembranous organ located within the pelvic cavity behind the symphysis pubis. In the male, it lies against the rectum, and in the female it lies against the vagina and uterus. When filled it may contain 17 fluid ounces (500 ml) of urine and it pushes upward, indenting the abdominal cavity. The trigone area is the floor of the bladder formed by three points, the two ureteral orifices and the urethral orifice. The dome is the expandable superior surface of the bladder. The ureteric orifice is that area surrounding the ureteral openings. The urachus in the adult forms the middle umbilical ligament of the bladder. PHYSIOLOGY – The urinary bladder functions as a reservoir for the urine produced by the kidneys until the individual expels the urine (micturition). Micturition occurs when the bladder becomes distended with urine and stretch receptor nerves signal the micturition center in the sacral spinal cord. Parasympathetic nerve impulses start rhythmically contracting the bladder and the individual senses an urgency to urinate. Following the midbrain decision to urinate, the external urethral sphincter is relaxed, and urination begins as the bladder muscle contracts.

Bladder Neck – The bladder neck is that area surrounding the urethral orifice.

Kidney – ANATOMY – The kidneys are reddish-brown, bean-shaped organs about 4.7 inches (12 cm) long, 2.3 inches (6 cm) wide, and 1.2 inches (3 cm) thick, located on either side of the vertebral column in the retroperitoneal space. The kidneys are supplied with arterial blood from the renal arteries which branch off from the aorta, and are drained by the renal veins which connect with the inferior vena cava. PHYSIOLOGY – The kidneys function to remove metabolic wastes from the blood by transferring them into the urine. They also regulate red blood cell production, blood pressure, calcium absorption, and the pH level of the blood.

Kidney Pelvis – The kidney (renal) pelvis is the funnel-shaped urinary collecting system of the kidney at the upper end of the ureter.

Ureter – The ureter is the musculomembranous tube extending from the renal pelvis to the bladder that transports the urine from the kidney to the bladder using gravity and peristaltic contraction.

Urethra – The urethra is the musculomembranous tube which extends and carries urine from the bladder to the external urethral opening (meatus).

Anatomical Illustrations of Urinary System

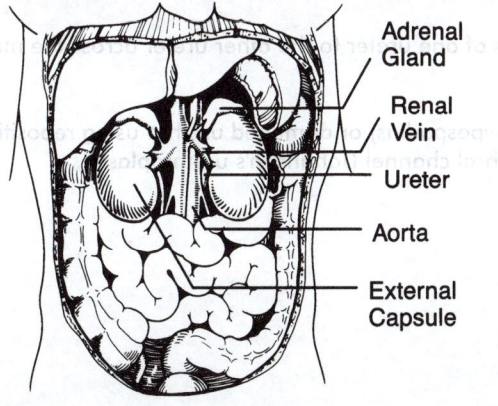

KIDNEY — ANTERIOR VIEW

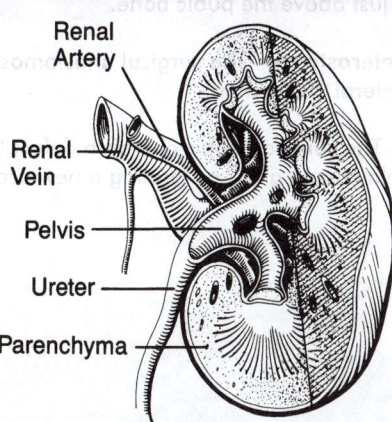

KIDNEY — (CUT AWAY VIEW)

Continued on next page

Educational Annotations | T – Urinary System

Anatomical Illustrations of Urinary System

Continued from previous page

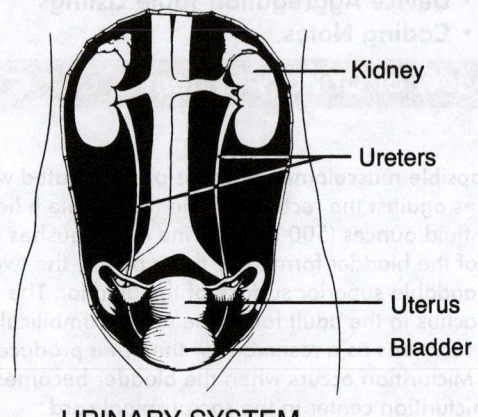

URINARY SYSTEM

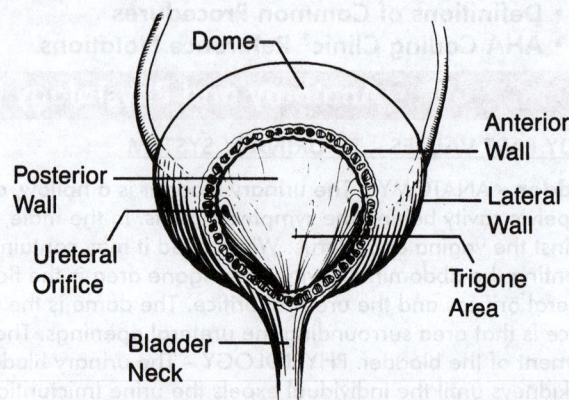

BLADDER — ANTERIOR (CUT-AWAY) VIEW

Definitions of Common Procedures of Urinary System

Bladder neck suspension – The surgical procedure to reposition and support the bladder neck using sutures or a sling of tissue that attaches each end of the sling to pelvic tissue (fascia) or the abdominal wall using stitches.

Cystoscopy – The insertion of an endoscope (cystoscope) through the urethra and into the bladder for visual examination and often to perform procedures on the bladder and urethra.

Extracorporeal shock wave lithotripsy (ESWL) on kidney stone – The breaking apart of kidney stones by using high-energy sound shock waves.

Kidney transplant – The surgical replacement of an end-stage diseased kidney using a donor kidney (living or non-living donor), and sometimes from a genetically identical twin (syngeneic).

Nephrectomy – The surgical removal of a kidney.

Nephropexy – The surgical fixation of a kidney to treat a floating kidney (nephroptosis).

Suprapubic cystostomy – The surgical bypass of the urine from the bladder to outside the body via an implanted catheter placed just above the pubic bone.

Transureteroureterostomy – The surgical anastomosis of one ureter to the other ureter across the midline to bypass distal ureteral obstruction.

Urethroplasty – The surgical repair of a birth defect (hypospadias) or damaged urethra using repositioning, anastomosis, onlay tissue graft, or forming a new urethral channel (Johanson's urethroplasty).

Educational Annotations | T – Urinary System

AHA Coding Clinic® Reference Notations of Urinary System

ROOT OPERATION SPECIFIC - T - URINARY SYSTEM
BYPASS - 1
CHANGE - 2
DESTRUCTION - 5
DILATION - 7
    Insertion (dilation) of ureteral stent..AHA 15:2Q:p8
    Insertion of UroLift® System into prostate ....AHA 13:4Q:p123
DIVISION - 8
DRAINAGE - 9
EXCISION - B
    Polyp excision in ileal loop (neobladder)..AHA 14:2Q:p8
EXTIRPATION - C
    Extirpation with fragmentation of renal pelvis stone ....AHA 15:2Q:p7
    Fragmentation and removal of kidney, ureteral, and bladder stones ....AHA 15:2Q:p8
    Ureteroscopic laser lithotripsy with removal of stone fragments.................AHA 13:4Q:p122
EXTRACTION - D
FRAGMENTATION - F
    Extracorporeal shock wave lithotripsy (ESWL) on kidney stone ....AHA 13:4Q:p122
INSERTION - H
INSPECTION - J
OCCLUSION - L
REATTACHMENT - M
RELEASE - N
REMOVAL - P
REPAIR - Q
REPLACEMENT - R
REPOSITION - S
RESECTION - T
    Complete nephroureterectomy..AHA 14:3Q:p16
SUPPLEMENT - U
RESTRICTION - V
    Deflux injection into bladder at ureteral orifices ....AHA 15:2Q:p11
REVISION - W
TRANSPLANTATION - Y

Body Part Key Listings of Urinary System

See also Body Part Key in Appendix C

Bulbourethral (Cowper's) gland	*use* Urethra
Cowper's (bulbourethral) gland	*use* Urethra
External urethral sphincter	*use* Urethra
Internal urethral sphincter	*use* Urethra
Membranous urethra	*use* Urethra
Penile urethra	*use* Urethra
Prostatic urethra	*use* Urethra
Renal calyx	*use* Kidney, Bilateral/Left/Right
Renal capsule	*use* Kidney, Bilateral/Left/Right
Renal cortex	*use* Kidney, Bilateral/Left/Right
Renal segment	*use* Kidney, Bilateral/Left/Right
Trigone of bladder	*use* Bladder
Ureteral orifice	*use* Ureter, Bilateral/Left/Right
Ureteropelvic junction (UPJ)	*use* Kidney Pelvis, Left/Right
Ureterovesical orifice	*use* Ureter, Bilateral/Left/Right

0T

MEDICAL AND SURGICAL SECTION – 2016 ICD-10-PCS

[2016.PCS]

Educational Annotations | T – Urinary System

Device Key Listings of Urinary System

See also Device Key in Appendix D

AMS 800® Urinary Control System	*use* Artificial Sphincter in Urinary System
Artificial urinary sphincter (AUS)	*use* Artificial Sphincter in Urinary System
Autograft	*use* Autologous Tissue Substitute
Cystostomy tube	*use* Drainage Device
Foley catheter	*use* Drainage Device
Percutaneous nephrostomy catheter	*use* Drainage Device
Sacral nerve modulation (SNM) lead	*use* Stimulator Lead in Urinary System
Sacral neuromodulation lead	*use* Stimulator Lead in Urinary System
Stent, intraluminal (cardiovascular) (gastrointestinal) (hepatobiliary) (urinary)	*use* Intraluminal Device *use* Intraluminal Device
Tissue bank graft	*use* Nonautologous Tissue Substitute
Urinary incontinence stimulator lead	*use* Stimulator Lead in Urinary System

Device Aggregation Table Listings of Urinary System

See also Device Aggregation Table in Appendix E

Specific Device	For Operation	In Body System	General Device
None Listed in Device Aggregation Table for this Body System			

Coding Notes of Urinary System

Body System Specific PCS Reference Manual Exercises

PCS CODE	T – URINARY SYSTEM EXERCISES
0T170ZC	Open urinary diversion, left ureter, using ileal conduit to skin.
0T2BX0Z	Foley urinary catheter exchange. (This is coded to Drainage Device because urine is being drained.)
0T778DZ	Cystoscopy with dilation of left ureteral stricture, with stent placement.
0T7C8ZZ	Cystoscopy with intraluminal dilation of bladder neck stricture.
0T9B70Z	Routine Foley catheter placement.
0TB03ZX	Percutaneous needle core biopsy of right kidney.
0TCB8ZZ	Transurethral cystoscopy with removal of bladder stone.
0TF6XZZ 0TF7XZZ	Extracorporeal shock-wave lithotripsy (ESWL), bilateral ureters. (The bilateral ureter body part value is not available for the root operation Fragmentation, so the procedures are coded separately.)
0TFB8ZZ	Transurethral cystoscopy with fragmentation of bladder calculus.
0TJB8ZZ	Transurethral diagnostic cystoscopy.
0TN60ZZ	Laparotomy with exploration and adhesiolysis of right ureter.
0TP98DZ	Cystoscopy with retrieval of left ureteral stent.
0TT10ZZ	Explantation of left failed kidney, open.
0TY10Z0	Left kidney/pancreas organ bank transplant.
0FYG0Z0	

T – URINARY SYSTEM 0T1

TUBULAR GROUP: Bypass, Dilation, Occlusion, Restriction
Root Operations that alter the diameter/route of a tubular body part.

1ST – **0** Medical and Surgical
2ND – **T** Urinary System
3RD – **1 BYPASS**

EXAMPLE: Ileal conduit urinary diversion   CMS Ex: Coronary artery bypass

BYPASS: Altering the route of passage of the contents of a tubular body part.

EXPLANATION: Rerouting contents to a downstream part ...

Body Part – 4TH	Approach – 5TH	Device – 6TH	Qualifier – 7TH
3 Kidney Pelvis, Right 4 Kidney Pelvis, Left	0 Open 4 Percutaneous endoscopic	7 Autologous tissue substitute J Synthetic substitute K Nonautologous tissue substitute Z No device	3 Kidney Pelvis, Right 4 Kidney Pelvis, Left 6 Ureter, Right 7 Ureter, Left 8 Colon 9 Colocutaneous A Ileum B Bladder C Ileocutaneous D Cutaneous
3 Kidney Pelvis, Right 4 Kidney Pelvis, Left	3 Percutaneous	J Synthetic substitute	D Cutaneous
6 Ureter, Right 7 Ureter, Left 8 Ureters, Bilateral	0 Open 4 Percutaneous endoscopic	7 Autologous tissue substitute J Synthetic substitute K Nonautologous tissue substitute Z No device	6 Ureter, Right 7 Ureter, Left 8 Colon 9 Colocutaneous A Ileum B Bladder C Ileocutaneous D Cutaneous
6 Ureter, Right 7 Ureter, Left 8 Ureters, Bilateral	3 Percutaneous	J Synthetic substitute	D Cutaneous
B Bladder	0 Open 4 Percutaneous endoscopic	7 Autologous tissue substitute J Synthetic substitute K Nonautologous tissue substitute Z No device	9 Colocutaneous C Ileocutaneous D Cutaneous
B Bladder	3 Percutaneous	J Synthetic substitute	D Cutaneous

0T2

MEDICAL AND SURGICAL SECTION – 2016 ICD-10-PCS

[2016.PCS]

DEVICE GROUP: Change, Insertion, Removal, Replacement, Revision, Supplement
Root Operations that always involve a device.

- 1ST – **0** Medical and Surgical
- 2ND – **T** Urinary System
- 3RD – **2 CHANGE**

EXAMPLE: Exchange Foley catheter | CMS Ex: Changing urinary catheter

CHANGE: Taking out or off a device from a body part and putting back an identical or similar device in or on the same body part without cutting or puncturing the skin or a mucous membrane.

EXPLANATION: ALL Changes use EXTERNAL approach only ...

Body Part – 4TH	Approach – 5TH	Device – 6TH	Qualifier – 7TH
5 Kidney 9 Ureter B Bladder D Urethra	X External	0 Drainage device Y Other device	Z No qualifier

---

EXCISION GROUP: Excision, Resection, Destruction, Extraction, (Detachment)
Root Operations that take out some or all of a body part.

- 1ST – **0** Medical and Surgical
- 2ND – **T** Urinary System
- 3RD – **5 DESTRUCTION**

EXAMPLE: Cystoscopic laser ablation | CMS Ex: Fulguration polyp

DESTRUCTION: Physical eradication of all or a portion of a body part by the direct use of energy, force, or a destructive agent.

EXPLANATION: None of the body part is physically taken out

Body Part – 4TH	Approach – 5TH	Device – 6TH	Qualifier – 7TH
0 Kidney, Right 1 Kidney, Left 3 Kidney Pelvis, Right 4 Kidney Pelvis, Left 6 Ureter, Right 7 Ureter, Left B Bladder C Bladder Neck	0 Open 3 Percutaneous 4 Percutaneous endoscopic 7 Via natural or artificial opening 8 Via natural or artificial opening endoscopic	Z No device	Z No qualifier
D Urethra	0 Open 3 Percutaneous 4 Percutaneous endoscopic 7 Via natural or artificial opening 8 Via natural or artificial opening endoscopic X External	Z No device	Z No qualifier

T – URINARY SYSTEM 0T8

TUBULAR GROUP: Bypass, Dilation, Occlusion, Restriction
Root Operations that alter the diameter/route of a tubular body part.

- 1ST – **0** Medical and Surgical
- 2ND – **T** Urinary System
- 3RD – **7 DILATION**

EXAMPLE: Urethral dilation CMS Ex: Transluminal angioplasty

DILATION: Expanding an orifice or the lumen of a tubular body part.

EXPLANATION: By force (stretching) or cutting ...

Body Part – 4TH	Approach – 5TH	Device – 6TH	Qualifier – 7TH
3 Kidney Pelvis, Right	0 Open	D Intraluminal device	Z No qualifier
4 Kidney Pelvis, Left	3 Percutaneous	Z No device	
6 Ureter, Right	4 Percutaneous endoscopic		
7 Ureter, Left	7 Via natural or artificial opening		
8 Ureters, Bilateral	8 Via natural or artificial opening endoscopic		
B Bladder			
C Bladder Neck			
D Urethra			

DIVISION GROUP: Division, Release
Root Operations involving cutting or separation only.

- 1ST – **0** Medical and Surgical
- 2ND – **T** Urinary System
- 3RD – **8 DIVISION**

EXAMPLE: Division bladder neck CMS Ex: Osteotomy

DIVISION: Cutting into a body part without draining fluids and/or gases from the body part in order to separate or transect a body part.

EXPLANATION: Separated into two or more portions ...

Body Part – 4TH	Approach – 5TH	Device – 6TH	Qualifier – 7TH
2 Kidneys, Bilateral	0 Open	Z No device	Z No qualifier
C Bladder Neck	3 Percutaneous		
	4 Percutaneous endoscopic		

595

0T9 MEDICAL AND SURGICAL SECTION – 2016 ICD-10-PCS

DRAINAGE GROUP: Drainage, Extirpation, Fragmentation
Root Operations that take out solids/fluids/gases from a body part.

- 1ST - **0** Medical and Surgical
- 2ND - **T** Urinary System
- 3RD - **9 DRAINAGE**

EXAMPLE: Foley catheter placement   CMS Ex: Thoracentesis

DRAINAGE: Taking or letting out fluids and/or gases from a body part.

EXPLANATION: Qualifier "X Diagnostic" indicates biopsy ...

Body Part – 4TH	Approach – 5TH	Device – 6TH	Qualifier – 7TH
0 Kidney, Right 1 Kidney, Left 3 Kidney Pelvis, Right 4 Kidney Pelvis, Left 6 Ureter, Right 7 Ureter, Left 8 Ureters, Bilateral B Bladder C Bladder Neck	0 Open 3 Percutaneous 4 Percutaneous endoscopic 7 Via natural or artificial opening 8 Via natural or artificial opening endoscopic	0 Drainage device	Z No qualifier
0 Kidney, Right 1 Kidney, Left 3 Kidney Pelvis, Right 4 Kidney Pelvis, Left 6 Ureter, Right 7 Ureter, Left 8 Ureters, Bilateral B Bladder C Bladder Neck	0 Open 3 Percutaneous 4 Percutaneous endoscopic 7 Via natural or artificial opening 8 Via natural or artificial opening endoscopic	Z No device	X Diagnostic Z No qualifier
D Urethra	0 Open 3 Percutaneous 4 Percutaneous endoscopic 7 Via natural or artificial opening 8 Via natural or artificial opening endoscopic X External	0 Drainage device	Z No qualifier
D Urethra	0 Open 3 Percutaneous 4 Percutaneous endoscopic 7 Via natural or artificial opening 8 Via natural or artificial opening endoscopic X External	Z No device	X Diagnostic Z No qualifier

0TB
T – URINARY SYSTEM

EXCISION GROUP: Excision, Resection, Destruction, Extraction, (Detachment)
Root Operations that take out some or all of a body part.

- 1ST – **0** Medical and Surgical
- 2ND – **T** Urinary System
- 3RD – **B** EXCISION

EXAMPLE: Needle core biopsy kidney   **CMS Ex:** Liver biopsy

EXCISION: Cutting out or off, without replacement, a portion of a body part.

EXPLANATION: Qualifier "X Diagnostic" indicates biopsy …

Body Part – 4TH	Approach – 5TH	Device – 6TH	Qualifier – 7TH
0 Kidney, Right 1 Kidney, Left 3 Kidney Pelvis, Right 4 Kidney Pelvis, Left 6 Ureter, Right 7 Ureter, Left B Bladder C Bladder Neck	0 Open 3 Percutaneous 4 Percutaneous endoscopic 7 Via natural or artificial opening 8 Via natural or artificial opening endoscopic	Z No device	X Diagnostic Z No qualifier
D Urethra	0 Open 3 Percutaneous 4 Percutaneous endoscopic 7 Via natural or artificial opening 8 Via natural or artificial opening endoscopic X External	Z No device	X Diagnostic Z No qualifier

0TC
MEDICAL AND SURGICAL SECTION – 2016 ICD-10-PCS
[2016.PCS]

DRAINAGE GROUP: Drainage, Extirpation, Fragmentation
Root Operations that take out solids/fluids/gases from a body part.

1ST - **0** Medical and Surgical
2ND - **T** Urinary System
3RD - **C EXTIRPATION**

EXAMPLE: Removal bladder stone CMS Ex: Choledocholithotomy

EXTIRPATION: Taking or cutting out solid matter from a body part.

EXPLANATION: Abnormal byproduct or foreign body ...

Body Part – 4TH	Approach – 5TH	Device – 6TH	Qualifier – 7TH
0 Kidney, Right 1 Kidney, Left 3 Kidney Pelvis, Right 4 Kidney Pelvis, Left 6 Ureter, Right 7 Ureter, Left B Bladder C Bladder Neck	0 Open 3 Percutaneous 4 Percutaneous endoscopic 7 Via natural or artificial opening 8 Via natural or artificial opening endoscopic	Z No device	Z No qualifier
D Urethra	0 Open 3 Percutaneous 4 Percutaneous endoscopic 7 Via natural or artificial opening 8 Via natural or artificial opening endoscopic X External	Z No device	Z No qualifier

EXCISION GROUP: Excision, Resection, Destruction, Extraction, (Detachment)
Root Operations that take out some or all of a body part.

1ST - **0** Medical and Surgical
2ND - **T** Urinary System
3RD - **D EXTRACTION**

EXAMPLE: Kidney extraction CMS Ex: D&C

EXTRACTION: Pulling or stripping out or off all or a portion of a body part by the use of force.

EXPLANATION: None for this Body System

Body Part – 4TH	Approach – 5TH	Device – 6TH	Qualifier – 7TH
0 Kidney, Right 1 Kidney, Left	0 Open 3 Percutaneous 4 Percutaneous endoscopic	Z No device	Z No qualifier

T – URINARY SYSTEM 0 T F

DRAINAGE GROUP: Drainage, Extirpation, Fragmentation
Root Operations that take out solids/fluids/gases from a body part.

1ST - **0** Medical and Surgical
2ND - **T** Urinary System
3RD - **F** FRAGMENTATION

EXAMPLE: Extracorporeal shockwave lithotripsy CMS Ex: ESWL

FRAGMENTATION: Breaking solid matter in a body part into pieces.

EXPLANATION: Pieces are not taken out during procedure ...

Body Part – 4TH	Approach – 5TH	Device – 6TH	Qualifier – 7TH
3 Kidney Pelvis, Right 4 Kidney Pelvis, Left 6 Ureter, Right 7 Ureter, Left B Bladder C Bladder Neck D Urethra NC*	0 Open 3 Percutaneous 4 Percutaneous endoscopic 7 Via natural or artificial opening 8 Via natural or artificial opening endoscopic X External	Z No device	Z No qualifier

NC* – Some procedures are considered non-covered by Medicare. See current Medicare Code Editor for details.

0TH — MEDICAL AND SURGICAL SECTION – 2016 ICD-10-PCS

DEVICE GROUP: Change, Insertion, Removal, Replacement, Revision, Supplement
Root Operations that always involve a device.

1ST – **0** Medical and Surgical
2ND – **T** Urinary System
3RD – **H** INSERTION

EXAMPLE: Artificial bladder sphincter   CMS Ex: Central venous catheter

INSERTION: Putting in a nonbiological appliance that monitors, assists, performs, or prevents a physiological function but does not physically take the place of a body part.

EXPLANATION: None

Body Part – 4TH	Approach – 5TH	Device – 6TH	Qualifier – 7TH
5 Kidney	0 Open 3 Percutaneous 4 Percutaneous endoscopic 7 Via natural or artificial opening 8 Via natural or artificial opening endoscopic	2 Monitoring device 3 Infusion device	Z No qualifier
9 Ureter	0 Open 3 Percutaneous 4 Percutaneous endoscopic 7 Via natural or artificial opening 8 Via natural or artificial opening endoscopic	2 Monitoring device 3 Infusion device M Stimulator lead	Z No qualifier
B Bladder	0 Open 3 Percutaneous 4 Percutaneous endoscopic 7 Via natural or artificial opening 8 Via natural or artificial opening endoscopic	2 Monitoring device 3 Infusion device L Artificial sphincter M Stimulator lead NC*	Z No qualifier
C Bladder Neck	0 Open 3 Percutaneous 4 Percutaneous endoscopic 7 Via natural or artificial opening 8 Via natural or artificial opening endoscopic	L Artificial sphincter	Z No qualifier
D Urethra	0 Open 3 Percutaneous 4 Percutaneous endoscopic 7 Via natural or artificial opening 8 Via natural or artificial opening endoscopic X External	2 Monitoring device 3 Infusion device L Artificial sphincter	Z No qualifier

NC* – Non-covered by Medicare. See current Medicare Code Editor for details.

T – URINARY SYSTEM 0TL

EXAMINATION GROUP: Inspection, (Map)
Root Operations involving examination only.

- 1ST – **0** Medical and Surgical
- 2ND – **T** Urinary System
- 3RD – **J** INSPECTION

EXAMPLE: Ureteroscopy
CMS Ex: Colonoscopy

INSPECTION: Visually and/or manually exploring a body part.

EXPLANATION: Direct or instrumental visualization ...

Body Part – 4TH	Approach – 5TH	Device – 6TH	Qualifier – 7TH
5 Kidney 9 Ureter B Bladder D Urethra	0 Open 3 Percutaneous 4 Percutaneous endoscopic 7 Via natural or artificial opening 8 Via natural or artificial opening endoscopic X External	Z No device	Z No qualifier

TUBULAR GROUP: Bypass, Dilation, Occlusion, Restriction
Root Operations that alter the diameter/route of a tubular body part.

- 1ST – **0** Medical and Surgical
- 2ND – **T** Urinary System
- 3RD – **L** OCCLUSION

EXAMPLE: Occlusion kidney pelvis
CMS Ex: Fallopian tube ligation

OCCLUSION: Completely closing an orifice or lumen of a tubular body part.

EXPLANATION: Natural or artificially created orifice ...

Body Part – 4TH	Approach – 5TH	Device – 6TH	Qualifier – 7TH
3 Kidney Pelvis, Right 4 Kidney Pelvis, Left 6 Ureter, Right 7 Ureter, Left B Bladder C Bladder Neck	0 Open 3 Percutaneous 4 Percutaneous endoscopic	C Extraluminal device D Intraluminal device Z No device	Z No qualifier
3 Kidney Pelvis, Right 4 Kidney Pelvis, Left 6 Ureter, Right 7 Ureter, Left B Bladder C Bladder Neck	7 Via natural or artificial opening 8 Via natural or artificial opening endoscopic	D Intraluminal device Z No device	Z No qualifier
D Urethra	0 Open 3 Percutaneous 4 Percutaneous endoscopic X External	C Extraluminal device D Intraluminal device Z No device	Z No qualifier
D Urethra	7 Via natural or artificial opening 8 Via natural or artificial opening endoscopic	D Intraluminal device Z No device	Z No qualifier

0TM — MEDICAL AND SURGICAL SECTION – 2016 ICD-10-PCS

MOVE GROUP: Reattachment, Reposition, (Transfer), Transplantation
Root Operations that put in/put back or move some/all of a body part.

- 1ST - **0** Medical and Surgical
- 2ND - **T** Urinary System
- 3RD - **M** REATTACHMENT

EXAMPLE: Replantation avulsed kidney
CMS Ex: Reattachment hand

REATTACHMENT: Putting back in or on all or a portion of a separated body part to its normal location or other suitable location.

EXPLANATION: With/without reconnection of vessels/nerves…

Body Part – 4TH	Approach – 5TH	Device – 6TH	Qualifier – 7TH
0 Kidney, Right	0 Open	Z No device	Z No qualifier
1 Kidney, Left	4 Percutaneous endoscopic		
2 Kidneys, Bilateral			
3 Kidney Pelvis, Right			
4 Kidney Pelvis, Left			
6 Ureter, Right			
7 Ureter, Left			
8 Ureters, Bilateral			
B Bladder			
C Bladder Neck			
D Urethra			

DIVISION GROUP: Division, Release
Root Operations involving cutting or separation only.

- 1ST - **0** Medical and Surgical
- 2ND - **T** Urinary System
- 3RD - **N** RELEASE

EXAMPLE: Adhesiolysis ureter
CMS Ex: Carpal tunnel release

RELEASE: Freeing a body part from an abnormal physical constraint by cutting or by the use of force.

EXPLANATION: None of the body part is taken out …

Body Part – 4TH	Approach – 5TH	Device – 6TH	Qualifier – 7TH
0 Kidney, Right	0 Open	Z No device	Z No qualifier
1 Kidney, Left	3 Percutaneous		
3 Kidney Pelvis, Right	4 Percutaneous endoscopic		
4 Kidney Pelvis, Left	7 Via natural or artificial opening		
6 Ureter, Right	8 Via natural or artificial opening endoscopic		
7 Ureter, Left			
B Bladder			
C Bladder Neck			
D Urethra	0 Open	Z No device	Z No qualifier
	3 Percutaneous		
	4 Percutaneous endoscopic		
	7 Via natural or artificial opening		
	8 Via natural or artificial opening endoscopic		
	X External		

T – URINARY SYSTEM 0 T P

DEVICE GROUP: Change, Insertion, Removal, Replacement, Revision, Supplement
Root Operations that always involve a device.

1ST - **0** Medical and Surgical
2ND - **T** Urinary System
3RD - **P** REMOVAL

EXAMPLE: Removal ureteral stent CMS Ex: Chest tube removal

REMOVAL: Taking out or off a device from a body part.

EXPLANATION: Removal device without reinsertion ...

Body Part – 4TH	Approach – 5TH	Device – 6TH	Qualifier – 7TH
5 Kidney	0 Open 3 Percutaneous 4 Percutaneous endoscopic 7 Via natural or artificial opening 8 Via natural or artificial opening endoscopic	0 Drainage device 2 Monitoring device 3 Infusion device 7 Autologous tissue substitute C Extraluminal device D Intraluminal device J Synthetic substitute K Nonautologous tissue substitute	Z No qualifier
5 Kidney	X External	0 Drainage device 2 Monitoring device 3 Infusion device D Intraluminal device	Z No qualifier
9 Ureter	0 Open 3 Percutaneous 4 Percutaneous endoscopic 7 Via natural or artificial opening 8 Via natural or artificial opening endoscopic	0 Drainage device 2 Monitoring device 3 Infusion device 7 Autologous tissue substitute C Extraluminal device D Intraluminal device J Synthetic substitute K Nonautologous tissue substitute M Stimulator lead	Z No qualifier
9 Ureter	X External	0 Drainage device 2 Monitoring device 3 Infusion device D Intraluminal device M Stimulator lead	Z No qualifier

continued ⇨

0TP REMOVAL – continued

Body Part – 4ᵀᴴ	Approach – 5ᵀᴴ	Device – 6ᵀᴴ	Qualifier – 7ᵀᴴ
B Bladder	0 Open 3 Percutaneous 4 Percutaneous endoscopic 7 Via natural or artificial opening 8 Via natural or artificial opening endoscopic	0 Drainage device 2 Monitoring device 3 Infusion device 7 Autologous tissue substitute C Extraluminal device D Intraluminal device J Synthetic substitute K Nonautologous tissue substitute L Artificial sphincter M Stimulator lead NC*	Z No qualifier
B Bladder	X External	0 Drainage device 2 Monitoring device 3 Infusion device D Intraluminal device L Artificial sphincter M Stimulator lead	Z No qualifier
D Urethra	0 Open 3 Percutaneous 4 Percutaneous endoscopic 7 Via natural or artificial opening 8 Via natural or artificial opening endoscopic	0 Drainage device 2 Monitoring device 3 Infusion device 7 Autologous tissue substitute C Extraluminal device D Intraluminal device J Synthetic substitute K Nonautologous tissue substitute L Artificial sphincter	Z No qualifier
D Urethra	X External	0 Drainage device 2 Monitoring device 3 Infusion device D Intraluminal device L Artificial sphincter	Z No qualifier

NC* – Non-covered by Medicare. See current Medicare Code Editor for details.

T – URINARY SYSTEM 0TR

OTHER REPAIRS GROUP: (Control), Repair
Root Operations that define other repairs.

1ST - 0 Medical and Surgical
2ND - T Urinary System
3RD - Q REPAIR

EXAMPLE: Suture lacerated kidney   CMS Ex: Suture laceration

REPAIR: Restoring, to the extent possible, a body part to its normal anatomic structure and function.

EXPLANATION: Only when no other root operation applies ...

Body Part – 4TH	Approach – 5TH	Device – 6TH	Qualifier – 7TH
0 Kidney, Right 1 Kidney, Left 3 Kidney Pelvis, Right 4 Kidney Pelvis, Left 6 Ureter, Right 7 Ureter, Left B Bladder C Bladder Neck	0 Open 3 Percutaneous 4 Percutaneous endoscopic 7 Via natural or artificial opening 8 Via natural or artificial opening endoscopic	Z No device	Z No qualifier
D Urethra	0 Open 3 Percutaneous 4 Percutaneous endoscopic 7 Via natural or artificial opening 8 Via natural or artificial opening endoscopic X External	Z No device	Z No qualifier

DEVICE GROUP: Change, Insertion, Removal, Replacement, Revision, Supplement
Root Operations that always involve a device.

1ST - 0 Medical and Surgical
2ND - T Urinary System
3RD - R REPLACEMENT

EXAMPLE: Segmental ureteral replacement   CMS Ex: Total hip

REPLACEMENT: Putting in or on a biological or synthetic material that physically takes the place and/or function of all or a portion of a body part.

EXPLANATION: Includes taking out body part, or eradication...

Body Part – 4TH	Approach – 5TH	Device – 6TH	Qualifier – 7TH
3 Kidney Pelvis, Right 4 Kidney Pelvis, Left 6 Ureter, Right 7 Ureter, Left B Bladder C Bladder Neck	0 Open 4 Percutaneous endoscopic 7 Via natural or artificial opening 8 Via natural or artificial opening endoscopic	7 Autologous tissue substitute J Synthetic substitute K Nonautologous tissue substitute	Z No qualifier
D Urethra	0 Open 4 Percutaneous endoscopic 7 Via natural or artificial opening 8 Via natural or artificial opening endoscopic X External	7 Autologous tissue substitute J Synthetic substitute K Nonautologous tissue substitute	Z No qualifier

0TS — MEDICAL AND SURGICAL SECTION – 2016 ICD-10-PCS

MOVE GROUP: Reattachment, Reposition, (Transfer), Transplantation
Root Operations that put in/put back or move some/all of a body part.

- 1ST – **0** Medical and Surgical
- 2ND – **T** Urinary System
- 3RD – **S** REPOSITION

EXAMPLE: Bladder neck (sling) suspension **CMS Ex:** FX reduction

REPOSITION: Moving to its normal location, or other suitable location, all or a portion of a body part.

EXPLANATION: May or may not be cut to be moved …

Body Part – 4TH		Approach – 5TH	Device – 6TH	Qualifier – 7TH
0 Kidney, Right	6 Ureter, Right	0 Open	Z No device	Z No qualifier
1 Kidney, Left	7 Ureter, Left	4 Percutaneous endoscopic		
2 Kidneys, Bilateral	8 Ureters, Bilateral			
3 Kidney Pelvis, Right	B Bladder			
4 Kidney Pelvis, Left	C Bladder Neck			
	D Urethra			

EXCISION GROUP: Excision, Resection, Destruction, Extraction, (Detachment)
Root Operations that take out some or all of a body part.

- 1ST – **0** Medical and Surgical
- 2ND – **T** Urinary System
- 3RD – **T** RESECTION

EXAMPLE: Nephrectomy **CMS Ex:** Cholecystectomy

RESECTION: Cutting out or off, without replacement, all of a body part.

EXPLANATION: None

Body Part – 4TH	Approach – 5TH	Device – 6TH	Qualifier – 7TH
0 Kidney, Right	0 Open	Z No device	Z No qualifier
1 Kidney, Left	4 Percutaneous endoscopic		
2 Kidneys, Bilateral			
3 Kidney Pelvis, Right	0 Open	Z No device	Z No qualifier
4 Kidney Pelvis, Left	4 Percutaneous endoscopic		
6 Ureter, Right	7 Via natural or artificial opening		
7 Ureter, Left	8 Via natural or artificial opening endoscopic		
B Bladder			
C Bladder Neck			
D Urethra			

T – URINARY SYSTEM 0TU

DEVICE GROUP: Change, Insertion, Removal, Replacement, Revision, Supplement
Root Operations that always involve a device.

1ST - 0 Medical and Surgical	EXAMPLE: Repair bladder defect with graft	CMS Ex: Hernia repair mesh
2ND - T Urinary System	**SUPPLEMENT:** Putting in or on biological or synthetic material that physically reinforces and/or augments the function of a portion of a body part.	
3RD - U SUPPLEMENT	EXPLANATION: Biological material from same individual ...	

Body Part – 4TH	Approach – 5TH	Device – 6TH	Qualifier – 7TH
3 Kidney Pelvis, Right 4 Kidney Pelvis, Left 6 Ureter, Right 7 Ureter, Left B Bladder C Bladder Neck	0 Open 4 Percutaneous endoscopic 7 Via natural or artificial opening 8 Via natural or artificial opening endoscopic	7 Autologous tissue substitute J Synthetic substitute K Nonautologous tissue substitute	Z No qualifier
D Urethra	0 Open 4 Percutaneous endoscopic 7 Via natural or artificial opening 8 Via natural or artificial opening endoscopic X External	7 Autologous tissue substitute J Synthetic substitute K Nonautologous tissue substitute	Z No qualifier

URINARY 0TU

607

0TV

MEDICAL AND SURGICAL SECTION – 2016 ICD-10-PCS

TUBULAR GROUP: Bypass, Dilation, Occlusion, Restriction
Root Operations that alter the diameter/route of a tubular body part.

1ST - **0** Medical and Surgical
2ND - **T** Urinary System
3RD - **V** RESTRICTION

EXAMPLE: Ureteral restrictive stent   CMS Ex: Cervical cerclage

RESTRICTION: Partially closing an orifice or the lumen of a tubular body part.

EXPLANATION: Natural or artificially created orifice …

Body Part – 4TH	Approach – 5TH	Device – 6TH	Qualifier – 7TH
3 Kidney Pelvis, Right 4 Kidney Pelvis, Left 6 Ureter, Right 7 Ureter, Left B Bladder C Bladder Neck	0 Open 3 Percutaneous 4 Percutaneous endoscopic	C Extraluminal device D Intraluminal device Z No device	Z No qualifier
3 Kidney Pelvis, Right 4 Kidney Pelvis, Left 6 Ureter, Right 7 Ureter, Left B Bladder C Bladder Neck	7 Via natural or artificial opening 8 Via natural or artificial opening endoscopic	D Intraluminal device Z No device	Z No qualifier
D Urethra	0 Open 3 Percutaneous 4 Percutaneous endoscopic	C Extraluminal device D Intraluminal device Z No device	Z No qualifier
D Urethra	7 Via natural or artificial opening 8 Via natural or artificial opening endoscopic	D Intraluminal device Z No device	Z No qualifier
D Urethra	X External	Z No device	Z No qualifier

0TW — T – URINARY SYSTEM

DEVICE GROUP: Change, Insertion, Removal, Replacement, Revision, Supplement
Root Operations that always involve a device.

- 1ST – **0** Medical and Surgical
- 2ND – **T** Urinary System
- 3RD – **W** REVISION

EXAMPLE: Reposition stimulator lead | CMS Ex: Adjustment pacemaker lead

REVISION: Correcting, to the extent possible, a portion of a malfunctioning device or the position of a displaced device.

EXPLANATION: May replace components of a device …

Body Part – 4TH	Approach – 5TH	Device – 6TH	Qualifier – 7TH
5 Kidney	0 Open 3 Percutaneous 4 Percutaneous endoscopic 7 Via natural or artificial opening 8 Via natural or artificial opening endoscopic X External	0 Drainage device 2 Monitoring device 3 Infusion device 7 Autologous tissue substitute C Extraluminal device D Intraluminal device J Synthetic substitute K Nonautologous tissue substitute	Z No qualifier
9 Ureter	0 Open 3 Percutaneous 4 Percutaneous endoscopic 7 Via natural or artificial opening 8 Via natural or artificial opening endoscopic X External	0 Drainage device 2 Monitoring device 3 Infusion device 7 Autologous tissue substitute C Extraluminal device D Intraluminal device J Synthetic substitute K Nonautologous tissue substitute M Stimulator lead	Z No qualifier
B Bladder	0 Open 3 Percutaneous 4 Percutaneous endoscopic 7 Via natural or artificial opening 8 Via natural or artificial opening endoscopic X External	0 Drainage device 2 Monitoring device 3 Infusion device 7 Autologous tissue substitute C Extraluminal device D Intraluminal device J Synthetic substitute K Nonautologous tissue substitute L Artificial sphincter M Stimulator lead	Z No qualifier
D Urethra	0 Open 3 Percutaneous 4 Percutaneous endoscopic 7 Via natural or artificial opening 8 Via natural or artificial opening endoscopic X External	0 Drainage device 2 Monitoring device 3 Infusion device 7 Autologous tissue substitute C Extraluminal device D Intraluminal device J Synthetic substitute K Nonautologous tissue substitute L Artificial sphincter	Z No qualifier

0TY

MEDICAL AND SURGICAL SECTION – 2016 ICD-10-PCS [2016.PCS]

MOVE GROUP: Reattachment, Reposition, (Transfer), **Transplantation**
Root Operations that put in/put back or move some/all of a body part.

1ST – 0	Medical and Surgical
2ND – T	Urinary System
3RD – Y	TRANSPLANTATION

EXAMPLE: Kidney transplant   **CMS Ex:** Kidney transplant

TRANSPLANTATION: Putting in or on all or a portion of a living body part taken from another individual or animal to physically take the place and/or function of all or a portion of a similar body part.

EXPLANATION: May take over all or part of its function ...

Body Part – 4TH	Approach – 5TH	Device – 6TH	Qualifier – 7TH
0 Kidney, Right LC*	0 Open	Z No device	0 Allogenic
1 Kidney, Left LC*			1 Syngeneic
			2 Zooplastic

LC* – Some procedures are considered limited coverage by Medicare. See current Medicare Code Editor for details.

Educational Annotations | U – Female Reproductive System

Body System Specific Educational Annotations for the Female Reproductive System include:
- Anatomy and Physiology Review
- Anatomical Illustrations
- Definitions of Common Procedures
- AHA Coding Clinic® Reference Notations
- Body Part Key Listings
- Device Key Listings
- Device Aggregation Table Listings
- Coding Notes

Anatomy and Physiology Review of Female Reproductive System

BODY PART VALUES – U - FEMALE REPRODUCTIVE SYSTEM

Cervix – The cervix is the lower portion of the uterus that extends downward into the vagina.

Clitoris – ANATOMY – The highly innervated, sensitive female sex organ that is located above the urethral opening (meatus) and at the junction of the labia minora. PHYSIOLOGY – It is generally accepted as the primary anatomical source of female sexual pleasure.

Cul-de-sac – The deep peritoneal recess between the rectum and back wall of the uterus (also known as the pouch of Douglas and rectouterine pouch).

Endometrium – The mucous membrane interior lining of the uterus that lies upon the thick muscular myometrium of the body.

Fallopian Tube – ANATOMY – The fallopian tubes (also known as oviducts, uterine tubes, and salpinges) are the tubular canals from each side of the uterus to the area immediately next to each ovary (fimbriae). PHYSIOLOGY – The fallopian tubes serve to transport the ova to the uterus.

Hymen – The hymen is a membrane of tissue that surrounds or partially covers the vaginal opening.

Ova – The human reproductive egg(s).

Ovary – ANATOMY – The ovaries are the paired, flat, ovoid female reproductive glands located on each side of the uterus, attached to the broad ligament, and are approximately 1.4 inches (3.5 cm) in length and 0.8 inches (2 cm) in width. PHYSIOLOGY – The ovaries function to produce the human reproductive egg cell (ova, ovum), and to produce hormones. The ovaries secrete estrogen, testosterone, and progesterone.

Uterine Supporting Structure – The ligaments, fibromuscular bands, and connective tissue that support the uterus, ovaries, and fallopian tubes. The broad ligament is the double-layered fold of the peritoneum with the loose connective tissue between its layers, called the parametrium. The round ligaments are the fibromuscular bands attached to the uterus below the fallopian tube orifices and to the pelvic wall.

Uterus – ANATOMY – The uterus is the pear-shaped, hollow, muscular female reproductive organ that is about 2.8 inches (7 cm) in length and up to 2 inches (5 cm) in width, located within the pelvic cavity, and resting slightly above the bladder. The fallopian tubes enter into the upper portion. The cervix is the lower portion that extends downward into the vagina. The isthmus is the narrowed lower end of the body of the uterus. The body is the bulky upper portion with the dome above the fallopian tube orifices (also known as the fundus or corpus uteri). The endometrium is the mucous membrane interior lining lying upon the thick muscular myometrium of the body. The ovarian and uterine arteries supply blood to the uterus. PHYSIOLOGY – The uterus functions to receive the embryo, serve as attachment for the placenta, stretch and enlarge to allow for the fetus to grow, and to rhythmically contract for delivery of the fetus.

Vagina – ANATOMY – The vagina is the elastic, musculomembranous canal extending from the uterus to the vulva, passing in front of the rectum and behind the bladder, attached by loose connective tissue, and is approximately 3-4 inches (7.5-10 cm) in length. PHYSIOLOGY – The vagina functions to receive the penis and ejaculated sperm during intercourse, pass the fetus to birth during delivery, and convey the menstrual discharge out of the body.

Vestibular Gland – The vestibular glands (also known as paraurethral, Bartholin's, and Skene's glands) are small mucous-secreting glands that open on either side of the urethral orifice and vaginal opening.

Vulva – ANATOMY – The vulva is the group of external female genital organs comprising the labia majora, labia minora, clitoris, and vestibular glands. PHYSIOLOGY – The vulva functions to protect the genital organs at the entrance of the vagina, and aid in sexual stimulation and lubrication during intercourse.

0U

MEDICAL AND SURGICAL SECTION – 2016 ICD-10-PCS

Educational Annotations | U – Female Reproductive System

Anatomical Illustrations of Female Reproductive System

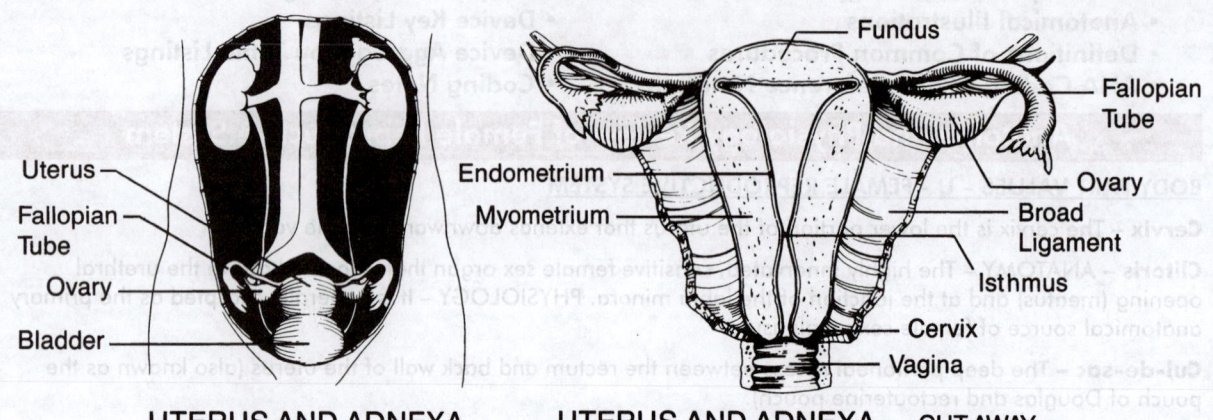

UTERUS AND ADNEXA

UTERUS AND ADNEXA — CUT-AWAY

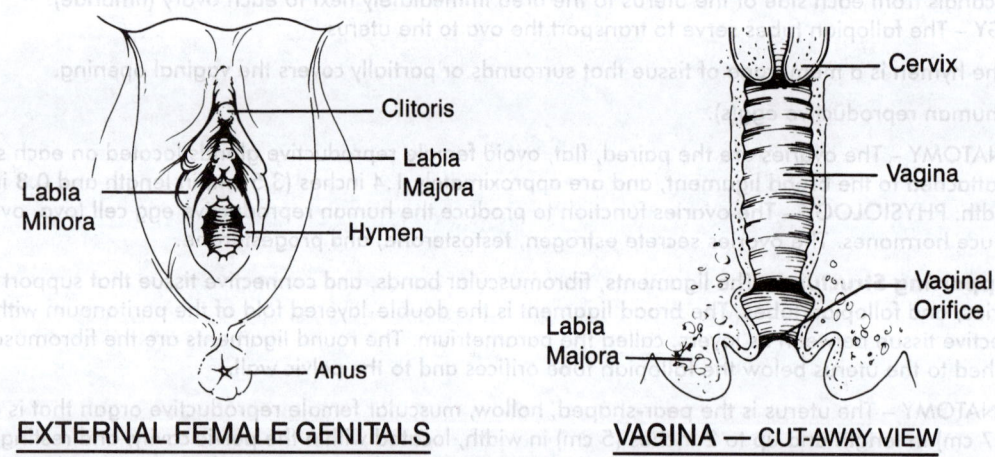

EXTERNAL FEMALE GENITALS

VAGINA — CUT-AWAY VIEW

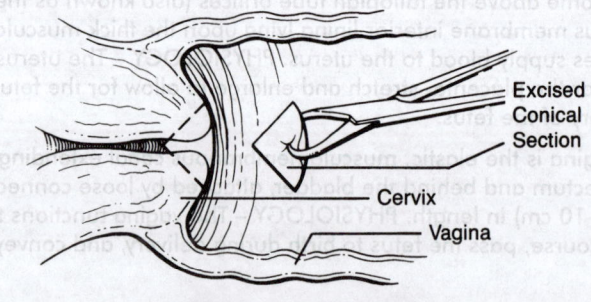

CONIZATION OF CERVIX

Educational Annotations | U – Female Reproductive System

Definitions of Common Procedures of Female Reproductive System

Cervical cerclage – The placement of an encircling suture in the cervix to prevent a miscarriage or premature birth.

Hysterectomy – The surgical removal of the uterus (subtotal) and often the cervix (total).

Oophorectomy – The surgical removal of one or both ovaries.

Ovarian cystectomy – The surgical removal of an ovarian cyst leaving the ovary intact.

Salpingectomy – The surgical removal of one or both fallopian tubes.

Vaginoplasty – The plastic surgical restoration of vaginal defects or deformities.

AHA Coding Clinic® Reference Notations of Female Reproductive System

ROOT OPERATION SPECIFIC - U - FEMALE REPRODUCTIVE SYSTEM
BYPASS - 1
CHANGE - 2
DESTRUCTION - 5
DILATION - 7
DIVISION - 8
DRAINAGE - 9
EXCISION - B
    Excision of labia majora skin tags..AHA 14:3Q:p12
    Uterine fibroids, multiple...AHA 14:4Q:p16
EXTIRPATION - C
    Clot evacuation from uterus post delivery.....................................AHA 13:2Q:p38
EXTRACTION - D
FRAGMENTATION - F
INSERTION - H
    IUD insertion during cesarean section..AHA 13:2Q:p34
INSPECTION - J
    Laparoscopic procedure converted to open..................................AHA 15:1Q:p33
OCCLUSION - L
REATTACHMENT - M
RELEASE - N
REMOVAL - P
REPAIR - Q
    Periurethral obstetric laceration repair...AHA 14:4Q:p18
    Repair of lacerated clitoris..AHA 13:4Q:p120
REPOSITION - S
RESECTION - T
    Bilateral oophorectomy..AHA 15:1Q:p33
    Bilateral salpingectomy..AHA 15:1Q:p33
    Hysterectomy..AHA 15:1Q:p33
    Removal of cervix..AHA 15:1Q:p33
    Removal of remaining portion of ovary...AHA 13:1Q:p24
    Total (open) hysterectomy..AHA 13:3Q:p28
SUPPLEMENT - U
RESTRICTION - V
REVISION - W
TRANSPLANTATION - Y

Educational Annotations | U – Female Reproductive System

Body Part Key Listings of Female Reproductive System

See also Body Part Key in Appendix C

Bartholin's (greater vestibular) gland	*use* Vestibular Gland
Broad ligament	*use* Uterine Supporting Structure
Fundus uteri	*use* Uterus
Greater vestibular (Bartholin's) gland	*use* Vestibular Gland
Infundibulopelvic ligament	*use* Uterine Supporting Structure
Labia majora	*use* Vulva
Labia minora	*use* Vulva
Myometrium	*use* Uterus
Ovarian ligament	*use* Uterine Supporting Structure
Oviduct	*use* Fallopian Tube, Left/Right
Paraurethral (Skene's) gland	*use* Vestibular Gland
Perimetrium	*use* Uterus
Round ligament of uterus	*use* Uterine Supporting Structure
Salpinx	*use* Fallopian Tube, Left/Right
Skene's (paraurethral) gland	*use* Vestibular Gland
Uterine cornu	*use* Uterus
Uterine tube	*use* Fallopian Tube, Left/Right

Device Key Listings of Female Reproductive System

See also Device Key in Appendix D

Autograft	*use* Autologous Tissue Substitute
Brachytherapy seeds	*use* Radioactive Element
Intrauterine device (IUD)	*use* Contraceptive Device in Female Reproductive System
Pessary ring	*use* Intraluminal Device, Pessary in Female Reproductive System
Tissue bank graft	*use* Nonautologous Tissue Substitute
Vaginal pessary	*use* Intraluminal Device, Pessary in Female Reproductive System

Device Aggregation Table Listings of Female Reproductive System

See also Device Aggregation Table in Appendix E

Specific Device	For Operation	In Body System	General Device
Intraluminal Device, Pessary	All applicable	Female Reproductive System	D Intraluminal Device

Educational Annotations | U – Female Reproductive System

Coding Notes of Female Reproductive System

Body System Specific PCS Reference Manual Exercises

PCS CODE	U – FEMALE REPRODUCTIVE SYSTEM EXERCISES
0U524ZZ	Laparoscopy with destruction of endometriosis, bilateral ovaries.
0U778ZZ	Hysteroscopy with balloon dilation of bilateral fallopian tubes.
0U914ZZ	Laparoscopy with left ovarian cystotomy and drainage.
0UB14ZZ	Laparoscopy with excision of endometrial implant from left ovary.
0UCG7ZZ	Non-incisional removal of intraluminal foreign body from vagina. (The approach "External" is also a possibility. It is assumed here that since the patient went to the doctor to have the object removed, that it was not in the vaginal orifice.)
0UDB8ZX	Hysteroscopy with D&C, diagnostic.
0UDN4ZZ	Laparoscopy with needle aspiration of ova for in-vitro fertilization.
0UF68ZZ	Hysteroscopy with intraluminal lithotripsy of left fallopian tube calcification.
0UJD8ZZ	Colposcopy with diagnostic hysteroscopy.
0UL74CZ	Laparoscopy with bilateral occlusion of fallopian tubes using Hulka extraluminal clips.
0UN14ZZ	Laparoscopy with freeing of left ovary and fallopian tube.
0UN64ZZ	
0UPH71Z	Transvaginal removal of brachytherapy seeds.
0UT9FZZ	Laparoscopic-assisted vaginal hysterectomy, supracervical resection.
0UVC7ZZ	Cervical cerclage using Shirodkar technique.

Educational Annotations

U – Female Reproductive System

NOTES

U – FEMALE REPRODUCTIVE SYSTEM 0U2

TUBULAR GROUP: Bypass, Dilation, Occlusion, Restriction
Root Operations that alter the diameter/route of a tubular body part.

- 1ST – **0** Medical and Surgical
- 2ND – **U** Female Reproductive System ♀
- 3RD – **1 BYPASS**

EXAMPLE: Fallopian tube bypass CMS Ex: Coronary artery bypass

BYPASS: Altering the route of passage of the contents of a tubular body part.

EXPLANATION: Rerouting contents to a downstream part …

Body Part – 4TH	Approach – 5TH	Device – 6TH	Qualifier – 7TH
5 Fallopian Tube, Right 6 Fallopian Tube, Left	0 Open 4 Percutaneous endoscopic	7 Autologous tissue substitute J Synthetic substitute K Nonautologous tissue substitute Z No device	5 Fallopian Tube, Right 6 Fallopian Tube, Left 9 Uterus

DEVICE GROUP: Change, Insertion, Removal, (Replacement), Revision, Supplement
Root Operations that always involve a device.

- 1ST – **0** Medical and Surgical
- 2ND – **U** Female Reproductive System ♀
- 3RD – **2 CHANGE**

EXAMPLE: Exchange drain tube CMS Ex: Changing urinary catheter

CHANGE: Taking out or off a device from a body part and putting back an identical or similar device in or on the same body part without cutting or puncturing the skin or a mucous membrane.

EXPLANATION: ALL Changes use EXTERNAL approach only …

Body Part – 4TH	Approach – 5TH	Device – 6TH	Qualifier – 7TH
3 Ovary 8 Fallopian Tube M Vulva	X External	0 Drainage device Y Other device	Z No qualifier
D Uterus and Cervix	X External	0 Drainage device H Contraceptive device Y Other device	Z No qualifier
H Vagina and Cul-de-sac	X External	0 Drainage device G Intraluminal device, pessary Y Other device	Z No qualifier

0U5

MEDICAL AND SURGICAL SECTION – 2016 ICD-10-PCS

EXCISION GROUP: Excision, Resection, Destruction, Extraction, (Detachment)
Root Operations that take out some or all of a body part.

- 1ST - **0** Medical and Surgical
- 2ND - **U** Female Reproductive System ♀
- 3RD - **5 DESTRUCTION**

EXAMPLE: Fulguration endometriosis   **CMS Ex:** Fulguration polyp

DESTRUCTION: Physical eradication of all or a portion of a body part by the direct use of energy, force, or a destructive agent.

EXPLANATION: None of the body part is physically taken out

Body Part – 4TH	Approach – 5TH	Device – 6TH	Qualifier – 7TH
0 Ovary, Right 1 Ovary, Left 2 Ovaries, Bilateral 4 Uterine Supporting Structure	0 Open 3 Percutaneous 4 Percutaneous endoscopic	Z No device	Z No qualifier
5 Fallopian Tube, Right 6 Fallopian Tube, Left 7 Fallopian Tubes, Bilateral NC* 9 Uterus B Endometrium C Cervix F Cul-de-sac	0 Open 3 Percutaneous 4 Percutaneous endoscopic 7 Via natural or artificial opening 8 Via natural or artificial opening endoscopic	Z No device	Z No qualifier
G Vagina K Hymen	0 Open 3 Percutaneous 4 Percutaneous endoscopic 7 Via natural or artificial opening 8 Via natural or artificial opening endoscopic X External	Z No device	Z No qualifier
J Clitoris L Vestibular Gland M Vulva	0 Open X External	Z No device	Z No qualifier

NC* – Non-covered by Medicare. See current Medicare Code Editor for details.

U – FEMALE REPRODUCTIVE SYSTEM — 0U8

TUBULAR GROUP: Bypass, Dilation, Occlusion, Restriction
Root Operations that alter the diameter/route of a tubular body part.

- 1ST – **0** Medical and Surgical
- 2ND – **U** Female Reproductive System ♀
- 3RD – **7 DILATION**

EXAMPLE: Dilation fallopian tubes   CMS Ex: Transluminal angioplasty

DILATION: Expanding an orifice or the lumen of a tubular body part.

EXPLANATION: By force (stretching) or cutting ...

Body Part – 4TH	Approach – 5TH	Device – 6TH	Qualifier – 7TH
5 Fallopian Tube, Right 6 Fallopian Tube, Left 7 Fallopian Tubes, Bilateral 9 Uterus C Cervix G Vagina	0 Open 3 Percutaneous 4 Percutaneous endoscopic 7 Via natural or artificial opening 8 Via natural or artificial opening endoscopic	D Intraluminal device Z No device	Z No qualifier
K Hymen	0 Open 3 Percutaneous 4 Percutaneous endoscopic 7 Via natural or artificial opening 8 Via natural or artificial opening endoscopic X External	D Intraluminal device Z No device	Z No qualifier

DIVISION GROUP: Division, Release
Root Operations involving cutting or separation only.

- 1ST – **0** Medical and Surgical
- 2ND – **U** Female Reproductive System ♀
- 3RD – **8 DIVISION**

EXAMPLE: Hymenotomy   CMS Ex: Osteotomy

DIVISION: Cutting into a body part without draining fluids and/or gases from the body part in order to separate or transect a body part.

EXPLANATION: Separated into two or more portions ...

Body Part – 4TH	Approach – 5TH	Device – 6TH	Qualifier – 7TH
0 Ovary, Right 1 Ovary, Left 2 Ovaries, Bilateral 4 Uterine Supporting Structure	0 Open 3 Percutaneous 4 Percutaneous endoscopic	Z No device	Z No qualifier
K Hymen	7 Via natural or artificial opening 8 Via natural or artificial opening endoscopic X External	Z No device	Z No qualifier

0U9

MEDICAL AND SURGICAL SECTION – 2016 ICD-10-PCS [2016.PCS]

DRAINAGE GROUP: Drainage, Extirpation, Fragmentation
Root Operations that take out solids/fluids/gases from a body part.

1ST - **0** Medical and Surgical
2ND - **U** Female Reproductive System ♀
3RD - **9 DRAINAGE**

EXAMPLE: Drainage ovarian cyst   CMS Ex: Thoracentesis

DRAINAGE: Taking or letting out fluids and/or gases from a body part.

EXPLANATION: Qualifier "X Diagnostic" indicates biopsy ...

Body Part – 4TH	Approach – 5TH	Device – 6TH	Qualifier – 7TH
0 Ovary, Right 1 Ovary, Left 2 Ovaries, Bilateral	0 Open 3 Percutaneous 4 Percutaneous endoscopic	0 Drainage device	Z No qualifier
0 Ovary, Right 1 Ovary, Left 2 Ovaries, Bilateral	0 Open 3 Percutaneous 4 Percutaneous endoscopic	Z No device	X Diagnostic Z No qualifier
0 Ovary, Right 1 Ovary, Left 2 Ovaries, Bilateral	X External	Z No device	Z No qualifier
4 Uterine Supporting Structure	0 Open 3 Percutaneous 4 Percutaneous endoscopic	0 Drainage device	Z No qualifier
4 Uterine Supporting Structure	0 Open 3 Percutaneous 4 Percutaneous endoscopic	Z No device	X Diagnostic Z No qualifier
5 Fallopian Tube, Right 6 Fallopian Tube, Left 7 Fallopian Tubes, Bilateral 9 Uterus C Cervix F Cul-de-sac	0 Open 3 Percutaneous 4 Percutaneous endoscopic 7 Via natural or artificial opening 8 Via natural or artificial opening endoscopic	0 Drainage device	Z No qualifier
5 Fallopian Tube, Right 6 Fallopian Tube, Left 7 Fallopian Tubes, Bilateral 9 Uterus C Cervix F Cul-de-sac	0 Open 3 Percutaneous 4 Percutaneous endoscopic 7 Via natural or artificial opening 8 Via natural or artificial opening endoscopic	Z No device	X Diagnostic Z No qualifier

continued ⇨

0 U 9 DRAINAGE – continued

U – FEMALE REPRODUCTIVE SYSTEM

Body Part – 4ᵀᴴ	Approach – 5ᵀᴴ	Device – 6ᵀᴴ	Qualifier – 7ᵀᴴ
G Vagina K Hymen	0 Open 3 Percutaneous 4 Percutaneous endoscopic 7 Via natural or artificial opening 8 Via natural or artificial opening endoscopic X External	0 Drainage device	Z No qualifier
G Vagina K Hymen	0 Open 3 Percutaneous 4 Percutaneous endoscopic 7 Via natural or artificial opening 8 Via natural or artificial opening endoscopic X External	Z No device	X Diagnostic Z No qualifier
J Clitoris L Vestibular Gland M Vulva	0 Open X External	0 Drainage device	Z No qualifier
J Clitoris L Vestibular Gland M Vulva	0 Open X External	Z No device	X Diagnostic Z No qualifier

0UB — MEDICAL AND SURGICAL SECTION – 2016 ICD-10-PCS

EXCISION GROUP: Excision, Resection, Destruction, Extraction, (Detachment)
Root Operations that take out some or all of a body part.

- 1ST – **0** Medical and Surgical
- 2ND – **U** Female Reproductive System ♀
- 3RD – **B** EXCISION

EXAMPLE: Excision uterine fibroids
CMS Ex: Liver biopsy

EXCISION: Cutting out or off, without replacement, a portion of a body part.

EXPLANATION: Qualifier "X Diagnostic" indicates biopsy ...

Body Part – 4TH	Approach – 5TH	Device – 6TH	Qualifier – 7TH
0 Ovary, Right 1 Ovary, Left 2 Ovaries, Bilateral 4 Uterine Supporting Structure 5 Fallopian Tube, Right 6 Fallopian Tube, Left 7 Fallopian Tubes, Bilateral 9 Uterus C Cervix F Cul-de-sac	0 Open 3 Percutaneous 4 Percutaneous endoscopic 7 Via natural or artificial opening 8 Via natural or artificial opening endoscopic	Z No device	X Diagnostic Z No qualifier
G Vagina K Hymen	0 Open 3 Percutaneous 4 Percutaneous endoscopic 7 Via natural or artificial opening 8 Via natural or artificial opening endoscopic X External	Z No device	X Diagnostic Z No qualifier
J Clitoris L Vestibular Gland M Vulva	0 Open X External	Z No device	X Diagnostic Z No qualifier

U – FEMALE REPRODUCTIVE SYSTEM — 0UC

DRAINAGE GROUP: Drainage, Extirpation, Fragmentation
Root Operations that take out solids/fluids/gases from a body part.

- 1ST – **0** Medical and Surgical
- 2ND – **U** Female Reproductive System ♀
- 3RD – **C** EXTIRPATION

EXAMPLE: Clot evacuation post delivery   **CMS Ex:** Choledocholithotomy

EXTIRPATION: Taking or cutting out solid matter from a body part.

EXPLANATION: Abnormal byproduct or foreign body ...

Body Part – 4TH	Approach – 5TH	Device – 6TH	Qualifier – 7TH
0 Ovary, Right 1 Ovary, Left 2 Ovaries, Bilateral 4 Uterine Supporting Structure	0 Open 3 Percutaneous 4 Percutaneous endoscopic	Z No device	Z No qualifier
5 Fallopian Tube, Right 6 Fallopian Tube, Left 7 Fallopian Tubes, Bilateral 9 Uterus B Endometrium C Cervix F Cul-de-sac	0 Open 3 Percutaneous 4 Percutaneous endoscopic 7 Via natural or artificial opening 8 Via natural or artificial opening endoscopic	Z No device	Z No qualifier
G Vagina K Hymen	0 Open 3 Percutaneous 4 Percutaneous endoscopic 7 Via natural or artificial opening 8 Via natural or artificial opening endoscopic X External	Z No device	Z No qualifier
J Clitoris L Vestibular Gland M Vulva	0 Open X External	Z No device	Z No qualifier

0 U D

MEDICAL AND SURGICAL SECTION – 2016 ICD-10-PCS

EXCISION GROUP: Excision, Resection, Destruction, Extraction, (Detachment)
Root Operations that take out some or all of a body part.

- 1ST – **0** Medical and Surgical
- 2ND – **U** Female Reproductive System ♀
- 3RD – **D** EXTRACTION

EXAMPLE: Dilation and curettage — CMS Ex: D&C

EXTRACTION: Pulling or stripping out or off all or a portion of a body part by the use of force.

EXPLANATION: Qualifier "X Diagnostic" indicates biopsy ...

Body Part – 4TH	Approach – 5TH	Device – 6TH	Qualifier – 7TH
B Endometrium	7 Via natural or artificial opening 8 Via natural or artificial opening endoscopic	Z No device	X Diagnostic Z No qualifier
N Ova	0 Open 3 Percutaneous 4 Percutaneous endoscopic	Z No device	Z No qualifier

DRAINAGE GROUP: Drainage, Extirpation, Fragmentation
Root Operations that take out solids/fluids/gases from a body part.

- 1ST – **0** Medical and Surgical
- 2ND – **U** Female Reproductive System ♀
- 3RD – **F** FRAGMENTATION

EXAMPLE: Lithotripsy fallopian tube calcification — CMS Ex: ESWL

FRAGMENTATION: Breaking solid matter in a body part into pieces.

EXPLANATION: Pieces are not taken out during procedure ...

Body Part – 4TH	Approach – 5TH	Device – 6TH	Qualifier – 7TH
5 Fallopian Tube, Right 6 Fallopian Tube, Left 7 Fallopian Tubes, Bilateral 9 Uterus	0 Open 3 Percutaneous 4 Percutaneous endoscopic 7 Via natural or artificial opening 8 Via natural or artificial opening endoscopic X External NC*	Z No device	Z No qualifier

NC* – Non-covered by Medicare. See current Medicare Code Editor for details.

0UH

U – FEMALE REPRODUCTIVE SYSTEM

DEVICE GROUP: Change, Insertion, Removal, (Replacement), Revision, Supplement
Root Operations that always involve a device.

1ST – **0** Medical and Surgical
2ND – **U** Female Reproductive System ♀
3RD – **H** INSERTION

EXAMPLE: Insertion of IUD   CMS Ex: Insertion central venous catheter

INSERTION: Putting in a nonbiological appliance that monitors, assists, performs, or prevents a physiological function but does not physically take the place of a body part.

EXPLANATION: None

Body Part – 4TH	Approach – 5TH	Device – 6TH	Qualifier – 7TH
3 Ovary	0 Open 3 Percutaneous 4 Percutaneous endoscopic	3 Infusion device	Z No qualifier
8 Fallopian Tube D Uterus and Cervix H Vagina and Cul-de-sac	0 Open 3 Percutaneous 4 Percutaneous endoscopic 7 Via natural or artificial opening 8 Via natural or artificial opening endoscopic	3 Infusion device	Z No qualifier
9 Uterus	7 Via natural or artificial opening 8 Via natural or artificial opening endoscopic	H Contraceptive device	Z No qualifier
C Cervix	0 Open 3 Percutaneous 4 Percutaneous endoscopic	1 Radioactive element	Z No qualifier
C Cervix	7 Via natural or artificial opening 8 Via natural or artificial opening endoscopic	1 Radioactive element H Contraceptive device	Z No qualifier
F Cul-de-sac	7 Via natural or artificial opening 8 Via natural or artificial opening endoscopic	G Intraluminal device, pessary	Z No qualifier
G Vagina	0 Open 3 Percutaneous 4 Percutaneous endoscopic X External	1 Radioactive element	Z No qualifier
G Vagina	7 Via natural or artificial opening 8 Via natural or artificial opening endoscopic	1 Radioactive element G Intraluminal device, pessary	Z No qualifier

0UJ

MEDICAL AND SURGICAL SECTION – 2016 ICD-10-PCS

[2016.PCS]

EXAMINATION GROUP: Inspection, (Map)
Root Operations involving examination only.

1ST – **0** Medical and Surgical
2ND – **U** Female Reproductive System ♀
3RD – **J** INSPECTION

EXAMPLE: Hysteroscopy   CMS Ex: Colonoscopy

INSPECTION: Visually and/or manually exploring a body part.

EXPLANATION: Direct or instrumental visualization ...

Body Part – 4TH	Approach – 5TH	Device – 6TH	Qualifier – 7TH
3 Ovary	0 Open 3 Percutaneous 4 Percutaneous endoscopic X External	Z No device	Z No qualifier
8 Fallopian Tube D Uterus and Cervix H Vagina and Cul-de-sac	0 Open 3 Percutaneous 4 Percutaneous endoscopic 7 Via natural or artificial opening 8 Via natural or artificial opening endoscopic X External	Z No device	Z No qualifier
M Vulva	0 Open X External	Z No device	Z No qualifier

FEMALE OUJ

U – FEMALE REPRODUCTIVE SYSTEM — 0 U M

TUBULAR GROUP: Bypass, Dilation, Occlusion, Restriction
Root Operations that alter the diameter/route of a tubular body part.

1ST - 0 Medical and Surgical
2ND - U Female Reproductive System ♀
3RD - L OCCLUSION

EXAMPLE: Fallopian tube clipping CMS Ex: Fallopian tube ligation

OCCLUSION: Completely closing an orifice or lumen of a tubular body part.

EXPLANATION: Natural or artificially created orifice ...

Body Part – 4TH	Approach – 5TH	Device – 6TH	Qualifier – 7TH
5 Fallopian Tube, Right 6 Fallopian Tube, Left 7 Fallopian Tubes, Bilateral NC*	0 Open 3 Percutaneous 4 Percutaneous endoscopic	C Extraluminal device D Intraluminal device Z No device	Z No qualifier
5 Fallopian Tube, Right 6 Fallopian Tube, Left 7 Fallopian Tubes, Bilateral NC*	7 Via natural or artificial opening 8 Via natural or artificial opening endoscopic	D Intraluminal device Z No device	Z No qualifier
F Cul-de-sac G Vagina	7 Via natural or artificial opening 8 Via natural or artificial opening endoscopic	D Intraluminal device Z No device	Z No qualifier

NC* – Non-covered by Medicare. See current Medicare Code Editor for details.

MOVE GROUP: Reattachment, Reposition, (Transfer), Transplantation
Root Operations that put in/put back or move some/all of a body part.

1ST - 0 Medical and Surgical
2ND - U Female Reproductive System ♀
3RD - M REATTACHMENT

EXAMPLE: Reattach avulsed round ligament CMS Ex: Reattachment hand

REATTACHMENT: Putting back in or on all or a portion of a separated body part to its normal location or other suitable location.

EXPLANATION: With/without reconnection of vessels/nerves...

Body Part – 4TH		Approach – 5TH	Device – 6TH	Qualifier – 7TH
0 Ovary, Right 1 Ovary, Left 2 Ovaries, Bilateral 4 Uterine Supporting Structure 5 Fallopian Tube, Right	6 Fallopian Tube, Left 7 Fallopian Tubes, Bilateral 9 Uterus C Cervix F Cul-de-sac G Vagina	0 Open 4 Percutaneous endoscopic	Z No device	Z No qualifier
J Clitoris M Vulva		X External	Z No device	Z No qualifier
K Hymen		0 Open 4 Percutaneous endoscopic X External	Z No device	Z No qualifier

0 U N

MEDICAL AND SURGICAL SECTION – 2016 ICD-10-PCS

DIVISION GROUP: Division, Release
Root Operations involving cutting or separation only.

1ST - **0** Medical and Surgical
2ND - **U** Female Reproductive System ♀
3RD - **N RELEASE**

EXAMPLE: Adhesiolysis ovary and tube CMS Ex: Carpal tunnel release

RELEASE: Freeing a body part from an abnormal physical constraint by cutting or by the use of force.

EXPLANATION: None of the body part is taken out …

Body Part – 4TH	Approach – 5TH	Device – 6TH	Qualifier – 7TH
0 Ovary, Right 1 Ovary, Left 2 Ovaries, Bilateral 4 Uterine Supporting Structure	0 Open 3 Percutaneous 4 Percutaneous endoscopic	Z No device	Z No qualifier
5 Fallopian Tube, Right 6 Fallopian Tube, Left 7 Fallopian Tubes, Bilateral 9 Uterus C Cervix F Cul-de-sac	0 Open 3 Percutaneous 4 Percutaneous endoscopic 7 Via natural or artificial opening 8 Via natural or artificial opening endoscopic	Z No device	Z No qualifier
G Vagina K Hymen	0 Open 3 Percutaneous 4 Percutaneous endoscopic 7 Via natural or artificial opening 8 Via natural or artificial opening endoscopic X External	Z No device	Z No qualifier
J Clitoris L Vestibular Gland M Vulva	0 Open X External	Z No device	Z No qualifier

U – FEMALE REPRODUCTIVE SYSTEM

0UP

DEVICE GROUP: Change, Insertion, Removal, (Replacement), Revision, Supplement
Root Operations that always involve a device.

1ST – **0** Medical and Surgical
2ND – **U** Female Reproductive System ♀
3RD – **P REMOVAL**

EXAMPLE: Removal IUD
CMS Ex: Chest tube removal

REMOVAL: Taking out or off a device from a body part.

EXPLANATION: Removal device without reinsertion ...

Body Part – 4TH	Approach – 5TH	Device – 6TH	Qualifier – 7TH
3 Ovary	0 Open 3 Percutaneous 4 Percutaneous endoscopic X External	0 Drainage device 3 Infusion device	Z No qualifier
8 Fallopian Tube	0 Open 3 Percutaneous 4 Percutaneous endoscopic 7 Via natural or artificial opening 8 Via natural or artificial opening endoscopic	0 Drainage device 3 Infusion device 7 Autologous tissue substitute C Extraluminal device D Intraluminal device J Synthetic substitute K Nonautologous tissue substitute	Z No qualifier
8 Fallopian Tube	X External	0 Drainage device 3 Infusion device D Intraluminal device	Z No qualifier
D Uterus and Cervix	0 Open 3 Percutaneous 4 Percutaneous endoscopic 7 Via natural or artificial opening 8 Via natural or artificial opening endoscopic	0 Drainage device 1 Radioactive element 3 Infusion device 7 Autologous tissue substitute C Extraluminal device D Intraluminal device H Contraceptive device J Synthetic substitute K Nonautologous tissue substitute	Z No qualifier
D Uterus and Cervix	X External	0 Drainage device 3 Infusion device D Intraluminal device H Contraceptive device	Z No qualifier

continued ⇨

0UP REMOVAL – continued

Body Part – 4TH	Approach – 5TH	Device – 6TH	Qualifier – 7TH
H Vagina and Cul-de-sac	0 Open 3 Percutaneous 4 Percutaneous endoscopic 7 Via natural or artificial opening 8 Via natural or artificial opening endoscopic	0 Drainage device 1 Radioactive element 3 Infusion device 7 Autologous tissue substitute D Intraluminal device J Synthetic substitute K Nonautologous tissue substitute	Z No qualifier
H Vagina and Cul-de-sac	X External	0 Drainage device 1 Radioactive element 3 Infusion device D Intraluminal device	Z No qualifier
M Vulva	0 Open	0 Drainage device 7 Autologous tissue substitute J Synthetic substitute K Nonautologous tissue substitute	Z No qualifier
M Vulva	X External	0 Drainage device	Z No qualifier

U – FEMALE REPRODUCTIVE SYSTEM

OTHER REPAIRS GROUP: (Control), Repair
Root Operations that define other repairs.

1ST - 0 Medical and Surgical
2ND - U Female Reproductive System ♀
3RD - Q REPAIR

EXAMPLE: Repair vulvar laceration
CMS Ex: Suture laceration

REPAIR: Restoring, to the extent possible, a body part to its normal anatomic structure and function.

EXPLANATION: Only when no other root operation applies …

Body Part – 4TH	Approach – 5TH	Device – 6TH	Qualifier – 7TH
0 Ovary, Right 1 Ovary, Left 2 Ovaries, Bilateral 4 Uterine Supporting Structure	0 Open 3 Percutaneous 4 Percutaneous endoscopic	Z No device	Z No qualifier
5 Fallopian Tube, Right 6 Fallopian Tube, Left 7 Fallopian Tubes, Bilateral 9 Uterus C Cervix F Cul-de-sac	0 Open 3 Percutaneous 4 Percutaneous endoscopic 7 Via natural or artificial opening 8 Via natural or artificial opening endoscopic	Z No device	Z No qualifier
G Vagina K Hymen	0 Open 3 Percutaneous 4 Percutaneous endoscopic 7 Via natural or artificial opening 8 Via natural or artificial opening endoscopic X External	Z No device	Z No qualifier
J Clitoris L Vestibular Gland M Vulva	0 Open X External	Z No device	Z No qualifier

MOVE GROUP: Reattachment, Reposition, (Transfer), Transplantation
Root Operations that put in/put back or move some/all of a body part.

1ST - 0 Medical and Surgical
2ND - U Female Reproductive System ♀
3RD - S REPOSITION

EXAMPLE: Relocation fallopian tube
CMS Ex: Fracture reduction

REPOSITION: Moving to its normal location, or other suitable location, all or a portion of a body part.

EXPLANATION: May or may not be cut to be moved …

Body Part – 4TH	Approach – 5TH	Device – 6TH	Qualifier – 7TH
0 Ovary, Right 6 Fallopian Tube, Left 1 Ovary, Left 7 Fallopian Tubes, Bilateral 2 Ovaries, Bilateral C Cervix 4 Uterine Supporting Structure F Cul-de-sac 5 Fallopian Tube, Right	0 Open 4 Percutaneous endoscopic	Z No device	Z No qualifier
9 Uterus G Vagina	0 Open 4 Percutaneous endoscopic X External	Z No device	Z No qualifier

0UT

MEDICAL AND SURGICAL SECTION – 2016 ICD-10-PCS

EXCISION GROUP: Excision, Resection, Destruction, Extraction, (Detachment)
Root Operations that take out some or all of a body part.

1ST - 0	Medical and Surgical
2ND - U	Female Reproductive System ♀
3RD - T	**RESECTION**

EXAMPLE: Bilateral oophorectomy

CMS Ex: Cholecystectomy

RESECTION: Cutting out or off, without replacement, all of a body part.

EXPLANATION: None

Body Part – 4TH	Approach – 5TH	Device – 6TH	Qualifier – 7TH
0 Ovary, Right 1 Ovary, Left 2 Ovaries, Bilateral 5 Fallopian Tube, Right 6 Fallopian Tube, Left 7 Fallopian Tubes, Bilateral 9 Uterus	0 Open 4 Percutaneous endoscopic 7 Via natural or artificial opening 8 Via natural or artificial opening endoscopic F Via natural or artificial opening with percutaneous endoscopic assistance	Z No device	Z No qualifier
4 Uterine Supporting Structure C Cervix F Cul-de-sac G Vagina	0 Open 4 Percutaneous endoscopic 7 Via natural or artificial opening 8 Via natural or artificial opening endoscopic	Z No device	Z No qualifier
J Clitoris L Vestibular Gland M Vulva	0 Open X External	Z No device	Z No qualifier
K Hymen	0 Open 4 Percutaneous endoscopic 7 Via natural or artificial opening 8 Via natural or artificial opening endoscopic X External	Z No device	Z No qualifier

U – FEMALE REPRODUCTIVE SYSTEM

DEVICE GROUP: Change, Insertion, Removal, (Replacement), Revision, Supplement
Root Operations that always involve a device.

1ST - 0 Medical and Surgical
2ND - U Female Reproductive System ♀
3RD - U SUPPLEMENT

EXAMPLE: Colporrhaphy with mesh CMS Ex: Hernia repair with mesh

SUPPLEMENT: Putting in or on biological or synthetic material that physically reinforces and/or augments the function of a portion of a body part.

EXPLANATION: Biological material from same individual ...

Body Part – 4TH	Approach – 5TH	Device – 6TH	Qualifier – 7TH
4 Uterine Supporting Structure	0 Open 4 Percutaneous endoscopic	7 Autologous tissue substitute J Synthetic substitute K Nonautologous tissue substitute	Z No qualifier
5 Fallopian Tube, Right 6 Fallopian Tube, Left 7 Fallopian Tubes, Bilateral F Cul-de-sac	0 Open 4 Percutaneous endoscopic 7 Via natural or artificial opening 8 Via natural or artificial opening endoscopic	7 Autologous tissue substitute J Synthetic substitute K Nonautologous tissue substitute	Z No qualifier
G Vagina K Hymen	0 Open 4 Percutaneous endoscopic 7 Via natural or artificial opening 8 Via natural or artificial opening endoscopic X External	7 Autologous tissue substitute J Synthetic substitute K Nonautologous tissue substitute	Z No qualifier
J Clitoris M Vulva	0 Open X External	7 Autologous tissue substitute J Synthetic substitute K Nonautologous tissue substitute	Z No qualifier

0 U V — MEDICAL AND SURGICAL SECTION – 2016 ICD-10-PCS

TUBULAR GROUP: Bypass, Dilation, Occlusion, Restriction
Root Operations that alter the diameter/route of a tubular body part.

- 1ST – **0** Medical and Surgical
- 2ND – **U** Female Reproductive System ♀
- 3RD – **V** RESTRICTION

EXAMPLE: Cervical cerclage **CMS Ex:** Cervical cerclage

RESTRICTION: Partially closing an orifice or the lumen of a tubular body part.

EXPLANATION: Natural or artificially created orifice ...

Body Part – 4TH	Approach – 5TH	Device – 6TH	Qualifier – 7TH
C Cervix	0 Open 3 Percutaneous 4 Percutaneous endoscopic	C Extraluminal device D Intraluminal device Z No device	Z No qualifier
C Cervix	7 Via natural or artificial opening 8 Via natural or artificial opening endoscopic	D Intraluminal device Z No device	Z No qualifier

U – FEMALE REPRODUCTIVE SYSTEM 0UW

DEVICE GROUP: Change, Insertion, Removal, (Replacement), Revision, Supplement
Root Operations that always involve a device.

1ST - 0	Medical and Surgical
2ND - U	Female Reproductive System ♀
3RD - W	REVISION

EXAMPLE: Reposition intrauterine device **CMS Ex:** Adjustment lead

REVISION: Correcting, to the extent possible, a portion of a malfunctioning device or the position of a displaced device.

EXPLANATION: May replace components of a device ...

Body Part – 4TH	Approach – 5TH	Device – 6TH	Qualifier – 7TH
3 Ovary	0 Open 3 Percutaneous 4 Percutaneous endoscopic X External	0 Drainage device 3 Infusion device	Z No qualifier
8 Fallopian Tube	0 Open 3 Percutaneous 4 Percutaneous endoscopic 7 Via natural or artificial opening 8 Via natural or artificial opening endoscopic X External	0 Drainage device 3 Infusion device 7 Autologous tissue substitute C Extraluminal device D Intraluminal device J Synthetic substitute K Nonautologous tissue substitute	Z No qualifier
D Uterus and Cervix	0 Open 3 Percutaneous 4 Percutaneous endoscopic 7 Via natural or artificial opening 8 Via natural or artificial opening endoscopic	0 Drainage device 1 Radioactive element 3 Infusion device 7 Autologous tissue substitute C Extraluminal device D Intraluminal device H Contraceptive device J Synthetic substitute K Nonautologous tissue substitute	Z No qualifier
D Uterus and Cervix	X External	0 Drainage device 3 Infusion device 7 Autologous tissue substitute C Extraluminal device D Intraluminal device H Contraceptive device J Synthetic substitute K Nonautologous tissue substitute	Z No qualifier

continued ⇨

0 U W REVISION – continued

Body Part – 4TH	Approach – 5TH	Device – 6TH	Qualifier – 7TH
H Vagina and Cul-de-sac	0 Open 3 Percutaneous 4 Percutaneous endoscopic 7 Via natural or artificial opening 8 Via natural or artificial opening endoscopic	0 Drainage device 1 Radioactive element 3 Infusion device 7 Autologous tissue substitute D Intraluminal device J Synthetic substitute K Nonautologous tissue substitute	Z No qualifier
H Vagina and Cul-de-sac	X External	0 Drainage device 3 Infusion device 7 Autologous tissue substitute D Intraluminal device J Synthetic substitute K Nonautologous tissue substitute	Z No qualifier
M Vulva	0 Open X External	0 Drainage device 7 Autologous tissue substitute J Synthetic substitute K Nonautologous tissue substitute	Z No qualifier

MOVE GROUP: Reattachment, Reposition, (Transfer), Transplantation
Root Operations that put in/put back or move some/all of a body part.

- 1ST – **0** Medical and Surgical
- 2ND – **U** Female Reproductive System ♀
- 3RD – **Y** TRANSPLANTATION

EXAMPLE: Ovarian transplant   CMS Ex: Kidney transplant

TRANSPLANTATION: Putting in or on all or a portion of a living body part taken from another individual or animal to physically take the place and/or function of all or a portion of a similar body part.

EXPLANATION: May take over all or part of its function ...

Body Part – 4TH	Approach – 5TH	Device – 6TH	Qualifier – 7TH
0 Ovary, Right 1 Ovary, Left	0 Open	Z No device	0 Allogenic 1 Syngeneic 2 Zooplastic

Educational Annotations | V – Male Reproductive System

Body System Specific Educational Annotations for the Male Reproductive System include:
- Anatomy and Physiology Review
- Anatomical Illustrations
- Definitions of Common Procedures
- AHA Coding Clinic® Reference Notations
- Body Part Key Listings
- Device Key Listings
- Device Aggregation Table Listings
- Coding Notes

Anatomy and Physiology Review of Male Reproductive System

BODY PART VALUES – V - MALE REPRODUCTIVE SYSTEM

Epididymis – ANATOMY – The epididymis is a tightly coiled, threadlike tube that is about 20 feet (6 m) long. It is connected to ducts within the testis and emerges from the top of the testis, descends along its posterior surface, and then courses upward to become the vas deferens. PHYSIOLOGY – The epididymis functions to store and mature sperm cells, and to transport the sperm from the testicular ducts to the vas deferens.

Penis – ANATOMY – The penis is the cylindrical male sexual organ which contains the urethra and is located at the base of the male perineum. The body (shaft) is composed of 3 columns of erectile tissue, including a pair of dorsally located corpora cavernosa and a single corpus spongiosum below. The corpus spongiosum, through which the urethra extends, is enlarged at its distal end to form a sensitive, cone-shaped glans penis. A loose fold of skin, called the prepuce (foreskin) covers the glans penis, unless removed by circumcision. PHYSIOLOGY – The penis functions as the specialized sexual organ in the male that when erect is inserted into the female vagina for sexual intercourse. It also functions to convey urine and seminal fluid through the urethra to the outside at the urethral opening (meatus). Erection is obtained by sexual excitement, stimulating parasympathetic nerve impulses causing blood engorgement of the corpora cavernosa and corpus spongiosum.

Prepuce – The loose fold of skin (foreskin) that covers the glans penis, unless removed by circumcision.

Prostate – ANATOMY – The walnut-shaped male reproductive organ that surrounds the urethra just below the bladder. PHYSIOLOGY – The prostate secretes a slightly alkaline fluid that constitutes approximately one-third of the volume of the semen. The alkalinity of semen helps neutralize the acidity of the vaginal tract, prolonging the lifespan of sperm.

Scrotum – ANATOMY – The scrotum is a pouch of skin, subcutaneous, and muscular tissue that hangs from the lower abdominal region behind the penis. PHYSIOLOGY – The scrotum protects the testis and spermatic cord by contracting and relaxing the dartos muscle.

Seminal Vesicle – ANATOMY – A pair of tubular male reproductive glands that are located above the prostate and below the bladder. They pass into the prostatic tissue and their excretory ducts open into the vas deferens and form the ejaculatory ducts. PHYSIOLOGY – The seminal vesicles secrete approximately two-thirds of the ejaculated semen volume. The nutrient-rich seminal fluid provides energy for the sperm cells.

Spermatic Cord – ANATOMY – The spermatic cord is a canal of peritoneal tissue about 18 inches (45 cm) long beginning at the testis and ending in the ejaculatory duct, and is externally contained along with the testis in the scrotum. PHYSIOLOGY – The spermatic cord contains and protects the vas deferens, arteries, nerves, and lymphatic vessels.

Testis – ANATOMY – The testes are the male reproductive organs that are ovoid structures in the scrotum, suspended by a spermatic cord, and approximately 2 inches (5 cm) in length and 1.2 inches (3 cm) in diameter. Each testis is enclosed by a tough, white fibrous capsule called the tunica albuginea. PHYSIOLOGY – The testes function to produce sperm cells for human reproduction and secrete male hormones, primarily testosterone.

Tunica Vaginalis – The serous membrane covering of the testes that is comprised of two layers, visceral and parietal.

Vas Deferens – ANATOMY – The vas deferens (ductus deferens) is a muscular tube that begins at the epididymis and ends at the union of the seminal vesicle and forms the ejaculatory duct within the prostatic tissue. PHYSIOLOGY – The vas deferens transports the sperm using peristalsis from the testis/epididymis to the ejaculatory duct.

Educational Annotations | 0V – Male Reproductive System

Anatomical Illustrations of Male Reproductive System

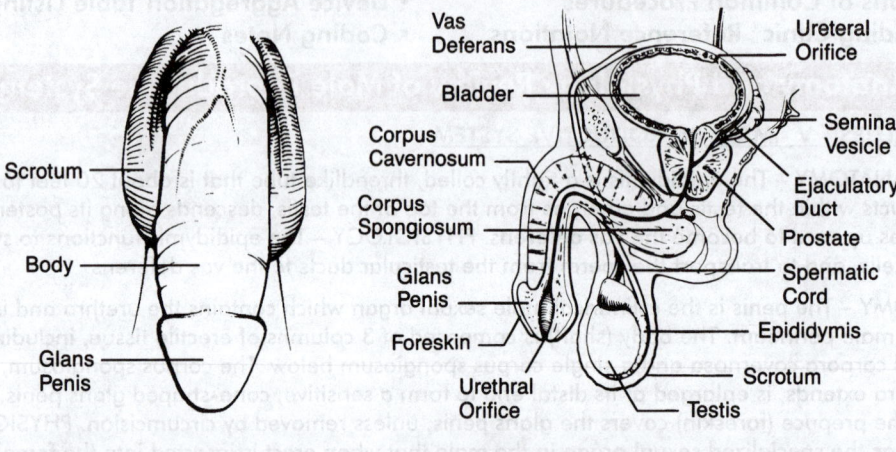

PENIS — FRONTAL VIEW

MALE GENITAL ORGANS — SAGITTAL VIEW

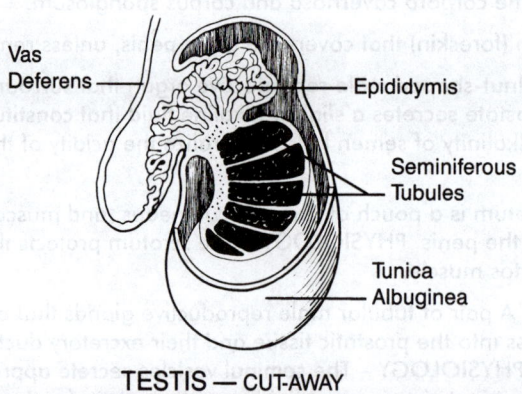

TESTIS — CUT-AWAY

Definitions of Common Procedures of Male Reproductive System

Orchiectomy – The surgical removal of one or both of the testicles.

Orchiopexy – The surgical procedure to move an undescended testicle into the scrotum and secure it in place.

Radical retropubic prostatectomy – The surgical removal of the entire prostate gland and some surrounding tissues that is performed through an open approach between the belly button and pubic bone.

TUNA (transurethral needle ablation of prostate) – The transurethral endoscopic destruction of prostate tissue using radiofrequency (RF) needles that delivers heat to reduce benign prostatic hyperplasia.

TURP (transurethral resection of prostate) – The surgical removal of part or all (total) of the prostate gland through an endoscopic approach.

Vasoepididymostomy – The microsurgical anastomosis of the epididymis to the vas deferens to reverse a vasectomy or to overcome an epididymal obstruction.

Vasovasostomy – The surgical re-anastomosis of the severed vas deferens to reverse a vasectomy.

Educational Annotations | V – Male Reproductive System

AHA Coding Clinic® Reference Notations of Male Reproductive System

ROOT OPERATION SPECIFIC - V - MALE REPRODUCTIVE SYSTEM
BYPASS - 1
CHANGE - 2
DESTRUCTION - 5
DILATION - 7
DRAINAGE - 9
EXCISION - B
EXTIRPATION - C
INSERTION - H
INSPECTION - J
OCCLUSION - L
REATTACHMENT - M
RELEASE - N
REMOVAL - P
REPAIR - Q
REPLACEMENT - R
REPOSITION - S
RESECTION - T
    Radical prostatectomy, robotic-assisted, with bilateral resection of
    vas deferens and seminal vesicles ....AHA 14:4Q:p33
SUPPLEMENT - U
REVISION - W

Body Part Key Listings of Male Reproductive System

See also Body Part Key in Appendix C

Corpus cavernosum	*use* Penis
Corpus spongiosum	*use* Penis
Ductus deferens	*use* Vas Deferens, Bilateral/Left/Right
Ejaculatory duct	*use* Vas Deferens, Bilateral/Left/Right
Foreskin	*use* Prepuce
Glans penis	*use* Prepuce

Device Key Listings of Male Reproductive System

See also Device Key in Appendix D

Autograft	*use* Autologous Tissue Substitute
Brachytherapy seeds	*use* Radioactive Element
Tissue bank graft	*use* Nonautologous Tissue Substitute

Device Aggregation Table Listings of Male Reproductive System

See also Device Aggregation Table in Appendix E

Specific Device	For Operation	In Body System	General Device
None Listed in Device Aggregation Table for this Body System			

Educational Annotations

V – Male Reproductive System

Coding Notes of Male Reproductive System

Body System Specific PCS Reference Manual Exercises

PCS CODE	V – MALE REPRODUCTIVE SYSTEM EXERCISES
0V508ZZ	Transurethral endoscopic laser ablation of prostate.
0VH081Z	Cystoscopy with placement of brachytherapy seeds in prostate gland.
0VT00ZZ	Total retropubic prostatectomy, open.

V – MALE PREPRODUCTIVE SYSTEM   0 V 2

TUBULAR GROUP: Bypass, Dilation, Occlusion, (Restriction)
Root Operations that alter the diameter/route of a tubular body part.

1ST - **0** Medical and Surgical
2ND - **V** Male Reproductive System ♂
3RD - **1 BYPASS**

EXAMPLE: Vasoepididymostomy CMS Ex: Coronary artery bypass

BYPASS: Altering the route of passage of the contents of a tubular body part.

EXPLANATION: Rerouting contents to a downstream part ...

Body Part – 4TH	Approach – 5TH	Device – 6TH	Qualifier – 7TH
N Vas Deferens, Right	0 Open	7 Autologous tissue substitute	J Epididymis, Right
P Vas Deferens, Left	4 Percutaneous endoscopic	J Synthetic substitute	K Epididymis, Left
Q Vas Deferens, Bilateral		K Nonautologous tissue substitute	N Vas Deferens, Right
		Z No device	P Vas Deferens, Left

DEVICE GROUP: Change, Insertion, Removal, Replacement, Revision, Supplement
Root Operations that always involve a device.

1ST - **0** Medical and Surgical
2ND - **V** Male Reproductive System ♂
3RD - **2 CHANGE**

EXAMPLE: Exchange drain tube CMS Ex: Changing urinary catheter

CHANGE: Taking out or off a device from a body part and putting back an identical or similar device in or on the same body part without cutting or puncturing the skin or a mucous membrane.

EXPLANATION: ALL Changes use EXTERNAL approach only ...

Body Part – 4TH	Approach – 5TH	Device – 6TH	Qualifier – 7TH
4 Prostate and Seminal Vesicles	X External	0 Drainage device	Z No qualifier
8 Scrotum and Tunica Vaginalis		Y Other device	
D Testis			
M Epididymis and Spermatic Cord			
R Vas Deferens			
S Penis			

0V5

EXCISION GROUP: Excision, Resection, Destruction, (Extraction), (Detachment)
Root Operations that take out some or all of a body part.

1ST - 0	Medical and Surgical
2ND - V	Male Reproductive System ♂
3RD - 5	DESTRUCTION

EXAMPLE: Needle ablation (TUNA) prostate | CMS Ex: Fulguration polyp

DESTRUCTION: Physical eradication of all or a portion of a body part by the direct use of energy, force, or a destructive agent.

EXPLANATION: None of the body part is physically taken out

Body Part – 4TH	Approach – 5TH	Device – 6TH	Qualifier – 7TH
0 Prostate	0 Open 3 Percutaneous 4 Percutaneous endoscopic 7 Via natural or artificial opening 8 Via natural or artificial opening endoscopic	Z No device	Z No qualifier
1 Seminal Vesicle, Right 2 Seminal Vesicle, Left 3 Seminal Vesicles, Bilateral 6 Tunica Vaginalis, Right 7 Tunica Vaginalis, Left 9 Testis, Right B Testis, Left C Testes, Bilateral F Spermatic Cord, Right G Spermatic Cord, Left H Spermatic Cords, Bilateral J Epididymis, Right K Epididymis, Left L Epididymis, Bilateral N Vas Deferens, Right NC* P Vas Deferens, Left NC* Q Vas Deferens, Bilateral NC*	0 Open 3 Percutaneous 4 Percutaneous endoscopic	Z No device	Z No qualifier
5 Scrotum S Penis T Prepuce	0 Open 3 Percutaneous 4 Percutaneous endoscopic X External	Z No device	Z No qualifier

NC* – Non-covered by Medicare. See current Medicare Code Editor for details.

TUBULAR GROUP: Bypass, Dilation, Occlusion, (Restriction)
Root Operations that alter the diameter/route of a tubular body part.

1ST - 0	Medical and Surgical
2ND - V	Male Reproductive System ♂
3RD - 7	DILATION

EXAMPLE: Dilation vas deferens | CMS Ex: Transluminal angioplasty

DILATION: Expanding an orifice or the lumen of a tubular body part.

EXPLANATION: By force (stretching) or cutting ...

Body Part – 4TH	Approach – 5TH	Device – 6TH	Qualifier – 7TH
N Vas Deferens, Right P Vas Deferens, Left Q Vas Deferens, Bilateral	0 Open 3 Percutaneous 4 Percutaneous endoscopic	D Intraluminal device Z No device	Z No qualifier

0V9

V – MALE PREPRODUCTIVE SYSTEM

DRAINAGE GROUP: Drainage, Extirpation, (Fragmentation)
Root Operations that take out solids/fluids/gases from a body part.

- 1ST - **0** Medical and Surgical
- 2ND - **V** Male Reproductive System ♂
- 3RD - **9** DRAINAGE

EXAMPLE: Drainage epididymal cyst
CMS Ex: Thoracentesis

DRAINAGE: Taking or letting out fluids and/or gases from a body part.

EXPLANATION: Qualifier "X Diagnostic" indicates biopsy ...

Body Part – 4TH			Approach – 5TH	Device – 6TH	Qualifier – 7TH
0 Prostate			0 Open 3 Percutaneous 4 Percutaneous endoscopic 7 Via natural or artificial opening 8 Via natural or artificial opening endoscopic	0 Drainage device	Z No qualifier
0 Prostate			0 Open 3 Percutaneous 4 Percutaneous endoscopic 7 Via natural or artificial opening 8 Via natural or artificial opening endoscopic	Z No device	X Diagnostic Z No qualifier
1 Seminal Vesicle, Right 2 Seminal Vesicle, Left 3 Seminal Vesicles, Bilateral 6 Tunica Vaginalis, Right 7 Tunica Vaginalis, Left 9 Testis, Right B Testis, Left C Testes, Bilateral	F Spermatic Cord, Right G Spermatic Cord, Left H Spermatic Cords, Bilateral J Epididymis, Right K Epididymis, Left L Epididymis, Bilateral N Vas Deferens, Right P Vas Deferens, Left Q Vas Deferens, Bilateral		0 Open 3 Percutaneous 4 Percutaneous endoscopic	0 Drainage device	Z No qualifier
1 Seminal Vesicle, Right 2 Seminal Vesicle, Left 3 Seminal Vesicles, Bilateral 6 Tunica Vaginalis, Right 7 Tunica Vaginalis, Left 9 Testis, Right B Testis, Left C Testes, Bilateral	F Spermatic Cord, Right G Spermatic Cord, Left H Spermatic Cords, Bilateral J Epididymis, Right K Epididymis, Left L Epididymis, Bilateral N Vas Deferens, Right P Vas Deferens, Left Q Vas Deferens, Bilateral		0 Open 3 Percutaneous 4 Percutaneous endoscopic	Z No device	X Diagnostic Z No qualifier
5 Scrotum S Penis T Prepuce			0 Open 3 Percutaneous 4 Percutaneous endoscopic X External	0 Drainage device	Z No qualifier
5 Scrotum S Penis T Prepuce			0 Open 3 Percutaneous 4 Percutaneous endoscopic X External	Z No device	X Diagnostic Z No qualifier

0VB

MEDICAL AND SURGICAL SECTION – 2016 ICD-10-PCS

EXCISION GROUP: Excision, Resection, Destruction, (Extraction), (Detachment)
Root Operations that take out some or all of a body part.

1ST - **0** Medical and Surgical
2ND - **V** Male Reproductive System ♂
3RD - **B** EXCISION

EXAMPLE: TURP (non-total) **CMS Ex:** Liver biopsy

EXCISION: Cutting out or off, without replacement, a portion of a body part.

EXPLANATION: Qualifier "X Diagnostic" indicates biopsy ...

Body Part – 4TH	Approach – 5TH	Device – 6TH	Qualifier – 7TH
0 Prostate	0 Open 3 Percutaneous 4 Percutaneous endoscopic 7 Via natural or artificial opening 8 Via natural or artificial opening endoscopic	Z No device	X Diagnostic Z No qualifier
1 Seminal Vesicle, Right 2 Seminal Vesicle, Left 3 Seminal Vesicles, Bilateral 6 Tunica Vaginalis, Right 7 Tunica Vaginalis, Left 9 Testis, Right B Testis, Left C Testes, Bilateral F Spermatic Cord, Right G Spermatic Cord, Left H Spermatic Cords, Bilateral J Epididymis, Right K Epididymis, Left L Epididymis, Bilateral N Vas Deferens, Right NC* P Vas Deferens, Left NC* Q Vas Deferens, Bilateral NC*	0 Open 3 Percutaneous 4 Percutaneous endoscopic	Z No device	X Diagnostic Z No qualifier
5 Scrotum S Penis T Prepuce	0 Open 3 Percutaneous 4 Percutaneous endoscopic X External	Z No device	X Diagnostic Z No qualifier

NC* – Some procedures are considered non-covered by Medicare. See current Medicare Code Editor for details.

V – MALE PREPRODUCTIVE SYSTEM 0VC

DRAINAGE GROUP: Drainage, Extirpation, (Fragmentation)
Root Operations that take out solids/fluids/gases from a body part.

1ST - **0** Medical and Surgical
2ND - **V** Male Reproductive System ♂
3RD - **C EXTIRPATION**

EXAMPLE: Removal foreign body   CMS Ex: Choledocholithotomy

EXTIRPATION: Taking or cutting out solid matter from a body part.

EXPLANATION: Abnormal byproduct or foreign body …

Body Part – 4TH		Approach – 5TH	Device – 6TH	Qualifier – 7TH
0 Prostate		0 Open 3 Percutaneous 4 Percutaneous endoscopic 7 Via natural or artificial opening 8 Via natural or artificial opening endoscopic	Z No device	Z No qualifier
1 Seminal Vesicle, Right 2 Seminal Vesicle, Left 3 Seminal Vesicles, Bilateral 6 Tunica Vaginalis, Right 7 Tunica Vaginalis, Left 9 Testis, Right B Testis, Left C Testes, Bilateral	F Spermatic Cord, Right G Spermatic Cord, Left H Spermatic Cords, Bilateral J Epididymis, Right K Epididymis, Left L Epididymis, Bilateral N Vas Deferens, Right P Vas Deferens, Left Q Vas Deferens, Bilateral	0 Open 3 Percutaneous 4 Percutaneous endoscopic	Z No device	Z No qualifier
5 Scrotum S Penis T Prepuce		0 Open 3 Percutaneous 4 Percutaneous endoscopic X External	Z No device	Z No qualifier

0VH

DEVICE GROUP: Change, Insertion, Removal, Replacement, Revision, Supplement
Root Operations that always involve a device.

- 1ST – **0** Medical and Surgical
- 2ND – **V** Male Reproductive System ♂
- 3RD – **H** INSERTION

EXAMPLE: Insertion radioactive element | CMS Ex: Central venous catheter

INSERTION: Putting in a nonbiological appliance that monitors, assists, performs, or prevents a physiological function but does not physically take the place of a body part.

EXPLANATION: None

Body Part – 4TH	Approach – 5TH	Device – 6TH	Qualifier – 7TH
0 Prostate	0 Open 3 Percutaneous 4 Percutaneous endoscopic 7 Via natural or artificial opening 8 Via natural or artificial opening endoscopic	1 Radioactive element	Z No qualifier
4 Prostate and Seminal Vesicles 8 Scrotum and Tunica Vaginalis D Testis M Epididymis and Spermatic Cord R Vas Deferens	0 Open 3 Percutaneous 4 Percutaneous endoscopic 7 Via natural or artificial opening 8 Via natural or artificial opening endoscopic	3 Infusion device	Z No qualifier
S Penis	0 Open 3 Percutaneous 4 Percutaneous endoscopic X External	3 Infusion device	Z No qualifier

EXAMINATION GROUP: Inspection (Map)
Root Operations involving examination only.

- 1ST – **0** Medical and Surgical
- 2ND – **V** Male Reproductive System ♂
- 3RD – **J** INSPECTION

EXAMPLE: Prostate exam | CMS Ex: Colonoscopy

INSPECTION: Visually and/or manually exploring a body part.

EXPLANATION: Direct or instrumental visualization ...

Body Part – 4TH	Approach – 5TH	Device – 6TH	Qualifier – 7TH
4 Prostate and Seminal Vesicles 8 Scrotum and Tunica Vaginalis D Testis M Epididymis and Spermatic Cord R Vas Deferens S Penis	0 Open 3 Percutaneous 4 Percutaneous endoscopic X External	Z No device	Z No qualifier

V – MALE PREPRODUCTIVE SYSTEM   0VM

[2016.PCS]

TUBULAR GROUP: Bypass, Dilation, Occlusion, (Restriction)
Root Operations that alter the diameter/route of a tubular body part.

1ST - **0** Medical and Surgical	EXAMPLE: Vasectomy	CMS Ex: Fallopian tube ligation
2ND - **V** Male Reproductive System ♂	**OCCLUSION:** Completely closing an orifice or lumen of a tubular body part.	
3RD - **L OCCLUSION**	EXPLANATION: Natural or artificially created orifice …	

Body Part – 4TH	Approach – 5TH	Device – 6TH	Qualifier – 7TH
F Spermatic Cord, Right NC* G Spermatic Cord, Left NC* H Spermatic Cords, Bilateral NC* N Vas Deferens, Right NC* P Vas Deferens, Left NC* Q Vas Deferens, Bilateral NC*	0 Open 3 Percutaneous 4 Percutaneous endoscopic	C Extraluminal device D Intraluminal device Z No device	Z No qualifier

NC* – Some procedures are considered non-covered by Medicare. See current Medicare Code Editor for details.

MOVE GROUP: Reattachment, Reposition, (Transfer), (Transplantation)
Root Operations that put in/put back or move some/all of a body part.

1ST - **0** Medical and Surgical	EXAMPLE: Penis reattachment	CMS Ex: Reattachment hand
2ND - **V** Male Reproductive System ♂	**REATTACHMENT:** Putting back in or on all or a portion of a separated body part to its normal location or other suitable location.	
3RD - **M REATTACHMENT**	EXPLANATION: With/without reconnection of vessels/nerves…	

Body Part – 4TH	Approach – 5TH	Device – 6TH	Qualifier – 7TH
5 Scrotum S Penis	X External	Z No device	Z No qualifier
6 Tunica Vaginalis, Right F Spermatic Cord, Right 7 Tunica Vaginalis, Left G Spermatic Cord, Left 9 Testis, Right H Spermatic Cords, Bilateral B Testis, Left C Testes, Bilateral	0 Open 4 Percutaneous endoscopic	Z No device	Z No qualifier

0VN

MEDICAL AND SURGICAL SECTION – 2016 ICD-10-PCS

DIVISION GROUP: (Division), Release
Root Operations involving cutting or separation only.

1ST - **0** Medical and Surgical
2ND - **V** Male Reproductive System ♂
3RD - **N** RELEASE

EXAMPLE: Adhesiolysis spermatic cord   CMS Ex: Carpal tunnel release

RELEASE: Freeing a body part from an abnormal physical constraint by cutting or by the use of force.

EXPLANATION: None of the body part is taken out ...

Body Part – 4TH		Approach – 5TH	Device – 6TH	Qualifier – 7TH
0 Prostate		0 Open 3 Percutaneous 4 Percutaneous endoscopic 7 Via natural or artificial opening 8 Via natural or artificial opening endoscopic	Z No device	Z No qualifier
1 Seminal Vesicle, Right 2 Seminal Vesicle, Left 3 Seminal Vesicles, Bilateral 6 Tunica Vaginalis, Right 7 Tunica Vaginalis, Left 9 Testis, Right B Testis, Left C Testes, Bilateral	F Spermatic Cord, Right G Spermatic Cord, Left H Spermatic Cords, Bilateral J Epididymis, Right K Epididymis, Left L Epididymis, Bilateral N Vas Deferens, Right P Vas Deferens, Left Q Vas Deferens, Bilateral	0 Open 3 Percutaneous 4 Percutaneous endoscopic	Z No device	Z No qualifier
5 Scrotum S Penis T Prepuce		0 Open 3 Percutaneous 4 Percutaneous endoscopic X External	Z No device	Z No qualifier

648

V – MALE PREPRODUCTIVE SYSTEM

0VP

DEVICE GROUP: Change, Insertion, Removal, Replacement, Revision, Supplement
Root Operations that always involve a device.

1ST - **0** Medical and Surgical
2ND - **V** Male Reproductive System ♂
3RD - **P** REMOVAL

EXAMPLE: Removal drain tube

CMS Ex: Chest tube removal

REMOVAL: Taking out or off a device from a body part.

EXPLANATION: Removal device without reinsertion ...

Body Part – 4TH	Approach – 5TH	Device – 6TH	Qualifier – 7TH
4 Prostate and Seminal Vesicles	0 Open 3 Percutaneous 4 Percutaneous endoscopic 7 Via natural or artificial opening 8 Via natural or artificial opening endoscopic	0 Drainage device 1 Radioactive element 3 Infusion device 7 Autologous tissue substitute J Synthetic substitute K Nonautologous tissue substitute	Z No qualifier
4 Prostate and Seminal Vesicles	X External	0 Drainage device 1 Radioactive element 3 Infusion device	Z No qualifier
8 Scrotum and Tunica Vaginalis D Testis S Penis	0 Open 3 Percutaneous 4 Percutaneous endoscopic 7 Via natural or artificial opening 8 Via natural or artificial opening endoscopic	0 Drainage device 3 Infusion device 7 Autologous tissue substitute J Synthetic substitute K Nonautologous tissue substitute	Z No qualifier
8 Scrotum and Tunica Vaginalis D Testis S Penis	X External	0 Drainage device 3 Infusion device	Z No qualifier
M Epididymis and Spermatic Cord	0 Open 3 Percutaneous 4 Percutaneous endoscopic 7 Via natural or artificial opening 8 Via natural or artificial opening endoscopic	0 Drainage device 3 Infusion device 7 Autologous tissue substitute C Extraluminal device J Synthetic substitute K Nonautologous tissue substitute	Z No qualifier
M Epididymis and Spermatic Cord	X External	0 Drainage device 3 Infusion device	Z No qualifier
R Vas Deferens	0 Open 3 Percutaneous 4 Percutaneous endoscopic 7 Via natural or artificial opening 8 Via natural or artificial opening endoscopic	0 Drainage device 3 Infusion device 7 Autologous tissue substitute C Extraluminal device D Intraluminal device J Synthetic substitute K Nonautologous tissue substitute	Z No qualifier
R Vas Deferens	X External	0 Drainage device 3 Infusion device D Intraluminal device	Z No qualifier

0VQ

MEDICAL AND SURGICAL SECTION – 2016 ICD-10-PCS

OTHER REPAIRS GROUP: (Control), Repair
Root Operations that define other repairs.

- 1ST – **0** Medical and Surgical
- 2ND – **V** Male Reproductive System ♂
- 3RD – **Q REPAIR**

EXAMPLE: Repair laceration scrotum   CMS Ex: Suture laceration

REPAIR: Restoring, to the extent possible, a body part to its normal anatomic structure and function.

EXPLANATION: Only when no other root operation applies …

Body Part – 4TH	Approach – 5TH	Device – 6TH	Qualifier – 7TH
0 Prostate	0 Open 3 Percutaneous 4 Percutaneous endoscopic 7 Via natural or artificial opening 8 Via natural or artificial opening endoscopic	Z No device	Z No qualifier
1 Seminal Vesicle, Right 2 Seminal Vesicle, Left 3 Seminal Vesicles, Bilateral 6 Tunica Vaginalis, Right 7 Tunica Vaginalis, Left 9 Testis, Right B Testis, Left C Testes, Bilateral F Spermatic Cord, Right G Spermatic Cord, Left H Spermatic Cords, Bilateral J Epididymis, Right K Epididymis, Left L Epididymis, Bilateral N Vas Deferens, Right P Vas Deferens, Left Q Vas Deferens, Bilateral	0 Open 3 Percutaneous 4 Percutaneous endoscopic	Z No device	Z No qualifier
5 Scrotum S Penis T Prepuce	0 Open 3 Percutaneous 4 Percutaneous endoscopic X External	Z No device	Z No qualifier

---

DEVICE GROUP: Change, Insertion, Removal, Replacement, Revision, Supplement
Root Operations that always involve a device.

- 1ST – **0** Medical and Surgical
- 2ND – **V** Male Reproductive System ♂
- 3RD – **R REPLACEMENT**

EXAMPLE: Testis removal with replacement   CMS Ex: Total hip

REPLACEMENT: Putting in or on a biological or synthetic material that physically takes the place and/or function of all or a portion of a body part.

EXPLANATION: Includes taking out body part, or eradication…

Body Part – 4TH	Approach – 5TH	Device – 6TH	Qualifier – 7TH
9 Testis, Right B Testis, Left C Testes, Bilateral	0 Open	J Synthetic substitute	Z No qualifier

V – MALE REPRODUCTIVE SYSTEM

0VT

MOVE GROUP: Reattachment, Reposition, (Transfer), (Transplantation)
Root Operations that put in/put back or move some/all of a body part.

- 1ST – **0** Medical and Surgical
- 2ND – **V** Male Reproductive System ♂
- 3RD – **S** REPOSITION

EXAMPLE: Relocation undescended testis **CMS Ex:** Fracture reduction

REPOSITION: Moving to its normal location, or other suitable location, all or a portion of a body part.

EXPLANATION: May or may not be cut to be moved …

Body Part – 4TH		Approach – 5TH	Device – 6TH	Qualifier – 7TH
9 Testis, Right	F Spermatic Cord, Right	0 Open	Z No device	Z No qualifier
B Testis, Left	G Spermatic Cord, Left	3 Percutaneous		
C Testes, Bilateral	H Spermatic Cords, Bilateral	4 Percutaneous endoscopic		

EXCISION GROUP: Excision, Resection, Destruction, (Extraction), (Detachment)
Root Operations that take out some or all of a body part.

- 1ST – **0** Medical and Surgical
- 2ND – **V** Male Reproductive System ♂
- 3RD – **T** RESECTION

EXAMPLE: Total retropubic prostatectomy **CMS Ex:** Cholecystectomy

RESECTION: Cutting out or off, without replacement, all of a body part.

EXPLANATION: None

Body Part – 4TH		Approach – 5TH	Device – 6TH	Qualifier – 7TH
0 Prostate		0 Open 4 Percutaneous endoscopic 7 Via natural or artificial opening 8 Via natural or artificial opening endoscopic	Z No device	Z No qualifier
1 Seminal Vesicle, Right	F Spermatic Cord, Right	0 Open	Z No device	Z No qualifier
2 Seminal Vesicle, Left	G Spermatic Cord, Left	4 Percutaneous endoscopic		
3 Seminal Vesicles, Bilateral	H Spermatic Cords, Bilateral			
6 Tunica Vaginalis, Right	J Epididymis, Right			
7 Tunica Vaginalis, Left	K Epididymis, Left			
9 Testis, Right	L Epididymis, Bilateral			
B Testis, Left	N Vas Deferens, Right NC*			
C Testes, Bilateral	P Vas Deferens, Left NC*			
	Q Vas Deferens, Bilateral NC*			
5 Scrotum		0 Open	Z No device	Z No qualifier
S Penis		4 Percutaneous endoscopic		
T Prepuce		X External		

NC* – Non-covered by Medicare. See current Medicare Code Editor for details.

0VU

MEDICAL AND SURGICAL SECTION – 2016 ICD-10-PCS

DEVICE GROUP: Change, Insertion, Removal, Replacement, Revision, Supplement
Root Operations that always involve a device.

1ST – **0** Medical and Surgical
2ND – **V** Male Reproductive System ♂
3RD – **U** SUPPLEMENT

EXAMPLE: Tunica vaginalis repair with graft   **CMS Ex:** Hernia with mesh

SUPPLEMENT: Putting in or on biological or synthetic material that physically reinforces and/or augments the function of a portion of a body part.

EXPLANATION: Biological material from same individual ...

Body Part – 4TH		Approach – 5TH	Device – 6TH	Qualifier – 7TH
1 Seminal Vesicle, Right 2 Seminal Vesicle, Left 3 Seminal Vesicles, Bilateral 6 Tunica Vaginalis, Right 7 Tunica Vaginalis, Left F Spermatic Cord, Right G Spermatic Cord, Left H Spermatic Cords, Bilateral	J Epididymis, Right K Epididymis, Left L Epididymis, Bilateral N Vas Deferens, Right P Vas Deferens, Left Q Vas Deferens, Bilateral	0 Open 4 Percutaneous endoscopic	7 Autologous tissue substitute J Synthetic substitute K Nonautologous tissue substitute	Z No qualifier
5 Scrotum S Penis T Prepuce		0 Open 4 Percutaneous endoscopic X External	7 Autologous tissue substitute J Synthetic substitute K Nonautologous tissue substitute	Z No qualifier
9 Testis, Right B Testis, Left C Testes, Bilateral		0 Open	7 Autologous tissue substitute J Synthetic substitute K Nonautologous tissue substitute	Z No qualifier

V – MALE PREPRODUCTIVE SYSTEM   0VW

DEVICE GROUP: Change, Insertion, Removal, Replacement, Revision, Supplement
Root Operations that always involve a device.

1ST - **0** Medical and Surgical
2ND - **V** Male Reproductive System ♂
3RD - **W REVISION**

EXAMPLE: Reposition drain tube   CMS Ex: Adjustment pacemaker lead

REVISION: Correcting, to the extent possible, a portion of a malfunctioning device or the position of a displaced device.

EXPLANATION: May replace components of a device …

Body Part – 4TH	Approach – 5TH	Device – 6TH	Qualifier – 7TH
4 Prostate and Seminal Vesicles 8 Scrotum and Tunica Vaginalis D Testis S Penis	0 Open 3 Percutaneous 4 Percutaneous endoscopic 7 Via natural or artificial opening 8 Via natural or artificial opening endoscopic X External	0 Drainage device 3 Infusion device 7 Autologous tissue substitute J Synthetic substitute K Nonautologous tissue substitute	Z No qualifier
M Epididymis and Spermatic Cord	0 Open 3 Percutaneous 4 Percutaneous endoscopic 7 Via natural or artificial opening 8 Via natural or artificial opening endoscopic X External	0 Drainage device 3 Infusion device 7 Autologous tissue substitute C Extraluminal device J Synthetic substitute K Nonautologous tissue substitute	Z No qualifier
R Vas Deferens	0 Open 3 Percutaneous 4 Percutaneous endoscopic 7 Via natural or artificial opening 8 Via natural or artificial opening endoscopic X External	0 Drainage device 3 Infusion device 7 Autologous tissue substitute C Extraluminal device D Intraluminal device J Synthetic substitute K Nonautologous tissue substitute	Z No qualifier

MEDICAL AND SURGICAL SECTION – 2016 ICD-10-PCS

NOTES

Educational Annotations | W – Anatomical Regions, General

Body System Specific Educational Annotations for the Anatomical Regions, General include:
- Anatomy and Physiology Review
- Anatomical Illustrations
- Definitions of Common Procedures
- AHA Coding Clinic® Reference Notations
- Body Part Key Listings
- Device Key Listings
- Device Aggregation Table Listings
- Coding Notes

Anatomy and Physiology Review of Anatomical Regions, General

BODY PART VALUES – W - ANATOMICAL REGIONS, GENERAL

Coding Guideline B2.1a - Body System, General Guideline – The procedure codes in the general anatomical regions body systems should only be used when the procedure is performed on an anatomical region rather than a specific body part (e.g., root operations Control and Detachment, Drainage of a body cavity) or the rare occasion when no information is available to support assignment of a code to a specific body part. Example: Control of postoperative hemorrhage is coded to the root operation Control, which is found in the general anatomical regions body systems.

Abdominal Wall – The multi-tissue-layered covering of the abdominal and pelvic portions of the trunk.

Back – The multi-tissue-layered covering of the back portion of the trunk.

Chest Wall – The multi-tissue-layered covering of the thoracic portion of the trunk.

Cranial Cavity – The space inside the skull.

Face – The multi-tissue-layered covering of the anterior portion of the head.

Gastrointestinal Tract – The alimenatary tract from the esophagus to the anus.

Genitourinary Tract – The organs and structures of the urinary and reproductive systems.

Head – The portion of the human body above the neck.

Jaw – The anterior, lower, movable, articulated portion of the head.

Mediastinum – The central portion of the thoracic cavity that lies between the right pleura, left pleura, sternum, and vertebral column and contains the heart, great vessels, esophagus, bronchi, and thymus.

Neck – The portion of the human body above the trunk and below the head.

Oral Cavity and Throat – The space formed by the mouth, pharynx, and larynx.

Pelvic Cavity – The lower abdominal space containing the rectum, bladder, and reproductive organs.

Pericardial Cavity – The thoracic, fluid-filled space formed by the double-walled peritoneal sac that contains the heart.

Perineum, Female – The multi-tissue-layered area between the vulva and the anus.

Perineum, Male – The multi-tissue-layered area between the scrotum and the anus.

Peritoneal Cavity – The abdominal space between the parietal peritoneum and visceral peritoneum.

Pleural Cavity – The thoracic, fluid-filled space between the visceral pleura and parietal pleura.

Respiratory Tract – The organs and structures involved in respiration.

Retroperitoneum – The space behind the peritoneum that borders the deep muscles of the back and contains the kidneys, adrenals, most of the duodenum, ascending and descending colon, and the pancreas.

Anatomical Illustrations of Anatomical Regions, General

None for the Anatomical Regions, General Body System

Educational Annotations | W – Anatomical Regions, General

Definitions of Common Procedures of Anatomical Regions, General

Abdominoplasty (tummy tuck) – The cosmetic plastic surgical procedure to remove excess fat and skin from the abdominal wall area.

Chest tube for pneumothorax – The surgical insertion of a plastic tube through the chest wall and into the pleural space to remove the air of a pneumothorax.

Episiotomy – The surgical incision of the perineum (with subsequent closure) to expand the opening of the vagina and prevent tearing of the perineal tissues during delivery.

Face lift (rhytidectomy) – The cosmetic plastic surgical procedure to remove the visible signs of aging in the face and neck including removing excess skin and fat with resulting tightening of the facial skin. The procedure often includes a cosmetic blepharoplasty of the eyelids.

Paracentesis – The procedural insertion of a needle or catheter through the abdominal wall and into the peritoneal cavity to drain excess fluid.

Pleuroperitoneal shunt – The shunting redirection of excessive pleural fluid by placing a catheter into the pleural space and tunneling it into the peritoneal cavity.

Thoracentesis – The procedural insertion of a needle or catheter through the chest wall and into the pleural space to drain fluid (pleural effusion, empyema, blood, chyle).

AHA Coding Clinic® Reference Notations of Anatomical Regions, General

ROOT OPERATION SPECIFIC - W - ANATOMICAL REGIONS, GENERAL

ALTERATION - 0
    Browpexy ....AHA 15:1Q:p31

BYPASS - 1
    Creation of percutaneous cutaneoperitoneal fistula for peritoneal
        dialysis ....AHA 13:4Q:p126
        Official Correction of 13:4Q:p126 & 127 ....AHA 15:2Q:p36
    Creation of percutaneous cutaneoperitoneal fistula
        laparoscopically for peritoneal dialysis ....AHA 13:4Q:p127
        Official Correction of 13:4Q:p126 & 127 ....AHA 15:2Q:p36

CHANGE - 2

CONTROL - 3
    Control of post vaginal delivery bleeding ....AHA 14:4Q:p44

CREATION - 4

DIVISION - 8

DRAINAGE - 9

EXCISION - B
    Excision of inclusion cyst of perineum ....AHA 13:4Q:p119

EXTIRPATION - C

FRAGMENTATION - F

INSERTION - H
    Placement of peritoneal dialysis device ....AHA 15:2Q:p36

INSPECTION - J
    Ventriculoperitoneal (VP) shunt with laparoscopic assistance ....AHA 13:2Q:p36

REATTACHMENT - M

REMOVAL - P

REPAIR - Q
    Abdominoplasty of ventral hernia ....AHA 14:4Q:p38
    Parastomal hernia repair ....AHA 14:3Q:p28

SUPPLEMENT - U
    Reconstruction of chest wall using Marlex overlay plate ....AHA 12:4Q:p101
    Repair of incisional hernia with component release and mesh ....AHA 14:4Q:p39

REVISION - W
    Replacement of disconnected abdominal portion of VP shunt ....AHA 15:2Q:p9

Educational Annotations | W – Anatomical Regions, General

Body Part Key Listings of Anatomical Regions, General

See also Body Part Key in Appendix C

Retroperitoneal space	*use* Retroperitoneum
Retropubic space	*use* Pelvic Cavity

Device Key Listings of Anatomical Regions, General

See also Device Key in Appendix D

Autograft	*use* Autologous Tissue Substitute
Bard® Composix® Kugel® patch	*use* Synthetic Substitute
Bard® Ventralex™ hernia patch	*use* Synthetic Substitute
Bard® Composix® (E/X)(LP) mesh	*use* Synthetic Substitute
Bard® Dulex™ mesh	*use* Synthetic Substitute
Brachytherapy seeds	*use* Radioactive Element
Flexible Composite Mesh	*use* Synthetic Substitute
GORE® DUALMESH®	*use* Synthetic Substitute
Nitinol framed polymer mesh	*use* Synthetic Substitute
Partially absorbable mesh	*use* Synthetic Substitute
PHYSIOMESH™ Flexible Composite Mesh	*use* Synthetic Substitute
Polypropylene mesh	*use* Synthetic Substitute
PROCEED™ Ventral Patch	*use* Synthetic Substitute
PROLENE Polypropylene Hernia System (PHS)	*use* Synthetic Substitute
Rebound HRD® (Hernia Repair Device)	*use* Synthetic Substitute
Thoracostomy tube	*use* Drainage Device
Tissue bank graft	*use* Nonautologous Tissue Substitute
ULTRAPRO Hernia System (UHS)	*use* Synthetic Substitute
ULTRAPRO Partially Absorbable Lightweight Mesh	*use* Synthetic Substitute
ULTRAPRO Plug	*use* Synthetic Substitute
Ventrio™ Hernia Patch	*use* Synthetic Substitute

Aggregation Key Listings of Anatomical Regions, General

See also Device Aggregation Table in Appendix E

Specific Device	For Operation	In Body System	General Device
None Listed in Device Aggregation Table for this Body System			

Educational Annotations

W – Anatomical Regions, General

Coding Notes of Anatomical Regions, General

Body System Relevant Coding Guidelines

Control vs. more definitive root operations
 B3.7
  The root operation Control is defined as, "Stopping, or attempting to stop, postprocedural bleeding." If an attempt to stop postprocedural bleeding is initially unsuccessful, and to stop the bleeding requires performing any of the definitive root operations Bypass, Detachment, Excision, Extraction, Reposition, Replacement, or Resection, then that root operation is coded instead of Control.
  Example: Resection of spleen to stop postprocedural bleeding is coded to Resection instead of Control.

Body System Specific PCS Reference Manual Exercises

PCS CODE	W – ANATOMICAL REGIONS, GENERAL EXERCISES
0W020ZZ	Cosmetic face lift, open, no other information available.
0W0F0ZZ	Abdominoplasty (tummy tuck), open.
0W190JG	Open pleuroperitoneal shunt, right pleural cavity, using synthetic device.
0W2BX0Z	Change chest tube for left pneumothorax.
0W3D0ZZ	Reopening of thoracotomy site with drainage and control of post-op hemopericardium.
0W3H0ZZ	Control of post-operative retroperitoneal bleeding via laparotomy.
0W3R8ZZ	Hysteroscopy with cautery of post-hysterectomy oozing and evacuation of clot.
0W4M0J0	Creation of vagina in male patient using synthetic material.
0W4N0K1	Creation of penis in female patient using tissue bank donor graft.
0W9930Z	Percutaneous chest tube placement for right pneumothorax.
0W9B3ZZ	Thoracentesis of left pleural effusion. (This is drainage of the pleural cavity.)
0W9G3ZZ	Percutaneous drainage of ascites. (This is drainage of the cavity and not the peritoneal membrane itself.)
0WJ90ZZ	Thoracotomy with exploration of right pleural cavity.
0WQF0ZZ	Closure of abdominal wall stab wound.
0WQN0ZZ	Perineoplasty with repair of old obstetric laceration, open.
0WUF0JZ	Abdominal wall herniorrhaphy, open, using synthetic mesh.

W – ANATOMICAL REGIONS, GENERAL 0W1

OTHER OBJECTIVES GROUP: Alteration, Creation, (Fusion)
Root Operations that define other objectives.

1ST - **0** Medical and Surgical
2ND - **W** Anatomical Regions, General
3RD - **0** ALTERATION

EXAMPLE: Abdominoplasty (tummy tuck) CMS Ex: Face lift

ALTERATION: Modifying the anatomic structure of a body part without affecting the function of the body part.

EXPLANATION: Principal purpose is to improve appearance

Body Part – 4TH	Approach – 5TH	Device – 6TH	Qualifier – 7TH
0 Head	0 Open	7 Autologous tissue substitute	Z No qualifier
2 Face	3 Percutaneous	J Synthetic substitute	
4 Upper Jaw	4 Percutaneous endoscopic	K Nonautologous tissue substitute	
5 Lower Jaw		Z No device	
6 Neck			
8 Chest Wall			
F Abdominal Wall			
K Upper Back			
L Lower Back			
M Perineum, Male ♂			
N Perineum, Female ♀			

TUBULAR GROUP: Bypass, (Dilation), (Occlusion), (Restriction)
Root Operations that alter the diameter/route of a tubular body part.

1ST - **0** Medical and Surgical
2ND - **W** Anatomical Regions, General
3RD - **1** BYPASS

EXAMPLE: Pleuroperitoneal shunt CMS Ex: Coronary artery bypass

BYPASS: Altering the route of passage of the contents of a tubular body part.

EXPLANATION: Rerouting contents to a downstream part ...

Body Part – 4TH	Approach – 5TH	Device – 6TH	Qualifier – 7TH
1 Cranial Cavity	0 Open	J Synthetic substitute	9 Pleural Cavity, Right
			B Pleural Cavity, Left
			G Peritoneal Cavity
			J Pelvic Cavity
9 Pleural Cavity, Right	0 Open	J Synthetic substitute	4 Cutaneous
B Pleural Cavity, Left	4 Percutaneous endoscopic		9 Pleural Cavity, Right
G Peritoneal Cavity			B Pleural Cavity, Left
J Pelvic Cavity			G Peritoneal Cavity
			J Pelvic Cavity
			Y Lower Vein
9 Pleural Cavity, Right	3 Percutaneous	J Synthetic substitute	4 Cutaneous
B Pleural Cavity, Left			
G Peritoneal Cavity			
J Pelvic Cavity			

0W2

MEDICAL AND SURGICAL SECTION – 2016 ICD-10-PCS

DEVICE GROUP: Change, Insertion, Removal, (Replacement), Revision, Supplement
Root Operations that always involve a device.

- 1ST – **0** Medical and Surgical
- 2ND – **W** Anatomical Regions, General
- 3RD – **2** CHANGE

EXAMPLE: Exchange chest tube   **CMS Ex:** Changing urinary catheter

CHANGE: Taking out or off a device from a body part and putting back an identical or similar device in or on the same body part without cutting or puncturing the skin or a mucous membrane.

EXPLANATION: ALL Changes use EXTERNAL approach only ...

Body Part – 4TH		Approach – 5TH	Device – 6TH	Qualifier – 7TH
0 Head	D Pericardial Cavity	X External	0 Drainage device	Z No qualifier
1 Cranial Cavity	F Abdominal Wall		Y Other device	
2 Face	G Peritoneal Cavity			
4 Upper Jaw	H Retroperitoneum			
5 Lower Jaw	J Pelvic Cavity			
6 Neck	K Upper Back			
8 Chest Wall	L Lower Back			
9 Pleural Cavity, Right	M Perineum, Male ♂			
B Pleural Cavity, Left	N Perineum, Female ♀			
C Mediastinum				

REGIONS GENERAL 0W2

W – ANATOMICAL REGIONS, GENERAL 0W3

OTHER REPAIRS GROUP: Control, Repair
Root Operations that define other repairs.

1ST - **0** Medical and Surgical
2ND - **W** Anatomical Regions, General
3RD - **3 CONTROL**

EXAMPLE: Cautery post-op oozing   CMS Ex: Control post-op hemorrhage

CONTROL: Stopping, or attempting to stop, postprocedural bleeding.

EXPLANATION: Bleeding site coded to an anatomical region...

Body Part – 4TH		Approach – 5TH	Device – 6TH	Qualifier – 7TH
0 Head 1 Cranial Cavity 2 Face 4 Upper Jaw 5 Lower Jaw 6 Neck 8 Chest Wall 9 Pleural Cavity, Right B Pleural Cavity, Left C Mediastinum	D Pericardial Cavity F Abdominal Wall G Peritoneal Cavity H Retroperitoneum J Pelvic Cavity K Upper Back L Lower Back M Perineum, Male ♂ N Perineum, Female ♀	0 Open 3 Percutaneous 4 Percutaneous endoscopic	Z No device	Z No qualifier
3 Oral Cavity and Throat		0 Open 3 Percutaneous 4 Percutaneous endoscopic 7 Via natural or artificial opening 8 Via natural or artificial opening endoscopic X External	Z No device	Z No qualifier
P Gastrointestinal Tract Q Respiratory Tract R Genitourinary Tract		0 Open 3 Percutaneous 4 Percutaneous endoscopic 7 Via natural or artificial opening 8 Via natural or artificial opening endoscopic	Z No device	Z No qualifier

0W4 MEDICAL AND SURGICAL SECTION – 2016 ICD-10-PCS

OTHER OBJECTIVES GROUP: Alteration, Creation, (Fusion)
Root Operations that define other objectives.

- 1ST – **0** Medical and Surgical
- 2ND – **W** Anatomical Regions, General
- 3RD – **4 CREATION**

EXAMPLE: Creation penis in female CMS Ex: Creation vagina in male

CREATION: Making a new genital structure that does not take over the function of a body part.

EXPLANATION: Used only for sex change operations

Body Part – 4TH	Approach – 5TH	Device – 6TH	Qualifier – 7TH
M Perineum, Male ♂ NC*	0 Open	7 Autologous tissue substitute J Synthetic substitute K Nonautologous tissue substitute Z No device	0 Vagina
N Perineum, Female ♀ NC*	0 Open	7 Autologous tissue substitute J Synthetic substitute K Nonautologous tissue substitute Z No device	1 Penis

NC* – Non-covered by Medicare. See current Medicare Code Editor for details.

DIVISION GROUP: Division, (Release)
Root Operations involving cutting or separation only.

- 1ST – **0** Medical and Surgical
- 2ND – **W** Anatomical Regions, General
- 3RD – **8 DIVISION**

EXAMPLE: Episiotomy CMS Ex: Osteotomy

DIVISION: Cutting into a body part without draining fluids and/or gases from the body part in order to separate or transect a body part.

EXPLANATION: Separated into two or more portions ...

Body Part – 4TH	Approach – 5TH	Device – 6TH	Qualifier – 7TH
N Perineum, Female ♀	X External	Z No device	Z No qualifier

W – ANATOMICAL REGIONS, GENERAL — 0W9

DRAINAGE GROUP: Drainage, Extirpation, Fragmentation
Root Operations that take out solids/fluids/gases from a body part.

1ST – **0** Medical and Surgical
2ND – **W** Anatomical Regions, General
3RD – **9** DRAINAGE

EXAMPLE: Paracentesis for ascites
CMS Ex: Thoracentesis

DRAINAGE: Taking or letting out fluids and/or gases from a body part.

EXPLANATION: Qualifier "X Diagnostic" indicates biopsy …

Body Part – 4TH		Approach – 5TH	Device – 6TH	Qualifier – 7TH
0 Head	C Mediastinum	0 Open	0 Drainage device	Z No qualifier
1 Cranial Cavity	D Pericardial Cavity	3 Percutaneous		
2 Face	F Abdominal Wall	4 Percutaneous endoscopic		
3 Oral Cavity and Throat	G Peritoneal Cavity			
4 Upper Jaw	H Retroperitoneum			
5 Lower Jaw	J Pelvic Cavity			
6 Neck	K Upper Back			
8 Chest Wall	L Lower Back			
9 Pleural Cavity, Right	M Perineum, Male ♂			
B Pleural Cavity, Left	N Perineum, Female ♀			
0 Head	C Mediastinum	0 Open	Z No device	X Diagnostic
1 Cranial Cavity	D Pericardial Cavity	3 Percutaneous		Z No qualifier
2 Face	F Abdominal Wall	4 Percutaneous endoscopic		
3 Oral Cavity and Throat	G Peritoneal Cavity			
4 Upper Jaw	H Retroperitoneum			
5 Lower Jaw	J Pelvic Cavity			
6 Neck	K Upper Back			
8 Chest Wall	L Lower Back			
9 Pleural Cavity, Right	M Perineum, Male ♂			
B Pleural Cavity, Left	N Perineum, Female ♀			

0WB

MEDICAL AND SURGICAL SECTION – 2016 ICD-10-PCS

EXCISION GROUP: Excision, (Resection), (Destruction), (Extraction), (Detachment)
Root Operations that take out some or all of a body part.

1ST - **0** Medical and Surgical
2ND - **W** Anatomical Regions, General
3RD - **B** EXCISION

EXAMPLE: Excision perineal inclusion cyst
CMS Ex: Liver biopsy

EXCISION: Cutting out or off, without replacement, a portion of a body part.

EXPLANATION: Qualifier "X Diagnostic" indicates biopsy …

Body Part – 4TH	Approach – 5TH	Device – 6TH	Qualifier – 7TH
0 Head 2 Face 4 Upper Jaw 5 Lower Jaw 8 Chest Wall	K Upper Back L Lower Back M Perineum, Male ♂ N Perineum, Female ♀	0 Open 3 Percutaneous 4 Percutaneous endoscopic X External	Z No device	X Diagnostic Z No qualifier
6 Neck F Abdominal Wall		0 Open 3 Percutaneous 4 Percutaneous endoscopic	Z No device	X Diagnostic Z No qualifier
6 Neck F Abdominal Wall		X External	Z No device	2 Stoma X Diagnostic Z No qualifier
C Mediastinum H Retroperitoneum		0 Open 3 Percutaneous 4 Percutaneous endoscopic	Z No device	X Diagnostic Z No qualifier

REGIONS GENERAL 0WB

0WF

W – ANATOMICAL REGIONS, GENERAL

DRAINAGE GROUP: Drainage, Extirpation, Fragmentation
Root Operations that take out solids/fluids/gases from a body part.

- 1ST – **0** Medical and Surgical
- 2ND – **W** Anatomical Regions, General
- 3RD – **C** EXTIRPATION

EXAMPLE: Evacuation clot cranial cavity | CMS Ex: Choledocholithotomy

EXTIRPATION: Taking or cutting out solid matter from a body part.

EXPLANATION: Abnormal byproduct or foreign body …

Body Part – 4TH	Approach – 5TH	Device – 6TH	Qualifier – 7TH
1 Cranial Cavity 3 Oral Cavity and Throat 9 Pleural Cavity, Right B Pleural Cavity, Left C Mediastinum D Pericardial Cavity G Peritoneal Cavity J Pelvic Cavity	0 Open 3 Percutaneous 4 Percutaneous endoscopic X External	Z No device	Z No qualifier
P Gastrointestinal Tract Q Respiratory Tract R Genitourinary Tract	0 Open 3 Percutaneous 4 Percutaneous endoscopic 7 Via natural or artificial opening 8 Via natural or artificial opening endoscopic X External	Z No device	Z No qualifier

DRAINAGE GROUP: Drainage, Extirpation, Fragmentation
Root Operations that take out solids/fluids/gases from a body part.

- 1ST – **0** Medical and Surgical
- 2ND – **W** Anatomical Regions, General
- 3RD – **F** FRAGMENTATION

EXAMPLE: Lithotripsy pericardial cavity | CMS Ex: EWSL

FRAGMENTATION: Breaking solid matter in a body part into pieces.

EXPLANATION: Pieces are not taken out during procedure …

Body Part – 4TH	Approach – 5TH	Device – 6TH	Qualifier – 7TH
1 Cranial Cavity 3 Oral Cavity and Throat 9 Pleural Cavity, Right B Pleural Cavity, Left C Mediastinum D Pericardial Cavity G Peritoneal Cavity J Pelvic Cavity	0 Open 3 Percutaneous 4 Percutaneous endoscopic X External NC*	Z No device	Z No qualifier
P Gastrointestinal Tract Q Respiratory Tract R Genitourinary Tract	0 Open 3 Percutaneous 4 Percutaneous endoscopic 7 Via natural or artificial opening 8 Via natural or artificial opening endoscopic X External NC*	Z No device	Z No qualifier

NC* – Some procedures are considered non-covered by Medicare. See current Medicare Code Editor for details.

0WH MEDICAL AND SURGICAL SECTION – 2016 ICD-10-PCS

DEVICE GROUP: Change, Insertion, Removal, (Replacement), Revision, Supplement
Root Operations that always involve a device.

1ST - 0	Medical and Surgical
2ND - W	Anatomical Regions, General
3RD - H	INSERTION

EXAMPLE: Implantation infusion pump **CMS Ex:** Central venous catheter

INSERTION: Putting in a nonbiological appliance that monitors, assists, performs, or prevents a physiological function but does not physically take the place of a body part.

EXPLANATION: None

Body Part – 4TH	Approach – 5TH	Device – 6TH	Qualifier – 7TH
0 Head 1 Cranial Cavity 2 Face 3 Oral Cavity and Throat 4 Upper Jaw 5 Lower Jaw 6 Neck 8 Chest Wall 9 Pleural Cavity, Right B Pleural Cavity, Left C Mediastinum D Pericardial Cavity F Abdominal Wall G Peritoneal Cavity H Retroperitoneum J Pelvic Cavity K Upper Back L Lower Back M Perineum, Male ♂ N Perineum, Female ♀	0 Open 3 Percutaneous 4 Percutaneous endoscopic	1 Radioactive element 3 Infusion device Y Other device	Z No qualifier
P Gastrointestinal Tract Q Respiratory Tract R Genitourinary Tract	0 Open 3 Percutaneous 4 Percutaneous endoscopic 7 Via natural or artificial opening 8 Via natural or artificial opening endoscopic	1 Radioactive element 3 Infusion device Y Other device	Z No qualifier

666

W – ANATOMICAL REGIONS, GENERAL — 0WM

EXAMINATION GROUP: Inspection, (Map)
Root Operations involving examination only.

- 1ST – **0** Medical and Surgical
- 2ND – **W** Anatomical Regions, General
- 3RD – **J** INSPECTION

EXAMPLE: Exploration peritoneal cavity   CMS Ex: Colonoscopy

INSPECTION: Visually and/or manually exploring a body part.

EXPLANATION: Direct or instrumental visualization ...

Body Part – 4TH		Approach – 5TH	Device – 6TH	Qualifier – 7TH
0 Head	8 Chest Wall	0 Open	Z No device	Z No qualifier
2 Face	F Abdominal Wall	3 Percutaneous		
3 Oral Cavity and Throat	K Upper Back	4 Percutaneous endoscopic		
4 Upper Jaw	L Lower Back			
5 Lower Jaw	M Perineum, Male ♂	X External		
6 Neck	N Perineum, Female ♀			
1 Cranial Cavity	D Pericardial Cavity	0 Open	Z No device	Z No qualifier
9 Pleural Cavity, Right	G Peritoneal Cavity	3 Percutaneous		
B Pleural Cavity, Left	H Retroperitoneum	4 Percutaneous endoscopic		
C Mediastinum	J Pelvic Cavity			
P Gastrointestinal Tract		0 Open	Z No device	Z No qualifier
Q Respiratory Tract		3 Percutaneous		
R Genitourinary Tract		4 Percutaneous endoscopic		
		7 Via natural or artificial opening		
		8 Via natural or artificial opening endoscopic		

MOVE GROUP: Reattachment, (Reposition), (Transfer), (Transplantation)
Root Operations that put in/put back or move some/all of a body part.

- 1ST – **0** Medical and Surgical
- 2ND – **W** Anatomical Regions, General
- 3RD – **M** REATTACHMENT

EXAMPLE: Replantation avulsed perineum   CMS Ex: Reattachment hand

REATTACHMENT: Putting back in or on all or a portion of a separated body part to its normal location or other suitable location.

EXPLANATION: With/without reconnection of vessels/nerves...

Body Part – 4TH		Approach – 5TH	Device – 6TH	Qualifier – 7TH
2 Face	F Abdominal Wall	0 Open	Z No device	Z No qualifier
4 Upper Jaw	K Upper Back			
5 Lower Jaw	L Lower Back			
6 Neck	M Perineum, Male ♂			
8 Chest Wall	N Perineum, Female ♀			

0WP

MEDICAL AND SURGICAL SECTION – 2016 ICD-10-PCS

DEVICE GROUP: Change, Insertion, Removal, (Replacement), Revision, Supplement
Root Operations that always involve a device.

- 1ST – **0** Medical and Surgical
- 2ND – **W** Anatomical Regions, General
- 3RD – **P** REMOVAL

EXAMPLE: Removal infusion pump

CMS Ex: Chest tube removal

REMOVAL: Taking out or off a device from a body part.

EXPLANATION: Removal device without reinsertion ...

Body Part – 4TH		Approach – 5TH	Device – 6TH	Qualifier – 7TH
0 Head 2 Face 4 Upper Jaw 5 Lower Jaw 6 Neck 8 Chest Wall	C Mediastinum F Abdominal Wall K Upper Back L Lower Back M Perineum, Male ♂ N Perineum, Female ♀	0 Open 3 Percutaneous 4 Percutaneous endoscopic X External	0 Drainage device 1 Radioactive element 3 Infusion device 7 Autologous tissue substitute J Synthetic substitute K Nonautologous tissue substitute Y Other device	Z No qualifier
1 Cranial Cavity 9 Pleural Cavity, Right B Pleural Cavity, Left G Peritoneal Cavity J Pelvic Cavity		0 Open 3 Percutaneous 4 Percutaneous endoscopic	0 Drainage device 1 Radioactive element 3 Infusion device J Synthetic substitute Y Other device	Z No qualifier
1 Cranial Cavity 9 Pleural Cavity, Right B Pleural Cavity, Left G Peritoneal Cavity J Pelvic Cavity		X External	0 Drainage device 1 Radioactive element 3 Infusion device	Z No qualifier
D Pericardial Cavity H Retroperitoneum		0 Open 3 Percutaneous 4 Percutaneous endoscopic	0 Drainage device 1 Radioactive element 3 Infusion device Y Other device	Z No qualifier
D Pericardial Cavity H Retroperitoneum		X External	0 Drainage device 1 Radioactive element 3 Infusion device	Z No qualifier
P Gastrointestinal Tract Q Respiratory Tract R Genitourinary Tract		0 Open 3 Percutaneous 4 Percutaneous endoscopic 7 Via natural or artificial opening 8 Via natural or artificial opening endoscopic X External	1 Radioactive element 3 Infusion device Y Other device	Z No qualifier

W – ANATOMICAL REGIONS, GENERAL 0W0

OTHER REPAIRS GROUP: Control, Repair
Root Operations that define other repairs.

1ST – 0 Medical and Surgical
2ND – W Anatomical Regions, General
3RD – Q REPAIR

EXAMPLE: Parastomal hernia repair   CMS Ex: Suture laceration

REPAIR: Restoring, to the extent possible, a body part to its normal anatomic structure and function.

EXPLANATION: Only when no other root operation applies …

Body Part – 4TH		Approach – 5TH	Device – 6TH	Qualifier – 7TH
0 Head 2 Face 4 Upper Jaw 5 Lower Jaw 8 Chest Wall	K Upper Back L Lower Back M Perineum, Male ♂ N Perineum, Female ♀	0 Open 3 Percutaneous 4 Percutaneous endoscopic X External	Z No device	Z No qualifier
6 Neck F Abdominal Wall		0 Open 3 Percutaneous 4 Percutaneous endoscopic	Z No device	Z No qualifier
6 Neck F Abdominal Wall		X External	Z No device	2 Stoma Z No qualifier
C Mediastinum		0 Open 3 Percutaneous 4 Percutaneous endoscopic	Z No device	Z No qualifier

DEVICE GROUP: Change, Insertion, Removal, (Replacement), Revision, Supplement
Root Operations that always involve a device.

1ST – 0 Medical and Surgical
2ND – W Anatomical Regions, General
3RD – U SUPPLEMENT

EXAMPLE: Parastomal hernia repair with mesh   CMS Ex: With mesh

SUPPLEMENT: Putting in or on biological or synthetic material that physically reinforces and/or augments the function of a portion of a body part.

EXPLANATION: Biological material from same individual …

Body Part – 4TH		Approach – 5TH	Device – 6TH	Qualifier – 7TH
0 Head 2 Face 4 Upper Jaw 5 Lower Jaw 6 Neck 8 Chest Wall	C Mediastinum F Abdominal Wall K Upper Back L Lower Back M Perineum, Male ♂ N Perineum, Female ♀	0 Open 4 Percutaneous endoscopic	7 Autologous tissue substitute J Synthetic substitute K Nonautologous tissue substitute	Z No qualifier

0WW

MEDICAL AND SURGICAL SECTION – 2016 ICD-10-PCS

DEVICE GROUP: Change, Insertion, Removal, (Replacement), Revision, Supplement
Root Operations that always involve a device.

1ST – **0** Medical and Surgical
2ND – **W** Anatomical Regions, General
3RD – **W** REVISION

EXAMPLE: Reposition infusion pump | **CMS Ex:** Adjustment pacemaker lead

REVISION: Correcting, to the extent possible, a portion of a malfunctioning device or the position of a displaced device.

EXPLANATION: May replace components of a device ...

Body Part – 4TH	Approach – 5TH	Device – 6TH	Qualifier – 7TH
0 Head 2 Face 4 Upper Jaw 5 Lower Jaw 6 Neck 8 Chest Wall C Mediastinum F Abdominal Wall K Upper Back L Lower Back M Perineum, Male ♂ N Perineum, Female ♀	0 Open 3 Percutaneous 4 Percutaneous endoscopic X External	0 Drainage device 1 Radioactive element 3 Infusion device 7 Autologous tissue substitute J Synthetic substitute K Nonautologous tissue substitute Y Other device	Z No qualifier
1 Cranial Cavity 9 Pleural Cavity, Right B Pleural Cavity, Left G Peritoneal Cavity J Pelvic Cavity	0 Open 3 Percutaneous 4 Percutaneous endoscopic X External	0 Drainage device 1 Radioactive element 3 Infusion device J Synthetic substitute Y Other device	Z No qualifier
D Pericardial Cavity H Retroperitoneum	0 Open 3 Percutaneous 4 Percutaneous endoscopic X External	0 Drainage device 1 Radioactive element 3 Infusion device Y Other device	Z No qualifier
P Gastrointestinal Tract Q Respiratory Tract R Genitourinary Tract	0 Open 3 Percutaneous 4 Percutaneous endoscopic 7 Via natural or artificial opening 8 Via natural or artificial opening endoscopic X External	1 Radioactive element 3 Infusion device Y Other device	Z No qualifier

Educational Annotations | X – Anatomical Regions, Upper Extremities

Body System Specific Educational Annotations for the Anatomical Regions, Upper Extremities include:

- Anatomy and Physiology Review
- Anatomical Illustrations
- Definitions of Common Procedures
- AHA Coding Clinic® Reference Notations
- Body Part Key Listings
- Device Key Listings
- Device Aggregation Table Listings
- Coding Notes

Anatomy and Physiology Review of Anatomical Regions, Upper Extremities

BODY PART VALUES – X - ANATOMICAL REGIONS, UPPER EXTREMITIES

Coding Guideline B2.1a - Body System, General Guideline – The procedure codes in the general anatomical regions body systems should only be used when the procedure is performed on an anatomical region rather than a specific body part (e.g., root operations Control and Detachment, Drainage of a body cavity) or the rare occasion when no information is available to support assignment of a code to a specific body part. Example: Control of postoperative hemorrhage is coded to the root operation Control, which is found in the general anatomical regions body systems.

1st Ray – The first digit of the hand and its associated first metacarpal bone.

2nd Ray – The second digit of the hand and its associated second metacarpal bone.

3rd Ray – The third digit of the hand and its associated third metacarpal bone.

4th Ray – The fourth digit of the hand and its associated fourth metacarpal bone.

5th Ray – The fifth digit of the hand and its associated fifth metacarpal bone.

Axilla – The multi-tissue-layered area at the junction of the arm and trunk on the underside of the shoulder joint.

Elbow Region – The multi-tissue-layered elbow joint area.

Forequarter – The portion of the body including the upper extremity, scapula, and clavicle.

Hand – The portion of the upper extermity distal to the forearm.

Index Finger – The second digit of the hand.

Little Finger – The fifth digit of the hand.

Lower Arm – The portion of the upper extermity distal to the elbow.

Middle Finger – The third digit of the hand.

Ring Finger – The fourth digit of the hand.

Shoulder Region – The multi-tissue-layered shoulder joint area.

Thumb – The first digit of the hand.

Upper Arm – The portion of the upper extermity distal to the shoulder and proximal to the elbow.

Upper Extremity – The entire upper extremity (arm).

Wrist Region – The multi-tissue-layered wrist joint area.

Educational Annotations

X – Anatomical Regions, Upper Extremities

Anatomical Illustrations of Anatomical Regions, Upper Extremities

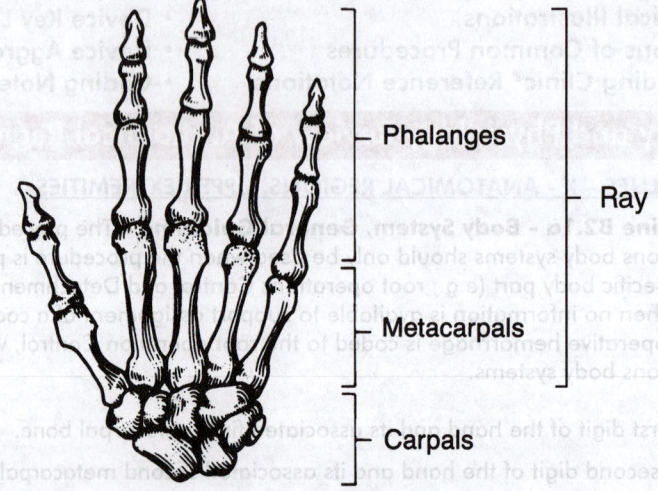

RIGHT HAND — DORSAL VIEW

Definitions of Common Procedures of Anatomical Regions, Upper Extremities

Amputation through elbow – The surgical detachment and removal of the lower arm including the entire radius and ulna that is performed through the elbow joint.

Forequarter amputation – The surgical detachment and removal of the entire arm including part or all of the scapula and clavicle.

Reattachment of severed thumb – The surgical reconnection of a thumb that has been traumatically amputated.

Transfer of index finger to thumb – The surgical dissection and migration of the index finger, including division of the metacarpal index ray bone that is positioned to function as the thumb.

Transplantation of toe to thumb – The surgical detachment of the great toe or second toe and microsurgical connection at the thumb site to function as the thumb.

Educational Annotations | X – Anatomical Regions, Upper Extremities

AHA Coding Clinic® Reference Notations of Anatomical Regions, Upper Extremities

ROOT OPERATION SPECIFIC - X - ANATOMICAL REGIONS, UPPER EXTREMITIES
ALTERATION - 0
CHANGE - 2
CONTROL - 3
    Control of post arterial bypass bleeding .... AHA 15:1Q:p35
DETACHMENT - 6
DRAINAGE - 9
EXCISION - B
INSERTION - H
INSPECTION - J
REATTACHMENT - M
REMOVAL - P
REPAIR - Q
REPLACEMENT - R
SUPPLEMENT - U
REVISION - W
TRANSFER - X

Body Part Key Listings of Anatomical Regions, Upper Extremities

See also Body Part Key in Appendix C
None for the Anatomical Regions, Upper Extremities Body System

Device Key Listings of Anatomical Regions, Upper Extremities

See also Device Key in Appendix D
Autograft .... *use* Autologous Tissue Substitute
Brachytherapy seeds .... *use* Radioactive Element
Tissue bank graft .... *use* Nonautologous Tissue Substitute

Device Aggregation Table Listings of Anatomical Regions, Upper Extremities

See also Device Aggregation Table in Appendix E

Specific Device	For Operation	In Body System	General Device
None Listed in Device Aggregation Table for this Body System			

Educational Annotations | X – Anatomical Regions, Upper Extremities

Coding Notes of Anatomical Regions, Upper Extremities

Body System Relevant Coding Guidelines

Control vs. more definitive root operations
  B3.7
    The root operation Control is defined as, "Stopping, or attempting to stop, postprocedural bleeding." If an attempt to stop postprocedural bleeding is initially unsuccessful, and to stop the bleeding requires performing any of the definitive root operations Bypass, Detachment, Excision, Extraction, Reposition, Replacement, or Resection, then that root operation is coded instead of Control.
  Example: Resection of spleen to stop postprocedural bleeding is coded to Resection instead of Control.

Body System Specific PCS Reference Manual Exercises

PCS CODE	X – ANATOMICAL REGIONS, UPPER EXTREMITIES EXERCISES
0X3F0ZZ	Open exploration and ligation of post-op arterial bleeder, left forearm.
0X600ZZ	Right forequarter amputation. (The Forequarter body part includes amputation along any part of the scapula and clavicle.)
0X680Z2	Mid-shaft amputation, right humerus.
0X6B0ZZ	Amputation at right elbow level.
0X6J0Z0	Right wrist joint amputation. (Amputation at the wrist joint is actually complete amputation of the hand.)
0X6K0Z8	Fifth ray carpometacarpal joint amputation, left hand. (A "Complete" ray amputation is through the carpometacarpal joint.)
0X6L0Z3	DIP joint amputation of right thumb. (The qualifier "Low" here means through the distal interphalangeal joint.)
0XMK0ZZ	Reattachment of severed left hand.
0XXP0ZM	Transfer left index finger to left thumb position, open.

X – ANATOMICAL REGIONS, UPPER EXTREMITIES   0 X 3

OTHER OBJECTIVES GROUP: Alteration, (Creation), (Fusion)
Root Operations that define other objectives.

- **1ST - 0** Medical and Surgical
- **2ND - X** Anatomical Regions, Upper Extremities
- **3RD - 0** ALTERATION

EXAMPLE: Cosmetic deltoid augmentation   CMS Ex: Face lift

ALTERATION: Modifying the anatomic structure of a body part without affecting the function of the body part.

EXPLANATION: Principal purpose is to improve appearance

Body Part – 4TH		Approach – 5TH	Device – 6TH	Qualifier – 7TH
2 Shoulder Region, Right	B Elbow Region, Right	0 Open	7 Autologous tissue substitute	Z No qualifier
3 Shoulder Region, Left	C Elbow Region, Left	3 Percutaneous	J Synthetic substitute	
4 Axilla, Right	D Lower Arm, Right	4 Percutaneous endoscopic	K Nonautologous tissue substitute	
5 Axilla, Left	F Lower Arm, Left		Z No device	
6 Upper Extremity, Right	G Wrist Region, Right			
7 Upper Extremity, Left	H Wrist Region, Left			
8 Upper Arm, Right				
9 Upper Arm, Left				

DEVICE GROUP: Change, Insertion, Removal, Replacement, Revision, Supplement
Root Operations that always involve a device.

- **1ST - 0** Medical and Surgical
- **2ND - X** Anatomical Regions, Upper Extremities
- **3RD - 2** CHANGE

EXAMPLE: Exchange drain tube   CMS Ex: Changing urinary catheter

CHANGE: Taking out or off a device from a body part and putting back an identical or similar device in or on the same body part without cutting or puncturing the skin or a mucous membrane.

EXPLANATION: ALL Changes use EXTERNAL approach only ...

Body Part – 4TH	Approach – 5TH	Device – 6TH	Qualifier – 7TH
6 Upper Extremity, Right	X External	0 Drainage device	Z No qualifier
7 Upper Extremity, Left		Y Other device	

OTHER REPAIRS GROUP: Control, Repair
Root Operations that define other repairs.

- **1ST - 0** Medical and Surgical
- **2ND - X** Anatomical Regions, Upper Extremities
- **3RD - 3** CONTROL

EXAMPLE: Ligation post-op bleeder   CMS Ex: Control post-op hemorrhage

CONTROL: Stopping, or attempting to stop, postprocedural bleeding.

EXPLANATION: Bleeding site coded to an anatomical region...

Body Part – 4TH		Approach – 5TH	Device – 6TH	Qualifier – 7TH
2 Shoulder Region, Right	B Elbow Region, Right	0 Open	Z No device	Z No qualifier
3 Shoulder Region, Left	C Elbow Region, Left	3 Percutaneous		
4 Axilla, Right	D Lower Arm, Right	4 Percutaneous endoscopic		
5 Axilla, Left	F Lower Arm, Left			
6 Upper Extremity, Right	G Wrist Region, Right			
7 Upper Extremity, Left	H Wrist Region, Left			
8 Upper Arm, Right	J Hand, Right			
9 Upper Arm, Left	K Hand, Left			

0X6

MEDICAL AND SURGICAL SECTION – 2016 ICD-10-PCS

EXCISION GROUP: Excision, (Resection), (Destruction), (Extraction), Detachment
Root Operations that take out some or all of a body part.

1ST - **0** Medical and Surgical	EXAMPLE: Amputation hand CMS Ex: Leg amputation
2ND - **X** Anatomical Regions, Upper Extremities	**DETACHMENT:** Cutting off all or portion of the upper or lower extremities.
3RD - **6** DETACHMENT	EXPLANATION: Qualifier specifies amputation level ...

REGIONS UPPER EXT 0 X 6

Body Part – 4TH		Approach – 5TH	Device – 6TH	Qualifier – 7TH
0 Forequarter, Right 1 Forequarter, Left 2 Shoulder Region, Right	3 Shoulder Region, Left B Elbow Region, Right C Elbow Region, Left	0 Open	Z No device	Z No qualifier
8 Upper Arm, Right 9 Upper Arm, Left D Lower Arm, Right F Lower Arm, Left		0 Open	Z No device	1 High 2 Mid 3 Low
J Hand, Right K Hand, Left		0 Open	Z No device	0 Complete 4 Complete 1st Ray 5 Complete 2nd Ray 6 Complete 3rd Ray 7 Complete 4th Ray 8 Complete 5th Ray 9 Partial 1st Ray B Partial 2nd Ray C Partial 3rd Ray D Partial 4th Ray F Partial 5th Ray
L Thumb, Right M Thumb, Left N Index Finger, Right P Index Finger, Left Q Middle Finger, Right R Middle Finger, Left	S Ring Finger, Right T Ring Finger, Left V Little Finger, Right W Little Finger, Left	0 Open	Z No device	0 Complete 1 High 2 Mid 3 Low

X – ANATOMICAL REGIONS, UPPER EXTREMITIES — 0XB

DRAINAGE GROUP: Drainage, (Extirpation), (Fragmentation)
Root Operations that take out solids/fluids/gases from a body part.

- 1ST - **0** Medical and Surgical
- 2ND - **X** Anatomical Regions, Upper Extremities
- 3RD - **9 DRAINAGE**

EXAMPLE: I&D deep wound infection
CMS Ex: Thoracentesis

DRAINAGE: Taking or letting out fluids and/or gases from a body part.

EXPLANATION: Qualifier "X Diagnostic" indicates biopsy …

Body Part – 4TH		Approach – 5TH	Device – 6TH	Qualifier – 7TH
2 Shoulder Region, Right	B Elbow Region, Right	0 Open	0 Drainage device	Z No qualifier
3 Shoulder Region, Left	C Elbow Region, Left	3 Percutaneous		
4 Axilla, Right	D Lower Arm, Right	4 Percutaneous endoscopic		
5 Axilla, Left	F Lower Arm, Left			
6 Upper Extremity, Right	G Wrist Region, Right			
7 Upper Extremity, Left	H Wrist Region, Left			
8 Upper Arm, Right	J Hand, Right			
9 Upper Arm, Left	K Hand, Left			

Body Part – 4TH		Approach – 5TH	Device – 6TH	Qualifier – 7TH
2 Shoulder Region, Right	B Elbow Region, Right	0 Open	Z No device	X Diagnostic
3 Shoulder Region, Left	C Elbow Region, Left	3 Percutaneous		Z No qualifier
4 Axilla, Right	D Lower Arm, Right	4 Percutaneous endoscopic		
5 Axilla, Left	F Lower Arm, Left			
6 Upper Extremity, Right	G Wrist Region, Right			
7 Upper Extremity, Left	H Wrist Region, Left			
8 Upper Arm, Right	J Hand, Right			
9 Upper Arm, Left	K Hand, Left			

EXCISION GROUP: Excision, (Resection), (Destruction), (Extraction), Detachment
Root Operations that take out some or all of a body part.

- 1ST - **0** Medical and Surgical
- 2ND - **X** Anatomical Regions, Upper Extremities
- 3RD - **B EXCISION**

EXAMPLE: Excision tumor axilla region
CMS Ex: Liver biopsy

EXCISION: Cutting out or off, without replacement, a portion of a body part.

EXPLANATION: Qualifier "X Diagnostic" indicates biopsy …

Body Part – 4TH		Approach – 5TH	Device – 6TH	Qualifier – 7TH
2 Shoulder Region, Right	B Elbow Region, Right	0 Open	Z No device	X Diagnostic
3 Shoulder Region, Left	C Elbow Region, Left	3 Percutaneous		Z No qualifier
4 Axilla, Right	D Lower Arm, Right	4 Percutaneous endoscopic		
5 Axilla, Left	F Lower Arm, Left			
6 Upper Extremity, Right	G Wrist Region, Right			
7 Upper Extremity, Left	H Wrist Region, Left			
8 Upper Arm, Right	J Hand, Right			
9 Upper Arm, Left	K Hand, Left			

0XH — MEDICAL AND SURGICAL SECTION – 2016 ICD-10-PCS

DEVICE GROUP: Change, Insertion, Removal, Replacement, Revision, Supplement
Root Operations that always involve a device.

- 1ST – **0** Medical and Surgical
- 2ND – **X** Anatomical Regions, Upper Extremities
- 3RD – **H** INSERTION

EXAMPLE: Implant infusion device CMS Ex: Central venous catheter

INSERTION: Putting in a nonbiological appliance that monitors, assists, performs, or prevents a physiological function but does not physically take the place of a body part.

EXPLANATION: None

Body Part – 4TH	Approach – 5TH	Device – 6TH	Qualifier – 7TH
2 Shoulder Region, Right B Elbow Region, Right	0 Open	1 Radioactive element	Z No qualifier
3 Shoulder Region, Left C Elbow Region, Left	3 Percutaneous	3 Infusion device	
4 Axilla, Right D Lower Arm, Right	4 Percutaneous endoscopic	Y Other device	
5 Axilla, Left F Lower Arm, Left			
6 Upper Extremity, Right G Wrist Region, Right			
7 Upper Extremity, Left H Wrist Region, Left			
8 Upper Arm, Right J Hand, Right			
9 Upper Arm, Left K Hand, Left			

EXAMINATION GROUP: Inspection, (Map)
Root Operations involving examination only.

- 1ST – **0** Medical and Surgical
- 2ND – **X** Anatomical Regions, Upper Extremities
- 3RD – **J** INSPECTION

EXAMPLE: Exploration axilla region CMS Ex: Colonoscopy

INSPECTION: Visually and/or manually exploring a body part.

EXPLANATION: Direct or instrumental visualization ...

Body Part – 4TH	Approach – 5TH	Device – 6TH	Qualifier – 7TH
2 Shoulder Region, Right B Elbow Region, Right	0 Open	Z No device	Z No qualifier
3 Shoulder Region, Left C Elbow Region, Left	3 Percutaneous		
4 Axilla, Right D Lower Arm, Right	4 Percutaneous endoscopic		
5 Axilla, Left F Lower Arm, Left	X External		
6 Upper Extremity, Right G Wrist Region, Right			
7 Upper Extremity, Left H Wrist Region, Left			
8 Upper Arm, Right J Hand, Right			
9 Upper Arm, Left K Hand, Left			

X – ANATOMICAL REGIONS, UPPER EXTREMITIES 0XP

MOVE GROUP: Reattachment, (Reposition), Transfer, (Transplantation)
Root Operations that put in/put back or move some/all of a body part.

- 1ST – **0** Medical and Surgical
- 2ND – **X** Anatomical Regions, Upper Extremities
- 3RD – **M REATTACHMENT**

EXAMPLE: Reattachment severed thumb CMS Ex: Reattachment hand

REATTACHMENT: Putting back in or on all or a portion of a separated body part to its normal location or other suitable location.

EXPLANATION: With/without reconnection of vessels/nerves...

Body Part – 4TH		Approach – 5TH	Device – 6TH	Qualifier – 7TH
0 Forequarter, Right	G Wrist Region, Right	0 Open	Z No device	Z No qualifier
1 Forequarter, Left	H Wrist Region, Left			
2 Shoulder Region, Right	J Hand, Right			
3 Shoulder Region, Left	K Hand, Left			
4 Axilla, Right	L Thumb, Right			
5 Axilla, Left	M Thumb, Left			
6 Upper Extremity, Right	N Index Finger, Right			
7 Upper Extremity, Left	P Index Finger, Left			
8 Upper Arm, Right	Q Middle Finger, Right			
9 Upper Arm, Left	R Middle Finger, Left			
B Elbow Region, Right	S Ring Finger, Right			
C Elbow Region, Left	T Ring Finger, Left			
D Lower Arm, Right	V Little Finger, Right			
F Lower Arm, Left	W Little Finger, Left			

DEVICE GROUP: Change, Insertion, Removal, Replacement, Revision, Supplement
Root Operations that always involve a device.

- 1ST – **0** Medical and Surgical
- 2ND – **X** Anatomical Regions, Upper Extremities
- 3RD – **P REMOVAL**

EXAMPLE: Removal drain tube CMS Ex: Chest tube removal

REMOVAL: Taking out or off a device from a body part.

EXPLANATION: Removal device without reinsertion ...

Body Part – 4TH	Approach – 5TH	Device – 6TH	Qualifier – 7TH
6 Upper Extremity, Right	0 Open	0 Drainage device	Z No qualifier
7 Upper Extremity, Left	3 Percutaneous	1 Radioactive element	
	4 Percutaneous endoscopic	3 Infusion device	
	X External	7 Autologous tissue substitute	
		J Synthetic substitute	
		K Nonautologous tissue substitute	
		Y Other device	

679

0XQ

MEDICAL AND SURGICAL SECTION – 2016 ICD-10-PCS   [2016.PCS]

OTHER REPAIRS GROUP: Control, Repair
Root Operations that define other repairs.

1ST - **0** Medical and Surgical 2ND - **X** Anatomical Regions, Upper Extremities 3RD - **Q REPAIR**	EXAMPLE: Repair lower arm	CMS Ex: Suture laceration
	REPAIR: Restoring, to the extent possible, a body part to its normal anatomic structure and function.	
	EXPLANATION: Only when no other root operation applies ...	

Body Part – 4TH	Approach – 5TH	Device – 6TH	Qualifier – 7TH
2 Shoulder Region, Right J Hand, Right 3 Shoulder Region, Left K Hand, Left 4 Axilla, Right L Thumb, Right 5 Axilla, Left M Thumb, Left 6 Upper Extremity, Right N Index Finger, Right 7 Upper Extremity, Left P Index Finger, Left 8 Upper Arm, Right Q Middle Finger, Right 9 Upper Arm, Left R Middle Finger, Left B Elbow Region, Right S Ring Finger, Right C Elbow Region, Left T Ring Finger, Left D Lower Arm, Right V Little Finger, Right F Lower Arm, Left W Little Finger, Left G Wrist Region, Right H Wrist Region, Left	0 Open 3 Percutaneous 4 Percutaneous endoscopic X External	Z No device	Z No qualifier

DEVICE GROUP: Change, Insertion, Removal, Replacement, Revision, Supplement
Root Operations that always involve a device.

1ST - **0** Medical and Surgical 2ND - **X** Anatomical Regions, Upper Extremities 3RD - **R REPLACEMENT**	EXAMPLE: Replacement thumb with toe	CMS Ex: Total hip
	REPLACEMENT: Putting in or on a biological or synthetic material that physically takes the place and/or function of all or a portion of a body part.	
	EXPLANATION: Includes taking out body part, or eradication...	

Body Part – 4TH	Approach – 5TH	Device – 6TH	Qualifier – 7TH
L Thumb, Right M Thumb, Left	0 Open 4 Percutaneous endoscopic	7 Autologous tissue substitute	N Toe, Right P Toe, Left

X – ANATOMICAL REGIONS, UPPER EXTREMITIES   0XW

DEVICE GROUP: Change, Insertion, Removal, Replacement, Revision, Supplement
Root Operations that always involve a device.

1ST - **0** Medical and Surgical
2ND - **X** Anatomical Regions, Upper Extremities
3RD - **U SUPPLEMENT**

EXAMPLE: Augmentation graft axilla | CMS Ex: Hernia repair with mesh

SUPPLEMENT: Putting in or on biological or synthetic material that physically reinforces and/or augments the function of a portion of a body part.

EXPLANATION: Biological material from same individual ...

Body Part – 4TH	Approach – 5TH	Device – 6TH	Qualifier – 7TH
2 Shoulder Region, Right J Hand, Right	0 Open	7 Autologous tissue substitute	Z No qualifier
3 Shoulder Region, Left K Hand, Left	4 Percutaneous endoscopic	J Synthetic substitute	
4 Axilla, Right L Thumb, Right		K Nonautologous tissue substitute	
5 Axilla, Left M Thumb, Left			
6 Upper Extremity, Right N Index Finger, Right			
7 Upper Extremity, Left P Index Finger, Left			
8 Upper Arm, Right Q Middle Finger, Right			
9 Upper Arm, Left R Middle Finger, Left			
B Elbow Region, Right S Ring Finger, Right			
C Elbow Region, Left T Ring Finger, Left			
D Lower Arm, Right V Little Finger, Right			
F Lower Arm, Left W Little Finger, Left			
G Wrist Region, Right			
H Wrist Region, Left			

DEVICE GROUP: Change, Insertion, Removal, Replacement, Revision, Supplement
Root Operations that always involve a device.

1ST - **0** Medical and Surgical
2ND - **X** Anatomical Regions, Upper Extremities
3RD - **W REVISION**

EXAMPLE: Reposition drain tube | CMS Ex: Adjustment pacemaker lead

REVISION: Correcting, to the extent possible, a portion of a malfunctioning device or the position of a displaced device.

EXPLANATION: May replace components of a device ...

Body Part – 4TH	Approach – 5TH	Device – 6TH	Qualifier – 7TH
6 Upper Extremity, Right	0 Open	0 Drainage device	Z No qualifier
7 Upper Extremity, Left	3 Percutaneous	3 Infusion device	
	4 Percutaneous endoscopic	7 Autologous tissue substitute	
	X External	J Synthetic substitute	
		K Nonautologous tissue substitute	
		Y Other device	

0XX

MEDICAL AND SURGICAL SECTION – 2016 ICD-10-PCS

MOVE GROUP: Reattachment, (Reposition), Transfer, (Transplantation)
Root Operations that put in/put back or move some/all of a body part.

- 1ST – **0** Medical and Surgical
- 2ND – **X** Anatomical Regions, Upper Extremities
- 3RD – **X** TRANSFER

EXAMPLE: Transfer index finger to thumb **CMS Ex:** Tendon transfer

TRANSFER: Moving, without taking out, all or a portion of a body part to another location to take over the function of all or a portion of a body part.

EXPLANATION: The body part remains connected ...

Body Part – 4TH	Approach – 5TH	Device – 6TH	Qualifier – 7TH
N Index Finger, Right	0 Open	Z No device	L Thumb, Right
P Index Finger, Left	0 Open	Z No device	M Thumb, Left

REGIONS UPPER EXT 0XX

Educational Annotations | Y – Anatomical Regions, Lower Extremities

Body System Specific Educational Annotations for the Anatomical Regions, Lower Extremities include:
- Anatomy and Physiology Review
- Anatomical Illustrations
- Definitions of Common Procedures
- AHA Coding Clinic® Reference Notations
- Body Part Key Listings
- Device Key Listings
- Device Aggregation Table Listings
- Coding Notes

Anatomy and Physiology Review of Anatomical Regions, Lower Extremities

BODY PART VALUES – Y - ANATOMICAL REGIONS, LOWER EXTREMITIES

Coding Guideline B2.1a - Body System, General Guideline – The procedure codes in the general anatomical regions body systems should only be used when the procedure is performed on an anatomical region rather than a specific body part (e.g., root operations Control and Detachment, Drainage of a body cavity) or the rare occasion when no information is available to support assignment of a code to a specific body part. Example: Control of postoperative hemorrhage is coded to the root operation Control, which is found in the general anatomical regions body systems.

1st Ray – The first digit of the foot and its associated first metatarsal bone.

2nd Ray – The second digit of the foot and its associated second metatarsal bone.

3rd Ray – The third digit of the foot and its associated third metatarsal bone.

4th Ray – The fourth digit of the foot and its associated fourth metatarsal bone.

5th Ray – The fifth digit of the foot and its associated fifth metatarsal bone.

1st Toe – The first digit of the foot.

2nd Toe – The second digit of the foot.

3rd Toe – The third digit of the foot.

4th Toe – The fourth digit of the foot.

5th Toe – The fifth digit of the foot.

Ankle Region – The multi-tissue-layered ankle joint area.

Buttock – The rounded lower portions of the posterior trunk including the gluteus muscles.

Femoral Region – The multi-tissue-layered area of the anterior upper inner portion of the thigh (also known as the femoral triangle). See also the body part "Upper Leg."

Foot – The portion of the lower extermity distal to the lower end of the tibia and fibula.

Hindquarter – The portion of the body including the lower extremity, buttock, and pelvis.

Inguinal Region – The multi-tissue-layered area between the lower abdomen, thigh, and pubic bone.

Knee Region – The multi-tissue-layered knee joint area.

Lower Extremity – The entire lower extremity (leg).

Lower Leg – The portion of the lower extermity distal to the knee.

Upper Leg – The portion of the lower extermity distal to the hip and proximal to the knee.

Educational Annotations | Y – Anatomical Regions, Lower Extremities

Anatomical Illustrations of Anatomical Regions, Lower Extremities

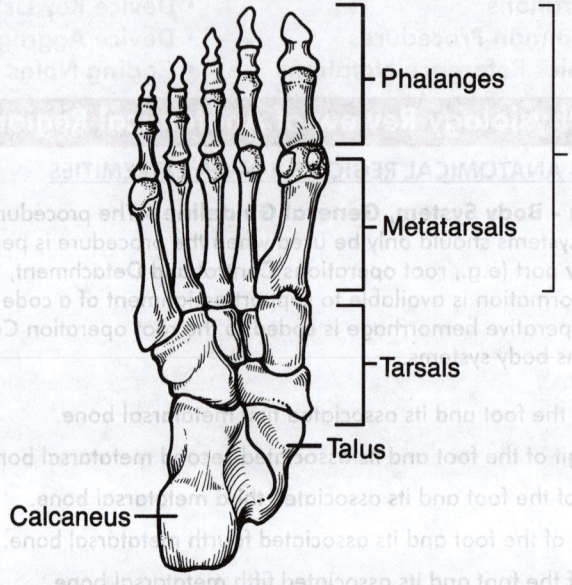

RIGHT FOOT — PLANTAR VIEW

Definitions of Common Procedures of Anatomical Regions, Lower Extremities

Buttock implants – The plastic surgical enhancement of the buttocks usually using solid silicone implants or by fat transfers.

Hindquarter amputation – The surgical detachment and removal of the entire leg including part or all of the buttock and pelvis.

Midfoot amputation – The surgical detachment and removal of the distal foot that is performed through the tarsal-metatarsal joints.

Educational Annotations | Y – Anatomical Regions, Lower Extremities

AHA Coding Clinic® Reference Notations of Anatomical Regions, Lower Extremities

ROOT OPERATION SPECIFIC - Y - ANATOMICAL REGIONS, LOWER EXTREMITIES
ALTERATION - 0
CHANGE - 2
CONTROL - 3
DETACHMENT - 6
    Amputation of 1st toe at the interphalangeal joint ....AHA 15:2Q:p2
    Midfoot amputation ....AHA 15:1Q:p28
DRAINAGE - 9
    Incision and drainage of femoral region wound infection ....AHA 15:1Q:p22
    Incision and drainage of inguinal region wound infection ....AHA 15:1Q:p22
EXCISION - B
INSERTION - H
INSPECTION - J
REATTACHMENT - M
REMOVAL - P
REPAIR - Q
SUPPLEMENT - U
REVISION - W

Body Part Key Listings of Anatomical Regions, Lower Extremities

See also Body Part Key in Appendix C
Hallux ....*use* 1st Toe, Left/Right
Inguinal canal ....*use* Inguinal Region, Bilateral/Left/Right
Inguinal triangle ....*use* Inguinal Region, Bilateral/Left/Right

Device Key Listings of Anatomical Regions, Lower Extremities

See also Device Key in Appendix D
Autograft ....*use* Autologous Tissue Substitute
Brachytherapy seeds ....*use* Radioactive Element
Tissue bank graft ....*use* Nonautologous Tissue Substitute

Device Aggregation Table Listings of Anatomical Regions, Lower Extremities

See also Device Aggregation Table in Appendix E

Specific Device	For Operation	In Body System	General Device
None Listed in Device Aggregation Table for this Body System			

Educational Annotations

Y – Anatomical Regions, Lower Extremities

Coding Notes of Anatomical Regions, Lower Extremities

Body System Relevant Coding Guidelines

Control vs. more definitive root operations
  B3.7
  The root operation Control is defined as, "Stopping, or attempting to stop, postprocedural bleeding." If an attempt to stop postprocedural bleeding is initially unsuccessful, and to stop the bleeding requires performing any of the definitive root operations Bypass, Detachment, Excision, Extraction, Reposition, Replacement, or Resection, then that root operation is coded instead of Control.
  Example: Resection of spleen to stop postprocedural bleeding is coded to Resection instead of Control.

Body System Specific PCS Reference Manual Exercises

PCS CODE	Y – ANATOMICAL REGIONS, LOWER EXTREMITIES EXERCISES
0Y3F4ZZ	Arthroscopy with drainage of hemarthrosis at previous operative site, right knee.
0Y620ZZ	Right leg and hip amputation through ischium. (The "Hindquarter" body part includes amputation along any part of the hip bone.)
0Y6C0Z3	Right above-knee amputation, distal femur.
0Y6H0Z1	Right below-knee amputation, proximal tibia/fibula. (The qualifier "High" here means the portion of the tibia/fibula closest to the knee.)
0Y6N0Z9	Trans-metatarsal amputation of foot at left big toe. (A "Partial" amputation is through the shaft of the metatarsal bone.)
0Y6W0Z1	Left fourth toe amputation, mid-proximal phalanx. (The qualifier "High" here means anywhere along the proximal phalanx.)
0YU64JZ	Laparoscopic repair of left inguinal hernia with marlex plug.

Y – ANATOMICAL REGIONS, LOWER EXTREMITIES

OTHER OBJECTIVES GROUP: Alteration, (Creation), (Fusion)
Root Operations that define other objectives.

1ST - 0 Medical and Surgical
2ND - Y Anatomical Regions, Lower Extremities
3RD - 0 ALTERATION

EXAMPLE: Cosmetic buttock augmentation   CMS Ex: Face lift

ALTERATION: Modifying the anatomic structure of a body part without affecting the function of the body part.

EXPLANATION: Principal purpose is to improve appearance

Body Part – 4TH		Approach – 5TH	Device – 6TH	Qualifier – 7TH
0 Buttock, Right	F Knee Region, Right	0 Open	7 Autologous tissue substitute	Z No qualifier
1 Buttock, Left	G Knee Region, Left	3 Percutaneous	J Synthetic substitute	
9 Lower Extremity, Right	H Lower Leg, Right	4 Percutaneous endoscopic	K Nonautologous tissue substitute	
B Lower Extremity, Left	J Lower Leg, Left		Z No device	
C Upper Leg, Right	K Ankle Region, Right			
D Upper Leg, Left	L Ankle Region, Left			

DEVICE GROUP: Change, Insertion, Removal, (Replacement), Revision, Supplement
Root Operations that always involve a device.

1ST - 0 Medical and Surgical
2ND - Y Anatomical Regions, Lower Extremities
3RD - 2 CHANGE

EXAMPLE: Exchange drain tube   CMS Ex: Changing urinary catheter

CHANGE: Taking out or off a device from a body part and putting back an identical or similar device in or on the same body part without cutting or puncturing the skin or a mucous membrane.

EXPLANATION: ALL Changes use EXTERNAL approach only ...

Body Part – 4TH	Approach – 5TH	Device – 6TH	Qualifier – 7TH
9 Lower Extremity, Right	X External	0 Drainage device	Z No qualifier
B Lower Extremity, Left		Y Other device	

OTHER REPAIRS GROUP: Control, Repair
Root Operations that define other repairs.

1ST - 0 Medical and Surgical
2ND - Y Anatomical Regions, Lower Extremities
3RD - 3 CONTROL

EXAMPLE: Ligation post-op bleeder   CMS Ex: Control post-op hemorrhage

CONTROL: Stopping, or attempting to stop, postprocedural bleeding.

EXPLANATION: Bleeding site coded to an anatomical region...

Body Part – 4TH		Approach – 5TH	Device – 6TH	Qualifier – 7TH
0 Buttock, Right	F Knee Region, Right	0 Open	Z No device	Z No qualifier
1 Buttock, Left	G Knee Region, Left	3 Percutaneous		
5 Inguinal Region, Right	H Lower Leg, Right	4 Percutaneous endoscopic		
6 Inguinal Region, Left	J Lower Leg, Left			
7 Femoral Region, Right	K Ankle Region, Right			
8 Femoral Region, Left	L Ankle Region, Left			
9 Lower Extremity, Right	M Foot, Right			
B Lower Extremity, Left	N Foot, Left			
C Upper Leg, Right				
D Upper Leg, Left				

0Y6

MEDICAL AND SURGICAL SECTION – 2016 ICD-10-PCS

EXCISION GROUP: Excision, (Resection), (Destruction), (Extraction), **Detachment**
Root Operations that take out some or all of a body part.

1ST - **0** Medical and Surgical	EXAMPLE: Below knee amputation	CMS Ex: Leg amputation
2ND - **Y** Anatomical Regions, Lower Extremities	**DETACHMENT:** Cutting off all or portion of the upper or lower extremities.	
3RD - **6 DETACHMENT**	EXPLANATION: Qualifier specifies amputation level …	

REGIONS LOWER EXT 0Y6

Body Part – 4TH		Approach – 5TH	Device – 6TH	Qualifier – 7TH
2 Hindquarter, Right 3 Hindquarter, Left 4 Hindquarter, Bilateral	7 Femoral Region, Right 8 Femoral Region, Left F Knee Region, Right G Knee Region, Left	0 Open	Z No device	Z No qualifier
C Upper Leg, Right D Upper Leg, Left H Lower Leg, Right J Lower Leg, Left		0 Open	Z No device	1 High 2 Mid 3 Low
M Foot, Right N Foot, Left		0 Open	Z No device	0 Complete 4 Complete 1st Ray 5 Complete 2nd Ray 6 Complete 3rd Ray 7 Complete 4th Ray 8 Complete 5th Ray 9 Partial 1st Ray B Partial 2nd Ray C Partial 3rd Ray D Partial 4th Ray F Partial 5th Ray
P 1st Toe, Right Q 1st Toe, Left R 2nd Toe, Right S 2nd Toe, Left T 3rd Toe, Right	U 3rd Toe, Left V 4th Toe, Right W 4th Toe, Left X 5th Toe, Right Y 5th Toe, Left	0 Open	Z No device	0 Complete 1 High 2 Mid 3 Low

688

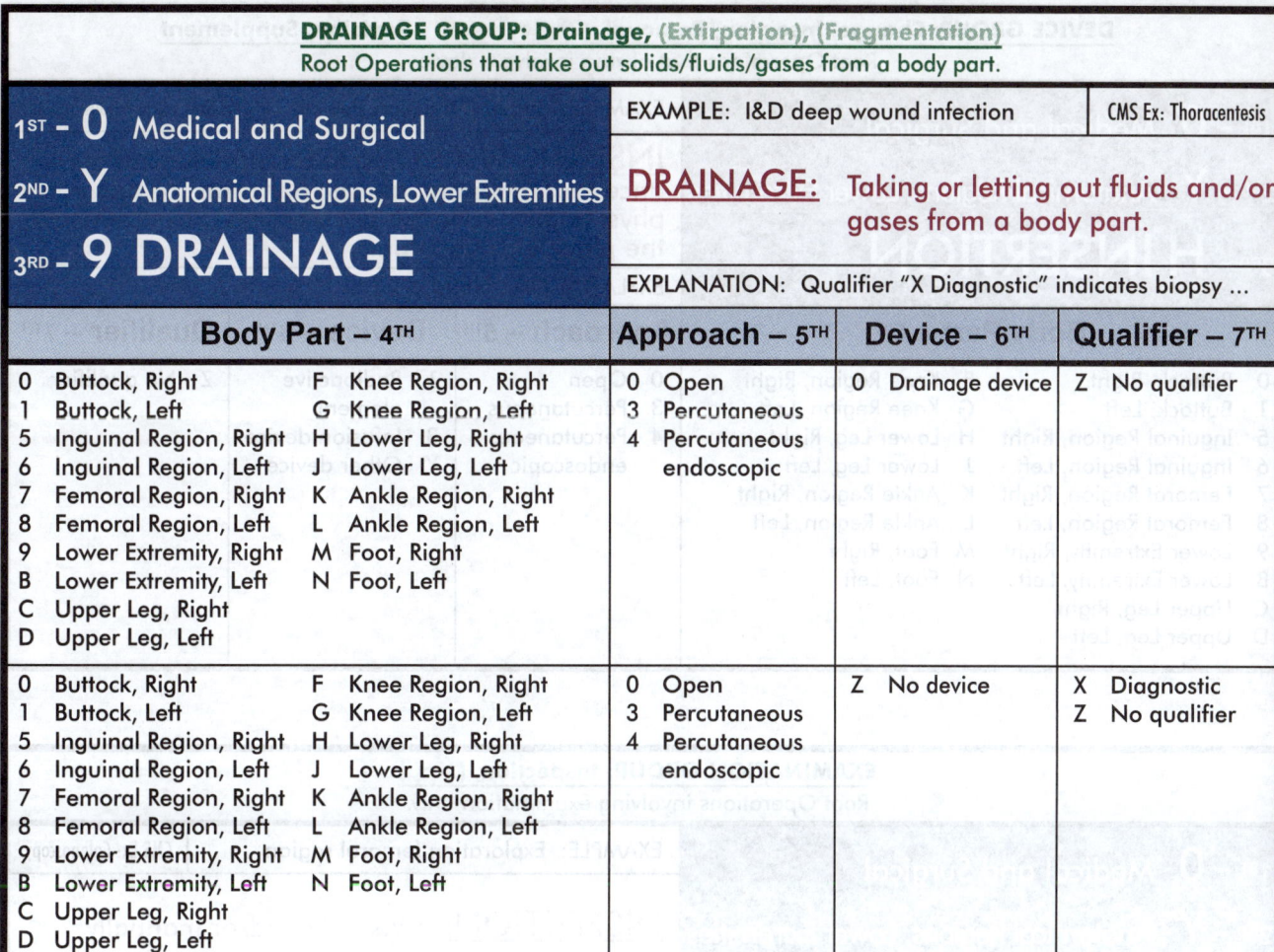

0YH

MEDICAL AND SURGICAL SECTION – 2016 ICD-10-PCS

DEVICE GROUP: Change, Insertion, Removal, (Replacement), Revision, Supplement
Root Operations that always involve a device.

| 1ST - **0** Medical and Surgical |
| 2ND - **Y** Anatomical Regions, Lower Extremities |
| 3RD - **H** INSERTION |

EXAMPLE: Implant infusion device **CMS Ex:** Central venous catheter

INSERTION: Putting in a nonbiological appliance that monitors, assists, performs, or prevents a physiological function but does not physically take the place of a body part.

EXPLANATION: None

Body Part – 4TH		Approach – 5TH	Device – 6TH	Qualifier – 7TH
0 Buttock, Right	F Knee Region, Right	0 Open	1 Radioactive element	Z No qualifier
1 Buttock, Left	G Knee Region, Left	3 Percutaneous	3 Infusion device	
5 Inguinal Region, Right	H Lower Leg, Right	4 Percutaneous endoscopic	Y Other device	
6 Inguinal Region, Left	J Lower Leg, Left			
7 Femoral Region, Right	K Ankle Region, Right			
8 Femoral Region, Left	L Ankle Region, Left			
9 Lower Extremity, Right	M Foot, Right			
B Lower Extremity, Left	N Foot, Left			
C Upper Leg, Right				
D Upper Leg, Left				

EXAMINATION GROUP: Inspection, (Map)
Root Operations involving examination only.

| 1ST - **0** Medical and Surgical |
| 2ND - **Y** Anatomical Regions, Lower Extremities |
| 3RD - **J** INSPECTION |

EXAMPLE: Exploration femoral region **CMS Ex:** Colonoscopy

INSPECTION: Visually and/or manually exploring a body part.

EXPLANATION: Direct or instrumental visualization ...

Body Part – 4TH		Approach – 5TH	Device – 6TH	Qualifier – 7TH
0 Buttock, Right	E Femoral Region, Bilateral	0 Open	Z No device	Z No qualifier
1 Buttock, Left	F Knee Region, Right	3 Percutaneous		
5 Inguinal Region, Right	G Knee Region, Left	4 Percutaneous endoscopic		
6 Inguinal Region, Left	H Lower Leg, Right	X External		
7 Femoral Region, Right	J Lower Leg, Left			
8 Femoral Region, Left	K Ankle Region, Right			
9 Lower Extremity, Right	L Ankle Region, Left			
A Inguinal Region, Bilateral	M Foot, Right			
B Lower Extremity, Left	N Foot, Left			
C Upper Leg, Right				
D Upper Leg, Left				

Y – ANATOMICAL REGIONS, LOWER EXTREMITIES — 0YP

MOVE GROUP: Reattachment, (Reposition), (Transfer), (Transplantation)
Root Operations that put in/put back or move some/all of a body part.

- 1ST – **0** Medical and Surgical
- 2ND – **Y** Anatomical Regions, Lower Extremities
- 3RD – **M REATTACHMENT**

EXAMPLE: Reattachment severed 1st toe   CMS Ex: Reattachment hand

REATTACHMENT: Putting back in or on all or a portion of a separated body part to its normal location or other suitable location.

EXPLANATION: With/without reconnection of vessels/nerves...

Body Part – 4TH		Approach – 5TH	Device – 6TH	Qualifier – 7TH
0 Buttock, Right	H Lower Leg, Right	0 Open	Z No device	Z No qualifier
1 Buttock, Left	J Lower Leg, Left			
2 Hindquarter, Right	K Ankle Region, Right			
3 Hindquarter, Left	L Ankle Region, Left			
4 Hindquarter, Bilateral	M Foot, Right			
5 Inguinal Region, Right	N Foot, Left			
6 Inguinal Region, Left	P 1st Toe, Right			
7 Femoral Region, Right	Q 1st Toe, Left			
8 Femoral Region, Left	R 2nd Toe, Right			
9 Lower Extremity, Right	S 2nd Toe, Left			
B Lower Extremity, Left	T 3rd Toe, Right			
C Upper Leg, Right	U 3rd Toe, Left			
D Upper Leg, Left	V 4th Toe, Right			
F Knee Region, Right	W 4th Toe, Left			
G Knee Region, Left	X 5th Toe, Right			
	Y 5th Toe, Left			

DEVICE GROUP: Change, Insertion, Removal, (Replacement), Revision, Supplement
Root Operations that always involve a device.

- 1ST – **0** Medical and Surgical
- 2ND – **Y** Anatomical Regions, Lower Extremities
- 3RD – **P REMOVAL**

EXAMPLE: Removal drain tube   CMS Ex: Chest tube removal

REMOVAL: Taking out or off a device from a body part.

EXPLANATION: Removal device without reinsertion ...

Body Part – 4TH	Approach – 5TH	Device – 6TH	Qualifier – 7TH
9 Lower Extremity, Right	0 Open	0 Drainage device	Z No qualifier
B Lower Extremity, Left	3 Percutaneous	1 Radioactive element	
	4 Percutaneous endoscopic	3 Infusion device	
	X External	7 Autologous tissue substitute	
		J Synthetic substitute	
		K Nonautologous tissue substitute	
		Y Other device	

0YQ — MEDICAL AND SURGICAL SECTION – 2016 ICD-10-PCS

OTHER REPAIRS GROUP: Control, Repair
Root Operations that define other repairs.

- 1ST – **0** Medical and Surgical
- 2ND – **Y** Anatomical Regions, Lower Extremities
- 3RD – **Q** REPAIR

EXAMPLE: Repair upper leg
CMS Ex: Suture laceration

REPAIR: Restoring, to the extent possible, a body part to its normal anatomic structure and function.

EXPLANATION: Only when no other root operation applies ...

Body Part – 4TH		Approach – 5TH	Device – 6TH	Qualifier – 7TH
0 Buttock, Right	K Ankle Region, Right	0 Open	Z No device	Z No qualifier
1 Buttock, Left	L Ankle Region, Left	3 Percutaneous		
5 Inguinal Region, Right	M Foot, Right	4 Percutaneous endoscopic		
6 Inguinal Region, Left	N Foot, Left	X External		
7 Femoral Region, Right	P 1st Toe, Right			
8 Femoral Region, Left	Q 1st Toe, Left			
9 Lower Extremity, Right	R 2nd Toe, Right			
A Inguinal Region, Bilateral	S 2nd Toe, Left			
B Lower Extremity, Left	T 3rd Toe, Right			
C Upper Leg, Right	U 3rd Toe, Left			
D Upper Leg, Left	V 4th Toe, Right			
E Femoral Region, Bilateral	W 4th Toe, Left			
F Knee Region, Right	X 5th Toe, Right			
G Knee Region, Left	Y 5th Toe, Left			
H Lower Leg, Right				
J Lower Leg, Left				

DEVICE GROUP: Change, Insertion, Removal, (Replacement), Revision, Supplement
Root Operations that always involve a device.

- 1ST – **0** Medical and Surgical
- 2ND – **Y** Anatomical Regions, Lower Extremities
- 3RD – **U** SUPPLEMENT

EXAMPLE: Inguinal hernia repair with mesh
CMS Ex: Hernia with mesh

SUPPLEMENT: Putting in or on biological or synthetic material that physically reinforces and/or augments the function of a portion of a body part.

EXPLANATION: Biological material from same individual ...

Body Part – 4TH		Approach – 5TH	Device – 6TH	Qualifier – 7TH
0 Buttock, Right	K Ankle Region, Right	0 Open	7 Autologous tissue substitute	Z No qualifier
1 Buttock, Left	L Ankle Region, Left	4 Percutaneous endoscopic	J Synthetic substitute	
5 Inguinal Region, Right	M Foot, Right		K Nonautologous tissue substitute	
6 Inguinal Region, Left	N Foot, Left			
7 Femoral Region, Right	P 1st Toe, Right			
8 Femoral Region, Left	Q 1st Toe, Left			
9 Lower Extremity, Right	R 2nd Toe, Right			
A Inguinal Region, Bilateral	S 2nd Toe, Left			
B Lower Extremity, Left	T 3rd Toe, Right			
C Upper Leg, Right	U 3rd Toe, Left			
D Upper Leg, Left	V 4th Toe, Right			
E Femoral Region, Bilateral	W 4th Toe, Left			
F Knee Region, Right	X 5th Toe, Right			
G Knee Region, Left	Y 5th Toe, Left			
H Lower Leg, Right				
J Lower Leg, Left				

Y – ANATOMICAL REGIONS, LOWER EXTREMITIES — 0YW

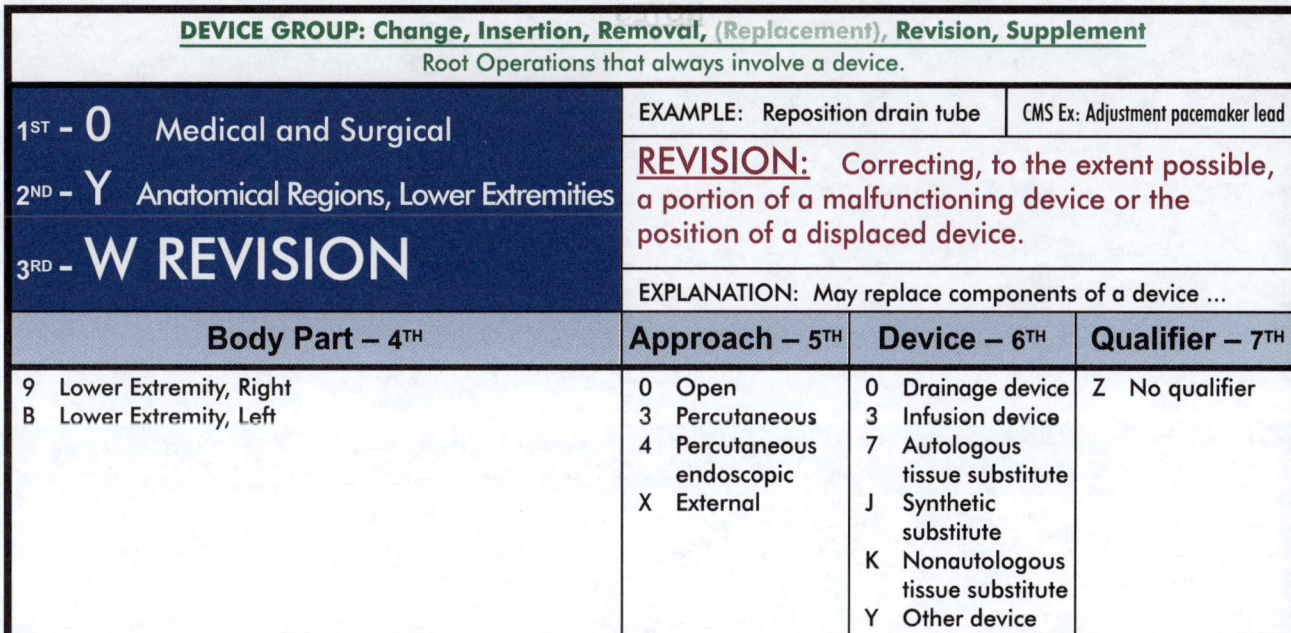

DEVICE GROUP: Change, Insertion, Removal, (Replacement), Revision, Supplement
Root Operations that always involve a device.

- 1ST – **0** Medical and Surgical
- 2ND – **Y** Anatomical Regions, Lower Extremities
- 3RD – **W REVISION**

EXAMPLE: Reposition drain tube
CMS Ex: Adjustment pacemaker lead

REVISION: Correcting, to the extent possible, a portion of a malfunctioning device or the position of a displaced device.

EXPLANATION: May replace components of a device ...

Body Part – 4TH	Approach – 5TH	Device – 6TH	Qualifier – 7TH
9 Lower Extremity, Right	0 Open	0 Drainage device	Z No qualifier
B Lower Extremity, Left	3 Percutaneous	3 Infusion device	
	4 Percutaneous endoscopic	7 Autologous tissue substitute	
	X External	J Synthetic substitute	
		K Nonautologous tissue substitute	
		Y Other device	

MEDICAL AND SURGICAL SECTION – 2016 ICD-10-PCS

NOTES

Educational Annotations | Section 1 – Obstetrics

Section Specific Educational Annotations for the Obstetrics Section include:
- Anatomy and Physiology Review
- Anatomical Illustrations
- Definitions of Common Procedures
- AHA Coding Clinic® Reference Notations
- Body Part Key Listings
- Device Key Listings
- Device Aggregation Table Listings
- Coding Notes

Anatomy and Physiology Review of Obstetrics

BODY PART VALUES – 0 - Obstetrics

Products of Conception – The fetus, placenta, and other tissue derived from a fertilized gestation.

Products of Conception, Ectopic – Products of conception that develop outside the uterus.

Products of Conception, Retained – Products of conception that remain in the uterus following delivery, termination of pregnancy, or miscarriage.

Anatomical Illustrations of Obstetrics

None for the Obstetrics Section

Definitions of Common Procedures of Obstetrics

Amniocentesis – The medical procedure of inserting a needle with ultrasound guidance through the abdominal wall and uterine wall, and then puncturing the amniotic sac to withdraw a small amount of amniotic fluid that is used for testing for fetal abnormalities, usually done early in the second trimester.

Amnioscopy – The instrumental visualization of the fetus and lower amniotic sac by using an amnioscope that is inserted into the vaginal canal and used in late pregnancy or during labor.

Cesarean section (C-section) – The surgical delivery of the fetus through an incision in the uterine wall. The classical c-section incision is a vertical incision in the abdomen and in the mid to upper portion of the uterus. The low cervical c-section incision is a transverse (horizontal) or vertical incision in the abdomen just above the pubis and in the lower portion of the uterus just above the cervix.

Forceps-assisted vaginal delivery – The use of special tools that are curved and shallow cup-shaped to assist delivering a fetus that is having difficulty passing through the birth canal. The descriptions of low, mid, or high forceps are based on the stage of fetal head engagement and station of progress entering and passing through the birth canal.

Removal of tubal pregnancy – The open or laparoscopic-approach surgical removal of an ectopic pregnancy (embryo attaches outside the uterus) that is attached in a fallopian tube. The fallopian tube may be incised (salpingostomy) or a segment may need to be excised (salpingectomy).

Vacuum-assisted vaginal delivery – The use of a special vacuum extractor with a soft plastic cup that attaches to the fetal head with suction to help deliver the fetus through the birth canal.

Educational Annotations | Section 1 – Obstetrics

AHA Coding Clinic® Reference Notations of Obstetrics

ROOT OPERATION SPECIFIC - OBSTETRICS - Section 1

MISC
- Induction of labor, IV oxytocin, peripheral vein .... AHA 14:4Q:p17
- Induction of labor with Cervidil dinoprostone vaginal tampon .... AHA 14:2Q:p8
- Pitocin to augment active labor .... AHA 14:2Q:p9

CHANGE - 2

DRAINAGE - 9
- Artificial rupture of membranes .... AHA 14:2Q:p9
- Laser microseptostomy for twin-twin transfusion syndrome .... AHA 14:3Q:p12

ABORTION - A

EXTRACTION - D
- Cesarean section with vacuum assistance .... AHA 14:4Q:p43
- Vacuum D&C for blighted ovum .... AHA 14:4Q:p43

DELIVERY - E
- Assisted vaginal delivery .... AHA 14:2Q:p9

INSERTION - H
- Intrauterine pressure monitoring during labor .... AHA 13:2Q:p36

INSPECTION - J

REMOVAL - P

REPAIR - Q
- Fetoscopic laser photocoagulation of vascular connections .... AHA 14:3Q:p12

REPOSITION - S

RESECTION - T

TRANSPLANTATION - Y

Body Part Key Listings of Obstetrics

None for the Obstetrics Section

Device Key Listings of Obstetrics

None for the Obstetrics Section

Device Aggregation Table Listings of Obstetrics

None for the Obstetrics Section

Educational Annotations | Section 1 – Obstetrics

Coding Notes of Obstetrics

Body System Relevant Coding Guidelines

C. Obstetrics Section

Products of conception
 C1
  Procedures performed on the products of conception are coded to the Obstetrics section. Procedures performed on the pregnant female other than the products of conception are coded to the appropriate root operation in the Medical and Surgical section.
  Example: Amniocentesis is coded to the products of conception body part in the Obstetrics section. Repair of obstetric urethral laceration is coded to the urethra body part in the Medical and Surgical section.

Procedures following delivery or abortion
 C2
  Procedures performed following a delivery or abortion for curettage of the endometrium or evacuation of retained products of conception are all coded in the Obstetrics section, to the root operation Extraction and the body part Products of Conception, Retained. Diagnostic or therapeutic dilation and curettage performed during times other than the postpartum or post-abortion period are all coded in the Medical and Surgical section, to the root operation Extraction and the body part Endometrium.

Med/Surg Related Section Specific PCS Reference Manual Exercises

PCS CODE	1 – OBSTETRICS EXERCISES
10903ZA	Fetal spinal tap, percutaneous.
10A07ZW	Abortion by dilation and evacuation following laminaria insertion.
10A07ZX	Abortion by abortifacient insertion.
10D00Z2	Extraperitoneal c-section, low transverse incision.
10E0XZZ	Manually assisted spontaneous abortion. (Since the pregnancy was not artificially terminated, this is coded to Delivery, because it captures the procedure objective. The fact that it was an abortion will be identified in the diagnosis code.)
10J07ZZ	Bimanual pregnancy examination.
10P073Z	Transvaginal removal of fetal monitoring electrode.
10Q00ZK	Open in utero repair of congenital diaphragmatic hernia. (Diaphragm is classified to the Respiratory body system in the Medical and Surgical section.)
10T24ZZ	Laparoscopy with total excision of tubal pregnancy.
10Y04ZS	Fetal kidney transplant, laparoscopic.

Educational Annotations

Section 1 – Obstetrics

NOTES

1 – OBSTETRICS

OBSTETRICS SECTION:
Change, Drainage, Abortion, Extraction, Delivery, Insertion, Inspection, Removal, Repair, Reposition, Resection, Transplantation
Root Operations that are performed on the products of conception.

1ST – **1** Obstetrics
2ND – **0** Pregnancy ♀
3RD – **2 CHANGE**

EXAMPLE: Exchanging intrauterine pressure monitor

CHANGE: Taking out or off a device from a body part and putting back an identical or similar device in or on the same body part without cutting or puncturing the skin or a mucous membrane.

EXPLANATION: None

Body Part – 4TH	Approach – 5TH	Device – 6TH	Qualifier – 7TH
0 Products of Conception	7 Via natural or artificial opening	3 Monitoring electrode Y Other device	Z No qualifier

---

OBSTETRICS SECTION:
Change, Drainage, Abortion, Extraction, Delivery, Insertion, Inspection, Removal, Repair, Reposition, Resection, Transplantation
Root Operations that are performed on the products of conception.

1ST – **1** Obstetrics
2ND – **0** Pregnancy ♀
3RD – **9 DRAINAGE**

EXAMPLE: Amniocentesis, artificial rupture of membranes

DRAINAGE: Taking or letting out fluids and/or gases from a body part.

EXPLANATION: Qualifier identifies type of fluid

Body Part – 4TH	Approach – 5TH	Device – 6TH	Qualifier – 7TH
0 Products of Conception	0 Open 3 Percutaneous 4 Percutaneous endoscopic 7 Via natural or artificial opening 8 Via natural or artificial opening endoscopic	Z No device	9 Fetal blood A Fetal cerebrospinal fluid B Fetal fluid, other C Amniotic fluid, therapeutic D Fluid, other U Amniotic fluid, diagnostic

OBSTETRICS SECTION:
Change, Drainage, Abortion, Extraction, Delivery, Insertion, Inspection, Removal, Repair, Reposition, Resection, Transplantation
Root Operations that are performed on the products of conception.

- 1ˢᵗ – **1** Obstetrics
- 2ⁿᵈ – **0** Pregnancy ♀
- 3ʳᵈ – **A** ABORTION

EXAMPLE: Therapeutic abortion

ABORTION: Artificially terminating a pregnancy.

EXPLANATION: None

Body Part – 4ᵀᴴ	Approach – 5ᵀᴴ	Device – 6ᵀᴴ	Qualifier – 7ᵀᴴ
0 Products of Conception	0 Open 3 Percutaneous 4 Percutaneous endoscopic 8 Via natural or artificial opening endoscopic	Z No device	Z No qualifier
0 Products of Conception	7 Via natural or artificial opening	Z No device	6 Vacuum W Laminaria X Abortifacient Z No qualifier

OBSTETRICS SECTION:
Change, Drainage, Abortion, Extraction, Delivery, Insertion, Inspection, Removal, Repair, Reposition, Resection, Transplantation
Root Operations that are performed on the products of conception.

- 1ˢᵗ – **1** Obstetrics
- 2ⁿᵈ – **0** Pregnancy ♀
- 3ʳᵈ – **D** EXTRACTION

EXAMPLE: Cesarean or forceps-assisted delivery

EXTRACTION: Pulling or stripping out or off all or a portion of a body part by the use of force.

EXPLANATION: Qualifier - type of instrumentation/assistance

Body Part – 4ᵀᴴ	Approach – 5ᵀᴴ	Device – 6ᵀᴴ	Qualifier – 7ᵀᴴ
0 Products of Conception	0 Open	Z No device	0 Classical 1 Low cervical 2 Extraperitoneal
0 Products of Conception	7 Via natural or artificial opening	Z No device	3 Low forceps 4 Mid forceps 5 High forceps 6 Vacuum 7 Internal version 8 Other
1 Products of Conception, Retained 2 Products of Conception, Ectopic	7 Via natural or artificial opening 8 Via natural or artificial opening endoscopic	Z No device	Z No qualifier

1 – OBSTETRICS   10H

OBSTETRICS SECTION:
Change, Drainage, Abortion, Extraction, Delivery, Insertion, Inspection, Removal, Repair, Reposition, Resection, Transplantation
Root Operations that are performed on the products of conception.

- 1ST – **1** Obstetrics
- 2ND – **0** Pregnancy ♀
- 3RD – **E DELIVERY**

EXAMPLE: Spontaneous vaginal delivery

DELIVERY: Assisting the passage of the products of conception from the genital canal.

EXPLANATION: Manually assisted delivery without instruments

Body Part – 4TH	Approach – 5TH	Device – 6TH	Qualifier – 7TH
0 Products of Conception	X External	Z No device	Z No qualifier

---

OBSTETRICS SECTION:
Change, Drainage, Abortion, Extraction, Delivery, Insertion, Inspection, Removal, Repair, Reposition, Resection, Transplantation
Root Operations that are performed on the products of conception.

- 1ST – **1** Obstetrics
- 2ND – **0** Pregnancy ♀
- 3RD – **H INSERTION**

EXAMPLE: Insertion intrauterine pressure monitor

INSERTION: Putting in a nonbiological appliance that monitors, assists, performs, or prevents a physiological function but does not physically take the place of a body part.

EXPLANATION: None

Body Part – 4TH	Approach – 5TH	Device – 6TH	Qualifier – 7TH
0 Products of Conception	0 Open 7 Via natural or artificial opening	3 Monitoring electrode Y Other device	Z No qualifier

10J

MEDICAL/SURGICAL RELATED SECTIONS – 2016 ICD-10-PCS [2016.PCS]

OBSTETRICS SECTION:
Change, Drainage, Abortion, Extraction, Delivery, Insertion, Inspection, Removal, Repair, Reposition, Resection, Transplantation
Root Operations that are performed on the products of conception.

- 1ST – **1** Obstetrics
- 2ND – **0** Pregnancy ♀
- 3RD – **J** INSPECTION

EXAMPLE: Amnioscopy, bimanual pregnancy examination

INSPECTION: Visually and/or manually exploring a body part.

EXPLANATION: Direct or instrumental visualization …

Body Part – 4TH	Approach – 5TH	Device – 6TH	Qualifier – 7TH
0 Products of Conception 1 Products of Conception, Retained 2 Products of Conception, Ectopic	0 Open 3 Percutaneous 4 Percutaneous endoscopic 7 Via natural or artificial opening 8 Via natural or artificial opening endoscopic X External	Z No device	Z No qualifier

OBSTETRICS SECTION:
Change, Drainage, Abortion, Extraction, Delivery, Insertion, Inspection, Removal, Repair, Reposition, Resection, Transplantation
Root Operations that are performed on the products of conception.

- 1ST – **1** Obstetrics
- 2ND – **0** Pregnancy ♀
- 3RD – **P** REMOVAL

EXAMPLE: Removal fetal monitoring electrode

REMOVAL: Taking out or off a device from a body part, region or orifice.

EXPLANATION: Removal device without reinsertion …

Body Part – 4TH	Approach – 5TH	Device – 6TH	Qualifier – 7TH
0 Products of Conception	0 Open 7 Via natural or artificial opening	3 Monitoring electrode Y Other device	Z No qualifier

OBSTETRICS 10J

1 – OBSTETRICS — 10S

OBSTETRICS SECTION:
Change, Drainage, Abortion, Extraction, Delivery, Insertion, Inspection, Removal, Repair, Reposition, Resection, Transplanation
Root Operations that are performed on the products of conception.

- 1ST – **1** Obstetrics
- 2ND – **0** Pregnancy ♀
- 3RD – **Q REPAIR**

EXAMPLE: In utero repair congenital diaphragmatic hernia

REPAIR: Restoring, to the extent possible, a body part to its normal anatomic structure and function.

EXPLANATION: Only when no other root operation applies …

Body Part – 4TH	Approach – 5TH	Device – 6TH	Qualifier – 7TH
0 Products of Conception	0 Open 3 Percutaneous 4 Percutaneous endoscopic 7 Via natural or artificial opening 8 Via natural or artificial opening endoscopic	Y Other device Z No device	E Nervous system F Cardiovascular system G Lymphatics and hemic H Eye J Ear, nose and sinus K Respiratory system L Mouth and throat M Gastrointestinal system N Hepatobiliary and pancreas P Endocrine system Q Skin R Musculoskeletal system S Urinary system T Female reproductive system V Male reproductive system Y Other body system

---

OBSTETRICS SECTION:
Change, Drainage, Abortion, Extraction, Delivery, Insertion, Inspection, Removal, Repair, Reposition, Resection, Transplanation
Root Operations that are performed on the products of conception.

- 1ST – **1** Obstetrics
- 2ND – **0** Pregnancy ♀
- 3RD – **S REPOSITION**

EXAMPLE: Manual external version of fetus

REPOSITION: Moving to its normal location, or other suitable location, all or a portion of a body part.

EXPLANATION: May or may not be cut to be moved …

Body Part – 4TH	Approach – 5TH	Device – 6TH	Qualifier – 7TH
0 Products of Conception	7 Via natural or artificial opening X External	Z No device	Z No qualifier
2 Products of Conception, Ectopic	0 Open 3 Percutaneous 4 Percutaneous endoscopic 7 Via natural or artificial opening 8 Via natural or artificial opening endoscopic	Z No device	Z No qualifier

10T

OBSTETRICS SECTION:
Change, Drainage, Abortion, Extraction, Delivery, Insertion, Inspection, Removal, Repair, Reposition, Resection, Transplantation
Root Operations that are performed on the products of conception.

- 1ST – **1** Obstetrics
- 2ND – **0** Pregnancy ♀
- 3RD – **T** RESECTION

EXAMPLE: Surgical removal ectopic pregnancy

RESECTION: Cutting out or off, without replacement, all of a body part.

EXPLANATION: None

Body Part – 4TH	Approach – 5TH	Device – 6TH	Qualifier – 7TH
2 Products of Conception, Ectopic	0 Open 3 Percutaneous 4 Percutaneous endoscopic 7 Via natural or artificial opening 8 Via natural or artificial opening endoscopic	Z No device	Z No qualifier

---

OBSTETRICS SECTION:
Change, Drainage, Abortion, Extraction, Delivery, Insertion, Inspection, Removal, Repair, Reposition, Resection, Transplantation
Root Operations that are performed on the products of conception.

- 1ST – **1** Obstetrics
- 2ND – **0** Pregnancy ♀
- 3RD – **Y** TRANSPLANTATION

EXAMPLE: Fetal kidney transplant

TRANSPLANTATION: Putting in or on all or a portion of a living body part taken from another individual or animal to physically take the place and/or function of all or a portion of a similar body part.

EXPLANATION: May take over all or part of its function ...

Body Part – 4TH	Approach – 5TH	Device – 6TH	Qualifier – 7TH	
0 Products of Conception	3 Percutaneous 4 Percutaneous endoscopic 7 Via natural or artificial opening	Z No device	E Nervous system F Cardiovascular system G Lymphatics and hemic H Eye J Ear, nose and sinus K Respiratory system L Mouth and throat M Gastrointestinal system	N Hepatobiliary and pancreas P Endocrine system Q Skin R Musculoskeletal system S Urinary system T Female reproductive system V Male reproductive system Y Other body system

Educational Annotations | Section 2 – Placement

Section Specific Educational Annotations for the Placement Section include:
- Anatomy and Physiology Review
- Anatomical Illustrations
- AHA Coding Clinic® Reference Notations
- Body Part Key Listings
- Device Key Listings
- Device Aggregation Table Listings
- Coding Notes

Anatomy and Physiology Review of Placement

BODY REGION VALUES – 2 - Placement

Abdominal Wall – The multi-tissue-layered covering of the abdominal and pelvic portions of the trunk.

Anorectal – The multi-tissue-layered area containing the anus and rectum.

Back – The multi-tissue-layered covering of the back portion of the trunk.

Chest Wall – The multi-tissue-layered covering of the thoracic portion of the trunk.

Ear – The organ of hearing comprised of the external ear (auricle or pinna), middle ear (malleus, incus, and stapes bones), and inner ear (cochlea).

Face – The multi-tissue-layered covering of the anterior portion of the head.

Female Genital Tract – The organs and structures of the reproductive systems.

Finger – A digit of the hand.

Foot – The portion of the lower extermity distal to the lower end of the tibia and fibula.

Hand – The portion of the upper extermity distal to the forearm.

Head – The portion of the human body above the neck.

Inguinal Region – The multi-tissue-layered area between the lower abdomen, thigh, and pubic bone.

Lower Arm – The portion of the upper extermity distal to the elbow.

Lower Extremity – The entire lower extremity (leg).

Lower Leg – The portion of the lower extermity distal to the knee.

Mouth and Pharynx – The portion of the head formed by the oral cavity and pharynx.

Nasal – The multi-tissue-layered area of the nose in the anterior portion of the head.

Neck – The portion of the human body above the trunk and below the head.

Thumb – The first digit of the hand.

Toe – A digit of the foot.

Upper Arm – The portion of the upper extermity distal to the shoulder and proximal to the elbow.

Upper Extremity – The entire upper extremity (arm).

Upper Leg – The portion of the lower extermity distal to the hip and proximal to the knee.

Urethra – The urethra is the musculomembranous tube which extends and carries urine from the bladder to the external urethral opening (meatus).

Anatomical Illustrations of Placement

None for the Placement Section

Educational Annotations | Section 2 – Placement

AHA Coding Clinic® Reference Notations of Placement

ROOT OPERATION SPECIFIC - PLACEMENT - Section 2
CHANGE - 0
COMPRESSION - 1
DRESSING - 2
IMMOBILIZATION - 3
PACKING - 4
REMOVAL - 5
TRACTION - 6
  Tongs used to stabilize cervical fracture .... AHA 13:2Q:p39

Body Part Key Listings of Placement

See also Body Part Key in Appendix C
Hallux .... *use* 1st Toe, Left/Right
Inguinal canal .... *use* Inguinal Region, Bilateral/Left/Right
Inguinal triangle .... *use* Inguinal Region, Bilateral/Left/Right

Device Key Listings of Placement

None for the Placement Section

Device Aggregation Table Listings of Placement

None for the Placement Section

Coding Notes of Placement

Med/Surg Related Section Specific PCS Reference Manual Exercises

PCS CODE	2 – PLACEMENT EXERCISES
2W0PX6Z	Exchange of pressure dressing to left thigh.
2W18X7Z	Placement of intermittent pneumatic compression device, covering entire right arm.
2W27X4Z	Sterile dressing placement to left groin region.
2W32X3Z	Placement of neck brace.
2W44X5Z	Packing of wound, chest wall.
2W5AX1Z	Removal of splint, right shoulder.
2W6MX0Z	Mechanical traction of entire left leg.
2Y04X5Z	Change of vaginal packing.
2Y42X5Z	Placement of packing material, right ear.
2Y50X5Z	Removal of packing material from pharynx.

2 – PLACEMENT 2W0

PLACEMENT SECTION: Change, Compression, Dressing, Immobilization, Packing, Removal, Traction
Root Operations include only those that are performed without an incision or a puncture.

1ST - **2** Placement
2ND - **W** Anatomical Regions
3RD - **0** CHANGE

EXAMPLE: Changing a cast

CHANGE: Taking out or off a device from a body part and putting back an identical or similar device in or on the same body part without cutting or puncturing the skin or a mucous membrane.

EXPLANATION: Performed without an incision or a puncture ...

Body Region – 4TH		Approach – 5TH	Device – 6TH	Qualifier – 7TH
0 Head	G Thumb, Right	X External	0 Traction apparatus	Z No qualifier
2 Neck	H Thumb, Left		1 Splint	
3 Abdominal Wall	J Finger, Right		2 Cast	
4 Chest Wall	K Finger, Left		3 Brace	
5 Back	L Lower Extremity, Right		4 Bandage	
6 Inguinal Region, Right	M Lower Extremity, Left		5 Packing material	
7 Inguinal Region, Left	N Upper Leg, Right		6 Pressure dressing	
8 Upper Extremity, Right	P Upper Leg, Left		7 Intermittent pressure device	
9 Upper Extremity, Left	Q Lower Leg, Right		Y Other device	
A Upper Arm, Right	R Lower Leg, Left			
B Upper Arm, Left	S Foot, Right			
C Lower Arm, Right	T Foot, Left			
D Lower Arm, Left	U Toe, Right			
E Hand, Right	V Toe, Left			
F Hand, Left				
1 Face		X External	0 Traction apparatus	Z No qualifier
			1 Splint	
			2 Cast	
			3 Brace	
			4 Bandage	
			5 Packing material	
			6 Pressure dressing	
			7 Intermittent pressure device	
			9 Wire	
			Y Other device	

2W1

PLACEMENT SECTION: Change, Compression, Dressing, Immobilization, Packing, Removal, Traction
Root Operations include only those that are performed without an incision or a puncture.

- 1ST – **2** Placement
- 2ND – **W** Anatomical Regions
- 3RD – **1** COMPRESSION

EXAMPLE: Application of pressure dressing

COMPRESSION: Putting pressure on a body region.

EXPLANATION: Performed without an incision or puncture ...

Body Region – 4TH		Approach – 5TH	Device – 6TH	Qualifier – 7TH
0 Head	G Thumb, Right	X External	6 Pressure dressing	Z No qualifier
1 Face	H Thumb, Left		7 Intermittent pressure device	
2 Neck	J Finger, Right			
3 Abdominal Wall	K Finger, Left			
4 Chest Wall	L Lower Extremity, Right			
5 Back	M Lower Extremity, Left			
6 Inguinal Region, Right	N Upper Leg, Right			
7 Inguinal Region, Left	P Upper Leg, Left			
8 Upper Extremity, Right	Q Lower Leg, Right			
9 Upper Extremity, Left	R Lower Leg, Left			
A Upper Arm, Right	S Foot, Right			
B Upper Arm, Left	T Foot, Left			
C Lower Arm, Right	U Toe, Right			
D Lower Arm, Left	V Toe, Left			
E Hand, Right				
F Hand, Left				

PLACEMENT SECTION: Change, Compression, Dressing, Immobilization, Packing, Removal, Traction
Root Operations include only those that are performed without an incision or a puncture.

- 1ST – **2** Placement
- 2ND – **W** Anatomical Regions
- 3RD – **2** DRESSING

EXAMPLE: Bandage-type dressing

DRESSING: Putting material on a body region for protection.

EXPLANATION: Performed without an incision or puncture ...

Body Region – 4TH		Approach – 5TH	Device – 6TH	Qualifier – 7TH
0 Head	G Thumb, Right	X External	4 Bandage	Z No qualifier
1 Face	H Thumb, Left			
2 Neck	J Finger, Right			
3 Abdominal Wall	K Finger, Left			
4 Chest Wall	L Lower Extremity, Right			
5 Back	M Lower Extremity, Left			
6 Inguinal Region, Right	N Upper Leg, Right			
7 Inguinal Region, Left	P Upper Leg, Left			
8 Upper Extremity, Right	Q Lower Leg, Right			
9 Upper Extremity, Left	R Lower Leg, Left			
A Upper Arm, Right	S Foot, Right			
B Upper Arm, Left	T Foot, Left			
C Lower Arm, Right	U Toe, Right			
D Lower Arm, Left	V Toe, Left			
E Hand, Right				
F Hand, Left				

2W4

[2016 PCS] — 2 – PLACEMENT

PLACEMENT SECTION: Change, Compression, Dressing, Immobilization, Packing, Removal, Traction
Root Operations include only those that are performed without an incision or a puncture.

| 1ST - **2** Placement |
| 2ND - **W** Anatomical Regions |
| 3RD - **3 IMMOBILIZATION** |

EXAMPLE: Application of brace or splint

IMMOBILIZATION: Limiting or preventing motion of a body region.

EXPLANATION: Performed without an incision or puncture …

Body Region – 4TH		Approach – 5TH	Device – 6TH	Qualifier – 7TH
0 Head 2 Neck 3 Abdominal Wall 4 Chest Wall 5 Back 6 Inguinal Region, Right 7 Inguinal Region, Left 8 Upper Extremity, Right 9 Upper Extremity, Left A Upper Arm, Right B Upper Arm, Left C Lower Arm, Right D Lower Arm, Left E Hand, Right F Hand, Left	G Thumb, Right H Thumb, Left J Finger, Right K Finger, Left L Lower Extremity, Right M Lower Extremity, Left N Upper Leg, Right P Upper Leg, Left Q Lower Leg, Right R Lower Leg, Left S Foot, Right T Foot, Left U Toe, Right V Toe, Left	X External	1 Splint 2 Cast 3 Brace Y Other device	Z No qualifier
1 Face		X External	1 Splint 2 Cast 3 Brace 9 Wire Y Other device	Z No qualifier

---

PLACEMENT SECTION: Change, Compression, Dressing, Immobilization, Packing, Removal, Traction
Root Operations include only those that are performed without an incision or a puncture.

| 1ST - **2** Placement |
| 2ND - **W** Anatomical Regions |
| 3RD - **4 PACKING** |

EXAMPLE: Open wound packing

PACKING: Putting material in a body region or orifice.

EXPLANATION: Performed without an incision or puncture …

Body Region – 4TH		Approach – 5TH	Device – 6TH	Qualifier – 7TH
0 Head 1 Face 2 Neck 3 Abdominal Wall 4 Chest Wall 5 Back 6 Inguinal Region, Right 7 Inguinal Region, Left 8 Upper Extremity, Right 9 Upper Extremity, Left A Upper Arm, Right B Upper Arm, Left C Lower Arm, Right D Lower Arm, Left E Hand, Right F Hand, Left	G Thumb, Right H Thumb, Left J Finger, Right K Finger, Left L Lower Extremity, Right M Lower Extremity, Left N Upper Leg, Right P Upper Leg, Left Q Lower Leg, Right R Lower Leg, Left S Foot, Right T Foot, Left U Toe, Right V Toe, Left	X External	5 Packing material	Z No qualifier

2W5 MEDICAL/SURGICAL RELATED SECTIONS – 2016 ICD-10-PCS [2016.PCS]

PLACEMENT SECTION: Change, Compression, Dressing, Immobilization, Packing, Removal, Traction
Root Operations include only those that are performed without an incision or a puncture.

1ST - **2** Placement
2ND - **W** Anatomical Regions
3RD - **5 REMOVAL**

EXAMPLE: Cast removal

REMOVAL: Taking out or off a device from a body part.

EXPLANATION: Performed without an incision or puncture …

Body Region – 4TH		Approach – 5TH	Device – 6TH	Qualifier – 7TH
0 Head 2 Neck 3 Abdominal Wall 4 Chest Wall 5 Back 6 Inguinal Region, Right 7 Inguinal Region, Left 8 Upper Extremity, Right 9 Upper Extremity, Left A Upper Arm, Right B Upper Arm, Left C Lower Arm, Right D Lower Arm, Left E Hand, Right F Hand, Left	G Thumb, Right H Thumb, Left J Finger, Right K Finger, Left L Lower Extremity, Right M Lower Extremity, Left N Upper Leg, Right P Upper Leg, Left Q Lower Leg, Right R Lower Leg, Left S Foot, Right T Foot, Left U Toe, Right V Toe, Left	X External	0 Traction apparatus 1 Splint 2 Cast 3 Brace 4 Bandage 5 Packing material 6 Pressure dressing 7 Intermittent pressure device Y Other device	Z No qualifier
1 Face		X External	0 Traction apparatus 1 Splint 2 Cast 3 Brace 4 Bandage 5 Packing material 6 Pressure dressing 7 Intermittent pressure device 9 Wire Y Other device	Z No qualifier

2 – PLACEMENT

2W6

PLACEMENT SECTION: Change, Compression, Dressing, Immobilization, Packing, Removal, Traction
Root Operations include only those that are performed without an incision or a puncture.

1ST – **2** Placement
2ND – **W** Anatomical Regions
3RD – **6** TRACTION

EXAMPLE: Lumbar traction using traction table

TRACTION: Exerting a pulling force on a body region in a distal direction.

EXPLANATION: Performed without an incision or puncture ...

Body Region – 4TH		Approach – 5TH	Device – 6TH	Qualifier – 7TH
0 Head	G Thumb, Right	X External	0 Traction apparatus	Z No qualifier
1 Face	H Thumb, Left		Z No device	
2 Neck	J Finger, Right			
3 Abdominal Wall	K Finger, Left			
4 Chest Wall	L Lower Extremity, Right			
5 Back	M Lower Extremity, Left			
6 Inguinal Region, Right	N Upper Leg, Right			
7 Inguinal Region, Left	P Upper Leg, Left			
8 Upper Extremity, Right	Q Lower Leg, Right			
9 Upper Extremity, Left	R Lower Leg, Left			
A Upper Arm, Right	S Foot, Right			
B Upper Arm, Left	T Foot, Left			
C Lower Arm, Right	U Toe, Right			
D Lower Arm, Left	V Toe, Left			
E Hand, Right				
F Hand, Left				

PLACEMENT SECTION: Change, Compression, Dressing, Immobilization, Packing, Removal, Traction
Root Operations include only those that are performed without an incision or a puncture.

1ST - 2 Placement
2ND - Y Anatomical Orifices
3RD - 0 CHANGE

EXAMPLE: Replacing nasal packing

CHANGE: Taking out or off a device from a body part and putting back an identical or similar device in or on the same body part without cutting or puncturing the skin or a mucous membrane.

EXPLANATION: Performed without an incision or puncture ...

Body Region – 4TH	Approach – 5TH	Device – 6TH	Qualifier – 7TH
0 Mouth and Pharynx 1 Nasal 2 Ear 3 Anorectal 4 Female Genital Tract ♀ 5 Urethra	X External	5 Packing material	Z No qualifier

PLACEMENT SECTION: Change, Compression, Dressing, Immobilization, Packing, Removal, Traction
Root Operations include only those that are performed without an incision or a puncture.

1ST - 2 Placement
2ND - Y Anatomical Orifices
3RD - 4 PACKING

EXAMPLE: Insertion of nasal packing

PACKING: Putting material in a body region or orifice.

EXPLANATION: Performed without an incision or puncture ...

Body Region – 4TH	Approach – 5TH	Device – 6TH	Qualifier – 7TH
0 Mouth and Pharynx 1 Nasal 2 Ear 3 Anorectal 4 Female Genital Tract ♀ 5 Urethra	X External	5 Packing material	Z No qualifier

PLACEMENT SECTION: Change, Compression, Dressing, Immobilization, Packing, Removal, Traction
Root Operations include only those that are performed without an incision or a puncture.

1ST - 2 Placement
2ND - Y Anatomical Orifices
3RD - 5 REMOVAL

EXAMPLE: Removal of nasal packing

REMOVAL: Taking out or off a device from a body part.

EXPLANATION: Performed without an incision or puncture ...

Body Region – 4TH	Approach – 5TH	Device – 6TH	Qualifier – 7TH
0 Mouth and Pharynx 1 Nasal 2 Ear 3 Anorectal 4 Female Genital Tract ♀ 5 Urethra	X External	5 Packing material	Z No qualifier

Educational Annotations | Section 3 – Administration

Section Specific Educational Annotations for the Administration Section include:
- AHA Coding Clinic® Reference Notations
- Coding Notes

AHA Coding Clinic® Reference Notations of Administration

ROOT OPERATION SPECIFIC - ADMINISTRATION - Section 3
INTRODUCTION - 0
Chemoembolization of hepatic artery	AHA 15:1Q:p38
Glucagon to flush bile duct stones	AHA 14:3Q:p11
Imaging report to identify the body part of an infusion device	AHA 14:3Q:p5
Immune globulin (Rh-D, anti-D), injection, intramuscular	AHA 14:4Q:p16
Induction of labor, IV oxytocin, peripheral vein	AHA 14:4Q:p17
Induction of labor with Cervidil dinoprostone vaginal tampon	AHA 14:2Q:p8
Infusion of thrombolytic therapy	AHA 14:4Q:p19
Injection of combination of drugs	AHA 14:4Q:p45
Injection of intrathecal chemotherapy	AHA 15:1Q:p31
Injection of Ovation® (extracellular matrix) into amputation wound	AHA 15:2Q:p27
Injection of sclerosing agent into an esophageal varix	AHA 13:1Q:p27
Injection of substances with vitrectomy	AHA 15:2Q:p24
Injection of talc in pleura for pleurodesis	AHA 15:2Q:p31
Instillation of saline and Sepra film solution	AHA 14:4Q:p38
Intraoperative (open) placement of chemotherapy wafers	AHA 14:4Q:p34
Nasogastric (NG) tube used for both drainage and feeding	AHA 15:2Q:p29
Neulasta injection to prevent infection	AHA 14:2Q:p10
tPA administration	AHA 13:4Q:p124

IRRIGATION - 1
TRANSFUSION - 2

Coding Notes of Administration

Med/Surg Related Section Specific PCS Reference Manual Exercises

PCS CODE	3 – ADMINISTRATION EXERCISES
30243G0	Autologous bone marrow transplant via central venous line.
30263V1	Transfusion of antihemophilic factor, (nonautologous) via arterial central line.
3E0102A	Implantation of anti-microbial envelope with cardiac defibrillator placement, open.
3E03317	Systemic infusion of recombinant tissue plasminogen activator (r-tPA) via peripheral venous catheter.
3E0436Z	Infusion of total parenteral nutrition via central venous catheter.
3E0G8GC	Esophagogastroscopy with botox injection into esophageal sphincter. (Botulinum toxin is a paralyzing agent with temporary effects; it does not sclerose or destroy the nerve.)
3E0P3Q1	Transabdominal in-vitro fertilization, implantation of donor ovum.
3E0P7LZ	Transvaginal artificial insemination.
3E1M39Z	Peritoneal dialysis via indwelling catheter.
3E1U38Z	Percutaneous irrigation of knee joint.

Educational Annotations | Section 3 – Administration

NOTES

3 – ADMINISTRATION 3C1

ADMINISTRATION SECTION: Introduction, Irrigation, Transfusion
Root Operations that define procedures where a diagnostic or therapeutic substance is given to the patient.

1ST - 3 Administration
2ND - 0 Circulatory
3RD - 2 TRANSFUSION

EXAMPLE: Whole blood transfusion

TRANSFUSION: Putting in blood or blood products.

EXPLANATION: Blood products, bone marrow, and stem cells

Body System Region – 4TH	Approach – 5TH	Substance – 6TH		Qualifier – 7TH
3 Peripheral Vein 4 Central Vein	0 Open 3 Percutaneous	A Stem cells, embryonic NC*		Z No qualifier
3 Peripheral Vein 4 Central Vein	0 Open 3 Percutaneous	G Bone marrow NC* H Whole blood J Serum albumin K Frozen plasma L Fresh plasma M Plasma cryoprecipitate N Red blood cells P Frozen red cells	Q White cells R Platelets S Globulin T Fibrinogen V Antihemophilic factors W Factor IX X Stem cells, cord blood Y Stem cells, hematopoietic NC*	0 Autologous 1 Nonautologous
5 Peripheral Artery 6 Central Artery	0 Open 3 Percutaneous	G Bone marrow NC* H Whole blood J Serum albumin K Frozen plasma L Fresh plasma M Plasma cryoprecipitate N Red blood cells P Frozen red cells	Q White cells R Platelets S Globulin T Fibrinogen V Antihemophilic factors W Factor IX X Stem cells, cord blood Y Stem cells, hematopoietic NC*	0 Autologous 1 Nonautologous
7 Products of Conception, Circulatory ♀	3 Percutaneous 7 Via natural or artificial opening	H Whole blood J Serum albumin K Frozen plasma L Fresh plasma M Plasma cryoprecipitate N Red blood cells P Frozen red cells	Q White cells R Platelets S Globulin T Fibrinogen V Antihemophilic factors W Factor IX	1 Nonautologous
8 Vein	0 Open 3 Percutaneous	B 4-Factor prothrombin complex concentrate		1 Nonautologous

NC* – Some procedures are considered non-covered by Medicare. See current Medicare Code Editor for details.

ADMINISTRATION SECTION: Introduction, Irrigation, Transfusion
Root Operations that define procedures where a diagnostic or therapeutic substance is given to the patient.

1ST - 3 Administration
2ND - C Indwelling Device
3RD - 1 IRRIGATION

EXAMPLE: Irrigation of catheter port

IRRIGATION: Putting in or on a cleansing substance.

EXPLANATION: Cleansing substance

Body System/Region – 4TH	Approach – 5TH	Substance – 6TH	Qualifier – 7TH
Z None	X External	8 Irrigating substance	Z No qualifier

3E0

ADMINISTRATION SECTION: Introduction, Irrigation, Transfusion
Root Operations that define procedures where a diagnostic or therapeutic substance is given to the patient.

- **1ST – 3** Administration
- **2ND – E** Physiological Systems and Anatomical Regions
- **3RD – 0** INTRODUCTION

EXAMPLE: Infusion of chemotherapy agent

INTRODUCTION: Putting in or on a therapeutic, diagnostic, nutritional, physiological, or prophylactic substance except blood or blood products.

EXPLANATION: Substances other than blood and cleansing ...

Body System/Region – 4TH	Approach – 5TH	Substance – 6TH	Qualifier – 7TH
0 Skin and Mucous Membranes	X External	0 Antineoplastic	5 Other antineoplastic M Monoclonal antibody
0 Skin and Mucous Membranes	X External	2 Anti-infective	8 Oxazolidinones 9 Other anti-infective
0 Skin and Mucous Membranes	X External	3 Anti-inflammatory 4 Serum, toxoid and vaccine B Local anesthetic K Other diagnostic substance M Pigment N Analgesics, hypnotics, sedatives T Destructive agent	Z No qualifier
0 Skin and Mucous Membranes	X External	G Other therapeutic substance	C Other substance
1 Subcutaneous Tissue	0 Open	2 Anti-infective	A Anti-infective envelope
1 Subcutaneous Tissue	3 Percutaneous	0 Antineoplastic	5 Other antineoplastic M Monoclonal antibody
1 Subcutaneous Tissue	3 Percutaneous	2 Anti-infective	8 Oxazolidinones 9 Other anti-infective A Anti-infective envelope
1 Subcutaneous Tissue	3 Percutaneous	3 Anti-inflammatory 4 Serum, toxoid and vaccine 6 Nutritional substance 7 Electrolytic and water balance substance B Local anesthetic H Radioactive substance K Other diagnostic substance N Analgesics, hypnotics, sedatives T Destructive agent	Z No qualifier
1 Subcutaneous Tissue	3 Percutaneous	G Other therapeutic substance	C Other substance
1 Subcutaneous Tissue	3 Percutaneous	V Hormone	G Insulin J Other hormone
2 Muscle	3 Percutaneous	0 Antineoplastic	5 Other antineoplastic M Monoclonal antibody
2 Muscle	3 Percutaneous	2 Anti-infective	8 Oxazolidinones 9 Other anti-infective

continued

3E0 INTRODUCTION – continued

Body System/Region – 4TH	Approach – 5TH	Substance – 6TH	Qualifier – 7TH
2 Muscle	3 Percutaneous	3 Anti-inflammatory 4 Serum, toxoid and vaccine 6 Nutritional substance 7 Electrolytic and water balance substance B Local anesthetic H Radioactive substance K Other diagnostic substance N Analgesics, hypnotics, sedatives T Destructive agent	Z No qualifier
2 Muscle	3 Percutaneous	G Other therapeutic substance	C Other substance
3 Peripheral Vein	0 Open	0 Antineoplastic	2 High-dose interleukin-2 3 Low-dose interleukin-2 5 Other antineoplastic M Monoclonal antibody P Clofarabine
3 Peripheral Vein	0 Open	1 Thrombolytic	6 Recombinant human-activated protein C 7 Other thrombolytic
3 Peripheral Vein	0 Open	2 Anti-infective	8 Oxazolidinones 9 Other anti-infective
3 Peripheral Vein	0 Open	3 Anti-inflammatory 4 Serum, toxoid and vaccine 6 Nutritional substance 7 Electrolytic and water balance substance F Intracirculatory anesthetic H Radioactive substance K Other diagnostic substance N Analgesics, hypnotics, sedatives P Platelet inhibitor R Antiarrhythmic T Destructive agent X Vasopressor	Z No qualifier
3 Peripheral Vein	0 Open	G Other therapeutic substance	C Other substance N Blood brain barrier disruption
3 Peripheral Vein	0 Open	U Pancreatic islet cells	0 Autologous 1 Nonautologous
3 Peripheral Vein	0 Open	V Hormone	G Insulin H Human B-type natriuretic peptide J Other hormone

continued

3 E 0 INTRODUCTION – continued

Body System/Region – 4TH	Approach – 5TH	Substance – 6TH	Qualifier – 7TH
3 Peripheral Vein	0 Open	W Immunotherapeutic	K Immunostimulator L Immunosuppressive
3 Peripheral Vein	3 Percutaneous	0 Antineoplastic	2 High-dose interleukin-2 3 Low-dose interleukin-2 5 Other antineoplastic M Monoclonal antibody P Clofarabine
3 Peripheral Vein	3 Percutaneous	1 Thrombolytic	6 Recombinant human-activated protein C 7 Other thrombolytic
3 Peripheral Vein	3 Percutaneous	2 Anti-infective	8 Oxazolidinones 9 Other anti-infective
3 Peripheral Vein	3 Percutaneous	3 Anti-inflammatory 4 Serum, toxoid and vaccine 6 Nutritional substance 7 Electrolytic and water balance substance F Intracirculatory anesthetic H Radioactive substance K Other diagnostic substance N Analgesics, hypnotics, sedatives P Platelet inhibitor R Antiarrhythmic T Destructive agent X Vasopressor	Z No qualifier
3 Peripheral Vein	3 Percutaneous	G Other therapeutic substance	C Other substance N Blood brain barrier disruption Q Glucarpidase
3 Peripheral Vein	3 Percutaneous	U Pancreatic islet cells	0 Autologous 1 Nonautologous
3 Peripheral Vein	3 Percutaneous	V Hormone	G Insulin H Human B-type natriuretic peptide J Other hormone
3 Peripheral Vein	3 Percutaneous	W Immunotherapeutic	K Immunostimulator L Immunosuppressive

continued ⇨

3 E 0 INTRODUCTION—continued

Body System/Region – 4TH	Approach – 5TH	Substance – 6TH	Qualifier – 7TH
4 Central Vein	0 Open	0 Antineoplastic	2 High-dose interleukin-2 3 Low-dose interleukin-2 5 Other antineoplastic M Monoclonal antibody P Clofarabine
4 Central Vein	0 Open	1 Thrombolytic	6 Recombinant human-activated protein C 7 Other thrombolytic
4 Central Vein	0 Open	2 Anti-infective	8 Oxazolidinones 9 Other anti-infective
4 Central Vein	0 Open	3 Anti-inflammatory 4 Serum, toxoid and vaccine 6 Nutritional substance 7 Electrolytic and water balance substance F Intracirculatory anesthetic H Radioactive substance K Other diagnostic substance N Analgesics, hypnotics, sedatives P Platelet inhibitor R Antiarrhythmic T Destructive agent X Vasopressor	Z No qualifier
4 Central Vein	0 Open	G Other therapeutic substance	C Other substance N Blood brain barrier disruption
4 Central Vein	0 Open	V Hormone	G Insulin H Human B-type natriuretic peptide J Other hormone
4 Central Vein	0 Open	W Immunotherapeutic	K Immunostimulator L Immunosuppressive

continued ➡

3E0 INTRODUCTION – continued

ADMINISTRATION 3E0

Body System/Region – 4TH	Approach – 5TH	Substance – 6TH	Qualifier – 7TH
4 Central Vein	3 Percutaneous	0 Antineoplastic	2 High-dose interleukin-2 3 Low-dose interleukin-2 5 Other antineoplastic M Monoclonal antibody P Clofarabine
4 Central Vein	3 Percutaneous	1 Thrombolytic	6 Recombinant human-activated protein C 7 Other thrombolytic
4 Central Vein	3 Percutaneous	2 Anti-infective	8 Oxazolidinones 9 Other anti-infective
4 Central Vein	3 Percutaneous	3 Anti-inflammatory 4 Serum, toxoid and vaccine 6 Nutritional substance 7 Electrolytic and water balance substance F Intracirculatory anesthetic H Radioactive substance K Other diagnostic substance N Analgesics, hypnotics, sedatives P Platelet inhibitor R Antiarrhythmic T Destructive agent X Vasopressor	Z No qualifier
4 Central Vein	3 Percutaneous	G Other therapeutic substance	C Other substance N Blood brain barrier disruption Q Glucarpidase
4 Central Vein	3 Percutaneous	V Hormone	G Insulin H Human B-type natriuretic peptide J Other hormone
4 Central Vein	3 Percutaneous	W Immunotherapeutic	K Immunostimulator L Immunosuppressive

continued ⇨

3 E 0 INTRODUCTION—continued

Body System/Region – 4TH	Approach – 5TH	Substance – 6TH	Qualifier – 7TH
5 Peripheral Artery 6 Central Artery	0 Open 3 Percutaneous	0 Antineoplastic	2 High-dose interleukin-2 3 Low-dose interleukin-2 5 Other antineoplastic M Monoclonal antibody P Clofarabine
5 Peripheral Artery 6 Central Artery	0 Open 3 Percutaneous	1 Thrombolytic	6 Recombinant human-activated protein C 7 Other thrombolytic
5 Peripheral Artery 6 Central Artery	0 Open 3 Percutaneous	2 Anti-infective	8 Oxazolidinones 9 Other anti-infective
5 Peripheral Artery 6 Central Artery	0 Open 3 Percutaneous	3 Anti-inflammatory 4 Serum, toxoid and vaccine 6 Nutritional substance 7 Electrolytic and water balance substance F Intracirculatory anesthetic H Radioactive substance K Other diagnostic substance N Analgesics, hypnotics, sedatives P Platelet inhibitor R Antiarrhythmic T Destructive agent X Vasopressor	Z No qualifier
5 Peripheral Artery 6 Central Artery	0 Open 3 Percutaneous	G Other therapeutic substance	C Other substance N Blood brain barrier disruption
5 Peripheral Artery 6 Central Artery	0 Open 3 Percutaneous	V Hormone	G Insulin H Human B-type natriuretic peptide J Other hormone
5 Peripheral Artery 6 Central Artery	0 Open 3 Percutaneous	W Immunotherapeutic	K Immunostimulator L Immunosuppressive

continued ⇨

3E0 INTRODUCTION – continued

Body System/Region – 4TH	Approach – 5TH	Substance – 6TH	Qualifier – 7TH
7 Coronary Artery 8 Heart	0 Open 3 Percutaneous	1 Thrombolytic	6 Recombinant human-activated protein C 7 Other thrombolytic
7 Coronary Artery 8 Heart	0 Open 3 Percutaneous	G Other therapeutic substance	C Other substance
7 Coronary Artery 8 Heart	0 Open 3 Percutaneous	K Other diagnostic substance P Platelet inhibitor	Z No qualifier
9 Nose	3 Percutaneous 7 Via natural or artificial opening X External	0 Antineoplastic	5 Other antineoplastic M Monoclonal antibody
9 Nose	3 Percutaneous 7 Via natural or artificial opening X External	2 Anti-infective	8 Oxazolidinones 9 Other anti-infective
9 Nose	3 Percutaneous 7 Via natural or artificial opening X External	3 Anti-inflammatory 4 Serum, toxoid and vaccine B Local anesthetic H Radioactive substance K Other diagnostic substance N Analgesics, hypnotics, sedatives T Destructive agent	Z No qualifier
9 Nose	3 Percutaneous 7 Via natural or artificial opening X External	G Other therapeutic substance	C Other substance
A Bone Marrow	3 Percutaneous	0 Antineoplastic	5 Other antineoplastic M Monoclonal antibody
A Bone Marrow	3 Percutaneous	G Other therapeutic substance	C Other substance

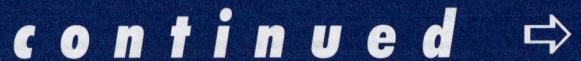

3E0 INTRODUCTION – continued

Body System/Region – 4ᵀᴴ	Approach – 5ᵀᴴ	Substance – 6ᵀᴴ	Qualifier – 7ᵀᴴ
B Ear	3 Percutaneous 7 Via natural or artificial opening X External	0 Antineoplastic	4 Liquid brachytherapy radioisotope 5 Other antineoplastic M Monoclonal antibody
B Ear	3 Percutaneous 7 Via natural or artificial opening X External	2 Anti-infective	8 Oxazolidinones 9 Other anti-infective
B Ear	3 Percutaneous 7 Via natural or artificial opening X External	3 Anti-inflammatory B Local anesthetic H Radioactive substance K Other diagnostic substance N Analgesics, hypnotics, sedatives T Destructive agent	Z No qualifier
B Ear	3 Percutaneous 7 Via natural or artificial opening X External	G Other therapeutic substance	C Other substance
C Eye	3 Percutaneous 7 Via natural or artificial opening X External	0 Antineoplastic	4 Liquid brachytherapy radioisotope 5 Other antineoplastic M Monoclonal antibody
C Eye	3 Percutaneous 7 Via natural or artificial opening X External	2 Anti-infective	8 Oxazolidinones 9 Other anti-infective
C Eye	3 Percutaneous 7 Via natural or artificial opening X External	3 Anti-inflammatory B Local anesthetic H Radioactive substance K Other diagnostic substance M Pigment N Analgesics, hypnotics, sedatives T Destructive agent	Z No qualifier
C Eye	3 Percutaneous 7 Via natural or artificial opening X External	G Other therapeutic substance	C Other substance
C Eye	3 Percutaneous 7 Via natural or artificial opening X External	S Gas	F Other gas

continued ⇨

3E0 INTRODUCTION – continued

Body System/Region – 4TH	Approach – 5TH	Substance – 6TH	Qualifier – 7TH
D Mouth and Pharynx	3 Percutaneous 7 Via natural or artificial opening X External	0 Antineoplastic	4 Liquid brachytherapy radioisotope 5 Other antineoplastic M Monoclonal antibody
D Mouth and Pharynx	3 Percutaneous 7 Via natural or artificial opening X External	2 Anti-infective	8 Oxazolidinones 9 Other anti-infective
D Mouth and Pharynx	3 Percutaneous 7 Via natural or artificial opening X External	3 Anti-inflammatory 4 Serum, toxoid and vaccine 6 Nutritional substance 7 Electrolytic and water balance substance B Local anesthetic H Radioactive substance K Other diagnostic substance N Analgesics, hypnotics, sedatives R Antiarrhythmic T Destructive agent	Z No qualifier
D Mouth and Pharynx	3 Percutaneous 7 Via natural or artificial opening X External	G Other therapeutic substance	C Other substance
E Products of Conception ♀ G Upper GI H Lower GI K Genitourinary Tract N Male Reproductive ♂	3 Percutaneous 7 Via natural or artificial opening 8 Via natural or artificial opening endoscopic	0 Antineoplastic	4 Liquid brachytherapy radioisotope 5 Other antineoplastic M Monoclonal antibody
E Products of Conception ♀ G Upper GI H Lower GI K Genitourinary Tract N Male Reproductive ♂	3 Percutaneous 7 Via natural or artificial opening 8 Via natural or artificial opening endoscopic	2 Anti-infective	8 Oxazolidinones 9 Other anti-infective
E Products of Conception ♀ G Upper GI H Lower GI K Genitourinary Tract N Male Reproductive ♂	3 Percutaneous 7 Via natural or artificial opening 8 Via natural or artificial opening endoscopic	3 Anti-inflammatory 6 Nutritional substance 7 Electrolytic and water balance substance B Local anesthetic H Radioactive substance K Other diagnostic substance N Analgesics, hypnotics, sedatives T Destructive agent	Z No qualifier

continued ➪

3 E 0 INTRODUCTION – continued

Body System/Region – 4TH	Approach – 5TH	Substance – 6TH	Qualifier – 7TH
E Products of Conception ♀ G Upper GI H Lower GI K Genitourinary Tract N Male Reproductive ♂	3 Percutaneous 7 Via natural or artificial opening 8 Via natural or artificial opening endoscopic	G Other therapeutic substance	C Other substance
E Products of Conception ♀ G Upper GI H Lower GI K Genitourinary Tract N Male Reproductive ♂	3 Percutaneous 7 Via natural or artificial opening 8 Via natural or artificial opening endoscopic	S Gas	F Other gas
F Respiratory Tract	3 Percutaneous	0 Antineoplastic	4 Liquid brachytherapy radioisotope 5 Other antineoplastic M Monoclonal antibody
F Respiratory Tract	3 Percutaneous	2 Anti-infective	8 Oxazolidinones 9 Other anti-infective
F Respiratory Tract	3 Percutaneous	3 Anti-inflammatory 6 Nutritional substance 7 Electrolytic and water balance substance B Local anesthetic H Radioactive substance K Other diagnostic substance N Analgesics, hypnotics, sedatives T Destructive agent	Z No qualifier
F Respiratory Tract	3 Percutaneous	G Other therapeutic substance	C Other substance
F Respiratory Tract	3 Percutaneous	S Gas	D Nitric oxide F Other gas
F Respiratory Tract	7 Via natural or artificial opening 8 Via natural or artificial opening endoscopic	0 Antineoplastic	4 Liquid brachytherapy radioisotope 5 Other antineoplastic M Monoclonal antibody
F Respiratory Tract	7 Via natural or artificial opening 8 Via natural or artificial opening endoscopic	2 Anti-infective	8 Oxazolidinones 9 Other anti-infective

continued ⇨

3 E 0 INTRODUCTION – continued

Body System/Region – 4TH	Approach – 5TH	Substance – 6TH	Qualifier – 7TH
F Respiratory Tract	7 Via natural or artificial opening 8 Via natural or artificial opening endoscopic	3 Anti-inflammatory 6 Nutritional substance 7 Electrolytic and water balance substance B Local anesthetic D Inhalation anesthetic H Radioactive substance K Other diagnostic substance N Analgesics, hypnotics, sedatives T Destructive agent	Z No qualifier
F Respiratory Tract	7 Via natural or artificial opening 8 Via natural or artificial opening endoscopic	G Other therapeutic substance	C Other substance
F Respiratory Tract	7 Via natural or artificial opening 8 Via natural or artificial opening endoscopic	S Gas	D Nitric oxide F Other gas
J Biliary and Pancreatic Tract	3 Percutaneous 7 Via natural or artificial opening 8 Via natural or artificial opening endoscopic	0 Antineoplastic	4 Liquid brachytherapy radioisotope 5 Other antineoplastic M Monoclonal antibody
J Biliary and Pancreatic Tract	3 Percutaneous 7 Via natural or artificial opening 8 Via natural or artificial opening endoscopic	2 Anti-infective	8 Oxazolidinones 9 Other anti-infective
J Biliary and Pancreatic Tract	3 Percutaneous 7 Via natural or artificial opening 8 Via natural or artificial opening endoscopic	3 Anti-inflammatory 6 Nutritional substance 7 Electrolytic and water balance substance B Local anesthetic H Radioactive substance K Other diagnostic substance N Analgesics, hypnotics, sedatives T Destructive agent	Z No qualifier
J Biliary and Pancreatic Tract	3 Percutaneous 7 Via natural or artificial opening 8 Via natural or artificial opening endoscopic	G Other therapeutic substance	C Other substance

continued ⇨

3E0 INTRODUCTION – continued

Body System/Region – 4TH	Approach – 5TH	Substance – 6TH	Qualifier – 7TH
J Biliary and Pancreatic Tract	3 Percutaneous 7 Via natural or artificial opening 8 Via natural or artificial opening endoscopic	S Gas	F Other gas
J Biliary and Pancreatic Tract	3 Percutaneous 7 Via natural or artificial opening 8 Via natural or artificial opening endoscopic	U Pancreatic islet cells	0 Autologous 1 Nonautologous
L Pleural Cavity M Peritoneal Cavity	0 Open	5 Adhesion barrier	Z No qualifier
L Pleural Cavity M Peritoneal Cavity	3 Percutaneous	0 Antineoplastic	4 Liquid brachytherapy radioisotope 5 Other antineoplastic M Monoclonal antibody
L Pleural Cavity M Peritoneal Cavity	3 Percutaneous	2 Anti-infective	8 Oxazolidinones 9 Other anti-infective
L Pleural Cavity M Peritoneal Cavity	3 Percutaneous	3 Anti-inflammatory 6 Nutritional substance 7 Electrolytic and water balance substance B Local anesthetic H Radioactive substance K Other diagnostic substance N Analgesics, hypnotics, sedatives T Destructive agent	Z No qualifier
L Pleural Cavity M Peritoneal Cavity	3 Percutaneous	G Other therapeutic substance	C Other substance
L Pleural Cavity M Peritoneal Cavity	3 Percutaneous	S Gas	F Other gas
L Pleural Cavity M Peritoneal Cavity	7 Via natural or artificial opening	0 Antineoplastic	4 Liquid brachytherapy radioisotope 5 Other antineoplastic M Monoclonal antibody
L Pleural Cavity M Peritoneal Cavity	7 Via natural or artificial opening	S Gas	F Other gas

continued ⇨

3E0 INTRODUCTION – continued

Body System/Region – 4ᵀᴴ	Approach – 5ᵀᴴ	Substance – 6ᵀᴴ	Qualifier – 7ᵀᴴ
P Female Reproductive ♀	0 Open	5 Adhesion barrier	Z No qualifier
P Female Reproductive ♀	3 Percutaneous 7 Via natural or artificial opening	0 Antineoplastic	4 Liquid brachytherapy radioisotope 5 Other antineoplastic M Monoclonal antibody
P Female Reproductive ♀	3 Percutaneous 7 Via natural or artificial opening	2 Anti-infective	8 Oxazolidinones 9 Other anti-infective
P Female Reproductive ♀	3 Percutaneous 7 Via natural or artificial opening	3 Anti-inflammatory 6 Nutritional substance 7 Electrolytic and water balance substance B Local anesthetic H Radioactive substance K Other diagnostic substance L Sperm N Analgesics, hypnotics, sedatives T Destructive agent	Z No qualifier
P Female Reproductive ♀	3 Percutaneous 7 Via natural or artificial opening	G Other therapeutic substance	C Other substance
P Female Reproductive ♀	3 Percutaneous 7 Via natural or artificial opening	Q Fertilized ovum	0 Autologous 1 Nonautologous
P Female Reproductive ♀	3 Percutaneous 7 Via natural or artificial opening	S Gas	F Other gas
P Female Reproductive ♀	8 Via natural or artificial opening endoscopic	0 Antineoplastic	4 Liquid brachytherapy radioisotope 5 Other antineoplastic M Monoclonal antibody
P Female Reproductive ♀	8 Via natural or artificial opening endoscopic	2 Anti-infective	8 Oxazolidinones 9 Other anti-infective

continued ⇨

3 E 0 INTRODUCTION – continued

Body System/Region – 4TH	Approach – 5TH	Substance – 6TH	Qualifier – 7TH
P Female Reproductive ♀	8 Via natural or artificial opening endoscopic	3 Anti-inflammatory 6 Nutritional substance 7 Electrolytic and water balance substance B Local anesthetic H Radioactive substance K Other diagnostic substance N Analgesics, hypnotics, sedatives T Destructive agent	Z No qualifier
P Female Reproductive ♀	8 Via natural or artificial opening endoscopic	G Other therapeutic substance	C Other substance
P Female Reproductive ♀	8 Via natural or artificial opening endoscopic	S Gas	F Other gas
Q Cranial Cavity and Brain	0 Open	A Stem cells, embryonic	Z No qualifier
Q Cranial Cavity and Brain	0 Open	E Stem cells, somatic	0 Autologous 1 Nonautologous
Q Cranial Cavity and Brain	3 Percutaneous	0 Antineoplastic	4 Liquid brachytherapy radioisotope 5 Other antineoplastic M Monoclonal antibody
Q Cranial Cavity and Brain	3 Percutaneous	2 Anti-infective	8 Oxazolidinones 9 Other anti-infective
Q Cranial Cavity and Brain	3 Percutaneous	3 Anti-inflammatory 6 Nutritional substance 7 Electrolytic and water balance substance A Stem cells, embryonic B Local anesthetic H Radioactive substance K Other diagnostic substance N Analgesics, hypnotics, sedatives T Destructive agent	Z No qualifier
Q Cranial Cavity and Brain	3 Percutaneous	E Stem cells, somatic	0 Autologous 1 Nonautologous
Q Cranial Cavity and Brain	3 Percutaneous	G Other therapeutic substance	C Other substance
Q Cranial Cavity and Brain	3 Percutaneous	S Gas	F Other gas

continued

3E0 INTRODUCTION – continued

ADMINISTRATION 3E0

Body System/Region – 4TH	Approach – 5TH	Substance – 6TH	Qualifier – 7TH
Q Cranial Cavity and Brain	7 Via natural or artificial opening	0 Antineoplastic	4 Liquid brachytherapy radioisotope 5 Other antineoplastic M Monoclonal antibody
Q Cranial Cavity and Brain	7 Via natural or artificial opening	S Gas	F Other gas
R Spinal Canal	0 Open	A Stem cells, embryonic	Z No qualifier
R Spinal Canal	0 Open	E Stem cells, somatic	0 Autologous 1 Nonautologous
R Spinal Canal	3 Percutaneous	0 Antineoplastic	2 High-dose Interleukin-2 3 Low-dose Interleukin-2 4 Liquid brachytherapy radioisotope 5 Other antineoplastic M Monoclonal antibody
R Spinal Canal	3 Percutaneous	2 Anti-infective	8 Oxazolidinones 9 Other anti-infective
R Spinal Canal	3 Percutaneous	3 Anti-inflammatory 6 Nutritional substance 7 Electrolytic and water balance substance A Stem cells, embryonic B Local anesthetic C Regional anesthetic H Radioactive substance K Other diagnostic substance N Analgesics, hypnotics, sedatives T Destructive agent	Z No qualifier
R Spinal Canal	3 Percutaneous	E Stem cells, somatic	0 Autologous 1 Nonautologous
R Spinal Canal	3 Percutaneous	G Other therapeutic substance	C Other substance
R Spinal Canal	3 Percutaneous	S Gas	F Other gas
R Spinal Canal	7 Via natural or artificial opening	S Gas	F Other gas

continued ⇨

3 E 0 INTRODUCTION – continued

Body System/Region – 4TH	Approach – 5TH	Substance – 6TH	Qualifier – 7TH
S Epidural Space	3 Percutaneous	0 Antineoplastic	2 High-dose Interleukin-2 3 Low-dose Interleukin-2 4 Liquid brachytherapy radioisotope 5 Other antineoplastic M Monoclonal antibody
S Epidural Space	3 Percutaneous	2 Anti-infective	8 Oxazolidinones 9 Other anti-infective
S Epidural Space	3 Percutaneous	3 Anti-inflammatory 6 Nutritional substance 7 Electrolytic and water balance substance B Local anesthetic C Regional anesthetic H Radioactive substance K Other diagnostic substance N Analgesics, hypnotics, sedatives T Destructive agent	Z No qualifier
S Epidural Space	3 Percutaneous	G Other therapeutic substance	C Other substance
S Epidural Space	3 Percutaneous	S Gas	F Other gas
S Epidural Space	7 Via natural or artificial opening	S Gas	F Other gas
T Peripheral Nerves and Plexi X Cranial Nerves	3 Percutaneous	3 Anti-inflammatory B Local anesthetic C Regional anesthetic T Destructive agent	Z No qualifier
T Peripheral Nerves and Plexi X Cranial Nerves	3 Percutaneous	G Other therapeutic substance	C Other substance

continued ⇨

3E0 INTRODUCTION – continued

Body System/Region – 4TH	Approach – 5TH	Substance – 6TH	Qualifier – 7TH
U Joints	0 Open	2 Anti-infective	8 Oxazolidinones 9 Other anti-infective
U Joints	0 Open	G Other therapeutic substance	B Recombinant bone morphogenetic protein
U Joints	3 Percutaneous	0 Antineoplastic	4 Liquid brachytherapy radioisotope 5 Other antineoplastic M Monoclonal antibody
U Joints	3 Percutaneous	2 Anti-infective	8 Oxazolidinones 9 Other anti-infective
U Joints	3 Percutaneous	3 Anti-inflammatory 6 Nutritional substance 7 Electrolytic and water balance substance B Local anesthetic H Radioactive substance K Other diagnostic substance N Analgesics, hypnotics, sedatives T Destructive agent	Z No qualifier
U Joints	3 Percutaneous	G Other therapeutic substance	B Recombinant bone morphogenetic protein C Other substance
U Joints	3 Percutaneous	S Gas	F Other gas
V Bones	0 Open	G Other therapeutic substance	B Recombinant bone morphogenetic protein
V Bones	3 Percutaneous	0 Antineoplastic	5 Other antineoplastic M Monoclonal antibody
V Bones	3 Percutaneous	2 Anti-infective	8 Oxazolidinones 9 Other anti-infective
V Bones	3 Percutaneous	3 Anti-inflammatory 6 Nutritional substance 7 Electrolytic and water balance substance B Local anesthetic H Radioactive substance K Other diagnostic substance N Analgesics, hypnotics, sedatives T Destructive agent	Z No qualifier
V Bones	3 Percutaneous	G Other therapeutic substance	B Recombinant bone morphogenetic protein C Other substance

continued

3 E 0 INTRODUCTION – continued

Body System/Region – 4ᵀᴴ	Approach – 5ᵀᴴ	Substance – 6ᵀᴴ	Qualifier – 7ᵀᴴ
W Lymphatics	3 Percutaneous	0 Antineoplastic	5 Other antineoplastic M Monoclonal antibody
W Lymphatics	3 Percutaneous	2 Anti-infective	8 Oxazolidinones 9 Other anti-infective
W Lymphatics	3 Percutaneous	3 Anti-inflammatory 6 Nutritional substance 7 Electrolytic and water balance substance B Local anesthetic H Radioactive substance K Other diagnostic substance N Analgesics, hypnotics, sedatives T Destructive agent	Z No qualifier
W Lymphatics	3 Percutaneous	G Other therapeutic substance	C Other substance
Y Pericardial Cavity	3 Percutaneous	0 Antineoplastic	4 Liquid brachytherapy radioisotope 5 Other antineoplastic M Monoclonal antibody
Y Pericardial Cavity	3 Percutaneous	2 Anti-infective	8 Oxazolidinones 9 Other anti-infective
Y Pericardial Cavity	3 Percutaneous	3 Anti-inflammatory 6 Nutritional substance 7 Electrolytic and water balance substance B Local anesthetic H Radioactive substance K Other diagnostic substance N Analgesics, hypnotics, sedatives T Destructive agent	Z No qualifier
Y Pericardial Cavity	3 Percutaneous	G Other therapeutic substance	C Other substance
Y Pericardial Cavity	3 Percutaneous	S Gas	F Other gas
Y Pericardial Cavity	7 Via natural or artificial opening	0 Antineoplastic	4 Liquid brachytherapy radioisotope 5 Other antineoplastic M Monoclonal antibody
Y Pericardial Cavity	7 Via natural or artificial opening	S Gas	F Other gas

3E1

MEDICAL/SURGICAL RELATED SECTIONS – 2016 ICD-10-PCS

ADMINISTRATION SECTION: Introduction, Irrigation, Transfusion
Root Operations that define procedures where a diagnostic or therapeutic substance is given to the patient.

- 1ST – **3** Administration
- 2ND – **E** Physiological Systems and Anatomical Regions
- 3RD – **1** IRRIGATION

EXAMPLE: Flushing of eye

IRRIGATION: Putting in or on a cleansing substance.

EXPLANATION: Cleansing substance or dialysate

Body System/Region – 4TH	Approach – 5TH	Substance – 6TH	Qualifier – 7TH
0 Skin and Mucous Membranes C Eye	3 Percutaneous X External	8 Irrigating substance	X Diagnostic Z No qualifier
9 Nose B Ear F Respiratory Tract G Upper GI H Lower GI J Biliary and Pancreatic Tract K Genitourinary Tract N Male Reproductive ♂ P Female Reproductive ♀	3 Percutaneous 7 Via natural or artificial opening 8 Via natural or artificial opening endoscopic	8 Irrigating substance	X Diagnostic Z No qualifier
L Pleural Cavity Q Cranial Cavity and Brain R Spinal Canal S Epidural Space U Joints Y Pericardial Cavity	3 Percutaneous	8 Irrigating substance	X Diagnostic Z No qualifier
M Peritoneal Cavity	3 Percutaneous	8 Irrigating substance	X Diagnostic Z No qualifier
M Peritoneal Cavity	3 Percutaneous	9 Dialysate	Z No qualifier

Educational Annotations | Section 4 – Measurement and Monitoring

Section Specific Educational Annotations for the Measurement and Monitoring Section include:
- AHA Coding Clinic® Reference Notations
- Coding Notes

AHA Coding Clinic® Reference Notations of Measurement and Monitoring

ROOT OPERATION SPECIFIC - MEASUREMENT AND MONITORING - Section 4

MEASUREMENT - 0
Left heart cardiac catheterization .... AHA 13:3Q:p26

MONITORING - 1
EMG monitoring during surgery .... AHA 15:2Q:p14
Intraoperative neuromonitoring .... AHA 14:4Q:p28
.... AHA 15:1Q:p26

Coding Notes of Measurement and Monitoring

Med/Surg Related Section Specific PCS Reference Manual Exercises

PCS CODE	4 – MEASUREMENT AND MONITORING EXERCISES
4A023N8	Right and left heart cardiac catheterization with bilateral sampling and pressure measurements.
4A02XM4	Cardiac stress test, single measurement.
4A04XJ1	Peripheral venous pulse, external, single measurement.
4A07X7Z	Visual mobility test, single measurement.
4A08X0Z	Olfactory acuity test, single measurement.
4A09XCZ	Respiratory rate, external, single measurement.
4A0C85Z	EGD with biliary flow measurement.
4A1239Z	Left ventricular cardiac output monitoring from pulmonary artery wedge (Swan-Ganz) catheter.
4A12X45	Holter monitoring.
4A1H7CZ	Fetal heart rate monitoring, transvaginal.

Educational Annotations | Section 4 – Measurement and Monitoring

NOTES

Section Specific Educational Annotations on Measurement and Monitoring Section includes:
- AHA Coding Clinic Reference Notations
- Coding Notes

AHA Coding Clinic Reference Notations of Measurement and Monitoring

ROOT OPERATION SPECIFIC, MEASUREMENT AND MONITORING – Section 4

MEASUREMENT – 0
Left heart cardiac catheterization .... AHA 15:3Q:p26

MONITORING – 1
EMG monitoring during surgery .... AHA 15:2Q:p14
Intraoperative neuromonitoring .... AHA 14:4Q:p23
 .... AHA 15:1Q:p26

Coding Notes of Measurement and Monitoring

Med/Surg Related Section Specific PCS Reference Manual Exercises

PCS CODE	4 – MEASUREMENT AND MONITORING EXERCISES
4A023N8	Right and left heart cardiac catheterization with bilateral sampling and pressure measurements
4A02XM4	Cardiac stress test, single measurement
4A04XJ1	Peripheral venous pulse, external, single measurement
4A07XX2	Visual mobility test, single measurement
4A08X0Z	Olfactory acuity test, single measurement
4A09XCZ	Respiratory rate, external, single measurement
4A0C8SZ	EGD with biliary flow measurement
4A1239Z	Left ventricular cardiac output monitoring from pulmonary artery wedge (Swan-Ganz) catheter
4A12X45	Holter monitoring
4A1H7CZ	Fetal heart rate monitoring, transvaginal

MEASUREMENT AND MONITORING SECTION: Measurment, Monitoring

Root Operations that define one procedure/level and a series of procedures/levels obtained at intervals.

- 1ST – **4** Measurement and Monitoring
- 2ND – **A** Physiological Systems
- 3RD – **0** MEASUREMENT

EXAMPLE: EKG (single electrocardiogram)

MEASUREMENT: Determining the level of a physiological or physical function at a point in time.

EXPLANATION: Describes a single measurement

Body System – 4TH	Approach – 5TH	Function/Device – 6TH	Qualifier – 7TH
0 Central Nervous	0 Open	2 Conductivity 4 Electrical activity B Pressure	Z No qualifier
0 Central Nervous	3 Percutaneous	4 Electrical activity	Z No qualifier
0 Central Nervous	3 Percutaneous	B Pressure K Temperature R Saturation	D Intracranial
0 Central Nervous	7 Via natural or artificial opening	B Pressure K Temperature R Saturation	D Intracranial
0 Central Nervous	X External	2 Conductivity 4 Electrical activity	Z No qualifier
1 Peripheral Nervous	0 Open 3 Percutaneous X External	2 Conductivity	9 Sensory B Motor
1 Peripheral Nervous	0 Open 3 Percutaneous X External	4 Electrical activity	Z No qualifier
2 Cardiac	0 Open 3 Percutaneous	4 Electrical activity 9 Output C Rate F Rhythm H Sound P Action currents	Z No qualifier
2 Cardiac	0 Open 3 Percutaneous	N Sampling and pressure	6 Right heart 7 Left heart 8 Bilateral
2 Cardiac	X External	4 Electrical activity	A Guidance Z No qualifier
2 Cardiac	X External	9 Output C Rate F Rhythm H Sound P Action currents	Z No qualifier
2 Cardiac	X External	M Total activity	4 Stress

continued ⇨

4 A 0 MEASUREMENT — continued

Body System – 4ᵀᴴ	Approach – 5ᵀᴴ	Function/Device – 6ᵀᴴ	Qualifier – 7ᵀᴴ
3 Arterial	0 Open 3 Percutaneous	5 Flow J Pulse	1 Peripheral 3 Pulmonary C Coronary
3 Arterial	0 Open 3 Percutaneous	B Pressure	1 Peripheral 3 Pulmonary C Coronary F Other thoracic
3 Arterial	0 Open 3 Percutaneous	H Sound R Saturation	1 Peripheral
3 Arterial	X External	5 Flow B Pressure H Sound J Pulse R Saturation	1 Peripheral
4 Venous	0 Open 3 Percutaneous	5 Flow B Pressure J Pulse	0 Central 1 Peripheral 2 Portal 3 Pulmonary
4 Venous	0 Open 3 Percutaneous	R Saturation	1 Peripheral
4 Venous	X External	5 Flow B Pressure J Pulse R Saturation	1 Peripheral
5 Circulatory	X External	L Volume	Z No qualifier
6 Lymphatic	0 Open 3 Percutaneous	5 Flow B Pressure	Z No qualifier
7 Visual	X External	0 Acuity 7 Mobility B Pressure	Z No qualifier
8 Olfactory	X External	0 Acuity	Z No qualifier
9 Respiratory	7 Via natural or artificial opening 8 Via natural or artificial opening endoscopic X External	1 Capacity 5 Flow C Rate D Resistance L Volume M Total activity	Z No qualifier
B Gastrointestinal	7 Via natural or artificial opening 8 Via natural or artificial opening endoscopic	8 Motility B Pressure G Secretion	Z No qualifier

continued

4 A 0 MEASUREMENT – continued

Body System – 4TH	Approach – 5TH	Function/Device – 6TH	Qualifier – 7TH
C Biliary	3 Percutaneous 4 Percutaneous endoscopic 7 Via natural or artificial opening 8 Via natural or artificial opening endoscopic	5 Flow B Pressure	Z No qualifier
D Urinary	7 Via natural or artificial opening	3 Contractility 5 Flow B Pressure D Resistance L Volume	Z No qualifier
F Musculoskeletal	3 Percutaneous X External	3 Contractility	Z No qualifier
H Products of Conception, Cardiac ♀	7 Via natural or artificial opening 8 Via natural or artificial opening endoscopic X External	4 Electrical activity C Rate F Rhythm H Sound	Z No qualifier
J Products of Conception, Nervous ♀	7 Via natural or artificial opening 8 Via natural or artificial opening endoscopic X External	2 Conductivity 4 Electrical activity B Pressure	Z No qualifier
Z None	7 Via natural or artificial opening	6 Metabolism K Temperature	Z No qualifier
Z None	X External	6 Metabolism K Temperature Q Sleep	Z No qualifier

4 A 1

MEDICAL/SURGICAL RELATED SECTIONS – 2016 ICD-10-PCS

MEASUREMENT AND MONITORING SECTION: Measurment, Monitoring
Root Operations that define one procedure/level and a series of procedures/levels obtained at intervals.

- 1ST – **4** Measurement and Monitoring
- 2ND – **A** Physiological Systems
- 3RD – **1 MONITORING**

EXAMPLE: Holter monitor

MONITORING: Determining the level of a physiological or physical function repetitively over a period of time.

EXPLANATION: Describes a series of measurements

Body System – 4TH	Approach – 5TH	Function/Device – 6TH	Qualifier – 7TH
0 Central Nervous	0 Open	2 Conductivity B Pressure	Z No qualifier
0 Central Nervous	0 Open	4 Electrical activity	G Intraoperative Z No qualifier
0 Central Nervous	3 Percutaneous	4 Electrical activity	G Intraoperative Z No qualifier
0 Central Nervous	3 Percutaneous	B Pressure K Temperature R Saturation	D Intracranial
0 Central Nervous	7 Via natural or artificial opening	B Pressure K Temperature R Saturation	D Intracranial
0 Central Nervous	X External	2 Conductivity	Z No qualifier
0 Central Nervous	X External	4 Electrical activity	G Intraoperative Z No qualifier
1 Peripheral Nervous	0 Open 3 Percutaneous X External	2 Conductivity	9 Sensory B Motor
1 Peripheral Nervous	0 Open 3 Percutaneous X External	4 Electrical activity	G Intraoperative Z No qualifier
2 Cardiac	0 Open 3 Percutaneous	4 Electrical activity 9 Output C Rate F Rhythm H Sound	Z No qualifier
2 Cardiac	X External	4 Electrical activity	5 Ambulatory Z No qualifier
2 Cardiac	X External	9 Output C Rate F Rhythm H Sound	Z No qualifier
2 Cardiac	X External	M Total activity	4 Stress
3 Arterial	0 Open 3 Percutaneous	5 Flow B Pressure J Pulse	1 Peripheral 3 Pulmonary C Coronary
3 Arterial	0 Open 3 Percutaneous	H Sound R Saturation	1 Peripheral

continued ⇒

4 A 1 MONITORING—continued

Body System – 4ᵀᴴ	Approach – 5ᵀᴴ	Function/Device – 6ᵀᴴ	Qualifier – 7ᵀᴴ
3 Arterial	X External	5 Flow B Pressure H Sound J Pulse R Saturation	1 Peripheral
4 Venous	0 Open 3 Percutaneous	5 Flow B Pressure J Pulse	0 Central 1 Peripheral 2 Portal 3 Pulmonary
4 Venous	0 Open 3 Percutaneous	R Saturation	0 Central 2 Portal 3 Pulmonary
4 Venous	X External	5 Flow B Pressure J Pulse	1 Peripheral
6 Lymphatic	0 Open 3 Percutaneous	5 Flow B Pressure	Z No qualifier
9 Respiratory	7 Via natural or artificial opening X External	1 Capacity 5 Flow C Rate D Resistance L Volume	Z No qualifier
B Gastrointestinal	7 Via natural or artificial opening 8 Via natural or artificial opening endoscopic	8 Motility B Pressure G Secretion	Z No qualifier
D Urinary	7 Via natural or artificial opening	3 Contractility 5 Flow B Pressure D Resistance L Volume	Z No qualifier
H Products of Conception, Cardiac ♀	7 Via natural or artificial opening 8 Via natural or artificial opening endoscopic X External	4 Electrical activity C Rate F Rhythm H Sound	Z No qualifier
J Products of Conception, Nervous ♀	7 Via natural or artificial opening 8 Via natural or artificial opening endoscopic X External	2 Conductivity 4 Electrical activity B Pressure	Z No qualifier
Z None	7 Via natural or artificial opening	K Temperature	Z No qualifier
Z None	X External	K Temperature Q Sleep	Z No qualifier

4B0

MEASUREMENT AND MONITORING SECTION: Measurment, Monitoring
Root Operations that define one procedure/level and a series of procedures/levels obtained at intervals.

1ST – **4** Measurement and Monitoring
2ND – **B** Physiological Devices
3RD – **0** MEASUREMENT

EXAMPLE: Pacemaker rate check

MEASUREMENT: Determining the level of a physiological or physical function at a point in time.

EXPLANATION: Describes a single measurement

Body System – 4TH	Approach – 5TH	Function/Device – 6TH	Qualifier – 7TH
0 Central Nervous 1 Peripheral Nervous F Musculoskeletal	X External	V Stimulator	Z No qualifier
2 Cardiac	X External	S Pacemaker T Defibrillator	Z No qualifier
9 Respiratory	X External	S Pacemaker	Z No qualifier

Educational Annotations | Section 5 – Extracorporeal Assistance and Performance

Section Specific Educational Annotations for the Extracorporeal Assistance and Performance Section include:
- AHA Coding Clinic® Reference Notations
- Coding Notes

AHA Coding Clinic® Reference Notations of Extracoporeal Assistance and Performance

ROOT OPERATION SPECIFIC - EXTRACORPOREAL ASSISTANCE AND PERFORMANCE - Section 5

ASSISTANCE - 0
BiPAP ventilatory support system	AHA 14:4Q:p9
Impella assistance/support	AHA 14:3Q:p19
Intra-aortic balloon pump	AHA 13:3Q:p18

PERFORMANCE - 1
Cardiopulmonary bypass	AHA 14:3Q:p17,20
	AHA 14:1Q:P10
	AHA 13:3Q:p18
Continuous cardiac pacing	AHA 13:3Q:p18
Mechanical ventilation	AHA 14:4Q:p3
Mechanical ventilation, at night for sleep apnea	AHA 14:4Q:p11

RESTORATION - 2

Coding Notes of Extracoporeal Assistance and Performance

Med/Surg Related Section Specific PCS Reference Manual Exercises

PCS CODE	5 – EXTRACORPOREAL ASSISTANCE AND PERFORMANCE EXERCISES
5A02115	Pulsatile compression boot with intermittent inflation. (This is coded to the function value Cardiac Output, because the purpose of such compression devices is to return blood to the heart faster.)
5A02210	IABP (intra-aortic balloon pump) continuous.
5A09358	IPPB (intermittent positive pressure breathing) for mobilization of secretions, 22 hours.
5A1223Z	Intra-operative cardiac pacing, continuous.
5A15223	ECMO (extracorporeal membrane oxygenation), continuous.
5A1935Z	Intermittent mechanical ventilation, 16 hours.
5A1945Z	Controlled mechanical ventilation (CMV), 45 hours.
5A1C00Z	Liver dialysis, single encounter.
5A1D60Z	Renal dialysis, series of encounters.
5A2204Z	Cardiac countershock with successful conversion to sinus rhythm.

Educational Annotations

Section 5 – Extracorporeal Assistance and Performance

NOTES

5 – EXTRACORPOREAL ASSISTANCE AND PERFORMANCE

EXTRACORPOREAL ASSISTANCE AND PERFORMANCE SECTION: Assistance, Performance, Restoration
Root Operations that use equipment to support a physiological function in some manner.

1ST - 5 Extracorporeal Assistance and Performance
2ND - A Physiological Systems
3RD - 0 ASSISTANCE

EXAMPLE: Intra-aortic balloon pump

ASSISTANCE: Taking over a portion of a physiological function by extracorporeal means.

EXPLANATION: Supports, but does not take over function ...

Body System – 4TH	Duration – 5TH	Function – 6TH	Qualifier – 7TH
2 Cardiac	1 Intermittent 2 Continuous	1 Output	0 Balloon pump 5 Pulsatile compression 6 Other pump D Impeller pump
5 Circulatory	1 Intermittent 2 Continuous	2 Oxygenation	1 Hyperbaric C Supersaturated
9 Respiratory	3 Less than 24 consecutive hours 4 24-96 consecutive hours 5 Greater than 96 consecutive hours	5 Ventilation	7 Continuous positive airway pressure 8 Intermittent positive airway pressure 9 Continuous negative airway pressure B Intermittent negative airway pressure Z No qualifier

EXTRACORPOREAL ASSISTANCE AND PERFORMANCE SECTION: Assistance, Performance, Restoration
Root Operations that use equipment to support a physiological function in some manner.

1ST - 5 Extracorporeal Assistance and Performance
2ND - A Physiological Systems
3RD - 1 PEFORMANCE

EXAMPLE: Cardiopulmonary bypass in CABG

PERFORMANCE: Completely taking over a physiological function by extracorporeal means.

EXPLANATION: Completely takes over function ...

Body System – 4TH	Duration – 5TH	Function – 6TH	Qualifier – 7TH
2 Cardiac	0 Single	1 Output	2 Manual
2 Cardiac	1 Intermittent	3 Pacing	Z No qualifier
2 Cardiac	2 Continuous	1 Output 3 Pacing	Z No qualifier
5 Circulatory	2 Continuous	2 Oxygenation	3 Membrane
9 Respiratory	0 Single	5 Ventilation	4 Nonmechanical
9 Respiratory	3 Less than 24 consecutive hours 4 24-96 consecutive hours 5 Greater than 96 consecutive hours LOS*	5 Ventilation	Z No qualifier
C Biliary D Urinary	0 Single 6 Multiple	0 Filtration	Z No qualifier

LOS* – Procedure Inconsistent with LOS Edit – Code only with length of stay of greater than four days. See current Medicare Code Editor for details.

5A2

MEDICAL/SURGICAL RELATED SECTIONS – 2016 ICD-10-PCS

EXTRACORPOREAL ASSISTANCE AND PERFORMANCE SECTION: Assistance, Performance, Restoration
Root Operations that use equipment to support a physiological function in some manner.

- 1ST – **5** Extracorporeal Assistance and Performance
- 2ND – **A** Physiological Systems
- 3RD – **2** RESTORATION

EXAMPLE: Cardiac defibrillation

RESTORATION: Returning, or attempting to return, a physiological function to its original state by extracorporeal means.

EXPLANATION: Defibrillation and cardioversion only ...

Body System – 4TH	Duration – 5TH	Function – 6TH	Qualifier – 7TH
2 Cardiac	0 Single	4 Rhythm	Z No qualifier

Educational Annotations | Section 6 – Extracorporeal Therapies

Section Specific Educational Annotations for the Extracorporeal Therapies Section include:
- AHA Coding Clinic® Reference Notations
- Coding Notes

AHA Coding Clinic® Reference Notations of Extracorporeal Therapies

ROOT OPERATION SPECIFIC - EXTRACORPOREAL THERAPIES - Section 6
ATMOSPHERIC CONTROL - 0
DECOMPRESSION - 1
ELECTROMAGNETIC THERAPY - 2
HYPERTHERMIA - 3
HYPOTHERMIA - 4
PHERESIS - 5
PHOTOTHERAPY - 6
ULTRASOUND THERAPY - 7
    Ultrasound accelerated thrombolysis ....AHA 14:4Q:p19
ULTRVIOLET LIGHT THERAPY - 8
SHOCK WAVE THERAPY - 9

Coding Notes of Extracorporeal Therapies

Med/Surg Related Section Specific PCS Reference Manual Exercises

PCS CODE	6 – EXTRACORPOREAL THERAPIES EXERCISES
6A0Z1ZZ	Antigen-free air conditioning, series treatment.
6A210ZZ	Extracorporeal electromagnetic stimulation (EMS) for urinary incontinence, single treatment.
6A221ZZ	TMS (transcranial magnetic stimulation), series treatment.
6A4Z0ZZ	Whole body hypothermia, single treatment.
6A550Z2	Donor thrombocytapheresis, single encounter.
6A551Z3	Plasmapheresis, series treatment.
6A650ZZ	Circulatory phototherapy, single encounter.
6A651ZZ	Bili-lite phototherapy, series treatment.
6A750ZZ	Therapeutic ultrasound of peripheral vessels, single treatment.
6A930ZZ	Shock wave therapy of plantar fascia, single treatment.

Section 6 – Extracorporeal Therapies

Educational Annotations

NOTES

Section Specific Educational Annotations for Extracorporeal Therapies Section Include:
- AHA Coding Clinic® Reference Notations
- Coding Notes

AHA Coding Clinic® Reference Notations for Extracorporeal Therapies

ROOT OPERATION SPECIFIC: EXTRACORPOREAL THERAPIES – Section 6

- ATMOSPHERIC CONTROL – 0
- DECOMPRESSION – 1
- ELECTROMAGNETIC THERAPY – 2
- HYPERTHERMIA – 3
- HYPOTHERMIA – 4
- PHERESIS – 5
- PHOTOTHERAPY – 6
- ULTRASOUND THERAPY – 7
  - Ultrasound accelerated thrombolysis .... AHA 14:4Q, p19
- ULTRAVIOLET LIGHT THERAPY – 8
- SHOCK WAVE THERAPY – 9

Coding Notes for Extracorporeal Therapies

Med/Surg Related Section Specific PCS Reference Manual Exercises

6 – EXTRACORPOREAL THERAPIES EXERCISES

PCS CODE	
6A0Z1ZZ	Antigen-free air conditioning, series treatment.
6A21022	Extracorporeal electromagnetic stimulation (EMS) for urinary incontinence, single treatment.
6A212ZZ	TMS (transcranial magnetic stimulation), series treatment.
6A4Z0ZZ	Whole body hypothermia, single treatment.
6A550ZZ	Donor thrombocytopheresis, single encounter.
6A551Z3	Plasmapheresis, series treatment.
6A650ZZ	Circulatory phototherapy, single encounter.
6A651ZZ	Bili-lite phototherapy, series treatment.
6A750ZZ	Therapeutic ultrasound of peripheral vessels, single treatment.
6A930ZZ	Shock wave therapy of plantar fascia, single treatment.

6 – EXTRACORPOREAL THERAPIES

EXTRACORPOREAL THERAPIES SECTION: Atmospheric Control, Decompression, Electromagnetic Therapy, Hyperthermia, Hypothermia, Pheresis, Phototherapy, Ultrasound Therapy, Ultraviolet Light Therapy, Shock Wave Therapy
Root Operations that describe other extracorporeal procedures that are not defined by Assistance and Performance in Section 5.

- 1ST – **6** Extracorporeal Therapies
- 2ND – **A** Physiological Systems
- 3RD – **0** ATMOSPHERIC CONTROL

EXAMPLE: Antigen-free air conditioning

ATMOSPHERIC CONTROL: Extracorporeal control of atmospheric pressure and composition.

EXPLANATION: Control of air composition and pressure …

Body System – 4TH	Duration – 5TH	Qualifier – 6TH	Qualifier – 7TH
Z None	0 Single 1 Multiple	Z No qualifier	Z No qualifier

EXTRACORPOREAL THERAPIES SECTION: Atmospheric Control, Decompression, Electromagnetic Therapy, Hyperthermia, Hypothermia, Pheresis, Phototherapy, Ultrasound Therapy, Ultraviolet Light Therapy, Shock Wave Therapy
Root Operations that describe other extracorporeal procedures that are not defined by Assistance and Performance in Section 5.

- 1ST – **6** Extracorporeal Therapies
- 2ND – **A** Physiological Systems
- 3RD – **1** DECOMPRESSION

EXAMPLE: Decompression chamber treatment

DECOMPRESSION: Extracorporeal elimination of undissolved gas from body fluids.

EXPLANATION: Used only to treat the "bends" …

Body System – 4TH	Duration – 5TH	Qualifier – 6TH	Qualifier – 7TH
5 Circulatory	0 Single 1 Multiple	Z No qualifier	Z No qualifier

---

EXTRACORPOREAL THERAPIES SECTION: Atmospheric Control, Decompression, Electromagnetic Therapy, Hyperthermia, Hypothermia, Pheresis, Phototherapy, Ultrasound Therapy, Ultraviolet Light Therapy, Shock Wave Therapy
Root Operations that describe other extracorporeal procedures that are not defined by Assistance and Performance in Section 5.

- 1ST – **6** Extracorporeal Therapies
- 2ND – **A** Physiological Systems
- 3RD – **2** ELECTROMAGNETIC THERAPY

EXAMPLE: Transcranial magnetic stimulation (TMS)

ELECTROMAGNETIC THERAPY: Extracorporeal treatment by electromagnetic rays.

EXPLANATION: Electromagnetic energy to stimulate cells

Body System – 4TH	Duration – 5TH	Qualifier – 6TH	Qualifier – 7TH
1 Urinary 2 Central Nervous	0 Single 1 Multiple	Z No qualifier	Z No qualifier

MEDICAL/SURGICAL RELATED SECTIONS – 2016 ICD-10-PCS

EXTRACORPOREAL THERAPIES SECTION: Atmospheric Control, Decompression, Electromagnetic Therapy, Hyperthermia, Hypothermia, Pheresis, Phototherapy, Ultrasound Therapy, Ultraviolet Light Therapy, Shock Wave Therapy
Root Operations that describe other extracorporeal procedures that are not defined by Assistance and Performance in Section 5.

1ST – **6** Extracorporeal Therapies
2ND – **A** Physiological Systems
3RD – **3** HYPERTHERMIA

EXAMPLE: Whole body hyperthermia

HYPERTHERMIA: Extracorporeal raising of body temperature.

EXPLANATION: Used to treat temperature imbalance ...

Body System – 4TH	Duration – 5TH	Qualifier – 6TH	Qualifier – 7TH
Z None	0 Single 1 Multiple	Z No qualifier	Z No qualifier

EXTRACORPOREAL THERAPIES SECTION: Atmospheric Control, Decompression, Electromagnetic Therapy, Hyperthermia, Hypothermia, Pheresis, Phototherapy, Ultrasound Therapy, Ultraviolet Light Therapy, Shock Wave Therapy
Root Operations that describe other extracorporeal procedures that are not defined by Assistance and Performance in Section 5.

1ST – **6** Extracorporeal Therapies
2ND – **A** Physiological Systems
3RD – **4** HYPOTHERMIA

EXAMPLE: Whole body hypothermia

HYPOTHERMIA: Extracorporeal lowering of body temperature.

EXPLANATION: Used to treat temperature imbalance ...

Body System – 4TH	Duration – 5TH	Qualifier – 6TH	Qualifier – 7TH
Z None	0 Single 1 Multiple	Z No qualifier	Z No qualifier

EXTRACORPOREAL THERAPIES SECTION: Atmospheric Control, Decompression, Electromagnetic Therapy, Hyperthermia, Hypothermia, Pheresis, Phototherapy, Ultrasound Therapy, Ultraviolet Light Therapy, Shock Wave Therapy
Root Operations that describe other extracorporeal procedures that are not defined by Assistance and Performance in Section 5.

1ST – **6** Extracorporeal Therapies
2ND – **A** Physiological Systems
3RD – **5** PHERESIS

EXAMPLE: Therapeutic leukapheresis

PHERESIS: Extracorporeal separation of blood products.

EXPLANATION: Used to separate and remove blood products

Body System – 4TH	Duration – 5TH	Qualifier – 6TH	Qualifier – 7TH
5 Circulatory	0 Single 1 Multiple	Z No qualifier	0 Erythrocytes 1 Leukocytes 2 Platelets 3 Plasma T Stem cells, cord blood V Stem cells, hematopoietic

6 – EXTRACORPOREAL THERAPIES   6 A 8

EXTRACORPOREAL THERAPIES SECTION: Atmospheric Control, Decompression, Electromagnetic Therapy, Hyperthermia, Hypothermia, Pheresis, Phototherapy, Ultrasound Therapy, Ultraviolet Light Therapy, Shock Wave Therapy
Root Operations that describe other extracorporeal procedures that are not defined by Assistance and Performance in Section 5.

- 1ST – **6** Extracorporeal Therapies
- 2ND – **A** Physiological Systems
- 3RD – **6** PHOTOTHERAPY

EXAMPLE: Phototherapy of circulatory system

PHOTOTHERAPY: Extracorporeal treatment by light rays.

EXPLANATION: Uses light rays for treatment …

Body System – 4TH	Duration – 5TH	Qualifier – 6TH	Qualifier – 7TH
0 Skin 5 Circulatory	0 Single 1 Multiple	Z No qualifier	Z No qualifier

---

EXTRACORPOREAL THERAPIES SECTION: Atmospheric Control, Decompression, Electromagnetic Therapy, Hyperthermia, Hypothermia, Pheresis, Phototherapy, Ultrasound Therapy, Ultraviolet Light Therapy, Shock Wave Therapy
Root Operations that describe other extracorporeal procedures that are not defined by Assistance and Performance in Section 5.

- 1ST – **6** Extracorporeal Therapies
- 2ND – **A** Physiological Systems
- 3RD – **7** ULTRASOUND THERAPY

EXAMPLE: Therapeutic ultrasound of vessels

ULTRASOUND THERAPY: Extracorporeal treatment by ultrasound.

EXPLANATION: Therapeutic use of ultrasound waves

Body System – 4TH	Duration – 5TH	Qualifier – 6TH	Qualifier – 7TH
5 Circulatory	0 Single 1 Multiple	Z No qualifier	4 Head and neck vessels 5 Heart 6 Peripheral vessels 7 Other vessels Z No qualifier

---

EXTRACORPOREAL THERAPIES SECTION: Atmospheric Control, Decompression, Electromagnetic Therapy, Hyperthermia, Hypothermia, Pheresis, Phototherapy, Ultrasound Therapy, Ultraviolet Light Therapy, Shock Wave Therapy
Root Operations that describe other extracorporeal procedures that are not defined by Assistance and Performance in Section 5.

- 1ST – **6** Extracorporeal Therapies
- 2ND – **A** Physiological Systems
- 3RD – **8** ULTRAVIOLET LIGHT THERAPY

EXAMPLE: Bililite phototherapy of newborns

ULTRAVIOLET LIGHT THERAPY: Extracorporeal treatment by ultraviolet light.

EXPLANATION: Uses ultraviolet light for treatment

Body System – 4TH	Duration – 5TH	Qualifier – 6TH	Qualifier – 7TH
0 Skin	0 Single 1 Multiple	Z No qualifier	Z No qualifier

6 A 9 MEDICAL/SURGICAL RELATED SECTIONS – 2016 ICD-10-PCS [2016.PCS]

EXTRACORPOREAL THERAPIES SECTION: Atmospheric Control, Decompression, Electromagnetic Therapy, Hyperthermia, Hypothermia, Pheresis, Phototherapy, Ultrasound Therapy, Ultraviolet Light Therapy, Shock Wave Therapy
Root Operations that describe other extracorporeal procedures that are not defined by Assistance and Performance in Section 5.

1ST – **6** Extracorporeal Therapies
2ND – **A** Physiological Systems
3RD – **9** SHOCK WAVE THERAPY

EXAMPLE: Shock wave treatment of fascia

SHOCK WAVE THERAPY: Extracorporeal treatment by shock waves.

EXPLANATION: Uses pulses of sound waves for treatment

Body System – 4TH	Duration – 5TH	Qualifier – 6TH	Qualifier – 7TH
3 Musculoskeletal	0 Single 1 Multiple	Z No qualifier	Z No qualifier

EXTRA THERAPIES 6 A 9

Educational Annotations | Section 7 – Osteopathic

Section Specific Educational Annotations for the Osteopathic Section include:
- AHA Coding Clinic® Reference Notations
- Coding Notes

AHA Coding Clinic® Reference Notations of Osteopathic

ROOT OPERATION SPECIFIC - OSTEOPATHIC - Section 7
TREATMENT - 0

Coding Notes of Osteopathic

Med/Surg Related Section Specific PCS Reference Manual Exercises

PCS CODE	7 – OSTEOPATHIC EXERCISES
7W00X5Z	Low velocity-high amplitude osteopathic treatment of head.
7W01X0Z	Articulatory osteopathic treatment of cervical region.
7W04X4Z	Indirect osteopathic treatment of sacrum.
7W06X8Z	Isotonic muscle energy treatment of right leg.
7W07X6Z	Lymphatic pump osteopathic treatment of left axilla.

Educational Annotations

Section 7 – Osteopathic

NOTES

OSTEOPATHIC SECTION: Treatment
Root Operation that defines osteopathic treatment.

1ST - 7 Osteopathic
2ND - W Anatomical Regions
3RD - 0 TREATMENT

EXAMPLE: Articulopathy osteopathic treatment

TREATMENT: Manual treatment to eliminate or alleviate somatic dysfunction and related disorders.

EXPLANATION: Uses only osteopathic methods and treatments

Body Region – 4TH	Approach – 5TH	Method – 6TH	Qualifier – 7TH
0 Head	X External	0 Articulatory-raising	Z None
1 Cervical		1 Fascial release	
2 Thoracic		2 General mobilization	
3 Lumbar		3 High velocity-low amplitude	
4 Sacrum		4 Indirect	
5 Pelvis		5 Low velocity-high amplitude	
6 Lower Extremities		6 Lymphatic pump	
7 Upper Extremities		7 Muscle energy-isometric	
8 Rib Cage		8 Muscle energy-isotonic	
9 Abdomen		9 Other method	

7 Osteopathic
W Anatomical Regions
0 Treatment

OSTEOPATHIC TREATMENT
0: of Operation that defines osteopathic treatment.

EXAMPLE: Articulatory osteopathic treatment

TREATMENT: Manual treatment to eliminate or alleviate somatic dysfunction and related disorders.

EXPLANATION: Uses only osteopathic methods and treatments

Body Region – 4th	Approach – 5th	Method – 6th	Qualifier – 7th
0 Head	X External	0 Articulatory-raising	Z None
1 Cervical		1 Fascial release	
2 Thoracic		2 General mobilization	
3 Lumbar		3 High velocity-low amplitude	
4 Sacrum		4 Indirect	
5 Pelvis		5 Low velocity-high amplitude	
6 Lower Extremities		6 Lymphatic pump	
7 Upper Extremities		7 Muscle energy-isometric	
8 Rib Cage		8 Muscle energy-isotonic	
9 Abdomen		9 Other method	

Educational Annotations | Section 8 – Other Procedures

Section Specific Educational Annotations for the Other Procedures Section include:
- AHA Coding Clinic® Reference Notations
- Coding Notes

AHA Coding Clinic® Reference Notations of Other Procedures

ROOT OPERATION SPECIFIC - OTHER PROCEDURES - Section 8
COLLECTION - 6
NEAR INFRARED SPECTROSCOPY - D
COMPUTER ASSISTED PROCEDURE - B
ROBOTIC ASSISTED PROCEDURE - C
    Radical prostatectomy, robotic-assisted, with bilateral resection of
        vas deferens and seminal vesicles .... AHA 14:4Q:p33
    Robotic assisted procedure .... AHA 15:1Q:p33
ACUPUNCTURE - 0
THERAPEUTIC MASSAGE - 1
OTHER METHOD - Y

Coding Notes of Other Procedures

Med/Surg Related Section Specific PCS Reference Manual Exercises

PCS CODE	8 – OTHER PROCEDURES EXERCISES
8E023DZ	Near infrared spectroscopy of leg vessels.
8E09XBG	CT computer assisted sinus surgery. (The primary procedure is coded separately.)
8E0W0CZ	Robotic assisted open prostatectomy. (The primary procedure is coded separately.)
8E0WXY8	Suture removal, abdominal wall.
8E0ZXY6	Isolation after infectious disease exposure.

Section 8 – Other Procedures

Educational Annotations

NOTES

8 – OTHER PROCEDURES 8E0

OTHER PROCEDURES SECTION: Other Procedures
Root Operation that defines procedures not included in the Medical and Medical/Surgical related sections.

- 1ST – **8** Other Procedures
- 2ND – **C** Indwelling Device
- 3RD – **0** OTHER PROCEDURES

EXAMPLE: None

OTHER PROCEDURES: Methodologies which attempt to remediate or cure a disorder or disease.

EXPLANATION: Procedures not included elsewhere

Body Region – 4TH	Approach – 5TH	Method – 6TH	Qualifier – 7TH
1 Nervous System	X External	6 Collection	J Cerebrospinal fluid L Other fluid
2 Circulatory System	X External	6 Collection	K Blood L Other fluid

OTHER PROCEDURES SECTION: Other Procedures
Root Operation that defines procedures not included in the Medical and Medical/Surgical related sections.

- 1ST – **8** Other Procedures
- 2ND – **E** Physiological Systems and Anatomical Regions
- 3RD – **0** OTHER PROCEDURES

EXAMPLE: Suture removal

OTHER PROCEDURES: Methodologies which attempt to remediate or cure a disorder or disease.

EXPLANATION: Procedures not included elsewhere

Body Region – 4TH	Approach – 5TH	Method – 6TH	Qualifier – 7TH
1 Nervous System U Female Reproductive System ♀	X External	Y Other method	7 Examination
2 Circulatory System	3 Percutaneous	D Near infrared spectroscopy	Z No qualifier
9 Head and Neck Region W Trunk Region	0 Open 3 Percutaneous 4 Percutaneous endoscopic 7 Via natural or artificial opening 8 Via natural or artificial opening endoscopic	C Robotic assisted procedure	Z No qualifier
9 Head and Neck Region W Trunk Region	X External	B Computer assisted procedure	F With fluoroscopy G With computerized tomography H With magnetic resonance imaging Z No qualifier
9 Head and Neck Region W Trunk Region	X External	C Robotic assisted procedure	Z No qualifier
9 Head and Neck Region W Trunk Region	X External	Y Other method	8 Suture removal

continued ➡

8E0 OTHER PROCEDURES—continued

Body Region – 4TH	Approach – 5TH	Method – 6TH	Qualifier – 7TH
H Integumentary System and Breast	3 Percutaneous	0 Acupuncture	0 Anesthesia Z No qualifier
H Integumentary System and Breast ♀	X External	6 Collection	2 Breast milk
H Integumentary System and Breast	X External	Y Other method	9 Piercing
K Musculoskeletal System	X External	1 Therapeutic massage	Z No qualifier
K Musculoskeletal System	X External	Y Other method	7 Examination
V Male Reproductive System	X External	1 Therapeutic massage	C Prostate ♂ D Rectum
V Male Reproductive System ♂	X External	6 Collection	3 Sperm
X Upper Extremity Y Lower Extremity	0 Open 3 Percutaneous 4 Percutaneous endoscopic	C Robotic assisted procedure	Z No qualifier
X Upper Extremity Y Lower Extremity	X External	B Computer assisted procedure	F With fluoroscopy G With computerized tomography H With magnetic resonance imaging Z No qualifier
X Upper Extremity Y Lower Extremity	X External	C Robotic assisted procedure	Z No qualifier
X Upper Extremity Y Lower Extremity	X External	Y Other method	8 Suture removal
Z None	X External	Y Other method	1 In vitro fertilization 4 Yoga therapy 5 Meditation 6 Isolation

Educational Annotations | Section 9 – Chiropractic

Section Specific Educational Annotations for the Chiropractic Section include:
- AHA Coding Clinic® Reference Notations
- Coding Notes

AHA Coding Clinic® Reference Notations of Chiropractic

ROOT OPERATION SPECIFIC - CHIROPRACTIC - Section 9
MANIPULATION - B

Coding Notes of Chiropractic

Med/Surg Related Section Specific PCS Reference Manual Exercises

PCS CODE	9 – CHIROPRACTIC EXERCISES
9WB0XKZ	Mechanically-assisted chiropractic manipulation of head.
9WB3XGZ	Chiropractic treatment of lumbar region using long lever specific contact.
9WB4XJZ	Chiropractic treatment of sacrum using long and short lever specific contact.
9WB6XDZ	Chiropractic extra-articular treatment of hip region.
9WB9XCZ	Chiropractic manipulation of abdominal region, indirect visceral.

Educational Annotations | Section 9 – Chiropractic

NOTES

CHIROPRACTIC SECTION: Manipulation
Root Operation that defines chiropractic procedures.

- 1ST – **9** Chiropractic
- 2ND – **W** Anatomical Regions
- 3RD – **B** MANIPULATION

EXAMPLE: Chiropractic manipulation of spine

MANIPULATION: Manual procedure that involves a directed thrust to move a joint past the physiological range of motion, without exceeding the anatomical limit.

EXPLANATION: None

Body Region – 4TH	Approach – 5TH	Method – 6TH	Qualifier – 7TH
0 Head	X External	B Non-manual	Z None
1 Cervical		C Indirect visceral	
2 Thoracic		D Extra-articular	
3 Lumbar		F Direct visceral	
4 Sacrum		G Long lever specific contact	
5 Pelvis		H Short lever specific contact	
6 Lower Extremities		J Long and short lever specific contact	
7 Upper Extremities		K Mechanically assisted	
8 Rib Cage		L Other method	
9 Abdomen			

NOTES

9: Chiropractic
W Anatomical Regions
B MANIPULATION

CHIROPRACTIC – Manipulation
Root Operation that defines & represents procedure

EXAMPLE: Chiropractic manipulation of spine

MANIPULATION: Manual procedure that involves a directed thrust to move a joint past the physiological range of motion, without exceeding the anatomical limit.

EXPLANATION: None

Body Region – 4th	Approach – 5th	Method – 6th	Qualifier – 7th
0 Head	X External	B Non-manual	Z None
1 Cervical		C Indirect visceral	
2 Thoracic		D Extra-articular	
3 Lumbar		F Direct visceral	
4 Sacrum		G Long lever specific contact	
5 Pelvis		H Short lever specific contact	
6 Lower Extremities		J Long and short lever specific contact	
7 Upper Extremities		K Mechanically assisted	
8 Rib Cage		L Other method	
9 Abdomen			

Educational Annotations | Section B – Imaging

Section Specific Educational Annotations for the Imaging Section include:
- AHA Coding Clinic® Reference Notations
- Coding Notes

AHA Coding Clinic® Reference Notations of Imaging

ROOT TYPE SPECIFIC - IMAGING - Section B
PLAIN RADIOGRAPHY - 0
FLUOROSCOPY - 1
COMPUTERIZED TOMOGRAPHY (CT SCAN) - 2
MAGNETIC RESONANCE IMAGING (MRI) - 3
ULTRASONOGRAPHY - 4
    Ultrasonic guidance during ERCP ....AHA 14:3Q:p15

Coding Notes of Imaging

Ancillary Section Specific PCS Reference Manual Exercises

PCS CODE	B – IMAGING EXERCISES
B2151ZZ	Left ventriculography using low osmolar contrast.
B342ZZ3	Intravascular ultrasound, left subclavian artery.
B41G1ZZ	Fluoroscopic guidance for percutaneous transluminal angioplasty (PTA) of left common femoral artery, low osmolar contrast.
B5181ZA	Fluoroscopic guidance for insertion of central venous catheter in SVC, low osmolar contrast.
BB240ZZ	CT scan of bilateral lungs, high osmolar contrast with densitometry.
BD11YZZ	Esophageal videofluoroscopy study with oral barium contrast.
BF43ZZZ	Endoluminal ultrasound of gallbladder and bile ducts.
BP0JZZZ	Portable X-ray study of right radius/ulna shaft, standard series.
BW21ZZZ	Non-contrast CT of abdomen and pelvis.
BY4DZZZ	Routine fetal ultrasound, second trimester twin gestation.

Section B – Imaging

Educational Annotations

NOTES

B – IMAGING

B02

1ST – **B** Imaging 2ND – **0** Central Nervous System 3RD – **0 PLAIN RADIOGRAPHY**	EXAMPLE: Chest X-ray **PLAIN RADIOGRAPHY:** Planar display of an image developed from the capture of external ionizing radiation on photographic or photoconductive plate.

Body Part – 4TH	Contrast – 5TH	Qualifier – 6TH	Qualifier – 7TH
B Spinal Cord	0 High osmolar 1 Low osmolar Y Other contrast Z None	Z None	Z None

1ST – **B** Imaging 2ND – **0** Central Nervous System 3RD – **1 FLUOROSCOPY**	EXAMPLE: Fluoroscopic guidance **FLUOROSCOPY:** Single plane or bi-plane real time display of an image developed from the capture of external ionizing radiation on a fluorescent screen. The image may also be stored by either digital or analog means.

Body Part – 4TH	Contrast – 5TH	Qualifier – 6TH	Qualifier – 7TH
B Spinal Cord	0 High osmolar 1 Low osmolar Y Other contrast Z None	Z None	Z None

1ST – **B** Imaging 2ND – **0** Central Nervous System 3RD – **2 COMPUTERIZED TOMOGRAPHY** (CT Scan)	EXAMPLE: CT Scan of head **COMPUTERIZED TOMOGRAPHY (CT Scan):** Computer reformatted digital display of multiplanar images developed from the capture of multiple exposures of external ionizing radiation.

Body Part – 4TH	Contrast – 5TH	Qualifier – 6TH	Qualifier – 7TH
0 Brain 7 Cisterna 8 Cerebral Ventricle(s) 9 Sella Turcica/Pituitary Gland B Spinal Cord	0 High osmolar 1 Low osmolar Y Other contrast	0 Unenhanced and enhanced Z None	Z None
0 Brain 7 Cisterna 8 Cerebral Ventricle(s) 9 Sella Turcica/Pituitary Gland B Spinal Cord	Z None	Z None	Z None

B03 ANCILLARY SECTIONS – 2016 ICD-10-PCS

1ST – B Imaging
2ND – 0 Central Nervous System
3RD – 3 MAGNETIC RESONANCE IMAGING (MRI)

EXAMPLE: MRI of knee

MAGNETIC RESONANCE IMAGING (MRI): Computer reformatted digital display of multiplanar images developed from the capture of radiofrequency signals emitted by nuclei in a body site excited within a magnetic field.

Body Part – 4TH	Contrast – 5TH	Qualifier – 6TH	Qualifier – 7TH
0 Brain 9 Sella Turcica/Pituitary Gland B Spinal Cord C Acoustic Nerves	Y Other contrast	0 Unenhanced and enhanced Z None	Z None
0 Brain 9 Sella Turcica/Pituitary Gland B Spinal Cord C Acoustic Nerves	Z None	Z None	Z None

---

1ST – B Imaging
2ND – 0 Central Nervous System
3RD – 4 ULTRASONOGRAPHY

EXAMPLE: Abdominal ultrasound

ULTRASONOGRAPHY: Real time display of images of anatomy or flow information developed from the capture of reflected and attenuated high frequency sound waves.

Body Part – 4TH	Contrast – 5TH	Qualifier – 6TH	Qualifier – 7TH
0 Brain B Spinal Cord	Z None	Z None	Z None

1ST – B Imaging
2ND – 2 Heart
3RD – 0 PLAIN RADIOGRAPHY

EXAMPLE: Chest X-ray

PLAIN RADIOGRAPHY: Planar display of an image developed from the capture of external ionizing radiation on photographic or photoconductive plate.

Body Part – 4TH	Contrast – 5TH	Qualifier – 6TH	Qualifier – 7TH
0 Coronary Artery, Single 1 Coronary Arteries, Multiple 2 Coronary Artery Bypass Graft, Single 3 Coronary Artery Bypass Grafts, Multiple 4 Heart, Right 5 Heart, Left 6 Heart, Right and Left 7 Internal Mammary Bypass Graft, Right 8 Internal Mammary Bypass Graft, Left F Bypass Graft, Other	0 High osmolar 1 Low osmolar Y Other contrast	Z None	Z None

B – IMAGING

1ST - **B** Imaging 2ND - **2** Heart 3RD - **1** FLUOROSCOPY	EXAMPLE: Fluoroscopic guidance **FLUOROSCOPY:** Single plane or bi-plane real time display of an image developed from the capture of external ionizing radiation on a fluorescent screen. The image may also be stored by either digital or analog means.			
Body Part – 4TH	**Contrast – 5TH**	**Qualifier – 6TH**	**Qualifier – 7TH**	
0 Coronary Artery, Single 1 Coronary Arteries, Multiple 2 Coronary Artery Bypass Graft, Single 3 Coronary Artery Bypass Grafts, Multiple	0 High osmolar 1 Low osmolar Y Other contrast	1 Laser	0 Intraoperative	
0 Coronary Artery, Single 1 Coronary Arteries, Multiple 2 Coronary Artery Bypass Graft, Single 3 Coronary Artery Bypass Grafts, Multiple	0 High osmolar 1 Low osmolar Y Other contrast	Z None	Z None	
4 Heart, Right 5 Heart, Left 6 Heart, Right and Left 7 Internal Mammary Bypass Graft, Right 8 Internal Mammary Bypass Graft, Left F Bypass Graft, Other	0 High osmolar 1 Low osmolar Y Other contrast	Z None	Z None	

1ST - **B** Imaging 2ND - **2** Heart 3RD - **2** COMPUTERIZED TOMOGRAPHY (CT Scan)	EXAMPLE: CT Scan of head **COMPUTERIZED TOMOGRAPHY (CT Scan):** Computer reformatted digital display of multiplanar images developed from the capture of multiple exposures of external ionizing radiation.			
Body Part – 4TH	**Contrast – 5TH**	**Qualifier – 6TH**	**Qualifier – 7TH**	
1 Coronary Arteries, Multiple 3 Coronary Artery Bypass Grafts, Multiple 6 Heart, Right and Left	0 High osmolar 1 Low osmolar Y Other contrast	0 Unenhanced and enhanced Z None	Z None	
1 Coronary Arteries, Multiple 3 Coronary Artery Bypass Grafts, Multiple 6 Heart, Right and Left	Z None	2 Intravascular optical coherence Z None	Z None	

1ST - **B** Imaging 2ND - **2** Heart 3RD - **3** MAGNETIC RESONANCE IMAGING (MRI)	EXAMPLE: MRI of knee **MAGNETIC RESONANCE IMAGING (MRI):** Computer reformatted digital display of multiplanar images developed from the capture of radiofrequency signals emitted by nuclei in a body site excited within a magnetic field.			
Body Part – 4TH	**Contrast – 5TH**	**Qualifier – 6TH**	**Qualifier – 7TH**	
1 Coronary Arteries, Multiple 3 Coronary Artery Bypass Grafts, Multiple 6 Heart, Right and Left	Y Other contrast	0 Unenhanced and enhanced Z None	Z None	
1 Coronary Arteries, Multiple 3 Coronary Artery Bypass Grafts, Multiple 6 Heart, Right and Left	Z None	Z None	Z None	

B24 ANCILLARY SECTIONS – 2016 ICD-10-PCS

1ST - **B** Imaging 2ND - **2** Heart 3RD - **4** ULTRASONOGRAPHY	EXAMPLE: Abdominal ultrasound **ULTRASONOGRAPHY:** Real time display of images of anatomy or flow information developed from the capture of reflected and attenuated high frequency sound waves.		
Body Part – 4TH	**Contrast – 5TH**	**Qualifier – 6TH**	**Qualifier – 7TH**
0 Coronary Artery, Single 1 Coronary Arteries, Multiple 4 Heart, Right 5 Heart, Left 6 Heart, Right and Left B Heart with Aorta C Pericardium D Pediatric Heart	Y Other contrast	Z None	Z None
0 Coronary Artery, Single 1 Coronary Arteries, Multiple 4 Heart, Right 5 Heart, Left 6 Heart, Right and Left B Heart with Aorta C Pericardium D Pediatric Heart	Z None	Z None	3 Intravascular 4 Trans esophageal Z None

1ST - **B** Imaging 2ND - **3** Upper Arteries 3RD - **0** PLAIN RADIOGRAPHY	EXAMPLE: Chest X-ray **PLAIN RADIOGRAPHY:** Planar display of an image developed from the capture of external ionizing radiation on photographic or photoconductive plate.		
Body Part – 4TH	**Contrast – 5TH**	**Qualifier – 6TH**	**Qualifier – 7TH**
0 Thoracic Aorta 1 Brachiocephalic-Subclavian Artery, Right 2 Subclavian Artery, Left 3 Common Carotid Artery, Right 4 Common Carotid Artery, Left 5 Common Carotid Arteries, Bilateral 6 Internal Carotid Artery, Right 7 Internal Carotid Artery, Left 8 Internal Carotid Arteries, Bilateral 9 External Carotid Artery, Right B External Carotid Artery, Left C External Carotid Arteries, Bilateral D Vertebral Artery, Right F Vertebral Artery, Left G Vertebral Arteries, Bilateral H Upper Extremity Arteries, Right J Upper Extremity Arteries, Left K Upper Extremity Arteries, Bilateral L Intercostal and Bronchial Arteries M Spinal Arteries N Upper Arteries, Other P Thoraco-Abdominal Aorta Q Cervico-Cerebral Arch R Intracranial Arteries S Pulmonary Artery, Right T Pulmonary Artery, Left	0 High osmolar 1 Low osmolar Y Other contrast Z None	Z None	Z None

B – IMAGING

B 3 1

1ST - **B** Imaging 2ND - **3** Upper Arteries 3RD - **1** FLUOROSCOPY	EXAMPLE: Fluoroscopic guidance **FLUOROSCOPY:** Single plane or bi-plane real time display of an image developed from the capture of external ionizing radiation on a fluorescent screen. The image may also be stored by either digital or analog means.		
Body Part – 4TH	**Contrast – 5TH**	**Qualifier – 6TH**	**Qualifier – 7TH**
0 Thoracic Aorta 1 Brachiocephalic-Subclavian Artery, Right 2 Subclavian Artery, Left 3 Common Carotid Artery, Right 4 Common Carotid Artery, Left 5 Common Carotid Arteries, Bilateral 6 Internal Carotid Artery, Right 7 Internal Carotid Artery, Left 8 Internal Carotid Arteries, Bilateral 9 External Carotid Artery, Right B External Carotid Artery, Left C External Carotid Arteries, Bilateral D Vertebral Artery, Right F Vertebral Artery, Left G Vertebral Arteries, Bilateral H Upper Extremity Arteries, Right J Upper Extremity Arteries, Left K Upper Extremity Arteries, Bilateral L Intercostal and Bronchial Arteries M Spinal Arteries N Upper Arteries, Other R Intracranial Arteries P Thoraco-Abdominal Aorta S Pulmonary Artery, Right Q Cervico-Cerebral Arch T Pulmonary Artery, Left	0 High osmolar 1 Low osmolar Y Other contrast	1 Laser	0 Intraoperative
0 Thoracic Aorta 1 Brachiocephalic-Subclavian Artery, Right 2 Subclavian Artery, Left 3 Common Carotid Artery, Right 4 Common Carotid Artery, Left 5 Common Carotid Arteries, Bilateral 6 Internal Carotid Artery, Right 7 Internal Carotid Artery, Left 8 Internal Carotid Arteries, Bilateral 9 External Carotid Artery, Right B External Carotid Artery, Left C External Carotid Arteries, Bilateral D Vertebral Artery, Right F Vertebral Artery, Left G Vertebral Arteries, Bilateral H Upper Extremity Arteries, Right J Upper Extremity Arteries, Left K Upper Extremity Arteries, Bilateral L Intercostal and Bronchial Arteries M Spinal Arteries N Upper Arteries, Other R Intracranial Arteries P Thoraco-Abdominal Aorta S Pulmonary Artery, Right Q Cervico-Cerebral Arch T Pulmonary Artery, Left	0 High osmolar 1 Low osmolar Y Other contrast	Z None	Z None

continued ⇨

B31 FLUOROSCOPY—continued

Body Part – 4ᵀᴴ	Contrast – 5ᵀᴴ	Qualifier – 6ᵀᴴ	Qualifier – 7ᵀᴴ
0 Thoracic Aorta	Z None	Z None	Z None
1 Brachiocephalic-Subclavian Artery, Right			
2 Subclavian Artery, Left			
3 Common Carotid Artery, Right			
4 Common Carotid Artery, Left			
5 Common Carotid Arteries, Bilateral			
6 Internal Carotid Artery, Right			
7 Internal Carotid Artery, Left			
8 Internal Carotid Arteries, Bilateral			
9 External Carotid Artery, Right			
B External Carotid Artery, Left			
C External Carotid Arteries, Bilateral			
D Vertebral Artery, Right			
F Vertebral Artery, Left			
G Vertebral Arteries, Bilateral			
H Upper Extremity Arteries, Right			
J Upper Extremity Arteries, Left			
K Upper Extremity Arteries, Bilateral			
L Intercostal and Bronchial Arteries			
M Spinal Arteries			
N Upper Arteries, Other R Intracranial Arteries			
P Thoraco-Abdominal Aorta S Pulmonary Artery, Right			
Q Cervico-Cerebral Arch T Pulmonary Artery, Left			

1ˢᵀ - **B** Imaging
2ᴺᴰ - **3** Upper Arteries
3ᴿᴰ - **2** COMPUTERIZED TOMOGRAPHY (CT Scan)

EXAMPLE: CT Scan of head

COMPUTERIZED TOMOGRAPHY (CT Scan): Computer reformatted digital display of multiplanar images developed from the capture of multiple exposures of external ionizing radiation.

Body Part – 4ᵀᴴ	Contrast – 5ᵀᴴ	Qualifier – 6ᵀᴴ	Qualifier – 7ᵀᴴ
0 Thoracic Aorta	0 High osmolar	Z None	Z None
5 Common Carotid Arteries, Bilateral	1 Low osmolar		
8 Internal Carotid Arteries, Bilateral	Y Other contrast		
G Vertebral Arteries, Bilateral			
R Intracranial Arteries			
S Pulmonary Artery, Right			
T Pulmonary Artery, Left			
0 Thoracic Aorta	Z None	2 Intravascular optical coherence	Z None
5 Common Carotid Arteries, Bilateral		Z None	
8 Internal Carotid Arteries, Bilateral			
G Vertebral Arteries, Bilateral			
R Intracranial Arteries			
S Pulmonary Artery, Right			
T Pulmonary Artery, Left			

B – IMAGING

1ST - **B**	Imaging
2ND - **3**	Upper Arteries
3RD - **3**	**MAGNETIC RESONANCE IMAGING (MRI)**

EXAMPLE: MRI of knee

MAGNETIC RESONANCE IMAGING (MRI): Computer reformatted digital display of multiplanar images developed from the capture of radiofrequency signals emitted by nuclei in a body site excited within a magnetic field.

Body Part – 4TH	Contrast – 5TH	Qualifier – 6TH	Qualifier – 7TH
0 Thoracic Aorta 5 Common Carotid Arteries, Bilateral 8 Internal Carotid Arteries, Bilateral G Vertebral Arteries, Bilateral H Upper Extremity Arteries, Right J Upper Extremity Arteries, Left K Upper Extremity Arteries, Bilateral M Spinal Arteries Q Cervico-Cerebral Arch R Intracranial Arteries	Y Other contrast	0 Unenhanced and enhanced Z None	Z None
0 Thoracic Aorta 5 Common Carotid Arteries, Bilateral 8 Internal Carotid Arteries, Bilateral G Vertebral Arteries, Bilateral H Upper Extremity Arteries, Right J Upper Extremity Arteries, Left K Upper Extremity Arteries, Bilateral M Spinal Arteries Q Cervico-Cerebral Arch R Intracranial Arteries	Z None	Z None	Z None

1ST - **B**	Imaging
2ND - **3**	Upper Arteries
3RD - **4**	**ULTRASONOGRAPHY**

EXAMPLE: Abdominal ultrasound

ULTRASONOGRAPHY: Real time display of images of anatomy or flow information developed from the capture of reflected and attenuated high frequency sound waves.

Body Part – 4TH	Contrast – 5TH	Qualifier – 6TH	Qualifier – 7TH
0 Thoracic Aorta 1 Brachiocephalic-Subclavian Artery, Right 2 Subclavian Artery, Left 3 Common Carotid Artery, Right 4 Common Carotid Artery, Left 5 Common Carotid Arteries, Bilateral 6 Internal Carotid Artery, Right 7 Internal Carotid Artery, Left 8 Internal Carotid Arteries, Bilateral H Upper Extremity Arteries, Right J Upper Extremity Arteries, Left K Upper Extremity Arteries, Bilateral R Intracranial Arteries S Pulmonary Artery, Right T Pulmonary Artery, Left V Ophthalmic Arteries	Z None	Z None	3 Intravascular Z None

B40

ANCILLARY SECTIONS – 2016 ICD-10-PCS

1ST - **B** Imaging
2ND - **4** Lower Arteries
3RD - **0** PLAIN RADIOGRAPHY

EXAMPLE: Chest X-ray

PLAIN RADIOGRAPHY: Planar display of an image developed from the capture of external ionizing radiation on photographic or photoconductive plate.

Body Part – 4TH	Contrast – 5TH	Qualifier – 6TH	Qualifier – 7TH
0 Abdominal Aorta	0 High osmolar	Z None	Z None
2 Hepatic Artery	1 Low osmolar		
3 Splenic Arteries	Y Other contrast		
4 Superior Mesenteric Artery			
5 Inferior Mesenteric Artery			
6 Renal Artery, Right			
7 Renal Artery, Left			
8 Renal Arteries, Bilateral			
9 Lumbar Arteries			
B Intra-Abdominal Arteries, Other			
C Pelvic Arteries			
D Aorta and Bilateral Lower Extremity Arteries			
F Lower Extremity Arteries, Right			
G Lower Extremity Arteries, Left			
J Lower Arteries, Other			
M Renal Artery Transplant			

IMAGING

B40

B – IMAGING

B41

1ST - **B** Imaging
2ND - **4** Lower Arteries
3RD - **1** FLUOROSCOPY

EXAMPLE: Fluoroscopic guidance

FLUOROSCOPY: Single plane or bi-plane real time display of an image developed from the capture of external ionizing radiation on a fluorescent screen. The image may also be stored by either digital or analog means.

Body Part – 4TH	Contrast – 5TH	Qualifier – 6TH	Qualifier – 7TH
0 Abdominal Aorta 2 Hepatic Artery 3 Splenic Arteries 4 Superior Mesenteric Artery 5 Inferior Mesenteric Artery 6 Renal Artery, Right 7 Renal Artery, Left 8 Renal Arteries, Bilateral 9 Lumbar Arteries B Intra-Abdominal Arteries, Other C Pelvic Arteries D Aorta and Bilateral Lower Extremity Arteries F Lower Extremity Arteries, Right G Lower Extremity Arteries, Left J Lower Arteries, Other	0 High osmolar 1 Low osmolar Y Other contrast	1 Laser	0 Intraoperative
0 Abdominal Aorta 2 Hepatic Artery 3 Splenic Arteries 4 Superior Mesenteric Artery 5 Inferior Mesenteric Artery 6 Renal Artery, Right 7 Renal Artery, Left 8 Renal Arteries, Bilateral 9 Lumbar Arteries B Intra-Abdominal Arteries, Other C Pelvic Arteries D Aorta and Bilateral Lower Extremity Arteries F Lower Extremity Arteries, Right G Lower Extremity Arteries, Left J Lower Arteries, Other	0 High osmolar 1 Low osmolar Y Other contrast	Z None	Z None
0 Abdominal Aorta 2 Hepatic Artery 3 Splenic Arteries 4 Superior Mesenteric Artery 5 Inferior Mesenteric Artery 6 Renal Artery, Right 7 Renal Artery, Left 8 Renal Arteries, Bilateral 9 Lumbar Arteries B Intra-Abdominal Arteries, Other C Pelvic Arteries D Aorta and Bilateral Lower Extremity Arteries F Lower Extremity Arteries, Right G Lower Extremity Arteries, Left J Lower Arteries, Other	Z None	Z None	Z None

ANCILLARY SECTIONS – 2016 ICD-10-PCS

B42

1ST – B Imaging
2ND – 4 Lower Arteries
3RD – 2 COMPUTERIZED TOMOGRAPHY (CT Scan)

EXAMPLE: CT Scan of head

COMPUTERIZED TOMOGRAPHY (CT Scan): Computer reformatted digital display of multiplanar images developed from the capture of multiple exposures of external ionizing radiation.

Body Part – 4TH	Contrast – 5TH	Qualifier – 6TH	Qualifier – 7TH
0 Abdominal Aorta 1 Celiac Artery 4 Superior Mesenteric Artery 8 Renal Arteries, Bilateral C Pelvic Arteries F Lower Extremity Arteries, Right G Lower Extremity Arteries, Left H Lower Extremity Arteries, Bilateral M Renal Artery Transplant	0 High osmolar 1 Low osmolar Y Other contrast	Z None	Z None
0 Abdominal Aorta 1 Celiac Artery 4 Superior Mesenteric Artery 8 Renal Arteries, Bilateral C Pelvic Arteries F Lower Extremity Arteries, Right G Lower Extremity Arteries, Left H Lower Extremity Arteries, Bilateral M Renal Artery Transplant	Z None	2 Intravascular optical coherence Z None	Z None

1ST – B Imaging
2ND – 4 Lower Arteries
3RD – 3 MAGNETIC RESONANCE IMAGING (MRI)

EXAMPLE: MRI of knee

MAGNETIC RESONANCE IMAGING (MRI): Computer reformatted digital display of multiplanar images developed from the capture of radiofrequency signals emitted by nuclei in a body site excited within a magnetic field.

Body Part – 4TH	Contrast – 5TH	Qualifier – 6TH	Qualifier – 7TH
0 Abdominal Aorta 1 Celiac Artery 4 Superior Mesenteric Artery 8 Renal Arteries, Bilateral C Pelvic Arteries F Lower Extremity Arteries, Right G Lower Extremity Arteries, Left H Lower Extremity Arteries, Bilateral	Y Other contrast	0 Unenhanced and enhanced Z None	Z None
0 Abdominal Aorta 1 Celiac Artery 4 Superior Mesenteric Artery 8 Renal Arteries, Bilateral C Pelvic Arteries F Lower Extremity Arteries, Right G Lower Extremity Arteries, Left H Lower Extremity Arteries, Bilateral	Z None	Z None	Z None

B – IMAGING

B50

1ST - **B** Imaging
2ND - **4** Lower Arteries
3RD - **4** ULTRASONOGRAPHY

EXAMPLE: Abdominal ultrasound

ULTRASONOGRAPHY: Real time display of images of anatomy or flow information developed from the capture of reflected and attenuated high frequency sound waves.

Body Part – 4TH	Contrast – 5TH	Qualifier – 6TH	Qualifier – 7TH
0 Abdominal Aorta 4 Superior Mesenteric Artery 5 Inferior Mesenteric Artery 6 Renal Artery, Right 7 Renal Artery, Left 8 Renal Arteries, Bilateral B Intra-Abdominal Arteries, Other F Lower Extremity Arteries, Right G Lower Extremity Arteries, Left H Lower Extremity Arteries, Bilateral K Celiac and Mesenteric Arteries L Femoral Artery N Penile Arteries	Z None	Z None	3 Intravascular Z None

1ST - **B** Imaging
2ND - **5** Veins
3RD - **0** PLAIN RADIOGRAPHY

EXAMPLE: Chest X-ray

PLAIN RADIOGRAPHY: Planar display of an image developed from the capture of external ionizing radiation on photographic or photoconductive plate.

Body Part – 4TH		Contrast – 5TH	Qualifier – 6TH	Qualifier – 7TH
0 Epidural Veins 1 Cerebral and Cerebellar Veins 2 Intracranial Sinuses 3 Jugular Veins, Right 4 Jugular Veins, Left 5 Jugular Veins, Bilateral 6 Subclavian Vein, Right 7 Subclavian Vein, Left 8 Superior Vena Cava 9 Inferior Vena Cava B Lower Extremity Veins, Right C Lower Extremity Veins, Left D Lower Extremity Veins, Bilateral F Pelvic (Iliac) Veins, Right	G Pelvic (Iliac) Veins, Left H Pelvic (Iliac) Veins, Bilateral J Renal Vein, Right K Renal Vein, Left L Renal Veins, Bilateral M Upper Extremity Veins, Right N Upper Extremity Veins, Left P Upper Extremity Veins, Bilateral Q Pulmonary Vein, Right R Pulmonary Vein, Left S Pulmonary Veins, Bilateral T Portal and Splanchnic Veins V Veins, Other W Dialysis Shunt/Fistula	0 High osmolar 1 Low osmolar Y Other contrast	Z None	Z None

B51 ANCILLARY SECTIONS – 2016 ICD-10-PCS [2016.PCS]

Fluoroscopy

- 1ST – **B** Imaging
- 2ND – **5** Veins
- 3RD – **1 FLUOROSCOPY**

EXAMPLE: Fluoroscopic guidance

FLUOROSCOPY: Single plane or bi-plane real time display of an image developed from the capture of external ionizing radiation on a fluorescent screen. The image may also be stored by either digital or analog means.

Body Part – 4TH	Contrast – 5TH	Qualifier – 6TH	Qualifier – 7TH
0 Epidural Veins 1 Cerebral and Cerebellar Veins 2 Intracranial Sinuses 3 Jugular Veins, Right 4 Jugular Veins, Left 5 Jugular Veins, Bilateral 6 Subclavian Vein, Right 7 Subclavian Vein, Left 8 Superior Vena Cava 9 Inferior Vena Cava B Lower Extremity Veins, Right C Lower Extremity Veins, Left D Lower Extremity Veins, Bilateral F Pelvic (Iliac) Veins, Right G Pelvic (Iliac) Veins, Left H Pelvic (Iliac) Veins, Bilateral J Renal Vein, Right K Renal Vein, Left L Renal Veins, Bilateral M Upper Extremity Veins, Right N Upper Extremity Veins, Left P Upper Extremity Veins, Bilateral Q Pulmonary Vein, Right R Pulmonary Vein, Left S Pulmonary Veins, Bilateral T Portal and Splanchnic Veins V Veins, Other W Dialysis Shunt/Fistula	0 High osmolar 1 Low osmolar Y Other contrast Z None	Z None	A Guidance Z None

Computerized Tomography

- 1ST – **B** Imaging
- 2ND – **5** Veins
- 3RD – **2 COMPUTERIZED TOMOGRAPHY (CT Scan)**

EXAMPLE: CT Scan of head

COMPUTERIZED TOMOGRAPHY (CT Scan): Computer reformatted digital display of multiplanar images developed from the capture of multiple exposures of external ionizing radiation.

Body Part – 4TH	Contrast – 5TH	Qualifier – 6TH	Qualifier – 7TH
2 Intracranial Sinuses 8 Superior Vena Cava 9 Inferior Vena Cava F Pelvic (Iliac) Veins, Right G Pelvic (Iliac) Veins, Left H Pelvic (Iliac) Veins, Bilateral J Renal Vein, Right K Renal Vein, Left L Renal Veins, Bilateral Q Pulmonary Vein, Right R Pulmonary Vein, Left S Pulmonary Veins, Bilateral T Portal and Splanchnic Veins	0 High osmolar 1 Low osmolar Y Other contrast	0 Unenhanced and enhanced Z None	Z None
2 Intracranial Sinuses 8 Superior Vena Cava 9 Inferior Vena Cava F Pelvic (Iliac) Veins, Right G Pelvic (Iliac) Veins, Left H Pelvic (Iliac) Veins, Bilateral J Renal Vein, Right K Renal Vein, Left L Renal Veins, Bilateral Q Pulmonary Vein, Right R Pulmonary Vein, Left S Pulmonary Veins, Bilateral T Portal and Splanchnic Veins	Z None	2 Intravascular optical coherence Z None	Z None

B – IMAGING

1ST - **B** Imaging	EXAMPLE: MRI of knee
2ND - **5** Veins	**MAGNETIC RESONANCE IMAGING (MRI):** Computer reformatted digital display of multiplanar images developed from the capture of radiofrequency signals emitted by nuclei in a body site excited within a magnetic field.
3RD - **3** MAGNETIC RESONANCE IMAGING (MRI)	

Body Part – 4TH		Contrast – 5TH	Qualifier – 6TH	Qualifier – 7TH
1 Cerebral and Cerebellar Veins 2 Intracranial Sinuses 5 Jugular Veins, Bilateral 8 Superior Vena Cava 9 Inferior Vena Cava B Lower Extremity Veins, Right C Lower Extremity Veins, Left D Lower Extremity Veins, Bilateral	H Pelvic (Iliac) Veins, Bilateral L Renal Veins, Bilateral M Upper Extremity Veins, Right N Upper Extremity Veins, Left P Upper Extremity Veins, Bilateral S Pulmonary Veins, Bilateral T Portal and Splanchnic Veins V Veins, Other	Y Other contrast	0 Unenhanced and enhanced Z None	Z None
1 Cerebral and Cerebellar Veins 2 Intracranial Sinuses 5 Jugular Veins, Bilateral 8 Superior Vena Cava 9 Inferior Vena Cava B Lower Extremity Veins, Right C Lower Extremity Veins, Left D Lower Extremity Veins, Bilateral	H Pelvic (Iliac) Veins, Bilateral L Renal Veins, Bilateral M Upper Extremity Veins, Right N Upper Extremity Veins, Left P Upper Extremity Veins, Bilateral S Pulmonary Veins, Bilateral T Portal and Splanchnic Veins V Veins, Other	Z None	Z None	Z None

1ST - **B** Imaging	EXAMPLE: Abdominal ultrasound
2ND - **5** Veins	**ULTRASONOGRAPHY:** Real time display of images of anatomy or flow information developed from the capture of reflected and attenuated high frequency sound waves.
3RD - **4** ULTRASONOGRAPHY	

Body Part – 4TH		Contrast – 5TH	Qualifier – 6TH	Qualifier – 7TH
3 Jugular Veins, Right 4 Jugular Veins, Left 6 Subclavian Vein, Right 7 Subclavian Vein, Left 8 Superior Vena Cava 9 Inferior Vena Cava B Lower Extremity Veins, Right C Lower Extremity Veins, Left	D Lower Extremity Veins, Bilateral J Renal Vein, Right K Renal Vein, Left L Renal Veins, Bilateral M Upper Extremity Veins, Right N Upper Extremity Veins, Left P Upper Extremity Veins, Bilateral T Portal and Splanchnic Veins	Z None	Z None	3 Intravascular A Guidance Z None

B70

Imaging — Lymphatic System — Plain Radiography

- 1ST – **B** Imaging
- 2ND – **7** Lymphatic System
- 3RD – **0** PLAIN RADIOGRAPHY

EXAMPLE: Chest X-ray

PLAIN RADIOGRAPHY: Planar display of an image developed from the capture of external ionizing radiation on photographic or photoconductive plate.

Body Part – 4TH	Contrast – 5TH	Qualifier – 6TH	Qualifier – 7TH
0 Abdominal/Retroperitoneal Lymphatics, Unilateral 1 Abdominal/Retroperitoneal Lymphatics, Bilateral 4 Lymphatics, Head and Neck 5 Upper Extremity Lymphatics, Right 6 Upper Extremity Lymphatics, Left 7 Upper Extremity Lymphatics, Bilateral 8 Lower Extremity Lymphatics, Right 9 Lower Extremity Lymphatics, Left B Lower Extremity Lymphatics, Bilateral C Lymphatics, Pelvic	0 High osmolar 1 Low osmolar Y Other contrast	Z None	Z None

Imaging — Eye — Plain Radiography

- 1ST – **B** Imaging
- 2ND – **8** Eye
- 3RD – **0** PLAIN RADIOGRAPHY

EXAMPLE: Chest X-ray

PLAIN RADIOGRAPHY: Planar display of an image developed from the capture of external ionizing radiation on photographic or photoconductive plate.

Body Part – 4TH	Contrast – 5TH	Qualifier – 6TH	Qualifier – 7TH
0 Lacrimal Duct, Right 1 Lacrimal Duct, Left 2 Lacrimal Ducts, Bilateral	0 High osmolar 1 Low osmolar Y Other contrast	Z None	Z None
3 Optic Foramina, Right 4 Optic Foramina, Left 5 Eye, Right 6 Eye, Left 7 Eyes, Bilateral	Z None	Z None	Z None

Imaging — Eye — Computerized Tomography (CT Scan)

- 1ST – **B** Imaging
- 2ND – **8** Eye
- 3RD – **2** COMPUTERIZED TOMOGRAPHY (CT Scan)

EXAMPLE: CT Scan of head

COMPUTERIZED TOMOGRAPHY (CT Scan): Computer reformatted digital display of multiplanar images developed from the capture of multiple exposures of external ionizing radiation.

Body Part – 4TH	Contrast – 5TH	Qualifier – 6TH	Qualifier – 7TH
5 Eye, Right 6 Eye, Left 7 Eyes, Bilateral	0 High osmolar 1 Low osmolar Y Other contrast	0 Unenhanced and enhanced Z None	Z None
5 Eye, Right 6 Eye, Left 7 Eyes, Bilateral	Z None	Z None	Z None

B – IMAGING

B90

1ST - B	Imaging			
2ND - 8	Eye			
3RD - 3	MAGNETIC RESONANCE IMAGING (MRI)			

EXAMPLE: MRI of knee

MAGNETIC RESONANCE IMAGING (MRI): Computer reformatted digital display of multiplanar images developed from the capture of radiofrequency signals emitted by nuclei in a body site excited within a magnetic field.

Body Part – 4TH	Contrast – 5TH	Qualifier – 6TH	Qualifier – 7TH
5 Eye, Right 6 Eye, Left 7 Eyes, Bilateral	Y Other contrast	0 Unenhanced and enhanced Z None	Z None
5 Eye, Right 6 Eye, Left 7 Eyes, Bilateral	Z None	Z None	Z None

1ST - B	Imaging
2ND - 8	Eye
3RD - 4	ULTRASONOGRAPHY

EXAMPLE: Abdominal ultrasound

ULTRASONOGRAPHY: Real time display of images of anatomy or flow information developed from the capture of reflected and attenuated high frequency sound waves.

Body Part – 4TH	Contrast – 5TH	Qualifier – 6TH	Qualifier – 7TH
5 Eye, Right 6 Eye, Left 7 Eyes, Bilateral	Z None	Z None	Z None

1ST - B	Imaging
2ND - 9	Ear, Nose, Mouth and Throat
3RD - 0	PLAIN RADIOGRAPHY

EXAMPLE: Chest X-ray

PLAIN RADIOGRAPHY: Planar display of an image developed from the capture of external ionizing radiation on photographic or photoconductive plate.

Body Part – 4TH	Contrast – 5TH	Qualifier – 6TH	Qualifier – 7TH
2 Paranasal Sinuses F Nasopharynx/Oropharynx H Mastoids	Z None	Z None	Z None
4 Parotid Gland, Right 5 Parotid Gland, Left 6 Parotid Glands, Bilateral 7 Submandibular Gland, Right 8 Submandibular Gland, Left 9 Submandibular Glands, Bilateral B Salivary Gland, Right C Salivary Gland, Left D Salivary Glands, Bilateral	0 High osmolar 1 Low osmolar Y Other contrast	Z None	Z None

B91 ANCILLARY SECTIONS – 2016 ICD-10-PCS [2016.PCS]

1ST – **B** Imaging 2ND – **9** Ear, Nose, Mouth and Throat 3RD – **1** FLUOROSCOPY	EXAMPLE: Fluoroscopic guidance **FLUOROSCOPY:** Single plane or bi-plane real time display of an image developed from the capture of external ionizing radiation on a fluorescent screen. The image may also be stored by either digital or analog means.		
Body Part – 4TH	**Contrast – 5TH**	**Qualifier – 6TH**	**Qualifier – 7TH**
G Pharynx and Epiglottis J Larynx	Y Other contrast Z None	Z None	Z None

1ST – **B** Imaging 2ND – **9** Ear, Nose, Mouth and Throat 3RD – **2** COMPUTERIZED TOMOGRAPHY (CT Scan)	EXAMPLE: CT Scan of head **COMPUTERIZED TOMOGRAPHY (CT Scan):** Computer reformatted digital display of multiplanar images developed from the capture of multiple exposures of external ionizing radiation.		
Body Part – 4TH	**Contrast – 5TH**	**Qualifier – 6TH**	**Qualifier – 7TH**
0 Ear 2 Paranasal Sinuses 6 Parotid Glands, Bilateral 9 Submandibular Glands, Bilateral D Salivary Glands, Bilateral F Nasopharynx/Oropharynx J Larynx	0 High osmolar 1 Low osmolar Y Other contrast	0 Unenhanced and enhanced Z None	Z None
0 Ear 2 Paranasal Sinuses 6 Parotid Glands, Bilateral 9 Submandibular Glands, Bilateral D Salivary Glands, Bilateral F Nasopharynx/Oropharynx J Larynx	Z None	Z None	Z None

1ST – **B** Imaging 2ND – **9** Ear, Nose, Mouth and Throat 3RD – **3** MAGNETIC RESONANCE IMAGING (MRI)	EXAMPLE: MRI of knee **MAGNETIC RESONANCE IMAGING (MRI):** Computer reformatted digital display of multiplanar images developed from the capture of radiofrequency signals emitted by nuclei in a body site excited within a magnetic field.		
Body Part – 4TH	**Contrast – 5TH**	**Qualifier – 6TH**	**Qualifier – 7TH**
0 Ear 2 Paranasal Sinuses 6 Parotid Glands, Bilateral 9 Submandibular Glands, Bilateral D Salivary Glands, Bilateral F Nasopharynx/Oropharynx J Larynx	Y Other contrast	0 Unenhanced and enhanced Z None	Z None
0 Ear 2 Paranasal Sinuses 6 Parotid Glands, Bilateral 9 Submandibular Glands, Bilateral D Salivary Glands, Bilateral F Nasopharynx/Oropharynx J Larynx	Z None	Z None	Z None

B – IMAGING

BB2

1ST - **B** Imaging 2ND - **B** Respiratory System 3RD - **0** PLAIN RADIOGRAPHY	EXAMPLE: Chest X-ray **PLAIN RADIOGRAPHY:** Planar display of an image developed from the capture of external ionizing radiation on photographic or photoconductive plate.

Body Part – 4TH	Contrast – 5TH	Qualifier – 6TH	Qualifier – 7TH
7 Tracheobronchial Tree, Right 8 Tracheobronchial Tree, Left 9 Tracheobronchial Trees, Bilateral	Y Other contrast	Z None	Z None
D Upper Airways	Z None	Z None	Z None

1ST - **B** Imaging 2ND - **B** Respiratory System 3RD - **1** FLUOROSCOPY	EXAMPLE: Fluoroscopic guidance **FLUOROSCOPY:** Single plane or bi-plane real time display of an image developed from the capture of external ionizing radiation on a fluorescent screen. The image may also be stored by either digital or analog means.

Body Part – 4TH	Contrast – 5TH	Qualifier – 6TH	Qualifier – 7TH
2 Lung, Right 3 Lung, Left 4 Lungs, Bilateral 6 Diaphragm C Mediastinum D Upper Airways	Z None	Z None	Z None
7 Tracheobronchial Tree, Right 8 Tracheobronchial Tree, Left 9 Tracheobronchial Trees, Bilateral	Y Other contrast	Z None	Z None

1ST - **B** Imaging 2ND - **B** Respiratory System 3RD - **2** COMPUTERIZED TOMOGRAPHY (CT Scan)	EXAMPLE: CT Scan of head **COMPUTERIZED TOMOGRAPHY (CT Scan):** Computer reformatted digital display of multiplanar images developed from the capture of multiple exposures of external ionizing radiation.

Body Part – 4TH	Contrast – 5TH	Qualifier – 6TH	Qualifier – 7TH
4 Lungs, Bilateral 7 Tracheobronchial Tree, Right 8 Tracheobronchial Tree, Left 9 Tracheobronchial Trees, Bilateral F Trachea/Airways	0 High osmolar 1 Low osmolar Y Other contrast	0 Unenhanced and enhanced Z None	Z None
4 Lungs, Bilateral 7 Tracheobronchial Tree, Right 8 Tracheobronchial Tree, Left 9 Tracheobronchial Trees, Bilateral F Trachea/Airways	Z None	Z None	Z None

BB3 ANCILLARY SECTIONS – 2016 ICD-10-PCS [2016.PCS]

1ST – **B** Imaging 2ND – **B** Respiratory System 3RD – **3** MAGNETIC RESONANCE IMAGING (MRI)	EXAMPLE: MRI of knee **MAGNETIC RESONANCE IMAGING (MRI):** Computer reformatted digital display of multiplanar images developed from the capture of radiofrequency signals emitted by nuclei in a body site excited within a magnetic field.		
Body Part – 4TH	**Contrast – 5TH**	**Qualifier – 6TH**	**Qualifier – 7TH**
G Lung Apices	Y Other contrast	0 Unenhanced and enhanced Z None	Z None
G Lung Apices	Z None	Z None	Z None

1ST – **B** Imaging 2ND – **B** Respiratory System 3RD – **4** ULTRASONOGRAPHY	EXAMPLE: Abdominal ultrasound **ULTRASONOGRAPHY:** Real time display of images of anatomy or flow information developed from the capture of reflected and attenuated high frequency sound waves.		
Body Part – 4TH	**Contrast – 5TH**	**Qualifier – 6TH**	**Qualifier – 7TH**
B Pleura C Mediastinum	Z None	Z None	Z None

1ST – **B** Imaging 2ND – **D** Gastrointestinal System 3RD – **1** FLUOROSCOPY	EXAMPLE: Fluoroscopic guidance **FLUOROSCOPY:** Single plane or bi-plane real time display of an image developed from the capture of external ionizing radiation on a fluorescent screen. The image may also be stored by either digital or analog means.		
Body Part – 4TH	**Contrast – 5TH**	**Qualifier – 6TH**	**Qualifier – 7TH**
1 Esophagus 5 Upper GI 2 Stomach 6 Upper GI and Small Bowel 3 Small Bowel 9 Duodenum 4 Colon B Mouth/Oropharynx	Y Other contrast Z None	Z None	Z None

B – IMAGING

BF0

1ST - **B** Imaging 2ND - **D** Gastrointestinal System 3RD - **2** COMPUTERIZED TOMOGRAPHY (CT Scan)	EXAMPLE: CT Scan of head **COMPUTERIZED TOMOGRAPHY (CT Scan):** Computer reformatted digital display of multiplanar images developed from the capture of multiple exposures of external ionizing radiation.		
Body Part – 4TH	**Contrast – 5TH**	**Qualifier – 6TH**	**Qualifier – 7TH**
4 Colon	0 High osmolar 1 Low osmolar Y Other contrast	0 Unenhanced and enhanced Z None	Z None
4 Colon	Z None	Z None	Z None

1ST - **B** Imaging 2ND - **D** Gastrointestinal System 3RD - **4** ULTRASONOGRAPHY	EXAMPLE: Abdominal ultrasound **ULTRASONOGRAPHY:** Real time display of images of anatomy or flow information developed from the capture of reflected and attenuated high frequency sound waves.		
Body Part – 4TH	**Contrast – 5TH**	**Qualifier – 6TH**	**Qualifier – 7TH**
1 Esophagus 2 Stomach 7 Gastrointestinal Tract 8 Appendix 9 Duodenum C Rectum	Z None	Z None	Z None

1ST - **B** Imaging 2ND - **F** Hepatobiliary System and Pancreas 3RD - **0** PLAIN RADIOGRAPHY	EXAMPLE: Chest X-ray **PLAIN RADIOGRAPHY:** Planar display of an image developed from the capture of external ionizing radiation on photographic or photoconductive plate.		
Body Part – 4TH	**Contrast – 5TH**	**Qualifier – 6TH**	**Qualifier – 7TH**
0 Bile Ducts 3 Gallbladder and Bile Ducts C Hepatobiliary System, All	0 High osmolar 1 Low osmolar Y Other contrast	Z None	Z None

BF1

B F 1 — FLUOROSCOPY

- 1ST – **B** Imaging
- 2ND – **F** Hepatobiliary System and Pancreas
- 3RD – **1** FLUOROSCOPY

EXAMPLE: Fluoroscopic guidance

FLUOROSCOPY: Single plane or bi-plane real time display of an image developed from the capture of external ionizing radiation on a fluorescent screen. The image may also be stored by either digital or analog means.

Body Part – 4TH	Contrast – 5TH	Qualifier – 6TH	Qualifier – 7TH
0 Bile Ducts 1 Biliary and Pancreatic Ducts 2 Gallbladder 3 Gallbladder and Bile Ducts 4 Gallbladder, Bile Ducts and Pancreatic Ducts 8 Pancreatic Ducts	0 High osmolar 1 Low osmolar Y Other contrast	Z None	Z None

B F 2 — COMPUTERIZED TOMOGRAPHY (CT Scan)

- 1ST – **B** Imaging
- 2ND – **F** Hepatobiliary System and Pancreas
- 3RD – **2** COMPUTERIZED TOMOGRAPHY (CT Scan)

EXAMPLE: CT Scan of head

COMPUTERIZED TOMOGRAPHY (CT Scan): Computer reformatted digital display of multiplanar images developed from the capture of multiple exposures of external ionizing radiation.

Body Part – 4TH	Contrast – 5TH	Qualifier – 6TH	Qualifier – 7TH
5 Liver 6 Liver and Spleen 7 Pancreas C Hepatobiliary System, All	0 High osmolar 1 Low osmolar Y Other contrast	0 Unenhanced and enhanced Z None	Z None
5 Liver 6 Liver and Spleen 7 Pancreas C Hepatobiliary System, All	Z None	Z None	Z None

B F 3 — MAGNETIC RESONANCE IMAGING (MRI)

- 1ST – **B** Imaging
- 2ND – **F** Hepatobiliary System and Pancreas
- 3RD – **3** MAGNETIC RESONANCE IMAGING (MRI)

EXAMPLE: MRI of knee

MAGNETIC RESONANCE IMAGING (MRI): Computer reformatted digital display of multiplanar images developed from the capture of radiofrequency signals emitted by nuclei in a body site excited within a magnetic field.

Body Part – 4TH	Contrast – 5TH	Qualifier – 6TH	Qualifier – 7TH
5 Liver 6 Liver and Spleen 7 Pancreas	Y Other contrast	0 Unenhanced and enhanced Z None	Z None
5 Liver 6 Liver and Spleen 7 Pancreas	Z None	Z None	Z None

B – IMAGING

1ST - **B** Imaging 2ND - **F** Hepatobiliary System and Pancreas 3RD - **4** ULTRASONOGRAPHY	EXAMPLE: Abdominal ultrasound **ULTRASONOGRAPHY:** Real time display of images of anatomy or flow information developed from the capture of reflected and attenuated high frequency sound waves.		
Body Part – 4TH	**Contrast – 5TH**	**Qualifier – 6TH**	**Qualifier – 7TH**
0 Bile Ducts 2 Gallbladder 3 Gallbladder and Bile Ducts 5 Liver 6 Liver and Spleen 7 Pancreas C Hepatobiliary System, All	Z None	Z None	Z None

1ST - **B** Imaging 2ND - **G** Endocrine System 3RD - **2** COMPUTERIZED TOMOGRAPHY (CT Scan)	EXAMPLE: CT Scan of head **COMPUTERIZED TOMOGRAPHY (CT Scan):** Computer reformatted digital display of multiplanar images developed from the capture of multiple exposures of external ionizing radiation.		
Body Part – 4TH	**Contrast – 5TH**	**Qualifier – 6TH**	**Qualifier – 7TH**
2 Adrenal Glands, Bilateral 3 Parathyroid Glands 4 Thyroid Gland	0 High osmolar 1 Low osmolar Y Other contrast	0 Unenhanced and enhanced Z None	Z None
2 Adrenal Glands, Bilateral 3 Parathyroid Glands 4 Thyroid Gland	Z None	Z None	Z None

1ST - **B** Imaging 2ND - **G** Endocrine System 3RD - **3** MAGNETIC RESONANCE IMAGING (MRI)	EXAMPLE: MRI of knee **MAGNETIC RESONANCE IMAGING (MRI):** Computer reformatted digital display of multiplanar images developed from the capture of radiofrequency signals emitted by nuclei in a body site excited within a magnetic field.		
Body Part – 4TH	**Contrast – 5TH**	**Qualifier – 6TH**	**Qualifier – 7TH**
2 Adrenal Glands, Bilateral 3 Parathyroid Glands 4 Thyroid Gland	Y Other contrast	0 Unenhanced and enhanced Z None	Z None
2 Adrenal Glands, Bilateral 3 Parathyroid Glands 4 Thyroid Gland	Z None	Z None	Z None

BG4

ANCILLARY SECTIONS – 2016 ICD-10-PCS

1ST - B Imaging
2ND - G Endocrine System
3RD - 4 ULTRASONOGRAPHY

EXAMPLE: Abdominal ultrasound

ULTRASONOGRAPHY: Real time display of images of anatomy or flow information developed from the capture of reflected and attenuated high frequency sound waves.

Body Part – 4TH	Contrast – 5TH	Qualifier – 6TH	Qualifier – 7TH
0 Adrenal Gland, Right 1 Adrenal Gland, Left 2 Adrenal Glands, Bilateral 3 Parathyroid Glands 4 Thyroid Gland	Z None	Z None	Z None

---

1ST - B Imaging
2ND - H Skin, Subcutaneous Tissue and Breast
3RD - 0 PLAIN RADIOGRAPHY

EXAMPLE: Chest X-ray

PLAIN RADIOGRAPHY: Planar display of an image developed from the capture of external ionizing radiation on photographic or photoconductive plate.

Body Part – 4TH	Contrast – 5TH	Qualifier – 6TH	Qualifier – 7TH
0 Breast, Right 1 Breast, Left 2 Breasts, Bilateral	Z None	Z None	Z None
3 Single Mammary Duct, Right 4 Single Mammary Duct, Left 5 Multiple Mammary Ducts, Right 6 Multiple Mammary Ducts, Left	0 High osmolar 1 Low osmolar Y Other contrast Z None	Z None	Z None

B – IMAGING

BH4

1ST - **B** Imaging	EXAMPLE: MRI of knee
2ND - **H** Skin, Subcutaneous Tissue and Breast	**MAGNETIC RESONANCE IMAGING (MRI):** Computer reformatted digital display of multiplanar images developed from the capture of radiofrequency signals emitted by nuclei in a body site excited within a magnetic field.
3RD - **3** MAGNETIC RESONANCE IMAGING (MRI)	

Body Part – 4TH	Contrast – 5TH	Qualifier – 6TH	Qualifier – 7TH
0 Breast, Right 1 Breast, Left 2 Breasts, Bilateral D Subcutaneous Tissue, Head/Neck F Subcutaneous Tissue, Upper Extremity G Subcutaneous Tissue, Thorax H Subcutaneous Tissue, Abdomen and Pelvis J Subcutaneous Tissue, Lower Extremity	Y Other contrast	0 Unenhanced and enhanced Z None	Z None
0 Breast, Right 1 Breast, Left 2 Breasts, Bilateral D Subcutaneous Tissue, Head/Neck F Subcutaneous Tissue, Upper Extremity G Subcutaneous Tissue, Thorax H Subcutaneous Tissue, Abdomen and Pelvis J Subcutaneous Tissue, Lower Extremity	Z None	Z None	Z None

1ST - **B** Imaging	EXAMPLE: Abdominal ultrasound
2ND - **H** Skin, Subcutaneous Tissue and Breast	**ULTRASONOGRAPHY:** Real time display of images of anatomy or flow information developed from the capture of reflected and attenuated high frequency sound waves.
3RD - **4** ULTRASONOGRAPHY	

Body Part – 4TH		Contrast – 5TH	Qualifier – 6TH	Qualifier – 7TH
0 Breast, Right 1 Breast, Left 2 Breasts, Bilateral 7 Extremity, Upper	8 Extremity, Lower 9 Abdominal Wall B Chest Wall C Head and Neck	Z None	Z None	Z None

B L 3

MRI - Connective Tissue

- 1ST – **B** Imaging
- 2ND – **L** Connective Tissue
- 3RD – **3** MAGNETIC RESONANCE IMAGING (MRI)

EXAMPLE: MRI of knee

MAGNETIC RESONANCE IMAGING (MRI): Computer reformatted digital display of multiplanar images developed from the capture of radiofrequency signals emitted by nuclei in a body site excited within a magnetic field.

Body Part – 4TH	Contrast – 5TH	Qualifier – 6TH	Qualifier – 7TH
0 Connective Tissue, Upper Extremity 1 Connective Tissue, Lower Extremity 2 Tendons, Upper Extremity 3 Tendons, Lower Extremity	Y Other contrast	0 Unenhanced and enhanced Z None	Z None
0 Connective Tissue, Upper Extremity 1 Connective Tissue, Lower Extremity 2 Tendons, Upper Extremity 3 Tendons, Lower Extremity	Z None	Z None	Z None

Ultrasonography - Connective Tissue

- 1ST – **B** Imaging
- 2ND – **L** Connective Tissue
- 3RD – **4** ULTRASONOGRAPHY

EXAMPLE: Abdominal ultrasound

ULTRASONOGRAPHY: Real time display of images of anatomy or flow information developed from the capture of reflected and attenuated high frequency sound waves.

Body Part – 4TH	Contrast – 5TH	Qualifier – 6TH	Qualifier – 7TH
0 Connective Tissue, Upper Extremity 1 Connective Tissue, Lower Extremity 2 Tendons, Upper Extremity 3 Tendons, Lower Extremity	Z None	Z None	Z None

Plain Radiography - Skull and Facial Bones

- 1ST – **B** Imaging
- 2ND – **N** Skull and Facial Bones
- 3RD – **0** PLAIN RADIOGRAPHY

EXAMPLE: Chest X-ray

PLAIN RADIOGRAPHY: Planar display of an image developed from the capture of external ionizing radiation on photographic or photoconductive plate.

Body Part – 4TH	Contrast – 5TH	Qualifier – 6TH	Qualifier – 7TH
0 Skull 1 Orbit, Right 2 Orbit, Left 3 Orbits, Bilateral 4 Nasal Bones 5 Facial Bones 6 Mandible B Zygomatic Arch, Right C Zygomatic Arch, Left D Zygomatic Arches, Bilateral G Tooth, Single H Teeth, Multiple J Teeth, All	Z None	Z None	Z None
7 Temporomandibular Joint, Right 8 Temporomandibular Joint, Left 9 Temporomandibular Joints, Bilateral	0 High osmolar 1 Low osmolar Y Other contrast Z None	Z None	Z None

B – IMAGING

BN1 — Imaging, Skull and Facial Bones, Fluoroscopy

- 1ST – **B** Imaging
- 2ND – **N** Skull and Facial Bones
- 3RD – **1** FLUOROSCOPY

EXAMPLE: Fluoroscopic guidance

FLUOROSCOPY: Single plane or bi-plane real time display of an image developed from the capture of external ionizing radiation on a fluorescent screen. The image may also be stored by either digital or analog means.

Body Part – 4TH	Contrast – 5TH	Qualifier – 6TH	Qualifier – 7TH
7 Temporomandibular Joint, Right 8 Temporomandibular Joint, Left 9 Temporomandibular Joints, Bilateral	0 High osmolar 1 Low osmolar Y Other contrast Z None	Z None	Z None

BN2 — Imaging, Skull and Facial Bones, Computerized Tomography (CT Scan)

- 1ST – **B** Imaging
- 2ND – **N** Skull and Facial Bones
- 3RD – **2** COMPUTERIZED TOMOGRAPHY (CT Scan)

EXAMPLE: CT Scan of head

COMPUTERIZED TOMOGRAPHY (CT Scan): Computer reformatted digital display of multiplanar images developed from the capture of multiple exposures of external ionizing radiation.

Body Part – 4TH	Contrast – 5TH	Qualifier – 6TH	Qualifier – 7TH
0 Skull 3 Orbits, Bilateral 5 Facial Bones 6 Mandible 9 Temporomandibular Joints, Bilateral F Temporal Bones	0 High osmolar 1 Low osmolar Y Other contrast Z None	Z None	Z None

BN3 — Imaging, Skull and Facial Bones, Magnetic Resonance Imaging (MRI)

- 1ST – **B** Imaging
- 2ND – **N** Skull and Facial Bones
- 3RD – **3** MAGNETIC RESONANCE IMAGING (MRI)

EXAMPLE: MRI of knee

MAGNETIC RESONANCE IMAGING (MRI): Computer reformatted digital display of multiplanar images developed from the capture of radiofrequency signals emitted by nuclei in a body site excited within a magnetic field.

Body Part – 4TH	Contrast – 5TH	Qualifier – 6TH	Qualifier – 7TH
9 Temporomandibular Joints, Bilateral	Y Other contrast Z None	Z None	Z None

B P 0

ANCILLARY SECTIONS – 2016 ICD-10-PCS

1ST – B Imaging
2ND – P Non-Axial Upper Bones
3RD – 0 PLAIN RADIOGRAPHY

EXAMPLE: Chest X-ray

PLAIN RADIOGRAPHY: Planar display of an image developed from the capture of external ionizing radiation on photographic or photoconductive plate.

Body Part – 4TH		Contrast – 5TH	Qualifier – 6TH	Qualifier – 7TH
0 Sternoclavicular Joint, Right 1 Sternoclavicular Joint, Left 2 Sternoclavicular Joints, Bilateral 3 Acromioclavicular Joints, Bilateral 4 Clavicle, Right 5 Clavicle, Left 6 Scapula, Right 7 Scapula, Left	A Humerus, Right B Humerus, Left E Upper Arm, Right F Upper Arm, Left J Forearm, Right K Forearm, Left N Hand, Right P Hand, Left R Finger(s), Right S Finger(s), Left X Ribs, Right Y Ribs, Left	Z None	Z None	Z None
8 Shoulder, Right 9 Shoulder, Left C Hand/Finger Joint, Right D Hand/Finger Joint, Left	G Elbow, Right H Elbow, Left L Wrist, Right M Wrist, Left	0 High osmolar 1 Low osmolar Y Other contrast Z None	Z None	Z None

1ST – B Imaging
2ND – P Non-Axial Upper Bones
3RD – 1 FLUOROSCOPY

EXAMPLE: Fluoroscopic guidance

FLUOROSCOPY: Single plane or bi-plane real time display of an image developed from the capture of external ionizing radiation on a fluorescent screen. The image may also be stored by either digital or analog means.

Body Part – 4TH		Contrast – 5TH	Qualifier – 6TH	Qualifier – 7TH
0 Sternoclavicular Joint, Right 1 Sternoclavicular Joint, Left 2 Sternoclavicular Joints, Bilateral 3 Acromioclavicular Joints, Bilateral 4 Clavicle, Right 5 Clavicle, Left 6 Scapula, Right 7 Scapula, Left	A Humerus, Right B Humerus, Left E Upper Arm, Right F Upper Arm, Left J Forearm, Right K Forearm, Left N Hand, Right P Hand, Left R Finger(s), Right S Finger(s), Left X Ribs, Right Y Ribs, Left	Z None	Z None	Z None
8 Shoulder, Right 9 Shoulder, Left L Wrist, Right M Wrist, Left		0 High osmolar 1 Low osmolar Y Other contrast Z None	Z None	Z None
C Hand/Finger Joint, Right D Hand/Finger Joint, Left G Elbow, Right H Elbow, Left		0 High osmolar 1 Low osmolar Y Other contrast	Z None	Z None

COMPUTERIZED TOMOGRAPHY (CT Scan)

- 1ST – **B** Imaging
- 2ND – **P** Non-Axial Upper Bones
- 3RD – **2** COMPUTERIZED TOMOGRAPHY (CT Scan)

EXAMPLE: CT Scan of head

COMPUTERIZED TOMOGRAPHY (CT Scan): Computer reformatted digital display of multiplanar images developed from the capture of multiple exposures of external ionizing radiation.

Body Part – 4TH	Contrast – 5TH	Qualifier – 6TH	Qualifier – 7TH
0 Sternoclavicular Joint, Right 1 Sternoclavicular Joint, Left W Thorax	0 High osmolar 1 Low osmolar Y Other contrast	Z None	Z None
2 Sternoclavicular Joints, Bilateral 3 Acromioclavicular Joints, Bilateral 4 Clavicle, Right 5 Clavicle, Left 6 Scapula, Right 7 Scapula, Left 8 Shoulder, Right 9 Shoulder, Left A Humerus, Right B Humerus, Left E Upper Arm, Right F Upper Arm, Left G Elbow, Right H Elbow, Left J Forearm, Right K Forearm, Left L Wrist, Right M Wrist, Left N Hand, Right P Hand, Left Q Hands and Wrists, Bilateral R Finger(s), Right S Finger(s), Left T Upper Extremity, Right U Upper Extremity, Left V Upper Extremities, Bilateral X Ribs, Right Y Ribs, Left	0 High osmolar 1 Low osmolar Y Other contrast Z None	Z None	Z None
C Hand/Finger Joint, Right D Hand/Finger Joint, Left	Z None	Z None	Z None

MAGNETIC RESONANCE IMAGING (MRI)

- 1ST – **B** Imaging
- 2ND – **P** Non-Axial Upper Bones
- 3RD – **3** MAGNETIC RESONANCE IMAGING (MRI)

EXAMPLE: MRI of knee

MAGNETIC RESONANCE IMAGING (MRI): Computer reformatted digital display of multiplanar images developed from the capture of radiofrequency signals emitted by nuclei in a body site excited within a magnetic field.

Body Part – 4TH	Contrast – 5TH	Qualifier – 6TH	Qualifier – 7TH
8 Shoulder, Right 9 Shoulder, Left C Hand/Finger Joint, Right D Hand/Finger Joint, Left E Upper Arm, Right F Upper Arm, Left G Elbow, Right H Elbow, Left J Forearm, Right K Forearm, Left L Wrist, Right M Wrist, Left	Y Other contrast	0 Unenhanced and enhanced Z None	Z None
8 Shoulder, Right 9 Shoulder, Left C Hand/Finger Joint, Right D Hand/Finger Joint, Left E Upper Arm, Right F Upper Arm, Left G Elbow, Right H Elbow, Left J Forearm, Right K Forearm, Left L Wrist, Right M Wrist, Left	Z None	Z None	Z None

BP4 — ANCILLARY SECTIONS – 2016 ICD-10-PCS

1ST - B Imaging
2ND - P Non-Axial Upper Bones
3RD - 4 ULTRASONOGRAPHY

EXAMPLE: Abdominal ultrasound

ULTRASONOGRAPHY: Real time display of images of anatomy or flow information developed from the capture of reflected and attenuated high frequency sound waves.

Body Part – 4TH	Contrast – 5TH	Qualifier – 6TH	Qualifier – 7TH
8 Shoulder, Right L Wrist, Right 9 Shoulder, Left M Wrist, Left G Elbow, Right N Hand, Right H Elbow, Left P Hand, Left	Z None	Z None	1 Densitometry Z None

---

1ST - B Imaging
2ND - Q Non-Axial Lower Bones
3RD - 0 PLAIN RADIOGRAPHY

EXAMPLE: Chest X-ray

PLAIN RADIOGRAPHY: Planar display of an image developed from the capture of external ionizing radiation on photographic or photoconductive plate.

Body Part – 4TH	Contrast – 5TH	Qualifier – 6TH	Qualifier – 7TH
0 Hip, Right 1 Hip, Left	0 High osmolar 1 Low osmolar Y Other contrast	Z None	Z None
0 Hip, Right 1 Hip, Left	Z None	Z None	1 Densitometry Z None
3 Femur, Right 4 Femur, Left	Z None	Z None	1 Densitometry Z None
7 Knee, Right 8 Knee, Left G Ankle, Right H Ankle, Left	0 High osmolar 1 Low osmolar Y Other contrast Z None	Z None	Z None
D Lower Leg, Right M Foot, Left F Lower Leg, Left P Toe(s), Right J Calcaneus, Right Q Toe(s), Left K Calcaneus, Left V Patella, Right L Foot, Right W Patella, Left	Z None	Z None	Z None
X Foot/Toe Joint, Right Y Foot/Toe Joint, Left	0 High osmolar 1 Low osmolar Y Other contrast	Z None	Z None

B – IMAGING

BQ2

1ST – **B** Imaging
2ND – **Q** Non-Axial Lower Bones
3RD – **1** FLUOROSCOPY

EXAMPLE: Fluoroscopic guidance

FLUOROSCOPY: Single plane or bi-plane real time display of an image developed from the capture of external ionizing radiation on a fluorescent screen. The image may also be stored by either digital or analog means.

Body Part – 4TH		Contrast – 5TH	Qualifier – 6TH	Qualifier – 7TH
0 Hip, Right 1 Hip, Left 7 Knee, Right 8 Knee, Left	G Ankle, Right H Ankle, Left X Foot/Toe Joint, Right Y Foot/Toe Joint, Left	0 High osmolar 1 Low osmolar Y Other contrast Z None	Z None	Z None
3 Femur, Right 4 Femur, Left D Lower Leg, Right F Lower Leg, Left J Calcaneus, Right K Calcaneus, Left	L Foot, Right M Foot, Left P Toe(s), Right Q Toe(s), Left V Patella, Right W Patella, Left	Z None	Z None	Z None

---

1ST – **B** Imaging
2ND – **Q** Non-Axial Lower Bones
3RD – **2** COMPUTERIZED TOMOGRAPHY (CT Scan)

EXAMPLE: CT Scan of head

COMPUTERIZED TOMOGRAPHY (CT Scan): Computer reformatted digital display of multiplanar images developed from the capture of multiple exposures of external ionizing radiation.

Body Part – 4TH		Contrast – 5TH	Qualifier – 6TH	Qualifier – 7TH
0 Hip, Right 1 Hip, Left 3 Femur, Right 4 Femur, Left 7 Knee, Right 8 Knee, Left D Lower Leg, Right F Lower Leg, Left G Ankle, Right H Ankle, Left J Calcaneus, Right	K Calcaneus, Left L Foot, Right M Foot, Left P Toe(s), Right Q Toe(s), Left R Lower Extremity, Right S Lower Extremity, Left V Patella, Right W Patella, Left X Foot/Toe Joint, Right Y Foot/Toe Joint, Left	0 High osmolar 1 Low osmolar Y Other contrast Z None	Z None	Z None
B Tibia/Fibula, Right C Tibia/Fibula, Left		0 High osmolar 1 Low osmolar Y Other contrast	Z None	Z None

795

BQ3

ANCILLARY SECTIONS – 2016 ICD-10-PCS

1ST – **B** Imaging
2ND – **Q** Non-Axial Lower Bones
3RD – **3** MAGNETIC RESONANCE IMAGING (MRI)

EXAMPLE: MRI of knee

MAGNETIC RESONANCE IMAGING (MRI): Computer reformatted digital display of multiplanar images developed from the capture of radiofrequency signals emitted by nuclei in a body site excited within a magnetic field.

Body Part – 4TH		Contrast – 5TH	Qualifier – 6TH	Qualifier – 7TH
0 Hip, Right	H Ankle, Left	Y Other contrast	0 Unenhanced and enhanced	Z None
1 Hip, Left	J Calcaneus, Right		Z None	
3 Femur, Right	K Calcaneus, Left			
4 Femur, Left	L Foot, Right			
7 Knee, Right	M Foot, Left			
8 Knee, Left	P Toe(s), Right			
D Lower Leg, Right	Q Toe(s), Left			
F Lower Leg, Left	V Patella, Right			
G Ankle, Right	W Patella, Left			
0 Hip, Right	H Ankle, Left	Z None	Z None	Z None
1 Hip, Left	J Calcaneus, Right			
3 Femur, Right	K Calcaneus, Left			
4 Femur, Left	L Foot, Right			
7 Knee, Right	M Foot, Left			
8 Knee, Left	P Toe(s), Right			
D Lower Leg, Right	Q Toe(s), Left			
F Lower Leg, Left	V Patella, Right			
G Ankle, Right	W Patella, Left			

1ST – **B** Imaging
2ND – **Q** Non-Axial Lower Bones
3RD – **4** ULTRASONOGRAPHY

EXAMPLE: Abdominal ultrasound

ULTRASONOGRAPHY: Real time display of images of anatomy or flow information developed from the capture of reflected and attenuated high frequency sound waves.

Body Part – 4TH		Contrast – 5TH	Qualifier – 6TH	Qualifier – 7TH
0 Hip, Right	7 Knee, Right	Z None	Z None	Z None
1 Hip, Left	8 Knee, Left			
2 Hips, Bilateral	9 Knees, Bilateral			

B – IMAGING

BR1

1ST - B Imaging
2ND - R Axial Skeleton, Except Skull and Facial Bones
3RD - 0 PLAIN RADIOGRAPHY

EXAMPLE: Chest X-ray

PLAIN RADIOGRAPHY: Planar display of an image developed from the capture of external ionizing radiation on photographic or photoconductive plate.

Body Part – 4TH		Contrast – 5TH	Qualifier – 6TH	Qualifier – 7TH
0 Cervical Spine 7 Thoracic Spine	9 Lumbar Spine G Whole Spine	Z None	Z None	1 Densitometry Z None
1 Cervical Disc(s) 2 Thoracic Disc(s) 3 Lumbar Disc(s)	4 Cervical Facet Joint(s) 5 Thoracic Facet Joint(s) 6 Lumbar Facet Joint(s) D Sacroiliac Joints	0 High osmolar 1 Low osmolar Y Other contrast Z None	Z None	Z None
8 Thoracolumbar Joint B Lumbosacral Joint	C Pelvis F Sacrum and Coccyx H Sternum	Z None	Z None	Z None

1ST - B Imaging
2ND - R Axial Skeleton, Except Skull and Facial Bones
3RD - 1 FLUOROSCOPY

EXAMPLE: Fluoroscopic guidance

FLUOROSCOPY: Single plane or bi-plane real time display of an image developed from the capture of external ionizing radiation on a fluorescent screen. The image may also be stored by either digital or analog means.

Body Part – 4TH		Contrast – 5TH	Qualifier – 6TH	Qualifier – 7TH
0 Cervical Spine 1 Cervical Disc(s) 2 Thoracic Disc(s) 3 Lumbar Disc(s) 4 Cervical Facet Joint(s) 5 Thoracic Facet Joint(s) 6 Lumbar Facet Joint(s) 7 Thoracic Spine	8 Thoracolumbar Joint 9 Lumbar Spine B Lumbosacral Joint C Pelvis D Sacroiliac Joints F Sacrum and Coccyx G Whole Spine H Sternum	0 High osmolar 1 Low osmolar Y Other contrast Z None	Z None	Z None

797

BR2 ANCILLARY SECTIONS – 2016 ICD-10-PCS [2016.PCS]

1ST - **B** Imaging 2ND - **R** Axial Skeleton, Except Skull and Facial Bones 3RD - **2 COMPUTERIZED TOMOGRAPHY (CT Scan)**	EXAMPLE: CT Scan of head **COMPUTERIZED TOMOGRAPHY (CT Scan):** Computer reformatted digital display of multiplanar images developed from the capture of multiple exposures of external ionizing radiation.

Body Part – 4TH		Contrast – 5TH	Qualifier – 6TH	Qualifier – 7TH
0 Cervical Spine 7 Thoracic Spine 9 Lumbar Spine	C Pelvis D Sacroiliac Joints F Sacrum and Coccyx	0 High osmolar 1 Low osmolar Y Other contrast Z None	Z None	Z None

1ST - **B** Imaging 2ND - **R** Axial Skeleton, Except Skull and Facial Bones 3RD - **3 MAGNETIC RESONANCE IMAGING (MRI)**	EXAMPLE: MRI of knee **MAGNETIC RESONANCE IMAGING (MRI):** Computer reformatted digital display of multiplanar images developed from the capture of radiofrequency signals emitted by nuclei in a body site excited within a magnetic field.

Body Part – 4TH		Contrast – 5TH	Qualifier – 6TH	Qualifier – 7TH
0 Cervical Spine 1 Cervical Disc(s) 2 Thoracic Disc(s) 3 Lumbar Disc(s)	7 Thoracic Spine 9 Lumbar Spine C Pelvis F Sacrum and Coccyx	Y Other contrast	0 Unenhanced and enhanced Z None	Z None
0 Cervical Spine 1 Cervical Disc(s) 2 Thoracic Disc(s) 3 Lumbar Disc(s)	7 Thoracic Spine 9 Lumbar Spine C Pelvis F Sacrum and Coccyx	Z None	Z None	Z None

1ST - **B** Imaging 2ND - **R** Axial Skeleton, Except Skull and Facial Bones 3RD - **4 ULTRASONOGRAPHY**	EXAMPLE: Abdominal ultrasound **ULTRASONOGRAPHY:** Real time display of images of anatomy or flow information developed from the capture of reflected and attenuated high frequency sound waves.

Body Part – 4TH	Contrast – 5TH	Qualifier – 6TH	Qualifier – 7TH
0 Cervical Spine 7 Thoracic Spine 9 Lumbar Spine F Sacrum and Coccyx	Z None	Z None	Z None

B – IMAGING

BT2

1ST - B Imaging	EXAMPLE: Chest X-ray
2ND - T Urinary System	**PLAIN RADIOGRAPHY:** Planar display of an image developed from the capture of external ionizing radiation on photographic or photoconductive plate.
3RD - 0 PLAIN RADIOGRAPHY	

Body Part – 4TH		Contrast – 5TH	Qualifier – 6TH	Qualifier – 7TH
0 Bladder	5 Urethra	0 High osmolar	Z None	Z None
1 Kidney, Right	6 Ureter, Right	1 Low osmolar		
2 Kidney, Left	7 Ureter, Left	Y Other contrast		
3 Kidneys, Bilateral	8 Ureters, Bilateral	Z None		
4 Kidneys, Ureters and Bladder	B Bladder and Urethra			
	C Ileal Diversion Loop			

1ST - B Imaging	EXAMPLE: Fluoroscopic guidance
2ND - T Urinary System	**FLUOROSCOPY:** Single plane or bi-plane real time display of an image developed from the capture of external ionizing radiation on a fluorescent screen. The image may also be stored by either digital or analog means.
3RD - 1 FLUOROSCOPY	

Body Part – 4TH		Contrast – 5TH	Qualifier – 6TH	Qualifier – 7TH
0 Bladder	B Bladder and Urethra	0 High osmolar	Z None	Z None
1 Kidney, Right	C Ileal Diversion Loop	1 Low osmolar		
2 Kidney, Left	D Kidney, Ureter and Bladder, Right	Y Other contrast		
3 Kidneys, Bilateral	F Kidney, Ureter and Bladder, Left	Z None		
4 Kidneys, Ureters and Bladder	G Ileal Loop, Ureters and Kidneys			
5 Urethra				
6 Ureter, Right				
7 Ureter, Left				

1ST - B Imaging	EXAMPLE: CT Scan of head
2ND - T Urinary System	**COMPUTERIZED TOMOGRAPHY (CT Scan):** Computer reformatted digital display of multiplanar images developed from the capture of multiple exposures of external ionizing radiation.
3RD - 2 COMPUTERIZED TOMOGRAPHY (CT Scan)	

Body Part – 4TH		Contrast – 5TH	Qualifier – 6TH	Qualifier – 7TH
0 Bladder	3 Kidneys, Bilateral	0 High osmolar	0 Unenhanced and enhanced	Z None
1 Kidney, Right	9 Kidney Transplant	1 Low osmolar	Z None	
2 Kidney, Left		Y Other contrast		
0 Bladder	3 Kidneys, Bilateral	Z None	Z None	Z None
1 Kidney, Right	9 Kidney Transplant			
2 Kidney, Left				

BT3 — ANCILLARY SECTIONS – 2016 ICD-10-PCS [2016.PCS]

1ST - B Imaging
2ND - T Urinary System
3RD - 3 MAGNETIC RESONANCE IMAGING (MRI)

EXAMPLE: MRI of knee

MAGNETIC RESONANCE IMAGING (MRI): Computer reformatted digital display of multiplanar images developed from the capture of radiofrequency signals emitted by nuclei in a body site excited within a magnetic field.

Body Part – 4TH		Contrast – 5TH	Qualifier – 6TH	Qualifier – 7TH
0 Bladder	3 Kidneys, Bilateral	Y Other contrast	0 Unenhanced and enhanced	Z None
1 Kidney, Right	9 Kidney Transplant		Z None	
2 Kidney, Left				
0 Bladder	3 Kidneys, Bilateral	Z None	Z None	Z None
1 Kidney, Right	9 Kidney Transplant			
2 Kidney, Left				

1ST - B Imaging
2ND - T Urinary System
3RD - 4 ULTRASONOGRAPHY

EXAMPLE: Abdominal ultrasound

ULTRASONOGRAPHY: Real time display of images of anatomy or flow information developed from the capture of reflected and attenuated high frequency sound waves.

Body Part – 4TH		Contrast – 5TH	Qualifier – 6TH	Qualifier – 7TH
0 Bladder	6 Ureter, Right	Z None	Z None	Z None
1 Kidney, Right	7 Ureter, Left			
2 Kidney, Left	8 Ureters, Bilateral			
3 Kidneys, Bilateral	9 Kidney Transplant			
5 Urethra	J Kidneys and Bladder			

1ST - B Imaging
2ND - U Female Reproductive System ♀
3RD - 0 PLAIN RADIOGRAPHY

EXAMPLE: Chest X-ray

PLAIN RADIOGRAPHY: Planar display of an image developed from the capture of external ionizing radiation on photographic or photoconductive plate.

Body Part – 4TH		Contrast – 5TH	Qualifier – 6TH	Qualifier – 7TH
0 Fallopian Tube, Right	6 Uterus	0 High osmolar	Z None	Z None
1 Fallopian Tube, Left	8 Uterus and Fallopian Tubes	1 Low osmolar		
2 Fallopian Tubes, Bilateral		Y Other contrast		
	9 Vagina			

B – IMAGING

BU4

1ST - **B** Imaging 2ND - **U** Female Reproductive System ♀ 3RD - **1** FLUOROSCOPY	EXAMPLE: Fluoroscopic guidance **FLUOROSCOPY:** Single plane or bi-plane real time display of an image developed from the capture of external ionizing radiation on a fluorescent screen. The image may also be stored by either digital or analog means.		
Body Part – 4TH	**Contrast – 5TH**	**Qualifier – 6TH**	**Qualifier – 7TH**
0 Fallopian Tube, Right 6 Uterus 1 Fallopian Tube, Left 8 Uterus and Fallopian 2 Fallopian Tubes, Bilateral Tubes 9 Vagina	0 High osmolar 1 Low osmolar Y Other contrast Z None	Z None	Z None

1ST - **B** Imaging 2ND - **U** Female Reproductive System ♀ 3RD - **3** MAGNETIC RESONANCE IMAGING (MRI)	EXAMPLE: MRI of knee **MAGNETIC RESONANCE IMAGING (MRI):** Computer reformatted digital display of multiplanar images developed from the capture of radiofrequency signals emitted by nuclei in a body site excited within a magnetic field.		
Body Part – 4TH	**Contrast – 5TH**	**Qualifier – 6TH**	**Qualifier – 7TH**
3 Ovary, Right 9 Vagina 4 Ovary, Left B Pregnant Uterus 5 Ovaries, Bilateral C Uterus and Ovaries 6 Uterus	Y Other contrast	0 Unenhanced and enhanced Z None	Z None
3 Ovary, Right 9 Vagina 4 Ovary, Left B Pregnant Uterus 5 Ovaries, Bilateral C Uterus and Ovaries 6 Uterus	Z None	Z None	Z None

1ST - **B** Imaging 2ND - **U** Female Reproductive System ♀ 3RD - **4** ULTRASONOGRAPHY	EXAMPLE: Abdominal ultrasound **ULTRASONOGRAPHY:** Real time display of images of anatomy or flow information developed from the capture of reflected and attenuated high frequency sound waves.		
Body Part – 4TH	**Contrast – 5TH**	**Qualifier – 6TH**	**Qualifier – 7TH**
0 Fallopian Tube, Right 4 Ovary, Left 1 Fallopian Tube, Left 5 Ovaries, Bilateral 2 Fallopian Tubes, Bilateral 6 Uterus 3 Ovary, Right C Uterus and Ovaries	Y Other contrast Z None	Z None	Z None

BV0 ANCILLARY SECTIONS – 2016 ICD-10-PCS [2016.PCS]

1ST - B Imaging
2ND - V Male Reproductive System ♂
3RD - 0 PLAIN RADIOGRAPHY

EXAMPLE: Chest X-ray

PLAIN RADIOGRAPHY: Planar display of an image developed from the capture of external ionizing radiation on photographic or photoconductive plate.

Body Part – 4TH	Contrast – 5TH	Qualifier – 6TH	Qualifier – 7TH
0 Corpora Cavernosa 5 Testicle, Right	0 High osmolar	Z None	Z None
1 Epididymis, Right 6 Testicle, Left	1 Low osmolar		
2 Epididymis, Left 8 Vasa Vasorum	Y Other contrast		
3 Prostate			

1ST - B Imaging
2ND - V Male Reproductive System ♂
3RD - 1 FLUOROSCOPY

EXAMPLE: Fluoroscopic guidance

FLUOROSCOPY: Single plane or bi-plane real time display of an image developed from the capture of external ionizing radiation on a fluorescent screen. The image may also be stored by either digital or analog means.

Body Part – 4TH	Contrast – 5TH	Qualifier – 6TH	Qualifier – 7TH
0 Corpora Cavernosa	0 High osmolar	Z None	Z None
8 Vasa Vasorum	1 Low osmolar		
	Y Other contrast		
	Z None		

1ST - B Imaging
2ND - V Male Reproductive System ♂
3RD - 2 COMPUTERIZED TOMOGRAPHY (CT Scan)

EXAMPLE: CT Scan of head

COMPUTERIZED TOMOGRAPHY (CT Scan): Computer reformatted digital display of multiplanar images developed from the capture of multiple exposures of external ionizing radiation.

Body Part – 4TH	Contrast – 5TH	Qualifier – 6TH	Qualifier – 7TH
3 Prostate	0 High osmolar	0 Unenhanced and enhanced	Z None
	1 Low osmolar	Z None	
	Y Other contrast		
3 Prostate	Z None	Z None	Z None

B – IMAGING

BW0

Section 1: Magnetic Resonance Imaging (MRI)

- **1ST** – **B** Imaging
- **2ND** – **V** Male Reproductive System ♂
- **3RD** – **3** MAGNETIC RESONANCE IMAGING (MRI)

EXAMPLE: MRI of knee

MAGNETIC RESONANCE IMAGING (MRI): Computer reformatted digital display of multiplanar images developed from the capture of radiofrequency signals emitted by nuclei in a body site excited within a magnetic field.

Body Part – 4TH		Contrast – 5TH	Qualifier – 6TH	Qualifier – 7TH
0 Corpora Cavernosa 3 Prostate 4 Scrotum	5 Testicle, Right 6 Testicle, Left 7 Testicles, Bilateral	Y Other contrast	0 Unenhanced and enhanced Z None	Z None
0 Corpora Cavernosa 3 Prostate 4 Scrotum	5 Testicle, Right 6 Testicle, Left 7 Testicles, Bilateral	Z None	Z None	Z None

Section 2: Ultrasonography

- **1ST** – **B** Imaging
- **2ND** – **V** Male Reproductive System ♂
- **3RD** – **4** ULTRASONOGRAPHY

EXAMPLE: Abdominal ultrasound

ULTRASONOGRAPHY: Real time display of images of anatomy or flow information developed from the capture of reflected and attenuated high frequency sound waves.

Body Part – 4TH	Contrast – 5TH	Qualifier – 6TH	Qualifier – 7TH
4 Scrotum 9 Prostate and Seminal Vesicles B Penis	Z None	Z None	Z None

Section 3: Plain Radiography

- **1ST** – **B** Imaging
- **2ND** – **W** Anatomical regions
- **3RD** – **0** PLAIN RADIOGRAPHY

EXAMPLE: Chest X-ray

PLAIN RADIOGRAPHY: Planar display of an image developed from the capture of external ionizing radiation on photographic or photoconductive plate.

Body Part – 4TH		Contrast – 5TH	Qualifier – 6TH	Qualifier – 7TH
0 Abdomen 1 Abdomen and Pelvis 3 Chest B Long Bones, All	C Lower Extremity J Upper Extremity K Whole Body L Whole Skeleton M Whole Body, Infant	Z None	Z None	Z None

BW1 — ANCILLARY SECTIONS – 2016 ICD-10-PCS

- 1ST – **B** Imaging
- 2ND – **W** Anatomical Regions
- 3RD – **1** FLUOROSCOPY

EXAMPLE: Fluoroscopic guidance

FLUOROSCOPY: Single plane or bi-plane real time display of an image developed from the capture of external ionizing radiation on a fluorescent screen. The image may also be stored by either digital or analog means.

Body Part – 4TH	Contrast – 5TH	Qualifier – 6TH	Qualifier – 7TH
1 Abdomen and Pelvis 9 Head and Neck C Lower Extremity J Upper Extremity	0 High osmolar 1 Low osmolar Y Other contrast Z None	Z None	Z None

---

- 1ST – **B** Imaging
- 2ND – **W** Anatomical Regions
- 3RD – **2** COMPUTERIZED TOMOGRAPHY (CT Scan)

EXAMPLE: CT Scan of head

COMPUTERIZED TOMOGRAPHY (CT Scan): Computer reformatted digital display of multiplanar images developed from the capture of multiple exposures of external ionizing radiation.

Body Part – 4TH		Contrast – 5TH	Qualifier – 6TH	Qualifier – 7TH
0 Abdomen 1 Abdomen and Pelvis 4 Chest and Abdomen 5 Chest, Abdomen and Pelvis	8 Head 9 Head and Neck F Neck G Pelvic Region	0 High osmolar 1 Low osmolar Y Other contrast	0 Unenhanced and enhanced Z None	Z None
0 Abdomen 1 Abdomen and Pelvis 4 Chest and Abdomen 5 Chest, Abdomen and Pelvis	8 Head 9 Head and Neck F Neck G Pelvic Region	Z None	Z None	Z None

---

- 1ST – **B** Imaging
- 2ND – **W** Anatomical Regions
- 3RD – **3** MAGNETIC RESONANCE IMAGING (MRI)

EXAMPLE: MRI of knee

MAGNETIC RESONANCE IMAGING (MRI): Computer reformatted digital display of multiplanar images developed from the capture of radiofrequency signals emitted by nuclei in a body site excited within a magnetic field.

Body Part – 4TH		Contrast – 5TH	Qualifier – 6TH	Qualifier – 7TH
0 Abdomen 8 Head F Neck	G Pelvic Region H Retroperitoneum P Brachial Plexus	Y Other contrast	0 Unenhanced and enhanced Z None	Z None
0 Abdomen 8 Head F Neck	G Pelvic Region H Retroperitoneum P Brachial Plexus	Z None	Z None	Z None
3 Chest		Y Other contrast	0 Unenhanced and enhanced Z None	Z None

B – IMAGING

BY4

1ST - **B** Imaging 2ND - **W** Anatomical Regions 3RD - **4** ULTRASONOGRAPHY	EXAMPLE: Abdominal ultrasound
	ULTRASONOGRAPHY: Real time display of images of anatomy or flow information developed from the capture of reflected and attenuated high frequency sound waves.

Body Part – 4TH	Contrast – 5TH	Qualifier – 6TH	Qualifier – 7TH
0 Abdomen 1 Abdomen and Pelvis F Neck G Pelvic Region	Z None	Z None	Z None

---

1ST - **B** Imaging 2ND - **Y** Fetus and Obstetrical ♀ 3RD - **3** MAGNETIC RESONANCE IMAGING (MRI)	EXAMPLE: MRI of knee
	MAGNETIC RESONANCE IMAGING (MRI): Computer reformatted digital display of multiplanar images developed from the capture of radiofrequency signals emitted by nuclei in a body site excited within a magnetic field.

Body Part – 4TH	Contrast – 5TH	Qualifier – 6TH	Qualifier – 7TH
0 Fetal Head 4 Fetal Spine 1 Fetal Heart 5 Fetal Extremities 2 Fetal Thorax 6 Whole Fetus 3 Fetal Abdomen	Y Other contrast	0 Unenhanced and enhanced Z None	Z None
0 Fetal Head 4 Fetal Spine 1 Fetal Heart 5 Fetal Extremities 2 Fetal Thorax 6 Whole Fetus 3 Fetal Abdomen	Z None	Z None	Z None

---

1ST - **B** Imaging 2ND - **Y** Fetus and Obstetrical ♀ 3RD - **4** ULTRASONOGRAPHY	EXAMPLE: Abdominal ultrasound
	ULTRASONOGRAPHY: Real time display of images of anatomy or flow information developed from the capture of reflected and attenuated high frequency sound waves.

Body Part – 4TH	Contrast – 5TH	Qualifier – 6TH	Qualifier – 7TH
7 Fetal Umbilical Cord 8 Placenta 9 First Trimester, Single Fetus B First Trimester, Multiple Gestation C Second Trimester, Single Fetus D Second Trimester, Multiple Gestation F Third Trimester, Single Fetus G Third Trimester, Multiple Gestation	Z None	Z None	Z None

NOTES

Educational Annotations | Section C – Nuclear Medicine

Section Specific Educational Annotations for the Nuclear Medicine Section include:
- AHA Coding Clinic® Reference Notations
- Coding Notes

AHA Coding Clinic® Reference Notations of Nuclear Medicine

ROOT TYPE SPECIFIC - NUCLEAR MEDICINE - Section C
PLANAR NUCLEAR MEDICINE IMAGING - 1
TOMOGRAPHIC (TOMO) NUCLEAR MEDICINE IMAGING - 2
POSITRON EMMISION TOMOGRAPHY (PET) - 3
NONIMAGING NUCLEAR MEDICINE UPTAKE - 4
NONIMAGING NUCLEAR MEDICINE PROBE - 5
NONIMAGING NUCLEAR MEDICINE ASSAY - 6
SYSTEMIC NUCLEAR MEDICINE THERAPY - 7

Coding Notes of Nuclear Medicine

Ancillary Section Specific PCS Reference Manual Exercises

PCS CODE	C – NUCLEAR MEDICINE EXERCISES
C030BZZ	Carbon 11 PET scan of brain with quantification.
C050VZZ	Xenon gas nonimaging probe of brain.
C226YZZ	Tomo scan of right and left heart, unspecified radiopharmaceutical, qualitative gated rest.
C23GQZZ	PET scan of myocardium using rubidium.
C763HZZ	Iodinated albumin nuclear medicine assay, blood plasma volume study.
CD15YZZ	Upper GI scan, radiopharmaceutical unspecified, for gastric emptying.
CH22SZZ	Thallous chloride tomographic scan of bilateral breasts.
CP151ZZ	Uniplanar scan of spine using technetium oxidronate, with first pass study.
CT631ZZ	Technetium pentetate assay of kidneys, ureters, and bladder.
CW1BLZZ	Gallium citrate scan of head and neck, single plane imaging.

Educational Annotations

Section C – Nuclear Medicine

NOTES

C – NUCLEAR MEDICINE

| 1ST - **C** Nuclear Medicine |
| 2ND - **0** Central Nervous System |
| 3RD - **1** PLANAR NUCLEAR MEDICINE IMAGING |

EXAMPLE: Gallium scan, single plane image

PLANAR NUCLEAR MEDICINE IMAGING: Introduction of radioactive materials into the body for single plane display of images developed from the capture of radioactive emissions.

Body Part – 4TH	Radionuclide – 5TH	Qualifier – 6TH	Qualifier – 7TH
0 Brain	1 Technetium 99m (Tc-99m) Y Other radionuclide	Z None	Z None
5 Cerebrospinal Fluid	D Indium 111 (In-111) Y Other radionuclide	Z None	Z None
Y Central Nervous System	Y Other radionuclide	Z None	Z None

| 1ST - **C** Nuclear Medicine |
| 2ND - **0** Central Nervous System |
| 3RD - **2** TOMOGRAPHIC (TOMO) NUCLEAR MEDICINE IMAGING |

EXAMPLE: Tomo scan of breast

TOMOGRAPHIC (TOMO) NUCLEAR MEDICINE IMAGING: Introduction of radioactive materials into the body for three dimensional display of images developed from the capture of radioactive emissions.

Body Part – 4TH	Radionuclide – 5TH	Qualifier – 6TH	Qualifier – 7TH
0 Brain	1 Technetium 99m (Tc-99m) F Iodine 123 (I-123) S Thallium 201 (Tl-201) Y Other radionuclide	Z None	Z None
5 Cerebrospinal Fluid	D Indium 111 (In-111) Y Other radionuclide	Z None	Z None
Y Central Nervous System	Y Other radionuclide	Z None	Z None

| 1ST - **C** Nuclear Medicine |
| 2ND - **0** Central Nervous System |
| 3RD - **3** POSITRON EMISSION (PET) TOMOGRAPHIC IMAGING |

EXAMPLE: PET scan of brain

POSITRON EMISSION TOMOGRAPHIC (PET) IMAGING: Introduction of radioactive materials into the body for three dimensional display of images developed from the simultaneous capture, 180 degrees apart, of radioactive emissions.

Body Part – 4TH	Radionuclide – 5TH	Qualifier – 6TH	Qualifier – 7TH
0 Brain	B Carbon 11 (C-11) K Fluorine 18 (F-18) M Oxygen 15 (O-15) Y Other radionuclide	Z None	Z None
Y Central Nervous System	Y Other radionuclide	Z None	Z None

C05 — ANCILLARY SECTIONS – 2016 ICD-10-PCS

1ST - C Nuclear Medicine
2ND - 0 Central Nervous System
3RD - 5 NONIMAGING NUCLEAR MEDICINE PROBE

EXAMPLE: Xenon gas nonimaging probe of brain

NONIMAGING NUCLEAR MEDICINE PROBE: Introduction of radioactive materials into the body for the study of distribution and fate of certain substances by the detection of radioactive emissions; or, alternatively, measurement of absorption of radioactive emissions from an external source.

Body Part – 4TH	Radionuclide – 5TH	Qualifier – 6TH	Qualifier – 7TH
0 Brain	V Xenon 133 (Xe-133) Y Other radionuclide	Z None	Z None
Y Central Nervous System	Y Other radionuclide	Z None	Z None

1ST - C Nuclear Medicine
2ND - 2 Heart
3RD - 1 PLANAR NUCLEAR MEDICINE IMAGING

EXAMPLE: Gallium scan, single plane image

PLANAR NUCLEAR MEDICINE IMAGING: Introduction of radioactive materials into the body for single plane display of images developed from the capture of radioactive emissions.

Body Part – 4TH	Radionuclide – 5TH	Qualifier – 6TH	Qualifier – 7TH
6 Heart, Right and Left	1 Technetium 99m (Tc-99m) Y Other radionuclide	Z None	Z None
G Myocardium	1 Technetium 99m (Tc-99m) D Indium 111 (In-111) S Thallium 201 (Tl-201) Y Other radionuclide Z None	Z None	Z None
Y Heart	Y Other radionuclide	Z None	Z None

1ST - C Nuclear Medicine
2ND - 2 Heart
3RD - 2 TOMOGRAPHIC (TOMO) NUCLEAR MEDICINE IMAGING

EXAMPLE: Tomo scan of breast

TOMOGRAPHIC (TOMO) NUCLEAR MEDICINE IMAGING: Introduction of radioactive materials into the body for three dimensional display of images developed from the capture of radioactive emissions.

Body Part – 4TH	Radionuclide – 5TH	Qualifier – 6TH	Qualifier – 7TH
6 Heart, Right and Left	1 Technetium 99m (Tc-99m) Y Other radionuclide	Z None	Z None
G Myocardium	1 Technetium 99m (Tc-99m) D Indium 111 (In-111) K Fluorine 18 (F-18) S Thallium 201 (Tl-201) Y Other radionuclide Z None	Z None	Z None
Y Heart	Y Other radionuclide	Z None	Z None

C – NUCLEAR MEDICINE

C 51

1ST – **C** Nuclear Medicine 2ND – **2** Heart 3RD – **3** POSITRON EMISSION (PET) TOMOGRAPHIC IMAGING	EXAMPLE: PET scan of brain **POSITRON EMISSION TOMOGRAPHIC (PET) IMAGING:** Introduction of radioactive materials into the body for three dimensional display of images developed from the simultaneous capture, 180 degrees apart, of radioactive emissions.

Body Part – 4TH	Radionuclide – 5TH	Qualifier – 6TH	Qualifier – 7TH
G Myocardium	K Fluorine 18 (F-18) M Oxygen 15 (O-15) Q Rubidium 82 (Rb-82) R Nitrogen 13 (N-13) Y Other radionuclide	Z None	Z None
Y Heart	Y Other radionuclide	Z None	Z None

1ST – **C** Nuclear Medicine 2ND – **2** Heart 3RD – **5** NONIMAGING NUCLEAR MEDICINE PROBE	EXAMPLE: Xenon gas nonimaging probe of brain **NONIMAGING NUCLEAR MEDICINE PROBE:** Introduction of radioactive materials into the body for the study of distribution and fate of certain substances by the detection of radioactive emissions; or, alternatively, measurement of absorption of radioactive emissions from an external source.

Body Part – 4TH	Radionuclide – 5TH	Qualifier – 6TH	Qualifier – 7TH
6 Heart, Right and Left	1 Technetium 99m (Tc-99m) Y Other radionuclide	Z None	Z None
Y Heart	Y Other radionuclide	Z None	Z None

1ST – **C** Nuclear Medicine 2ND – **5** Veins 3RD – **1** PLANAR NUCLEAR MEDICINE IMAGING	EXAMPLE: Gallium scan, single plane image **PLANAR NUCLEAR MEDICINE IMAGING:** Introduction of radioactive materials into the body for single plane display of images developed from the capture of radioactive emissions.

Body Part – 4TH	Radionuclide – 5TH	Qualifier – 6TH	Qualifier – 7TH
B Lower Extremity Veins, Right C Lower Extremity Veins, Left D Lower Extremity Veins, Bilateral N Upper Extremity Veins, Right P Upper Extremity Veins, Left Q Upper Extremity Veins, Bilateral R Central Veins	1 Technetium 99m (Tc-99m) Y Other radionuclide	Z None	Z None
Y Veins	Y Other radionuclide	Z None	Z None

C71

Nuclear Medicine — Lymphatic and Hematologic System — Planar Nuclear Medicine Imaging

- 1ST – **C** Nuclear Medicine
- 2ND – **7** Lymphatic and Hematologic System
- 3RD – **1** PLANAR NUCLEAR MEDICINE IMAGING

EXAMPLE: Gallium scan, single plane image

PLANAR NUCLEAR MEDICINE IMAGING: Introduction of radioactive materials into the body for single plane display of images developed from the capture of radioactive emissions.

Body Part – 4TH	Radionuclide – 5TH	Qualifier – 6TH	Qualifier – 7TH
0 Bone Marrow	1 Technetium 99m (Tc-99m) D Indium 111 (In-111) Y Other radionuclide	Z None	Z None
2 Spleen 5 Lymphatics, Head and Neck D Lymphatics, Pelvic J Lymphatics, Head K Lymphatics, Neck L Lymphatics, Upper Chest M Lymphatics, Trunk N Lymphatics, Upper Extremity P Lymphatics, Lower Extremity	1 Technetium 99m (Tc-99m) Y Other radionuclide	Z None	Z None
3 Blood	D Indium 111 (In-111) Y Other radionuclide	Z None	Z None
Y Lymphatic and Hematologic System	Y Other radionuclide	Z None	Z None

Nuclear Medicine — Lymphatic and Hematologic System — Tomographic (Tomo) Nuclear Medicine Imaging

- 1ST – **C** Nuclear Medicine
- 2ND – **7** Lymphatic and Hematologic System
- 3RD – **2** TOMOGRAPHIC (TOMO) NUCLEAR MEDICINE IMAGING

EXAMPLE: Tomo scan of breast

TOMOGRAPHIC (TOMO) NUCLEAR MEDICINE IMAGING: Introduction of radioactive materials into the body for three dimensional display of images developed from the capture of radioactive emissions.

Body Part – 4TH	Radionuclide – 5TH	Qualifier – 6TH	Qualifier – 7TH
2 Spleen	1 Technetium 99m (Tc-99m) Y Other radionuclide	Z None	Z None
Y Lymphatic and Hematologic System	Y Other radionuclide	Z None	Z None

Nuclear Medicine — Lymphatic and Hematologic System — Nonimaging Nuclear Medicine Probe

- 1ST – **C** Nuclear Medicine
- 2ND – **7** Lymphatic and Hematologic System
- 3RD – **5** NONIMAGING NUCLEAR MEDICINE PROBE

EXAMPLE: Xenon gas nonimaging probe of brain

NONIMAGING NUCLEAR MEDICINE PROBE: Introduction of radioactive materials into the body for the study of distribution and fate of certain substances by the detection of radioactive emissions; or, alternatively, measurement of absorption of radioactive emissions from an external source.

Body Part – 4TH	Radionuclide – 5TH	Qualifier – 6TH	Qualifier – 7TH
5 Lymphatics, Head and Neck D Lymphatics, Pelvic J Lymphatics, Head K Lymphatics, Neck L Lymphatics, Upper Chest M Lymphatics, Trunk N Lymphatics, Upper Extremity P Lymphatics, Lower Extremity	1 Technetium 99m (Tc-99m) Y Other radionuclide	Z None	Z None
Y Lymphatic and Hematologic System	Y Other radionuclide	Z None	Z None

C – NUCLEAR MEDICINE

C91

- 1ST – **C** Nuclear Medicine
- 2ND – **7** Lymphatic and Hematologic System
- 3RD – **6** NONIMAGING NUCLEAR MEDICINE ASSAY

EXAMPLE: Technetium assay of kidneys

NONIMAGING NUCLEAR MEDICINE ASSAY: Introduction of radioactive materials into the body for the study of body fluids and blood elements, by the detection of radioactive emissions.

Body Part – 4TH	Radionuclide – 5TH	Qualifier – 6TH	Qualifier – 7TH
3 Blood	1 Technetium 99m (Tc-99m) 7 Cobalt 58 (Co-58) C Cobalt 57 (Co-57) D Indium 111 (In-111) H Iodine 125 (I-125) W Chromium (Cr-51) Y Other radionuclide	Z None	Z None
Y Lymphatic and Hematologic System	Y Other radionuclide	Z None	Z None

---

- 1ST – **C** Nuclear Medicine
- 2ND – **8** Eye
- 3RD – **1** PLANAR NUCLEAR MEDICINE IMAGING

EXAMPLE: Gallium scan, single plane image

PLANAR NUCLEAR MEDICINE IMAGING: Introduction of radioactive materials into the body for single plane display of images developed from the capture of radioactive emissions.

Body Part – 4TH	Radionuclide – 5TH	Qualifier – 6TH	Qualifier – 7TH
9 Lacrimal Ducts, Bilateral	1 Technetium 99m (Tc-99m) Y Other radionuclide	Z None	Z None
Y Eye	Y Other radionuclide	Z None	Z None

- 1ST – **C** Nuclear Medicine
- 2ND – **9** Ear, Nose, Mouth and Throat
- 3RD – **1** PLANAR NUCLEAR MEDICINE IMAGING

EXAMPLE: Gallium scan, single plane image

PLANAR NUCLEAR MEDICINE IMAGING: Introduction of radioactive materials into the body for single plane display of images developed from the capture of radioactive emissions.

Body Part – 4TH	Radionuclide – 5TH	Qualifier – 6TH	Qualifier – 7TH
B Salivary Glands, Bilateral	1 Technetium 99m (Tc-99m) Y Other radionuclide	Z None	Z None
Y Ear, Nose, Mouth and Throat	Y Other radionuclide	Z None	Z None

ANCILLARY SECTIONS – 2016 ICD-10-PCS

CB1

1ST -	C	Nuclear Medicine
2ND -	B	Respiratory System
3RD -	1	PLANAR NUCLEAR MEDICINE IMAGING

EXAMPLE: Gallium scan, single plane image

PLANAR NUCLEAR MEDICINE IMAGING: Introduction of radioactive materials into the body for single plane display of images developed from the capture of radioactive emissions.

Body Part – 4TH	Radionuclide – 5TH	Qualifier – 6TH	Qualifier – 7TH
2 Lungs and Bronchi	1 Technetium 99m (Tc-99m) 9 Krypton (Kr-81m) T Xenon 127 (Xe-127) V Xenon 133 (Xe-133) Y Other radionuclide	Z None	Z None
Y Respiratory System	Y Other radionuclide	Z None	Z None

1ST -	C	Nuclear Medicine
2ND -	B	Respiratory System
3RD -	2	TOMOGRAPHIC (TOMO) NUCLEAR MEDICINE IMAGING

EXAMPLE: Tomo scan of breast

TOMOGRAPHIC (TOMO) NUCLEAR MEDICINE IMAGING: Introduction of radioactive materials into the body for three dimensional display of images developed from the capture of radioactive emissions.

Body Part – 4TH	Radionuclide – 5TH	Qualifier – 6TH	Qualifier – 7TH
2 Lungs and Bronchi	1 Technetium 99m (Tc-99m) 9 Krypton (Kr-81m) Y Other radionuclide	Z None	Z None
Y Respiratory System	Y Other radionuclide	Z None	Z None

1ST -	C	Nuclear Medicine
2ND -	B	Respiratory System
3RD -	3	POSITRON EMISSION (PET) TOMOGRAPHIC IMAGING

EXAMPLE: PET scan of brain

POSITRON EMISSION TOMOGRAPHIC (PET) IMAGING: Introduction of radioactive materials into the body for three dimensional display of images developed from the simultaneous capture, 180 degrees apart, of radioactive emissions.

Body Part – 4TH	Radionuclide – 5TH	Qualifier – 6TH	Qualifier – 7TH
2 Lungs and Bronchi	K Fluorine 18 (F-18) Y Other radionuclide	Z None	Z None
Y Respiratory System	Y Other radionuclide	Z None	Z None

C – NUCLEAR MEDICINE

1ST - **C** Nuclear Medicine 2ND - **D** Gastrointestinal System 3RD - **1** PLANAR NUCLEAR MEDICINE IMAGING	EXAMPLE: Gallium scan, single plane image **PLANAR NUCLEAR MEDICINE IMAGING:** Introduction of radioactive materials into the body for single plane display of images developed from the capture of radioactive emissions.

Body Part – 4TH	Radionuclide – 5TH	Qualifier – 6TH	Qualifier – 7TH
5 Upper Gastrointestinal Tract 7 Gastrointestinal Tract	1 Technetium 99m (Tc-99m) D Indium 111 (In-111) Y Other radionuclide	Z None	Z None
Y Digestive System	Y Other radionuclide	Z None	Z None

1ST - **C** Nuclear Medicine 2ND - **D** Gastrointestinal System 3RD - **2** TOMOGRAPHIC (TOMO) NUCLEAR MEDICINE IMAGING	EXAMPLE: Tomo scan of breast **TOMOGRAPHIC (TOMO) NUCLEAR MEDICINE IMAGING:** Introduction of radioactive materials into the body for three dimensional display of images developed from the capture of radioactive emissions.

Body Part – 4TH	Radionuclide – 5TH	Qualifier – 6TH	Qualifier – 7TH
7 Gastrointestinal Tract	1 Technetium 99m (Tc-99m) D Indium 111 (In-111) Y Other radionuclide	Z None	Z None
Y Digestive System	Y Other radionuclide	Z None	Z None

1ST - **C** Nuclear Medicine 2ND - **F** Hepatobiliary System and Pancreas 3RD - **1** PLANAR NUCLEAR MEDICINE IMAGING	EXAMPLE: Gallium scan, single plane image **PLANAR NUCLEAR MEDICINE IMAGING:** Introduction of radioactive materials into the body for single plane display of images developed from the capture of radioactive emissions.

Body Part – 4TH	Radionuclide – 5TH	Qualifier – 6TH	Qualifier – 7TH
4 Gallbladder 5 Liver 6 Liver and Spleen C Hepatobiliary System, All	1 Technetium 99m (Tc-99m) Y Other radionuclide	Z None	Z None
Y Hepatobiliary System and Pancreas	Y Other radionuclide	Z None	Z None

CF2

ANCILLARY SECTIONS – 2016 ICD-10-PCS

- 1ST – **C** Nuclear Medicine
- 2ND – **F** Hepatobiliary System and Pancreas
- 3RD – **2** TOMOGRAPHIC (TOMO) NUCLEAR MEDICINE IMAGING

EXAMPLE: Tomo scan of breast

TOMOGRAPHIC (TOMO) NUCLEAR MEDICINE IMAGING: Introduction of radioactive materials into the body for three dimensional display of images developed from the capture of radioactive emissions.

Body Part – 4TH	Radionuclide – 5TH	Qualifier – 6TH	Qualifier – 7TH
4 Gallbladder 5 Liver 6 Liver and Spleen	1 Technetium 99m (Tc-99m) Y Other radionuclide	Z None	Z None
Y Hepatobiliary System and Pancreas	Y Other radionuclide	Z None	Z None

---

- 1ST – **C** Nuclear Medicine
- 2ND – **G** Endocrine System
- 3RD – **1** PLANAR NUCLEAR MEDICINE IMAGING

EXAMPLE: Gallium scan, single plane image

PLANAR NUCLEAR MEDICINE IMAGING: Introduction of radioactive materials into the body for single plane display of images developed from the capture of radioactive emissions.

Body Part – 4TH	Radionuclide – 5TH	Qualifier – 6TH	Qualifier – 7TH
1 Parathyroid Glands	1 Technetium 99m (Tc-99m) S Thallium 201 (Tl-201) Y Other radionuclide	Z None	Z None
2 Thyroid Gland	1 Technetium 99m (Tc-99m) F Iodine 123 (I-123) G Iodine 131 (I-131) Y Other radionuclide	Z None	Z None
4 Adrenal Glands, Bilateral	G Iodine 131 (I-131) Y Other radionuclide	Z None	Z None
Y Endocrine System	Y Other radionuclide	Z None	Z None

- 1ST – **C** Nuclear Medicine
- 2ND – **G** Endocrine System
- 3RD – **2** TOMOGRAPHIC (TOMO) NUCLEAR MEDICINE IMAGING

EXAMPLE: Tomo scan of breast

TOMOGRAPHIC (TOMO) NUCLEAR MEDICINE IMAGING: Introduction of radioactive materials into the body for three dimensional display of images developed from the capture of radioactive emissions.

Body Part – 4TH	Radionuclide – 5TH	Qualifier – 6TH	Qualifier – 7TH
1 Parathyroid Glands	1 Technetium 99m (Tc-99m) S Thallium 201 (Tl-201) Y Other radionuclide	Z None	Z None
Y Endocrine System	Y Other radionuclide	Z None	Z None

C – NUCLEAR MEDICINE

CH2

1ST -	C	Nuclear Medicine
2ND -	G	Endocrine System
3RD -	4	NONIMAGING NUCLEAR MEDICINE UPTAKE

EXAMPLE: Iodine uptake test of thyroid

NONIMAGING NUCLEAR MEDICINE UPTAKE: Introduction of radioactive materials into the body for measurements of organ function, from the detection of radioactive emissions.

Body Part – 4TH	Radionuclide – 5TH	Qualifier – 6TH	Qualifier – 7TH
2 Thyroid Gland	1 Technetium 99m (Tc-99m) F Iodine 123 (I-123) G Iodine 131 (I-131) Y Other radionuclide	Z None	Z None
Y Endocrine System	Y Other radionuclide	Z None	Z None

1ST -	C	Nuclear Medicine
2ND -	H	Skin, Subcutaneous Tissue and Breast
3RD -	1	PLANAR NUCLEAR MEDICINE IMAGING

EXAMPLE: Gallium scan, single plane image

PLANAR NUCLEAR MEDICINE IMAGING: Introduction of radioactive materials into the body for single plane display of images developed from the capture of radioactive emissions.

Body Part – 4TH	Radionuclide – 5TH	Qualifier – 6TH	Qualifier – 7TH
0 Breast, Right 1 Breast, Left 2 Breasts, Bilateral	1 Technetium 99m (Tc-99m) S Thallium 201 (Tl-201) Y Other radionuclide	Z None	Z None
Y Skin, Subcutaneous Tissue and Breast	Y Other radionuclide	Z None	Z None

---

1ST -	C	Nuclear Medicine
2ND -	H	Skin, Subcutaneous Tissue and Breast
3RD -	2	TOMOGRAPHIC (TOMO) NUCLEAR MEDICINE IMAGING

EXAMPLE: Tomo scan of breast

TOMOGRAPHIC (TOMO) NUCLEAR MEDICINE IMAGING: Introduction of radioactive materials into the body for three dimensional display of images developed from the capture of radioactive emissions.

Body Part – 4TH	Radionuclide – 5TH	Qualifier – 6TH	Qualifier – 7TH
0 Breast, Right 1 Breast, Left 2 Breasts, Bilateral	1 Technetium 99m (Tc-99m) S Thallium 201 (Tl-201) Y Other radionuclide	Z None	Z None
Y Skin, Subcutaneous Tissue and Breast	Y Other radionuclide	Z None	Z None

ANCILLARY SECTIONS – 2016 ICD-10-PCS

CP1

1ST – C Nuclear Medicine
2ND – P Musculoskeletal System
3RD – 1 PLANAR NUCLEAR MEDICINE IMAGING

EXAMPLE: Gallium scan, single plane image

PLANAR NUCLEAR MEDICINE IMAGING: Introduction of radioactive materials into the body for single plane display of images developed from the capture of radioactive emissions.

Body Part – 4TH	Radionuclide – 5TH	Qualifier – 6TH	Qualifier – 7TH
1 Skull 4 Thorax 5 Spine 6 Pelvis 7 Spine and Pelvis 8 Upper Extremity, Right 9 Upper Extremity, Left B Upper Extremities, Bilateral C Lower Extremity, Right D Lower Extremity, Left F Lower Extremities, Bilateral Z Musculoskeletal System, All	1 Technetium 99m (Tc-99m) Y Other radionuclide	Z None	Z None
Y Musculoskeletal System, Other	Y Other radionuclide	Z None	Z None

---

1ST – C Nuclear Medicine
2ND – P Musculoskeletal System
3RD – 2 TOMOGRAPHIC (TOMO) NUCLEAR MEDICINE IMAGING

EXAMPLE: Tomo scan of breast

TOMOGRAPHIC (TOMO) NUCLEAR MEDICINE IMAGING: Introduction of radioactive materials into the body for three dimensional display of images developed from the capture of radioactive emissions.

Body Part – 4TH	Radionuclide – 5TH	Qualifier – 6TH	Qualifier – 7TH
1 Skull 2 Cervical Spine 3 Skull and Cervical Spine 4 Thorax 6 Pelvis 7 Spine and Pelvis 8 Upper Extremity, Right 9 Upper Extremity, Left B Upper Extremities, Bilateral C Lower Extremity, Right D Lower Extremity, Left F Lower Extremities, Bilateral G Thoracic Spine H Lumbar Spine J Thoracolumbar Spine	1 Technetium 99m (Tc-99m) Y Other radionuclide	Z None	Z None
Y Musculoskeletal System, Other	Y Other radionuclide	Z None	Z None

C – NUCLEAR MEDICINE

1ST - C Nuclear Medicine
2ND - P Musculoskeletal System
3RD - 5 NONIMAGING NUCLEAR MEDICINE PROBE

EXAMPLE: Xenon gas nonimaging probe of brain

NONIMAGING NUCLEAR MEDICINE PROBE: Introduction of radioactive materials into the body for the study of distribution and fate of certain substances by the detection of radioactive emissions; or, alternatively, measurement of absorption of radioactive emissions from an external source.

Body Part – 4TH	Radionuclide – 5TH	Qualifier – 6TH	Qualifier – 7TH
5 Spine N Upper Extremities P Lower Extremities	Z None	Z None	Z None
Y Musculoskeletal System, Other	Y Other radionuclide	Z None	Z None

1ST - C Nuclear Medicine
2ND - T Urinary System
3RD - 1 PLANAR NUCLEAR MEDICINE IMAGING

EXAMPLE: Gallium scan, single plane image

PLANAR NUCLEAR MEDICINE IMAGING: Introduction of radioactive materials into the body for single plane display of images developed from the capture of radioactive emissions.

Body Part – 4TH	Radionuclide – 5TH	Qualifier – 6TH	Qualifier – 7TH
3 Kidneys, Ureters and Bladder	1 Technetium 99m (Tc-99m) F Iodine 123 (I-123) G Iodine 131 (I-131) Y Other radionuclide	Z None	Z None
H Bladder and Ureters	1 Technetium 99m (Tc-99m) Y Other radionuclide	Z None	Z None
Y Urinary System	Y Other radionuclide	Z None	Z None

1ST - C Nuclear Medicine
2ND - T Urinary System
3RD - 2 TOMOGRAPHIC (TOMO) NUCLEAR MEDICINE IMAGING

EXAMPLE: Tomo scan of breast

TOMOGRAPHIC (TOMO) NUCLEAR MEDICINE IMAGING: Introduction of radioactive materials into the body for three dimensional display of images developed from the capture of radioactive emissions.

Body Part – 4TH	Radionuclide – 5TH	Qualifier – 6TH	Qualifier – 7TH
3 Kidneys, Ureters and Bladder	1 Technetium 99m (Tc-99m) Y Other radionuclide	Z None	Z None
Y Urinary System	Y Other radionuclide	Z None	Z None

CT6 ANCILLARY SECTIONS – 2016 ICD-10-PCS [2016.PCS]

1ST – **C** Nuclear Medicine 2ND – **T** Urinary System 3RD – **6** NONIMAGING NUCLEAR MEDICINE ASSAY	EXAMPLE: Technetium assay of kidneys **NONIMAGING NUCLEAR MEDICINE ASSAY:** Introduction of radioactive materials into the body for the study of body fluids and blood elements, by the detection of radioactive emissions.

Body Part – 4TH	Radionuclide – 5TH	Qualifier – 6TH	Qualifier – 7TH
3 Kidneys, Ureters and Bladder	1 Technetium 99m (Tc-99m) F Iodine 123 (I-123) G Iodine 131 (I-131) H Iodine 125 (I-125) Y Other radionuclide	Z None	Z None
Y Urinary System	Y Other radionuclide	Z None	Z None

1ST – **C** Nuclear Medicine 2ND – **V** Male Reproductive System 3RD – **1** PLANAR NUCLEAR MEDICINE IMAGING	EXAMPLE: Gallium scan, single plane image **PLANAR NUCLEAR MEDICINE IMAGING:** Introduction of radioactive materials into the body for single plane display of images developed from the capture of radioactive emissions.

Body Part – 4TH	Radionuclide – 5TH	Qualifier – 6TH	Qualifier – 7TH
9 Testicles, Bilateral ♂	1 Technetium 99m (Tc-99m) Y Other radionuclide	Z None	Z None
Y Male Reproductive System ♂	Y Other radionuclide	Z None	Z None

820

C – NUCLEAR MEDICINE

CW2

1ST - C Nuclear Medicine
2ND - W Anatomical Regions
3RD - 1 PLANAR NUCLEAR MEDICINE IMAGING

EXAMPLE: Gallium scan, single plane image

PLANAR NUCLEAR MEDICINE IMAGING: Introduction of radioactive materials into the body for single plane display of images developed from the capture of radioactive emissions.

Body Part – 4TH	Radionuclide – 5TH	Qualifier – 6TH	Qualifier – 7TH
0 Abdomen 1 Abdomen and Pelvis 4 Chest and Abdomen 6 Chest and Neck B Head and Neck D Lower Extremity J Pelvic Region M Upper Extremity N Whole Body	1 Technetium 99m (Tc-99m) D Indium 111 (In-111) F Iodine 123 (I-123) G Iodine 131 (I-131) L Gallium 67 (Ga-67) S Thallium 201 (Tl-201) Y Other radionuclide	Z None	Z None
3 Chest	1 Technetium 99m (Tc-99m) D Indium 111 (In-111) F Iodine 123 (I-123) G Iodine 131 (I-131) K Fluorine 18 (F-18) L Gallium 67 (Ga-67) S Thallium 201 (Tl-201) Y Other radionuclide	Z None	Z None
Y Anatomical Regions, Multiple	Y Other radionuclide	Z None	Z None
Z Anatomical Region, Other	Z None	Z None	Z None

1ST - C Nuclear Medicine
2ND - W Anatomical Regions
3RD - 2 TOMOGRAPHIC (TOMO) NUCLEAR MEDICINE IMAGING

EXAMPLE: Tomo scan of breast

TOMOGRAPHIC (TOMO) NUCLEAR MEDICINE IMAGING: Introduction of radioactive materials into the body for three dimensional display of images developed from the capture of radioactive emissions.

Body Part – 4TH	Radionuclide – 5TH	Qualifier – 6TH	Qualifier – 7TH
0 Abdomen 1 Abdomen and Pelvis 3 Chest 4 Chest and Abdomen 6 Chest and Neck B Head and Neck D Lower Extremity J Pelvic Region M Upper Extremity	1 Technetium 99m (Tc-99m) D Indium 111 (In-111) F Iodine 123 (I-123) G Iodine 131 (I-131) K Fluorine 18 (F-18) L Gallium 67 (Ga-67) S Thallium 201 (Tl-201) Y Other radionuclide	Z None	Z None
Y Anatomical Regions, Multiple	Y Other radionuclide	Z None	Z None

CW3 — ANCILLARY SECTIONS – 2016 ICD-10-PCS

1ST – C Nuclear Medicine
2ND – W Anatomical Regions
3RD – 3 POSITRON EMISSION (PET) TOMOGRAPHIC IMAGING

EXAMPLE: PET scan of brain

POSITRON EMISSION TOMOGRAPHIC (PET) IMAGING: Introduction of radioactive materials into the body for three dimensional display of images developed from the simultaneous capture, 180 degrees apart, of radioactive emissions.

Body Part – 4TH	Radionuclide – 5TH	Qualifier – 6TH	Qualifier – 7TH
N Whole Body	Y Other radionuclide	Z None	Z None

1ST – C Nuclear Medicine
2ND – W Anatomical Regions
3RD – 5 NONIMAGING NUCLEAR MEDICINE PROBE

EXAMPLE: Xenon gas nonimaging probe of brain

NONIMAGING NUCLEAR MEDICINE PROBE: Introduction of radioactive materials into the body for the study of distribution and fate of certain substances by the detection of radioactive emissions; or, alternatively, measurement of absorption of radioactive emissions from an external source.

Body Part – 4TH	Radionuclide – 5TH	Qualifier – 6TH	Qualifier – 7TH
0 Abdomen 1 Abdomen and Pelvis 3 Chest 4 Chest and Abdomen 6 Chest and Neck B Head and Neck D Lower Extremity J Pelvic Region M Upper Extremity	1 Technetium 99m (Tc-99m) D Indium 111 (In-111) Y Other radionuclide	Z None	Z None

---

1ST – C Nuclear Medicine
2ND – W Anatomical Regions
3RD – 7 SYSTEMIC NUCLEAR MEDICINE THERAPY

EXAMPLE: None

SYSTEMIC NUCLEAR MEDICINE THERAPY: Introduction of unsealed radioactive materials into the body for treatment.

Body Part – 4TH	Radionuclide – 5TH	Qualifier – 6TH	Qualifier – 7TH
0 Abdomen 3 Chest	N Phosphorus 32 (P-32) Y Other radionuclide	Z None	Z None
G Thyroid	G Iodine 131 (I-131) Y Other radionuclide	Z None	Z None
N Whole Body	8 Samarium 153 (Sm-153) G Iodine 131 (I-131) N Phosphorus 32 (P-32) P Strontium 89 (Sr-89) Y Other radionuclide	Z None	Z None
Y Anatomical Regions, Multiple	Y Other radionuclide	Z None	Z None

Educational Annotations

Section D – Radiation Therapy

Section Specific Educational Annotations for the Radiation Therapy Section include:
- AHA Coding Clinic® Reference Notations
- Coding Notes

AHA Coding Clinic® Reference Notations of Radiation Therapy

ROOT TYPE SPECIFIC - RADIATION THERAPY - Section D
BEAM RADIATION - 0
BRACHYTHERAPY - 1
STEREOTACTIC RADIOSURGERY - 3
OTHER RADIATION - Y

Coding Notes of Radiation Therapy

Ancillary Section Specific PCS Reference Manual Exercises

PCS CODE	D – RADIATION THERAPY EXERCISES
D 0 0 1 1 Z Z	8 MeV photon beam radiation to brain.
D 0 1 6 B 9 Z	LDR brachytherapy to spinal cord using iodine.
D 8 Y 0 F Z Z	Plaque radiation of left eye, single port.
D 9 Y 5 7 Z Z	Contact radiation of tongue.
D D Y 5 C Z Z	IORT of colon, 3 ports.
D F 0 3 4 Z Z	Heavy particle radiation treatment of pancreas, four risk sites.
D M 0 1 3 Z Z	Electron radiation treatment of right breast, custom device.
D V 1 0 9 B Z	HDR Brachytherapy of prostate using Palladium 103.
D W Y 5 G F Z	Whole body Phosphorus 32 administration with risk to hematopoetic system.
D W Y 6 8 Z Z	Hyperthermia oncology treatment of pelvic region.

Educational Annotations

Section D – Radiation Therapy

NOTES

Section Specific Educational Annotations – Radiation Therapy Section include:
- AHA Coding Clinic® Reference Notations
- Coding Notes

AHA Coding Clinic® Reference Notations of Radiation Therapy

ROOT TYPE SPECIFIC – RADIATION THERAPY – Section D
- BEAM RADIATION – 0
- BRACHYTHERAPY – 1
- STEREOTACTIC RADIOSURGERY – 3
- OTHER RADIATION – Y

Coding Notes of Radiation Therapy

Ancillary Section Specific PCS Reference Manual Exercises.

D – RADIATION THERAPY EXERCISES

PCS CODE	
D0011ZZ	8 MeV photon beam radiation to brain.
D0168ZZ	LDR brachytherapy to spinal cord using iodine.
D8Y0FZZ	Plaque radiation of left eye, single port.
D9Y57ZZ	Contact radiation of tongue.
DDY5CZZ	IORT of colon, 3 ports.
DF034ZZ	Heavy particle radiation treatment of pancreas, four risk sites.
DM013ZZ	Electron radiation treatment of right breast, custom device.
DV109BZ	HDR Brachytherapy of prostate using Palladium 103.
DWY5GFZ	Whole body Phosphorus 32 administration with risk to hematopoietic system.
DWY68ZZ	Hyperthermia oncology treatment of pelvic region.

D – RADIATION THERAPY

MODALITY: BEAM RADIATION

- 1ST - **D** Radiation Therapy
- 2ND - **0** Central and Peripheral Nervous System
- 3RD - **0** BEAM RADIATION

EXAMPLE: External beam radiation

Treatment Site – 4TH	Modality Qualifier – 5TH	Isotope – 6TH	Qualifier – 7TH
0 Brain 1 Brain Stem 6 Spinal Cord 7 Peripheral Nerve	0 Photons <1 MeV 1 Photons 1 - 10 MeV 2 Photons >10 MeV 4 Heavy particles (protons, ions) 5 Neutrons 6 Neutron capture	Z None	Z None
0 Brain 1 Brain Stem 6 Spinal Cord 7 Peripheral Nerve	3 Electrons	Z None	0 Intraoperative Z None

MODALITY: BRACHYTHERAPY

- 1ST - **D** Radiation Therapy
- 2ND - **0** Central and Peripheral Nervous System
- 3RD - **1** BRACHYTHERAPY

EXAMPLE: Insertion of radioactive material

Treatment Site – 4TH	Modality Qualifier – 5TH	Isotope – 6TH	Qualifier – 7TH
0 Brain 1 Brain Stem 6 Spinal Cord 7 Peripheral Nerve	9 High dose rate (HDR) B Low dose rate (LDR)	7 Cesium 137 (Cs-137) 8 Iridium 192 (Ir-192) 9 Iodine 125 (I-125) B Palladium 103 (Pd-103) C Californium 252 (Cf-252) Y Other isotope	Z None

MODALITY: STEREOTACTIC RADIOSURGERY

- 1ST - **D** Radiation Therapy
- 2ND - **0** Central and Peripheral Nervous System
- 3RD - **2** STEREOTACTIC RADIOSURGERY

EXAMPLE: Particulate stereotactic radiosurgery

Treatment Site – 4TH	Modality Qualifier – 5TH	Isotope – 6TH	Qualifier – 7TH
0 Brain 1 Brain Stem 6 Spinal Cord 7 Peripheral Nerve	D Stereotactic other photon radiosurgery H Stereotactic particulate radiosurgery J Stereotactic gamma beam radiosurgery	Z None	Z None

ANCILLARY SECTIONS – 2016 ICD-10-PCS

D 0 Y

1ST - D Radiation Therapy
2ND - 0 Central and Peripheral Nervous System
3RD - Y OTHER RADIATION

EXAMPLE: Laser interstitial thermal therapy
MODALITY: OTHER RADIATION

Treatment Site – 4TH	Modality Qualifier – 5TH	Isotope – 6TH	Qualifier – 7TH
0 Brain 1 Brain Stem 6 Spinal Cord 7 Peripheral Nerve	7 Contact radiation 8 Hyperthermia F Plaque radiation K Laser interstitial thermal therapy	Z None	Z None

D 7 0

1ST - D Radiation Therapy
2ND - 7 Lymphatic and Hematologic System
3RD - 0 BEAM RADIATION

EXAMPLE: External beam radiation
MODALITY: BEAM RADIATION

Treatment Site – 4TH	Modality Qualifier – 5TH	Isotope – 6TH	Qualifier – 7TH
0 Bone Marrow 1 Thymus 2 Spleen 3 Lymphatics, Neck 4 Lymphatics, Axillary 5 Lymphatics, Thorax 6 Lymphatics, Abdomen 7 Lymphatics, Pelvis 8 Lymphatics, Inguinal	0 Photons <1 MeV 1 Photons 1 - 10 MeV 2 Photons >10 MeV 4 Heavy particles (protons, ions) 5 Neutrons 6 Neutron capture	Z None	Z None
0 Bone Marrow 1 Thymus 2 Spleen 3 Lymphatics, Neck 4 Lymphatics, Axillary 5 Lymphatics, Thorax 6 Lymphatics, Abdomen 7 Lymphatics, Pelvis 8 Lymphatics, Inguinal	3 Electrons	Z None	0 Intraoperative Z None

D – RADIATION THERAPY

D7Y

[2016.PCS]

1ST - D Radiation Therapy
2ND - 7 Lymphatic and Hematologic System
3RD - 1 BRACHYTHERAPY

EXAMPLE: Insertion of radioactive material
MODALITY: BRACHYTHERAPY

Treatment Site – 4TH	Modality Qualifier – 5TH	Isotope – 6TH	Qualifier – 7TH
0 Bone Marrow 1 Thymus 2 Spleen 3 Lymphatics, Neck 4 Lymphatics, Axillary 5 Lymphatics, Thorax 6 Lymphatics, Abdomen 7 Lymphatics, Pelvis 8 Lymphatics, Inguinal	9 High dose rate (HDR) B Low dose rate (LDR)	7 Cesium 137 (Cs-137) 8 Iridium 192 (Ir-192) 9 Iodine 125 (I-125) B Palladium 103 (Pd-103) C Californium 252 (Cf-252) Y Other isotope	Z None

---

1ST - D Radiation Therapy
2ND - 7 Lymphatic and Hematologic System
3RD - 2 STEREOTACTIC RADIOSURGERY

EXAMPLE: Particulate stereotactic radiosurgery
MODALITY: STEREOTACTIC RADIOSURGERY

Treatment Site – 4TH	Modality Qualifier – 5TH	Isotope – 6TH	Qualifier – 7TH
0 Bone Marrow 1 Thymus 2 Spleen 3 Lymphatics, Neck 4 Lymphatics, Axillary 5 Lymphatics, Thorax 6 Lymphatics, Abdomen 7 Lymphatics, Pelvis 8 Lymphatics, Inguinal	D Stereotactic other photon radiosurgery H Stereotactic particulate radiosurgery J Stereotactic gamma beam radiosurgery	Z None	Z None

---

1ST - D Radiation Therapy
2ND - 7 Lymphatic and Hematologic System
3RD - Y OTHER RADIATION

EXAMPLE: Laser interstitial thermal therapy
MODALITY: OTHER RADIATION

Treatment Site – 4TH	Modality Qualifier – 5TH	Isotope – 6TH	Qualifier – 7TH
0 Bone Marrow 1 Thymus 2 Spleen 3 Lymphatics, Neck 4 Lymphatics, Axillary 5 Lymphatics, Thorax 6 Lymphatics, Abdomen 7 Lymphatics, Pelvis 8 Lymphatics, Inguinal	8 Hyperthermia F Plaque radiation	Z None	Z None

RADIATION THERAPY D80

MODALITY: BEAM RADIATION

- 1ST – **D** Radiation Therapy
- 2ND – **8** Eye
- 3RD – **0** BEAM RADIATION

EXAMPLE: External beam radiation

Treatment Site – 4TH	Modality Qualifier – 5TH	Isotope – 6TH	Qualifier – 7TH
0 Eye	0 Photons <1 MeV 1 Photons 1 - 10 MeV 2 Photons >10 MeV 4 Heavy particles (protons, ions) 5 Neutrons 6 Neutron capture	Z None	Z None
0 Eye	3 Electrons	Z None	0 Intraoperative Z None

MODALITY: BRACHYTHERAPY

- 1ST – **D** Radiation Therapy
- 2ND – **8** Eye
- 3RD – **1** BRACHYTHERAPY

EXAMPLE: Insertion of radioactive material

Treatment Site – 4TH	Modality Qualifier – 5TH	Isotope – 6TH	Qualifier – 7TH
0 Eye	9 High dose rate (HDR) B Low dose rate (LDR)	7 Cesium 137 (Cs-137) 8 Iridium 192 (Ir-192) 9 Iodine 125 (I-125) B Palladium 103 (Pd-103) C Californium 252 (Cf-252) Y Other isotope	Z None

MODALITY: STEREOTACTIC RADIOSURGERY

- 1ST – **D** Radiation Therapy
- 2ND – **8** Eye
- 3RD – **2** STEREOTACTIC RADIOSURGERY

EXAMPLE: Particulate stereotactic radiosurgery

Treatment Site – 4TH	Modality Qualifier – 5TH	Isotope – 6TH	Qualifier – 7TH
0 Eye	D Stereotactic other photon radiosurgery H Stereotactic particulate radiosurgery J Stereotactic gamma beam radiosurgery	Z None	Z None

D – RADIATION THERAPY

1ST - D Radiation Therapy
2ND - 8 Eye
3RD - Y OTHER RADIATION

EXAMPLE: Laser interstitial thermal therapy
MODALITY: OTHER RADIATION

Treatment Site – 4TH	Modality Qualifier – 5TH	Isotope – 6TH	Qualifier – 7TH
0 Eye	7 Contact radiation 8 Hyperthermia F Plaque radiation	Z None	Z None

1ST - D Radiation Therapy
2ND - 9 Ear, Nose, Mouth and Throat
3RD - 0 BEAM RADIATION

EXAMPLE: External beam radiation
MODALITY: BEAM RADIATION

Treatment Site – 4TH	Modality Qualifier – 5TH	Isotope – 6TH	Qualifier – 7TH
0 Ear 7 Sinuses 1 Nose 8 Hard Palate 3 Hypopharynx 9 Soft Palate 4 Mouth B Larynx 5 Tongue D Nasopharynx 6 Salivary Glands F Oropharynx	0 Photons <1 MeV 1 Photons 1 - 10 MeV 2 Photons >10 MeV 4 Heavy particles (protons, ions) 5 Neutrons 6 Neutron capture	Z None	Z None
0 Ear 7 Sinuses 1 Nose 8 Hard Palate 3 Hypopharynx 9 Soft Palate 4 Mouth B Larynx 5 Tongue D Nasopharynx 6 Salivary Glands F Oropharynx	3 Electrons	Z None	0 Intraoperative Z None

1ST - D Radiation Therapy
2ND - 9 Ear, Nose, Mouth and Throat
3RD - 1 BRACHYTHERAPY

EXAMPLE: Insertion of radioactive material
MODALITY: BRACHYTHERAPY

Treatment Site – 4TH	Modality Qualifier – 5TH	Isotope – 6TH	Qualifier – 7TH
0 Ear 7 Sinuses 1 Nose 8 Hard Palate 3 Hypopharynx 9 Soft Palate 4 Mouth B Larynx 5 Tongue D Nasopharynx 6 Salivary Glands F Oropharynx	9 High dose rate (HDR) B Low dose rate (LDR)	7 Cesium 137 (Cs-137) 8 Iridium 192 (Ir-192) 9 Iodine 125 (I-125) B Palladium 103 (Pd-103) C Californium 252 (Cf-252) Y Other isotope	Z None

D92

ANCILLARY SECTIONS – 2016 ICD-10-PCS

1ST - D Radiation Therapy
2ND - 9 Ear, Nose, Mouth and Throat
3RD - 2 STEREOTACTIC RADIOSURGERY

EXAMPLE: Particulate stereotactic radiosurgery
MODALITY: STEREOTACTIC RADIOSURGERY

Treatment Site – 4TH	Modality Qualifier – 5TH	Isotope – 6TH	Qualifier – 7TH
0 Ear 8 Hard Palate 1 Nose 9 Soft Palate 4 Mouth B Larynx 5 Tongue C Pharynx 6 Salivary Glands D Nasopharynx 7 Sinuses	D Stereotactic other photon radiosurgery H Stereotactic particulate radiosurgery J Stereotactic gamma beam radiosurgery	Z None	Z None

1ST - D Radiation Therapy
2ND - 9 Ear, Nose, Mouth and Throat
3RD - Y OTHER RADIATION

EXAMPLE: Laser interstitial thermal therapy
MODALITY: OTHER RADIATION

Treatment Site – 4TH	Modality Qualifier – 5TH	Isotope – 6TH	Qualifier – 7TH
0 Ear 7 Sinuses 1 Nose 8 Hard Palate 5 Tongue 9 Soft Palate 6 Salivary Glands	7 Contact radiation 8 Hyperthermia F Plaque radiation	Z None	Z None
3 Hypopharynx F Oropharynx	7 Contact radiation 8 Hyperthermia	Z None	Z None
4 Mouth B Larynx D Nasopharynx	7 Contact radiation 8 Hyperthermia C Intraoperative radiation therapy (IORT) F Plaque radiation	Z None	Z None
C Pharynx	C Intraoperative radiation therapy (IORT) F Plaque radiation	Z None	Z None

1ST - D Radiation Therapy
2ND - B Respiratory System
3RD - 0 BEAM RADIATION

EXAMPLE: External beam radiation
MODALITY: BEAM RADIATION

Treatment Site – 4TH	Modality Qualifier – 5TH	Isotope – 6TH	Qualifier – 7TH
0 Trachea 6 Mediastinum 1 Bronchus 7 Chest Wall 2 Lung 8 Diaphragm 5 Pleura	0 Photons <1 MeV 1 Photons 1 - 10 MeV 2 Photons >10 MeV 4 Heavy particles (protons, ions) 5 Neutrons 6 Neutron capture	Z None	Z None
0 Trachea 6 Mediastinum 1 Bronchus 7 Chest Wall 2 Lung 8 Diaphragm 5 Pleura	3 Electrons	Z None	0 Intraoperative Z None

D – RADIATION THERAPY

DBY

1ST -	D	Radiation Therapy
2ND -	B	Respiratory System
3RD -	1	BRACHYTHERAPY

EXAMPLE: Insertion of radioactive material

MODALITY: BRACHYTHERAPY

Treatment Site – 4TH	Modality Qualifier – 5TH	Isotope – 6TH	Qualifier – 7TH
0 Trachea 6 Mediastinum 1 Bronchus 7 Chest Wall 2 Lung 8 Diaphragm 5 Pleura	9 High dose rate (HDR) B Low dose rate (LDR)	7 Cesium 137 (Cs-137) 8 Iridium 192 (Ir-192) 9 Iodine 125 (I-125) B Palladium 103 (Pd-103) C Californium 252 (Cf-252) Y Other isotope	Z None

1ST -	D	Radiation Therapy
2ND -	B	Respiratory System
3RD -	2	STEREOTACTIC RADIOSURGERY

EXAMPLE: Particulate stereotactic radiosurgery

MODALITY: STEREOTACTIC RADIOSURGERY

Treatment Site – 4TH	Modality Qualifier – 5TH	Isotope – 6TH	Qualifier – 7TH
0 Trachea 6 Mediastinum 1 Bronchus 7 Chest Wall 2 Lung 8 Diaphragm 5 Pleura	D Stereotactic other photon radiosurgery H Stereotactic particulate radiosurgery J Stereotactic gamma beam radiosurgery	Z None	Z None

1ST -	D	Radiation Therapy
2ND -	B	Respiratory System
3RD -	Y	OTHER RADIATION

EXAMPLE: Laser interstitial thermal therapy

MODALITY: OTHER RADIATION

Treatment Site – 4TH	Modality Qualifier – 5TH	Isotope – 6TH	Qualifier – 7TH
0 Trachea 6 Mediastinum 1 Bronchus 7 Chest Wall 2 Lung 8 Diaphragm 5 Pleura	7 Contact radiation 8 Hyperthermia F Plaque radiation K Laser interstitial thermal therapy	Z None	Z None

DD0 — ANCILLARY SECTIONS – 2016 ICD-10-PCS

1ST - D Radiation Therapy
2ND - D Gastrointestinal System
3RD - 0 BEAM RADIATION

EXAMPLE: External beam radiation
MODALITY: BEAM RADIATION

Treatment Site – 4TH	Modality Qualifier – 5TH	Isotope – 6TH	Qualifier – 7TH
0 Esophagus 4 Ileum 1 Stomach 5 Colon 2 Duodenum 7 Rectum 3 Jejunum	0 Photons <1 MeV 1 Photons 1 - 10 MeV 2 Photons >10 MeV 4 Heavy particles (protons, ions) 5 Neutrons 6 Neutron capture	Z None	Z None
0 Esophagus 4 Ileum 1 Stomach 5 Colon 2 Duodenum 7 Rectum 3 Jejunum	3 Electrons	Z None	0 Intraoperative Z None

1ST - D Radiation Therapy
2ND - D Gastrointestinal System
3RD - 1 BRACHYTHERAPY

EXAMPLE: Insertion of radioactive material
MODALITY: BRACHYTHERAPY

Treatment Site – 4TH	Modality Qualifier – 5TH	Isotope – 6TH	Qualifier – 7TH
0 Esophagus 4 Ileum 1 Stomach 5 Colon 2 Duodenum 7 Rectum 3 Jejunum	9 High dose rate (HDR) B Low dose rate (LDR)	7 Cesium 137 (Cs-137) 8 Iridium 192 (Ir-192) 9 Iodine 125 (I-125) B Palladium 103 (Pd-103) C Californium 252 (Cf-252) Y Other isotope	Z None

1ST - D Radiation Therapy
2ND - D Gastrointestinal System
3RD - 2 STEREOTACTIC RADIOSURGERY

EXAMPLE: Particulate stereotactic radiosurgery
MODALITY: STEREOTACTIC RADIOSURGERY

Treatment Site – 4TH	Modality Qualifier – 5TH	Isotope – 6TH	Qualifier – 7TH
0 Esophagus 4 Ileum 1 Stomach 5 Colon 2 Duodenum 7 Rectum 3 Jejunum	D Stereotactic other photon radiosurgery H Stereotactic particulate radiosurgery J Stereotactic gamma beam radiosurgery	Z None	Z None

D – RADIATION THERAPY

DF0

- 1ST – **D** Radiation Therapy
- 2ND – **D** Gastrointestinal System
- 3RD – **Y** OTHER RADIATION

EXAMPLE: Laser interstitial thermal therapy

MODALITY: OTHER RADIATION

Treatment Site – 4TH	Modality Qualifier – 5TH	Isotope – 6TH	Qualifier – 7TH
0 Esophagus	7 Contact radiation 8 Hyperthermia F Plaque radiation K Laser interstitial thermal therapy	Z None	Z None
1 Stomach 2 Duodenum 3 Jejunum 4 Ileum 5 Colon 7 Rectum	7 Contact radiation 8 Hyperthermia C Intraoperative radiation therapy (IORT) F Plaque radiation K Laser interstitial thermal therapy	Z None	Z None
8 Anus	C Intraoperative radiation therapy (IORT) F Plaque radiation K Laser interstitial thermal therapy	Z None	Z None

- 1ST – **D** Radiation Therapy
- 2ND – **F** Hepatobiliary System and Pancreas
- 3RD – **0** BEAM RADIATION

EXAMPLE: External beam radiation

MODALITY: BEAM RADIATION

Treatment Site – 4TH	Modality Qualifier – 5TH	Isotope – 6TH	Qualifier – 7TH
0 Liver 1 Gallbladder 2 Bile Ducts 3 Pancreas	0 Photons <1 MeV 1 Photons 1 - 10 MeV 2 Photons >10 MeV 4 Heavy particles (protons, ions) 5 Neutrons 6 Neutron capture	Z None	Z None
0 Liver 1 Gallbladder 2 Bile Ducts 3 Pancreas	3 Electrons	Z None	0 Intraoperative Z None

DF1 ANCILLARY SECTIONS – 2016 ICD-10-PCS

1ST - D Radiation Therapy
2ND - F Hepatobiliary System and Pancreas
3RD - 1 BRACHYTHERAPY

EXAMPLE: Insertion of radioactive material

MODALITY: BRACHYTHERAPY

Treatment Site – 4TH	Modality Qualifier – 5TH	Isotope – 6TH	Qualifier – 7TH
0 Liver 1 Gallbladder 2 Bile Ducts 3 Pancreas	9 High dose rate (HDR) B Low dose rate (LDR)	7 Cesium 137 (Cs-137) 8 Iridium 192 (Ir-192) 9 Iodine 125 (I-125) B Palladium 103 (Pd-103) C Californium 252 (Cf-252) Y Other isotope	Z None

1ST - D Radiation Therapy
2ND - F Hepatobiliary System and Pancreas
3RD - 2 STEREOTACTIC RADIOSURGERY

EXAMPLE: Particulate stereotactic radiosurgery

MODALITY: STEREOTACTIC RADIOSURGERY

Treatment Site – 4TH	Modality Qualifier – 5TH	Isotope – 6TH	Qualifier – 7TH
0 Liver 1 Gallbladder 2 Bile Ducts 3 Pancreas	D Stereotactic other photon radiosurgery H Stereotactic particulate radiosurgery J Stereotactic gamma beam radiosurgery	Z None	Z None

1ST - D Radiation Therapy
2ND - F Hepatobiliary System and Pancreas
3RD - Y OTHER RADIATION

EXAMPLE: Laser interstitial thermal therapy

MODALITY: OTHER RADIATION

Treatment Site – 4TH	Modality Qualifier – 5TH	Isotope – 6TH	Qualifier – 7TH
0 Liver 1 Gallbladder 2 Bile Ducts 3 Pancreas	7 Contact radiation 8 Hyperthermia C Intraoperative radiation therapy (IORT) F Plaque radiation K Laser interstitial thermal therapy	Z None	Z None

D – RADIATION THERAPY

DG2

1ST - D Radiation Therapy
2ND - G Endocrine System
3RD - 0 BEAM RADIATION

EXAMPLE: External beam radiation
MODALITY: BEAM RADIATION

Treatment Site – 4TH	Modality Qualifier – 5TH	Isotope – 6TH	Qualifier – 7TH
0 Pituitary Gland 1 Pineal Body 2 Adrenal Glands 4 Parathyroid Glands 5 Thyroid	0 Photons <1 MeV 1 Photons 1 - 10 MeV 2 Photons >10 MeV 5 Neutrons 6 Neutron capture	Z None	Z None
0 Pituitary Gland 1 Pineal Body 2 Adrenal Glands 4 Parathyroid Glands 5 Thyroid	3 Electrons	Z None	0 Intraoperative Z None

1ST - D Radiation Therapy
2ND - G Endocrine System
3RD - 1 BRACHYTHERAPY

EXAMPLE: Insertion of radioactive material
MODALITY: BRACHYTHERAPY

Treatment Site – 4TH	Modality Qualifier – 5TH	Isotope – 6TH	Qualifier – 7TH
0 Pituitary Gland 1 Pineal Body 2 Adrenal Glands 4 Parathyroid Glands 5 Thyroid	9 High dose rate (HDR) B Low dose rate (LDR)	7 Cesium 137 (Cs-137) 8 Iridium 192 (Ir-192) 9 Iodine 125 (I-125) B Palladium 103 (Pd-103) C Californium 252 (Cf-252) Y Other isotope	Z None

1ST - D Radiation Therapy
2ND - G Endocrine System
3RD - 2 STEREOTACTIC RADIOSURGERY

EXAMPLE: Particulate stereotactic radiosurgery
MODALITY: STEREOTACTIC RADIOSURGERY

Treatment Site – 4TH	Modality Qualifier – 5TH	Isotope – 6TH	Qualifier – 7TH
0 Pituitary Gland 1 Pineal Body 2 Adrenal Glands 4 Parathyroid Glands 5 Thyroid	D Stereotactic other photon radiosurgery H Stereotactic particulate radiosurgery J Stereotactic gamma beam radiosurgery	Z None	Z None

DGY

1ST - D Radiation Therapy
2ND - G Endocrine System
3RD - Y OTHER RADIATION

EXAMPLE: Laser interstitial thermal therapy

MODALITY: OTHER RADIATION

Treatment Site – 4TH	Modality Qualifier – 5TH	Isotope – 6TH	Qualifier – 7TH
0 Pituitary Gland 1 Pineal Body 2 Adrenal Glands 4 Parathyroid Glands 5 Thyroid	7 Contact radiation 8 Hyperthermia F Plaque radiation K Laser interstitial thermal therapy	Z None	Z None

1ST - D Radiation Therapy
2ND - H Skin
3RD - 0 BEAM RADIATION

EXAMPLE: External beam radiation

MODALITY: BEAM RADIATION

Treatment Site – 4TH	Modality Qualifier – 5TH	Isotope – 6TH	Qualifier – 7TH
2 Skin, Face 7 Skin, Back 3 Skin, Neck 8 Skin, Abdomen 4 Skin, Arm 9 Skin, Buttock 6 Skin, Chest B Skin, Leg	0 Photons <1 MeV 1 Photons 1 - 10 MeV 2 Photons >10 MeV 4 Heavy particles (protons, ions) 5 Neutrons 6 Neutron capture	Z None	Z None
2 Skin, Face 7 Skin, Back 3 Skin, Neck 8 Skin, Abdomen 4 Skin, Arm 9 Skin, Buttock 6 Skin, Chest B Skin, Leg	3 Electrons	Z None	0 Intraoperative Z None

1ST - D Radiation Therapy
2ND - H Skin
3RD - Y OTHER RADIATION

EXAMPLE: Laser interstitial thermal therapy

MODALITY: OTHER RADIATION

Treatment Site – 4TH	Modality Qualifier – 5TH	Isotope – 6TH	Qualifier – 7TH
2 Skin, Face 7 Skin, Back 3 Skin, Neck 8 Skin, Abdomen 4 Skin, Arm 9 Skin, Buttock 6 Skin, Chest B Skin, Leg	7 Contact radiation 8 Hyperthermia F Plaque radiation	Z None	Z None
5 Skin, Hand C Skin, Foot	F Plaque radiation	Z None	Z None

D – RADIATION THERAPY

DM2

1ST - D Radiation Therapy
2ND - M Breast
3RD - 0 BEAM RADIATION

EXAMPLE: External beam radiation

MODALITY: BEAM RADIATION

Treatment Site – 4TH	Modality Qualifier – 5TH	Isotope – 6TH	Qualifier – 7TH
0 Breast, Left 1 Breast, Right	0 Photons <1 MeV 1 Photons 1 - 10 MeV 2 Photons >10 MeV 4 Heavy particles (protons, ions) 5 Neutrons 6 Neutron capture	Z None	Z None
0 Breast, Left 1 Breast, Right	3 Electrons	Z None	0 Intraoperative Z None

---

1ST - D Radiation Therapy
2ND - M Breast
3RD - 1 BRACHYTHERAPY

EXAMPLE: Insertion of radioactive material

MODALITY: BRACHYTHERAPY

Treatment Site – 4TH	Modality Qualifier – 5TH	Isotope – 6TH	Qualifier – 7TH
0 Breast, Left 1 Breast, Right	9 High dose rate (HDR) B Low dose rate (LDR)	7 Cesium 137 (Cs-137) 8 Iridium 192 (Ir-192) 9 Iodine 125 (I-125) B Palladium 103 (Pd-103) C Californium 252 (Cf-252) Y Other isotope	Z None

---

1ST - D Radiation Therapy
2ND - M Breast
3RD - 2 STEREOTACTIC RADIOSURGERY

EXAMPLE: Particulate stereotactic radiosurgery

MODALITY: STEREOTACTIC RADIOSURGERY

Treatment Site – 4TH	Modality Qualifier – 5TH	Isotope – 6TH	Qualifier – 7TH
0 Breast, Left 1 Breast, Right	D Stereotactic other photon radiosurgery H Stereotactic particulate radiosurgery J Stereotactic gamma beam radiosurgery	Z None	Z None

DMY

ANCILLARY SECTIONS – 2016 ICD-10-PCS

1ST – D Radiation Therapy
2ND – M Breast
3RD – Y OTHER RADIATION

EXAMPLE: Laser interstitial thermal therapy
MODALITY: OTHER RADIATION

Treatment Site – 4TH	Modality Qualifier – 5TH	Isotope – 6TH	Qualifier – 7TH
0 Breast, Left 1 Breast, Right	7 Contact radiation 8 Hyperthermia F Plaque radiation K Laser interstitial thermal therapy	Z None	Z None

1ST – D Radiation Therapy
2ND – P Musculoskeletal System
3RD – 0 BEAM RADIATION

EXAMPLE: External beam radiation
MODALITY: BEAM RADIATION

Treatment Site – 4TH		Modality Qualifier – 5TH	Isotope – 6TH	Qualifier – 7TH
0 Skull 2 Maxilla 3 Mandible 4 Sternum 5 Rib(s) 6 Humerus	7 Radius/Ulna 8 Pelvic Bones 9 Femur B Tibia/Fibula C Other Bone	0 Photons <1 MeV 1 Photons 1 - 10 MeV 2 Photons >10 MeV 4 Heavy particles (protons, ions) 5 Neutrons 6 Neutron capture	Z None	Z None
0 Skull 2 Maxilla 3 Mandible 4 Sternum 5 Rib(s) 6 Humerus	7 Radius/Ulna 8 Pelvic Bones 9 Femur B Tibia/Fibula C Other Bone	3 Electrons	Z None	0 Intraoperative Z None

1ST – D Radiation Therapy
2ND – P Musculoskeletal System
3RD – Y OTHER RADIATION

EXAMPLE: Laser interstitial thermal therapy
MODALITY: OTHER RADIATION

Treatment Site – 4TH		Modality Qualifier – 5TH	Isotope – 6TH	Qualifier – 7TH
0 Skull 2 Maxilla 3 Mandible 4 Sternum 5 Rib(s) 6 Humerus	7 Radius/Ulna 8 Pelvic Bones 9 Femur B Tibia/Fibula C Other Bone	7 Contact radiation 8 Hyperthermia F Plaque radiation	Z None	Z None

RADIATION THERAPY DMY

D – RADIATION THERAPY

DT2

0 BEAM RADIATION

1ST - **D** Radiation Therapy
2ND - **T** Urinary System
3RD - **0** BEAM RADIATION

EXAMPLE: External beam radiation
MODALITY: BEAM RADIATION

Treatment Site – 4TH	Modality Qualifier – 5TH	Isotope – 6TH	Qualifier – 7TH
0 Kidney 1 Ureter 2 Bladder 3 Urethra	0 Photons <1 MeV 1 Photons 1 - 10 MeV 2 Photons >10 MeV 4 Heavy particles (protons, ions) 5 Neutrons 6 Neutron capture	Z None	Z None
0 Kidney 1 Ureter 2 Bladder 3 Urethra	3 Electrons	Z None	0 Intraoperative Z None

1 BRACHYTHERAPY

1ST - **D** Radiation Therapy
2ND - **T** Urinary System
3RD - **1** BRACHYTHERAPY

EXAMPLE: Insertion of radioactive material
MODALITY: BRACHYTHERAPY

Treatment Site – 4TH	Modality Qualifier – 5TH	Isotope – 6TH	Qualifier – 7TH
0 Kidney 1 Ureter 2 Bladder 3 Urethra	9 High dose rate (HDR) B Low dose rate (LDR)	7 Cesium 137 (Cs-137) 8 Iridium 192 (Ir-192) 9 Iodine 125 (I-125) B Palladium 103 (Pd-103) C Californium 252 (Cf-252) Y Other isotope	Z None

2 STEREOTACTIC RADIOSURGERY

1ST - **D** Radiation Therapy
2ND - **T** Urinary System
3RD - **2** STEREOTACTIC RADIOSURGERY

EXAMPLE: Particulate stereotactic radiosurgery
MODALITY: STEREOTACTIC RADIOSURGERY

Treatment Site – 4TH	Modality Qualifier – 5TH	Isotope – 6TH	Qualifier – 7TH
0 Kidney 1 Ureter 2 Bladder 3 Urethra	D Stereotactic other photon radiosurgery H Stereotactic particulate radiosurgery J Stereotactic gamma beam radiosurgery	Z None	Z None

ANCILLARY SECTIONS – 2016 ICD-10-PCS

1ST – D Radiation Therapy
2ND – T Urinary System
3RD – Y OTHER RADIATION

EXAMPLE: Laser interstitial thermal therapy
MODALITY: OTHER RADIATION

Treatment Site – 4TH	Modality Qualifier – 5TH	Isotope – 6TH	Qualifier – 7TH
0 Kidney 1 Ureter 2 Bladder 3 Urethra	7 Contact radiation 8 Hyperthermia C Intraoperative radiation therapy (IORT) F Plaque radiation	Z None	Z None

---

1ST – D Radiation Therapy
2ND – U Female Reproductive System ♀
3RD – 0 BEAM RADIATION

EXAMPLE: External beam radiation
MODALITY: BEAM RADIATION

Treatment Site – 4TH	Modality Qualifier – 5TH	Isotope – 6TH	Qualifier – 7TH
0 Ovary 1 Cervix 2 Uterus	0 Photons <1 MeV 1 Photons 1 - 10 MeV 2 Photons >10 MeV 4 Heavy particles (protons, ions) 5 Neutrons 6 Neutron capture	Z None	Z None
0 Ovary 1 Cervix 2 Uterus	3 Electrons	Z None	0 Intraoperative Z None

---

1ST – D Radiation Therapy
2ND – U Female Reproductive System ♀
3RD – 1 BRACHYTHERAPY

EXAMPLE: Insertion of radioactive material
MODALITY: BRACHYTHERAPY

Treatment Site – 4TH	Modality Qualifier – 5TH	Isotope – 6TH	Qualifier – 7TH
0 Ovary 1 Cervix 2 Uterus	9 High dose rate (HDR) B Low dose rate (LDR)	7 Cesium 137 (Cs-137) 8 Iridium 192 (Ir-192) 9 Iodine 125 (I-125) B Palladium 103 (Pd-103) C Californium 252 (Cf-252) Y Other isotope	Z None

D – RADIATION THERAPY

DV0

Modality: Stereotactic Radiosurgery

- 1ST – **D** Radiation Therapy
- 2ND – **U** Female Reproductive System ♀
- 3RD – **2** STEREOTACTIC RADIOSURGERY

EXAMPLE: Particulate stereotactic radiosurgery

Treatment Site – 4TH	Modality Qualifier – 5TH	Isotope – 6TH	Qualifier – 7TH
0 Ovary 1 Cervix 2 Uterus	D Stereotactic other photon radiosurgery H Stereotactic particulate radiosurgery J Stereotactic gamma beam radiosurgery	Z None	Z None

Modality: Other Radiation

- 1ST – **D** Radiation Therapy
- 2ND – **U** Female Reproductive System ♀
- 3RD – **Y** OTHER RADIATION

EXAMPLE: Laser interstitial thermal therapy

Treatment Site – 4TH	Modality Qualifier – 5TH	Isotope – 6TH	Qualifier – 7TH
0 Ovary 1 Cervix 2 Uterus	7 Contact radiation 8 Hyperthermia C Intraoperative radiation therapy (IORT) F Plaque radiation	Z None	Z None

Modality: Beam Radiation

- 1ST – **D** Radiation Therapy
- 2ND – **V** Male Reproductive System ♂
- 3RD – **0** BEAM RADIATION

EXAMPLE: External beam radiation

Treatment Site – 4TH	Modality Qualifier – 5TH	Isotope – 6TH	Qualifier – 7TH
0 Prostate 1 Testis	0 Photons <1 MeV 1 Photons 1 - 10 MeV 2 Photons >10 MeV 4 Heavy particles (protons, ions) 5 Neutrons 6 Neutron capture	Z None	Z None
0 Prostate 1 Testis	3 Electrons	Z None	0 Intraoperative Z None

DV1

BRACHYTHERAPY

- 1ST – **D** Radiation Therapy
- 2ND – **V** Male Reproductive System ♂
- 3RD – **1** BRACHYTHERAPY

EXAMPLE: Insertion of radioactive material

MODALITY: BRACHYTHERAPY

Treatment Site – 4TH	Modality Qualifier – 5TH	Isotope – 6TH	Qualifier – 7TH
0 Prostate 1 Testis	9 High dose rate (HDR) B Low dose rate (LDR)	7 Cesium 137 (Cs-137) 8 Iridium 192 (Ir-192) 9 Iodine 125 (I-125) B Palladium 103 (Pd-103) C Californium 252 (Cf-252) Y Other isotope	Z None

STEREOTACTIC RADIOSURGERY

- 1ST – **D** Radiation Therapy
- 2ND – **V** Male Reproductive System ♂
- 3RD – **2** STEREOTACTIC RADIOSURGERY

EXAMPLE: Particulate stereotactic radiosurgery

MODALITY: STEREOTACTIC RADIOSURGERY

Treatment Site – 4TH	Modality Qualifier – 5TH	Isotope – 6TH	Qualifier – 7TH
0 Prostate 1 Testis	D Stereotactic other photon radiosurgery H Stereotactic particulate radiosurgery J Stereotactic gamma beam radiosurgery	Z None	Z None

OTHER RADIATION

- 1ST – **D** Radiation Therapy
- 2ND – **V** Male Reproductive System ♂
- 3RD – **Y** OTHER RADIATION

EXAMPLE: Laser interstitial thermal therapy

MODALITY: OTHER RADIATION

Treatment Site – 4TH	Modality Qualifier – 5TH	Isotope – 6TH	Qualifier – 7TH
0 Prostate	7 Contact radiation 8 Hyperthermia C Intraoperative radiation therapy (IORT) F Plaque radiation K Laser interstitial thermal therapy	Z None	Z None
1 Testis	7 Contact radiation 8 Hyperthermia F Plaque radiation	Z None	Z None

D – RADIATION THERAPY

1ST - D Radiation Therapy
2ND - W Anatomical Regions
3RD - 0 BEAM RADIATION

EXAMPLE: External beam radiation
MODALITY: BEAM RADIATION

Treatment Site – 4TH	Modality Qualifier – 5TH	Isotope – 6TH	Qualifier – 7TH
1 Head and Neck 2 Chest 3 Abdomen 4 Hemibody 5 Whole Body 6 Pelvic Region	0 Photons <1 MeV 1 Photons 1 - 10 MeV 2 Photons >10 MeV 4 Heavy particles (protons, ions) 5 Neutrons 6 Neutron capture	Z None	Z None
1 Head and Neck 2 Chest 3 Abdomen 4 Hemibody 5 Whole Body 6 Pelvic Region	3 Electrons	Z None	0 Intraoperative Z None

1ST - D Radiation Therapy
2ND - W Anatomical Regions
3RD - 1 BRACHYTHERAPY

EXAMPLE: Insertion of radioactive material
MODALITY: BRACHYTHERAPY

Treatment Site – 4TH	Modality Qualifier – 5TH	Isotope – 6TH	Qualifier – 7TH
1 Head and Neck 2 Chest 3 Abdomen 6 Pelvic Region	9 High dose rate (HDR) B Low dose rate (LDR)	7 Cesium 137 (Cs-137) 8 Iridium 192 (Ir-192) 9 Iodine 125 (I-125) B Palladium 103 (Pd-103) C Californium 252 (Cf-252) Y Other isotope	Z None

1ST - D Radiation Therapy
2ND - W Anatomical Regions
3RD - 2 STEREOTACTIC RADIOSURGERY

EXAMPLE: Particulate stereotactic radiosurgery
MODALITY: STEREOTACTIC RADIOSURGERY

Treatment Site – 4TH	Modality Qualifier – 5TH	Isotope – 6TH	Qualifier – 7TH
1 Head and Neck 2 Chest 3 Abdomen 6 Pelvic Region	D Stereotactic other photon radiosurgery H Stereotactic particulate radiosurgery J Stereotactic gamma beam radiosurgery	Z None	Z None

DWY

ANCILLARY SECTIONS – 2016 ICD-10-PCS

- 1ST – **D** Radiation Therapy
- 2ND – **W** Anatomical Regions
- 3RD – **Y** OTHER RADIATION

EXAMPLE: Laser interstitial thermal therapy

MODALITY: OTHER RADIATION

Treatment Site – 4TH	Modality Qualifier – 5TH	Isotope – 6TH	Qualifier – 7TH
1 Head and Neck 2 Chest 3 Abdomen 4 Hemibody 6 Pelvic Region	7 Contact radiation 8 Hyperthermia F Plaque radiation	Z None	Z None
5 Whole Body	7 Contact radiation 8 Hyperthermia F Plaque radiation	Z None	Z None
5 Whole Body	G Isotope administration	D Iodine 131 (I-131) F Phosphorus 32 (P-32) G Strontium 89 (Sr-89) H Strontium 90 (Sr-90) Y Other isotope	Z None

844

Educational Annotations

Section F – Physical Rehabilitation and Diagnostic Audiology

Section Specific Educational Annotations for the Physical Rehabilitation and Diagnostic Audiology Section include:
- AHA Coding Clinic® Reference Notations
- Coding Notes

AHA Coding Clinic® Reference Notations of Physical Rehabilitation and Diagnostic Audiology

ROOT TYPE SPECIFIC - PHYSICAL REHABILITATION AND DIAGNOSTIC AUDIOLOGY - Section F

SPEECH ASSESSMENT - 0
MOTOR AND/OR NERVE FUNCTION ASSESSMENT - 1
ACTIVITIES OF DAILY LIVING ASSESSMENT - 2
HEARING ASSESSMENT - 3
HEARING AID ASSESSMENT - 4
VESTIBULAR ASSESSMENT - 5
SPEECH TREATMENT - 6
MOTOR TREATMENT - 7
ACTIVITIES OF DAILY LIVING TREATMENT - 8
HEARING TREATMENT - 9
COCHLEAR IMPLANT TREATMENT - B
VESTIBULAR TREATMENT - C
DEVICE FITTING - D
CAREGIVER TRAINING - F

Coding Notes of Physical Rehabilitation and Diagnostic Audiology

Ancillary Section Specific PCS Reference Manual Exercises

PCS CODE	F – PHYSICAL REHABILITATION AND DIAGNOSTIC AUDIOLOGY EXERCISES
F00ZHYZ	Bedside swallow assessment using assessment kit.
F02ZFZZ	Verbal assessment of patient's pain level.
F07L0ZZ	Physical therapy for range of motion and mobility, patient right hip, no special equipment.
F07M6ZZ	Group musculoskeletal balance training exercises, whole body, no special equipment. (Balance training is included in the Motor Treatment reference table under Therapeutic Exercise.)
F09Z2KZ	Individual therapy for auditory processing using tape recorder. (Tape recorder is listed in the equipment reference table under Audiovisual Equipment.)
F0DZ7EZ	Application of short arm cast in rehabilitation setting. (Inhibitory cast is listed in the equipment reference table under E, Orthosis.)
F0DZ8UZ	Individual fitting of left eye prosthesis.
F0FZ8ZZ	Caregiver training in airway clearance techniques.
F0FZJMZ	Caregiver training in communication skills using manual communication board. (Manual communication board is listed in the equipment reference table under M, Augmentative/Alternative Communication.)
F13Z31Z	Bekesy assessment using audiometer.

Educational Annotations

Section F – Physical Rehabilitation and Diagnostic Audiology

NOTES

F – PHYSICAL REHABILITATION AND DIAGNOSTIC AUDIOLOGY — F 0 0

1ST - F Physical Rehabilitation and Diagnostic Audiology
2ND - 0 Rehabilitation
3RD - 0 SPEECH ASSESSMENT

ROOT TYPE:
SPEECH ASSESSMENT: Measurement of speech and related functions.

Body System/Region – 4TH	Type Qualifier – 5TH	Equipment – 6TH	Qualifier 7TH
3 Neurological System - Whole Body	G Communicative/cognitive integration skills	K Audiovisual M Augmentative/alternative communication P Computer Y Other equipment Z None	Z None
Z None	0 Filtered speech 3 Staggered spondaic word Q Performance intensity phonetically balanced speech discrimination R Brief tone stimuli S Distorted speech T Dichotic stimuli V Temporal ordering of stimuli W Masking patterns	1 Audiometer 2 Sound field/booth K Audiovisual Z None	Z None
Z None	1 Speech threshold 2 Speech/word recognition	1 Audiometer 2 Sound field/booth 9 Cochlear implant K Audiovisual Z None	Z None
Z None	4 Sensorineural acuity level	1 Audiometer 2 Sound field/booth Z None	Z None
Z None	5 Synthetic sentence identification	1 Audiometer 2 Sound field/booth 9 Cochlear implant K Audiovisual	Z None
Z None	6 Speech and/or language screening 7 Nonspoken language 8 Receptive/expressive language C Aphasia G Communicative/cognitive integration skills L Augmentative/alternative communication system	K Audiovisual M Augmentative/alternative communication P Computer Y Other equipment Z None	Z None
Z None	9 Articulation/phonology	K Audiovisual P Computer Q Speech analysis Y Other equipment Z None	Z None

continued ⇨

F00 SPEECH ASSESSMENT — continued

Body System/Region – 4TH	Type Qualifier – 5TH	Equipment – 6TH	Qualifier 7TH
Z None	B Motor speech	K Audiovisual N Biosensory feedback P Computer Q Speech analysis T Aerodynamic function Y Other equipment Z None	Z None
Z None	D Fluency	K Audiovisual N Biosensory feedback P Computer Q Speech analysis S Voice analysis T Aerodynamic function Y Other equipment Z None	Z None
Z None	F Voice	K Audiovisual N Biosensory feedback P Computer S Voice analysis T Aerodynamic function Y Other equipment Z None	Z None
Z None	H Bedside swallowing and oral function P Oral peripheral mechanism	Y Other equipment Z None	Z None
Z None	J Instrumental swallowing and oral function	T Aerodynamic function W Swallowing Y Other equipment	Z None
Z None	K Orofacial myofunctional	K Audiovisual P Computer Y Other equipment Z None	Z None
Z None	M Voice prosthetic	K Audiovisual P Computer S Voice analysis V Speech prosthesis Y Other equipment Z None	Z None
Z None	N Non-invasive instrumental status	N Biosensory feedback P Computer Q Speech analysis S Voice analysis T Aerodynamic function Y Other equipment	Z None
Z None	X Other specified central auditory processing	Z None	Z None

F – PHYSICAL REHABILITATION AND DIAGNOSTIC AUDIOLOGY

1ST - F Physical Rehabilitation and Diagnostic Audiology
2ND - 0 Rehabilitation
3RD - 1 MOTOR AND/OR NERVE FUNCTION ASSESSMENT

ROOT TYPE:
MOTOR AND/OR NERVE FUNCTION ASSESSMENT: Measurement of motor, nerve, and related functions.

Body System/Region – 4TH	Type Qualifier – 5TH	Equipment – 6TH	Qualifier 7TH
0 Neurological System - Head and Neck 1 Neurological System - Upper Back / Upper Extremity 2 Neurological System - Lower Back / Lower Extremity 3 Neurological System - Whole Body	0 Muscle performance	E Orthosis F Assistive, adaptive, supportive or protective U Prosthesis Y Other equipment Z None	Z None
0 Neurological System - Head and Neck 1 Neurological System - Upper Back / Upper Extremity 2 Neurological System - Lower Back / Lower Extremity 3 Neurological System - Whole Body	1 Integumentary integrity 3 Coordination/dexterity 4 Motor function G Reflex integrity	Z None	Z None
0 Neurological System - Head and Neck 1 Neurological System - Upper Back / Upper Extremity 2 Neurological System - Lower Back / Lower Extremity 3 Neurological System - Whole Body	5 Range of motion and joint integrity 6 Sensory awareness/processing/integrity	Y Other equipment Z None	Z None

continued ⇨

F 0 1 MOTOR ASSESSMENT — continued

Body System/Region – 4TH	Type Qualifier – 5TH	Equipment – 6TH	Qualifier 7TH
D Integumentary System - Head and Neck F Integumentary System - Upper Back/Upper Extremity G Integumentary System - Lower Back/Lower Extremity H Integumentary System - Whole Body J Musculoskeletal System - Head and Neck K Musculoskeletal System - Upper Back/Upper Extremity L Musculoskeletal System - Lower Back/Lower Extremity M Musculoskeletal System - Whole Body	0 Muscle performance	E Orthosis F Assistive, adaptive, supportive or protective U Prosthesis Y Other equipment Z None	Z None
D Integumentary System - Head and Neck F Integumentary System - Upper Back/Upper Extremity G Integumentary System - Lower Back/Lower Extremity H Integumentary System - Whole Body J Musculoskeletal System - Head and Neck K Musculoskeletal System - Upper Back/Upper Extremity L Musculoskeletal System - Lower Back/Lower Extremity M Musculoskeletal System - Whole Body	1 Integumentary integrity	Z None	Z None

continued ⇨

F 0 1 MOTOR ASSESSMENT — continued

Body System/Region – 4ᵀᴴ	Type Qualifier – 5ᵀᴴ	Equipment – 6ᵀᴴ	Qualifier 7ᵀᴴ
D Integumentary System - Head and Neck F Integumentary System - Upper Back/Upper Extremity G Integumentary System - Lower Back/Lower Extremity H Integumentary System - Whole Body J Musculoskeletal System - Head and Neck K Musculoskeletal System - Upper Back/Upper Extremity L Musculoskeletal System - Lower Back/Lower Extremity M Musculoskeletal System - Whole Body	5 Range of motion and joint integrity 6 Sensory awareness/processing/integrity	Y Other equipment Z None	Z None
N Genitourinary System	0 Muscle performance	E Orthosis F Assistive, adaptive, supportive or protective U Prosthesis Y Other equipment Z None	Z None
Z None	2 Visual motor integration	K Audiovisual M Augmentative/alternative communication N Biosensory feedback P Computer Q Speech analysis S Voice analysis Y Other equipment Z None	Z None
Z None	7 Facial nerve function	7 Electrophysiologic	Z None
Z None	9 Somatosensory evoked potentials	J Somatosensory	Z None
Z None	B Bed Mobility C Transfer F Wheelchair mobility	E Orthosis F Assistive, adaptive, supportive or protective U Prosthesis Z None	Z None
Z None	D Gait and/or balance	E Orthosis F Assistive, adaptive, supportive or protective U Prosthesis Y Other equipment Z None	Z None

F02

ANCILLARY SECTIONS – 2016 ICD-10-PCS

- **1ST – F** Physical Rehabilitation and Diagnostic Audiology
- **2ND – 0** Rehabilitation
- **3RD – 2** ACTIVITIES OF DAILY LIVING ASSESSMENT

ROOT TYPE:
ACTIVITIES OF DAILY LIVING ASSESSMENT: Measurement of functional level for activities of daily living.

Body System/Region – 4TH	Type Qualifier – 5TH	Equipment – 6TH	Qualifier 7TH
0 Neurological System - Head and Neck	9 Cranial nerve integrity D Neuromotor development	Y Other equipment Z None	Z None
1 Neurological System - Upper Back/Upper Extremity 2 Neurological System - Lower Back/Lower Extremity 3 Neurological System - Whole Body	D Neuromotor development	Y Other equipment Z None	Z None
4 Circulatory System - Head and Neck 5 Circulatory System - Upper Back/Upper Extremity 6 Circulatory System - Lower Back/Lower Extremity 8 Respiratory System - Head and Neck 9 Respiratory System - Upper Back/Upper Extremity B Respiratory System - Lower Back/Lower Extremity	G Ventilation, respiration and circulation	C Mechanical G Aerobic endurance and conditioning Y Other equipment Z None	Z None
7 Circulatory System - Whole Body C Respiratory System - Whole Body	7 Aerobic capacity and endurance	E Orthosis G Aerobic endurance and conditioning U Prosthesis Y Other equipment Z None	Z None
7 Circulatory System - Whole Body C Respiratory System - Whole Body	G Ventilation, respiration and circulation	C Mechanical G Aerobic endurance and conditioning Y Other equipment Z None	Z None
Z None	0 Bathing/showering 1 Dressing 3 Grooming/personal hygiene 4 Home management	E Orthosis F Assistive, adaptive, supportive or protective U Prosthesis Z None	Z None
Z None	2 Feeding/eating 8 Anthropometric characteristics F Pain	Y Other equipment Z None	Z None

continued ➡

F02 ACTVITIES ASSESSMENT —continued

Body System/Region – 4TH	Type Qualifier – 5TH	Equipment – 6TH	Qualifier 7TH
Z None	5 Perceptual processing	K Audiovisual M Augmentative/alternative communication N Biosensory feedback P Computer Q Speech analysis S Voice analysis Y Other equipment Z None	Z None
Z None	6 Psychosocial skills	Z None	Z None
Z None	B Environmental, home and work barriers C Ergonomics and body mechanics	E Orthosis F Assistive, adaptive, supportive or protective U Prosthesis Y Other equipment Z None	Z None
Z None	H Vocational activities and functional community or work reintegration skills	E Orthosis F Assistive, adaptive, supportive or protective G Aerobic endurance and conditioning U Prosthesis Y Other equipment Z None	Z None

F 0 6

ANCILLARY SECTIONS – 2016 ICD-10-PCS

1ST - F Physical Rehabilitation and Diagnostic Audiology
2ND - 0 Rehabilitation
3RD - 6 SPEECH TREATMENT

ROOT TYPE:
SPEECH TREATMENT: Application of techniques to improve, augment, or compensate for speech and related functional impairment.

Body System/Region – 4TH	Type Qualifier – 5TH	Equipment – 6TH	Qualifier 7TH
3 Neurological System - Whole Body	6 Communicative/cognitive integration skills	K Audiovisual M Augmentative/alternative communication P Computer Y Other equipment Z None	Z None
Z None	0 Nonspoken language 3 Aphasia 6 Communicative/cognitive integration skills	K Audiovisual M Augmentative/alternative communication P Computer Y Other equipment Z None	Z None
Z None	1 Speech-language pathology and related disorders counseling 2 Speech-language pathology and related disorders prevention	K Audiovisual Z None	Z None
Z None	4 Articulation/phonology	K Audiovisual P Computer Q Speech analysis T Aerodynamic function Y Other equipment Z None	Z None
Z None	5 Aural rehabilitation	K Audiovisual L Assistive listening M Augmentative/alternative communication N Biosensory feedback P Computer Q Speech analysis S Voice analysis Y Other equipment Z None	Z None
Z None	7 Fluency	4 Electroacoustic immitance/acoustic reflex K Audiovisual N Biosensory feedback Q Speech analysis S Voice analysis T Aerodynamic function Y Other equipment Z None	Z None

continued ⇨

F 0 6 SPEECH TREATMENT — continued

Body System/Region – 4TH	Type Qualifier – 5TH	Equipment – 6TH	Qualifier 7TH
Z None	8 Motor speech	K Audiovisual N Biosensory feedback P Computer Q Speech analysis S Voice analysis T Aerodynamic function Y Other equipment Z None	Z None
Z None	9 Orofacial myofunctional	K Audiovisual P Computer Y Other equipment Z None	Z None
Z None	B Receptive/expressive language	K Audiovisual L Assistive listening M Augmentative/alternative communication P Computer Y Other equipment Z None	Z None
Z None	C Voice	K Audiovisual N Biosensory feedback P Computer S Voice analysis T Aerodynamic function V Speech prosthesis Y Other equipment Z None	Z None
Z None	D Swallowing dysfunction	M Augmentative/alternative communication T Aerodynamic function V Speech prosthesis Y Other equipment Z None	Z None

F07

ANCILLARY SECTIONS – 2016 ICD-10-PCS

- 1ST – **F** Physical Rehabilitation and Diagnostic Audiology
- 2ND – **0** Rehabilitation
- 3RD – **7** MOTOR TREATMENT

ROOT TYPE:

MOTOR TREATMENT: Exercise or activities to increase or facilitate motor function.

Body System/Region – 4TH	Type Qualifier – 5TH	Equipment – 6TH	Qualifier 7TH
0 Neurological System - Head and Neck	0 Range of motion and joint mobility	E Orthosis	Z None
1 Neurological System - Upper Back/Upper Extremity	1 Muscle performance	F Assistive, adaptive, supportive or protective	
2 Neurological System - Lower Back/Lower Extremity	2 Coordination/dexterity	U Prosthesis	
3 Neurological System - Whole Body	3 Motor function	Y Other equipment	
D Integumentary System - Head and Neck		Z None	
F Integumentary System - Upper Back/Upper Extremity			
G Integumentary System - Lower Back/Lower Extremity			
H Integumentary System - Whole Body			
J Musculoskeletal System - Head and Neck			
K Musculoskeletal System - Upper Back/Upper Extremity			
L Musculoskeletal System - Lower Back/Lower Extremity			
M Musculoskeletal System - Whole Body			

continued ⇨

F07 MOTOR TREATMENT — continued

Body System/Region – 4TH	Type Qualifier – 5TH	Equipment – 6TH	Qualifier 7TH
0 Neurological System - Head and Neck	6 Therapeutic exercise	B Physical Agents	Z None
1 Neurological System - Upper Back/Upper Extremity		C Mechanical	
2 Neurological System - Lower Back/Lower Extremity		D Electrotherapeutic	
3 Neurological System - Whole Body		E Orthosis	
D Integumentary System - Head and Neck		F Assistive, adaptive, supportive or protective	
F Integumentary System - Upper Back/Upper Extremity		G Aerobic endurance and conditioning	
G Integumentary System - Lower Back/Lower Extremity		H Mechanical or electromechanical	
H Integumentary System - Whole Body		U Prosthesis	
J Musculoskeletal System - Head and Neck		Y Other equipment	
K Musculoskeletal System - Upper Back/Upper Extremity		Z None	
L Musculoskeletal System - Lower Back/Lower Extremity			
M Musculoskeletal System - Whole Body			

continued ⇨

F07 MOTOR TREATMENT — continued

Body System/Region – 4TH	Type Qualifier – 5TH	Equipment – 6TH	Qualifier 7TH
0 Neurological System - Head and Neck 1 Neurological System - Upper Back/Upper Extremity 2 Neurological System - Lower Back/Lower Extremity 3 Neurological System - Whole Body D Integumentary System - Head and Neck F Integumentary System - Upper Back/Upper Extremity G Integumentary System - Lower Back/Lower Extremity H Integumentary System - Whole Body J Musculoskeletal System - Head and Neck K Musculoskeletal System - Upper Back/Upper Extremity L Musculoskeletal System - Lower Back/Lower Extremity M Musculoskeletal System - Whole Body	7 Manual therapy techniques	Z None	Z None
4 Circulatory System - Head and Neck 5 Circulatory System - Upper Back/Upper Extremity 6 Circulatory System - Lower Back/Lower Extremity 7 Circulatory System - Whole Body 8 Respiratory System - Head and Neck 9 Respiratory System - Upper Back/Upper Extremity B Respiratory System - Lower Back/Lower Extremity C Respiratory System - Whole Body	6 Therapeutic exercise	B Physical Agents C Mechanical D Electrotherapeutic E Orthosis F Assistive, adaptive, supportive or protective G Aerobic endurance and conditioning H Mechanical or electromechanical U Prosthesis Y Other equipment Z None	Z None

continued

F 07 MOTOR TREATMENT —continued

Body System/Region – 4TH	Type Qualifier – 5TH	Equipment – 6TH	Qualifier 7TH
N Genitourinary System	1 Muscle performance	E Orthosis F Assistive, adaptive, supportive or protective U Prosthesis Y Other equipment Z None	Z None
N Genitourinary System	6 Therapeutic exercise	B Physical Agents C Mechanical D Electrotherapeutic E Orthosis F Assistive, adaptive, supportive or protective G Aerobic endurance and conditioning H Mechanical or electromechanical U Prosthesis Y Other equipment Z None	Z None
Z None	4 Wheelchair mobility	D Electrotherapeutic E Orthosis F Assistive, adaptive, supportive or protective U Prosthesis Y Other equipment Z None	Z None
Z None	5 Bed mobility	C Mechanical E Orthosis F Assistive, adaptive, supportive or protective U Prosthesis Y Other equipment Z None	Z None
Z None	8 Transfer training	C Mechanical D Electrotherapeutic E Orthosis F Assistive, adaptive, supportive or protective U Prosthesis Y Other equipment Z None	Z None
Z None	9 Gait training/functional ambulation	C Mechanical D Electrotherapeutic E Orthosis F Assistive, adaptive, supportive or protective U Prosthesis Y Other equipment Z None	Z None

F08 ACTIVITIES OF DAILY LIVING TREATMENT

1ST – F Physical Rehabilitation and Diagnostic Audiology
2ND – 0 Rehabilitation
3RD – 8 ACTIVITIES OF DAILY LIVING TREATMENT

ROOT TYPE: ACTIVITIES OF DAILY LIVING TREATMENT: Exercise or activities to facilitate functional competence for activities of daily living.

Body System/Region – 4TH	Type Qualifier – 5TH	Equipment – 6TH	Qualifier 7TH
D Integumentary System - Head and Neck F Integumentary System - Upper Back/Upper Extremity G Integumentary System - Lower Back/Lower Extremity H Integumentary System - Whole Body J Musculoskeletal System - Head and Neck K Musculoskeletal System - Upper Back/Upper Extremity L Musculoskeletal System - Lower Back/Lower Extremity M Musculoskeletal System - Whole Body	5 Wound Management	B Physical Agents C Mechanical D Electrotherapeutic E Orthosis F Assistive, adaptive, supportive or protective U Prosthesis Y Other equipment Z None	Z None
Z None	0 Bathing/showering techniques 1 Dressing techniques 2 Grooming/personal hygiene	E Orthosis F Assistive, adaptive, supportive or protective U Prosthesis Y Other equipment Z None	Z None
Z None	3 Feeding/eating	C Mechanical D Electrotherapeutic E Orthosis F Assistive, adaptive, supportive or protective U Prosthesis Y Other equipment Z None	Z None
Z None	4 Home management	D Electrotherapeutic E Orthosis F Assistive, adaptive, supportive or protective U Prosthesis Y Other equipment Z None	Z None
Z None	6 Psychosocial skills	Z None	Z None
Z None	7 Vocational activities and functional community or work reintegration skills	B Physical Agents C Mechanical D Electrotherapeutic E Orthosis F Assistive, adaptive, supportive or protective G Aerobic endurance and conditioning U Prosthesis Y Other equipment Z None	Z None

F – PHYSICAL REHABILITATION AND DIAGNOSTIC AUDIOLOGY

1ST – F Physical Rehabilitation and Diagnostic Audiology
2ND – 0 Rehabilitation
3RD – 9 HEARING TREATMENT

ROOT TYPE:
HEARING TREATMENT: Application of techniques to improve, augment, or compensate for hearing and related functional impairment.

Body System/Region – 4TH	Type Qualifier – 5TH	Equipment – 6TH	Qualifier 7TH
Z None	0 Hearing and related disorders counseling 1 Hearing and related disorders prevention	K Audiovisual Z None	Z None
Z None	2 Auditory processing	K Audiovisual L Assistive listening P Computer Y Other equipment Z None	Z None
Z None	3 Cerumen management	X Cerumen management Z None	Z None

1ST – F Physical Rehabilitation and Diagnostic Audiology
2ND – 0 Rehabilitation
3RD – B COCHLEAR IMPLANT TREATMENT

ROOT TYPE:
COCHLEAR IMPLANT TREATMENT: Application of techniques to improve the communication abilities of individuals with cochlear implant.

Body System/Region – 4TH	Type Qualifier – 5TH	Equipment – 6TH	Qualifier 7TH
Z None	0 Cochlear implant rehabilitation	1 Audiometer 2 Sound field/booth 9 Cochlear implant K Audiovisual P Computer Y Other equipment	Z None

ANCILLARY SECTIONS – 2016 ICD-10-PCS

F 0 C

- 1ST – **F** Physical Rehabilitation and Diagnostic Audiology
- 2ND – **0** Rehabilitation
- 3RD – **C** VESTIBULAR TREATMENT

ROOT TYPE:

VESTIBULAR TREATMENT: Application of techniques to improve, augment, or compensate for vestibular and related functional impairment.

Body System/Region – 4TH	Type Qualifier – 5TH	Equipment – 6TH	Qualifier 7TH
3 Neurological System - Whole Body H Integumentary System - Whole Body M Musculoskeletal System - Whole Body	3 Postural control	E Orthosis F Assistive, adaptive, supportive or protective U Prosthesis Y Other equipment Z None	Z None
Z None	0 Vestibular	8 Vestibular/balance Z None	Z None
Z None	1 Perceptual processing 2 Visual motor integration	K Audiovisual L Assistive listening N Biosensory feedback P Computer Q Speech analysis S Voice analysis T Aerodynamic function Y Other equipment Z None	Z None

F 0 D

- 1ST – **F** Physical Rehabilitation and Diagnostic Audiology
- 2ND – **0** Rehabilitation
- 3RD – **D** DEVICE FITTING

ROOT TYPE:

DEVICE FITTING: Fitting of a device designed to facilitate or support achievement of a higher level of function.

Body System/Region – 4TH	Type Qualifier – 5TH	Equipment – 6TH	Qualifier 7TH
Z None	0 Tinnitus masker	5 Hearing aid selection/fitting/test Z None	Z None
Z None	1 Monaural hearing aid 2 Binaural hearing aid 5 Assistive listening device	1 Audiometer 2 Sound field/booth 5 Hearing aid selection/fitting/test K Audiovisual L Assistive listening Z None	Z None
Z None	3 Augmentative/alternative communication system	M Augmentative/alternative communication	Z None
Z None	4 Voice prosthetic	S Voice analysis V Speech prosthesis	Z None
Z None	6 Dynamic orthosis 7 Static orthosis 8 Prosthesis 9 Assistive, adaptive, supportive or protective devices	E Orthosis F Assistive, adaptive, supportive or protective U Prosthesis Z None	Z None

F – PHYSICAL REHABILITATION AND DIAGNOSTIC AUDIOLOGY

1ST - F Physical Rehabilitation and Diagnostic Audiology
2ND - 0 Rehabilitation
3RD - F CAREGIVER TRAINING

ROOT TYPE:
CAREGIVER TRAINING: Training in activities to support patient's optimal level of function.

Body System/Region – 4TH	Type Qualifier – 5TH	Equipment – 6TH	Qualifier 7TH
Z None	0 Bathing/showering technique 1 Dressing 2 Feeding and eating 3 Grooming/personal hygiene 4 Bed mobility 5 Transfer 6 Wheelchair mobility 7 Therapeutic exercise 8 Airway clearance techniques 9 Wound management B Vocational activities and functional community or work reintegration skills C Gait training/functional ambulation D Application, proper use and care of devices F Application, proper use and care of orthoses G Application, proper use and care of prosthesis H Home management	E Orthosis F Assistive, adaptive, supportive or protective U Prosthesis Z None	Z None
Z None	J Communication skills	K Audiovisual L Assistive Listening M Augmentative/alternative communication P Computer Z None	Z None

F13

ANCILLARY SECTIONS – 2016 ICD-10-PCS

- 1ST – **F** Physical Rehabilitation and Diagnostic Audiology
- 2ND – **1** Diagnostic Audiology
- 3RD – **3** HEARING ASSESSMENT

ROOT TYPE:

HEARING ASSESSMENT: Measurement of hearing and related functions.

Body System/Region – 4TH	Type Qualifier – 5TH	Equipment – 6TH	Qualifier 7TH
Z None	0 Hearing screening	0 Occupational hearing 1 Audiometer 2 Sound field/booth 3 Tympanometer 8 Vestibular/balance 9 Cochlear implant Z None	Z None
Z None	1 Pure tone audiometry, air 2 Pure tone audiometry, air and bone	0 Occupational hearing 1 Audiometer 2 Sound field/booth Z None	Z None
Z None	3 Bekesy audiometry 6 Visual reinforcement audiometry 9 Short increment sensitivity index B Stenger C Pure tone stenger	1 Audiometer 2 Sound field/booth Z None	Z None
Z None	4 Conditioned play audiometry 5 Select picture audiometry	1 Audiometer 2 Sound field/booth K Audiovisual Z None	Z None
Z None	7 Alternate binaural or monaural loudness balance	1 Audiometer K Audiovisual Z None	Z None
Z None	8 Tone decay D Tympanometry F Eustachian tube function G Acoustic reflex patterns H Acoustic reflex threshold J Acoustic reflex decay	3 Tympanometer 4 Electroacoustic immitance/acoustic reflex Z None	Z None
Z None	K Electrocochleography L Auditory evoked potentials	7 Electrophysiologic Z None	Z None
Z None	M Evoked otoacoustic emissions, screening N Evoked otoacoustic emissions, diagnostic	6 Otoacoustic emission (OAE) Z None	Z None
Z None	P Aural rehabilitation status	1 Audiometer 2 Sound field/booth 4 Electroacoustic immitance/acoustic reflex 9 Cochlear implant K Audiovisual L Assistive listening P Computer Z None	Z None
Z None	Q Auditory processing	K Audiovisual P Computer Y Other equipment Z None	Z None

REHAB & AUDIOLOGY F13

F – PHYSICAL REHABILITATION AND DIAGNOSTIC AUDIOLOGY

1ST - F Physical Rehabilitation and Diagnostic Audiology
2ND - 1 Diagnostic Audiology
3RD - 4 HEARING AID ASSESSMENT

ROOT TYPE:
HEARING AID ASSESSMENT: Measurement of the appropriateness and/or effectiveness of a hearing device.

Body System/Region – 4TH	Type Qualifier – 5TH	Equipment – 6TH	Qualifier 7TH
Z None	0 Cochlear implant	1 Audiometer 2 Sound field/booth 3 Tympanometer 4 Electroacoustic immitance/acoustic reflex 5 Hearing Aid Selection/fitting/test 7 Electrophysiologic 9 Cochlear implant K Audiovisual L Assistive listening P Computer Y Other equipment Z None	Z None
Z None	1 Ear canal probe microphone 6 Binaural electroacoustic hearing aid check 8 Monaural electroacoustic hearing aid check	5 Hearing Aid Selection/fitting/test Z None	Z None
Z None	2 Monaural hearing aid 3 Binaural hearing aid	1 Audiometer 2 Sound field/booth 3 Tympanometer 4 Electroacoustic immitance/acoustic reflex 5 Hearing Aid Selection/fitting/test K Audiovisual L Assistive listening P Computer Z None	Z None
Z None	4 Assistive listening system/device selection	1 Audiometer 2 Sound field/booth 3 Tympanometer 4 Electroacoustic immitance/acoustic reflex K Audiovisual L Assistive listening Z None	Z None
Z None	5 Sensory aids	1 Audiometer 2 Sound field/booth 3 Tympanometer 4 Electroacoustic immitance/acoustic reflex 5 Hearing Aid Selection/fitting/test K Audiovisual L Assistive listening Z None	Z None
Z None	7 Ear protector attenuation	0 Occupational hearing Z None	Z None

ANCILLARY SECTIONS – 2016 ICD-10-PCS

1ST - F Physical Rehabilitation and Diagnostic Audiology
2ND - 1 Diagnostic Audiology
3RD - 5 VESTIBULAR ASSESSMENT

ROOT TYPE:
VESTIBULAR ASSESSMENT: Measurement of the vestibular system and related functions.

Body System/Region – 4TH	Type Qualifier – 5TH	Equipment – 6TH	Qualifier 7TH
Z None	0 Bithermal, binaural caloric irrigation 1 Bithermal, monaural caloric irrigation 2 Unithermal binaural screen 3 Oscillating tracking 4 Sinusoidal vertical axis rotational 5 Dix-Hallpike dynamic 6 Computerized dynamic posturography	8 Vestibular/balance Z None	Z None
Z None	7 Tinnitus masker	5 Hearing aid selection/fitting/test Z None	Z None

866

Educational Annotations | Section G – Mental Health

Section Specific Educational Annotations for the Mental Health Section include:
- AHA Coding Clinic® Reference Notations
- Coding Notes

AHA Coding Clinic® Reference Notations of Mental Health

ROOT TYPE SPECIFIC - MENTAL HEALTH - Section G
PSYCHOLOGICAL TESTS - 1
CRISIS INTERVENTION - 2
INDIVIDUAL PSYCHOTHERAPY - 5
COUNSELING - 6
FAMILY PSYCHOTHERAPY - 7
ELECTROCONVULSIVE THERAPY - B
BIOFEEDBACK - C
HYPNOSIS - F
NARCOSYNTHESIS - G
GROUP THERAPY - H
LIGHT THERAPY - J

Coding Notes of Mental Health

Ancillary Section Specific PCS Reference Manual Exercises

PCS CODE	G – MENTAL HEALTH EXERCISES
GZ10ZZZ	Developmental testing.
GZ13ZZZ	Neuropsychological testing.
GZ2ZZZZ	Crisis intervention.
GZ58ZZZ	Cognitive-behavioral psychotherapy, individual.
GZ61ZZZ	Vocational counseling.
GZ72ZZZ	Family psychotherapy.
GZB1ZZZ	ECT (Electroconvulsive therapy), unilateral, multiple seizure.
GZFZZZZ	Hypnosis.
GZGZZZZ	Narcosynthesis.
GZJZZZZ	Light therapy.

Educational Annotations
Section G – Mental Health

NOTES

Section Specific Educational Annotations for Mental Health Section include:
- AHA Coding Clinic Reference Notations
- Coding Notes

AHA Coding Clinic Reference Notations of Mental Health

ROOT TYPE SPECIFIC - MENTAL HEALTH - Section G
PSYCHOLOGICAL TESTS - 1
CRISIS INTERVENTION - 2
INDIVIDUAL PSYCHOTHERAPY - 5
COUNSELING - 6
FAMILY PSYCHOTHERAPY - 7
ELECTROCONVULSIVE THERAPY - B
BIOFEEDBACK - C
HYPNOSIS - F
NARCOSYNTHESIS - G
GROUP THERAPY - H
LIGHT THERAPY - J

Coding Notes of Mental Health

Ancillary Section Specific PCS Reference Manual Exercises

PCS CODE	G - MENTAL HEALTH EXERCISES
GZ10ZZZ	Developmental testing.
GZ13ZZZ	Neuropsychological testing.
GZ2ZZZZ	Crisis intervention.
GZ58ZZZ	Cognitive-behavioral psychotherapy, individual.
GZ61ZZZ	Vocational counseling
GZ72ZZZ	Family psychotherapy.
GZ81ZZZ	ECT (Electroconvulsive therapy), unilateral, multiple seizure.
GZFZZZZ	Hypnosis.
GZGZZZZ	Narcosynthesis.
GZJZZZZ	Light therapy.

G – MENTAL HEALTH

GZ3

1ST – **G** Mental Health 2ND – **Z** None 3RD – **1 PSYCHOLOGICAL TESTS**	**ROOT TYPE:** **PSYCHOLOGICAL TESTS:** The administration and interpretation of standardized psychological tests and measurement instruments for the assessment of psychological function.

Qualifier – 4TH	Qualifier – 5TH	Qualifier – 6TH	Qualifier – 7TH
0 Developmental 1 Personality and behavioral 2 Intellectual and psychoeducational 3 Neuropsychological 4 Neurobehavioral and cognitive status	Z None	Z None	Z None

1ST – **G** Mental Health 2ND – **Z** None 3RD – **2 CRISIS INTERVENTION**	**ROOT TYPE:** **CRISIS INTERVENTION:** Treatment of a traumatized, acutely disturbed or distressed individual for the purpose of short-term stabilization.

Qualifier – 4TH	Qualifier – 5TH	Qualifier – 6TH	Qualifier – 7TH
Z None	Z None	Z None	Z None

1ST – **G** Mental Health 2ND – **Z** None 3RD – **3 MEDICATION MANAGEMENT**	**ROOT TYPE:** **MEDICATION MANAGEMENT:** Monitoring and adjusting the use of medications for the treatment of a mental health disorder.

Qualifier – 4TH	Qualifier – 5TH	Qualifier – 6TH	Qualifier – 7TH
Z None	Z None	Z None	Z None

ANCILLARY SECTIONS – 2016 ICD-10-PCS

1ST - **G** Mental Health 2ND - **Z** None 3RD - **5** INDIVIDUAL PSYCHOTHERAPY	**ROOT TYPE:** **INDIVIDUAL PSYCHOTHERAPY:** Treatment of an individual with a mental health disorder by behavioral, cognitive, psychoanalytic, psychodynamic or psychophysiological means to improve functioning or well-being.		
Qualifier – 4TH	**Qualifier – 5TH**	**Qualifier – 6TH**	**Qualifier – 7TH**
0 Interactive 1 Behavioral 2 Cognitive 3 Interpersonal 4 Psychoanalysis 5 Psychodynamic 6 Supportive 8 Cognitive-Behavioral 9 Psychophysiological	Z None	Z None	Z None

1ST - **G** Mental Health 2ND - **Z** None 3RD - **6** COUNSELING	**ROOT TYPE:** **COUNSELING:** The application of psychological methods to treat an individual with normal developmental issues and psychological problems in order to increase function, improve well-being, alleviate distress, maladjustment or resolve crises.		
Qualifier – 4TH	**Qualifier – 5TH**	**Qualifier – 6TH**	**Qualifier – 7TH**
0 Educational 1 Vocational 3 Other counseling	Z None	Z None	Z None

1ST - **G** Mental Health 2ND - **Z** None 3RD - **7** FAMILY PSYCHOTHERAPY	**ROOT TYPE:** **FAMILY PSYCHOTHERAPY:** Treatment that includes one or more family members of an individual with a mental health disorder by behavioral, cognitive, psychoanalytic, psychodynamic or psychophysiological means to improve functioning or well-being.		
Qualifier – 4TH	**Qualifier – 5TH**	**Qualifier – 6TH**	**Qualifier – 7TH**
2 Other family psychotherapy	Z None	Z None	Z None

G – MENTAL HEALTH — GZF

Electroconvulsive Therapy

- 1ST – **G** Mental Health
- 2ND – **Z** None
- 3RD – **B** ELECTROCONVULSIVE THERAPY

ROOT TYPE:

ELECTROCONVULSIVE THERAPY: The application of controlled electrical voltages to treat a mental health disorder.

Qualifier – 4TH	Qualifier – 5TH	Qualifier – 6TH	Qualifier – 7TH
0 Unilateral-single seizure 1 Unilateral-multiple seizure 2 Bilateral-single seizure 3 Bilateral-multiple seizure 4 Other electroconvulsive therapy	Z None	Z None	Z None

Biofeedback

- 1ST – **G** Mental Health
- 2ND – **Z** None
- 3RD – **C** BIOFEEDBACK

ROOT TYPE:

BIOFEEDBACK: Provision of information from the monitoring and regulating of physiological processes in conjunction with cognitive-behavioral techniques to improve patient functioning or well-being.

Qualifier – 4TH	Qualifier – 5TH	Qualifier – 6TH	Qualifier – 7TH
9 Other biofeedback	Z None	Z None	Z None

Hypnosis

- 1ST – **G** Mental Health
- 2ND – **Z** None
- 3RD – **F** HYPNOSIS

ROOT TYPE:

HYPNOSIS: Induction of a state of heightened suggestibility by auditory, visual and tactile techniques to elicit an emotional or behavioral response.

Qualifier – 4TH	Qualifier – 5TH	Qualifier – 6TH	Qualifier – 7TH
Z None	Z None	Z None	Z None

GZG

1ST - G Mental Health
2ND - Z None
3RD - G NARCOSYNTHESIS

ROOT TYPE:

NARCOSYNTHESIS: Administration of intravenous barbiturates in order to release suppressed or repressed thoughts.

Qualifier – 4TH	Qualifier – 5TH	Qualifier – 6TH	Qualifier – 7TH
Z None	Z None	Z None	Z None

1ST - G Mental Health
2ND - Z None
3RD - H GROUP PSYCHOTHERAPY

ROOT TYPE:

GROUP PSYCHOTHERAPY: Treatment of two or more individuals with a mental health disorder by behavioral, cognitive, psychoanalytic, psychodynamic or psychophysiological means to improve functioning or well-being.

Qualifier – 4TH	Qualifier – 5TH	Qualifier – 6TH	Qualifier – 7TH
Z None	Z None	Z None	Z None

1ST - G Mental Health
2ND - Z None
3RD - J LIGHT THERAPY

ROOT TYPE:

LIGHT THERAPY: Application of specialized light treatments to improve functioning or well-being.

Qualifier – 4TH	Qualifier – 5TH	Qualifier – 6TH	Qualifier – 7TH
Z None	Z None	Z None	Z None

Educational Annotations | Section H – Substance Abuse

Section Specific Educational Annotations for the Substance Abuse Section include:
- AHA Coding Clinic® Reference Notations
- Coding Notes

AHA Coding Clinic® Reference Notations of Substance Abuse

ROOT TYPE SPECIFIC - SUBSTANCE ABUSE TREATMENT - Section H
DETOXIFICATION SERVICES - 2
INDIVIDUAL COUNSELING - 3
GROUP COUNSELING - 4
INDIVIDUAL PSYCHOTHERAPY - 5
FAMILY COUNSELING - 6
MEDICATION MANAGEMENT - 8
PHARMACOTHERAPY - 9

Coding Notes of Substance Abuse

Ancillary Section Specific PCS Reference Manual Exercises

PCS CODE	H – SUBSTANCE ABUSE EXERCISES
HZ2ZZZZ	Patient in for alcohol detoxification treatment.
HZ3CZZZ	Post-test infectious disease counseling for IV drug abuser.
HZ42ZZZ	Group cognitive-behavioral counseling for substance abuse.
HZ47ZZZ	Group motivational counseling.
HZ53ZZZ	Individual 12-step psychotherapy for substance abuse.
HZ54ZZZ	Individual interpersonal psychotherapy for drug abuse.
HZ5CZZZ	Psychodynamic psychotherapy for drug dependent patient.
HZ63ZZZ	Substance abuse treatment family counseling.
HZ81ZZZ	Medication monitoring of patient on methadone maintenance.
HZ94ZZZ	Naltrexone treatment for drug dependency.

Educational Annotations

Section H – Substance Abuse

NOTES

Section Specific Educational Annotations - Substance Abuse Section include:
- AHA Coding Clinic® Reference Notations
- Coding Notes

AHA Coding Clinic® Reference Notations of Substance Abuse

ROOT TYPE SPECIFIC – SUBSTANCE ABUSE TREATMENT – Section H
DETOXIFICATION SERVICES – 2
INDIVIDUAL COUNSELING – 3
GROUP COUNSELING – 4
INDIVIDUAL PSYCHOTHERAPY – 5
FAMILY COUNSELING – 6
MEDICATION MANAGEMENT – 8
PHARMACOTHERAPY – 9

Coding Notes for Substance Abuse

Ancillary Section Specific PCS Reference Manual Exercises

PCS CODE	H – SUBSTANCE ABUSE EXERCISES
HZ2ZZZZ	Patient in for alcohol detoxification treatment.
HZ3CZZZ	Post-test infectious disease counseling for IV drug abuser.
HZ42ZZZ	Group cognitive-behavioral counseling for substance abuse.
HZ47ZZZ	Group motivational counseling.
HZ53ZZZ	Individual 12-step psychotherapy for substance abuse.
HZ54ZZZ	Individual interpersonal psychotherapy for drug abuse.
HZ5CZZZ	Psychodynamic psychotherapy for drug dependent patient.
HZ63ZZZ	Substance abuse treatment family counseling.
HZ81ZZZ	Medication monitoring of patient on methadone maintenance.
HZ94ZZZ	Naltrexone treatment for drug dependency.

H – SUBSTANCE ABUSE TREATMENT

HZ4

1ST - H Substance Abuse Treatment
2ND - Z None
3RD - 2 DETOXIFICATION SERVICES

ROOT TYPE:

DETOXIFICATION SERVICES: Detoxification from alcohol and/or drugs.

Qualifier – 4TH	Qualifier – 5TH	Qualifier – 6TH	Qualifier – 7TH
Z None	Z None	Z None	Z None

1ST - H Substance Abuse Treatment
2ND - Z None
3RD - 3 INDIVIDUAL COUNSELING

ROOT TYPE:

INDIVIDUAL COUNSELING: The application of psychological methods to treat an individual with addictive behavior.

Qualifier – 4TH	Qualifier – 5TH	Qualifier – 6TH	Qualifier – 7TH
0 Cognitive 1 Behavioral 2 Cognitive-behavioral 3 12-Step 4 Interpersonal 5 Vocational 6 Psychoeducation 7 Motivational enhancement 8 Confrontational 9 Continuing care B Spiritual C Pre/post-test infectious disease	Z None	Z None	Z None

---

1ST - H Substance Abuse Treatment
2ND - Z None
3RD - 4 GROUP COUNSELING

ROOT TYPE:

GROUP COUNSELING: The application of psychological methods to treat two or more individuals with addictive behavior.

Qualifier – 4TH	Qualifier – 5TH	Qualifier – 6TH	Qualifier – 7TH
0 Cognitive 1 Behavioral 2 Cognitive-behavioral 3 12-Step 4 Interpersonal 5 Vocational 6 Psychoeducation 7 Motivational enhancement 8 Confrontational 9 Continuing care B Spiritual C Pre/post-test infectious disease	Z None	Z None	Z None

HZ5

Substance Abuse

- 1ST – **H** Substance Abuse Treatment
- 2ND – **Z** None
- 3RD – **5** INDIVIDUAL PSYCHOTHERAPY

ROOT TYPE:

INDIVIDUAL PSYCHOTHERAPY: Treatment of an individual with addictive behavior by behavioral, cognitive, psychoanalytic, psychodynamic or psychophysiological means.

Qualifier – 4TH	Qualifier – 5TH	Qualifier – 6TH	Qualifier – 7TH
0 Cognitive	Z None	Z None	Z None
1 Behavioral			
2 Cognitive-behavioral			
3 12-Step			
4 Interpersonal			
5 Interactive			
6 Psychoeducation			
7 Motivational enhancement			
8 Confrontational			
9 Supportive			
B Psychoanalysis			
C Psychodynamic			
D Psychophysiological			

- 1ST – **H** Substance Abuse Treatment
- 2ND – **Z** None
- 3RD – **6** FAMILY COUNSELING

ROOT TYPE:

FAMILY COUNSELING: The application of psychological methods that includes one or more family members to treat an individual with addictive behavior.

Qualifier – 4TH	Qualifier – 5TH	Qualifier – 6TH	Qualifier – 7TH
3 Other family counseling	Z None	Z None	Z None

- 1ST – **H** Substance Abuse Treatment
- 2ND – **Z** None
- 3RD – **8** MEDICATION MANAGEMENT

ROOT TYPE:

MEDICATION MANAGEMENT: Monitoring and adjusting the use of replacement medications for the treatment of addiction.

Qualifier – 4TH	Qualifier – 5TH	Qualifier – 6TH	Qualifier – 7TH
0 Nicotine replacement	Z None	Z None	Z None
1 Methadone maintenance			
2 Levo-alpha-acetyl-methadol (LAAM)			
3 Antabuse			
4 Naltrexone			
5 Naloxone			
6 Clonidine			
7 Bupropion			
8 Psychiatric medication			
9 Other replacement medication			

1ST - H Substance Abuse Treatment 2ND - Z None 3RD - 9 PHARMACOTHERAPY	**ROOT TYPE:** **PHARMACOTHERAPY:** The use of replacement medications for the treatment of addiction.		
Qualifier – 4TH	**Qualifier – 5TH**	**Qualifier – 6TH**	**Qualifier – 7TH**
0 Nicotine replacement 1 Methadone maintenance 2 Levo-alpha-acetyl-methadol (LAAM) 3 Antabuse 4 Naltrexone 5 Naloxone 6 Clonidine 7 Bupropion 8 Psychiatric medication 9 Other replacement medication	Z None	Z None	Z None

ANCILLARY SECTIONS – 2016 ICD-10-PCS

NOTES

Educational Annotations | Section X – New Technology

Section Specific Educational Annotations for the New Technology Section include:
- AHA Coding Clinic® Reference Notations
- Coding Notes

NEW TECHNOLOGY – SECTION X

Section X New Technology is the section in ICD-10-PCS for codes that uniquely identify procedures requested via the New Technology Application Process, and for codes that capture new technologies not currently classified in ICD-10-PCS.

This section may include codes for medical and surgical procedures, medical and surgical-related procedures, or ancillary procedures designated as new technology.

In section X, the seven characters are defined as follows:
- First character: section (X)
- Second character: body system
- Third character: operation
- Fourth character: body part
- Fifth character: approach
- Sixth character: device/substance/technology
- Seventh character: new technology group

The New Technology section includes infusions of new technology drugs, and can potentially include a wide range of other new technology medical, surgical, and ancillary procedures. The example below is for infusion of a new technology drug.

Coding Note: Seventh Character New Technology Group
In ICD-10-PCS, the type of information specified in the seventh character is called the qualifier, and the information specified depends on the section. In this section, the seventh character is used exclusively to indicate the new technology group.

The New Technology Group is a number or letter that changes each year that new technology codes are added to the system. For example, Section X codes added for the first year have the seventh character value 1, New Technology Group 1, and the next year that Section X codes are added have the seventh character value 2 New Technology Group 2, and so on.

Changing the seventh character New Technology Group to a unique value every year that there are new codes in this section allows the ICD-10-PCS to "recycle" the values in the third, fourth, and sixth characters as needed. This avoids the creation of duplicate codes, because the root operation, body part, and device/substance/technology values can specify a different meaning with every new technology group, if needed. Having a unique value for the New Technology Group maximizes the flexibility and capacity of section X over its lifespan, and allows it to evolve as medical technology evolves.

Body System Values
Second character body systems in this section do not change from year to year. They are a fixed set of values that combine the uses of body system, body region, and physiological system as specified in other sections in ICD-10-PCS. As a result, the second character body system values are broader values. This allows body part values to be as general or specific as they need to be to efficiently represent the body part applicable to a new technology.

Root Operations
Third character root operations in this section use the same root operation values as their counterparts in other sections of ICD-10-PCS. The example above uses the root operation value Introduction. This root operation has the same definition as its counterpart in section 3 of ICD-10-PCS, as given below.

- 0 – Introduction: Putting in or on a therapeutic, diagnostic, nutritional, physiological, or prophylactic substance except blood or blood products

Continued on next page

Educational Annotations | Section X – New Technology

Continued from previous page

Body Part Values
Fourth character body part values in this section use the same body part values as their closest counterparts in other sections of ICD-10-PCS. The example above uses the body part value 4 Central Vein. This is its closest counterpart in section 3 of ICD-10-PCS.

Device/Substance/Technology Values
In this section, the sixth character contains a general description of the key feature of the new technology. The example above uses the device/substance/technology value 2 Ceftazidime-Avibactam Anti-infective.

AHA Coding Clinic® Reference Notations of New Technology

ROOT OPERATION SPECIFIC - NEW TECHNOLOGY - Section X
MISC

Coding Notes of New Technology

Ancillary Section Specific PCS Reference Manual Exercises

PCS CODE	X – NEW TECHNOLOGY EXERCISES
X W 0 3 3 2 1	Infusion of ceftazidime via peripheral venous catheter.

Body System Relevant Coding Guidelines

D. New Technology Section – Section X

General guidelines

D1
Section X codes are standalone codes. They are not supplemental codes. Section X codes fully represent the specific procedure described in the code title, and do not require any additional codes from other sections of ICD-10-PCS. When section X contains a code title which describes a specific new technology procedure, only that X code is reported for the procedure. There is no need to report a broader, non-specific code in another section of ICD-10-PCS.
Example: XW04321 Introduction of Ceftazidime-Avibactam Anti-infective into Central Vein, Percutaneous Approach, New Technology Group 1, can be coded to indicate that Ceftazidime-Avibactam Anti-infective was administered via a central vein. A separate code from table 3E0 in the Administration section of ICD-10-PCS is not coded in addition to this code.

X – NEW TECHNOLOGY

XW0

1ST - X New Technology 2ND - 2 Cardiovascular System 3RD - C EXTIRPATION	EXAMPLE: Removal coronary artery plaque
	EXTIRPATION: Taking or cutting out solid matter from a body part.
	EXPLANATION: Abnormal byproduct or foreign body ...

Body Part – 4TH	Approach – 5TH	Device/Substance/Technology – 6TH	Qualifier – 7TH
0 Coronary Artery, One Site 1 Coronary Artery, Two Sites 2 Coronary Artery, Three Sites 3 Coronary Artery, Four or More Sites	3 Percutaneous	6 Orbital atherectomy technology	1 New Technology Group 1

1ST - X New Technology 2ND - R Joints 3RD - 2 MONITORING	EXAMPLE: Holter monitor
	MONITORING: Determining the level of a physiological or physical function repetitively over a period of time.
	EXPLANATION: Describes a series of measurements

Body Part – 4TH	Approach – 5TH	Device/Substance/Technology – 6TH	Qualifier – 7TH
G Knee Joint, Right H Knee Joint, Left	0 Open	2 Intraoperative knee replacement sensor	1 New Technology Group 1

1ST - X New Technology 2ND - W Anatomical Regions 3RD - 0 INTRODUCTION	EXAMPLE: Infusion of substance
	INTRODUCTION: Putting in or on a therapeutic, diagnostic, nutritional, physiological, or prophylactic substance except blood or blood products.
	EXPLANATION: Substances other than blood ...

Body Part – 4TH	Approach – 5TH	Device/Substance/Technology – 6TH	Qualifier – 7TH
3 Peripheral Vein 4 Central Vein	3 Percutaneous	2 Ceftazidime-avibactam anti-infective 3 Idarucizumab, Dabigatran reversal agent 4 Isavuconazole anti-infective 5 Blinatumomab antineoplastic immunotherapy	1 New Technology Group 1

NOTES

APPENDIX A
ROOT OPERATIONS OF THE MEDICAL AND SURGICAL SECTION

APPENDIX A contains the following parts:
PART 1: Groups of Similar Root Operations (Medical and Surgical Section)
PART 2: Alphabetic Listing of Root Operations (Medical and Surgical Section)

PART 1: Groups of Similar Root Operations (Medical and Surgical Section)

The Root Operations of the Medical and Surgical section are divided into logical groups that share similar attributes. Each root operation chart group includes: root operation name, objective of the procedure, site of the procedure, and an example of that root operation. These root operation chart groups are:
- Root operations that take out some or all of a body part
- Root operations that take out solids/fluids/gases from a body part
- Root operations involving cutting or separation only
- Root operations that put in/put back or move some/all of a body part
- Root operations that alter the diameter/route of a tubular body part
- Root operations that always involve a device
- Root operations involving examination only
- Root operations that define other repairs
- Root operations that define other objectives

Bold word(s) within each chart identify the concept that help differentiate it from other root operations within that chart.

Root operations that take out some or all of a body part

Root Operation	Objective of Procedure	Site of Procedure	Example
Excision	Cutting out/off without replacement	**Some** of a body part	Breast lumpectomy
Resection	Cutting out/off without replacement	**All** of a body part	Total mastectomy
Detachment	Cutting out/off without replacement	**Extremity only**, any level	Amputation above elbow
Destruction	**Eradicating** without replacement	Some/all of a body part	Fulguration of endometrium
Extraction	**Pulling out** or off without replacement	Some/all of a body part	Suction D&C

Root operations that take out solids/fluids/gases from a body part

Root Operation	Objective of Procedure	Site of Procedure	Example
Drainage	Taking/letting out **fluids/gases**	Within a body part	Incision and drainage
Extirpation	Taking/cutting out **solid matter**	Within a body part	Thrombectomy
Fragmentation	**Breaking** solid matter into pieces	Within a body part	Lithotripsy

Root operations involving cutting or separation only

Root Operation	Objective of Procedure	Site of Procedure	Example
Division	Cutting into/**separating** a body part	Within a body part	Neurotomy
Release	**Freeing** a body part from constraint	Around a body part	Adhesiolysis

Root operations that put in/put back or move some/all of a body part

Root Operation	Objective of Procedure	Site of Procedure	Example
Transplantation	**Putting in** a living body part from a person/animal	Some/all of a body part	Kidney transplant
Reattachment	**Putting back** a detached body part	Some/all of a body part	Reattach finger
Transfer	**Moving** a body part to **function for** a similar body part	Some/all of a body part	Skin transfer flap
Reposition	**Moving** a body part to **normal** or other suitable location	Some/all of a body part	Move undescended testicle

Root operations that alter the diameter/route of a tubular body part

Root Operation	Objective of Procedure	Site of Procedure	Example
Restriction	**Partially** closing orifice/lumen	Tubular body part	Gastroesophageal fundoplication
Occlusion	**Completely** closing orifice/lumen	Tubular body part	Fallopian tube ligation
Dilation	**Expanding** orifice/lumen	Tubular body part	Percutaneous transluminal coronary angioplasty (PTCA)
Bypass	**Altering route** of passage	Tubular body part	Coronary artery bypass graft (CABG)

Root operations that always involve a device

Root Operation	Objective of Procedure	Site of Procedure	Example
Insertion	Putting in **non-biological** device	In/on a body part	Central line insertion
Replacement	Putting in device that **replaces** a body part	Some/all of a body part	Total hip replacement
Supplement	Putting in device that **reinforces** or augments a body part	In/on a body part	Abdominal wall herniorrhaphy using mesh
Change	**Exchanging** device without cutting/puncturing	In/on a body part	Drainage tube change
Removal	**Taking out** device	In/on a body part	Central line removal
Revision	**Correcting** a malfunctioning/displaced device	In/on a body part	Revision of pacemaker insertion

Root operations involving examination only

Root Operation	Objective of Procedure	Site of Procedure	Example
Inspection	Visual/manual **exploration**	Some/all of a body part	Diagnostic cystoscopy
Map	**Location** electrical impulses/functional areas	Brain/cardiac conduction mechanism	Cardiac mapping

Root operations that define other repairs

Root Operation	Objective of Procedure	Site of Procedure	Example
Control	Stopping/attempting to stop **postprocedural bleeding**	Anatomical region	Post-prostatectomy bleeding control
Repair	**Restoring** body part to its normal structure	Some/all of a body part	Suture laceration

Root operations that define other objectives

Root Operation	Objective of Procedure	Site of Procedure	Example
Fusion	Rendering joint **immobile**	Joint	Spinal fusion
Alteration	**Modifying** body part for cosmetic purposes without affecting function	Some/all of a body part	Face lift
Creation	Making new structure for **sex change** operation	Perineum	Artificial vagina/penis

Appendix A – Root Operations Med/Surg Section

PART 2: Alphabetic Listing of Root Operations (Medical and Surgical Section)

The Root Operations of the Medical and Surgical section are listed below in alphabetic order and include information detailing each root operation. Each root operation chart includes:
- Root Operation value and title
- Definition
- Explanation
- Examples

0 ALTERATION
DEFINITION: Modifying the anatomic structure of a body part without affecting the function of the body part
EXPLANATION: Principal purpose is to improve appearance
EXAMPLES: Face lift, breast augmentation

1 BYPASS
DEFINITION: Altering the route of passage of the contents of a tubular body part
EXPLANATION: Rerouting contents of a body part to a downstream area of the normal route, to a similar route and body part, or to an abnormal route and dissimilar body part. Includes one or more anastomoses, with or without the use of a device
EXAMPLES: Coronary artery bypass, colostomy formation

2 CHANGE
DEFINITION: Taking out or off a device from a body part and putting back an identical or similar device in or on the same body part without cutting or puncturing the skin or a mucous membrane
EXPLANATION: All CHANGE procedures are coded using the approach EXTERNAL
EXAMPLES: Urinary catheter change, gastrostomy tube change

3 CONTROL
DEFINITION: Stopping, or attempting to stop, postprocedural bleeding
EXPLANATION: The site of the bleeding is coded as an anatomical region and not to a specific body part
EXAMPLES: Control of post-prostatectomy hemorrhage, control of post-tonsillectomy hemorrhage

4 CREATION
DEFINITION: Making a new genital structure that does not take over the function of a body part
EXPLANATION: Used only for sex change operations
EXAMPLES: Creation of vagina in a male, creation of penis in a female

5 DESTRUCTION	**DEFINITION:** Physical eradication of all or a portion of a body part by the direct use of energy, force, or a destructive agent
EXPLANATION:	None of the body part is physically taken out
EXAMPLES:	Fulguration of rectal polyp, cautery of skin lesion

6 DETACHMENT	**DEFINITION:** Cutting off all or portion of the upper or lower extremities
EXPLANATION:	The body part value is the site of the detachment, with a qualifier if applicable to further specify the level where the extremity was detached
EXAMPLES:	Below knee amputation, disarticulation of shoulder

7 DILATION	**DEFINITION:** Expanding an orifice or the lumen of a tubular body part
EXPLANATION:	The orifice can be a natural orifice or an artificially created orifice. Accomplished by stretching a tubular body part using intraluminal pressure or by cutting part of the orifice or wall of the tubular body part.
EXAMPLES:	Percutaneous transluminal angioplasty, pyloromyotomy

8 DIVISION	**DEFINITION:** Cutting into a body part without draining fluids and/or gases from the body part in order to separate or transect a body part
EXPLANATION:	All or a portion of the body part is separated into two or more portions
EXAMPLES:	Spinal cordotomy, osteotomy

9 DRAINAGE	**DEFINITION:** Taking or letting out fluids and/or gases from a body part
EXPLANATION:	The qualifier DIAGNOSTIC is used to identify drainage procedures that are biopsies
EXAMPLES:	Thoracentesis, incision and drainage

B EXCISION	**DEFINITION:** Cutting out or off, without replacement, a portion of a body part
EXPLANATION:	The qualifier DIAGNOSTIC is used to identify excision procedures that are biopsies
EXAMPLES:	Partial nephrectomy, liver biopsy

C EXTIRPATION	**DEFINITION:** Taking or cutting out solid matter from a body part
EXPLANATION:	The solid matter may be an abnormal byproduct of a biological function or a foreign body; it may be imbedded in a body part or in the lumen of a tubular body part. The solid matter may or may not have been previously broken into pieces.
EXAMPLES:	Thrombectomy, choledocholithotomy

Appendix A – Root Operations Med/Surg Section

D EXTRACTION

DEFINITION: Pulling or stripping out or off all or a portion of a body part by the use of force

EXPLANATION: The qualifier DIAGNOSTIC is used to identify extraction procedures that are biopsies

EXAMPLES: Dilation and curettage, vein stripping

F FRAGMENTATION

DEFINITION: Breaking solid matter in a body part into pieces

EXPLANATION: Physical force (e.g., manual, ultrasonic) applied directly or indirectly is used to break the solid matter into pieces. The solid matter may be an abnormal byproduct of a biological function or a foreign body. The pieces of solid matter are not taken out.

EXAMPLES: Extracorporeal shockwave lithotripsy, transurethral lithotripsy

G FUSION

DEFINITION: Joining together portions of an articular body part rendering the articular body part immobile

EXPLANATION: The body part is joined together by fixation device, bone graft, or other means

EXAMPLES: Spinal fusion, ankle arthrodesis

H INSERTION

DEFINITION: Putting in a nonbiological appliance that monitors, assists, performs or prevents a physiological function but does not physically take the place of a body part

EXPLANATION: None

EXAMPLES: Insertion of radioactive implant, insertion of central venous catheter

J INSPECTION

DEFINITION: Visually and/or manually exploring a body part

EXPLANATION: Visual exploration may be performed with or without optical instrumentation. Manual exploration may be performed directly or through intervening body layers

EXAMPLES: Diagnostic arthroscopy, exploratory laparotomy

K MAP

DEFINITION: Locating the route of passage of electrical impulses and/or locating functional areas in a body part

EXPLANATION: Applicable only to the cardiac conduction mechanism and the central nervous system

EXAMPLES: Cardiac mapping, cortical mapping

L OCCLUSION

DEFINITION: Completely closing an orifice or the lumen of a tubular body part

EXPLANATION: The orifice can be a natural orifice or an artificially created orifice

EXAMPLES: Fallopian tube ligation, ligation of inferior vena cava

APPENDIX A – ROOT OPERATIONS MED/SURG SECTION

M REATTACHMENT

DEFINITION: Putting back in or on all or a portion of a separated body part to its normal location or other suitable location

EXPLANATION: Vascular circulation and nervous pathways may or may not be reestablished

EXAMPLES: Reattachment of hand, reattachment of avulsed kidney

N RELEASE

DEFINITION: Freeing a body part from an abnormal physical constraint by cutting or by the use of force

EXPLANATION: Some of the restraining tissue may be taken out but none of the body part is taken out

EXAMPLES: Adhesiolysis, carpal tunnel release

P REMOVAL

DEFINITION: Taking out or off a device from a body part

EXPLANATION: If a device is taken out and a similar device put in without cutting or puncturing the skin or mucous membrane, the procedure is coded to the root operation CHANGE. Otherwise, the procedure for taking out a device is coded to the root operation REMOVAL.

EXAMPLES: Drainage tube removal, cardiac pacemaker removal

Q REPAIR

DEFINITION: Restoring, to the extent possible, a body part to its normal anatomic structure and function

EXPLANATION: Used only when the method to accomplish the repair is not one of the other root operations

EXAMPLES: Colostomy takedown, suture of laceration

R REPLACEMENT

DEFINITION: Putting in or on biological or synthetic material that physically takes the place and/or function of all or a portion of a body part

EXPLANATION: The body part may have been taken out or replaced, or may be taken out, physically eradicated, or rendered non-functional during the REPLACEMENT procedure. A REMOVAL procedure is coded for taking out the device used in a previous replacement procedure.

EXAMPLES: Total hip replacement, bone graft, free skin graft

S REPOSITION

DEFINITION: Moving to its normal location, or other suitable location, all or a portion of a body part

EXPLANATION: The body part is moved to a new location from an abnormal location, or from a normal location where it is not functioning correctly. The body part may or may not be cut out or off to be moved to the new location.

EXAMPLES: Reposition of undescended testicle, fracture reduction

T RESECTION

DEFINITION: Cutting out or off, without replacement, all of a body part

EXPLANATION: None

EXAMPLES: Total nephrectomy, total lobectomy of lung

APPENDIX A – ROOT OPERATIONS MED/SURG SECTION

V RESTRICTION	DEFINITION: Partially closing an orifice or the lumen of a tubular body part
EXPLANATION:	The orifice can be a natural orifice or an artificially created orifice
EXAMPLES:	Esophagogastric fundoplication, cervical cerclage

W REVISION	DEFINITION: Correcting, to the extent possible, a portion of a malfunctioning device or the position of a displaced device
EXPLANATION:	Revision can include correcting a malfunctioning or displaced device by taking out or putting in components of the device such as a screw or pin
EXAMPLES:	Adjustment of position of pacemaker lead, recementing of hip prosthesis

U SUPPLEMENT	DEFINITION: Putting in or on biologic or synthetic material that physically reinforces and/or augments the function of a portion of a body part
EXPLANATION:	The biological material is non-living, or is living and from the same individual. The body part may have been previously replaced, and the Supplement procedure is performed to physically reinforce and/or augment the function of the replaced body part.
EXAMPLES:	Herniorrhaphy using mesh, free nerve graft, mitral valve ring annuloplasty, put a new acetabular liner in a previous hip replacement

X TRANSFER	DEFINITION: Moving, without taking out, all or a portion of a body part to another location to take over the function of all or a portion of a body part
EXPLANATION:	The body part transferred remains connected to its vascular and nervous supply
EXAMPLES:	Tendon transfer, skin pedicle flap transfer

Y TRANSPLANTATION	DEFINITION: Putting in or on all or a portion of a living body part taken from another individual or animal to physically take the place and/or function of all or a portion of a similar body part
EXPLANATION:	The native body part may or may not be taken out, and the transplanted body part may take over all or a portion of its function
EXAMPLES:	Kidney transplant, heart transplant

Root operation/type definitions, explanations, and examples of the Medical- and Surgical-Related Section and the Ancillary Section are found at the specific code tables in their respective sections.

APPENDIX B
APPROACH DEFINITIONS OF THE MEDICAL AND SURGICAL SECTION

0	OPEN	DEFINITION: Cutting through the skin or mucous membrane and any other body layers necessary to expose the site of the procedure
EXPLANATION:	Includes "laparoscopic-assisted" open approach procedures	
EXAMPLES:	Kidney tranplant, laparoscopic-assisted sigmoidectomy	

3	PERCUTANEOUS	DEFINITION: Entry, by puncture or minor incision, of instrumentation through the skin or mucous membrane and any other body layers necessary to reach the site of the procedure
EXPLANATION:	Includes procedures performed percutaneously via device placed for the procedure	
EXAMPLES:	Needle biopsy of liver, fragmentation of kidney stone performed via percutaneous nephrostomy	

4	PERCUTANEOUS ENDOSCOPIC	DEFINITION: Entry, by puncture or minor incision, of instrumentation through the skin or mucous membrane and any other body layers necessary to reach and visualize the site of the procedure
EXPLANATION:	Percutaneous procedures using visualization	
EXAMPLES:	Laparoscopic cholecystectomy, arthroscopy	

7	VIA NATURAL OR ARTIFICIAL OPENING	DEFINITION: Entry of instrumentation through a natural or artificial external opening to reach the site of the procedure
EXPLANATION:	Access entry through natural or artificial external opening WITHOUT visualization	
EXAMPLES:	Insertion of urinary catheter, insertion of endotracheal tube	

8	VIA NATURAL OR ARTIFICIAL OPENING ENDOSCOPIC	DEFINITION: Entry of instrumentation through a natural or artificial external opening to reach and visualize the site of the procedure
EXPLANATION:	Access entry through natural or artificial external opening using visualization	
EXAMPLES:	Bronchoscopy, colonoscopy with biopsy	

F	VIA NATURAL OR ARTIFICIAL OPENING WITH PERCUTANEOUS ENDOSCOPIC ASSISTANCE	DEFINITION: Entry of instrumentation through a natural or artificial external opening and entry, by puncture or minor incision, of instrumentation through the skin or mucous membrane and any other body layers necessary to aid in the performance of the procedure
EXPLANATION:	Access entry through natural or artificial external opening AND using a separate percutaneous visualization	
EXAMPLES:	Laparoscopic-assisted vaginal hysterectomy	

X	EXTERNAL	DEFINITION: Procedures performed directly on the skin or mucous membrane and procedures performed indirectly by the application of external force through the skin or mucous membrane
EXPLANATION:	Includes procedures performed within an orifice on structures that are visible without the aid of any instrumentation	
EXAMPLES:	Closed reduction of fracture, suture of laceration, tonsillectomy	

NOTES

APPENDIX C – BODY PART KEY

BODY PART	USE:
Abdominal aortic plexus	use Abdominal Sympathetic Nerve
Abdominal esophagus	use Esophagus, Lower
Abductor hallucis muscle	use Foot Muscle, Left/Right
Accessory cephalic vein	use Cephalic Vein, Left/Right
Accessory obturator nerve	use Lumbar Plexus
Accessory phrenic nerve	use Phrenic Nerve
Accessory spleen	use Spleen
Acetabulofemoral joint	use Hip Joint, Left/Right
Achilles tendon	use Lower Leg Tendon, Left/Right
Acromioclavicular ligament	use Shoulder Bursa and Ligament, Left/Right
Acromion (process)	use Scapula, Left/Right
Adductor brevis muscle	use Upper Leg Muscle, Left/Right
Adductor hallucis muscle	use Foot Muscle, Left/Right
Adductor longus muscle	use Upper Leg Muscle, Left/Right
Adductor magnus muscle	use Upper Leg Muscle, Left/Right
Adenohypophysis	use Pituitary Gland
Alar ligament of axis	use Head and Neck Bursa and Ligament
Alveolar process of mandible	use Mandible, Left/Right
Alveolar process of maxilla	use Maxilla, Left/Right
Anal orifice	use Anus
Anatomical snuffbox	use Lower Arm and Wrist Muscle, Left/Right
Angular artery	use Face Artery
Angular vein	use Face Vein, Left/Right
Annular ligament	use Elbow Bursa and Ligament, Left/Right
Anorectal junction	use Rectum
Ansa cervicalis	use Cervical Plexus
Antebrachial fascia	use Subcutaneous Tissue and Fascia, Lower Arm, Left/Right
Anterior (pectoral) lymph node	use Lymphatic, Axillary, Left/Right
Anterior cerebral artery	use Intracranial Artery
Anterior cerebral vein	use Intracranial Vein
Anterior choroidal artery	use Intracranial Artery
Anterior circumflex humeral artery	use Axillary Artery, Left/Right
Anterior communicating artery	use Intracranial Artery
Anterior cruciate ligament (ACL)	use Knee Bursa and Ligament, Left/Right
Anterior crural nerve	use Femoral Nerve
Anterior facial vein	use Face Vein, Left/Right
Anterior intercostal artery	use Internal Mammary Artery, Left/Right
Anterior interosseous nerve	use Median Nerve
Anterior lateral malleolar artery	use Anterior Tibial Artery, Left/Right
Anterior lingual gland	use Minor Salivary Gland
Anterior medial malleolar artery	use Anterior Tibial Artery, Left/Right
Anterior spinal artery	use Vertebral Artery, Left/Right

BODY PART	USE:
Anterior tibial recurrent artery	use Anterior Tibial Artery, Left/Right
Anterior ulnar recurrent artery	use Ulnar Artery, Left/Right
Anterior vagal trunk	use Vagus Nerve
Anterior vertebral muscle	use Neck Muscle, Left/Right
Antihelix	use External Ear, Bilateral/Left/Right
Antitragus	use External Ear, Bilateral/Left/Right
Antrum of Highmore	use Maxillary Sinus, Left/Right
Aortic annulus	use Aortic Valve
Aortic arch	use Thoracic Aorta
Aortic intercostal artery	use Thoracic Aorta
Apical (subclavicular) lymph node	use Lymphatic, Axillary, Left/Right
Apneustic center	use Pons
Aqueduct of Sylvius	use Cerebral Ventricle
Aqueous humour	use Anterior Chamber, Left/Right
Arachnoid mater, intracranial	use Cerebral Meninges
Arachnoid mater, spinal	use Spinal Meninges
Arcuate artery	use Foot Artery, Left/Right
Areola	use Nipple, Left/Right
Arterial canal (duct)	use Pulmonary Artery, Left
Aryepiglottic fold	use Larynx
Arytenoid cartilage	use Larynx
Arytenoid muscle	use Neck Muscle, Left/Right
Ascending aorta	use Thoracic Aorta
Ascending palatine artery	use Face Artery
Ascending pharyngeal artery	use External Carotid Artery, Left/Right
Atlantoaxial joint	use Cervical Vertebral Joint
Atrioventricular node	use Conduction Mechanism
Atrium dextrum cordis	use Atrium, Right
Atrium pulmonale	use Atrium, Left
Auditory tube	use Eustachian Tube, Left/Right
Auerbach's (myenteric) plexus	use Abdominal Sympathetic Nerve
Auricle	use External Ear, Bilateral/Left/Right
Auricularis muscle	use Head Muscle
Axillary fascia	use Subcutaneous Tissue and Fascia, Upper Arm, Left/Right
Axillary nerve	use Brachial Plexus
Bartholin's (greater vestibular) gland	use Vestibular Gland
Basal (internal) cerebral vein	use Intracranial Vein
Basal nuclei	use Basal Ganglia
Basilar artery	use Intracranial Artery
Basis pontis	use Pons
Biceps brachii muscle	use Upper Arm Muscle, Left/Right
Biceps femoris muscle	use Upper Leg Muscle, Left/Right
Bicipital aponeurosis	use Subcutaneous Tissue and Fascia, Lower Arm, Left/Right
Bicuspid valve	use Mitral Valve
Body of femur	use Femoral Shaft, Left/Right

BODY PART	USE:
Body of fibula	use Fibula, Left/Right
Bony labyrinth	use Inner Ear, Left/Right
Bony orbit	use Orbit, Left/Right
Bony vestibule	use Inner Ear, Left/Right
Botallo's duct	use Pulmonary Artery, Left
Brachial (lateral) lymph node	use Lymphatic, Axillary, Left/Right
Brachialis muscle	use Upper Arm Muscle, Left/Right
Brachiocephalic artery	use Innominate Artery
Brachiocephalic trunk	use Innominate Artery
Brachiocephalic vein	use Innominate Vein, Left/Right
Brachioradialis muscle	use Lower Arm and Wrist Muscle, Left/Right
Broad ligament	use Uterine Supporting Structure
Bronchial artery	use Thoracic Aorta
Buccal gland	use Buccal Mucosa
Buccinator lymph node	use Lymphatic, Head
Buccinator muscle	use Facial Muscle
Bulbospongiosus muscle	use Perineum Muscle
Bulbourethral (Cowper's) gland	use Urethra
Bundle of His	use Conduction Mechanism
Bundle of Kent	use Conduction Mechanism
Calcaneocuboid joint	use Tarsal Joint, Left/Right
Calcaneocuboid ligament	use Foot Bursa and Ligament, Left/Right
Calcaneofibular ligament	use Ankle Bursa and Ligament, Left/Right
Calcaneus	use Tarsal, Left/Right
Capitate bone	use Carpal, Left/Right
Cardia	use Esophagogastric Junction
Cardiac plexus	use Thoracic Sympathetic Nerve
Cardioesophageal junction	use Esophagogastric Junction
Caroticotympanic artery	use Internal Carotid Artery, Left/Right
Carotid glomus	use Carotid Body, Bilateral/Left/Right
Carotid sinus	use Internal Carotid Artery, Left/Right
Carotid sinus nerve	use Glossopharyngeal Nerve
Carpometacarpal (CMC) joint	use Metacarpocarpal Joint, Left/Right
Carpometacarpal ligament	use Hand Bursa and Ligament, Left/Right
Cauda equina	use Lumbar Spinal Cord
Cavernous plexus	use Head and Neck Sympathetic Nerve
Celiac (solar) plexus	use Abdominal Sympathetic Nerve
Celiac ganglion	use Abdominal Sympathetic Nerve
Celiac lymph node	use Lymphatic, Aortic
Celiac trunk	use Celiac Artery
Central axillary lymph node	use Lymphatic, Axillary, Left/Right
Cerebral aqueduct (Sylvius)	use Cerebral Ventricle
Cerebrum	use Brain
Cervical esophagus	use Esophagus, Upper
Cervical facet joint	use Cervical Vertebral Joint(s)
Cervical ganglion	use Head and Neck Sympathetic Nerve

BODY PART	USE:
Cervical interspinous ligament	use Head and Neck Bursa and Ligament
Cervical intertransverse ligament	use Head and Neck Bursa and Ligament
Cervical ligamentum flavum	use Head and Neck Bursa and Ligament
Cervical lymph node	use Lymphatic, Neck, Left/Right
Cervicothoracic facet joint	use Cervicothoracic Vertebral Joint
Choana	use Nasopharynx
Chondroglossus muscle	use Tongue, Palate, Pharynx Muscle
Chorda tympani	use Facial Nerve
Choroid plexus	use Cerebral Ventricle
Ciliary body	use Eye, Left/Right
Ciliary ganglion	use Head and Neck Sympathetic Nerve
Circle of Willis	use Intracranial Artery
Circumflex iliac artery	use Femoral Artery, Left/Right
Claustrum	use Basal Ganglia
Coccygeal body	use Coccygeal Glomus
Coccygeus muscle	use Trunk Muscle, Left/Right
Cochlea	use Inner Ear, Left/Right
Cochlear nerve	use Acoustic Nerve
Columella	use Nose
Common digital vein	use Foot Vein, Left/Right
Common facial vein	use Face Vein, Left/Right
Common fibular nerve	use Peroneal Nerve
Common hepatic artery	use Hepatic Artery
Common iliac (subaortic) lymph node	use Lymphatic, Pelvis
Common interosseous artery	use Ulnar Artery, Left/Right
Common peroneal nerve	use Peroneal Nerve
Condyloid process	use Mandible, Left/Right
Conus arteriosus	use Ventricle, Right
Conus medullaris	use Lumbar Spinal Cord
Coracoacromial ligament	use Shoulder Bursa and Ligament, Left/Right
Coracobrachialis muscle	use Upper Arm Muscle, Left/Right
Coracoclavicular ligament	use Shoulder Bursa and Ligament, Left/Right
Coracohumeral ligament	use Shoulder Bursa and Ligament, Left/Right
Coracoid process	use Scapula, Left/Right
Corniculate cartilage	use Larynx
Corpus callosum	use Brain
Corpus cavernosum	use Penis
Corpus spongiosum	use Penis
Corpus striatum	use Basal Ganglia
Corrugator supercilii muscle	use Facial Muscle
Costocervical trunk	use Subclavian Artery, Left/Right
Costoclavicular ligament	use Shoulder Bursa and Ligament, Left/Right
Costotransverse joint	use Thoracic Vertebral Joint
Costotransverse ligament	use Thorax Bursa and Ligament, Left/Right
Costovertebral joint	use Thoracic Vertebral Joint
Costoxiphoid ligament	use Thorax Bursa and Ligament, Left/Right

APPENDIX C – BODY PART KEY

BODY PART	USE:
Cowper's (bulbourethral) gland	use Urethra
Cremaster muscle	use Perineum Muscle
Cribriform plate	use Ethmoid Bone, Left/Right
Cricoid cartilage	use Trachea
Cricothyroid artery	use Thyroid Artery, Left/Right
Cricothyroid muscle	use Neck Muscle, Left/Right
Crural fascia	use Subcutaneous Tissue and Fascia, Upper Leg, Left/Right
Cubital lymph node	use Lymphatic, Upper Extremity, Left/Right
Cubital nerve	use Ulnar Nerve
Cuboid bone	use Tarsal, Left/Right
Cuboideonavicular joint	use Tarsal Joint, Left/Right
Culmen	use Cerebellum
Cuneiform cartilage	use Larynx
Cuneonavicular joint	use Tarsal Joint, Left/Right
Cuneonavicular ligament	use Foot Bursa and Ligament, Left/Right
Cutaneous (transverse) cervical nerve	use Cervical Plexus
Deep cervical fascia	use Subcutaneous Tissue and Fascia, Anterior Neck
Deep cervical vein	use Vertebral Vein, Left/Right
Deep circumflex iliac artery	use External Iliac Artery, Left/Right
Deep facial vein	use Face Vein, Left/Right
Deep femoral (profunda femoris) vein	use Femoral Vein, Left/Right
Deep femoral artery	use Femoral Artery, Left/Right
Deep palmar arch	use Hand Artery, Left/Right
Deep transverse perineal muscle	use Perineum Muscle
Deferential artery	use Internal Iliac Artery, Left/Right
Deltoid fascia	use Subcutaneous Tissue and Fascia, Upper Arm, Left/Right
Deltoid ligament	use Ankle Bursa and Ligament, Left/Right
Deltoid muscle	use Shoulder Muscle, Left/Right
Deltopectoral (infraclavicular) lymph node	use Lymphatic, Upper Extremity, Left/Right
Denticulate (dentate) ligament	use Spinal Meninges
Depressor anguli oris muscle	use Facial Muscle
Depressor labii inferioris muscle	
Depressor septi nasi muscle	
Depressor supercilii muscle	
Dermis	use Skin
Descending genicular artery	use Femoral Artery, Left/Right
Diaphragma sellae	use Dura Mater

BODY PART	USE:
Distal humerus	use Humeral Shaft, Left/Right
Distal humerus, involving joint	use Elbow Joint, Left/Right
Distal radioulnar joint	use Wrist Joint, Left/Right
Dorsal digital nerve	use Radial Nerve
Dorsal metacarpal vein	use Hand Vein, Left/Right
Dorsal metatarsal artery	use Foot Artery, Left/Right
Dorsal metatarsal vein	use Foot Vein, Left/Right
Dorsal scapular artery	use Subclavian Artery, Left/Right
Dorsal scapular nerve	use Brachial Plexus
Dorsal venous arch	use Foot Vein, Left/Right
Dorsalis pedis artery	use Anterior Tibial Artery, Left/Right
Duct of Santorini	use Pancreatic Duct, Accessory
Duct of Wirsung	use Pancreatic Duct
Ductus deferens	use Vas Deferens, Bilateral/Left/Right
Duodenal ampulla	use Ampulla of Vater
Duodenojejunal flexure	use Jejunum
Dura mater, intracranial	use Dura Mater
Dura mater, spinal	use Spinal Meninges
Dural venous sinus	use Intracranial Vein
Earlobe	use External Ear, Bilateral/Left/Right
Eighth cranial nerve	use Acoustic Nerve
Ejaculatory duct	use Vas Deferens, Bilateral/Left/Right
Eleventh cranial nerve	use Accessory Nerve
Encephalon	use Brain
Ependyma	use Cerebral Ventricle
Epidermis	use Skin
Epidural space intracranial	use Epidural Space
Epidural space, spinal	use Spinal Canal
Epiploic foramen	use Peritoneum
Epithalamus	use Thalamus
Epitrochlear lymph node	use Lymphatic, Upper Extremity, Left/Right
Erector spinae muscle	use Trunk Muscle, Left/Right
Esophageal artery	use Thoracic Aorta
Esophageal plexus	use Thoracic Sympathetic Nerve
Ethmoidal air cell	use Ethmoid Sinus, Left/Right
Extensor carpi radialis muscle	use Lower Arm and Wrist Muscle, Left/Right
Extensor carpi ulnaris muscle	
Extensor digitorum brevis muscle	use Foot Muscle, Left/Right
Extensor digitorum longus muscle	use Lower Leg Muscle, Left/Right
Extensor hallucis brevis muscle	use Foot Muscle, Left/Right
Extensor hallucis longus muscle	use Lower Leg Muscle, Left/Right
External anal sphincter	use Anal Sphincter
External auditory meatus	use External Auditory Canal, Left/Right
External maxillary artery	use Face Artery
External naris	use Nose

BODY PART	USE:
External oblique aponeurosis	use Subcutaneous Tissue and Fascia, Trunk
External oblique muscle	use Abdomen Muscle, Left/Right
External popliteal nerve	use Peroneal Nerve
External pudendal artery	use Femoral Artery, Left/Right
External pudendal vein	use Greater Saphenous Vein, Left/Right
External urethral sphincter	use Urethra
Extradural space, intracranial	use Epidural Space
Extradural space, spinal	use Spinal Canal
Facial artery	use Face Artery
False vocal cord	use Larynx
Falx cerebri	use Dura Mater
Fascia lata	use Subcutaneous Tissue and Fascia, Upper Leg, Left/Right
Femoral head	use Upper Femur, Left/Right
Femoral lymph node	use Lymphatic, Lower Extremity, Left/Right
Femoropatellar joint	use Knee Joint, Left/Right
	use Knee Joint, Femoral Surface, Left/Right
Femorotibial joint	use Knee Joint, Left/Right
	use Knee Joint, Tibial Surface, Left/Right
Fibular artery	use Peroneal Artery, Left/Right
Fibularis brevis muscle	use Lower Leg Muscle, Left/Right
Fibularis longus muscle	
Fifth cranial nerve	use Trigeminal Nerve
First cranial nerve	use Olfactory Nerve
First intercostal nerve	use Brachial Plexus
Flexor carpi radialis muscle	use Lower Arm and Wrist Muscle, Left/Right
Flexor carpi ulnaris muscle	
Flexor digitorum brevis muscle	use Foot Muscle, Left/Right
Flexor digitorum longus muscle	use Lower Leg Muscle, Left/Right
Flexor hallucis brevis muscle	use Foot Muscle, Left/Right
Flexor hallucis longus muscle	use Lower Leg Muscle, Left/Right
Flexor pollicis longus muscle	use Lower Arm and Wrist Muscle, Left/Right
Foramen magnum	use Occipital Bone, Left/Right
Foramen of Monro (intraventricular)	use Cerebral Ventricle
Foreskin	use Prepuce
Fossa of Rosenmuller	use Nasopharynx
Fourth cranial nerve	use Trochlear Nerve
Fourth ventricle	use Cerebral Ventricle
Fovea	use Retina, Left/Right
Frenulum labii inferioris	use Lower Lip
Frenulum labii superioris	use Upper Lip
Frenulum linguae	use Tongue
Frontal lobe	use Cerebral Hemisphere
Frontal vein	use Face Vein, Left/Right
Fundus uteri	use Uterus

BODY PART	USE:
Galea aponeurotica	use Subcutaneous Tissue and Fascia, Scalp
Ganglion impar (ganglion of Walther)	use Sacral Sympathetic Nerve
Gasserian ganglion	use Trigeminal Nerve
Gastric lymph node	use Lymphatic, Aortic
Gastric plexus	use Abdominal Sympathetic Nerve
Gastrocnemius muscle	use Lower Leg Muscle, Left/Right
Gastrocolic ligament	use Greater Omentum
Gastrocolic omentum	
Gastroduodenal artery	use Hepatic Artery
Gastroesophageal (GE) junction	use Esophagogastric Junction
Gastrohepatic omentum	use Lesser Omentum
Gastrophrenic ligament	use Greater Omentum
Gastrosplenic ligament	
Gemellus muscle	use Hip Muscle, Left/Right
Geniculate ganglion	use Facial Nerve
Geniculate nucleus	use Thalamus
Genioglossus muscle	use Tongue, Palate, Pharynx Muscle
Genitofemoral nerve	use Lumbar Plexus
Glans penis	use Prepuce
Glenohumeral joint	use Shoulder Joint, Left/Right
Glenohumeral ligament	use Shoulder Bursa and Ligament, Left/Right
Glenoid fossa (of scapula)	use Glenoid Cavity, Left/Right
Glenoid ligament (labrum)	use Shoulder Joint, Left/Right
Globus pallidus	use Basal Ganglia
Glossoepiglottic fold	use Epiglottis
Glottis	use Larynx
Gluteal lymph node	use Lymphatic, Pelvis
Gluteal vein	use Hypogastric Vein, Left/Right
Gluteus maximus muscle	use Hip Muscle, Left/Right
Gluteus medius muscle	
Gluteus minimus muscle	
Gracilis muscle	use Upper Leg Muscle, Left/Right
Great auricular nerve	use Cervical Plexus
Great cerebral vein	use Intracranial Vein
Great saphenous vein	use Greater Saphenous Vein, Left/Right
Greater alar cartilage	use Nose
Greater occipital nerve	use Cervical Nerve
Greater splanchnic nerve	use Thoracic Sympathetic Nerve
Greater superficial petrosal nerve	use Facial Nerve
Greater trochanter	use Upper Femur, Left/Right
Greater tuberosity	use Humeral Head, Left/Right
Greater vestibular (Bartholin's) gland	use Vestibular Gland
Greater wing	use Sphenoid Bone, Left/Right
Hallux	use 1st Toe, Left/Right
Hamate bone	use Carpal, Left/Right
Head of fibula	use Fibula, Left/Right
Helix	use External Ear, Bilateral/Left/Right
Hepatic artery proper	use Hepatic Artery
Hepatic flexure	use Ascending Colon

APPENDIX C – BODY PART KEY

BODY PART	USE:
Hepatic lymph node	use Lymphatic, Aortic
Hepatic plexus	use Abdominal Sympathetic Nerve
Hepatic portal vein	use Portal Vein
Hepatogastric ligament	use Lesser Omentum
Hepatopancreatic ampulla	use Ampulla of Vater
Humeroradial joint	use Elbow Joint, Left/Right
Humeroulnar joint	use Elbow Joint, Left/Right
Humerus, distal	use Humeral Shaft, Left/Right
Hyoglossus muscle	use Tongue, Palate, Pharynx Muscle
Hyoid artery	use Thyroid Artery, Left/Right
Hypogastric artery	use Internal Iliac Artery, Left/Right
Hypopharynx	use Pharynx
Hypophysis	use Pituitary Gland
Hypothenar muscle	use Hand Muscle, Left/Right
Ileal artery	use Superior Mesenteric Artery
Ileocolic artery	use Superior Mesenteric Artery
Ileocolic vein	use Colic Vein
Iliac crest	use Pelvic Bone, Left/Right
Iliac fascia	use Subcutaneous Tissue and Fascia, Upper Leg, Left/Right
Iliac lymph node	use Lymphatic, Pelvis
Iliacus muscle	use Hip Muscle, Left/Right
Iliofemoral ligament	use Hip Bursa and Ligament, Left/Right
Iliohypogastric nerve	use Lumbar Plexus
Ilioinguinal nerve	use Lumbar Plexus
Iliolumbar artery	use Internal Iliac Artery, Left/Right
Iliolumbar ligament	use Trunk Bursa and Ligament, Left/Right
Iliotibial tract (band)	use Subcutaneous Tissue and Fascia, Upper Leg, Left/Right
Ilium	use Pelvic Bone, Left/Right
Incus	use Auditory Ossicle, Left/Right
Inferior cardiac nerve	use Thoracic Sympathetic Nerve
Inferior cerebellar vein	use Intracranial Vein
Inferior cerebral vein	use Intracranial Vein
Inferior epigastric artery	use External Iliac Artery, Left/Right
Inferior epigastric lymph node	use Lymphatic, Pelvis
Inferior genicular artery	use Popliteal Artery, Left/Right
Inferior gluteal artery	use Internal Iliac Artery, Left/Right
Inferior gluteal nerve	use Sacral Plexus
Inferior hypogastric plexus	use Abdominal Sympathetic Nerve
Inferior labial artery	use Face Artery
Inferior longitudinal muscle	use Tongue, Palate, Pharynx Muscle
Inferior mesenteric ganglion	use Abdominal Sympathetic Nerve
Inferior mesenteric lymph node	use Lymphatic, Mesenteric
Inferior mesenteric plexus	use Abdominal Sympathetic Nerve
Inferior oblique muscle	use Extraocular Muscle, Left/Right
Inferior pancreaticoduodenal artery	use Superior Mesenteric Artery
Inferior phrenic artery	use Abdominal Aorta
Inferior rectus muscle	use Extraocular Muscle, Left/Right
Inferior suprarenal artery	use Renal Artery, Left/Right
Inferior tarsal plate	use Lower Eyelid, Left/Right
Inferior thyroid vein	use Innominate Vein, Left/Right
Inferior tibiofibular joint	use Ankle Joint, Left/Right
Inferior turbinate	use Nasal Turbinate
Inferior ulnar collateral artery	use Brachial Artery, Left/Right
Inferior vesical artery	use Internal Iliac Artery, Left/Right
Infraauricular lymph node	use Lymphatic, Head
Infraclavicular (deltopectoral) lymph node	use Lymphatic, Upper Extremity, Left/Right
Infrahyoid muscle	use Neck Muscle, Left/Right
Infraparotid lymph node	use Lymphatic, Head
Infraspinatus fascia	use Subcutaneous Tissue and Fascia, Upper Arm, Left/Right
Infraspinatus muscle	use Shoulder Muscle, Left/Right
Infundibulopelvic ligament	use Uterine Supporting Structure
Inguinal canal	use Inguinal Region, Bilateral/Left/Right
Inguinal triangle	use Inguinal Region, Bilateral/Left/Right
Interatrial septum	use Atrial Septum
Intercarpal joint	use Carpal Joint, Left/Right
Intercarpal ligament	use Hand Bursa and Ligament, Left/Right
Interclavicular ligament	use Shoulder Bursa and Ligament, Left/Right
Intercostal lymph node	use Lymphatic, Thorax
Intercostal muscle	use Thorax Muscle, Left/Right
Intercostal nerve	use Thoracic Nerve
Intercostobrachial nerve	use Thoracic Nerve
Intercuneiform joint	use Tarsal Joint, Left/Right
Intercuneiform ligament	use Foot Bursa and Ligament, Left/Right
Intermediate cuneiform bone	use Tarsal, Left/Right
Internal (basal) cerebral vein	use Intracranial Vein
Internal anal sphincter	use Anal Sphincter
Internal carotid plexus	use Head and Neck Sympathetic Nerve
Internal iliac vein	use Hypogastric Vein, Left/Right
Internal maxillary artery	use External Carotid Artery, Left/Right
Internal naris	use Nose
Internal oblique muscle	use Abdomen Muscle, Left/Right
Internal pudendal artery	use Internal Iliac Artery, Left/Right
Internal pudendal vein	use Hypogastric Vein, Left/Right
Internal thoracic artery	use Internal Mammary Artery, Left/Right Subclavian Artery, Left/Right
Internal urethral sphincter	use Urethra
Interphalangeal (IP) joint	use Finger Phalangeal Joint, Left/Right Toe Phalangeal Joint, Left/Right
Interphalangeal ligament	use Hand Bursa and Ligament, Left/Right Foot Bursa and Ligament, Left/Right
Interspinalis muscle	use Trunk Muscle, Left/Right
Interspinous ligament	use Head and Neck Bursa and Ligament use Trunk Bursa and Ligament, Left/Right

BODY PART	USE:
Intertransversarius muscle	use Trunk Muscle, Left/Right
Intertransverse ligament	use Trunk Bursa and Ligament, Left/Right
Interventricular foramen (Monro)	use Cerebral Ventricle
Interventricular septum	use Ventricular Septum
Intestinal lymphatic trunk	use Cisterna Chyli
Ischiatic nerve	use Sciatic Nerve
Ischiocavernosus muscle	use Perineum Muscle
Ischiofemoral ligament	use Hip Bursa and Ligament, Left/Right
Ischium	use Pelvic Bone, Left/Right
Jejunal artery	use Superior Mesenteric Artery
Jugular body	use Glomus Jugulare
Jugular lymph node	use Lymphatic, Neck, Left/Right
Labia majora	use Vulva
Labia minora	use Vulva
Labial gland	use Upper Lip, Lower Lip
Lacrimal canaliculus	use Lacrimal Duct, Left/Right
Lacrimal punctum	use Lacrimal Duct, Left/Right
Lacrimal sac	use Lacrimal Duct, Left/Right
Laryngopharynx	use Pharynx
Lateral (brachial) lymph node	use Lymphatic, Axillary, Left/Right
Lateral canthus	use Upper Eyelid, Left/Right
Lateral collateral ligament (LCL)	use Knee Bursa and Ligament, Left/Right
Lateral condyle of femur	use Lower Femur, Left/Right
Lateral condyle of tibia	use Tibia, Left/Right
Lateral cuneiform bone	use Tarsal, Left/Right
Lateral epicondyle of femur	use Lower Femur, Left/Right
Lateral epicondyle of humerus	use Humeral Shaft, Left/Right
Lateral femoral cutaneous nerve	use Lumbar Plexus
Lateral malleolus	use Fibula, Left/Right
Lateral meniscus	use Knee Joint, Left/Right
Lateral nasal cartilage	use Nose
Lateral plantar artery	use Foot Artery, Left/Right
Lateral plantar nerve	use Tibial Nerve
Lateral rectus muscle	use Extraocular Muscle, Left/Right
Lateral sacral artery	use Internal Iliac Artery, Left/Right
Lateral sacral vein	use Hypogastric Vein, Left/Right
Lateral sural cutaneous nerve	use Peroneal Nerve
Lateral tarsal artery	use Foot Artery, Left/Right
Lateral temporomandibular ligament	use Head and Neck Bursa and Ligament
Lateral thoracic artery	use Axillary Artery, Left/Right
Latissimus dorsi muscle	use Trunk Muscle, Left/Right
Least splanchnic nerve	use Thoracic Sympathetic Nerve
Left ascending lumbar vein	use Hemiazygos Vein
Left atrioventricular valve	use Mitral Valve

BODY PART	USE:
Left auricular appendix	use Atrium, Left
Left colic vein	use Colic Vein
Left coronary sulcus	use Heart, Left
Left gastric artery	use Gastric Artery
Left gastroepiploic artery	use Splenic Artery
Left gastroepiploic vein	use Splenic Vein
Left inferior phrenic vein	use Renal Vein, Left
Left inferior pulmonary vein	use Pulmonary Vein, Left
Left jugular trunk	use Thoracic Duct
Left lateral ventricle	use Cerebral Ventricle
Left ovarian vein	use Renal Vein, Left
Left second lumbar vein	use Renal Vein, Left
Left subclavian trunk	use Thoracic Duct
Left subcostal vein	use Hemiazygos Vein
Left superior pulmonary vein	use Pulmonary Vein, Left
Left suprarenal vein	use Renal Vein, Left
Left testicular vein	use Renal Vein, Left
Leptomeninges, intracranial	use Cerebral Meninges
Leptomeninges, spinal	use Spinal Meninges
Lesser alar cartilage	use Nose
Lesser occipital nerve	use Cervical Plexus
Lesser splanchnic nerve	use Thoracic Sympathetic Nerve
Lesser trochanter	use Upper Femur, Left/Right
Lesser tuberosity	use Humeral Head, Left/Right
Lesser wing	use Sphenoid Bone, Left/Right
Levator anguli oris muscle	use Facial Muscle
Levator ani muscle	use Trunk Muscle, Left/Right
Levator labii superioris alaeque nasi muscle	use Facial Muscle
Levator labii superioris muscle	use Facial Muscle
Levator palpebrae superioris muscle	use Upper Eyelid, Left/Right
Levator scapulae muscle	use Neck Muscle, Left/Right
Levator veli palatini muscle	use Tongue, Palate, Pharynx Muscle
Levatores costarum muscle	use Thorax Muscle, Left/Right
Ligament of head of fibula	use Knee Bursa and Ligament, Left/Right
Ligament of the lateral malleolus	use Ankle Bursa and Ligament, Left/Right
Ligamentum flavum	use Trunk Bursa and Ligament, Left/Right
Lingual artery	use External Carotid Artery, Left/Right
Lingual tonsil	use Tongue
Locus ceruleus	use Pons
Long thoracic nerve	use Brachial Plexus
Lumbar artery	use Abdominal Aorta
Lumbar facet joint	use Lumbar Vertebral Joint
Lumbar ganglion	use Lumbar Sympathetic Nerve
Lumbar lymph node	use Lymphatic, Aortic
Lumbar lymphatic trunk	use Cisterna Chyli

APPENDIX C – BODY PART KEY

BODY PART	USE:
Lumbar splanchnic nerve	use Lumbar Sympathetic Nerve
Lumbosacral facet joint	use Lumbosacral Joint
Lumbosacral trunk	use Lumbar Nerve
Lunate bone	use Carpal, Left/Right
Lunotriquetral ligament	use Hand Bursa and Ligament, Left/Right
Macula	use Retina, Left/Right
Malleus	use Auditory Ossicle, Left/Right
Mammary duct	use Breast, Bilateral/Left/Right
Mammary gland	
Mammillary body	use Hypothalamus
Mandibular nerve	use Trigeminal Nerve
Mandibular notch	use Mandible, Left/Right
Manubrium	use Sternum
Masseter muscle	use Head Muscle
Masseteric fascia	use Subcutaneous Tissue and Fascia, Face
Mastoid (postauricular) lymph node	use Lymphatic, Neck, Left/Right
Mastoid air cells	use Mastoid Sinus, Left/Right
Mastoid process	use Temporal Bone, Left/Right
Maxillary artery	use External Carotid Artery, Left/Right
Maxillary nerve	use Trigeminal Nerve
Medial canthus	use Lower Eyelid, Left/Right
Medial collateral ligament (MCL)	use Knee Bursa and Ligament, Left/Right
Medial condyle of femur	use Lower Femur, Left/Right
Medial condyle of tibia	use Tibia, Left/Right
Medial cuneiform bone	use Tarsal, Left/Right
Medial epicondyle of femur	use Lower Femur, Left/Right
Medial epicondyle of humerus	use Humeral Shaft, Left/Right
Medial malleolus	use Tibia, Left/Right
Medial meniscus	use Knee Joint, Left/Right
Medial plantar artery	use Foot Artery, Left/Right
Medial plantar nerve	use Tibial Nerve
Medial popliteal nerve	
Medial rectus muscle	use Extraocular Muscle, Left/Right
Medial sural cutaneous nerve	use Tibial Nerve
Median antebrachial vein	use Basilic Vein, Left/Right
Median cubital vein	
Median sacral artery	use Abdominal Aorta
Mediastinal lymph node	use Lymphatic, Thorax
Meissner's (submucous) plexus	use Abdominal Sympathetic Nerve
Membranous urethra	use Urethra
Mental foramen	use Mandible, Left/Right
Mentalis muscle	use Facial Muscle
Mesoappendix	use Mesentery
Mesocolon	
Metacarpal ligament	use Hand Bursa and Ligament, Left/Right
Metacarpophalangeal ligament	
Metatarsal ligament	use Foot Bursa and Ligament, Left/Right

BODY PART	USE:
Metatarsophalangeal (MTP) joint	use Metatarsal-Phalangeal Joint, Left/Right
Metatarsophalangeal ligament	use Foot Bursa and Ligament, Left/Right
Metathalamus	use Thalamus
Midcarpal joint	use Carpal Joint, Left/Right
Middle cardiac nerve	use Thoracic Sympathetic Nerve
Middle cerebral artery	use Intracranial Artery
Middle cerebral vein	use Intracranial Vein
Middle colic vein	use Colic Vein
Middle genicular artery	use Popliteal Artery, Left/Right
Middle hemorrhoidal vein	use Hypogastric Vein, Left/Right
Middle rectal artery	use Internal Iliac Artery, Left/Right
Middle suprarenal artery	use Abdominal Aorta
Middle temporal artery	use Temporal Artery, Left/Right
Middle turbinate	use Nasal Turbinate
Mitral annulus	use Mitral Valve
Molar gland	use Buccal Mucosa
Musculocutaneous nerve	use Brachial Plexus
Musculophrenic artery	use Internal Mammary Artery, Left/Right
Musculospiral nerve	use Radial Nerve
Myelencephalon	use Medulla Oblongata
Myenteric (Auerbach's) plexus	use Abdominal Sympathetic Nerve
Myometrium	use Uterus
Nail bed, Nail plate	use Finger Nail, Toe Nail
Nasal cavity	use Nose
Nasal concha	use Nasal Turbinate
Nasalis muscle	use Facial Muscle
Nasolacrimal duct	use Lacrimal Duct, Left/Right
Navicular bone	use Tarsal, Left/Right
Neck of femur	use Upper Femur, Left/Right
Neck of humerus (anatomical) (surgical)	use Humeral Head, Left/Right
Nerve to the stapedius	use Facial Nerve
Neurohypophysis	use Pituitary Gland
Ninth cranial nerve	use Glossopharyngeal Nerve
Nostril	use Nose
Obturator artery	use Internal Iliac Artery, Left/Right
Obturator lymph node	use Lymphatic, Pelvis
Obturator muscle	use Hip Muscle, Left/Right
Obturator nerve	use Lumbar Plexus
Obturator vein	use Hypogastric Vein, Left/Right
Obtuse margin	use Heart, Left
Occipital artery	use External Carotid Artery, Left/Right
Occipital lobe	use Cerebral Hemisphere
Occipital lymph node	use Lymphatic, Neck, Left/Right
Occipitofrontalis muscle	use Facial Muscle
Olecranon bursa	use Elbow Bursa and Ligament, Left/Right
Olecranon process	use Ulna, Left/Right
Olfactory bulb	use Olfactory Nerve
Ophthalmic artery	use Internal Carotid Artery, Left/Right
Ophthalmic nerve	use Trigeminal Nerve

BODY PART	USE:
Ophthalmic vein	use Intracranial Vein
Optic chiasma	use Optic Nerve
Optic disc	use Retina, Left/Right
Optic foramen	use Sphenoid Bone, Left/Right
Orbicularis oculi muscle	use Upper Eyelid, Left/Right
Orbicularis oris muscle	use Facial Muscle
Orbital fascia	use Subcutaneous Tissue and Fascia, Face
Orbital portion of: ethmoid bone, frontal bone, lacrimal bone, maxilla, palatine bone, sphenoid bone, zygomatic bone	use Orbit, Left/Right
Oropharynx	use Pharynx
Ossicular chain	use Auditory Ossicle, Left/Right
Otic ganglion	use Head and Neck Sympathetic Nerve
Oval window	use Middle Ear, Left/Right
Ovarian artery	use Abdominal Aorta
Ovarian ligament	use Uterine Supporting Structure
Oviduct	use Fallopian Tube, Left/Right
Palatine gland	use Buccal Mucosa
Palatine tonsil	use Tonsils
Palatine uvula	use Uvula
Palatoglossal muscle	use Tongue, Palate, Pharynx Muscle
Palatopharyngeal muscle	
Palmar (volar) digital vein	use Hand Vein, Left/Right
Palmar (volar) metacarpal vein	
Palmar cutaneous nerve	use Median Nerve, Radial Nerve
Palmar fascia (aponeurosis)	use Subcutaneous Tissue and Fascia, Hand, Left/Right
Palmar interosseous muscle	use Hand Muscle, Left/Right
Palmar ulnocarpal ligament	use Wrist Bursa and Ligament, Left/Right
Palmaris longus muscle	use Lower Arm and Wrist Muscle, Left/Right
Pancreatic artery	use Splenic Artery
Pancreatic plexus	use Abdominal Sympathetic Nerve
Pancreatic vein	use Splenic Vein
Pancreaticosplenic lymph node	use Lymphatic, Aortic
Paraaortic lymph node	
Pararectal lymph node	use Lymphatic, Mesenteric
Parasternal lymph node	use Lymphatic, Thorax
Paratracheal lymph node	
Paraurethral (Skene's) gland	use Vestibular Gland
Parietal lobe	use Cerebral Hemisphere
Parotid lymph node	use Lymphatic, Head
Parotid plexus	use Facial Nerve
Pars flaccida	use Tympanic Membrane, Left/Right
Patellar ligament	use Knee Bursa and Ligament, Left/Right
Patellar tendon	use Knee Tendon, Left/Right
Patellofemoral joint	use Knee Joint, Left/Right
	use Knee Joint, Femoral Surface, Left/Right

BODY PART	USE:
Pectineus muscle	use Upper Leg Muscle, Left/Right
Pectoral (anterior) lymph node	use Lymphatic, Axillary, Left/Right
Pectoral fascia	use Subcutaneous Tissue and Fascia, Chest
Pectoralis major muscle	use Thorax Muscle, Left/Right
Pectoralis minor muscle	
Pelvic splanchnic nerve	use Abdominal Sympathetic Nerve Sacral Sympathetic Nerve
Penile urethra	use Urethra
Pericardiophrenic artery	use Internal Mammary Artery, Left/Right
Perimetrium	use Uterus
Peroneus brevis muscle	use Lower Leg Muscle, Left/Right
Peroneus longus muscle	
Petrous part of temporal bone	use Temporal Bone, Left/Right
Pharyngeal constrictor muscle	use Tongue, Palate, Pharynx Muscle
Pharyngeal plexus	use Vagus Nerve
Pharyngeal recess	use Nasopharynx
Pharyngeal tonsil	use Adenoids
Pharyngotympanic tube	use Eustachian Tube, Left/Right
Pia mater, intracranial	use Cerebral Meninges
Pia mater, spinal	use Spinal Meninges
Pinna	use External Ear, Bilateral/Left/Right
Piriform recess (sinus)	use Pharynx
Piriformis muscle	use Hip Muscle, Left/Right
Pisiform bone	use Carpal, Left/Right
Pisohamate ligament	use Hand Bursa and Ligament, Left/Right
Pisometacarpal ligament	
Plantar digital vein	use Foot Vein, Left/Right
Plantar fascia (aponeurosis)	use Subcutaneous Tissue and Fascia, Foot, Left/Right
Plantar metatarsal vein	use Foot Vein, Left/Right
Plantar venous arch	
Platysma muscle	use Neck Muscle, Left/Right
Plica semilunaris	use Conjunctiva, Left/Right
Pneumogastric nerve	use Vagus Nerve
Pneumotaxic center	use Pons
Pontine tegmentum	
Popliteal ligament	use Knee Bursa and Ligament, Left/Right
Popliteal lymph node	use Lymphatic, Lower Extremity, Left/Right
Popliteal vein	use Femoral Vein, Left/Right
Popliteus muscle	use Lower Leg Muscle, Left/Right
Postauricular (mastoid) lymph node	use Lymphatic, Neck, Left/Right
Postcava	use Inferior Vena Cava
Posterior (subscapular) lymph node	use Lymphatic, Axillary, Left/Right
Posterior auricular artery	use External Carotid Artery, Left/Right
Posterior auricular nerve	use Facial Nerve
Posterior auricular vein	use External Jugular Vein, Left/Right
Posterior cerebral artery	use Intracranial Artery
Posterior chamber	use Eye, Left/Right

APPENDIX C – BODY PART KEY

BODY PART	USE:
Posterior circumflex humeral artery	use Axillary Artery, Left/Right
Posterior communicating artery	use Intracranial Artery
Posterior cruciate ligament (PCL)	use Knee Bursa and Ligament, Left/Right
Posterior facial (retromandibular) vein	use Face Vein, Left/Right
Posterior femoral cutaneous nerve	use Sacral Plexus
Posterior inferior cerebellar artery (PICA)	use Intracranial Artery
Posterior interosseous nerve	use Radial Nerve
Posterior labial nerve	use Pudendal Nerve
Posterior scrotal nerve	
Posterior spinal artery	use Vertebral Artery, Left/Right
Posterior tibial recurrent artery	use Anterior Tibial Artery, Left/Right
Posterior ulnar recurrent artery	use Ulnar Artery, Left/Right
Posterior vagal trunk	use Vagus Nerve
Preauricular lymph node	use Lymphatic, Head
Precava	use Superior Vena Cava
Prepatellar bursa	use Knee Bursa and Ligament, Left/Right
Pretracheal fascia	use Subcutaneous Tissue and Fascia, Anterior Neck
Prevertebral fascia	use Subcutaneous Tissue and Fascia, Posterior Neck
Princeps pollicis artery	use Hand Artery, Left/Right
Procerus muscle	use Facial Muscle
Profunda brachii	use Brachial Artery, Left/Right
Profunda femoris (deep femoral) vein	use Femoral Vein, Left/Right
Pronator quadratus muscle	use Lower Arm and Wrist Muscle, Left/Right
Pronator teres muscle	
Prostatic urethra	use Urethra
Proximal radioulnar joint	use Elbow Joint, Left/Right
Psoas muscle	use Hip Muscle, Left/Right
Pterygoid muscle	use Head Muscle
Pterygoid process	use Sphenoid Bone, Left/Right
Pterygopalatine (sphenopalatine) ganglion	use Head and Neck Sympathetic Nerve
Pubic ligament	use Trunk Bursa and Ligament, Left/Right
Pubis	use Pelvic Bone, Left/Right
Pubofemoral ligament	use Hip Bursa and Ligament, Left/Right
Pudendal nerve	use Sacral Plexus
Pulmoaortic canal	use Pulmonary Artery, Left
Pulmonary annulus	use Pulmonary Valve
Pulmonary plexus	use Vagus Nerve/Thoracic Sympathetic Nerve
Pulmonic valve	use Pulmonary Valve
Pulvinar	use Thalamus

BODY PART	USE:
Pyloric antrum	use Stomach, Pylorus
Pyloric canal	
Pyloric sphincter	
Pyramidalis muscle	use Abdomen Muscle, Left/Right
Quadrangular cartilage	use Nasal Septum
Quadrate lobe	use Liver
Quadratus femoris muscle	use Hip Muscle, Left/Right
Quadratus lumborum muscle	use Trunk Muscle, Left/Right
Quadratus plantae muscle	use Foot Muscle, Left/Right
Quadriceps (femoris)	use Upper Leg Muscle, Left/Right
Radial collateral carpal ligament	use Wrist Bursa and Ligament, Left/Right
Radial collateral ligament	use Elbow Bursa and Ligament, Left/Right
Radial notch	use Ulna, Left/Right
Radial recurrent artery	use Radial Artery, Left/Right
Radial vein	use Brachial Vein, Left/Right
Radialis indicis	use Hand Artery, Left/Right
Radiocarpal joint	use Wrist Joint, Left/Right
Radiocarpal ligament	use Wrist Bursa and Ligament, Left/Right
Radioulnar ligament	
Rectosigmoid junction	use Sigmoid Colon
Rectus abdominis muscle	use Abdomen Muscle, Left/Right
Rectus femoris muscle	use Upper Leg Muscle, Left/Right
Recurrent laryngeal nerve	use Vagus Nerve
Renal calyx	use Kidney, Bilateral/Left/Right
Renal capsule	
Renal cortex	
Renal plexus	use Abdominal Sympathetic Nerve
Renal segment	use Kidney, Bilateral/Left/Right
Renal segmental artery	use Renal Artery, Left/Right
Retroperitoneal lymph node	use Lymphatic, Aortic
Retroperitoneal space	use Retroperitoneum
Retropharyngeal lymph node	use Lymphatic, Neck, Left/Right
Retropubic space	use Pelvic Cavity
Rhinopharynx	use Nasopharynx
Rhomboid major muscle	use Trunk Muscle, Left/Right
Rhomboid minor muscle	
Right ascending lumbar vein	use Azygos Vein
Right atrioventricular valve	use Tricuspid Valve
Right auricular appendix	use Atrium, Right
Right colic vein	use Colic Vein
Right coronary sulcus	use Heart, Right
Right gastric artery	use Gastric Artery
Right gastroepiploic vein	use Superior Mesenteric Vein
Right inferior phrenic vein	use Inferior Vena Cava
Right inferior pulmonary vein	use Pulmonary Vein, Right
Right jugular trunk	use Lymphatic, Right Neck

BODY PART	USE:	BODY PART	USE:
Right lateral ventricle	use Cerebral Ventricle	Soleus muscle	use Lower Leg Muscle, Left/Right
Right lymphatic duct	use Lymphatic, Right Neck	Sphenomandibular ligament	use Head and Neck Bursa and Ligament
Right ovarian vein	use Inferior Vena Cava	Sphenopalatine (pterygopalatine) ganglion	use Head and Neck Sympathetic Nerve
Right second lumbar vein			
Right subclavian trunk	use Lymphatic, Right Neck	Spinal nerve, cervical	use Cervical Nerve
Right subcostal vein	use Azygos Vein	Spinal nerve, lumbar	use Lumbar Nerve
Right superior pulmonary vein	use Pulmonary Vein, Right	Spinal nerve, sacral	use Sacral Nerve
		Spinal nerve, thoracic	use Thoracic Nerve
Right suprarenal vein	use Inferior Vena Cava	Spinous process	use Cervical, Thoracic, Lumbar Vertebra
Right testicular vein		Spiral ganglion	use Acoustic Nerve
Rima glottidis	use Larynx	Splenic flexure	use Transverse Colon
Risorius muscle	use Facial Muscle	Splenic plexus	use Abdominal Sympathetic Nerve
Round ligament of uterus	use Uterine Supporting Structure	Splenius capitis muscle	use Head Muscle
Round window	use Inner Ear, Left/Right	Splenius cervicis muscle	use Neck Muscle, Left/Right
Sacral ganglion	use Sacral Sympathetic Nerve	Stapes	use Auditory Ossicle, Left/Right
Sacral lymph node	use Lymphatic, Pelvis	Stellate ganglion	use Head and Neck Sympathetic Nerve
Sacral splanchnic nerve	use Sacral Sympathetic Nerve	Stensen's duct	use Parotid Duct, Left/Right
Sacrococcygeal ligament	use Trunk Bursa and Ligament, Left/Right	Sternoclavicular ligament	use Shoulder Bursa and Ligament, Left/Right
Sacrococcygeal symphysis	use Sacrococcygeal Joint	Sternocleidomastoid artery	use Thyroid Artery, Left/Right
Sacroiliac ligament	use Trunk Bursa and Ligament, Left/Right		
Sacrospinous ligament		Sternocleidomastoid muscle	use Neck Muscle, Left/Right
Sacrotuberous ligament			
Salpingopharyngeus muscle	use Tongue, Palate, Pharynx Muscle	Sternocostal ligament	use Thorax Bursa and Ligament, Left/Right
		Styloglossus muscle	use Tongue, Palate, Pharynx Muscle
Salpinx	use Fallopian Tube, Left/Right	Stylomandibular ligament	use Head and Neck Bursa and Ligament
Saphenous nerve	use Femoral Nerve	Stylopharyngeus muscle	use Tongue, Palate, Pharynx Muscle
Sartorius muscle	use Upper Leg Muscle, Left/Right	Subacromial bursa	use Shoulder Bursa and Ligament, Left/Right
Scalene muscle	use Neck Muscle, Left/Right		
Scaphoid bone	use Carpal, Left/Right	Subaortic (common iliac) lymph node	use Lymphatic, Pelvis
Scapholunate ligament	use Hand Bursa and Ligament, Left/Right		
Scaphotrapezium ligament		Subarachnoid space, intracranial	use Subarachnoid Space
Scarpa's (vestibular) ganglion	use Acoustic Nerve	Subarachnoid space, spinal	use Spinal Canal
Sebaceous gland	use Skin	Subclavicular (apical) lymph node	use Lymphatic, Axillary, Left/Right
Second cranial nerve	use Optic Nerve		
Sella turcica	use Sphenoid Bone, Left/Right	Subclavius muscle	use Thorax Muscle, Left/Right
Semicircular canal	use Inner Ear, Left/Right	Subclavius nerve	use Brachial Plexus
Semimembranosus muscle	use Upper Leg Muscle, Left/Right	Subcostal artery	use Thoracic Aorta
Semitendinosus muscle		Subcostal muscle	use Thorax Muscle, Left/Right
Septal cartilage	use Nasal Septum	Subcostal nerve	use Thoracic Nerve
Serratus anterior muscle	use Thorax Muscle, Left/Right	Subdural space, intracranial	use Subdural Space
Serratus posterior muscle	use Trunk Muscle, Left/Right		
Seventh cranial nerve	use Facial Nerve	Subdural space, spinal	use Spinal Canal
Short gastric artery	use Splenic Artery	Submandibular ganglion	use Facial Nerve Head and Neck Sympathetic Nerve
Sigmoid artery	use Inferior Mesenteric Artery		
Sigmoid flexure	use Sigmoid Colon	Submandibular gland	use Submaxillary Gland, Left/Right
Sigmoid vein	use Inferior Mesenteric Vein	Submandibular lymph node	use Lymphatic, Head
Sinoatrial node	use Conduction Mechanism		
Sinus venosus	use Atrium, Right	Submaxillary ganglion	use Head and Neck Sympathetic Nerve
Sixth cranial nerve	use Abducens Nerve	Submaxillary lymph node	use Lymphatic, Head
Skene's (paraurethral) gland	use Vestibular Gland	Submental artery	use Face Artery
		Submental lymph node	use Lymphatic, Head
Small saphenous vein	use Lesser Saphenous Vein, Left/Right	Submucous (Meissner's) plexus	use Abdominal Sympathetic Nerve
Solar (celiac) plexus	use Abdominal Sympathetic Nerve		
		Suboccipital nerve	use Cervical Nerve

APPENDIX C – BODY PART KEY

BODY PART	USE:
Suboccipital venous plexus	use Vertebral Vein, Left/Right
Subparotid lymph node	use Lymphatic, Head
Subscapular (posterior) lymph node	use Lymphatic, Axillary, Left/Right
Subscapular aponeurosis	use Subcutaneous Tissue and Fascia, Upper Arm, Left/Right
Subscapular artery	use Axillary Artery, Left/Right
Subscapularis muscle	use Shoulder Muscle, Left/Right
Substantia nigra	use Basal Ganglia
Subtalar (talocalcaneal) joint	use Tarsal Joint, Left/Right
Subtalar ligament	use Foot Bursa and Ligament, Left/Right
Subthalamic nucleus	use Basal Ganglia
Superficial circumflex iliac vein	use Greater Saphenous Vein, Left/Right
Superficial epigastric artery	use Femoral Artery, Left/Right
Superficial epigastric vein	use Greater Saphenous Vein, Left/Right
Superficial palmar arch	use Hand Artery, Left/Right
Superficial palmar venous arch	use Hand Vein, Left/Right
Superficial temporal artery	use Temporal Artery, Left/Right
Superficial transverse perineal muscle	use Perineum Muscle
Superior cardiac nerve	use Thoracic Sympathetic Nerve
Superior cerebellar vein	use Intracranial Vein
Superior cerebral vein	
Superior clunic (cluneal) nerve	use Lumbar Nerve
Superior epigastric artery	use Internal Mammary Artery, Left/Right
Superior genicular artery	use Popliteal Artery, Left/Right
Superior gluteal artery	use Internal Iliac Artery, Left/Right
Superior gluteal nerve	use Lumbar Plexus
Superior hypogastric plexus	use Abdominal Sympathetic Nerve
Superior labial artery	use Face Artery
Superior laryngeal artery	use Thyroid Artery, Left/Right
Superior laryngeal nerve	use Vagus Nerve
Superior longitudinal muscle	use Tongue, Palate, Pharynx Muscle
Superior mesenteric ganglion	use Abdominal Sympathetic Nerve
Superior mesenteric lymph node	use Lymphatic, Mesenteric
Superior mesenteric plexus	use Abdominal Sympathetic Nerve
Superior oblique muscle	use Extraocular Muscle, Left/Right
Superior olivary nucleus	use Pons
Superior rectal artery	use Inferior Mesenteric Artery
Superior rectal vein	use Inferior Mesenteric Vein
Superior rectus muscle	use Extraocular Muscle, Left/Right
Superior tarsal plate	use Upper Eyelid, Left/Right
Superior thoracic artery	use Axillary Artery, Left/Right

BODY PART	USE:
Superior thyroid artery	use External Carotid Artery, Left/Right Thyroid Artery, Left/Right
Superior turbinate	use Nasal Turbinate
Superior ulnar collateral artery	use Brachial Artery, Left/Right
Supraclavicular (Virchow's) lymph node	use Lymphatic, Neck, Left/Right
Supraclavicular nerve	use Cervical Plexus
Suprahyoid lymph node	use Lymphatic, Head
Suprahyoid muscle	use Neck Muscle, Left/Right
Suprainguinal lymph node	use Lymphatic, Pelvis
Supraorbital vein	use Face Vein, Left/Right
Suprarenal gland	use Adrenal Gland, Bilateral/Left/Right
Suprarenal plexus	use Abdominal Sympathetic Nerve
Suprascapular nerve	use Brachial Plexus
Supraspinatus fascia	use Subcutaneous Tissue and Fascia, Upper Arm, Left/Right
Supraspinatus muscle	use Shoulder Muscle, Left/Right
Supraspinous ligament	use Trunk Bursa and Ligament, Left/Right
Suprasternal notch	use Sternum
Supratrochlear lymph node	use Lymphatic, Upper Extremity, Left/Right
Sural artery	use Popliteal Artery, Left/Right
Sweat gland	use Skin
Talocalcaneal (subtalar) joint	use Tarsal Joint, Left/Right
Talocalcaneal ligament	use Foot Bursa and Ligament, Left/Right
Talocalcaneonavicular joint	use Tarsal Joint, Left/Right
Talocalcaneonavicular ligament	use Foot Bursa and Ligament, Left/Right
Talocrural joint	use Ankle Joint, Left/Right
Talofibular ligament	use Ankle Bursa and Ligament, Left/Right
Talus bone	use Tarsal, Left/Right
Tarsometatarsal joint	use Metatarsal-Tarsal Joint, Left/Right
Tarsometatarsal ligament	use Foot Bursa and Ligament, Left/Right
Temporal lobe	use Cerebral Hemisphere
Temporalis muscle	use Head Muscle
Temporoparietalis muscle	
Tensor fasciae latae muscle	use Hip Muscle, Left/Right
Tensor veli palatini muscle	use Tongue, Palate, Pharynx Muscle
Tenth cranial nerve	use Vagus Nerve
Tentorium cerebelli	use Dura Mater
Teres major muscle	use Shoulder Muscle, Left/Right
Teres minor muscle	
Testicular artery	use Abdominal Aorta
Thenar muscle	use Hand Muscle, Left/Right
Third cranial nerve	use Oculomotor Nerve
Third occipital nerve	use Cervical Nerve
Third ventricle	use Cerebral Ventricle
Thoracic aortic plexus	use Thoracic Sympathetic Nerve

BODY PART	USE:
Thoracic esophagus	use Esophagus, Middle
Thoracic facet joint	use Thoracic Vertebral Joint
Thoracic ganglion	use Thoracic Sympathetic Nerve
Thoracoacromial artery	use Axillary Artery, Left/Right
Thoracolumbar facet joint	use Thoracolumbar Vertebral Joint
Thymus gland	use Thymus
Thyroarytenoid muscle	use Neck Muscle, Left/Right
Thyrocervical trunk	use Thyroid Artery, Left/Right
Thyroid cartilage	use Larynx
Tibialis anterior muscle	use Lower Leg Muscle, Left/Right
Tibialis posterior muscle	
Tibiofemoral joint	use Knee Joint, Left/Right
	use Knee Joint, Tibial Surface, Left/Right
Tracheobronchial lymph node	use Lymphatic, Thorax
Tragus	use External Ear, Bilateral/Left/Right
Transversalis fascia	use Subcutaneous Tissue and Fascia, Trunk
Transverse (cutaneous) cervical nerve	use Cervical Plexus
Transverse acetabular ligament	use Hip Bursa and Ligament, Left/Right
Transverse facial artery	use Temporal Artery, Left/Right
Transverse humeral ligament	use Shoulder Bursa and Ligament, Left/Right
Transverse ligament of atlas	use Head and Neck Bursa and Ligament
Transverse scapular ligament	use Shoulder Bursa and Ligament, Left/Right
Transverse thoracis muscle	use Thorax Muscle, Left/Right
Transversospinalis muscle	use Trunk Muscle, Left/Right
Transversus abdominis muscle	use Abdomen Muscle, Left/Right
Trapezium bone	use Carpal, Left/Right
Trapezius muscle	use Trunk Muscle, Left/Right
Trapezoid bone	use Carpal, Left/Right
Triceps brachii muscle	use Upper Arm Muscle, Left/Right
Tricuspid annulus	use Tricuspid Valve
Trifacial nerve	use Trigeminal Nerve
Trigone of bladder	use Bladder
Triquetral bone	use Carpal, Left/Right
Trochanteric bursa	use Hip Bursa and Ligament, Left/Right
Twelfth cranial nerve	use Hypoglossal Nerve
Tympanic cavity	use Middle Ear, Left/Right
Tympanic nerve	use Glossopharyngeal Nerve
Tympanic part of temporal bone	use Temporal Bone, Left/Right
Ulnar collateral carpal ligament	use Wrist Bursa and Ligament, Left/Right
Ulnar collateral ligament	use Elbow Bursa and Ligament, Left/Right
Ulnar notch	use Radius, Left/Right
Ulnar vein	use Brachial Vein, Left/Right
Umbilical artery	use Internal Iliac Artery, Left/Right
Ureteral orifice	use Ureter, Bilateral/Left/Right

BODY PART	USE:
Ureteropelvic junction (UPJ)	use Kidney Pelvis, Left/Right
Ureterovesical orifice	use Ureter, Bilateral/Left/Right
Uterine artery	use Internal Iliac Artery, Left/Right
Uterine cornu	use Uterus
Uterine tube	use Fallopian Tube, Left/Right
Uterine vein	use Hypogastric Vein, Left/Right
Vaginal artery	use Internal Iliac Artery, Left/Right
Vaginal vein	use Hypogastric Vein, Left/Right
Vastus intermedius muscle	use Upper Leg Muscle, Left/Right
Vastus lateralis muscle	
Vastus medialis muscle	
Ventricular fold	use Larynx
Vermiform appendix	use Appendix
Vermilion border	use Upper Lip, Lower Lip
Vertebral arch	use Cervical, Thoracic, Lumbar Vertebra
Vertebral canal	use Spinal Canal
Vertebral foramen	use Cervical, Thoracic, Lumbar Vertebra
Vertebral lamina	
Vertebral pedicle	
Vesical vein	use Hypogastric Vein, Left/Right
Vestibular (Scarpa's) ganglion	use Acoustic Nerve
Vestibular nerve	
Vestibulocochlear nerve	
Virchow's (supraclavicular) lymph node	use Lymphatic, Neck, Left/Right
Vitreous body	use Vitreous, Left/Right
Vocal fold	use Vocal Cord, Left/Right
Volar (palmar) digital vein	use Hand Vein, Left/Right
Volar (palmar) metacarpal vein	
Vomer bone	use Nasal Septum
Vomer of nasal septum	use Nasal Bone
Xiphoid process	use Sternum
Zonule of Zinn	use Lens, Left/Right
Zygomatic process of frontal bone	use Frontal Bone, Left/Right
Zygomatic process of temporal bone	use Temporal Bone, Left/Right
Zygomaticus muscle	use Facial Muscle

APPENDIX D – DEVICE KEY

DEVICE	USE:
3f (Aortic) Bioprosthesis valve	*use* Zooplastic Tissue in Heart and Great Vessels
AbioCor® Total Replacement Heart	*use* Synthetic Substitute
Absolute Pro Vascular (OTW) Self-Expanding Stent System	*use* Intraluminal Device
Acculink (RX) Carotid Stent System	*use* Intraluminal Device
Acellular Hydrated Dermis	*use* Nonautologous Tissue Substitute
Acetabular cup	*use* Liner in Lower Joints
Activa PC neurostimulator	*use* Stimulator Generator, Multiple Array for Insertion in Subcutaneous Tissue and Fascia
Activa RC neurostimulator	*use* Stimulator Generator, Multiple Array Rechargeable for Insertion in Subcutaneous Tissue and Fascia
Activa SC neurostimulator	*use* Stimulator Generator, Single Array for Insertion in Subcutaneous Tissue and Fascia
ACUITY™ Steerable Lead	*use* Cardiac Lead, Pacemaker for Insertion in Heart and Great Vessels Cardiac Lead, Defibrillator for Insertion in Heart and Great Vessels
Advisa (MRI)	*use* Pacemaker, Dual Chamber for Insertion in Subcutaneous Tissue and Fascia
AMPLATZER® Muscular VSD Occluder	*use* Synthetic Substitute
AMS 800® Urinary Control System	*use* Artificial Sphincter in Urinary System
AneuRx® AAA Advantage®	*use* Intraluminal Device
Annuloplasty ring	*use* Synthetic Substitute
Artificial anal sphincter (AAS)	*use* Artificial Sphincter in Gastrointestinal System
Artificial bowel sphincter (neosphincter)	*use* Artificial Sphincter in Gastrointestinal System
Artificial urinary sphincter (AUS)	*use* Artificial Sphincter in Urinary System
Ascenda Intrathecal Catheter	*use* Infusion Device
Assurant (Cobalt) stent	*use* Intraluminal Device
Attain Ability® lead	*use* Cardiac Lead, Pacemaker for Insertion in Heart and Great Vessels Cardiac Lead, Defibrillator for Insertion in Heart and Great Vessels
Attain StarFix® (OTW) lead	*use* Cardiac Lead, Pacemaker for Insertion in Heart and Great Vessels Cardiac Lead, Defibrillator for Insertion in Heart and Great Vessels
Autograft	*use* Autologous Tissue Substitute
Autologous artery graft	*use* Autologous Arterial Tissue in Heart and Great Vessels Autologous Arterial Tissue in Upper Arteries Autologous Arterial Tissue in Lower Arteries Autologous Arterial Tissue in Upper Veins Autologous Arterial Tissue in Lower Veins
Autologous vein graft	*use* Autologous Venous Tissue in Heart and Great Vessels Autologous Venous Tissue in Upper Arteries Autologous Venous Tissue in Lower Arteries Autologous Venous Tissue in Upper Veins Autologous Venous Tissue in Lower Veins
Axial Lumbar Interbody Fusion System	*use* Interbody Fusion Device in Lower Joints
AxiaLIF® System	*use* Interbody Fusion Device in Lower Joints
BAK/C® Interbody Cervical Fusion System	*use* Interbody Fusion Device in Upper Joints
Bard® Composix® (E/X)(LP) mesh	*use* Synthetic Substitute
Bard® Composix® Kugel® patch	*use* Synthetic Substitute
Bard® Dulex™ mesh	*use* Synthetic Substitute
Bard® Ventralex™ hernia patch	*use* Synthetic Substitute
Baroreflex Activation Therapy® (BAT®)	*use* Stimulator Lead in Upper Arteries Stimulator Generator in Subcutaneous Tissue and Fascia
Berlin Heart Ventricular Assist Device	*use* Implantable Heart Assist System in Heart and Great Vessels
Bioactive embolization coil(s)	*use* Intraluminal Device, Bioactive in Upper Arteries
Biventricular external heart assist system	*use* External Heart Assist System in Heart and Great Vessels
Blood glucose monitoring system	*use* Monitoring Device
Bone anchored hearing device	*use* Hearing Device, Bone Conduction for Insertion in Ear, Nose, Sinus Hearing Device in Head and Facial Bones
Bone bank bone graft	*use* Nonautologous Tissue Substitute
Bone screw (interlocking) (lag) (pedicle) (recessed)	*use* Internal Fixation Device in Head and Facial Bones, Upper Bones, Lower Bones
Bovine pericardial valve	*use* Zooplastic Tissue in Heart and Great Vessels
Bovine pericardium graft	*use* Zooplastic Tissue in Heart and Great Vessels

DEVICE	USE:
Brachytherapy seeds	use Radioactive Element
BRYAN® Cervical Disc System	use Synthetic Substitute
BVS 5000 Ventricular Assist Device	use External Heart Assist System in Heart and Great Vessels
Cardiac contractility modulation lead	use Cardiac Lead in Heart and Great Vessels
Cardiac event recorder	use Monitoring Device
Cardiac resynchronization therapy (CRT) lead	use Cardiac Lead, Pacemaker for Insertion in Heart and Great Vessels Cardiac Lead, Defibrillator for Insertion in Heart and Great Vessels
CardioMEMS® pressure sensor	use Monitoring Device, Pressure Sensor for Insertion in Heart and Great Vessels
Carotid (artery) sinus (baroreceptor) lead	use Stimulator Lead in Upper Arteries
Carotid WALLSTENT® Monorail® Endoprosthesis	use Intraluminal Device
Centrimag® Blood Pump	use External Heart Assist System in Heart and Great Vessels
Clamp and rod internal fixation system (CRIF)	use Internal Fixation Device in Upper Bones, Lower Bones
CoAxia NeuroFlo catheter	use Intraluminal Device
Cobalt/chromium head and polyethylene socket	use Synthetic Substitute, Metal on Polyethylene for Replacement in Lower Joints
Cobalt/chromium head and socket	use Synthetic Substitute, Metal for Replacement in Lower Joints
Cochlear implant (CI), multiple channel (electrode)	use Hearing Device, Multiple Channel Cochlear Prosthesis for Insertion in Ear, Nose, Sinus
Cochlear implant (CI), single channel (electrode)	use Hearing Device, Single Channel Cochlear Prosthesis for Insertion in Ear, Nose, Sinus
COGNIS® CRT-D	use Cardiac Resynchronization Defibrillator Pulse Generator for Insertion in Subcutaneous Tissue and Fascia
Colonic Z-Stent®	use Intraluminal Device
Complete (SE) stent	use Intraluminal Device
Concerto II CRT-D	use Cardiac Resynchronization Defibrillator Pulse Generator for Insertion in Subcutaneous Tissue and Fascia
CONSERVE® PLUS Total Resurfacing Hip System	use Resurfacing Device in Lower Joints
Consulta CRT-D	use Cardiac Resynchronization Defibrillator Pulse Generator for Insertion in Subcutaneous Tissue and Fascia
Consulta CRT-P	use Cardiac Resynchronization Pacemaker Pulse Generator for Insertion in Subcutaneous Tissue and Fascia
CONTAK RENEWAL® 3 RF (HE) CRT-D	use Cardiac Resynchronization Defibrillator Pulse Generator for Insertion in Subcutaneous Tissue and Fascia
Contegra Pulmonary Valved Conduit	use Zooplastic Tissue in Heart and Great Vessels
Continuous Glucose Monitoring (CGM) device	use Monitoring Device
CoreValve transcatheter aortic valve	use Zooplastic Tissue in Heart and Great Vessels
Cormet Hip Resurfacing System	use Resurfacing Device in Lower Joints
CoRoent® XL	use Interbody Fusion Device in Lower Joints
Corox OTW (Bipolar) Lead	use Cardiac Lead, Pacemaker for Insertion in Heart and Great Vessels Cardiac Lead, Defibrillator for Insertion in Heart and Great Vessels
Cortical strip neurostimulator lead	use Neurostimulator Lead in Central Nervous System
Cultured epidermal cell autograft	use Autologous Tissue Substitute
CYPHER® Stent	use Intraluminal Device, Drug-eluting in Heart and Great Vessels
Cystostomy tube	use Drainage Device
DBS lead	use Neurostimulator Lead in Central Nervous System
DeBakey Left Ventricular Assist Device	use Implantable Heart Assist System in Heart and Great Vessels
Deep brain neurostimulator lead	use Neurostimulator Lead in Central Nervous System
Delta frame external fixator	use External Fixation Device, Hybrid for Insertion in Upper Bones, Lower Bones External Fixation Device, Hybrid for Reposition in Upper Bones, Lower Bones
Delta III Reverse shoulder prosthesis	use Synthetic Substitute, Reverse Ball and Socket for Replacement in Upper Joints
Diaphragmatic pacemaker generator	use Stimulator Generator in Subcutaneous Tissue and Fascia
Direct Lateral Interbody Fusion (DLIF) device	use Interbody Fusion Device in Lower Joints
Driver stent (RX) (OTW)	use Intraluminal Device
DuraHeart Left Ventricular Assist System	use Implantable Heart Assist System in Heart and Great Vessels
Durata® Defibrillation Lead	use Cardiac Lead, Defibrillator for Insertion in Heart and Great Vessels
Dynesys® Dynamic Stabilization System	use Spinal Stabilization Device, Pedicle-Based for Insertion in Upper Joints, Lower Joints
E-Luminexx™ (Biliary) (Vascular) Stent	use Intraluminal Device
Electrical bone growth stimulator (EBGS)	use Bone Growth Stimulator in Head and Facial Bones, Upper Bones, Lower Bones
Electrical muscle stimulation (EMS) lead	use Stimulator Lead in Muscles
Electronic muscle stimulator lead	use Stimulator Lead in Muscles

APPENDIX D – DEVICE KEY

DEVICE	USE:
Embolization coil(s)	use Intraluminal Device
Endeavor® (III) (IV) (Sprint) Zotarolimus-eluting Coronary Stent System	use Intraluminal Device, Drug-eluting in Heart and Great Vessels
EndoSure® sensor	use Monitoring Device, Pressure Sensor for Insertion in Heart and Great Vessels
ENDOTAK RELIANCE® (G) Defibrillation Lead	use Cardiac Lead, Defibrillator for Insertion in Heart and Great Vessels
Endotracheal tube (cuffed) (double-lumen)	use Intraluminal Device, Endotracheal Airway in Respiratory System
Endurant® Endovascular Stent Graft	use Intraluminal Device
EnRhythm	use Pacemaker, Dual Chamber for Insertion in Subcutaneous Tissue and Fascia
Enterra gastric neurostimulator	use Stimulator Generator, Multiple Array for Insertion in Subcutaneous Tissue and Fascia
Epic™ Stented Tissue Valve (aortic)	use Zooplastic Tissue in Heart and Great Vessels
Epicel® cultured epidermal autograft	use Autologous Tissue Substitute
Esophageal obturator airway (EOA)	use Intraluminal Device, Airway in Gastrointestinal System
Esteem® implantable hearing system	use Hearing Device in Ear, Nose, Sinus
Evera (XT) (S) (DR/VR)	use Defibrillator Generator for Insertion in Subcutaneous Tissue and Fascia
Everolimus-eluting coronary stent	use Intraluminal Device, Drug-eluting in Heart and Great Vessels
Ex-PRESS™ mini glaucoma shunt	use Synthetic Substitute
Express® (LD) Premounted Stent System	use Intraluminal Device
Express® Biliary SD Monorail® Premounted Stent System	use Intraluminal Device
Express® SD Renal Monorail® Premounted Stent System	use Intraluminal Device
External fixator	use External Fixation Device in Head and Facial Bones, Upper Bones, Lower Bones, Upper Joints, Lower Joints
EXtreme Lateral Interbody Fusion (XLIF) device	use Interbody Fusion Device in Lower Joints
Facet replacement spinal stabilization device	use Spinal Stabilization Device, Facet Replacement for Insertion in Upper Joints, Lower Joints
FLAIR® Endovascular Stent Graft	use Intraluminal Device
Flexible Composite Mesh	use Synthetic Substitute
Foley catheter	use Drainage Device
Formula™ Balloon-Expandable Renal Stent System	use Intraluminal Device
Freestyle (Stentless) Aortic Root Bioprosthesis	use Zooplastic Tissue in Heart and Great Vessels
Fusion screw (compression) (lag) (locking)	use Internal Fixation Device in Upper Joints, Lower Joints
Gastric electrical stimulation (GES) lead	use Stimulator Lead in Gastrointestinal System
Gastric pacemaker lead	use Stimulator Lead in Gastrointestinal System
GORE® DUALMESH®	use Synthetic Substitute
Guedel airway	use Intraluminal Device, Airway in Mouth and Throat
Hancock Bioprosthesis (aortic) (mitral) valve	use Zooplastic Tissue in Heart and Great Vessels
Hancock Bioprosthetic Valved Conduit	use Zooplastic Tissue in Heart and Great Vessels
HeartMate II® Left Ventricular Assist Device (LVAD)	use Implantable Heart Assist System in Heart and Great Vessels
HeartMate XVE® Left Ventricular Assist Device (LVAD)	use Implantable Heart Assist System in Heart and Great Vessels
Herculink (RX) Elite Renal Stent System	use Intraluminal Device
Hip (joint) liner	use Liner in Lower Joints
Holter valve ventricular shunt	use Synthetic Substitute
Ilizarov external fixator	use External Fixation Device, Ring for Insertion in Upper Bones, Lower Bones External Fixation Device, Ring for Reposition in Upper Bones, Lower Bones
Ilizarov-Vecklich device	use External Fixation Device, Limb Lengthening for Insertion in Upper Bones, Lower Bones
Implantable cardioverter-defibrillator (ICD)	use Defibrillator Generator for Insertion in Subcutaneous Tissue and Fascia
Implantable drug infusion pump (anti-spasmodic) (chemotherapy) (pain)	use Infusion Device, Pump in Subcutaneous Tissue and Fascia
Implantable glucose monitoring device	use Monitoring Device
Implantable hemodynamic monitor (IHM)	use Monitoring Device, Hemodynamic for Insertion in Subcutaneous Tissue and Fascia
Implantable hemodynamic monitoring system (IHMS)	use Monitoring Device, Hemodynamic for Insertion in Subcutaneous Tissue and Fascia
Implantable Miniature Telescope™ (IMT)	use Synthetic Substitute, Intraocular Telescope for Replacement in Eye
Implanted (venous) (access) port	use Vascular Access Device, Reservoir in Subcutaneous Tissue and Fascia
InDura, intrathecal catheter (1P) (spinal)	use Infusion Device
Injection reservoir, port	use Vascular Access Device, Reservoir in Subcutaneous Tissue and Fascia
Injection reservoir, pump	use Infusion Device, Pump in Subcutaneous Tissue and Fascia
Interbody fusion (spine) cage	use Interbody Fusion Device in Upper Joints, Lower Joints

Appendix D – 2016 ICD-10-PCS

DEVICE	USE:
Interspinous process spinal stabilization device	use Spinal Stabilization Device, Interspinous Process for Insertion in Upper Joints, Lower Joints
InterStim® Therapy lead	use Neurostimulator Lead in Peripheral Nervous System
InterStim® Therapy neurostimulator	use Stimulator Generator, Single Array for Insertion in Subcutaneous Tissue and Fascia
Intramedullary (IM) rod (nail)	use Internal Fixation Device, Intramedullary in Upper Bones, Lower Bones
Intramedullary skeletal kinetic distractor (ISKD)	use Internal Fixation Device, Intramedullary in Upper Bones, Lower Bones
Intrauterine device (IUD)	use Contraceptive Device in Female Reproductive System
Itrel (3) (4) neurostimulator	use Stimulator Generator, Single Array for Insertion in Subcutaneous Tissue and Fascia
Joint fixation plate	use Internal Fixation Device in Upper Joints, Lower Joints
Joint liner (insert)	use Liner in Lower Joints
Joint spacer (antibiotic)	use Spacer in Upper Joints, Lower Joints
Kappa	use Pacemaker, Dual Chamber for Insertion in Subcutaneous Tissue and Fascia
Kirschner wire (K-wire)	use Internal Fixation Device in Head and Facial Bones, Upper Bones, Lower Bones, Upper Joints, Lower Joints
Knee (implant) insert	use Liner in Lower Joints
Kuntscher nail	use Internal Fixation Device, Intramedullary in Upper Bones, Lower Bones
LAP-BAND® adjustable gastric banding system	use Extraluminal Device
LifeStent® (Flexstar) (XL) Vascular Stent System	use Intraluminal Device
LIVIAN™ CRT-D	use Cardiac Resynchronization Defibrillator Pulse Generator for Insertion in Subcutaneous Tissue and Fascia
Loop recorder, implantable	use Monitoring Device
Mark IV Breathing Pacemaker System	use Stimulator Generator in Subcutaneous Tissue and Fascia
Maximo II DR (VR)	use Defibrillator Generator for Insertion in Subcutaneous Tissue and Fascia
Maximo II DR CRT-D	use Cardiac Resynchronization Defibrillator Pulse Generator for Insertion in Subcutaneous Tissue and Fascia
Melody® transcatheter pulmonary valve	use Zooplastic Tissue in Heart and Great Vessels
Micro-Driver stent (RX) (OTW)	use Intraluminal Device
MicroMed HeartAssist	use Implantable Heart Assist System in Heart and Great Vessels
Micrus CERECYTE microcoil	use Intraluminal Device, Bioactive in Upper Arteries
MitraClip valve repair system	use Synthetic Substitute
Mitroflow® Aortic Pericardial Heart Valve	use Zooplastic Tissue in Heart and Great Vessels
Mosaic Bioprosthesis (aortic) (mitral) valve	use Zooplastic Tissue in Heart and Great Vessels
MULTI-LINK (VISION) (MINI-VISION) (ULTRA) Coronary Stent System	use Intraluminal Device
Nasopharyngeal airway (NPA)	use Intraluminal Device, Airway in Ear, Nose, Sinus
Neuromuscular electrical stimulation (NEMS) lead	use Stimulator Lead in Muscles
Neurostimulator generator, multiple channel	use Stimulator Generator, Multiple Array for Insertion in Subcutaneous Tissue and Fascia
Neurostimulator generator, multiple channel rechargeable	use Stimulator Generator, Multiple Array Rechargeable for Insertion in Subcutaneous Tissue and Fascia
Neurostimulator generator, single channel	use Stimulator Generator, Single Array for Insertion in Subcutaneous Tissue and Fascia
Neurostimulator generator, single channel rechargeable	use Stimulator Generator, Single Array Rechargeable for Insertion in Subcutaneous Tissue and Fascia
Neutralization plate	use Internal Fixation Device in Head and Facial Bones, Upper Bones, Lower Bones
Nitinol framed polymer mesh	use Synthetic Substitute
Non-tunneled central venous catheter	use Infusion Device
Novacor Left Ventricular Assist Device	use Implantable Heart Assist System in Heart and Great Vessels
Novation® Ceramic AHS® (Articulation Hip System)	use Synthetic Substitute, Ceramic for Replacement in Lower Joints
Omnilink Elite Vascular Balloon Expandable Stent System	use Intraluminal Device
Open Pivot Aortic Valve Graft (AVG)	use Synthetic Substitute
Open Pivot (mechanical) valve	use Synthetic Substitute
Optimizer™ III implantable pulse generator	use Contractility Modulation Device for Insertion in Subcutaneous Tissue and Fascia
Oropharyngeal airway (OPA)	use Intraluminal Device, Airway in Mouth and Throat
Ovatio™ CRT-D	use Cardiac Resynchronization Defibrillator Pulse Generator for Insertion in Subcutaneous Tissue and Fascia
Oxidized zirconium ceramic hip bearing surface	use Synthetic Substitute, Ceramic on Polyethylene for Replacement in Lower Joints
Paclitaxel-eluting coronary stent	use Intraluminal Device, Drug-eluting in Heart and Great Vessels
Paclitaxel-eluting peripheral stent	use Intraluminal Device, Drug-eluting in Upper Arteries, Lower Arteries

APPENDIX D – DEVICE KEY

DEVICE	USE:
Partially absorbable mesh	*use* Synthetic Substitute
Pedicle-based dynamic stabilization device	*use* Spinal Stabilization Device, Pedicle-Based for Insertion in Upper Joints, Lower Joints
Percutaneous endoscopic gastrojejunostomy (PEG/J) tube	*use* Feeding Device in Gastrointestinal System
Percutaneous endoscopic gastrostomy (PEG) tube	*use* Feeding Device in Gastrointestinal System
Percutaneous nephrostomy catheter	*use* Drainage Device
Peripherally inserted central catheter (PICC)	*use* Infusion Device
Pessary ring	*use* Intraluminal Device, Pessary in Female Reproductive System
Phrenic nerve stimulator generator	*use* Stimulator Generator in Subcutaneous Tissue and Fascia
Phrenic nerve stimulator lead	*use* Diaphragmatic Pacemaker Lead in Respiratory System
PHYSIOMESH™ Flexible Composite Mesh	*use* Synthetic Substitute
Pipeline™ Embolization device (PED)	*use* Intraluminal Device
Polyethylene socket	*use* Synthetic Substitute, Polyethylene for Replacement in Lower Joints
Polymethylmethacrylate (PMMA)	*use* Synthetic Substitute
Polypropylene mesh	*use* Synthetic Substitute
Porcine (bioprosthetic) valve	*use* Zooplastic Tissue in Heart and Great Vessels
PRESTIGE® Cervical Disc	*use* Synthetic Substitute
PrimeAdvanced neurostimulator (SureScan) (MRI Safe)	*use* Stimulator Generator, Multiple Array for Insertion in Subcutaneous Tissue and Fascia
PROCEED™ Ventral Patch	*use* Synthetic Substitute
Prodisc-C	*use* Synthetic Substitute
Prodisc-L	*use* Synthetic Substitute
PROLENE Polypropylene Hernia System (PHS)	*use* Synthetic Substitute
Protecta XT CRT-D	*use* Cardiac Resynchronization Defibrillator Pulse Generator for Insertion in Subcutaneous Tissue and Fascia
Protecta XT DR (XT VR)	*use* Defibrillator Generator for Insertion in Subcutaneous Tissue and Fascia
Protégé® RX Carotid Stent System	*use* Intraluminal Device
Pump reservoir	*use* Infusion Device, Pump in Subcutaneous Tissue and Fascia
REALIZE® Adjustable Gastric Band	*use* Extraluminal Device
Rebound HRD® (Hernia Repair Device)	*use* Synthetic Substitute
RestoreAdvanced neurostimulator (SureScan) (MRI Safe)	*use* Stimulator Generator, Multiple Array Rechargeable for Insertion in Subcutaneous Tissue and Fascia
RestoreSensor neurostimulator (SureScan) (MRI Safe)	*use* Stimulator Generator, Multiple Array Rechargeable for Insertion in Subcutaneous Tissue and Fascia
RestoreUltra neurostimulator (SureScan) (MRI Safe)	*use* Stimulator Generator, Multiple Array Rechargeable for Insertion in Subcutaneous Tissue and Fascia
Reveal (DX) (XT)	*use* Monitoring Device
Reverse® Shoulder Prosthesis	*use* Synthetic Substitute, Reverse Ball and Socket for Replacement in Upper Joints
Revo MRI™ SureScan® pacemaker	*use* Pacemaker, Dual Chamber for Insertion in Subcutaneous Tissue and Fascia
Rheos® System device	*use* Stimulator Generator in Subcutaneous Tissue and Fascia
Rheos® System lead	*use* Stimulator Lead in Upper Arteries
RNS System lead	*use* Neurostimulator Lead in Central Nervous System
RNS system neurostimulator generator	*use* Neurostimulator Generator in Head and Facial Bones
Sacral nerve modulation (SNM) lead	*use* Stimulator Lead in Urinary System
Sacral neuromodulation lead	*use* Stimulator Lead in Urinary System
SAPIEN transcatheter aortic valve	*use* Zooplastic Tissue in Heart and Great Vessels
Secura (DR) (VR)	*use* Defibrillator Generator for Insertion in Subcutaneous Tissue and Fascia
Sheffield hybrid external fixator	*use* External Fixation Device, Hybrid for Insertion in Upper Bones, Lower Bones External Fixation Device, Hybrid for Reposition in Upper Bones, Lower Bones
Sheffield ring external fixator	*use* External Fixation Device, Ring for Insertion in Upper Bones, Lower Bones External Fixation Device, Ring for Reposition in Upper Bones, Lower Bones
Single lead pacemaker (atrium) (ventricle)	*use* Pacemaker, Single Chamber for Insertion in Subcutaneous Tissue and Fascia
Single lead rate responsive pacemaker (atrium) (ventricle)	*use* Pacemaker, Single Chamber Rate Responsive for Insertion in Subcutaneous Tissue and Fascia
Sirolimus-eluting coronary stent	*use* Intraluminal Device, Drug-eluting in Heart and Great Vessels
SJM Biocor® Stented Valve System	*use* Zooplastic Tissue in Heart and Great Vessels
Spinal cord neurostimulator lead	*use* Neurostimulator Lead in Central Nervous System
Spiration IBV™ Valve System	*use* Intraluminal Device, Endobronchial Valve in Respiratory System

DEVICE	USE:
Stent, intraluminal (cardiovascular) (gastrointestinal) (hepatobiliary) (urinary)	use Intraluminal Device
Stented tissue valve	use Zooplastic Tissue in Heart and Great Vessels
Stratos LV	use Cardiac Resynchronization Pacemaker Pulse Generator for Insertion in Subcutaneous Tissue and Fascia
Subcutaneous injection reservoir, port	use Vascular Access Device, Reservoir in Subcutaneous Tissue and Fascia
Subcutaneous injection reservoir, pump	use Infusion Device, Pump in Subcutaneous Tissue and Fascia
Subdermal progesterone implant	use Contraceptive Device in Subcutaneous Tissue and Fascia
SynCardia Total Artificial Heart	use Synthetic Substitute
Synchra CRT-P	use Cardiac Resynchronization Pacemaker Pulse Generator for Insertion in Subcutaneous Tissue and Fascia
SynchroMed pump	use Infusion Device, Pump in Subcutaneous Tissue and Fascia
Talent® Converter	use Intraluminal Device
Talent® Occluder	use Intraluminal Device
Talent® Stent Graft (abdominal) (thoracic)	use Intraluminal Device
TandemHeart® System	use External Heart Assist System in Heart and Great Vessels
TAXUS® Liberté® Paclitaxel-eluting Coronary Stent System	use Intraluminal Device, Drug-eluting in Heart and Great Vessels
Therapeutic occlusion coil(s)	use Intraluminal Device
Thoracostomy tube	use Drainage Device
Thoratec IVAD (Implantable Ventricular Assist Device)	use Implantable Heart Assist System in Heart and Great Vessels
Thoratec Paracorporeal Ventricular Assist Device	use External Heart Assist System in Heart and Great Vessels
Tibial insert	use Liner in Lower Joints
TigerPaw® system for closure of left atrial appendage	use Extraluminal Device
Tissue bank graft	use Nonautologous Tissue Substitute
Tissue expander (inflatable) (injectable)	use Tissue Expander in Skin and Breast Tissue Expander in Subcutaneous Tissue and Fascia
Titanium Sternal Fixation System (TSFS)	use Internal Fixation Device, Rigid Plate for Insertion in Upper Bones Internal Fixation Device, Rigid Plate for Reposition in Upper Bones
Total artificial (replacement) heart	use Synthetic Substitute
Tracheostomy tube	use Tracheostomy Device in Respiratory System
Trifecta™ Valve (aortic)	use Zooplastic Tissue in Heart and Great Vessels
Tunneled central venous catheter	use Vascular Access Device in Subcutaneous Tissue and Fascia
Tunneled spinal (intrathecal) catheter	use Infusion Device
Two lead pacemaker	use Pacemaker, Dual Chamber for Insertion in Subcutaneous Tissue and Fascia
Ultraflex™ Precision Colonic Stent System	use Intraluminal Device
ULTRAPRO Hernia System (UHS)	use Synthetic Substitute
ULTRAPRO Partially Absorbable Lightweight Mesh	use Synthetic Substitute
ULTRAPRO Plug	use Synthetic Substitute
Ultrasonic osteogenic stimulator	use Bone Growth Stimulator in Head and Facial Bones, Upper Bones, Lower Bones
Ultrasound bone healing system	use Bone Growth Stimulator in Head and Facial Bones, Upper Bones, Lower Bones
Uniplanar external fixator	use External Fixation Device, Monoplanar for Insertion in Upper Bones, Lower Bones External Fixation Device, Monoplanar for Reposition in Upper Bones, Lower Bones
Urinary incontinence stimulator lead	use Stimulator Lead in Urinary System
Vaginal pessary	use Intraluminal Device, Pessary in Female Reproductive System
Valiant Thoracic Stent Graft	use Intraluminal Device
Vectra® Vascular Access Graft	use Vascular Access Device in Subcutaneous Tissue and Fascia
Ventrio™ Hernia Patch	use Synthetic Substitute
Versa	use Pacemaker, Dual Chamber for Insertion in Subcutaneous Tissue and Fascia
Virtuoso (II) (DR) (VR)	use Defibrillator Generator for Insertion in Subcutaneous Tissue and Fascia
Viva (XT) (S)	use Cardiac Resynchronization Defibrillator Pulse Generator for Insertion in Subcutaneous Tissue and Fascia
WALLSTENT® Endoprosthesis	use Intraluminal Device
X-STOP® Spacer	use Spinal Stabilization Device, Interspinous Process for Insertion in Upper Joints, Lower Joints
Xact Carotid Stent System	use Intraluminal Device
Xenograft	use Zooplastic Tissue in Heart and Great Vessels

APPENDIX D – DEVICE KEY

DEVICE	USE:
XIENCE Everolimus Eluting Coronary Stent System	*use* Intraluminal Device, Drug-eluting in Heart and Great Vessels
XLIF® System	*use* Interbody Fusion Device in Lower Joints
Zenith Flex® AAA Endovascular Graft	*use* Intraluminal Device
Zenith TX2® TAA Endovascular Graft	*use* Intraluminal Device
Zenith® Renu™ AAA Ancillary Graft	*use* Intraluminal Device
Zilver® PTX® (paclitaxel) Drug-Eluting Peripheral Stent	*use* Intraluminal Device, Drug-eluting in Upper Arteries, Lower Arteries
Zimmer® NexGen® LPS Mobile Bearing Knee	*use* Synthetic Substitute
Zimmer® NexGen® LPS-Flex Mobile Knee	*use* Synthetic Substitute
Zotarolimus-eluting coronary stent	*use* Intraluminal Device, Drug-eluting in Heart and Great Vessels

Appendix E — 2016 ICD-10-PCS — Device Aggregation Table

Specific Device	For Operation	In Body System	General Device
Autologous Arterial Tissue	All applicable	Heart and Great Vessels Lower Arteries, Lower Veins Upper Arteries, Upper Veins	7 Autologous Tissue Substitute
Autologous Venous Tissue	All applicable	Heart and Great Vessels Lower Arteries, Lower Veins Upper Arteries, Upper Veins	7 Autologous Tissue Substitute
Cardiac Lead, Defibrillator	Insertion	Heart and Great Vessels	M Cardiac Lead
Cardiac Lead, Pacemaker	Insertion	Heart and Great Vessels	M Cardiac Lead
Cardiac Resynchronization Defibrillator Pulse Generator	Insertion	Subcutaneous Tissue and Fascia	P Cardiac Rhythm Related Device
Cardiac Resynchronization Pacemaker Pulse Generator	Insertion	Subcutaneous Tissue and Fascia	P Cardiac Rhythm Related Device
Contractility Modulation Device	Insertion	Subcutaneous Tissue and Fascia	P Cardiac Rhythm Related Device
Defibrillator Generator	Insertion	Subcutaneous Tissue and Fascia	P Cardiac Rhythm Related Device
Epiretinal Visual Prosthesis	All applicable	Eye	J Synthetic Substitute
External Fixation Device, Hybrid	Insertion	Lower Bones, Upper Bones	5 External Fixation Device
External Fixation Device, Hybrid	Reposition	Lower Bones, Upper Bones	5 External Fixation Device
External Fixation Device, Limb Lengthening	Insertion	Lower Bones, Upper Bones	5 External Fixation Device
External Fixation Device, Monoplanar	Insertion	Lower Bones, Upper Bones	5 External Fixation Device
External Fixation Device, Monoplanar	Reposition	Lower Bones, Upper Bones	5 External Fixation Device
External Fixation Device, Ring	Insertion	Lower Bones, Upper Bones	5 External Fixation Device
External Fixation Device, Ring	Reposition	Lower Bones, Upper Bones	5 External Fixation Device
Hearing Device, Bone Conduction	Insertion	Ear, Nose, Sinus	S Hearing Device
Hearing Device, Multiple Channel Cochlear Prosthesis	Insertion	Ear, Nose, Sinus	S Hearing Device
Hearing Device, Single Channel Cochlear Prosthesis	Insertion	Ear, Nose, Sinus	S Hearing Device
Internal Fixation Device, Intramedullary	All applicable	Lower Bones, Upper Bones	4 Internal Fixation Device
Internal Fixation Device, Rigid Plate	Insertion	Upper Bones	4 Internal Fixation Device
Internal Fixation Device, Rigid Plate	Reposition	Upper Bones	4 Internal Fixation Device
Intraluminal Device, Airway	All applicable	Ear, Nose, Sinus Gastrointestinal System Mouth and Throat	D Intraluminal Device
Intraluminal Device, Bioactive	All applicable	Upper Arteries	D Intraluminal Device
Intraluminal Device, Drug-eluting	All applicable	Heart and Great Vessels Lower Arteries, Upper Arteries	D Intraluminal Device
Intraluminal Device, Endobronchial Valve	All applicable	Respiratory System	D Intraluminal Device
Intraluminal Device, Endotracheal Airway	All applicable	Respiratory System	D Intraluminal Device
Intraluminal Device, Pessary	All applicable	Female Reproductive System	D Intraluminal Device
Intraluminal Device, Radioactive	All applicable	Heart and Great Vessels	D Intraluminal Device
Monitoring Device, Hemodynamic	Insertion	Subcutaneous Tissue and Fascia	2 Monitoring Device
Monitoring Device, Pressure Sensor	Insertion	Heart and Great Vessels	2 Monitoring Device
Pacemaker, Dual Chamber	Insertion	Subcutaneous Tissue and Fascia	P Cardiac Rhythm Related Device
Pacemaker, Single Chamber	Insertion	Subcutaneous Tissue and Fascia	P Cardiac Rhythm Related Device
Pacemaker, Single Chamber Rate Responsive	Insertion	Subcutaneous Tissue and Fascia	P Cardiac Rhythm Related Device
Spinal Stabilization Device, Facet Replacement	Insertion	Lower Joints, Upper Joints	4 Internal Fixation Device
Spinal Stabilization Device, Interspinous Process	Insertion	Lower Joints, Upper Joints	4 Internal Fixation Device
Spinal Stabilization Device, Pedicle-Based	Insertion	Lower Joints, Upper Joints	4 Internal Fixation Device
Stimulator Generator, Multiple Array	Insertion	Subcutaneous Tissue and Fascia	M Stimulator Generator
Stimulator Generator, Multiple Array Rechargeable	Insertion	Subcutaneous Tissue and Fascia	M Stimulator Generator
Stimulator Generator, Single Array	Insertion	Subcutaneous Tissue and Fascia	M Stimulator Generator
Stimulator Generator, Single Array Rechargeable	Insertion	Subcutaneous Tissue and Fascia	M Stimulator Generator
Synthetic Substitute, Ceramic	Replacement	Lower Joints	J Synthetic Substitute
Synthetic Substitute, Ceramic on Polyethylene	Replacement	Lower Joints	J Synthetic Substitute
Synthetic Substitute, Intraocular Telescope	Replacement	Eye	J Synthetic Substitute
Synthetic Substitute, Metal	Replacement	Lower Joints	J Synthetic Substitute
Synthetic Substitute, Metal on Polyethylene	Replacement	Lower Joints	J Synthetic Substitute
Synthetic Substitute, Polyethylene	Replacement	Lower Joints	J Synthetic Substitute
Synthetic Substitute, Reverse Ball and Socket	Replacement	Upper Joints	J Synthetic Substitute

APPENDIX F – QUALIFIER KEY
PHYSICAL REHABILITATION AND DIAGNOSTIC AUDIOLOGY

Acoustic Reflex Decay	Definition: Measures reduction in size/strength of acoustic reflex over time Includes/Examples: Includes site of lesion test
Acoustic Reflex Patterns	Definition: Defines site of lesion based upon presence/absence of acoustic reflexes with ipsilateral vs. contralateral stimulation
Acoustic Reflex Threshold	Definition: Determines minimal intensity that acoustic reflex occurs with ipsilateral and/or contralateral stimulation
Aerobic Capacity and Endurance	Definition: Measures autonomic responses to positional changes; perceived exertion, dyspnea or angina during activity; performance during exercise protocols; standard vital signs; and blood gas analysis or oxygen consumption
Alternate Binaural or Monaural Loudness Balance	Definition: Determines auditory stimulus parameter that yields the same objective sensation Includes/Examples: Sound intensities that yield same loudness perception
Anthropometric Characteristics	Definition: Measures edema, body fat composition, height, weight, length and girth
Aphasia (Assessment)	Definition: Measures expressive and receptive speech and language function including reading and writing
Aphasia (Treatment)	Definition: Applying techniques to improve, augment, or compensate for receptive/expressive language impairments
Articulation/Phonology (Assessment)	Definition: Measures speech production
Articulation/Phonology (Treatment)	Definition: Applying techniques to correct, improve, or compensate for speech productive impairment
Assistive Listening Device	Definition: Assists in use of effective and appropriate assistive listening device/system
Assistive Listening System/Device Selection	Definition: Measures the effectiveness and appropriateness of assistive listening systems/devices
Assistive, Adaptive, Supportive or Protective Devices	Explanation: Devices to facilitate or support achievement of a higher level of function in wheelchair mobility; bed mobility; transfer or ambulation ability; bath and showering ability; dressing; grooming; personal hygiene; play or leisure
Auditory Evoked Potentials	Definition: Measures electric responses produced by the VIIIth cranial nerve and brainstem following auditory stimulation
Auditory Processing (Assessment)	Definition: Evaluates ability to receive and process auditory information and comprehension of spoken language
Auditory Processing (Treatment)	Definition: Applying techniques to improve the receiving and processing of auditory information and comprehension of spoken language
Augmentative/Alternative Communication System (Assessment)	Definition: Determines the appropriateness of aids, techniques, symbols, and/or strategies to augment or replace speech and enhance communication Includes/Examples: Includes the use of telephones, writing equipment, emergency equipment, and TDD
Augmentative/Alternative Communication System (Treatment)	Includes/Examples: Includes augmentative communication devices and aids
Aural Rehabilitation	Definition: Applying techniques to improve the communication abilities associated with hearing loss
Aural Rehabilitation Status	Definition: Measures impact of a hearing loss including evaluation of receptive and expressive communication skills
Bathing/Showering	Includes/Examples: Includes obtaining and using supplies; soaping, rinsing, and drying body parts; maintaining bathing position; and transferring to and from bathing positions
Bathing/Showering Techniques	Definition: Activities to facilitate obtaining and using supplies, soaping, rinsing and drying body parts, maintaining bathing position, and transferring to and from bathing positions
Bed Mobility (Assessment)	Definition: Transitional movement within bed
Bed Mobility (Treatment)	Definition: Exercise or activities to facilitate transitional movements within bed
Bedside Swallowing and Oral Function	Includes/Examples: Bedside swallowing includes assessment of sucking, masticating, coughing, and swallowing. Oral function includes assessment of musculature for controlled movements, structures and functions to determine coordination and phonation

Appendix F – Qualifier Key Rehab and Audiology

Bekesy Audiometry	Definition: Uses an instrument that provides a choice of discrete or continuously varying pure tones; choice of pulsed or continuous signal
Binaural Electroacoustic Hearing Aid Check	Definition: Determines mechanical and electroacoustic function of bilateral hearing aids using hearing aid test box
Binaural Hearing Aid (Assessment)	Definition: Measures the candidacy, effectiveness, and appropriateness of hearing aids Explanation: Measures bilateral fit
Binaural Hearing Aid (Treatment)	Explanation: Assists in achieving maximum understanding and performance
Bithermal, Binaural Caloric Irrigation	Definition: Measures the rhythmic eye movements stimulated by changing the temperature of the vestibular system
Bithermal, Monaural Caloric Irrigation	Definition: Measures the rhythmic eye movements stimulated by changing the temperature of the vestibular system in one ear
Brief Tone Stimuli	Definition: Measures specific central auditory process
Cerumen Management	Definition: Includes examination of external auditory canal and tympanic membrane and removal of cerumen from external ear canal
Cochlear Implant	Definition: Measures candidacy for cochlear implant
Cochlear Implant Rehabilitation	Definition: Applying techniques to improve the communication abilities of individuals with cochlear implant; includes programming the device, providing patients/families with information
Communicative/Cognitive Integration Skills (Assessment)	Definition: Measures ability to use higher cortical functions Includes/Examples: Includes orientation, recognition, attention span, initiation and termination of activity, memory, sequencing, categorizing, concept formation, spatial operations, judgment, problem solving, generalization and pragmatic communication
Communicative/Cognitive Integration Skills (Treatment)	Definition: Activities to facilitate the use of higher cortical functions Includes/Examples: Includes level of arousal, orientation, recognition, attention span, initiation and termination of activity, memory sequencing, judgment and problem solving, learning and generalization, and pragmatic communication
Computerized Dynamic Posturography	Definition: Measures the status of the peripheral and central vestibular system and the sensory/motor component of balance; evaluates the efficacy of vestibular rehabilitation
Conditioned Play Audiometry	Definition: Behavioral measures using nonspeech and speech stimuli to obtain frequency-specific and ear-specific information on auditory status from the patient Explanation: Obtains speech reception threshold by having patient point to pictures of spondaic words
Coordination/Dexterity (Assessment)	Definition: Measures large and small muscle groups for controlled goal-directed movements Explanation: Dexterity includes object manipulation
Coordination/Dexterity (Treatment)	Definition: Exercise or activities to facilitate gross coordination and fine coordination
Cranial Nerve Integrity	Definition: Measures cranial nerve sensory and motor functions, including tastes, smell and facial expression
Dichotic Stimuli	Definition: Measures specific central auditory process
Distorted Speech	Definition: Measures specific central auditory process
Dix-Hallpike Dynamic	Definition: Measures nystagmus following Dix-Hallpike maneuver
Dressing	Includes/Examples: Includes selecting clothing and accessories, obtaining clothing from storage, dressing and, fastening and adjusting clothing and shoes, and applying and removing personal devices, prosthesis or orthosis
Dressing Techniques	Definition: Activities to facilitate selecting clothing and accessories, dressing and undressing, adjusting clothing and shoes, applying and removing devices, prostheses or orthoses
Dynamic Orthosis	Includes/Examples: Includes customized and prefabricated splints, inhibitory casts, spinal and other braces, and protective devices; allows motion through transfer of movement from other body parts or by use of outside forces
Ear Canal Probe Microphone	Definition: Real ear measures
Ear Protector Attentuation	Definition: Measures ear protector fit and effectiveness
Electrocochleography	Definition: Measures the VIIIth cranial nerve action potential
Environmental, Home and Work Barriers	Definition: Measures current and potential barriers to optimal function, including safety hazards, access problems and home or office design

Ergonomics and Body Mechanics	Definition: Ergonomic measurement of job tasks, work hardening or work conditioning needs; functional capacity; and body mechanics
Eustachian Tube Function	Definition: Measures eustachian tube function and patency of eustachian tube
Evoked Otoacoustic Emissions, Diagnostic	Definition: Measures auditory evoked potentials in a diagnostic format
Evoked Otoacoustic Emissions, Screening	Definition: Measures auditory evoked potentials in a screening format
Facial Nerve Function	Definition: Measures electrical activity of the VIIth cranial nerve (facial nerve)
Feeding/Eating (Assessment)	Includes/Examples: Includes setting up food, selecting and using utensils and tableware, bringing food or drink to mouth, cleaning face, hands, and clothing, and management of alternative methods of nourishment
Feeding/Eating (Treatment)	Definition: Exercise or activities to facilitate setting up food, selecting and using utensils and tableware, bringing food or drink to mouth, cleaning face, hands, and clothing, and management of alternative methods of nourishment
Filtered Speech	Definition: Uses high or low pass filtered speech stimuli to assess central auditory processing disorders, site of lesion testing
Fluency (Assessment)	Definition: Measures speech fluency or stuttering
Fluency (Treatment)	Definition: Applying techniques to improve and augment fluent speech
Gait and/or Balance	Definition: Measures biomechanical, arthrokinematic and other spatial and temporal characteristics of gait and balance
Gait Training/Functional Ambulation	Definition: Exercise or activities to facilitate ambulation on a variety of surfaces and in a variety of environments
Grooming/Personal Hygiene (Assessment)	Includes/Examples: Includes ability to obtain and use supplies in a sequential fashion, general grooming, oral hygiene, toilet hygiene, personal care devices, including care for artificial airways
Grooming/Personal Hygiene (Treatment)	Definition: Activities to facilitate obtaining and using supplies in a sequential fashion: general grooming, oral hygiene, toilet hygiene, cleaning body, and personal care devices, including artificial airways
Hearing and Related Disorders Counseling	Definition: Provides patients/families/caregivers with information, support, referrals to facilitate recovery from a communication disorder Includes/Examples: Includes strategies for psychosocial adjustment to hearing loss for clients and families/caregivers
Hearing and Related Disorders Prevention	Definition: Provides patients/families/caregivers with information and support to prevent communication disorders
Hearing Screening	Definition: Pass/refer measures designed to identify need for further audiologic assessment
Home Management (Assessment)	Definition: Obtaining and maintaining personal and household possessions and environment Includes/Examples: Includes clothing care, cleaning, meal preparation and cleanup, shopping, money management, household maintenance, safety procedures, and childcare/parenting
Home Management (Treatment)	Definition: Activities to facilitate obtaining and maintaining personal household possessions and environment Includes/Examples: Includes clothing care, cleaning, meal preparation and clean-up, shopping, money management, household maintenance, safety procedures, childcare/parenting
Instrumental Swallowing and Oral Function	Definition: Measures swallowing function using instrumental diagnostic procedures Explanation: Methods include videofluoroscopy, ultrasound, manometry, endoscopy
Integumentary Integrity	Includes/Examples: Includes burns, skin conditions, ecchymosis, bleeding, blisters, scar tissue, wounds and other traumas, tissue mobility, turgor and texture
Manual Therapy Techniques	Definition: Techniques in which the therapist uses his/her hands to administer skilled movements Includes/Examples: Includes connective tissue massage, joint mobilization and manipulation, manual lymph drainage, manual traction, soft tissue mobilization and manipulation
Masking Patterns	Definition: Measures central auditory processing status
Monaural Electroacoustic Hearing Aid Check	Definition: Determines mechanical and electroacoustic function of one hearing aid using hearing aid test box

APPENDIX F – QUALIFIER KEY REHAB AND AUDIOLOGY

Monaural Hearing Aid (Assessment)	Definition: Measures the candidacy, effectiveness, and appropriateness of a hearing aid Explanation: Measures unilateral fit
Monaural Hearing Aid (Treatment)	Explanation: Assists in achieving maximum understanding and performance
Motor Function (Assessment)	Definition: Measures the body's functional and versatile movement patterns Includes/Examples: Includes motor assessment scales, analysis of head, trunk and limb movement, and assessment of motor learning
Motor Function (Treatment)	Definition: Exercise or activities to facilitate crossing midline, laterality, bilateral integration, praxis, neuromuscular relaxation, inhibition, facilitation, motor function and motor learning
Motor Speech (Assessment)	Definition: Measures neurological motor aspects of speech production
Motor Speech (Treatment)	Definition: Applying techniques to improve and augment the impaired neurological motor aspects of speech production
Muscle Performance (Assessment)	Definition: Measures muscle strength, power and endurance using manual testing, dynamometry or computer-assisted electromechanical muscle test; functional muscle strength, power and endurance; muscle pain, tone, or soreness; or pelvic-floor musculature Explanation: Muscle endurance refers to the ability to contract a muscle repeatedly over time
Muscle Performance (Treatment)	Definition: Exercise or activities to increase the capacity of a muscle to do work in terms of strength, power, and/or endurance Explanation: Muscle strength is the force exerted to overcome resistance in one maximal effort. Muscle power is work produced per unit of time, or the product of strength and speed. Muscle endurance is the ability to contract a muscle repeatedly over time
Neuromotor Development	Definition: Measures motor development, righting and equilibrium reactions, and reflex and equilibrium reactions
Neurophysiologic Intraoperative	Definition: Monitors neural status during surgery
Non-invasive Instrumental Status	Definition: Instrumental measures of oral, nasal, vocal, and velopharyngeal functions as they pertain to speech production
Nonspoken Language (Assessment)	Definition: Measures nonspoken language (print, sign, symbols) for communication
Nonspoken Language (Treatment)	Definition: Applying techniques that improve, augment, or compensate spoken communication
Oral Peripheral Mechanism	Definition: Structural measures of face, jaw, lips, tongue, teeth, hard and soft palate, pharynx as related to speech production
Orofacial Myofunctional (Assessment)	Definition: Measures orofacial myofunctional patterns for speech and related functions
Orofacial Myofunctional (Treatment)	Definition: Applying techniques to improve, alter, or augment impaired orofacial myofunctional patterns and related speech production errors
Oscillating Tracking	Definition: Measures ability to visually track
Pain	Definition: Measures muscle soreness, pain and soreness with joint movement, and pain perception Includes/Examples: Includes questionnaires, graphs, symptom magnification scales or visual analog scales
Perceptual Processing (Assessment)	Definition: Measures stereognosis, kinesthesia, body schema, right-left discrimination, form constancy, position in space, visual closure, figure-ground, depth perception, spatial relations and topographical orientation
Perceptual Processing (Treatment)	Definition: Exercise and activities to facilitate perceptual processing Explanation: Includes stereognosis, kinesthesia, body schema, right-left discrimination, form constancy, position in space, visual closure, figure-ground, depth perception, spatial relations, and topographical orientation Includes/Examples: Includes stereognosis, kinesthesia, body schema, right-left discrimination, form constancy, position in space, visual closure, figure-ground, depth perception, spatial relations, and topographical orientation
Performance Intensity Phonetically Balanced Speech Discrimination	Definition: Measures word recognition over varying intensity levels
Postural Control	Definition: Exercise or activities to increase postural alignment and control
Prosthesis	Explanation: Artificial substitutes for missing body parts that augment performance or function

APPENDIX F – QUALIFIER KEY REHAB AND AUDIOLOGY

Psychosocial Skills (Assessment)	Definition: The ability to interact in society and to process emotions Includes/Examples: Includes psychological (values, interests, self-concept); social (role performance, social conduct, interpersonal skills, self expression); self-management (coping skills, time management, self-control)
Psychosocial Skills (Treatment)	Definition: The ability to interact in society and to process emotions Includes/Examples: Includes psychological (values, interests, self-concept); social (role performance, social conduct, interpersonal skills, self expression); self-management (coping skills, time management, self-control)
Pure Tone Audiometry, Air	Definition: Air-conduction pure tone threshold measures with appropriate masking
Pure Tone Audiometry, Air and Bone	Definition: Air-conduction and bone-conduction pure tone threshold measures with appropriate masking
Pure Tone Stenger	Definition: Measures unilateral nonorganic hearing loss based on simultaneous presentation of pure tones of differing volume
Range of Motion and Joint Integrity	Definition: Measures quantity, quality, grade, and classification of joint movement and/or mobility Explanation: Range of Motion is the space, distance or angle through which movement occurs at a joint or series of joints. Joint integrity is the conformance of joints to expected anatomic, biomechanical and kinematic norms
Range of Motion and Joint Mobility	Definition: Exercise or activities to increase muscle length and joint mobility
Receptive/Expressive Language (Assessment)	Definition: Measures receptive and expressive language
Receptive/Expressive Language (Treatment)	Definition: Applying techniques to improve and augment receptive/expressive language
Reflex Integrity	Definition: Measures the presence, absence, or exaggeration of developmentally appropriate, pathologic or normal reflexes
Select Picture Audiometry	Definition: Establishes hearing threshold levels for speech using pictures
Sensorineural Acuity Level	Definition: Measures sensorineural acuity masking presented via bone conduction
Sensory Aids	Definition: Determines the appropriateness of a sensory prosthetic device, other than a hearing aid or assistive listening system/device
Sensory Awareness/Processing/Integrity	Includes/Examples: Includes light touch, pressure, temperature, pain, sharp/dull, proprioception, vestibular, visual, auditory, gustatory, and olfactory
Short Increment Sensitivity Index	Definition: Measures the ear's ability to detect small intensity changes; site of lesion test requiring a behavioral response
Sinusoidal Vertical Axis Rotational	Definition: Measures nystagmus following rotation
Somatosensory Evoked Potentials	Definition: Measures neural activity from sites throughout the body
Speech and/or Language Screening	Definition: Identifies need for further speech and/or language evaluation
Speech Threshold	Definition: Measures minimal intensity needed to repeat spondaic words
Speech-Language Pathology and Related Disorders Counseling	Definition: Provides patients/families with information, support, referrals to facilitate recovery from a communication disorder
Speech-Language Pathology and Related Disorders Prevention	Definition: Applying techniques to avoid or minimize onset and/or development of a communication disorder
Speech/Word Recognition	Definition: Measures ability to repeat/identify single syllable words; scores given as a percentage; includes word recognition/speech discrimination
Staggered Spondaic Word	Definition: Measures central auditory processing site of lesion based upon dichotic presentation of spondaic words
Static Orthosis	Includes/Examples: Includes customized and prefabricated splints, inhibitory casts, spinal and other braces, and protective devices; has no moving parts, maintains joint(s) in desired position
Stenger	Definition: Measures unilateral nonorganic hearing loss based on simultaneous presentation of signals of differing volume
Swallowing Dysfunction	Definition: Activities to improve swallowing function in coordination with respiratory function Includes/Examples: Includes function and coordination of sucking, mastication, coughing, swallowing
Synthetic Sentence Identification	Definition: Measures central auditory dysfunction using identification of third order approximations of sentences and competing messages

Temporal Ordering of Stimuli	Definition: Measures specific central auditory process
Therapeutic Exercise	Definition: Exercise or activities to facilitate sensory awareness, sensory processing, sensory integration, balance training, conditioning, reconditioning Includes/Examples: Includes developmental activities, breathing exercises, aerobic endurance activities, aquatic exercises, stretching and ventilatory muscle training
Tinnitus Masker (Assessment)	Definition: Determines candidacy for tinnitus masker
Tinnitus Masker (Treatment)	Explanation: Used to verify physical fit, acoustic appropriateness, and benefit; assists in achieving maximum benefit
Tone Decay	Definition: Measures decrease in hearing sensitivity to a tone; site of lesion test requiring a behavioral response
Transfer	Definition: Transitional movement from one surface to another
Transfer Training	Definition: Exercise or activities to facilitate movement from one surface to another
Tympanometry	Definition: Measures the integrity of the middle ear; measures ease at which sound flows through the tympanic membrane while air pressure against the membrane is varied
Unithermal Binaural Screen	Definition: Measures the rhythmic eye movements stimulated by changing the temperature of the vestibular system in both ears using warm water, screening format
Ventilation, Respiration and Circulation	Definition: Measures ventilatory muscle strength, power and endurance, pulmonary function and ventilatory mechanics Includes/Examples: Includes ability to clear airway, activities that aggravate or relieve edema, pain, dyspnea or other symptoms, chest wall mobility, cardiopulmonary response to performance of ADL and IAD, cough and sputum, standard vital signs
Vestibular	Definition: Applying techniques to compensate for balance disorders; includes habituation, exercise therapy, and balance retraining
Visual Motor Integration (Assessment)	Definition: Coordinating the interaction of information from the eyes with body movement during activity
Visual Motor Integration (Treatment)	Definition: Exercise or activities to facilitate coordinating the interaction of information from eyes with body movement during activity
Visual Reinforcement Audiometry	Definition: Behavioral measures using nonspeech and speech stimuli to obtain frequency/ear-specific information on auditory status Includes/Examples: Includes a conditioned response of looking toward a visual reinforcer (e.g., lights, animated toy) every time auditory stimuli are heard
Vocational Activities and Functional Community or Work Reintegration Skills (Assessment)	Definition: Measures environmental, home, work (job/school/play) barriers that keep patients from functioning optimally in their environment Includes/Examples: Includes assessment of vocational skill and interests, environment of work (job/school/play), injury potential and injury prevention or reduction, ergonomic stressors, transportation skills, and ability to access and use community resources
Vocational Activities and Functional Community or Work Reintegration Skills (Treatment)	Definition: Activities to facilitate vocational exploration, body mechanics training, job acquisition, and environmental or work (job/school/play) task adaptation Includes/Examples: Includes injury prevention and reduction, ergonomic stressor reduction, job coaching and simulation, work hardening and conditioning, driving training, transportation skills, and use of community resources
Voice (Assessment)	Definition: Measures vocal structure, function and production
Voice (Treatment)	Definition: Applying techniques to improve voice and vocal function
Voice Prosthetic (Assessment)	Definition: Determines the appropriateness of voice prosthetic/adaptive device to enhance or facilitate communication
Voice Prosthetic (Treatment)	Includes/Examples: Includes electrolarynx, and other assistive, adaptive, supportive devices
Wheelchair Mobility (Assessment)	Definition: Measures fit and functional abilities within wheelchair in a variety of environments
Wheelchair Mobility (Treatment)	Definition: Management, maintenance and controlled operation of a wheelchair, scooter or other device, in and on a variety of surfaces and environments
Wound Management	Includes/Examples: Includes non-selective and selective debridement (enzymes, autolysis, sharp debridement), dressings (wound coverings, hydrogel, vacuum-assisted closure), topical agents, etc.

APPENDIX G – QUALIFIER KEY FOR MENTAL HEALTH

Behavioral	Definition: Primarily to modify behavior Includes/Examples: Includes modeling and role playing, positive reinforcement of target behaviors, response cost, and training of self-management skills
Cognitive	Definition: Primarily to correct cognitive distortions and errors
Cognitive-Behavioral	Definition: Combining cognitive and behavioral treatment strategies to improve functioning Explanation: Maladaptive responses are examined to determine how cognitions relate to behavior patterns in response to an event. Uses learning principles and information-processing models
Developmental	Definition: Age-normed developmental status of cognitive, social and adaptive behavior skills
Intellectual and Psychoeducational	Definition: Intellectual abilities, academic achievement and learning capabilities (including behaviors and emotional factors affecting learning)
Interactive	Definition: Uses primarily physical aids and other forms of non-oral interaction with a patient who is physically, psychologically or developmentally unable to use ordinary language for communication Includes/Examples: Includes the use of toys in symbolic play
Interpersonal	Definition: Helps an individual make changes in interpersonal behaviors to reduce psychological dysfunction Includes/Examples: Includes exploratory techniques, encouragement of affective expression, clarification of patient statements, analysis of communication patterns, use of therapy relationship and behavior change techniques
Neurobehavioral and Cognitive Status	Definition: Includes neurobehavioral status exam, interview(s), and observation for the clinical assessment of thinking, reasoning and judgment, acquired knowledge, attention, memory, visual spatial abilities, language functions, and planning
Neuropsychological	Definition: Thinking, reasoning and judgment, acquired knowledge, attention, memory, visual spatial abilities, language functions, planning
Personality and Behavioral	Definition: Mood, emotion, behavior, social functioning, psychopathological conditions, personality traits and characteristics
Psychoanalysis	Definition: Methods of obtaining a detailed account of past and present mental and emotional experiences to determine the source and eliminate or diminish the undesirable effects of unconscious conflicts Explanation: Accomplished by making the individual aware of their existence, origin, and inappropriate expression in emotions and behavior
Psychodynamic	Definition: Exploration of past and present emotional experiences to understand motives and drives using insight-oriented techniques to reduce the undesirable effects of internal conflicts on emotions and behavior Explanation: Techniques include empathetic listening, clarifying self-defeating behavior patterns, and exploring adaptive alternatives
Psychophysiological	Definition: Monitoring and alteration of physiological processes to help the individual associate physiological reactions combined with cognitive and behavioral strategies to gain improved control of these processes to help the individual cope more effectively
Supportive	Definition: Formation of therapeutic relationship primarily for providing emotional support to prevent further deterioration in functioning during periods of particular stress Explanation: Often used in conjunction with other therapeutic approaches
Vocational	Definition: Exploration of vocational interests, aptitudes and required adaptive behavior skills to develop and carry out a plan for achieving a successful vocational placement Includes/Examples: Includes enhancing work related adjustment and/or pursuing viable options in training education or preparation

APPENDIX G – 2016 ICD-10-PCS

NOTES

Behavioral	Definition: Primarily to modify behavior. Includes/Examples: Includes modeling and role playing, positive reinforcement of target behaviors, response cost, and training of self-management skills
Cognitive	Definition: Primarily to correct cognitive distortions and errors
Cognitive-behavioral	Definition: Combining cognitive and behavioral treatment strategies to improve functioning. Explanation: Maladaptive responses are examined to determine how cognitions relate to behavior patterns in response to an event. Uses learning principles and information-processing models
Developmental	Definition: Age-normed developmental status of cognitive, social and adaptive behavior skills
Intellectual and Psychoeducational	Definition: Intellectual abilities, academic achievement and learning capabilities (including behaviors and emotional factors affecting learning)
Interactive	Definition: Uses primarily physical aids and other forms of non-oral interaction with a patient who is physically, psychologically or developmentally unable to use ordinary language for communication. Includes/Examples: Includes the use of toys in symbolic play
Interpersonal	Definition: Helps an individual make changes in interpersonal behaviors to reduce psychological dysfunction. Includes/Examples: Includes exploratory techniques, encouragement of effective expression, clarification of patient statements, analysis of communication patterns, use of therapy relationship and behavior change techniques
Neurobehavioral and Cognitive Status	Definition: Includes neurobehavioral status exam, interview(s) and observation for the clinical assessment of thinking, reasoning and judgment, acquired knowledge, attention, memory, visual spatial abilities, language functions, and planning
Neuropsychological	Definition: Thinking, reasoning and judgment, acquired knowledge, attention, memory, visual spatial abilities, language functions, planning
Personality and Behavioral	Definition: Mood, emotion, behavior, social functioning, psychopathological conditions, personality traits and characteristics
Psychoanalysis	Definition: Methods of obtaining a detailed account of past and present mental and emotional experiences to determine the source and eliminate or diminish the undesirable effects of unconscious conflicts. Explanation: Accomplished by making the individual aware of their existence, origin, and inappropriate expression in emotions and behavior
Psychodynamic	Definition: Exploration of past and present emotional experiences to understand motives and drives using insight-oriented techniques to reduce the undesirable effects of internal conflicts on emotions and behavior. Explanation: Techniques include empathetic listening, clarifying self-defeating behavior patterns, and exploring adaptive alternatives
Psychophysiological	Definition: Monitoring and alteration of physiological processes to help the individual associate physiological reactions combined with cognitive and behavioral strategies to gain improved control of these processes to help the individual cope more effectively
Supportive	Definition: Formation of therapeutic relationship primarily for providing emotional support to prevent further deterioration in functioning during periods of particular stress. Explanation: Often used in conjunction with other therapeutic approaches
Vocational	Definition: Exploration of vocational interests, aptitudes and required adaptive behavior skills to develop and carry out a plan for achieving a successful vocational placement. Includes/Examples: Includes enhancing work related adjustment and/or pursuing viable options in training education or preparation

APPENDIX H – SUBSTANCE KEY

SUBSTANCE	USE:
AIGISRx Antibacterial Envelope	use Anti-Infective Envelope
Antimicrobial envelope	
Bone morphogenetic protein 2 (BMP 2)	use Recombinant Bone Morphogenetic Protein
Clolar	use Clofarabine
Kcentra	use 4-Factor Prothrombin Complex Concentrate
Nesiritide	use Human B-type Natriuretic Peptide
rhBMP-2	use Recombinant Bone Morphogenetic Protein
Seprafilm	use Adhesion Barrier
Tissue Plasminogen Activator (tPA) (r-tPA)	use Other Thrombolytic
Voraxaze	use Glucarpidase
Zyvox	use Oxazolidinones

APPENDIX I – NEW TECHNOLOGY KEY

ICD-10-PCS VALUE	DEFINITION
Root Operation: Extirpation	Definition: Taking or cutting out solid matter from a body part. Explanation: The solid matter may be an abnormal byproduct of a biological function or a foreign body; it may be imbedded in a body part or in the lumen of a tubular body part. The solid matter may or may not have been previously broken into pieces. Includes/Examples: Thrombectomy, choledocholithotomy
Root Operation: Introduction	Definition: Putting in or on a therapeutic, diagnostic, nutritional, physiological, or prophylactic substance except blood or blood products.
Root Operation: Monitoring	Definition: Determining the level of a physiological or physical function repetitively over a period of time.
Approach: External	Definition: Procedures performed directly on the skin or mucous membrane and procedures performed indirectly by the application of external force through the skin or mucous membrane.
Approach: Open	Definition: Cutting through the skin or mucous membrane and any other body layers necessary to expose the site of the procedure.
Approach: Percutaneous	Definition: Entry, by puncture or minor incision, of instrumentation through the skin or mucous membrane and any other body layers necessary to reach the site of the procedure.
Approach: Percutaneous Endoscopic	Definition: Entry, by puncture or minor incision, of instrumentation through the skin or mucous membrane and any other body layers necessary to reach and visualize the site of the procedure.